*Reprinted under authority
of Presidential Decree
No. 400 by*

JMC PRESS, INCORPORATED
388 Quezon Blvd. Ext.
Quezon City
Philippines

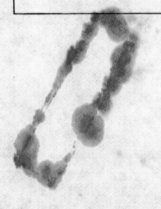

HUMAN NEUROANATOMY

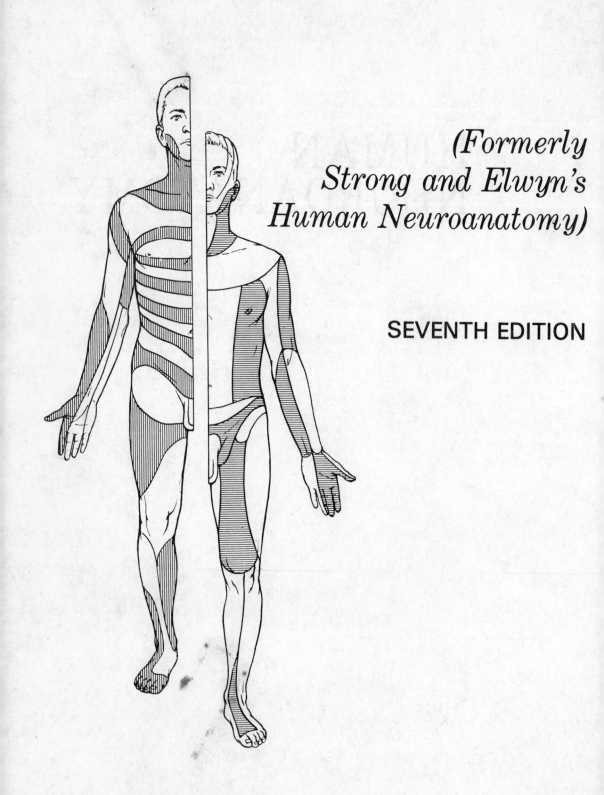

(Formerly Strong and Elwyn's Human Neuroanatomy)

SEVENTH EDITION

HUMAN
NEUROANATOMY

MALCOLM B. CARPENTER, A.B., M.D.

Professor of Anatomy, College of Physicians and Surgeons, Columbia University

THE WILLIAMS & WILKINS COMPANY
BALTIMORE

First Edition, May 1943
  Reprinted December 1943
  Reprinted December 1945
  Reprinted December 1946
Second Edition, 1948
  Reprinted June 1951
Third Edition, 1953
Fourth Edition, 1959
  Reprinted October 1960
  Reprinted August 1962
Fifth Edition, 1964
  Reprinted July 1965
Sixth Edition, 1969
  Reprinted April 1970
  Reprinted June 1971
  Reprinted May 1973

Made in the United States of America

Library of Congress Cataloging in Publication Data

Carpenter, Malcolm B
    Human Neuroanatomy = (formerly Strong and Elwyn's Human Neuroanatomy)

    Sixth ed. (1969) by R. C. Truex and M. B. Carpenter.
    1. Neuroanatomy. I. Strong, Oliver Smith, 1864–1951. Human Neuro-
anatomy. II. Truex, Raymond Carl, 1911–   . Human Neuroanatomy. III.
Title. [DNLM: 1. Nervous system—Anatomy and Histology. WL101 C296h]
QM451.T7 1976   611'.8   75-9956
ISBN 0-683-01460-9

Composed and Printed at
Waverly Press, Inc.
Mount Royal and Guilford Avenues
Baltimore, Maryland 21202 U.S.A.

Printed by J.M.C. Press Inc. with special agreement with
The Williams & Wilkins Company

Preface to the Seventh Edition

This edition, like the last, comes at a time when the curricula of many American medical schools are changing. After a period in which basic science teaching has been shortened, concentrated and fragmented, there appears to be renewed interest in more comprehensive course offerings that recognize the importance of broad integration. While appreciation of the basic sciences usually shows its strongest development after considerable clinical experience, even the beginning student recognizes that they form the foundation of a medical education, that they cannot be adequately taught, or comprehended, in a hurry, and that abbreviations usually are accomplished by serious omissions. In many medical schools new neuroscience programs have been developed and expanded in recognition of the importance of the nervous system in all clinical disciplines. Neuroanatomy is regarded as the most basic of the neurosciences because of the close correlation between structure and function, and its fundamental nature. As in all previous editions of this text attempts have been made to present clearly the structural organization of the nervous system together with interpretations of functional mechanisms and their clinical significance. Since few courses dealing with the structure and function of the nervous system will be identical, there appears to be a need for a reasonably comprehensive student textbook. The author has attempted to provide the student with a textbook of neuroanatomy that might meet these requirements.

The seventh edition has undergone extensive revisions and reorganization, which has resulted in consolidation of certain chapters and the addition of others. Material dealing with segmental and peripheral innervation has been combined in a single chapter. The chapter on the autonomic nervous system has been rewritten, and incorporates recent material on transmitter substances. Although the spinal cord is the simplest part of the central nervous system considerable revision of this section seemed necessary. The gross anatomy and internal structure of the spinal cord are presented as a unit, together with the basic principles of spinal reflexes. Spinal tracts and spinal cord syndromes are dealt with separately and new emphasis has been given to the analysis of spinal cord lesions. Experience has shown that a good understanding of the organization and function of spinal cord elements is essential before the student can appreciate the more complex organization of the brain stem. Presentation of the brain stem follows the format used in previous editions, except for rearrangements and additions designed to make reading and comprehension easier. The diencephalon, which represents the most difficult region for most students, has been divided into two main parts, the thalamus and the hypothalamus. The basal ganglia and related nuclei are discussed together; even though certain information is repeated, this seems to be the best context for understanding these structures. The amygdala has been grouped with the olfactory pathways and hippocampal formation. The cerebral cortex remains formidable, but the principal emphasis is upon clinical and functional concepts, rather than upon anatomical minutia. Each chapter dealing with the central nervous system has a section entitled, "Functional Considerations", in which attempts are made to: (1) relate structure and function, and (2) provide certain insight into clinical problems. Since details concerning regional blood supply have little meaning until the student understands the organization of the central nervous system, this chapter has been moved to the back of the book. This chapter and the atlas section, containing 24 full color plates, should be referred to frequently in the course of reading other chapters. In this revision the total number of chapters has been reduced by two and over one hundred and twenty new or revised illustrations have been added to various chapters, many of them in color. The Paris Nomina Anatomica (PNA) in its amended form as adopted by the International Anatomical Nomenclature Committee has been used.

The author has missed the wise and prudent counsel of his former co-author, Professor Raymond C. Truex of Temple University School of Medicine, who contributed so much to this text. The present author now accepts total responsibility for the contents of this text. Robert J. Demarest of the Department of Anatomy, College of Physicians and Surgeons, Columbia University, has been responsible for all new drawings in this edition. His unusual talents have contributed enormously to the success of this text. Dr. Fred A. Mettler has made available to the author

many superb illustrations from his *Neuroanatomy* (1948) which were drawn by Ivan Summer. I am grateful to Dr. Mettler and the C. V. Mosby Company for permission to publish these illustrations. The excellent technical assistance of Mrs. Greta Katzauer and Mr. Antonio B. Pereira who have worked closely with the author at Columbia for over fifteen years is acknowledged with special gratitude.

Colleagues at many medical schools have offered valuable suggestions, given generously of their time and complied graciously with my requests for illustrations. While the names of all individuals who supplied illustrations are cited in the figure legends, particular gratitude is expressed to the following: Drs. Ray C. Henrikson, Fred A. Mettler, Charles R. Noback, Roberta J. Pierson, Virginia Tennyson and Ernst Wood at Columbia University; Dr. David Bodian at Johns Hopkins University; Drs. Richard and Mary Bunge at Washington University; Dr. Milton W. Brightman at National Institutes of Health; Dr. William Bondareff at Northwestern University; Dr. Marc Colonnier at the University of Ottawa; Dr. David Felten at Indiana University; Dr. Clement A. Fox at Wayne State University; Dr. Torbjörn Malmfors, Karolinska Institutet, Sweden; Drs. Sanford L. Palay and Victoria Chan-Palay, Harvard Medical School; Dr. Alan Peters, Boston University; Dr. Joyce E. Shriver, Mt. Sinai Medical School; Dr. John E. Swett, University of Colorado; Dr. Constantino Sotelo, Laboratoire de Neuromorphologie, Paris; and Dr. James E. Vaughn, City of Hope National Medical Center. The cooperation of the C. V. Mosby Company, Rockefeller University Press, Oxford University Press, Elsevier Publishing Company and the Wistar Institute of Anatomy and Biology in granting permission to use certain illustrations is acknowledged with thanks.

Special acknowledgment must go to Mrs. Ruth Gutmann and Miss Anke Nolting for secretarial and editorial assistance. Finally, the author is grateful to the Publishers for their confidence, encouragement and numerous courtesies which have made the preparation of this book a satisfying experience.

Malcolm B. Carpenter

Preface to the First Edition

Neurology, more perhaps than any other branch of medicine, is dependent on an accurate knowledge of anatomy as a basis for the intelligent diagnosis and localization of neural disturbances. This book, the result of many years of neuroanatomical teaching, is intended to supply this basic anatomical need, to give the student and physician a thorough and clear presentation of the structural mechanisms of the human nervous system together with some understanding of their functional and clinical significance. It is an attempt to link structure and function into a dynamic pattern without sacrificing anatomical detail.

The book is a human neuroanatomy sufficiently rich in content to obviate the necessity of constantly consulting larger anatomical texts. It may be conveniently divided into two parts. The first part (Chapters I-VIII) is concerned with the general organization and meaning of the nervous system, its embryology and histological structure, and with some fundamental neurological problems as they apply to man. This is followed by a discussion of the organization and segmental distribution of the peripheral nerve elements, including an analysis of the functional components of the spinal nerves and of the various receptors and effectors. If these earlier chapters are perhaps more extensive than in most other texts, it is due

to the conviction that the book should be complete in itself, and also that a knowledge of these preliminaries is essential for an understanding of the complex machinery of the spinal cord and brain.

The second and larger part (Chapters IX-XX) is devoted to the architectonics of the central nervous system and may be regarded as "applied neuroanatomy." Special features of this part are the many fine photographs, both gross and microscopic, of the human brain and spinal cord, the great wealth of anatomical detail, and the discussion of the structural mechanisms in the light of clinical experience. While the individual portions of the nervous system are treated separately, an attempt has been made to achieve organic structural continuity by judicious repetition and overlapping and by constant reference to related topics already familiar to the student from previous chapters. The plan of exposition is substantially the same for each topic. The gross structure and relationships are concisely but thoroughly reviewed with the aid of clear and graphic illustrations. The internal structure is then presented in detail, usually based on a carefully graded series of fine and clearly labeled microphotographs of human material. At each level the student is familiarized with the exact location, extent and relationships of the various structures seen in the section. Finally the anatomical features of each part are reviewed more comprehensively as three-dimensional structural mechanisms, with a full discussion of their connections and clinical significance. We believe that this treatment will make the complicated structural details alive and interesting to the student. The illustrations are not segregated in the back of the book in the form of an atlas but are scattered in the text, in proper relation to the levels studied.

Besides the many original illustrations, a number of others selected from various and duly acknowledged sources have been completely redrawn and relabeled for the sake of clarity and simplicity. All the illustrations, whether original or borrowed, have been executed by Frances H. Elwyn to whose skill and patience the authors are deeply indebted. We are also indebted to

Dr. H. Alsop Riley for the use of several microphotographs; to Drs. R. C. Truex and Benjamin Salzer for the reading of several chapters; and especially to Dr. Otto Marburg for his many stimulating discussions and suggestions and for his critical reading of the chapters on the mesencephalon, diencephalon, and cerebral hemispheres. Thanks are also due to Rosette Spoerri for her competent help in preparing the manuscript and bibliography.

The authors cannot express too strongly their obligation to the publishers for their continuous courtesy and cooperation in all matters, and for their infinite patience in waiting for a manuscript long overdue.

Adolph Elwyn
Oliver S. Strong

Contents

PREFACE TO THE SEVENTH EDITION v
PREFACE TO THE FIRST EDITION ix

Chapter 1
MENINGES AND CEREBROSPINAL FLUID 1

Dura Mater 1
Pia Mater 7
Arachnoid ..., ... 9
  Arachnoid Granulations 11
Pia-Glia and the Perivascular
  Spaces 11

Cerebrospinal Fluid 14
Barriers Related to the Brain 16
  Blood-Brain Barrier 17
  Blood-Cerebrospinal Fluid Bar-
   rier 19
  Brain-Cerebrospinal Fluid Barrier 19

Chapter 2
GROSS ANATOMY OF THE BRAIN 19

The Cerebral Hemispheres 21
  Lateral Surface 22
   Frontal Lobe 23
   Parietal Lobe 23
   Temporal Lobe 24
   Occipital Lobe 24
   The Insula 24
  Medial Surface 26
   Limbic Lobe 27
  The Inferior Surface 28
  The White Matter 29
   Projection Fibers 29
   Association Fibers 31
   Commissural Fibers 32
The Basal Ganglia 32
  The Putamen 33
  The Globus Pallidus 33
  The Caudate Nucleus 33
  The Amygdaloid Nuclear
   Complex 33

The Lateral Ventricles 34
  The Anterior Horn 34
  The Body of the Lateral
   Ventricle 34
  The Inferior Horn 35
  The Posterior Horn 35
The Brain Stem 36
  The Medulla 38
   The Fourth Ventricle 39
  The Pons 41
  The Midbrain 42
   Crus Cerebri 42
   Substantia Nigra 43
  The Diencephalon 43
   The Epithalamus 43
   The Thalamus 43
   The Hypothalamus 45
   The Subthalamus 45
The Cerebellum 46

Chapter 3
DEVELOPMENT AND HISTOGENESIS OF THE NERVOUS SYSTEM ... 49

Formation of the Neural Tube 49
Neural Crest 49
Histogenesis of Neural Tube 50
Neurons 51
Glia Cells 52
Spinal Cord 53
   Neuron Differentiation 55
   Segmental Arrangement of Peripheral Nerve Elements 56
Brain 57

Myelencephalon 60
Metencephalon 61
Mesencephalon 63
Diencephalon 64
Telencephalon 65
   Corpus Striatum and Internal Capsule 66
   Cerebral Cortex 67
   Commissures 69

Chapter 4
THE NEURON ... 71

Neuroanatomical Methods 71
Functional Concept of Neurons 77
Varieties of Neurons 77
The Nerve Cell Body (Perikaryon) . 82
   Nucleus 84
   Nucleolus 84
   Chromophil Substance 84
   Neurofibrils 85
   Mitochondria 88
   Centrosome 88
   Golgi Apparatus 88
   Inclusions 90
   Neurosecretion 91
The Nerve Fiber 93
   Myelin 94

Nodes of Ranvier 96
Schmidt-Lantermann Clefts 97
Sheath of Schwann 99
Endoneurium 100
Perineurium 100
Epineurium 100
Unmyelinated Peripheral Nerve Fibers (Fibers of Remak) 100
   Fiber Size 101
Physical and Physiological Grouping of Nerve Fibers 101
The Synapse 103
   Degeneration of Nerve Fibers 105
   Retrograde Degeneration 107
   Regeneration 107

Chapter 5
NEUROGLIA, EPENDYMA AND CHOROID PLEXUS ... 115

Neuroglia 115
   Astrocytes 118
   Oligodendrocytes 122

Microglia 125
Ependyma 128
Choroid Epithelium 132

Chapter 6
RECEPTORS AND EFFECTORS ... 137

Receptors 138
   Classification 138
      Free Nerve Endings 142
      Diffuse Endings 143

   Encapsulated Endings 144
   Stretch Receptors 146
Relation of Receptors to Sensory Modalities 153

Referred Pain 155   Somatic Effectors 156
Effectors 156   Visceral Effectors 158

Chapter 7
SEGMENTAL AND PERIPHERAL INNERVATION 159

Spinal Nerve 159   Medial Brachial Cutaneous
Spinal Ganglia 161   Nerve 177
The Mixed Nerve 162   Injuries of the Brachial Plexus ... 177
Connective Tissue Sheaths 164   Lumbosacral Plexus 181
Segmental Innervation 164   Obturator Nerve 182
Peripheral Innervation 168   Femoral Nerve 182
Dorsal Rami 168   Lateral Femoral Cutaneous
Ventral Rami 169   Nerve 183
Cervical Plexus 169   Sciatic Nerve 184
Brachial Plexus 173   Tibial Nerve 184
Axillary Nerve 175   Common Peroneal Nerve 185
Radial Nerve 175   Gluteal Nerves 185
Musculocutaneous Nerve 176   Posterior Femoral Cutaneous
Median Nerve 176   Nerve 185
Ulnar Nerve 177   Functional Considerations 185
Medial Antebrachial Cuta-   Regeneration of Injured Peripheral
neous Nerve 177   Nerves 188

Chapter 8
THE AUTONOMIC NERVOUS SYSTEM 191

Pre- and Postganglionic Neurons 192   Chemical Mediation at Synapses . 200
The Sympathetic System 195   Denervation Sensitization 205
The Parasympathetic System ... 197   Central Autonomic Pathways 206
Visceral Afferent Fibers 199   Functional Considerations 208
Structure of Autonomic Ganglia . 199

Chapter 9
SPINAL CORD: GROSS ANATOMY AND INTERNAL
STRUCTURE 213

Gross Anatomy 213   Somatic Efferent Neurons 229
General Topography 214   Visceral Efferent Neurons 230
Internal Structure 216   Posterior Horn Neurons 231
Gray and White Substance 217   Arrangement of Entering Afferent
Spinal Cord Levels 218   Fibers 232
Nuclei and Cell Groups 221   Spinal Reflexes 235
Cytoarchitectural Lamination ... 222

Chapter 10
TRACTS OF THE SPINAL CORD 238

Long Ascending Spinal Tracts 238
  Posterior White Columns 238
  Anterior Spinothalamic Tract ... 242
  Lateral Spinothalamic Tract 245
  Spinotectal Tract 249
  Posterior Spinocerebellar Tract .. 249
  Anterior Spinocerebellar Tract .. 251
  Cuneocerebellar Tract 252
  Spinoreticular Fibers 253
  Other Ascending Fiber Systems in
  the Spinal Cord 253

Long Descending Spinal Tracts 255
  Corticospinal System 255
  Tectospinal Tract 261
  Rubrospinal Tract 261
  Vestibulospinal Tract 264
  Reticulospinal Tracts 267

Medial Longitudinal Fasciculus
(MLF) 269
Olivospinal Tract 270
Descending Autonomic Pathways 271
Ascending and Descending Spinal
Tracts 271
The Fasciculi Proprii 271
Upper and Lower Motor Neurons .. 272
Lesions of the Spinal Cord and
Nerve Roots 276
  Dorsal Root Lesions 277
  Ventral Root Lesions 277
  Spinal Cord Transection 278
  Spinal Hemisection 279
  Amyotrophic Lateral Sclerosis ... 280
  Combined System Disease 281
  Syringomyelia 282
  Other Spinal Syndromes 283

Chapter 11
THE MEDULLA 285

Spinomedullary Transition 286
  Corticospinal Decussation 287
  Posterior Column Nuclei 289
  Decussation of the Medial Lem-
  niscus 291
  Spinal Trigeminal Tract 293
  Spinal Trigeminal Nucleus 294
  Reticular Formation 296
  Area Postrema 296
  Cranial Nerve Nuclei 297
Olivary Levels of the Medulla 297
  Inferior Olivary Nuclear Complex 298
  Medullary Reticular Formation .. 300

Afferent Fibers to the Medullary
Reticular Formation 301
Efferent Fibers from the Medul-
lary Reticular Formation 302
Ascending and Descending Tracts 303
Inferior Cerebellar Peduncle 303
Cranial Nerves of the Medulla 304
  The Hypoglossal Nerve 305
  Spinal Accessory Nerve 308
  The Vagus Nerve 309
  The Glossopharyngeal Nerve 312
Corticobulbar Fibers 314
Medullary-Pontine Junction 318

Chapter 12
THE PONS 322

Caudal Pons 322
  Dorsal Portion 322
  Ventral Portion 323
Vestibulocochlear Nerve 325
  The Cochlea 326
  The Cochlear Nerve and Nuclei .. 326

Primary Auditory Fibers 327
Auditory Pathways 329
Efferent Cochlear Bundle 332
Lesions of the Auditory System ... 335
The Labyrinth 336
The Vestibular Nerve and Nuclei .. 337

Primary Vestibular Fibers 339
Secondary Vestibular Fibers 342
Medial Longitudinal Fasciculus
(MLF) 342
Functional Considerations 344
The Facial Nerve 346
Lesions of the Facial Nerve 348
The Abducens Nerve 349
Rostral Pons 351
The Pontine Reticular Formation 351
The Trigeminal Nerve 352
Trigeminal Ganglion 353

Spinal Trigeminal Tract and
Nucleus 354
The Principal Sensory Nucleus . 357
The Mesencephalic Nucleus ... 359
The Motor Nucleus 360
Secondary Trigeminal
Pathways 360
Trigeminal Reflexes 361
Isthmus of the Hindbrain 362
Superior Cerebellar Peduncle .. 363
Locus Ceruleus 364
Raphe Nuclei 365

Chapter 13
THE MESENCEPHALON 367

Inferior Collicular Level 367
The Inferior Colliculi 367
The Trochlear Nerve 369
Tegmental and Interpeduncular
Nuclei 369
Superior Collicular Level 370
Superior Colliculi 370
Functional Considerations 374
The Pretectal Region 374
The Posterior Commissure 376
The Oculomotor Nerve 377
The Oculomotor Nuclear
Complex 377
The Accessory Oculomotor
Nuclei 379

Afferent Connections of the
Oculomotor Complex 380
Lesions of the Third Nerve 382
Pupillary Reflexes 382
Nuclei of the Mesencephalic Teg-
mentum 384
The Red Nucleus 384
Lesions of the Red Nucleus ... 387
Mesencephalic Reticular Forma-
tion 388
Functional Considerations of the
Reticular Formation 388
Substantia Nigra 393
Crus Cerebri 397

Chapter 14
THE CEREBELLUM 399

Gross Anatomy 399
Cerebellar Cortex 401
The Molecular Layer 401
The Purkinje Cell Layer 401
The Granular Layer 402
Cortical Afferent Input 404
Structural Mechanisms 411
Neuroglia 412
The Deep Cerebellar Nuclei 414
The Dentate Nucleus 414
The Emboliform Nucleus 415
The Globose Nucleus 415

The Fastigial Nucleus 415
Cerebellar Connections 416
Afferent Fibers 416
Efferent Fibers 420
Cerebellar Organization 425
Functional Considerations 430
Neocerebellar Lesions 430
Archicerebellar Lesions 431
Anterior Lobe of the Cerebellum . 432
Modification of Cerebellar Dis-
turbances 433
Computer Functions 434

Chapter 15
THE DIENCEPHALON **435**

Midbrain-Diencephalic Junction . .   435
Caudal Diencephalon   437
The Epithalamus   438
The Thalamus   440
  The Anterior Nuclear Group   443
  The Dorsomedial Nucleus   444
  The Midline Nuclei   446
  The Intralaminar Nuclei   446
    The Centromedian Nucleus . . .   447
    The Parafascicular Nucleus . . .   447
  The Lateral Nuclear Group   451
    The Lateral Dorsal Nucleus . . .   451
    The Lateral Posterior Nucleus .   451
    The Pulvinar   451
  The Ventral Nuclear Mass   452
    The Ventral Anterior Nucleus .   452
    The Ventral Lateral Nucleus . .   454
    The Ventral Posterior Nucleus .   454
      The Ventral Posterolateral
      Nucleus   454
      The Ventral Posteromedial
      Nucleus   455

    The Ventral Posterior In-
    ferior Nucleus   456
    The Posterior Thalamic Zone . .   456
  The Medial Geniculate Body   457
  The Lateral Geniculate Body   458
  The Thalamic Reticular Nucleus   461
The Thalamic Radiations and Inter-
nal Capsule   462
The Visual Pathways   465
  The Retina   465
  The Optic Nerves   465
  The Optic Tract   466
  The Geniculocalcarine Tract   466
  Clinical Considerations   470
Functional Considerations of the
Thalamus   470
  The Specific Sensory Relay Nuclei   470
  The Cortical Relay Nuclei   473
  The Association Nuclei   474
  The Intralaminar and Midline Nu-
  clei   474

Chapter 16
THE HYPOTHALAMUS **478**

The Hypothalamic Nuclei   478
  The Lateral Hypothalamic Area .   478
  The Preoptic Area   479
  The Supraoptic Region   479
  The Tuberal Region   482
  The Mammillary Region   482
Connections of the Hypothalamus .   483
  The Afferent Connections of the
  Hypothalamus   483

The Efferent Connections of the
  Hypothalamus   487
    The Supraopticohypophysial
    Tract   488
    The Tuberohypophysial
    (Tuberoinfundibular) Tract . . .   488
Hypophysial Portal System   490
Supraoptic Decussations   490
Functional Considerations   491

Chapter 17
THE BASAL GANGLIA **496**

The Corpus Striatum   496
  The Caudate Nucleus   497
  The Lenticular Nucleus   497
    The Putamen   497
    The Globus Pallidus   498
    The Claustrum   499

Striatal Connections   499
  Striatal Afferent Fibers   499
    Corticostriate Fibers   499
    Thalamostriate Fibers   500
    Nigrostriate Fibers   501
  Striatal Efferent Fibers   504

Striopallidal Fibers 504
Strionigral Fibers 504
Pallidal Connections 504
Pallidal Afferent Fibers 504
Subthalamopallidal Fibers 504
Pallidofugal Fiber Systems 505
The Ansa Lenticularis 505
The Lenticular Fasciculus 505
The Thalamic Fasciculus 505
Pallidotegmental Fibers 507

The Subthalamic Fasciculus ... 508
The Subthalamic Region 509
The Subthalamic Nucleus 509
The Zona Incerta 511
Forel's Field H 511
Functional Considerations 512
Tremor 514
Athetosis 514
Chorea 515
Ballism 515

Chapter 18
OLFACTORY PATHWAYS, HIPPOCAMPAL FORMATION AND AMYGDALA **521**

Rhinencephalon 521
Olfactory Pathways 521
Olfactory Receptors 521
Olfactory Bulb 522
Olfactory Tract 523
Olfactory Lobe 524
Clinical Considerations 527
The Anterior Commissure 529
The Hippocampal Formation 530

Fornix 535
Functional Considerations 537
Amygdaloid Nuclear Complex 539
The Stria Terminalis 540
The Ventral Amygdalofugal Projection 541
Functional Considerations 542
Limbic System 543
Limbic Lobe 544

Chapter 19
THE CEREBRAL CORTEX **547**

Structure of the Cortex 547
Cortical Cells and Fibers 548
The Cortical Layers 550
The Interrelation of Cortical Neurons 551
Cortical Areas 556
Sensory Areas of the Cerebral Cortex 559
Primary Sensory Areas 559
Secondary Sensory Areas 559
The Primary Somesthetic Area .. 560
Somatic Sensory Area II 566
The Primary Visual Area 566
The Primary Auditory Area 574
The Gustatory Area 577
Vestibular Representation 578
Cortical Areas Concerned with Motor Function 578
The Primary Motor Area 578

The Premotor Area 582
Supplementary Motor Area 583
Cortical Eye Fields 585
Nonpyramidal Corticofugal Fibers . 586
Corticoreticular Fibers 586
Corticopontine Fibers 586
Corticothalamic Fibers 586
Phenomenon of Cortical Suppression 589
Considerations of Cortical Functions 589
Cerebral Dominance 589
Interhemispheric Transfer 591
Nonspecific Thalamocortical Relationships 592
Sleep 593
Higher Cortical Functions 595
Agnosia 596
Aphasia 596
Apraxia 597
Prefrontal Cortex 598

Chapter 20
BLOOD SUPPLY OF THE CENTRAL NERVOUS SYSTEM 600

Blood Supply of the Spinal Cord ... 600
Blood Supply of the Brain 603
  The Internal Carotid Artery 603
  The Vertebral Artery 605
  The Cerebral Arterial Circle 606
  The Cortical Branches 608
    The Anterior Cerebral Artery .. 608
    The Middle Cerebral Artery ... 609
    The Posterior Cerebral Arteries 609
  The Central Branches 612
    The Central or Ganglionic Arteries 612
    Choroidal Arteries 614

Blood Supply of Basal Ganglia, Internal Capsule and Diencephalon .. 615
Vertebral Basilar System 616
  Vertebral Artery 616
  Basilar Artery 616
  Medulla and Pons 616
  Mesencephalon 620
  Cerebellum 621
Arteries of the Dura 621
Cerebral Veins and Venous Sinuses . 622
  The Cerebral Veins 624
  The Superficial Cerebral Veins .. 626
  The Deep Cerebral Veins 627

BIBLIOGRAPHY 631
ATLAS OF BRAIN AND BRAIN STEM 673
INDEX 713

CHAPTER 1

Meninges and Cerebrospinal Fluid

The brain and spinal cord are delicate semisolid structures requiring protection and support. The brain is invested by various membranes, floated in a clear fluid and encased in a bony vault. Three membranes surround the brain. The most external is a dense connective tissue envelope known as the *dura mater* or *pachymeninx*. The innermost connective tissue membrane is the *pia mater*, a thin translucent membrane, adherent to the surface of the brain and spinal cord, which accurately follows every contour. Between these membranes is a delicate layer of reticular fibers forming a weblike membrane, the *arachnoid*. The pia mater and arachnoid have a similar structure and collectively are called the *leptomeninges*.

DURA MATER

The cranial dura consists of: (1) an outer *periosteal layer* adherent to the inner surface of the cranium which is rich in blood vessels and nerves, and (2) an inner *meningeal layer* lined with flat cells. At certain sites these layers are separated and form large venous sinuses (Fig. 1-1). The meningeal layer gives rise to several septa which divide the cranial cavity into compartments. The largest of these is the sickle-shaped *falx cerebri* which extends in the midline from the crista galli to the internal occipital protuberance (Fig. 1-2). Posteriorly this septum is continuous with other transverse dural septa arising from the superior crest of the petrous portion of the temporal bone. These septa form the *tentorium cerebelli* which roofs over the posterior fossa. The free borders of the tentorium form the *tentorial incisure* (Figs. 1-2 and 1-3), the only opening between these compartments. Thus these dura reflections divide the cranial cavity into paired lateral compartments for the cerebral hemispheres, and a single posterior compartment for the cerebellum and lower brain stem. The brain stem passes through the tentorial notch (Fig. 1-4). The occipital lobes lie on the superior surface of the tentorium. A small midsagittal septum below the tentorium forms the *falx cerebelli* (Fig. 1-2) which partially separates the cerebellar hemispheres. The *diaphragma sellae* roofs over the pituitary fossa and is perforated by the infundibulum. The dural sinuses are discussed in relationship with the cerebral veins in Chapter 20.

The major blood supply for the dura is provided by the middle meningeal artery, a branch of the maxillary artery, which enters the skull via the foramen spinosum (Figs. 1-3 and 20-3). The ophthalmic artery gives rise to anterior meningeal branches and the occipital and vertebral arteries provide posterior meningeal branches. Skull fractures lacerating these meningeal arteries produce space occupying epidural hemorrhages between the skull and the dura that require prompt surgical intervention.

1

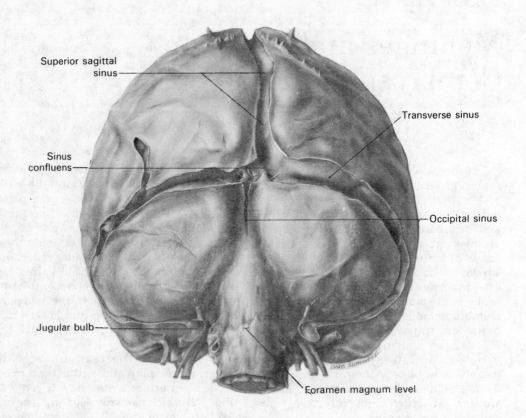

FIG. 1-1. Posterior view of the dura surrounding the brain. Prominent dural sinuses have been opened. The periosteal layer of the dura has been cut at the margins of the foramen magnum (from Mettler's *Neuroanatomy*, '48; courtesy of The C. V. Mosby Company).

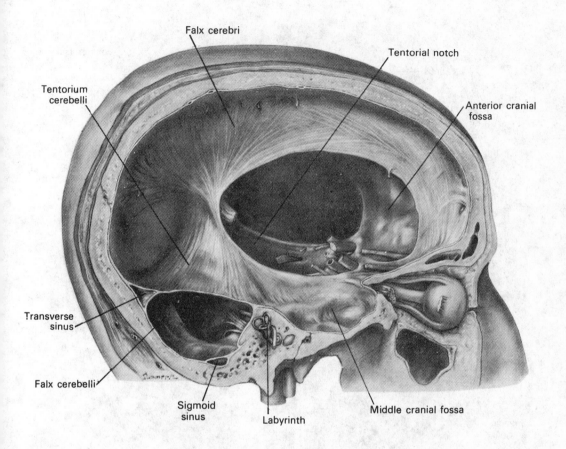

FIG. 1-2. Parasagittal section of the head showing the falx cerebri, the tentorium cerebelli and the falx cerebelli (from Mettler's *Neuroanatomy*, '48; courtesy of The C. V. Mosby Company).

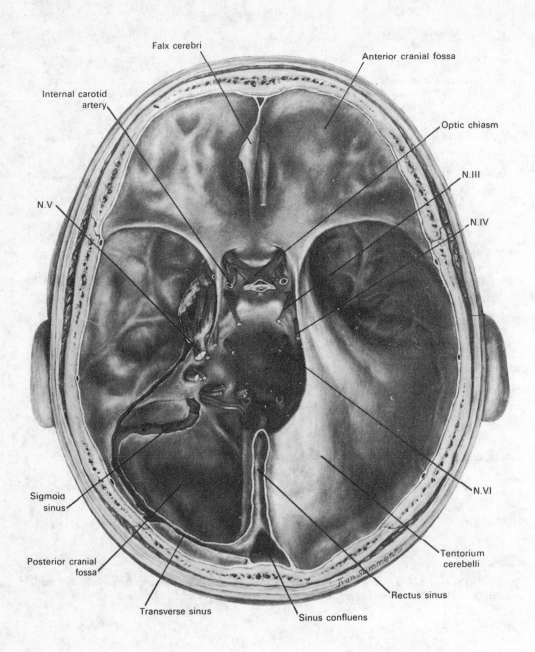

FIG. 1-3. View of the base of the skull with dura mater. The falx cerebri has been removed and the tentorium cerebelli has been cut away on the left to expose the posterior fossa (from Mettler's *Neuroanatomy*, '48; courtesy of The C. V. Mosby Company).

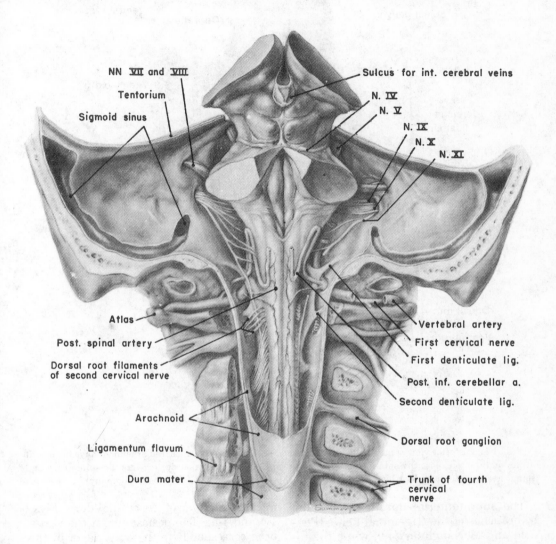

FIG. 1-4. Posterior view of the brain stem, upper cervical spinal cord and meninges (from Mettler's *Neuroanatomy*, '48; courtesy of The C. V. Mosby Company).

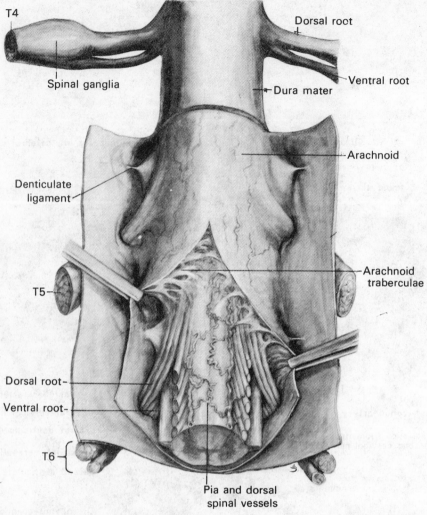

Fig. 1-5. Posterior view of part of the upper thoracic spinal cord. The dura and arachnoid have been split at the midline to expose the spinal cord and pial vessels. Above the intact dura covers the spinal cord and spinal nerve roots (from Mettler's *Neuroanatomy*, '48; courtesy of The C. V. Mosby Company).

The supratentorial dura is innervated by branches of the trigeminal nerve (Penfield and McNaughton, '40), while the infratentorial dura is supplied by branches of the upper cervical spinal nerves and the vagus nerve (Kimmel, '59, '61).

The innermost layer of the dura is composed of flattened mesothelial cells with a dense cytoplasm. This layer usually is in close contact with the arachnoid, suggesting that the *subdural space* is a potential space rather than an actual space (Davson, '67).

The *spinal dura* is a continuation of the meningeal layer of the cranial dura (Figs. 1-4 and 1-5). The periosteum of the vertebrae corresponds to the outer layer of the cranial dura. Inner and outer surfaces of the spinal dura are covered by a single layer of flat cells, and the dense membrane is separated from the periosteum by a narrow *epidural space*. The epidural space contains areolar tissue and the internal vertebral venous plexuses.

The spinal dura extends as a closed tube from the margins of the foramen magnum to the level of the second sacral vertebra (Fig. 1-6). At the caudal termination of the

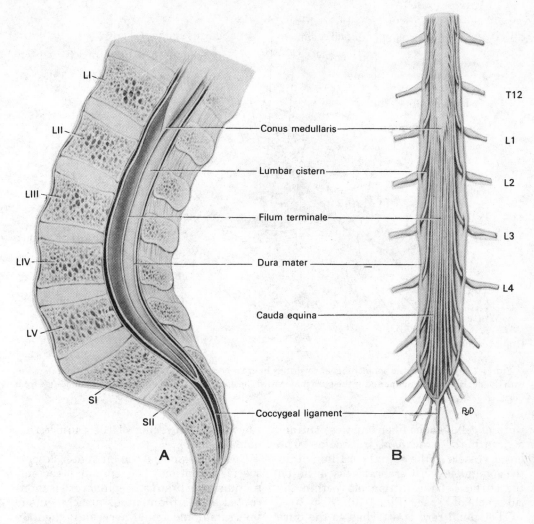

FIG. 1-6. Diagrammatic representation of the caudal part of the spinal cord and lumbar cistern. *A* is a sagittal view of the conus medullaris, lumbar cistern and lumbosacral vertebrae. *B* is a posterior view of the cauda equina and nerve roots.

dural sac the dura invests the filum terminale to form a thin fibrous cord, the *coccygeal ligament* (Fig. 1-6). This ligament extends caudally to the coccyx where it becomes continuous with the periosteum. The spinal cord ends at the lower border of the first lumbar vertebra. Extensions of the dura passing laterally around the spinal nerve roots form dural root sleeves (Figs. 1-5 and 1-7).

PIA MATER

This vascular membrane is composed of: (1) an inner membraneous layer, the *in-* *tima pia* (Key and Retzuis, 1875), and (2) a more superficial *epipial layer*. The intima pia, adherent to underlying nervous tissue, follows its contours closely and is composed of fine reticular and elastic fibers (Figs. 1-8 and 1-9). Where blood vessels enter and leave the central nervous system, the intima pia is invaginated forming a perivascular space (Fig. 1-14). The intima pia, like the arachnoid, is avascular and derives its nutrients by diffusion from the cerebrospinal fluid and the underlying nervous tissue (Millen and Woollam, '61, '62). The epipial layer is formed by a mesh-

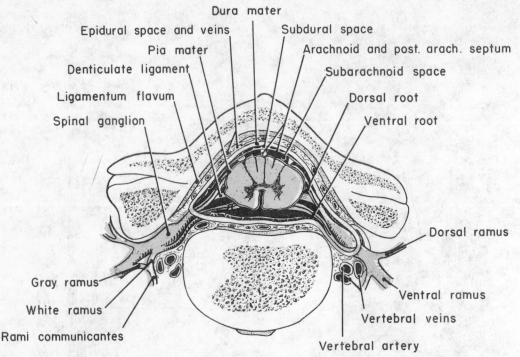

Dura mater

Epidural space and veins

Subdural space

Pia mater

Arachnoid and post. arach. septum

Denticulate ligament

Subarachnoid space

Ligamentum flavum

Dorsal root

Spinal ganglion

Ventral root

Dorsal ramus

Gray ramus

White ramus

Ventral ramus

Vertebral veins

Rami communicantes

Vertebral artery

Fig. 1-7. Spinal cord and its meningeal coverings in cross section. Note the continuity of the pia mater with the denticulate ligament and of the dura mater with the epineurium of the spinal nerves (modified from Corning, '22).

work of collagenous fiber bundles continuous with the arachnoid trabeculae. The blood vessels of the spinal cord lie within the epipial layer. Cerebral vessels lie on the surface of the intima pia within the subarachnoid space (Fig. 1-10).

The spinal cord is attached to the dura mater by a series of lateral flattened bands of epipial tissue known as the *denticulate ligaments* (Figs. 1-4, 1-5 and 1-7). Each triangular-shaped ligament is attached medially to the lateral surface of the spinal cord midway between the dorsal and ventral roots. The bases of these ligaments arise in the pia mater, and apices are firmly attached to the arachnoid and the inner surface of the dura. The denticulate ligaments alternate with the dural evaginations which mark the exits of the cervical, thoracic and first lumbar spinal nerves. On each lateral surface of the spinal cord 18 to 24 denticulate ligaments anchor the spinal cord to the dura. In the region of the conus medullaris epipial tis-

sue forms a covering of the filum terminale (Fig. 1-6).

Certain regions of the pia mater deserve special attention. The epipial layer surrounding the brain and spinal cord is interrupted at the filamentous attachments of the cranial and spinal nerves. As the individual nerve fibers enter or leave the brain and spinal cord they pierce the intima pia from which they derive an investment of squamous cells and fine reticular fibers (Fig. 1-8). The more fibrous intima pia is firmly anchored to the surface of the spinal cord by a thin but distinct *superficial glial membrane* (Fig. 1-9). The latter is composed of many fine processes of more deeply located fibrous astrocytes. Cell bodies of astrocytes can be observed in the glial membrane and many of the glial fibers possess bulbous expansions. The glial fibers and astrocytes are particularly prominent in the regions where the dorsal and ventral spinal roots penetrate the pia mater. In the region of the posterolateral sul-

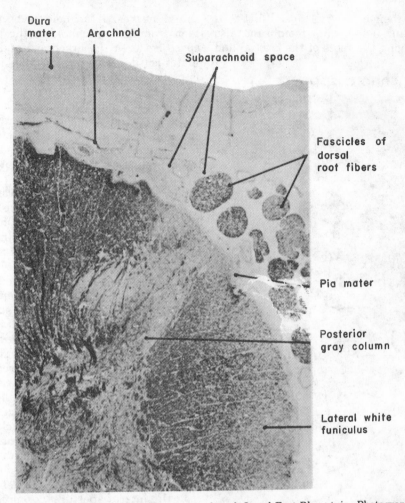

Fig. 1-8. Relations of meninges to the human spinal cord. Luxol Fast Blue stain. Photograph. ×28.

cus such glial elements constitute a barrier to the regenerating nerve fibers of avulsed or injured dorsal roots.

In the region of the ventricles the brain wall is formed by a single layer of ependymal cells, the outer surface of which is firmly adherent to the pia mater. In the roof of the third ventricle, in the lower part of the roof of the fourth ventricle and on the medial wall of the lateral ventricle (choroid fissure), the intima pia blends with the ependymal layer to form the *tela choroidea* (Fig. 5-14). The tela choroidea provides areas for the anchorage of the choroid plexuses in the ventricles. It has a triangular shape in the roof of the third and fourth ventricles, while the tela cho-roidea of the lateral ventricle (Fig. 2-22) is horse-shoe-shaped as it follows the choro-idal fissure (Fig. 18-8). The two layers of the pia mater in the transverse cerebral fissure, below the splenium of the corpus callosum and above the pineal body, form the *velum interpositum* (Fig. 2-22). The internal cerebral veins, branches of the posterior cerebral artery, and arteries to the choroid plexuses of the third and lat-eral ventricles lie between these two lay-ers (Figs. 20-19 and 20-20).

ARACHNOID

The arachnoid is a delicate nonvascular membrane between the dura and the pia mater which passes over the sulci without following their contours (Figs. 1-5, 1-8, 1-10, 1-12 and 1-14). This membrane also extends along the roots of the cranial and

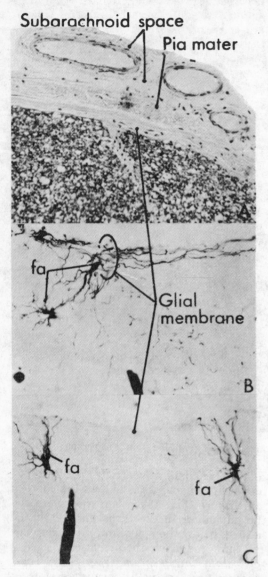

Subarachnoid space

Pia mater

Glial membrane

fa

fa

fa

A

B

C

FIG. 1-9. Photographs of human spinal cord that demonstrate the structure and relations of pia mater and external glial membrane. These layers form the covering of the spinal cord. A. Note that glial membrane is closely adherent to inner surface of pia mater. Luxol Fast Blue-cresyl violet stain. ×143. In B and C the processes and terminal enlargements of fibrous astrocytes (fa) are identified as they enter into the formation of the glial membrane. Golgi stain. ×263.

spinal nerves. Arachnoid trabeculae extend from the arachnoid to the pia. The space between the arachnoid and the pia mater is filled with cerebrospinal fluid and is called the *subarachnoid space* (Fig. 1-11). With certain cranial nerves, the olfactory, optic and acoustic, a subarachnoid space surrounds the nerves (Shanthaveerapa and Bourne, '64, '66; Davson,'67). A small subarachnoid space also surrounds the spinal nerve roots in the root sleeves (Fig. 1-7). In the spinal regions fewer arachnoid trabeculae are concentrated into several subarachnoid septa; hence the subarachnoid space is a more continuous cavity and the arachnoid a more distinct membrane (Figs. 1-7 and 1-8). The arachnoid, trabeculae and epipial surface are all covered with a single layer of flattened cells with large pale oval nuclei. When certain substances are injected into the subarachnoid space, these cells may swell and participate in phagocytic activity by ingesting particles of the foreign material. They may even become detached and form free macrophages.

The subarachnoid space is filled with cerebrospinal fluid and is in direct communication with the fourth ventricle of the brain by means of three apertures, one median and two lateral. The median aperture, or *foramen of Magendie*, is located in the caudal part of the thin ventricular roof; the lateral apertures, or *foramina of Luschka*, open into the pontine subarachnoid cistern posterior to the emerging fibers of the ninth cranial nerve (Fig. 1-10).

The extent of the subarachnoid space surrounding the brain shows local variations. Over the convexity of the cerebral hemisphere this space is narrow, except in the depths of the sulci. At the base of the brain and around the brain stem the pia and the arachnoid often are widely separated, creating what are called *subarachnoid cisterna* (Figs. 1-10 and 1-11). One of the largest cisterns is found between the medulla and the cerebellum. This is the *cerebellomedullary cistern* (cisterna magna) into which the foramina of the fourth ventricle open (Figs. 1-10 and 1-11). Cerebrospinal fluid from the fourth ventricle passes into the cerebellomedullary cistern via the median foramen of Magendie and the two lateral foramina of Luschka. Other cisterns of considerable size are the *pontine cistern*, the *interpeduncular cistern*, the *chiasmatic cistern* and the *superior cistern* (Figs. 1-10 and 1-11). The superior cistern, surrounding the posterior, superior and lateral surfaces of the midbrain, is referred to clinically as the *cisterna ambiens* (Davidoff and Dyke, '51; Taveras and Wood, '64). This cistern is of great importance because it contains the great vein of Galen, and the posterior cerebral and superior cerebellar arteries. Most of these cisterns can be visualized in pneumoencephalograms.

The *lumbar cistern* extends from the conus medullaris (lower border of the first lumbar vertebra) to about the level of the second lumbar vertebra (Fig. 1-6). It contains the filum terminale and nerve roots of the cauda equina. It is from this cistern that cerebrospinal fluid is withdrawn in a lumbar spinal tap.

Arachnoid Granulations. In regions adjacent to the superior sagittal sinus the cerebral pia-arachnoid gives rise to tufted prolongations which protrude through the meningeal layer of the dura into the superior sagittal sinus (Fig. 1-12). These granulations are variable in number and location and each consists of numerous arachnoid villi. These villi have a thin outer limiting membrane beneath which are bundles of collagenous and elastic fibers (Fig. 1-13). Cells similar to those of the pia-arachnoid are scattered among the fibers, and small oval epithelial cells cap the surface of the villi. Arachnoid granulations frequently are surrounded by a venous lacuna along the margin of the superior sagittal sinus. Arachnoid granulations are larger and more numerous at advanced age and tend to become calcified. The structure of a small granulation within a lateral lacuna of the superior sagittal sinus is shown in Figure 1-13. Although arachnoid villi are most numerous along the interhemispheric fissure, in relation to the superior longitudinal sinus, they are found also along the other venous sinuses within the skull. Arachnoid villi also have been described in the spinal arachnoid (Elman, '23) and along the optic nerve (Shanthaveerappa and Bourne, '64). In both the spinal and cerebral arachnoid, cell clusters are sometimes formed which become attached to the dura. These growths may become calcified or, under abnormal conditions, form the sites of neoplastic tumors. Arachnoid granulations more frequently occur with advancing age.

Such granulations are the major site of fluid transfer from the subarachnoid space to the venous system. The dural sinuses cannot collapse and the pressure within them is negative in the upright position. Venous pressure is therefore less than the hydrostatic pressure of the cerebrospinal fluid so that fluid moves from the subarachnoid space to the venous dural sinuses. Arachnoid granulations appear to function as passive, pressure-dependent, one-way-flow valves whose membranes are readily permeable to metabolites, Prussian blue reagents and even large molecular weight substances. For example, if plasma proteins, serum albumin or inulin are injected into the subarachnoid space, they rapidly appear in the venous blood (Davson, '60; Tschirgi, '60).

PIA-GLIA AND THE PERIVASCULAR SPACES

The intima pia or pia-glia is regarded as the external limiting membrane of the central nervous system (CNS). It has been suggested that the intima pia may be of ectodermal origin while the epipial tissue may be derived from mesoderm (Millen and Woollam, '61). As blood vessels enter and leave nervous tissue, they carry with them arachnoid and pia-glia which form a cuff around the vessel (Fig. 1-14). The space between the blood vessel and its "adventitial sheath" has long been called the *Virchow-Robin space*. It was suggested that these spaces might permit the flow of cerebrospinal fluid from the subarachnoid spaces into the depths of the tissue. Electron microscopic studies indicate that as blood vessels penetrate neural tissue from the subarachnoid space, reflections of the intima pia and arachnoid which form the

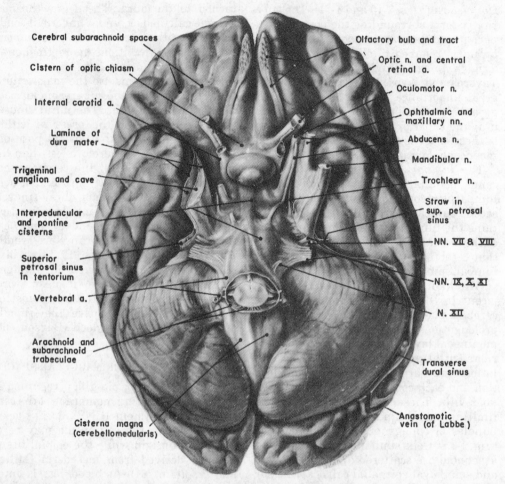

FIG. 1-10. Inferior view of brain, cranial nerves and meninges showing locations of subarachnoid cisterns (from Mettler's *Neuroanatomy*, '48; courtesy of The C. V. Mosby Company).

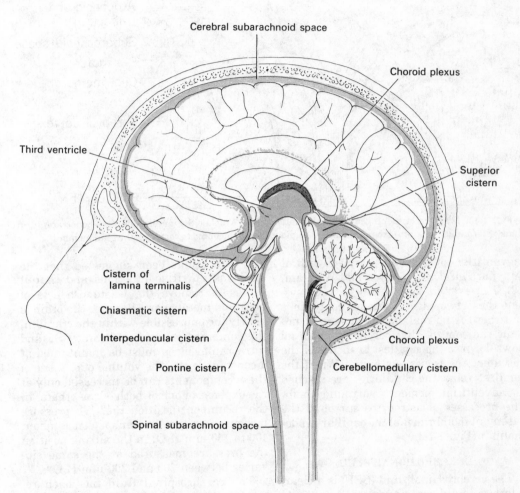

Fig. 1-11. Diagram of the subarachnoid cisterns as seen in a midsagittal view. The superior cistern is referred to clinically as the cisterna ambiens. The choroid plexus in the roof of the third ventricle and in the fourth ventricle is shown in *red*.

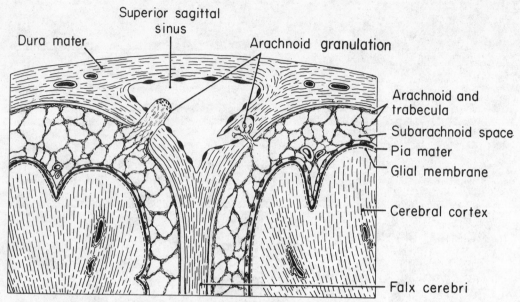

Fig. 1-12. Diagram of meningeal-cortical relationships. Arachnoid granulations may penetrate dural sinus or terminate in lateral lacuna of sinus. The pia is firmly anchored to cortex by the glial membrane.

"adventitial sheath" are carried with it (Maynard et al., '57; Millen and Woollam, '62). However in the central nervous system these two layers become continuous and there is no real space between them. Thus the concept that cerebrospinal fluid flows down to the smallest branches of the vascular tree is not sustained. When the smallest veins and capillaries are reached no adventitial elements surround them. The processes of astrocytes surround the basement membranes of the capillary endothelium (Fig. 1-15).

CEREBROSPINAL FLUID

The cerebrospinal fluid (CSF) is a clear, colorless liquid containing small amounts of protein, glucose and potassium and relatively large amounts of sodium chloride. There are no substances normally found in CSF which are not also found in blood plasma. No cellular component is found in CSF, although 1 to 5 cells/mm³ are considered to be within normal limits. The CSF serves to support and cushion the central nervous system against trauma. The buoyancy of CSF is indicated by the fact that a brain weighing 1500 g in air weighs only 50 g when immersed in CSF (Livings-

ton, '65). It has been suggested that the CSF has nutritive functions and that it serves to remove the waste products of neuronal metabolism. Because the brain is nearly incompressible within the cranium, the combined volumes of brain, CSF and intracranial blood must be maintained at a constant level. The volume of any one of these components can be increased only at the expense of one or both of the others. In the recumbent position the CSF pressure measured at the lumbar cistern is about 100 to 150 mm H_2O; in the sitting position the pressure measured at the same site varies between 200 and 300 mm H_2O.

The cerebrospinal fluid has been regarded as an ultrafiltrate of the blood plasma because of their resemblance, except for obvious differences in protein concentration (plasma, 6500 mg/100 g; CSF, 25 mg/100 g). The characteristic distribution of the number of ions and nonelectrolytes in CSF and plasma, however, is such that the CSF cannot be described as a simple filtrate or dialysate of the blood plasma. In general the CSF has higher Na^+, Cl^- and Mg^{++} concentrations and lower K^+, Ca^{++} and glucose concentrations than would be expected in a plasma dialysate. Finally the

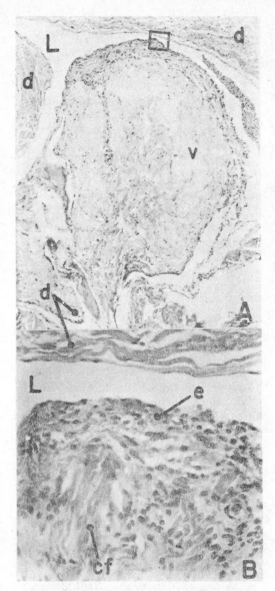

Fig. 1-13. *A*. Section of a human arachnoid granulation (*V*) in lateral lacuna of dural sinus (*L*). Relations of the dura (*d*) and area of enlargement are identified. ×28. *B*. Magnified area to demonstrate epithelial cap (*e*) and connective tissue fibers (*cf*) of granulation. Luxol Fast Blue-cresyl violet stain. Photograph. ×270.

osmotic pressure relationships are not sufficient to produce a virtually protein-free fluid from the blood plasma (Davson, '67). For these reasons, current evidence supports the theory that the CSF is a secre-tory product involving active transport mechanisms and the expenditure of energy. Na^+, K^+ and Cl^- are actively transported across epithelial cells of the choroid plexus into the ventricles (Woodbury, '65). Water, the principal constituent of the CSF, follows passively to maintain osmotic equilibrium. Smaller amounts of CSF are derived from the ependyma and subjacent glial elements as well as the capillary beds that supply the pia-arachnoid. The rate of CSF formation in man has been estimated to be between 600 and 700 ml/day (Davson, '67). Since the total volume of CSF in the subarachnoid spaces and ventricles in man is about 140 ml, of which only about 25 ml is in the ventricles, the daily turnover of the fluid is appreciable.

Cerebrospinal fluid formed in the lateral and third ventricles passes via the cerebral aqueduct into the fourth ventricle. The fluid enters the cerebellomedullary cistern via the medial and lateral apertures of the fourth ventricle. From this site the fluid circulates in the subarachnoid spaces surrounding both the brain and the spinal cord. The bulk of the CSF is passively returned to the venous system via the arachnoid villi. The hydrodynamic permeability of the arachnoid villi is large compared with that of peripheral capillaries. Large protein molecules leave the CSF by passage through the arachnoid villi at roughly the same rate as smaller molecules. The rate of exit of CSF via the arachnoid villi is pressure-dependent. The arachnoid villi serve as one-way valves. If the CSF pressure is greater than venous pressure, the leaflike valves open and CSF enters the dural sinuses. When venous pressure exceeds CSF pressure, the valves close and blood cannot enter the CSF. Small amounts of CSF may be taken up by the ependyma, arachnoid capillaries and lymphatics of the meninges and perivascular tissues.

An excessive amount of CSF produces an elevated pressure and in infants can cause hydrocephalus with enlargement of the ventricles, damage to neural tissue and changes in the neural cranium. Such increases in CSF may result from an over-

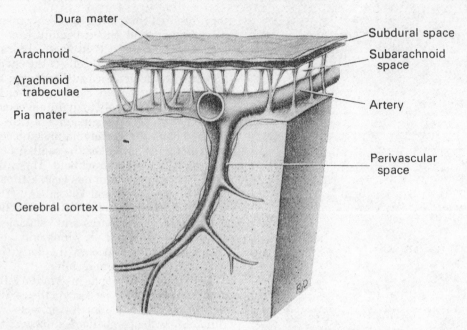

FIG. 1-14. Diagram of the meninges showing relationship of the membranes to the subarachnoid and perivascular spaces.

production of fluid, an obstruction to its flow or inadequate absorption. In most instances hydrocephalus results from obstruction within the ventricular system. Removal of the choroid plexus from one lateral ventricle usually causes that ventricle to collapse, while obstruction of one interventricular foramen causes dilatation of the ipsilateral lateral ventricle.

BARRIERS RELATED TO THE BRAIN

The functional capacity of all neurons of the brain and spinal cord are dependent upon the nature of the chemical milieu which surrounds them. To maintain an adequate ionic and oxygen atmosphere within the narrow limits of neuron survival requires the existence of a unique physiochemical system. Such a system, albeit ill-defined, does exist to regulate the transport of chemical substances between arterial blood, cerebrospinal fluid and the brain tissues. There is a striking difference in the concentration of various substances in the CSF in comparison to the plasma. There are also differences in the rate of transfer of these substances from the plasma to the CSF, and to the nerve cells. Some substances do not penetrate the cerebral capillary walls to reach the brain tissue; others do so only very slowly. These differential chemical pathways to the central nervous system neurons have been investigated extensively in laboratory animals and man. Microchemical assay, localization of isotopes, fluorescent dyes and electron microscopic methods, among others, have been utilized to elucidate some of the gaps in our knowledge concerning the structure and function of these pathways. Such barriers constitute regions where there is restricted diffusion of molecules across interfaces as compared to their rate of passage across other tissues (e.g., brain, skeletal muscle, liver, etc.). Blood-brain barrier, blood-CSF barrier and brain-CSF barrier are useful terms only if they are defined in terms of rate constants for diffusion across these tissue interfaces, or equated with the volume that a given substance occupies in the brain (Woodbury, '65). Evidence has been presented that the barriers develop at the time when blood vessels invade the brain

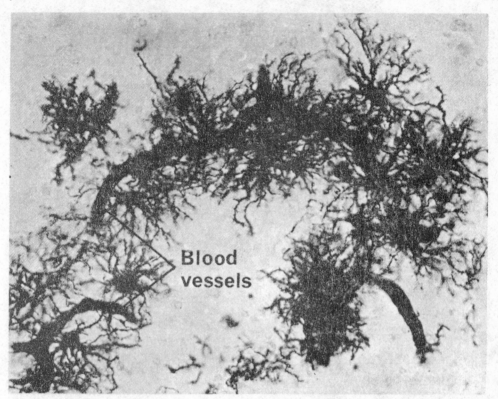

FIG. 1-15. Astrocytes and perivascular processes on blood vessels in the human cerebral cortex. Golgi stain. ×450.

(Grazer and Clemente, '57). Additional evidence suggests that the adult barriers react differently to the electric charge of various vital dyes (Friedmann and Elkeles, '32; Bakay, '52, '56). According to these authors the blood-brain barrier is more permeable to basic (positively charged) dyes, whereas the blood-CSF barrier is more permeable to acid (negatively charged) dyes. Such interfaces are both structural and functional entities which dynamically control the transfer of chemical substances into and out of the three fluid compartments of the brain (i.e., intercellular, intracellular and CSF). The relative importance of each of the components of the barriers shown in Figure 1-16 remains to be determined. For extensive presentations on this subject the student is referred to the excellent review articles (Rodriguez, '55, '57; Davson, '60, '67; Schmidt, '60; Sokoloff, '60; Tower, '60; Tschirgi, '60; Millen and Woollam, '62).

Blood-Brain Barrier. Arteries of the brain and spinal cord are invested with connective tissue of the pia-arachnoid as they lie in the subarachnoid space (Fig. 1-14). The pia and subjacent glial membrane blend with the vessel wall before it penetrates into the substance of the brain or spinal cord. The smaller branches of the arterial tree, within the nervous tissue, have only thin neuroglial membrane investments which persist down to the capillary level. The capillary endothelium, its continuous and homogeneous basement membrane and the numerous processes of the astrocytes are all that separate the plasma in the vessel from the intercellular spaces within the central nervous system (Fig. 1-15). These are the structures that have been equated by one or more investigators with the blood-brain barrier. Large numbers of astrocytes with perivascular feet are always present along the course of vessels in brain tissues stained by the

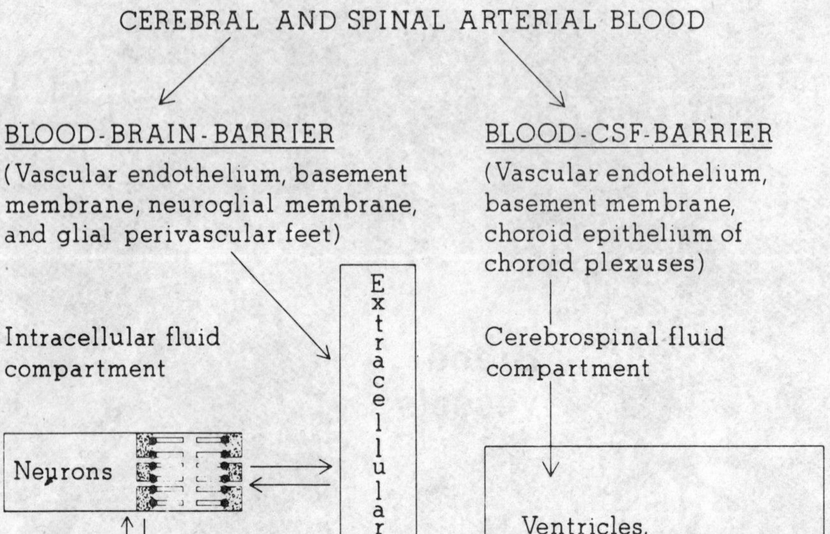

CEREBRAL AND SPINAL ARTERIAL BLOOD

BLOOD-BRAIN-BARRIER

(Vascular endothelium, basement membrane, neuroglial membrane, and glial perivascular feet)

BLOOD-CSF-BARRIER

(Vascular endothelium, basement membrane, choroid epithelium of choroid plexuses)

Intracellular fluid compartment

Extracellular compartment

Cerebrospinal fluid compartment

Neurons

Neuroglia

Ventricles, subarachnoid cisterns and spaces of CNS

Post-capillary venules and veins

BRAIN-CSF-BARRIER

(Ependyma, basement membrane, and sub-ependymal glial membrane)

Cerebral veins

Arachnoid villi

VENOUS BLOOD OF DURAL SINUSES AND SPINAL VEINS

FIG. 1-16. Diagram of the structural and functional relationships between the blood supply, cerebrospinal fluid and brain structures. Tissue elements that may participate in the formation of the so-called "barriers" are indicated in parentheses. Intercellular substances entering the neurons and neuroglial cells (i.e., intracellular compartment) must pass through the cell membrane, which is shown schematically as a protein-lipoid structure. *Solid arrows* indicate direction of fluid flow under normal and experimental conditions.

Golgi technic (Fig. 1-15). Maynard et al. ('57) observed that the expanded astrocytic processes form but a single incomplete layer around capillaries with only limited overlap. They estimate from electron micrographs that such astrocytic feet cover about 85% of total capillary surface. These authors also noted that the capillary endothelial cells of the central nervous system form a completely continuous layer without any suggestion of fenestrations such as those seen in the capillaries of the kidney. One or more of the components of the blood-brain barrier are stained after the intravenous injection of either aminoacridine dye proflavine HCl or the semicolloidal dye trypan blue, yet these dyes do not stain the adjacent neural tissue. However, several special structures within the central nervous system of adult animals do become stained after the intravenous injection of such vital dyes or they accumulate blood-borne radiotracers (e.g., P^{32}). These areas, presumably devoid of a blood-brain barrier, include the pineal body, pituitary gland, area postrema, subfornical organ, supraoptic crest and choroid plexus. All of these regions are highly vascular, and many are known or suspected to have a secretory function. Thus the blood-brain barrier, except in the special regions noted above, functions as a differential filter that permits the exchange of many substances from blood to the *extracellular compartment* (i.e., intercellular or interstitial fluid). It appears to be impermeable to other substances (e.g., vital dyes).

It will be noted in Figure 1-16 that the neurons and neuroglial cells comprise the *intracellular fluid compartment* of the brain. Passage of substances into, and out of, glial and neuronal cells takes place from the extracellular space and through cell membranes, not by direct entrance from the plasma. Estimates of the total extracellular space between neurons, neuroglia and capillaries of the brain vary widely with the different methods that have been used. Electron micrographic studies do not support the concept of widespread extracellular spaces in the CNS. Neurons, neuroglial cells and their processes take up essentially all the available room except for a fairly constant space of only 200 Å between adjacent elements (Schultz et al., '57; Farquhar and Hartmann, '57; Dempsey and Luse, '58). Neurochemical studies, on the other hand, assume that the chloride ion is essentially distributed in the extracellular fluid and have used brain chloride as a measure of the extent of the extracellular volume in the brain. Such values for brain extracellular space range between 25% (Woodbury, '58) and 40% (Elliott and Jasper, '49). Although the total extracellular space of the brain may be somewhat larger than the 4% determined from electron micrographs, it is probably less than 25%.

The narrow interstitial channels observed in electron micrographs can transport solutes between the plasma, interstitial fluid and cellular elements. There is evidence also that the interstitial fluid is not formed by an inward bulk movement of cerebrospinal fluid, but rather, that the subarachnoid CSF is formed in part, by a centrifugal flow of interstitial fluid out of the central nervous system (Davson, '60). The inflow and outflow of the interstitial fluids from the extracellular compartment are indicated by the arrows in Figure 1-16.

Blood-Cerebrospinal Fluid Barrier. The epithelium and adnexa of the choroid plexuses of the lateral, third and fourth ventricles are responsible for the actively secreted CSF as noted above (Fig. 1-16). Evidence that it is an effective barrier is attested to by the relatively higher concentration of sodium and chloride ions in CSF than in the plasma. In composition the CSF is the same as that of the interstitial tissue of the brain. It is interesting to note that P^{32} as inorganic phosphate when injected intravenously traversed the choroid plexus and then the CSF to reach the cerebral cortex (Bakay, '56). Thus the blood-CSF barrier is an effective one-way entry into the CSF fluid compartment of the brain, while the major drainage route is the arachnoid villus.

Brain-Cerebrospinal Fluid Barrier. The ependyma and subjacent glial tissues constitute a potential barrier between the

CSF and interstitial fluid of the brain. They are indeed structural entities, but the bulk of experimental evidence indicates that these elements pose little obstruction to the passage of fluids between the CSF and extracellular compartments. As noted above, the ependyma contributes to the CSF, while vital dyes, fluorescent dyes and isotopes injected into the CSF can gain access to the interstitial fluid and thence to the neuroglia and neurons of the brain. The path of such experimentally injected material is indicated schematically by the arrows in Figure 1-16. Attention is again called to the similarity in ionic composition of the CSF and interstitial fluids, for they play an important role in the maintenance and variation of membrane potentials in the central nervous system.

CHAPTER 2

Gross Anatomy of the Brain

The nervous system is composed of two parts, the central nervous system and the peripheral nervous system. The *peripheral nervous system* consists of the spinal and cranial nerves, while the *central nervous system* is represented by the brain and spinal cord. The autonomic nervous system, often considered as a separate functional entity, is part central and part peripheral.

The human brain is a relatively small structure weighing about 1400 g and constituting about 2% of the total body weight. The brain is commonly regarded as the organ solely concerned with thought, memory and consciousness and, while these are some of its functions, there are many others. All information we have concerning the world about us is conveyed centrally to the brain by an elaborate sensory system. Receptors of many kinds act as transducers which change physical and chemical stimuli in our environment into nerve impulses which the brain can read and give meaning to. The ability to discriminate between stimuli of the same and different types forms one of the bases for learning. Attention, consciousness, emotional experience and sleep are all central neural functions. Such higher functions as memory, imagination, thought and creative ability are poorly understood but must be related to complex neuronal activity. The brain also is concerned with all kinds of motor activity, with the regulation of visceral, endocrine and somatic functions and with the receptive and expressive use of symbols and signs that underlie communication. While the gross features of the human brain are not especially impressive, its versatility, potential capabilities, efficiency and self-programming nature put it in a class beyond any "electronic brain."

The brain consists of three basic subdivisions, the cerebral hemispheres, the brain stem, and the cerebellum. The massive paired *cerebral hemispheres* are derived from the *telencephalon*, the most rostral cerebral vesicle. The brain stem consists of four distinct parts: (1) the *diencephalon* (2) the *mesencephalon,* (3) the *metencephalon,* and (4) the *myelencephalon*. The diencephalon, the most rostral brain stem segment, is the part of the brain stem most intimately related to the forebrain (i.e., telencephalon). The mesencephalon, or midbrain, is the smallest and least differentiated division of the brain stem. The metencephalon (pons) and myelencephalon (medulla) together constitute the *rhombencephalon* or hindbrain. The cerebellum is a derivative of the metencephalon that develops from ectodermal thickenings about the rostral borders of the fourth ventricle, known as the rhombic lip.

THE CEREBRAL HEMISPHERES

The paired cerebral hemispheres are mirror image duplicates consisting of a highly convoluted gray cortex (pallium), an underlying white matter of considerable magnitude and a collection of deeply located neuronal masses, known as the basal ganglia. The cerebral hemispheres are partially separated from each other by

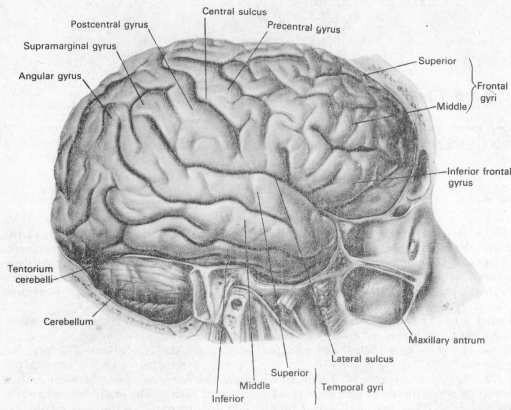

FIG. 2-1. Lateral view of the brain exposed in the skull to show topographical relationships (from Mettler's *Neuroanatomy*, '48; courtesy of The C. V. Mosby Company).

the *longitudinal fissure*. This fissure *in situ* contains the falx cerebri (Fig. 1-2). In frontal and occipital regions the separation of the hemispheres is complete, but in the central region the fissure extends only to fibers of the broad interhemispheric commissure, the corpus callosum (Fig. 2-4). Each cerebral hemisphere is subdivided into lobes by various sulci (Figs. 2-1 and 2-2). The major lobes of the brain are named for the bones of the skull which overlie them. Although the boundaries of the various lobes as seen in the gross specimen are somewhat arbitrary, multiple cortical areas in each lobe are histologically distinctive. The gray cellular mantle of the cerebral cortex in man is highly convoluted. The crest of a single convolution is referred to as a *gyrus*; *sulci* separate the various gyri, producing a pattern with more or less constant features. On the basis of the more constant sulci and gyri, the cerebrum is divided into six so-called lobes: (1) frontal, (2) temporal, (3) parietal, (4) occipital, (5) insular, and (6) limbic. Neither the insula nor the limbic lobe is a true lobe. The limbic lobe is a synthetic lobe on the medial aspect of the hemisphere consisting of portions of the frontal, parietal, occipital and temporal lobes which surround the upper part of the brain stem.

Lateral Surface

The two most important sulci for topographical orientation on the lateral convexity of the hemisphere are the lateral and central sulci (Figs. 2-1 and 2-2). The *lateral sulcus* begins inferiorly in the Sylvian fossa and extends posteriorly, separating the frontal and temporal lobes. Caudally this sulcus separates portions of the parietal and temporal lobes. The terminal ascending ramus of the sulcus extends into the inferior part of the parietal lobe. Por-

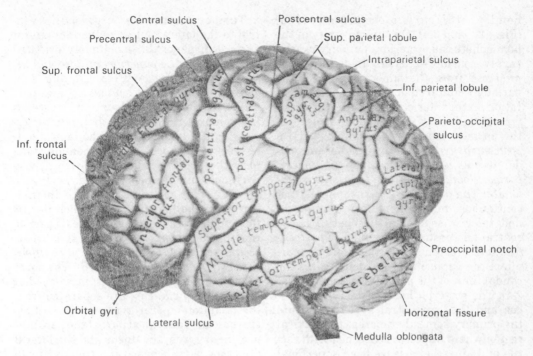

FIG. 2-2. Photograph of the lateral surface of the brain.

tions of the frontal, parietal and temporal lobes, adjacent to the lateral sulcus, which overlie the insular region are referred to as the *opercular portions* of these lobes (Fig. 2-3). The *central sulcus* is a prominent sulcus running from the superior margin of the hemisphere downward and forward toward the lateral sulcus (Figs. 2-1 and 2-2). Usually this sulcus is bowed in two locations and superiorly it does not extend onto the medial surface of the hemisphere for any distance. The depths of the sulcus constitute the boundary between the frontal and parietal lobes.

Frontal Lobe. This, the largest of all the lobes of the brain, comprises about one-third of the hemispheric surface. The frontal lobe extends rostrally from the central sulcus to the frontal pole; its inferior lateral boundary is the lateral sulcus. The convexity of the frontal lobe has four principal convolutions: (1) a *precentral* gyrus that parallels the central sulcus, and (2) three horizontally oriented convolutions, the *superior, middle* and *inferior frontal gyri* (Figs. 2-1 and 2-2). The anterior boundary of the precentral gyrus is the *precen-*

tral sulcus, which extends onto the medial surface of the hemisphere. The precentral gyrus and the anterior bank of the central sulcus comprise the *primary motor area*, where all parts of the body are represented in a distorted but topographical manner (Fig. 19-12). Regions of the frontal lobe rostral to the primary motor area are referred to as *premotor* and *prefrontal* areas. The broad middle frontal gyrus often is divided by a shallow horizontal sulcus into upper and lower tiers (Figs. 2-1 and 2-2). The inferior frontal gyrus is divided by anterior ascending rami of the lateral sulcus into three parts: (1) *pars orbitale*, (2) *pars triangularis*, and (3) *pars opercularis*. The pars triangularis and opercularis in the dominant hemisphere (usually the left in right-handed individuals) are referred to as *Broca's speech area*, a region concerned with the motor mechanisms of speech formulation.

Parietal Lobe. The boundaries of the parietal lobe are not precise, except for its anterior border on the lateral convexity formed by the central sulcus, and its posterior border on the medial aspect of the

hemisphere (*parieto-occipital sulcus*)
(Figs. 2-2 and 2-4). On the convexity of the
hemisphere the posterior boundary is arbi-
trarily considered as an imaginary line
projected from the superior limit of the
parieto-occipital sulcus to the small inden-
tation on the inferior surface known as the
preoccipital notch (Fig. 2-2). Three parts of
the parietal lobe are distinguished: (1) a
postcentral gyrus running parallel and caudal to the central sulcus, (2) a *superior
parietal lobule*, and (3) an *inferior parietal
lobule*. The postcentral gyrus, usually not
continuous, but broken up into superior
and inferior segments, lies between the
central and postcentral sulci. The *postcentral sulcus* extends over the superior margin of the hemisphere and demarcates the
caudal limit of the paracentral lobule (Fig.
2-4). The posterior bank of the central sulcus and the postcentral gyrus constitute
the primary somesthetic area, the cortical
region where impulses concerned with tactile and kinesthetic sense from superficial
and deep receptors converge and are somatotopically represented. The majority of
cortical neurons in the postcentral gyrus
are concerned with fixed receptive fields
on the contralateral side of the body that
are place-specific, modality-specific and related to discriminative aspects of sensation. The *intraparietal sulcus*, a horizontally oriented sulcus, divides portions of
the parietal lobe caudal to the postcentral
gyrus into superior and inferior parietal
lobules (Fig. 2-2). The *inferior parietal lobule* consists of two gyri, the *supramarginal*, about both banks of an ascending
ramus of the lateral sulcus, and the *angular*, which surrounds the ascending terminal part of the superior temporal sulcus
(Figs. 2-1 and 2-2). The inferior parietal
lobule represents a cortical association
area where various multisensory perceptions of a higher order from adjacent parietal, temporal and occipital regions overlap. This region is especially concerned
with mnemonic constellations that form
the basis for understanding and interpreting sensory signals. This is one region of
the cortex where different disturbances occur as a consequence of lesions in the dominant and nondominant hemisphere.

Temporal Lobe. This large lobe lies ventral to the lateral sulcus and on its lateral
surface displays three obliquely oriented
convolutions, the *superior, middle* and *inferior temporal gyri* (Figs. 2-1 and 2-2).
The *superior temporal sulcus* courses parallel with the lateral sulcus and its ascending ramus terminates in the angular gyrus. On the inner bank of the lateral sulcus several short, oblique convolutions
form the transverse gyri of Heschl; these
gyri constitute the *primary auditory cortex*
in man (Figs. 2-3 and 2-7). The inferior
surface of the temporal lobe which lies in
the middle fossa of the skull reveals part of
the *inferior temporal gyrus*, the broad
occipitotemporal gyrus and the *parahippocampal gyrus* (Figs. 2-5 and 2-6). The parahippocampal gyrus and its most medial
protrusion, the *uncus,* are separated from
the occipitotemporal gyrus by the collateral sulcus. The rostral part of the parahippocampal gyrus, the uncus and the lateral
olfactory stria constitute the pyriform
lobe, parts of which constitute the *primary
olfactory cortex* (Figs. 2-5 and 2-6).

Occipital Lobe. The small occipital lobe
rests on the tentorium cerebelli (Fig. 2-1).
The rostral boundary of this lobe is the
parieto-occipital sulcus on the medial aspect of the hemisphere (Fig. 2-4). The lateral surface of the occipital lobe is poorly
delimited from the parietal lobe and is
composed of a number of irregular *lateral
occipital gyri* which are separated into
groups by the *lateral occipital sulcus*.

On the medial aspect of the hemisphere
the occipital lobe is divided by the *calcarine sulcus* into the cuneus and the *lingual
gyrus* (Fig. 2-4). The calcarine sulcus joins
the parieto-occipital sulcus rostrally in a
"Y" shaped formation. The cortex on both
banks of the calcarine sulcus represents
the *primary visual cortex* (i.e., striate).
The visual cortex in each hemisphere receives impulses from the temporal half of
the ipsilateral retina and the nasal half of
the contralateral retina and is concerned
with perception from the contralateral half
of the visual field.

The Insula. This cortical area lies buried in the depths of the lateral sulcus and
can be seen only when the temporal and

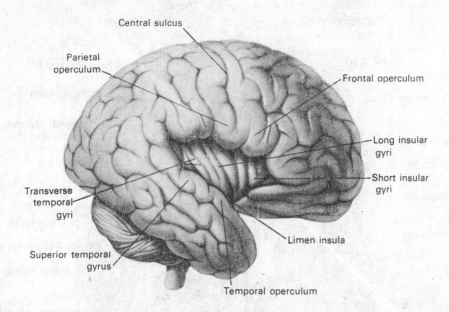

FIG. 2-3. View of the right cerebral hemisphere with the banks of the lateral sulcus drawn apart to expose the insula.

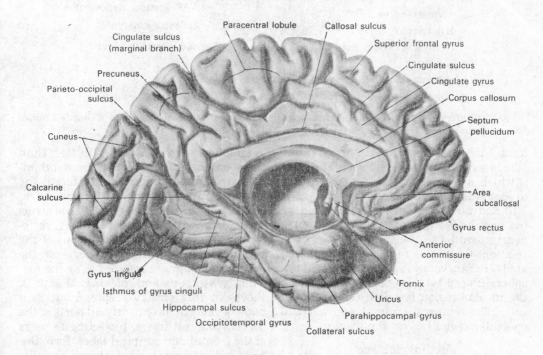

FIG. 2-4. Medial surface of the cerebral hemisphere with diencephalic structures removed (from Mettler's *Neuroanatomy*, '48; courtesy of The C. V. Mosby Company).

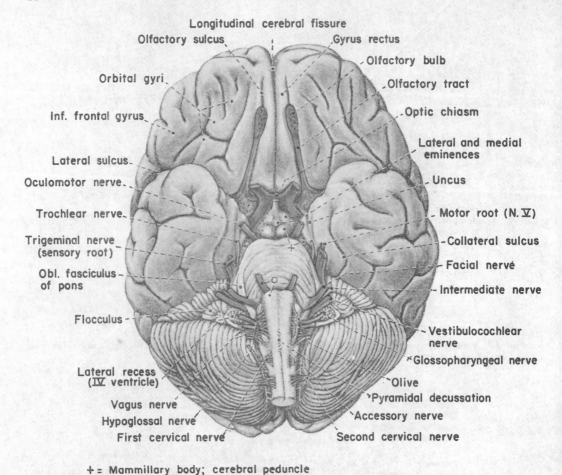

+ = Mammillary body; cerebral peduncle

O = Abducens nerve; pyramid of medulla

FIG. 2-5. Inferior surface of the brain showing the cranial nerves (from Truex and Kellner's *Detailed Atlas of the Head and Neck*, '58; courtesy of Oxford University Press).

frontal lobes are separated. This so-called lobe is a triangular cortical area, the apex of which is directed forward and downward to open into the lateral fossa (Figs. 2-3, 2-7, 2-10 and 2-11). The surface is covered by the *gyri breves* and *longus* which course nearly parallel to the lateral sulcus. The relationships of this region can be appreciated in transverse sections of the hemisphere (Fig. 2-14). The opening leading to the insular region is called the *limen insula*. The temporal, frontal and parietal opercular regions cover the insula.

Medial Surface

In a hemisected brain convolutions on the medial surface can be studied. The convolutions on the medial surface of the hemisphere are somewhat flatter than those on the convexity. The most prominent structure on the medial surface is the massive interhemispheric commissure, the *corpus callosum* (Fig. 2-4). This structure, composed of myelinated fibers, reciprocally interconnects broad regions of the two hemispheres. Different parts of the corpus callosum are referred to as the *rostrum, genu, body* and *splenium* (Fig. 2-7). Fibers in this structure spread out as a mass of radiations to nearly all parts of the cortex. Callosal fibers, projecting to parts of the frontal and occipital lobes, form the so-called *anterior* and *posterior forceps*, which are best appreciated in horizontal sections of the brain. The corpus callosum forms the floor of the longitudinal fissure,

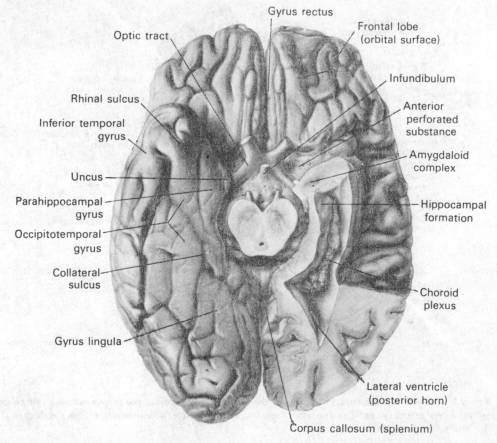

FIG. 2-6. View of the inferior surface of the brain following transection of the midbrain. The inferior and posterior horns of the left lateral ventricle have been opened and portions of the temporal lobe have been removed (from Mettler's *Neuroanatomy*, '48; courtesy of The C. V. Mosby Company).

as well as a good part of the roof of the lateral ventricle. The corpus callosum plays an important role in interhemispheric transfer of learned discriminations, sensory experience and memory.

The *callosal sulcus* separates the corpus callosum from the cingulate gyrus; posteriorly this sulcus curves around the splenium to be continued into the temporal lobe as the *hippocampal sulcus* (Fig. 2-4). The *cingulate gyrus*, dorsal to the callosal sulcus, encircles the corpus callosum and consists of two tiers. The *cingulate sulcus*, dorsal to the cingulate gyrus, runs parallel to the callosal sulcus, but near the splenium turns dorsally as the *marginal sulcus*. The anterior portion of cortex dorsal to the cingulate gyrus is the medial surface of the superior frontal gyrus. The *paracentral lobule* is formed by the precentral and post-

central gyri which extend onto the medial surface of the hemisphere, and is notched by the central sulcus (Fig. 2-4). The *paracentral sulcus*, continuous with the precentral sulcus, forms the rostral border of this lobule, while the *marginal sulcus*, continuous with the postcentral gyrus, forms the caudal border. The portion of the parietal lobe caudal to the paracentral lobule is known as the *precuneus;* this lobule lies immediately rostral to the parieto-occipital sulcus previously discussed.

Limbic Lobe. This is a synthetic lobe, consisting of large cortical convolutions or the medial aspect of the hemisphere which surround the rostral part of the brain stem and the interhemispheric commissure (Fig. 18-13). According to Broca (1878) the limbic lobe includes the *subcallosal, cingulate* and *parahippocampal gyri*, as well as

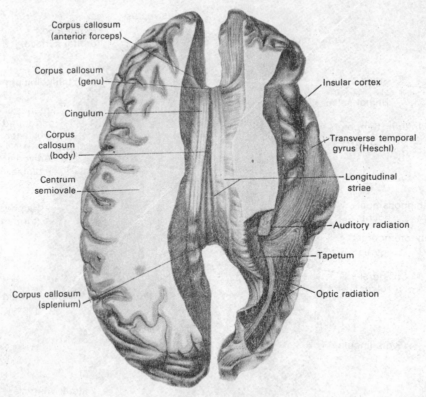

FIG. 2-7. Dissection of the superior surface of the hemispheres exposing the corpus callosum, cingulum, longitudinal striae and the optic and auditory radiations (from Mettler's *Neuroanatomy*; '48; courtesy of The C. V. Mosby Company).

primitive cortical derivatives, the *hippocampal formation* and the *dentate gyrus*, which in the course of development have become invaginated within the temporal lobe (Fig. 2-6). The parahippocampal gyrus is directly continuous with the cingulate gyrus by a narrow strip of cortex, posterior and inferior to the splenium, known as the *isthmus of the cingulate gyrus* (Fig. 2-4). The parahippocampal gyrus, the most medial convolution of the temporal lobe, is bounded laterally by the *rhinal* and *collateral sulci* and superiorly and medially by the *hippocampal sulcus* (Figs. 2-4, 2-5 and 2-6). Rostrally the parahippocampal gyrus hooks around the hippocampal sulcus to form a medially protruding convolution, the uncus. The proximity of the uncus to the cerebral peduncle should be noted.

There are wide differences of opinion concerning what should be lumped together as the so-called "limbic lobe" (Brodal, '69).

While all of these structures appear early in phylogenesis, physiological evidence suggests that wide functional differences exist between various components and separate functions are expressed by distinctive neural mechanisms.

The Inferior Surface

The inferior surface of the hemisphere consists of two parts: (1) a larger posterior portion, representing the inferior surfaces of the temporal and occipital lobes, and (2) the orbital surface of the frontal lobe (Figs. 2-5 and 2-6). The inferior surface of the occipital lobe and the posterior part of the temporal lobe lie on the tentorium cerebelli (Figs. 1-2 and 2-1), while rostral parts of the temporal lobe lie in the middle cranial fossa. Gyri present in this posterior part include: (1) the lingual gyrus, (2) the extensive occipitotemporal gyrus, and (3) the parahippocampal gyrus and uncus

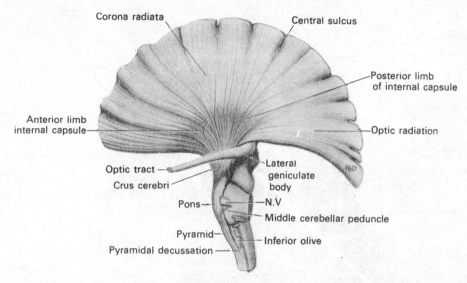

FIG. 2-8. Drawing of a dissection demonstrating the continuity and relationships of the corona radiata, the internal capsule, the crus cerebri and the medullary pyramid.

(Fig. 2-6). Part of the inferior temporal gyrus may be seen lateral to the occipito-temporal gyrus. A small part of the isthmus lies medially posterior to the splenium of the corpus callosum.

The orbital surface of the frontal lobe has a deep, straight sulcus medially, the olfactory sulcus, which contains both the olfactory bulb and tract (Fig. 2-5). The *gyrus rectus* lies along the ventromedial margin of the hemisphere medial to the olfactory sulcus. The region lateral to the olfactory sulcus contains the orbital gyri whose convolutional patterns are variable. Posteriorly the olfactory tract divides into *medial* and *lateral olfactory striae* (Figs. 2-5 and 2-6). Caudal to this is the olfactory trigone and the *anterior perforated substance,* a region studded with small openings through which numerous small blood vessels pass to deep regions (Figs. 2-5, 2-6, 2-17 and 20-9).

The White Matter

The massive white matter of the cerebral hemisphere forms the medullary core of the cortical convolutions and contains basically three types of fibers in prodigious quantity. Fibers within the white matter are classified as: (1) *projection fibers* that convey impulses either from the cortex to distant loci, or from distant loci to the cortex, (2) *association fibers* that interconnect various cortical regions of the same hemisphere, and (3) *commissural fibers* that interconnect corresponding cortical regions of the two hemispheres. The white matter extends from the cortex to the basal ganglia and the ventricular system. The common central mass of white matter, containing commissural, association and projection fibers, has an oval appearance in horizontal sections of the brain and is termed the *semioval center* (Fig. 2-7).

Projection Fibers. Afferent and efferent fibers conveying impulses to and from the entire cerebral cortex enter the white matter and are arranged as a radiating mass that converges toward the brain stem (Fig. 2-8). These radiating projection fibers are known as the *corona radiata.* Near the upper part of the brain stem these fibers form a compact band known as the *internal capsule,* which is flanked medially and laterally by nuclear masses (Figs. 2-9 and 2-10). Two distinct parts of the internal capsule are evident in horizontal sections of the hemispheres: (1) an anterior limb and (2) a posterior limb (Fig. 2-9). The *anterior limb* of the internal capsule

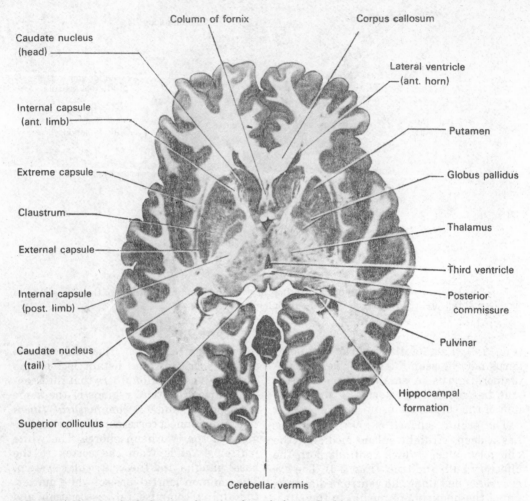

Caudate nucleus (head)

Column of fornix

Corpus callosum

Internal capsule (ant. limb)

Lateral ventricle (ant. horn)

Extreme capsule

Putamen

Claustrum

Globus pallidus

External capsule

Thalamus

Internal capsule (post. limb)

Third ventricle

Posterior commissure

Caudate nucleus (tail)

Pulvinar

Superior colliculus

Hippocampal formation

Cerebellar vermis

FIG. 2-9. Photograph of a horizontal section through the cerebral hemispheres showing relationships of internal structures.

partially separates two of the largest components of the basal ganglia, the caudate nucleus and the putamen. Fibers in the anterior limb of the internal capsule are directed horizontally, obliquely, laterally and upwards toward the frontal lobe, and in horizontal sections of the hemisphere appear to be cut in the longitudinal axis of the fiber bundles (Figs. 2-8, 2-9 and 2-10). In horizontal sections of the hemisphere the anterior and posterior limbs of the internal capsule meet at an obtuse angle with the apex directed medially. The larger and longer *posterior limb* of the internal capsule is flanked medially by the diencephalon and laterally by a part of the basal ganglia known as the lentiform nu-

cleus. The region of junction between the anterior and posterior limbs of the internal capsule is referred to as the *genu*. Fibers in the posterior limb of the internal capsule course in nearly a vertical plane toward the brain stem, and in horizontal sections fibers appear to be cut transversely. The most posterior component of the posterior limb of the internal capsule contains fibers, radiating toward the calcarine sulcus, known as the *optic radiation* (Figs. 2-7 and 2-8). Afferent fibers in the internal capsule arise mainly from the thalamus and project to nearly all regions of the cortex; these fibers are referred to as *thalamocortical radiations*. Efferent fibers in the internal capsule arise from cells in

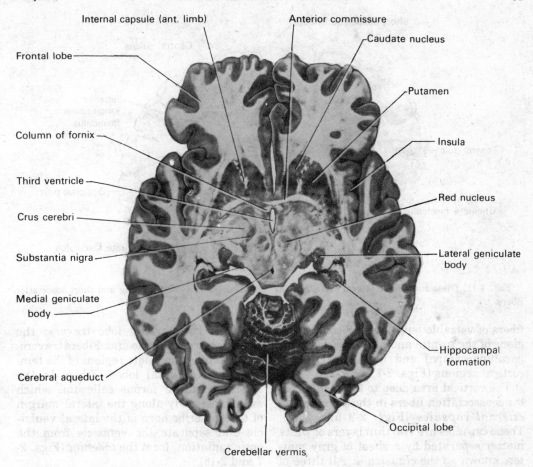

Internal capsule (ant. limb)

Anterior commissure

Caudate nucleus

Frontal lobe

Putamen

Column of fornix

Insula

Third ventricle

Crus cerebri

Red nucleus

Substantia nigra

Lateral geniculate body

Medial geniculate body

Cerebral aqueduct

Hippocampal formation

Occipital lobe

Cerebellar vermis

Fig. 2-10. Photograph of a horizontal section through the cerebral hemispheres passing through the anterior commissure and the crus cerebri.

various regions of the cerebral cortex and project to specific nuclear masses in the brain stem and spinal cord. These fibers are categorized as corticothalamic, cortico-pontine, corticobulbar and corticospinal.

Association Fibers. Fibers interconnecting various cortical regions within the same hemisphere are divided into long and short groups (Fig. 2-11). *Short association fibers* arch through the floor of each sulcus to connect adjacent convolutions; these fibers course transversely to the long axis of the sulci. *Long association fibers*, interconnecting cortical regions in different lobes within the same hemisphere, form three main bundles: (1) the uncinate fasciculus, (2) the arcuate fasciculus, and (3) the cingulum. The *uncinate fasciculus* is a compact bundle beneath the limen insula

which connects the orbital frontal gyri and parts of the inferior and middle frontal gyri with anterior portions of the temporal lobe. A deep placed part of this fasciculus is thought to connect the frontal and occipital lobes (i.e., inferior occipitofrontal fasciculus). The *arcuate fasciculus* sweeps around the insular region and its fan-shaped ends connect the superior and middle frontal gyri with parts of the temporal lobe. A group of superiorly situated fibers in this bundle extends caudally into portions of the parietal and occipital lobe, and is known as the *superior longitudinal fasciculus* (Fig. 2-11).

The principal association bundle on the medial aspect of the hemisphere lies in the white matter of the cingulate gyrus. This bundle, known as the *cingulum*, contains

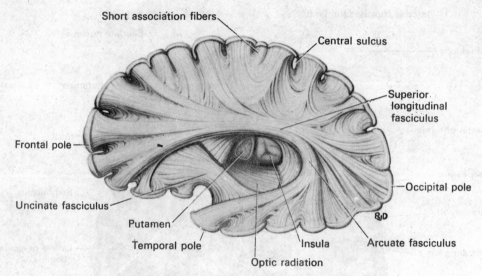

Short association fibers

Central sulcus

Superior
longitudinal
fasciculus

Frontal pole

Occipital pole

Uncinate fasciculus

Putamen

Temporal pole   Insula   Arcuate fasciculus

Optic radiation

FIG. 2-11. Dissection of the lateral surface of the left hemisphere to display long and short association
fibers.

fibers of variable length which connect regions of the frontal and parietal lobes with parahippocampal and adjacent temporal cortical regions (Figs. 2-7 and 2-12).

The cortical area deep to the insula contains association fibers in the *extreme* and *external capsules* (Figs. 2-9 and 2-13). These capsules are two thin layers of white matter separated by a sheet of gray matter, known as the *claustrum*. All three of these structures overlie the lateral aspect of the basal ganglia.

Commissural Fibers. Fibers interconnecting corresponding cortical regions of the two hemispheres are represented by two structures: (1) the corpus callosum, and (2) the anterior commissure. The *corpus callosum* is a broad thick plate of dense myelinated fibers that reciprocally interconnect broad regions of the cortex in all lobes with corresponding regions of the opposite hemisphere (Figs. 2-4, 2-7 and 2-12). These fibers traverse the floor of the hemispheric fissure, form most of the roof of the lateral ventricles and fan out in a massive callosal radiation as they are distributed to various cortical regions. The parts of the corpus callosum are designated as: (1) rostrum, (2) genu, (3) body, and (4) splenium. The genu contains fibers interconnecting anterior parts of the frontal lobes; fibers from the remaining parts of the frontal

lobe and the parietal lobe traverse the body of the corpus callosum. Fibers traversing the splenium relate regions of the temporal and occipital lobes. Fibers in the splenium of the corpus callosum, which sweep inferiorly along the lateral margin of the posterior horn of the lateral ventricle and separate the ventricle from the optic radiation, form the *tapetum* (Figs. 2-7 and 2-16).

The *anterior commissure* is a small compact bundle which crosses the midline rostral to the columns of the fornix (Figs. 2-4, 2-10, 2-12 and 2-13). This commissure has a general shape not unlike bicycle handlebars and consists of two parts that cannot be distinguished in the gross specimen (Fig. 18-7). A small anterior part of the commissure interconnects olfactory structures on the two sides (Fig. 18-3), while the larger posterior part mainly interconnects regions of the middle and inferior temporal gyri.

THE BASAL GANGLIA

The basal ganglia are subcortical nuclear masses derived from the telencephalon (Figs. 2-9, 2-10, 2-13 and 2-14). Structures composing the basal ganglia are the *caudate nucleus*, the *putamen*, the *globus pallidus* and the *amygdaloid nuclear complex*. The caudate nucleus, putamen and

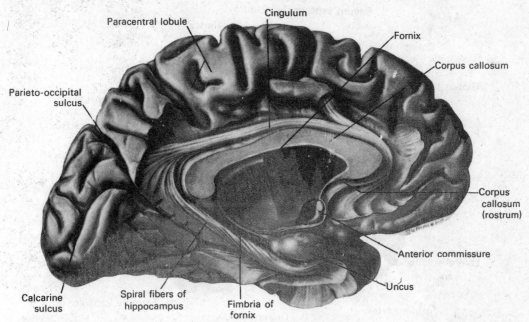

Paracentral lobule

Cingulum

Fornix

Corpus callosum

Parieto-occipital sulcus

Corpus callosum (rostrum)

Anterior commissure

Uncus

Calcarine sulcus

Spiral fibers of hippocampus

Fimbria of fornix

FIG. 2-12. Dissection of the medial surface of the left cerebral hemisphere exposing the cingulum. The diencephalon has been removed (from Mettler's *Neuroanatomy*, '48; courtesy of The C. V. Mosby Company).

globus pallidus constitute the *corpus striatum*. The term *lentiform nucleus* (lenticular nucleus) refers to the putamen and the globus pallidus. The lentiform nucleus, with the size and shape of a Brazil nut, in transverse sections appears as a wedge with the apex directed medially. This nuclear mass lies between the internal and the external capsules. A slightly curved vertical lamina of white matter divides the lentiform nucleus into an outer portion, the putamen, and an inner portion, the globus pallidus.

The Putamen. This is the largest and most lateral part of the basal ganglia; it lies between the lateral medullary lamina of the globus pallidus and the external capsule (Figs. 2-9, 2-10, 2-13 and 2-14). It is traversed by numerous fascicles of myelinated fibers directed ventromedially toward the globus pallidus, but these are seen clearly only in stained sections. The rostral part of the putamen is continuous with the head of the caudate nucleus (Fig. 17-4).

The Globus Pallidus. The globus pallidus, forming the most medial part of the lentiform nucleus, consists of two seg-

ments separated by the medial medullary lamina of the globus pallidus (Figs. 2-9, 2-13 and 2-14). The globus pallidus appears pale and homogeneous in freshly sectioned brains. Its medial border is formed largely by the fibers of the posterior limb of the internal capsule.

The Caudate Nucleus. This is an elongated arched gray mass related throughout its extent to the lateral cerebral ventricle (Figs. 2-9, 2-10, 2-13, 2-14 and 17-4). It consists of an enlarged rostral part, called the *head* of the caudate nucleus, which protrudes into the anterior horn of the lateral ventricle. The *tail* of the caudate nucaudate nucleus lies dorsolateral to the thalamus near the lateral wall of the lateral ventricle. The tail of the caudate nucleus follows the curvature of the inferior horn of the lateral ventricle and enters the temporal lobe (Fig. 2-9). The tail of the caudate nucleus terminates in the region of the amygdaloid nuclear complex (Fig. 2-14).

The Amygdaloid Nuclear Complex. This is a gray mass in the dorsomedial part of the temporal lobe which underlies the uncus (Figs. 2-6, 2-13 and 2-14). This

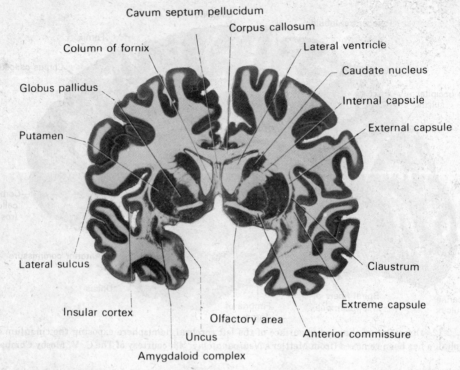

Cavum septum pellucidum

Corpus callosum

Column of fornix

Lateral ventricle

Caudate nucleus

Globus pallidus

Internal capsule

External capsule

Putamen

Lateral sulcus

Claustrum

Extreme capsule

Insular cortex

Olfactory area

Anterior commissure

Uncus

Amygdaloid complex

FIG. 2-13. Photograph of a frontal section of the brain passing through the columns of the fornix and the anterior commissure.

complex lies dorsal to the hippocampal formation and rostral to the tip of the inferior horn of the lateral ventricle. The amygdaloid complex gives rise to fibers of the *stria terminalis*, which arch along the entire medial border of the caudate nucleus and are especially evident near the junction of the caudate nucleus and thalamus (Figs. 2-18 and 2-22). The terminal vein lies near the stria terminalis.

THE LATERAL VENTRICLES

The ependymal-lined cavities of the cerebral hemisphere constitute the lateral ventricles. The arched-shaped lateral ventricles contain cerebrospinal fluid and conform to the general shape of the hemispheres (Fig. 2-15). The lateral ventricles can be divided into five parts: (1) the anterior (frontal) horn, (2) the ventricular body, (3) the collateral (atrium) trigone, (4) the inferior (temporal) horn, and (5) the posterior (occipital) horn. Each lateral ventricle communicates with the slit-shaped, midline third ventricle by two short chan-

nels, known as the interventricular foramina (Munro). These foramina serve as a basic reference point and are of great importance in radiographic studies.

The Anterior Horn. The anterior horn of the lateral ventricle lies rostral to the interventricular foramen, has a triangular shape in frontal section and extends forward, laterally and ventrally to end in a rounded termination in the substance of the frontal lobe (Figs. 2-9 and 2-13). The roof and rostral wall of this horn are formed by the corpus callosum, while its medial wall is the *septum pellucidum* which separates the ventricles of the two hemispheres (Fig. 2-4). The lateral wall of the ventricle is formed by the head of the caudate nucleus whose surface bulges convexly into the cavity (Figs. 2-9, 2-10, 2-13 and 2-22).

The Body of the Lateral Ventricle. This extends caudally from the interventricular foramen to an ill-defined point near the splenium of the corpus callosum. This narrower arched part of the ventricle

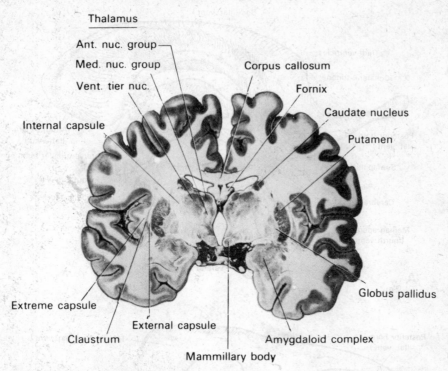

Thalamus
Ant. nuc. group
Med. nuc. group
Vent. tier nuc.
Internal capsule
Corpus callosum
Fornix
Caudate nucleus
Putamen
Extreme capsule
Claustrum
External capsule
Mammillary body
Amygdaloid complex
Globus pallidus

FIG. 2-14. Photograph of a frontal section of the brain at the level of the mammillary bodies. In this section the main nuclear groups of the thalamus are identified and portions of all components of the basal ganglia are present. The amygdaloid nuclear complex lies in the temporal lobe internal to the uncus and ventral to the lentiform nucleus.

continues until the ventricle begins to widen into the collateral trigone (referred to by neuroradiologists as the atrium). The *collateral trigone* comprises that part of the lateral ventricle near the splenium of the corpus callosum where the body of the lateral ventricle is confluent with the temporal and occipital horns.

The Inferior Horn. The inferior horn of the lateral ventricle curves downward and forward around the posterior aspect of the thalamus, and extends rostrally into the medial part of the temporal lobe to end approximately 3 cm from the temporal pole. The roof and lateral wall of the horn are formed by the tapetum (Figs. 2-7 and 2-16) and the optic radiation; the floor contains the *collateral eminence* caused by the deep collateral sulcus (Fig. 2-5). The inferior horn of the lateral ventricle contains the *hippocampal formation* in the medial wall of the horn which extends from the region of the splenium to the temporal tip of the ventricle (Figs. 2-6, 2-9 and 2-10).

The hippocampal formation, representing the phylogenetically oldest type of cortex, has become folded into the ventricle along the hippocampal sulcus. Along the superior and medial surfaces of the hippocampus is a flattened band of fibers, known as the fimbria, which extends from the region of the uncus toward the splenium of the corpus callosum. The fimbria extends under the corpus callosum and becomes the fornix (Figs. 2-12 and 2-22).

The Posterior Horn. The posterior horn of the lateral ventricle extends from the collateral trigone into the occipital lobe. This horn exhibits a high degree of variability in appearance and is often rudimentary. Often the occipital horn has the appearance of a small finger-like projection with a rounded tip. The roof and lateral wall of this horn are formed by tapetal fibers of the corpus callosum, while its floor is the white matter of the occipital lobe. The *calcar avis*, a longitudinal prominence, is produced by the deep penetration

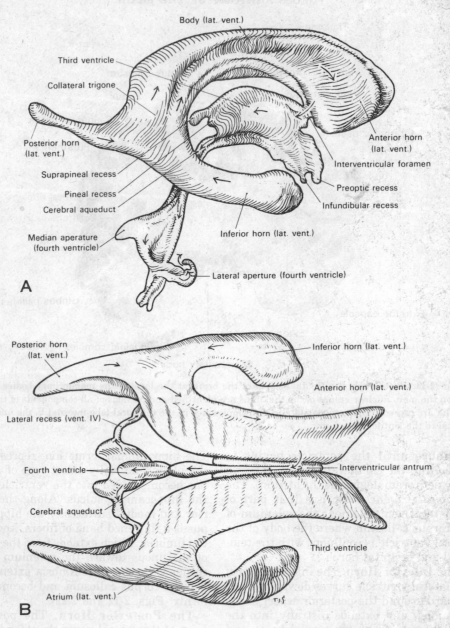

FIG. 2-15. Diagrams of the ventricular system in lateral (A) and superior (B) views (after Bailey, '48).

of the calcarine sulcus.

Portions of the lateral ventricles contain *choroid plexus* which is formed by the invagination of the ependymal roof plate into the ventricular cavities. Choroid plexus develops at sites where ependyma and pia mater containing blood vessels come together. This plexus is present in the body, collateral trigone and in the inferior horn of the lateral ventricle, and extends through the interventricular foramen to lie in the roof of the third ventricle (Fig. 2-22).

THE BRAIN STEM

In the intact brain only the anterior surface of the brain stem can be seen throughout its extent, because the cerebral hemi-

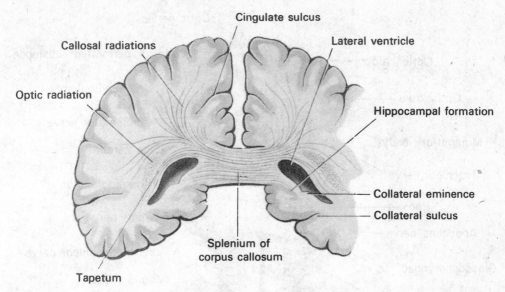

Cingulate sulcus

Callosal radiations

Lateral ventricle

Optic radiation

Hippocampal formation

Collateral eminence

Collateral sulcus

Splenium of
corpus callosum

Tapetum

FIG. 2-16. Drawing of a frontal section at the level of the splenium of the corpus callosum. Callosal fibers lateral to the ventricle are known as the tapetum. The optic radiations lie lateral to the tapetum.

spheres and cerebellum overlap the lateral and posterior surfaces. On the anterior surface of the brain stem the medulla, pons, midbrain and part of the *hypothalamus* (diencephalon) can be identified (Figs. 2-5 and 2-17). The most rostral portion of the brain stem, the diencephalon, is surrounded by hemispheric structures on all sides except for a small region between the *optic chiasm* and the *mammillary bodies*. The midbrain appears very small, but root fibers of the oculomotor nerve can be seen emerging between two massive fibers bundles, the *crura cerebri* (Figs. 2-5 and 2-7). The ventral surface of the pons produces a convex protrusion covered by transversely coursing fiber bundles which disappear laterally in the substance of the cerebellum. The medulla, caudal to the pons, reveals the large *medullary pyramids* medially and the oval *olivary eminences* dorsolaterally. The transition from medulla to spinal cord is characterized by the disappearance of the medullary pyramids, the development of the anterior median fissure of the spinal cord, a conspicuous reduction in size and the appearance of paired spinal nerves.

Removal of the cerebral hemispheres and cerebellum reveals the posterior and lateral surfaces of the brain stem (Figs. 2-18 and 2-19). The expanded diencephalon appears as two paired oval nuclear masses on each side of a vertical slitlike third ventricle (Fig. 2-18). The *thalamus* and *epithalamus*, seen in the posterior view of the brain stem, lie between the fibers of the internal capsule and are flanked dorsolaterally by the body and tail of the caudate nucleus. Along the dorsomedial margin of the thalamus is the *stria medullaris*, a band of fibers coursing posteriorly toward the base of the pineal gland. The most caudal part of the thalamus, the pulvinar, overlies part of the midbrain.

The dorsal aspect of the midbrain reveals the *superior* and *inferior colliculi* and their *brachia*, which relate these structures to particular parts of the thalamus. The trochlear nerve emerges from the dorsal part of the midbrain caudal to the inferior colliculus (Figs. 2-18 and 2-19).

The dorsal aspects of the hindbrain are revealed by removing the cerebellum (Fig. 2-18). This discloses the rhomboid fossa, an unpaired symmetrical ventricle that overlies the pons and medulla. The rhomboid-shaped fourth ventricle is surrounded by three paired cerebellar peduncles, which relate the three lowest brain stem segments to the cerebellum. The fourth ventricle contains several eminences which over-

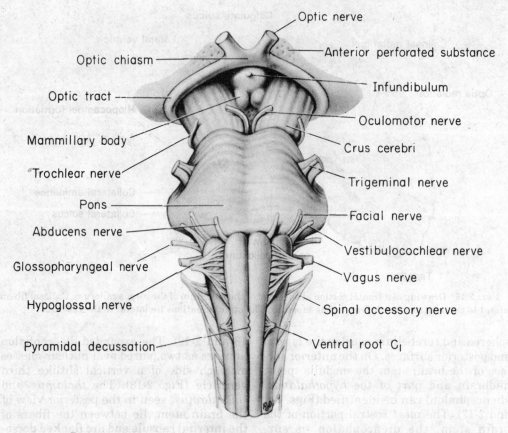

Optic nerve

Optic chiasm

Anterior perforated substance

Optic tract

Infundibulum

Oculomotor nerve

Mammillary body

Crus cerebri

Trochlear nerve

Trigeminal nerve

Pons

Facial nerve

Abducens nerve

Vestibulocochlear nerve

Glossopharyngeal nerve

Vagus nerve

Hypoglossal nerve

Spinal accessory nerve

Pyramidal decussation

Ventral root C_1

FIG. 2-17. Drawing of the anterior surface of the medulla, pons and midbrain.

lie nuclear masses, the most evident of which are the *facial colliculus* and the *hypoglossal eminence*. Caudal to the fourth ventricle on the dorsal surface of the medulla are nuclear masses related to ascending spinal systems, namely, the *cuneate* and *gracilis tubercles*.

Structurally the midbrain and hindbrain consist of three distinctive parts: (1) a roof plate dorsal to the ventricular system, (2) a central core of cells and fibers beneath the ventricular system known as the tegmentum, and (3) a massive collection of ventrally located fibers derived from cells of the cerebral cortex (Figs. 2-20 and 2-21). The *roof plate* of the midbrain is represented by the *tectum* or *quadrigeminal plate*, consisting of the superior and inferior colliculi; in the hindbrain the roof plate is more elaborate and is presented by the *cerebellum* and the *tela choroidea*. The *tegmentum* of the midbrain, pons and me-

dulla represents the brain stem *reticular formation,* a large collection of cells and intermingled fibers that subserves multiple functions. The *cortically derived ventral fiber system* forms the *crus cerebri* at midbrain levels, one of the principal constituents of the *ventral* or *basilar part* of the pons, and the *medullary pyramids* of the medulla. (Fig. 2-19). Both the reticular formation and the cortically derived ventral fiber system are continuous within the brain stem, but undergo change and modification at various levels (Fig. 2-8).

The Medulla

The medulla (myelencephalon), the most caudal basic subdivision of the brain stem, extends from the level of the foramen magnum to the caudal border of the pons. The transition from spinal cord to medulla is gradual and characterized by: (1) the obliteration of the anterior median

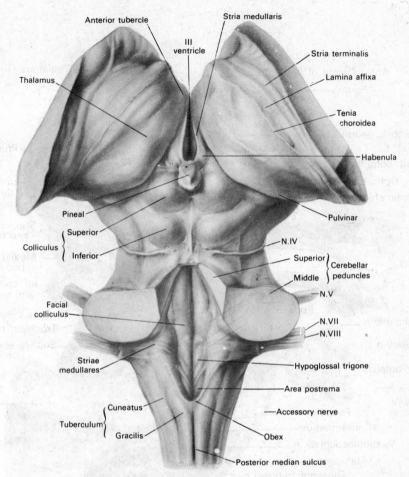

FIG. 2-18. Posterior aspect of the brain stem with the cerebellum removed (from Mettler's *Neuroanatomy*, '48; courtesy of The C. V. Mosby Company).

fissure ventrally and the decussation of the medullary pyramids, (2) the appearance of the gracilis and cuneate tubercles dorsally, (3) the disappearance of spinal nerves and the appearance of cranial nerves, and (4) the development of the fourth ventricle (Figs. 2-17, 2-18 and 2-19). The full development of the medullary pyramids, the appearance of the eminence of the inferior olivary complex, the widening of the fourth ventricle and the gradual increase in size of the inferior cerebellar peduncle give the medulla its characteristic configuration (Figs. 2-17 and 2-18). Cranial nerves associated with the medulla are: (1) the hypoglossal (N. XII) whose fibers emerge ventrolaterally between the pyramid and the inferior olivary complex, (2) the accessory (N. XI), the vagus (N. X) and the glossopharyngeal (N. IX) whose fibers emerge from the postolivary sulcus, and (3) the vestibulocochlear nerve (N. VIII) whose separate components enter the brain stem at the junction of the pons and medulla (Fig. 2-19). Auditory fibers are most dorsal and caudal and partially arch over the lateral aspect of the inferior cerebellar peduncle.

The Fourth Ventricle

The fourth ventricle is a broad shallow rhomboid-shaped cavity overlying the pons and medulla that extends from the central canal of the upper cervical spinal cord to the cerebral aqueduct of the midbrain (Figs. 2-15 and 2-18). Its roof is the

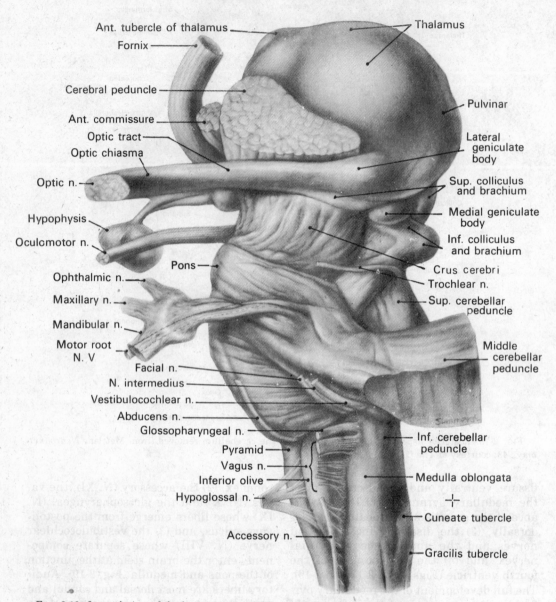

FIG. 2-19. Lateral view of the brain stem with the cerebellum removed showing the sites of emergence and entrance of most of the cranial nerves (from Mettler's *Neuroanatomy*, '48; courtesy of The C. V. Mosby Company).

cerebellum and the *superior* and *inferior medullary veli,* which extend toward an apex within the cerebellum known as the *fastigium* (Figs. 2-15, 2-20, 2-21 and 2-26). The superior medullary velum forms the roof of the pontine part of the ventricle, while the inferior medullary velum and the *tela choroidea* form the roof over the medullary part of this ventricle. *Choroid plexus* from the tela choroidea projects into the caudal part of the ventricle. The widest part of the fourth ventricle is immediately caudal to the *middle cerebellar peduncles.* In this region there is a *lateral recess* on each side, which extends over the surface of the inferior cerebellar peduncle to open into the *cerebellomedullary* (magna) *cistern* (Figs. 1-10 and 1-11). These small lateral recesses contain choroid plexus that protrudes through the *foramina of Luschka* into the subarachnoid space (Figs. 2-5 and 2-15). A small median aperture in the caudal part of the ventricle is known as the *foramen of Magendie.* Through these three apertures cerebrospinal fluid flows from the ventricular system into the subarachnoid spaces.

The *rhomboid fossa* which forms the floor of the fourth ventricle is divided by the *median sulcus* into symmetrical halves. The sulcus limitans divides each half into a *medial eminence* and a lateral region known as the *vestibular area* (Fig. 11-16). The vestibular nuclei lie beneath the vestibular area. The *facial colliculus* and the *hypoglossal trigone* lie within the medial eminence, with the latter near the caudal border of the ventricle. Transversely coursing fibers of the *striae medullares* run from the region of the lateral recess toward the midline and disappear in the median sulcus (Fig. 2-18); these strands of myelinated fibers lie rostral to the hypoglossal trigone. The *vagal trigone* lies lateral to the hypoglossal trigone. The most caudal end of the rhomboid fossa resembles a pen and is called the *calamus scriptorius.* The point of caudal junction of the walls of the fourth ventricle is known as the *obex* (Fig. 2-18). Immediately rostral to the obex on each side of the fourth ventricle is a slightly rounded eminence, the *area postrema.*

The Pons

The pons (metencephalon), representing the rostral part of the hindbrain, is well delimited on the anterior surface of the brain stem (Figs. 2-17, 2-19 and 2-20). The massive pontine protruberance covered by broad bands of transversely oriented fibers is separated from the crus cerebri of the midbrain by the superior pontine sulcus and from the anterior surface of the medulla by the inferior pontine sulcus. The predominantly transverse fibers in the ventral part of the pons form the *middle cerebellar peduncle* (Fig. 2-25). An anterior median depression, the *basilar sulcus,* indicates the position occupied by the basilar artery (Figs. 2-17 and 20-9).

Transverse sections of the pons reveal the basic organization (Fig. 12-1). The pons consists of a massive *ventral part* composed of: (1) longitudinal descending fiber bundles, (2) pontine nuclei, (3) transversely oriented fibers projecting to the cerebellum, and a smaller dorsal part, known as the *tegmentum.* The tegmental portion contains aggregations of cells and fibers which form a central core known as the reticular formation. The pontine tegmentum is continuous with the reticular formation of the medulla and midbrain. Cranial nerve nuclei, ascending sensory systems and older descending motor pathways are found within the tegmentum. Cranial nerves associated with the pons are the trigeminal (N. V), abducens (N. VI), facial (N. VII), and the two components of the vestibulocochlear nerve (N. VIII). The *abducens nucleus* lies in the floor of the fourth ventricle and is partially encircled by fibers of the facial nerve. Facial nerve fibers and cells of the abducens nucleus underlie the *facial colliculus* seen in the floor of the fourth ventricle (Fig. 2-18). Fibers of the abducens nerve emerge from the ventral surface of the brain stem at the junction of the pons and medulla. The facial and vestibulocochlear nerves emerge and enter the lateral surface of the pons at the *cerebellopontine angle,* formed by the junction of pons, medulla and cerebellum. The trigeminal nerve, consisting of motor and sensory fibers, passes

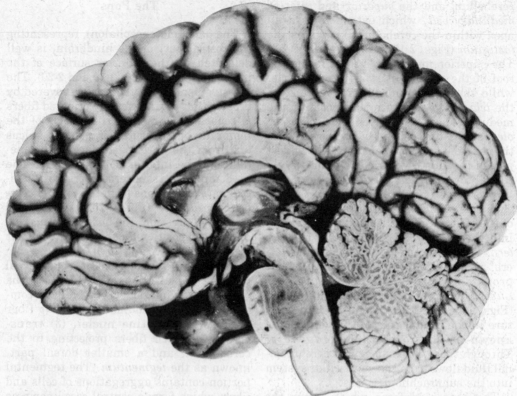

FIG. 2-20. Photograph of midsagittal section of the brain. Brain stem structures are identified in Figure 2-21.

through rostral parts of the middle cerebellar peduncle to reach nuclei in the dorsolateral pontine tegmentum (Fig. 2-19).

The *middle cerebellar peduncle* consists of a large number of fibers, arising from the pontine nuclei, which project to the cerebellum; this is the largest of the three cerebellar peduncles (Figs. 2-18 and 2-19).

The Midbrain

The midbrain (mesencephalon) is the smallest and least differentiated part of the brain stem (Figs. 2-18, 2-19 and 2-20). It consists of: (1) the *tectum,* represented by the superior and inferior colliculi, (2) the *tegmentum,* ventral to the cerebral aqueduct, and (3) the massive *crura cerebri* (Fig. 13-1). The tegmentum and *crura cerebri* are separated by a large pigmented nuclear mass, the *substantia nigra.* The superior colliculus and a region immediately rostal to it, known as the *pretectum,* are important relays in the visual system.

The inferior colliculus relays auditory impulses to thalamic nuclei that in turn project to specific cortical areas.

Two cranial nerves are associated with the midbrain, the oculomotor (N. III) and the trochlear (N. IV). The oculomotor nerve emerges from the *interpeduncular fossa,* between the massive crura cerebri Figs. 2-5, 2-17 and 2-19). The slender trochlear nerve exists from the dorsal surface of the brain stem, caudal to the inferior colliculus; fibers of this nerve cross in the superior medullary velum (Figs. 2-18 and 2-19). The fibers of the *superior cerebellar peduncle,* seen on each side of the upper part of the fourth ventricle (Figs. 2-18 and 2-19), decussate completely in the caudal midbrain tegmentum. Crossed fibers of this peduncle traverse and surround a discrete nuclear mass in the tegmentum called the *red nucleus* (Fig. 2-10).

Crus Cerebri. The crus cerebri on the ventral surface of the midbrain is collec-

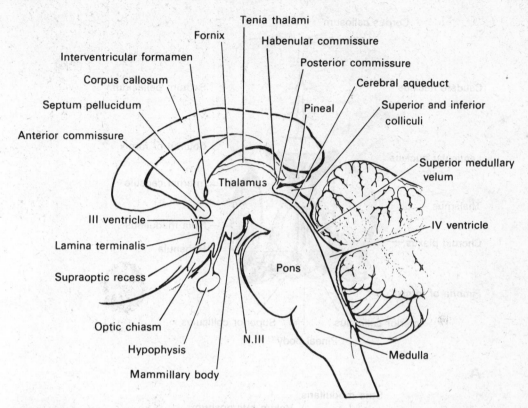

Fig. 2-21. Drawing of midsagittal section of the brain stem identifying structures shown in Figure 2-20.

tions of fibers originating in broad areas of the cerebral cortex that pass through the internal capsule (Figs. 2-8 and 2-17). These fibers project to: (1) spinal cord (i.e., corticospinal), (2) pontine nuclei (i.e., corticopontine), and (3) specific regions of the lower brain stem (i.e., corticobulbar). A large part of the corticobulbar fibers project to parts of the reticular formation.

Substantia Nigra. The pigmented substantia nigra, the largest single nuclear mass in the midbrain, has connections with parts of the basal ganglia and thalamus and is considered to subserve a motor function (Fig. 2-10).

The Diencephalon

The diencephalon, the most rostral part of the brain stem, is a paired structure on each side of the third ventricle (Figs. 2-9, 2-14, 2-18, 2-19, 2-20 and 2-21). The lateral ventricles, corpus callosum, fornix and velum interpositum lie superior to the di-

encephalon (Fig. 2-22). Fibers of the posterior limb of the internal capsule and the body and tail of the caudate nucleus constitute its lateral border. Caudally the diencephalon appears continuous with the tegmentum of the midbrain; the posterior commissure is regarded as the junctional zone between the diencephalon and mesencephalon (Figs. 2-9 and 2-21). The rostral boundary of the diencephalon is near the interventricular foramen, but portions of the hypothalamus extend almost to the *lamina terminalis* (Figs. 2-20 and 2-21). This complex consists of four parts: (1) the epithalamus, (2) the thalamus, (3) the hypothalamus, and (4) the subthalamus (Figs. 2-20, 2-21 and 2-22).

The Epithalamus. The epithalamus, evident on the dorsal surface of the diencephalon, consists of: (1) the pineal body, (2) the habenular nuclei, (3) the stria medullares, and (4) the tenia thalami (Fig. 2-18).

The Thalamus. The thalamus, the larg-

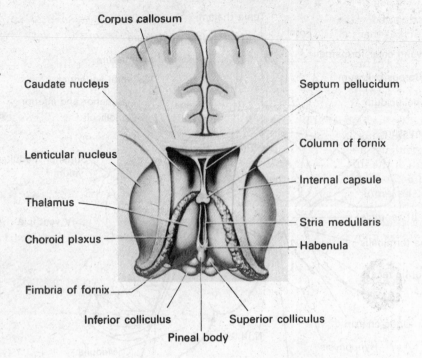

Corpus callosum

Caudate nucleus

Septum pellucidum

Column of fornix

Lenticular nucleus

Internal capsule

Thalamus

Stria medullaris

Choroid plexus

Habenula

Fimbria of fornix

Inferior colliculus   Superior colliculus

Pineal body

A

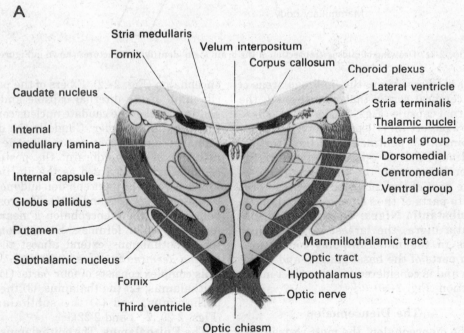

Stria medullaris   Velum interpositum

Fornix   Corpus callosum   Choroid plexus

Caudate nucleus   Lateral ventricle

Stria terminalis

Internal   Thalamic nuclei
medullary lamina   Lateral group

Dorsomedial

Internal capsule   Centromedian

Ventral group

Globus pallidus

Putamen   Mammillothalamic tract

Optic tract

Subthalamic nucleus   Hypothalamus

Fornix   Optic nerve

Third ventricle

Optic chiasm

B

FIG. 2-22. *A*. Posterior view of the diencephalon and related structures. *B*, Schematic drawing of a frontal section through the diencephalon (see Fig. 15-6) and adjacent structures indicating some of the major nuclear groups of the thalamus. The hypothalamus lies on both sides of the third ventricle below the hypothalamic sulcus.

est diencephalic subdivision, is an oblique egg-shaped nuclear mass at the rostral end of the brain stem (Figs. 2-9, 2-14, 2-18, 2-19, 2-20 and 2-22). This nuclear complex lies between the interventricular foramen and the posterior commissure and extends from the third ventricle to the medial border of the posterior limb of the internal capsule. The thalamus lies dorsal to the hypothalamic sulcus, a shallow groove on the lateral wall of the third ventricle (Figs. 2-20, 2-21 and 2-22). The lateral and caudal parts of the thalamus are enlarged and overlie midbrain structures. The superior surface of the thalamus is covered by a thin layer of fibers known as the *stratum zonale*. A narrow lateral strip of the superior surface, adjacent to the body and tail of the caudate nucleus, is covered by ependyma and forms part of the floor of the lateral ventricle. This strip is called the *lamina affixa* (Fig. 2-18). The *stria terminalis* and the *terminal vein* are present dorsally at the junction of thalamus and caudate nucleus. The *stria medullaris* extends along the dorsomedial margin of the thalamus near the roof of the third ventricle. The medial surfaces of thalami on each side of the third ventricle are partially fused in about 80% of human brains. This place of fusion is called the *interthalamic adhesion* or *massa intermedia* (Fig. 2-22).

Although most subdivisions of the thalamus are not evident in gross specimens, the *anterior tubercle* of the thalamus is discernible rostrally as a distinct swelling. The expanded posterior part of the thalamus that overhangs part of the midbrain is known as the *pulvinar* (Figs. 2-9 and 2-18). The *medial* and *lateral geniculate bodies,* important relay nuclei concerned with audition and vision, lie ventral to the pulvinar. These structures together are referred to as the *metathalamus*. The thalamus is divided into anterior, lateral, medial and ventral nuclear groups by a thin layer of myelinated fibers, known as the *internal medullary lamina* of the thalamus, which can be seen grossly in transverse sections of the brain (Figs. 2-14 and 2-22). Nuclear groups within the internal medullary lamina are collectively referred to as the *intralaminar thalamic nuclei*.

The thalamus is regarded as the neural structure whose relationships with other parts of the neuraxis provide the key to understanding the organization of the central nervous system. Like most keys it is small. This small part of the diencephalon is concerned with: (1) distributing most of the afferent input to the cerebral cortex, (2) the control of the electrocortical activity of the cerebral cortex, and (3) the integration of motor functions by providing the relays through which impulses from the basal ganglia and cerebellum can reach the motor cortex.

The Hypothalamus. The hypothalamus lies ventral to the hypothalamic sulcus and forms the inferior and lateral walls of the third ventricle (Figs. 2-20, 2-21 and 2-22). This subdivision of the diencephalon extends from the region of the optic chiasm to the caudal border of the mammillary bodies. The gross structures visible on the ventral surface include the *optic chiasm, infundibulum, tuber cinereum* and *mammillary bodies* (Fig. 2-6). The hypothalamus is divided into medial and lateral nuclear groups by fibers of the fornix which end in the mammillary body. Three rostrocaudal regions of the hypothalamus are recognized: (1) a supraoptic, dorsal to the optic chiasm, (2) a tuberal region centrally, and (3) a mammillary region caudally (Fig. 16-1).

The hypothalamus has a rostrocaudal extent of about 10 mm. This subdivision of the diencephalon is concerned with visceral, endocrine and metabolic activity, as well as with temperature regulation, sleep and emotion.

The Subthalamus. The subthalamus is a transitional zone ventral to the thalamus and lateral to the hypothalamus. It is bounded by the thalamus above, the hypothalamus medially and the internal capsule laterally (Figs. 2-14 and 2-22). The largest discrete nuclear mass is the *subthalamic nucleus,* a lens-shaped structure on the inner aspect of the internal capsule (Fig. 15-6). This region is traversed by many important fiber systems in their projection to thalamic nuclei. A small, relatively clear area, known as the *zona incerta,* serves as an important landmark in distinguishing certain fiber bundles. The subthalamic nucleus and pathways traversing this region are concerned with somatic motor function.

THE CEREBELLUM

The cerebellum overlies the posterior aspect of the pons and medulla and extends laterally under the tentorium to fill the greater part of the posterior fossa (Fig. 2-1). The superior surface is somewhat flattened, while the inferior surface is convex. A shallow *anterior cerebellar incisure* is present superiorly. A deeper and narrower *posterior cerebellar incisure* contains a fold of dura mater, the *falx cerebelli* (Fig. 1-2).

The cerebellum consists of a midline portion, the *vermis*, and two lateral lobes or *hemispheres*. This structure is essentially wedge-shaped, having a superior surface which is covered by the tentorium, a posterior surface in the suboccipital region and an inferior surface which overlies the fourth ventricle. On the superior surface the distinction between vermis and hemispheres is not sharp (Fig. 2-23). On the inferior surface two deep sulci clearly separate the vermis from the hemispheres. Inferiorly a deep median fossa, the *vallecula cerebelli*, is continuous with the posterior incisure. The floor of this fossa is formed by the inferior vermis (Fig. 2-24).

Structurally the cerebellum consists of a gray cortical mantle, the cerebellar cortex, a medullary core of white matter and four pairs of intrinsic nuclei. Three paired cerebellar peduncles connect the cerebellum with the three lower segments of the brain stem (Fig. 2-25).

The cerebellar cortex consists of a large number of narrow leaflike laminae known as cerebellar folia. Cerebellar folia on the surface are nearly parallel with each other and for the most part are transversely oriented. Each lamina contains several secondary and tertiary folia.

Five transversely oriented fissures divide the cerebellum into lobes and lobules (Fig. 14-1). These fissures and the various lobular subdivisions can be identified on the isolated cerebellum or in midsagittal section (Fig. 2-26). On the superior surface

of the cerebellum two fissures can be identified: (1) the *primary* and (2) the *posterior superior* (Fig. 2-23). The *horizontal fissure,* one of the most distinctive, roughly divides the cerebellum into superior and inferior halves. On the inferior surface the *prepyramidal* and *posterolateral fissures* are found (Fig. 2-26).

The cerebellar vermis is the key to understanding the gross organization of the cerebellum, but in this part there is no median raphe and the midline is difficult to establish. Portions of the cerebellum rostral to the primary fissure constitute the *anterior lobe of the cerebellum* (Figs. 2-23 and 14-1). In the vermis the lobules consist of the lingula, the central lobule and the culmen (Fig. 2-26); in the hemisphere the lingula has no corresponding part, but the *alar central lobule* and the *anterior quadrangular lobule* correspond to the central lobule and the culmen.

The *posterior lobe* of the cerebellum lies between the primary and posterolateral fissures and represents the largest subdivision of the cerebellum (Figs. 2-26 and 14-1). Vermal parts of the posterior lobe in sequence are the *declive, folium, tuber, pyramis,* and *uvula* (Fig. 2-26). The *simple lobule,* between the primary and posterior superior fissures, corresponds to the declive of the vermis (Fig. 14-1). The *ansiform lobule* is that part of the cerebellar hemisphere between the posterior superior fissure and the *gracile lobule*. The horizontal fissure divides the ansiform lobule into the *superior semilunar lobule* (crus I) and the *inferior semilunar lobule* (crus II). The vermal counterparts of the ansiform lobule are the folium and tuber. Between the prepyramidal and posterolateral fissures are the *pyramis* and *uvula* in the vermis and the *biventer lobule* and the *cerebellar tonsil* in the hemisphere (Figs. 2-25 and 2-26).

The *flocculonodular lobule* lies rostral to the posterolateral fissure and consists of the vermal nodulus and the paired flocculi (Fig. 2-25). The *nodulus* lies immediately caudal to the inferior medullary velum (Fig. 2-26).

In midsagittal section the relationships of the cerebellum to the brain stem are evident (Fig. 2-20). The complex branching

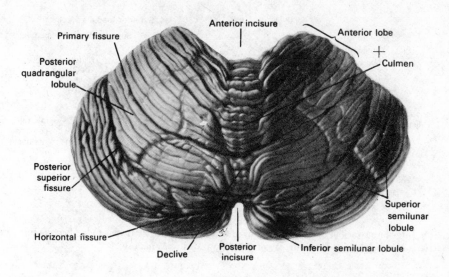

FIG. 2-23. Superior surface of cerebellum (from Mettler's *Neuroanatomy*, '48; courtesy of The C. V. Mosby Company).

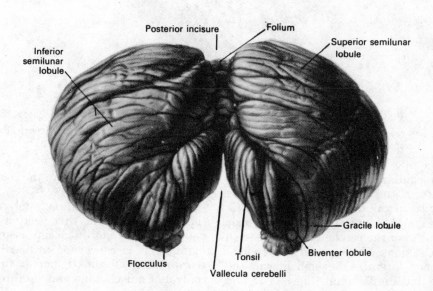

FIG. 2-24. Posteroinferior view of the cerebellum (from Mettler's *Neuroanatomy*, '48; courtesy of The C. V. Mosby Company).

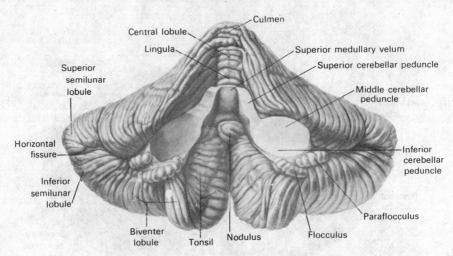

FIG. 2-25. Inferior surface of cerebellum removed from brain stem by transection of cerebellar peduncles (from Mettler's *Neuroanatomy*, '48; courtesy of The C. V. Mosby Company).

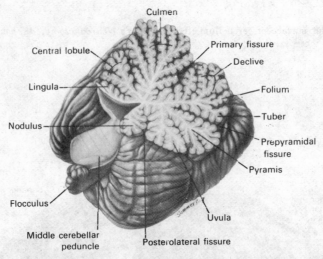

FIG. 2-26. View of the sagittally sectioned cerebellum showing the lobules of the cerebellar vermis. The primary fissure is the deepest of all cerebellar fissures (from Mettler's *Neuroanatomy*, '48; courtesy of The C. V. Mosby Company).

of the medullary core and the treelike appearance of the laminae and folia have given rise to the descriptive term, *arbor vitae* (Figs. 2-21 and 2-26). The intrinsic deep nuclei of the cerebellum can be seen only in sections. These nuclei are the dentate (most lateral), the emboliform, the globose and the fastigial (Figs. 14-12 and 14-13). The fastigial nuclei, commonly called the roof nuclei, lie in the roof of the fourth ventricle.

Although the cerebellum is derived from the metencephalon, this portion of the neuraxis functions in a suprasegmental manner. It is concerned primarily with coordination of somatic motor function, control of muscle tone and equilibrium.

CHAPTER 3

Development and Histogenesis of the Nervous System

FORMATION OF THE NEURAL TUBE

The central and peripheral nervous systems are derived from a thickened plate of ectoderm, known as the *neural plate*, which first appears late in the 3rd week of fetal life. The neural plate lies dorsally, rostral to the primitive streak and Hensen's node, and at first consists of a single layer of cells (Fig. 3-1). This ectoderm undergoes rapid proliferation and becomes stratified. The growth rate near the margins of the plate exceeds that in the midline, causing the formation of a *neural groove*, which is bounded on each side by an elevated *neural fold* (Fig. 3-2). As the primitive ectodermal cells proliferate, the neural groove deepens, and the neural folds thicken, become more prominent and ultimately fuse dorsally to form the *neural tube*. Closure of the neural tube begins in the region of the fourth somite (i.e., future cervical region) and proceeds in both cranial and caudal directions. During the formation of the neural tube its lumen has temporary cranial and caudal connections with the amniotic cavity via the *anterior* and *posterior neuropores* (Fig. 3-1). The anterior neuropore which represents the most rostral opening of the embryonic neural tube closes in embryos of 18 to 20 somites and ultimately becomes the *lamina terminalis*. The posterior neuropore usually closes later when the embryo has reached the 25 to 26 somite stage. At early stages in the formation of the neural tube, before closure is complete, rostral portions of the neural tube are enlarged and indicate the formation of primary brain vesicles. Three primary brain vesicles are evident by the time the neural tube is completely closed (Fig. 3-8). From these vesicles the brain is formed. Caudal portions of the neural tube which remain relatively small in diameter form the spinal cord.

The appearance of the neural folds heralds the segmentation of bilateral strips of paraxial mesoderm into somites (Fig. 3-1). New somites continue to be formed in a craniocaudal sequence; at the end of the 4th week 40 somites normally are present (Arey, '38).

NEURAL CREST

The lateral margins of the neural plate are thinner and continuous with the general body ectoderm. The thinned lateral margins of the neural plate (neural crest cells) are approximated as the neural folds meet and fuse. Neural crest cells form a temporary intermediate layer between the neural tube and the surface ectoderm (Fig. 3-2). This temporary layer extends from the level of the mesencephalon to the caudal somites and is for a time continuous across the midline. Neural crest cells divide in the midline, migrate laterally and become segmented into cell clusters between the neural tube and the somites

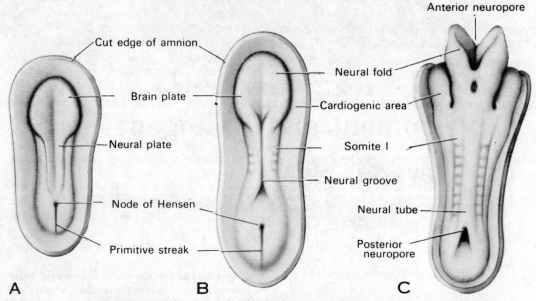

FIG. 3-1. Diagrams illustrating early development of human nervous system. *A*, Late presomite and early neural plate stage (modified from Davis, '23). *B*, Early somite and neural groove stage (modified from Ingalls, '20). *C*, Eight-somite and early neural tube stage (modified from Payne, '24).

(Fig. 3-2). These clusters of neural crest cells give rise to the primary sensory neurons of the dorsal root ganglia of spinal nerves. Similar cell clusters in the hindbrain give rise to sensory neurons which form cranial nerve ganglia (nerves V, VII, VIII, IX and X), but these are not segmentally arranged (Fig. 3-8).

The neural crest has a temporary existence as its cells migrate widely in the body and undergo various differentiations in different tissues (Horstadius, '50). All of the sensory cells and fibers of the peripheral nervous system (with a few exceptions) and most of the peripheral cells of the autonomic nervous system, are derived from the neural crest. Thus the neural crest gives rise to the unipolar spinal ganglion cells and their equivalent in the sensory ganglia of cranial nerves V, VII, IX and X. Some elements persisting as bipolar cells form the auditory nerve (Hamilton and Mossman, '72). Other derivatives of the neural crest include: (1) the neurolemmal sheath cells of all peripheral nerves, (2) capsule cells in ganglia, (3) sympathetic ganglia (4) chromaffin cells, and (5) pigment cells (Boyd, '60).

HISTOGENESIS OF NEURAL TUBE

The histogenetic changes whereby the columnar ectoderm is converted to nervous tissue are essentially the same in all parts of the neural tube. According to classic concepts, as the neural tube closes it is formed by a single layer of columnar cells. This epithelium proliferates forming a pseudostratified neuroepithelium several layers thick. Large ovoid cells near the central canal form a *germinal layer* in which rapid mitotic cell division takes place. Newly formed undifferentiated cells migrate peripherally so that the wall of the neural tube assumes a three-layered appearance. The three layers formed by these cells and their processes are: (1) an internal *ependymal layer* composed of columnar cells arranged radially around the central canal, and ovoid germinal cells undergoing mitosis, (2) a middle *mantle layer* of densely packed primitive neuroblasts derived from the germinal cells, and (3) an external *marginal layer* composed of the processes of cells in the mantle and ependymal layers (Fig. 3-3).

More recent studies based upon autoradi-

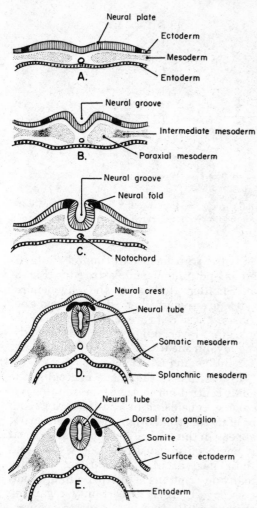

FIG. 3-2. Diagrams of transverse sections of embryos at different ages to show development of the spinal cord. *A*, Neural plate stage. *B*, Early neural groove stage. *C*, Late neural groove stage. *D*, Early neural tube and neural crest stage. *E*, Neural tube and dorsal root ganglion stage.

ographic and electron microscopic studies have challenged the classic concepts described above (Langman et al., '66; Langman, '68, '69; Lyser, '64, '68). These new data indicate that the wall of the recently closed neural tube consists of only one type of cell, the *neuroepithelial cell*. Neuroepithelial cells form a pseudostratified epithelium which extends from the *internal limiting membrane* to the *external limiting membrane*. Each neuroepithelial cell is wedge-shaped and possesses cytoplasmic processes which reach the internal limiting membrane and are attached to adjacent cells by *terminal bars* (Fig. 3-4). Nuclei of neuroepithelial cells have an oval shape and may be at variable distances from the external limiting membrane. Desoxyribonucleic acid (DNA) synthesis occurs only in nuclei near the external limiting membrane. When DNA synthesis is complete, the nucleus moves toward the lumen of the neural tube and the cell loses its contact with the external limiting membrane. Cells undergo mitosis when the nucleus has reached the innermost zone, and daughter cells remain attached by the terminal bars at the internal limiting membrane. After division the cells elongate and their nuclei migrate toward the external limiting membrane where further DNA synthesis occurs. Following closure of the neural tube, neuroepithelial cells give rise to another cell type characterized by a large round pale nucleus and dark-staining nucleolus. These cells no longer have the ability to synthesize DNA and constitute the primitive nerve cells or *neuroblasts* (Fig. 3-4). Neuroblasts, produced in increasing numbers, surround the neuroepithelial layer and form the *mantle layer*. The outermost layer containing the processes of the neuroblasts forms the *marginal layer* (Fig. 3-3).

NEURONS

Neuroblasts, arising from division of neuroepithelial cells, migrate into the mantle layer of the neural tube and increase in number as neuroepithelial cells continue to differentiate. These cells form rounded *apolar neuroblasts* (Fig. 3-5), which further differentiate into *bipolar neuroblasts* with two cytoplasmic processes on opposite sides of the cell body. One cytoplasm process elongates to form a *primitive axon*. The other cytoplasm process develops numerous small outgrowths which form arborizations known as *primitive dendrites*. At this stage the cell becomes a *multipolar neuroblast*. Further growth and differentiation results in the formation of an adult nerve cell or *neuron*. According to recent authors (Langman and Haden, '70), neuroblasts in the lateral

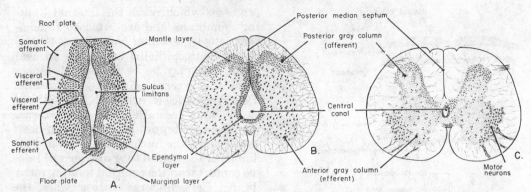

FIG. 3-3. Diagrams of differentiating layers of the spinal cord. *A*, Section through spinal cord of a 5-week human embryo. *B*, Cervical spinal cord of an 8-week human embryo. *C*, Cervical spinal cord of a 10-week human embryo (after Keibel and Mall, '12).

part of the anterior horn are formed first, and these are followed by those in the medial part of the anterior horn, the internuncial zone and posterior horn. Neuroblasts, once formed, lose their ability to divide.

GLIA CELLS

Some of the neuroepithelial cells differentiate into primitive *glioblasts* which form supporting cells. The majority of glioblasts are formed after the production of neuroblasts has ceased (Langman, '69). Glioblasts become spindle-shaped bipolar cells that extend the entire thickness of the neural tube. Their large nuclei are placed close to the lumen and their processes are attached to both the internal and external limiting membranes of the neural tube. Some glioblasts retain this position and become transformed into ependymal cells (Fig. 3-5). During maturation most ependymal cells lose their attachment to the external limiting membrane and their processes extend only a short distance from the central canal to become anchored in a subependymal glial membrane (Fig. 5-13). Ependymal cells in the adult form the lining of the central canal of the spinal cord and the ventricular surfaces of the brain. Epithelial cells of the choroid plexus (Fig. 5-15) are believed to be modified ependymal cells (i.e., of glioblast origin). Other glioblasts in the mantle layer lose their attachments with the limiting membrane and assume apolar or unipolar appearances. In later stages of development these detached stem cells send out new processes

and are transformed ultimately into fibrous and protoplasmic astrocytes (Fig. 3-5). Smaller glial cells, the oligodendrocytes, are thought to be derived from glioblasts. These cells are found mainly in the marginal layer and play a role in developing myelin sheaths (Fig. 5-9) (Bunge et al., '62; Bunge and Glass, '65).

In addition to the above neuroglia, the adult central nervous system contains *microglia*, considered by Rio-Hortega ('21) to be of mesodermal origin. These cells do not appear in the central nervous system until it has been invaded by blood vessels and their perivascular adventitia. Despite many descriptions of microglia in light microscopy, there is uncertainty regarding their identification in the electron microscope (Peters, et al., '70). Microglia are considered to serve a phagocytic function and may be derived from blood histiocytes.

In tissue culture neurons develop normally only when they are embedded in dense glia (Murray, '65). Glial cells retain a measure of motility in the adult, whereas neurons are immobile beyond the neuroblast stage. Glial cells also can divide and increase in number, while neurons do not divide after birth and remain in permanent interphase throughout life (Altman, '66). The latter is a significant point, for neural pathways, reflexes and storage of learned information all require a metabolically stable and permanent system of neurons. Structural and functional features of the neuroglial elements are presented in Chapter 5.

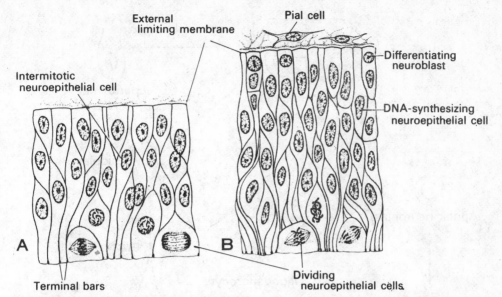

FIG. 3-4. Modern concepts of the development of the recently closed neural tube indicate only one cell type, the neuroepithelial cell. *A*, Wall of the recently closed neural tube with neuroepithelial cells which form a pseudostratified epithelium extending from the lumen to the external limiting membrane. *B*, Cross section of the wall of the neural tube at a more advanced stage than in *A*. Neuroepithelial cells are in phases of DNA synthesis or mitosis, except near the external limiting membrane where differentiating neuroblasts are found (after Langman, '69).

SPINAL CORD

Continued cell proliferation produces anterior and posterior thickenings in the mantle layer. Anterior thickenings form the larger *basal plates*, from which the anterior gray horn (motor) of the adult spinal cord is formed. Smaller posterior thickenings constitute the *alar plates*, from which the future posterior gray horn (sensory) of the spinal cord is formed. A longitudinal groove, the *sulcus limitans*, marks the lateral junction of basal and alar plates (Fig. 3-3). The sulcus limitans extends the length of the primitive spinal cord and continues into the brain stem; it remains as a prominent sulcus in the floor of the fourth ventricle in the adult brain (Fig. 11-16). In transverse sections of the neural tube the lumen is rhomboid-shaped with relatively thin *roof* and *floor plates* (Fig. 3-3). The roof and floor plates furnish only glioblastic elements.

Neuroblasts of the basal plates become the efferent peripheral neurons. Their axons penetrate the marginal layer and external limiting membrane and emerge from the spinal cord as ventral root fibers (Figs. 3-6 and 3-7). Fibers of the ventral root pass directly to skeletal muscle or to autonomic ganglia for the innervation of visceral structures (Figs. 3-7 and 9-22). All axons of cells of the alar plate remain within the central nervous system. Some arch anteriorly, cross through the basal plate to the opposite side, and reach the marginal layer, where they ascend or descend for variable distances (Fig. 3-6). Other axons remain on the same side and ascend or descend in the marginal layer. These neurons, whose processes are entirely confined to the central nervous system, constitute the *central*, or *intermediate, cells*. Those whose axons remain on the same side are known as *association cells*; those whose axons cross to the opposite side are *commissural cells*.

As development proceeds, the proliferation of the germinal cells gradually decreases and ultimately stops altogether. As more and more indifferent cells are transformed into neuroblasts, the nuclear layer progressively diminishes in size and ultimately is reduced to a single layer of

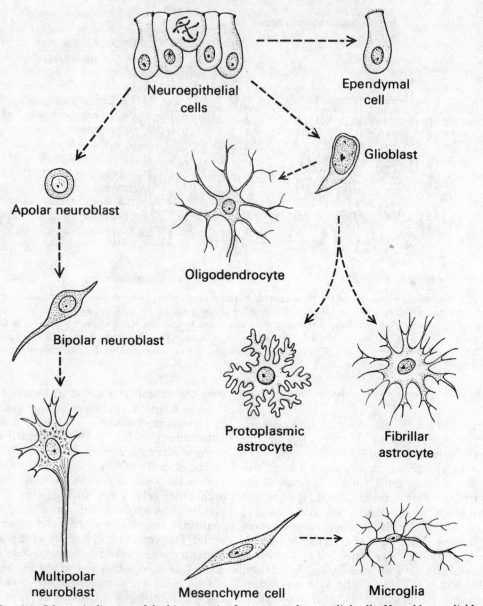

FIG. 3-5. Schematic diagram of the histogenesis of neurons and neuroglial cells. Neuroblasts, glioblasts and ependymal cells originate from neuroepithelial cells. The origin of the oligodendrocyte is obscure, but both protoplasmic and fibrillar astrocytes are derived from glioblasts. The microglia are considered to arise from mesenchyme.

columnar ependymal cells. In certain places, as in the anterior commissure of the spinal cord, some of the ependymal cells may retain their embryonal glioblastic character and extend the whole thickness of the neural wall (Fig. 3-6).

The mantle layer, on the other hand, progressively increases in size and becomes the gray matter of the spinal cord. It is surrounded by an expanding marginal layer which contains the descending and ascending axons of the central cells. At a much later period, most of the axons become myelinated and the marginal layer assumes the white, glistening appearance characteristic of the white matter of the adult spinal cord.

The expansion of the alar plates in a

medial direction brings these plates into close apposition. The *posterior median septum*, formed of glial processes and intima pia, marks the line of junction in the adult (Figs. 3-3 and 9-6). In the floor plate region, an invagination forms the anterior median fissure and greatly reduces the size of the central canal (Figs. 3-3 and 9-7). As a consequence of these changes, the embryonic neural tube is transformed into the spinal cord.

The spinal cord has a long cylindrical shape and is curved in the embryonic axis. There is an acute ventral flexure, *the cervical flexure*, at the junction of the spinal cord and hindbrain (rhombencephalon). Until the beginning of the 3rd month the spinal cord extends the entire length of the vertebral canal. After this time the mesodermal elements which have formed the cartilages and bones of the vertebral column grow more rapidly than the spinal cord, so that at birth the most caudal part of the spinal cord, the *conus medullaris*, lies at the level of the third lumbar vertebra. The sites of emergence of spinal nerves do not change, but there is a lengthening of root filaments between the intervertebral foramina and the spinal cord which is most marked for lumbar and sacral spinal roots. The large number of nerve roots surrounding the *filum terminale* (Fig. 1-6) constitute the *cauda equina*. In the adult the conus medullaris lies between the L1 and L2 vertebrae and the spinal cord occupies only the upper two-thirds of the vertebral canal (Fig. 9-3).

Neuron Differentiation. In the spinal ganglia, derived from the neural crest, a similar differentiation takes place. Many of the original polygonal or round cells become spindle-shaped and bipolar with the development of two neurofibrillar processes, one central and one peripheral (Figs. 3-6 and 4-6). The central processes enter the spinal cord as dorsal root fibers and there bifurcate into ascending and descending arms which contribute collaterals to the mantle layer or gray matter (Figs. 3-6 and 9-22).

In human embryos with a crown-to-rump length of 25 mm, many of the neuroblasts have attained the bipolar stage. A few neurons with greater amounts of cytoplasm and distinct neurofilaments appear transitional in shape and are referred to as pseudounipolar cells (Fig. 4-6). The cytoplasm of the cell body elongates, and the two processes become approximated. Ultimately the elongated cell cytoplasm forms the single stem of a T, while the top of the T is formed by the thin central and thicker peripheral processes (Truex, '39; Tennyson, '65). Many neurons are of the unipolar type in spinal ganglia of human 100 mm fetuses. Most of the spinal ganglia cells are true unipolar neurons in the newborn human infant. An occasional bipolar neuron or those in transitional stages may at times be observed in the adult dorsal root ganglia. It is interesting to note that a generous number of ganglionic neuroblasts may be produced initially. Thus, embryonic dorsal root and sympathetic ganglia appear to have an overabundance of neuroblasts when compared to the number of fully differentiated ganglion cells present at birth. For example, total cell counts of the submandibular ganglia in a graded series of human fetuses showed a progressive reduction from 12,128 cells at 17 weeks of gestation to 5,988 at full term (Crouse and Cucinotta, '65).

Not all of the cells in the spinal ganglia differentiate into neuroblasts. Some develop into *capsule* or *satellite cells* which form a capsule around the bodies of the spinal ganglion cells (Fig. 4-1A). Others wander out along the course of the growing peripheral nerve fibers, envelop them and ultimately become Schwann cells. These play an active role in the formation of myelin and may be considered as a peripheral type of neuroglia, perhaps most closely related to oligodendrocytes.

Besides the spinal ganglia, there are other peripheral aggregations of nerve cells known as *autonomic* or *sympathetic ganglia* (Figs. 3-7 and 8-2). Arising mainly from the neural crest, these cells form two ganglionic chains on the anterolateral aspect of the vertebral column (vertebral sympathetic ganglia). Others wander further to form the ganglia of the mesenteric plexuses (collateral or prevertebral ganglia), while some actually invade the walls of the viscera, or settle close to them, as the terminal or peripheral autonomic ganglia (Fig. 8-1). Here, too, differentiation occurs in several directions. Some cells en-

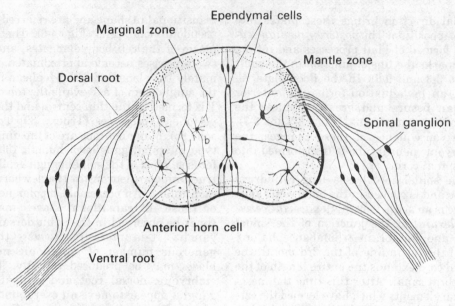

FIG. 3-6. Drawing of transverse section of spinal cord and spinal ganglia of a chick embryo. The mantle zone becomes the butterfly gray of the adult spinal cord, while the marginal zone develops into the white matter containing ascending and descending fiber tracts. *a* indicates afferent fiber with collaterals; *b* represents a column cell that projects contralaterally. Based upon silver impregnation.

large to form the multipolar sympathetic ganglion cells, whose axons terminate in visceral effectors, smooth muscle, heart muscle and glandular epithelium (Fig. 4-6). Others, as in the case of the spinal ganglia, give rise to satellite cells, which envelop the bodies of one or several ganglion cells. Finally, some differentiate into the chromaffin cells found in the adrenal medulla, carotid bodies and other portions of the body.

The origin of the autonomic ganglia is disputed. While some believe they are formed from the neural crest, others maintain that in part they are derived from the anterior part of the spinal cord, the cells migrating by way of the ventral roots. It is probable that in mammals, at least, both neural crest and spinal cord contribute to their formation. Inasmuch as the sympathetic cells are efferent in character, their origin would most likely be from the visceral efferent part of the spinal cord (Fig. 3-3).

Segmental Arrangement of Peripheral Nerve Elements. With the differentiation of the various types of nerve cells in

early stages of development, a neuronal mechanism adequate for complete, if simple, reflex arcs is established. Such arcs consist of afferent, intermediate and efferent neurons and their peripheral extensions. However, the synaptic junctions of these cells, which make such reflex arcs functional, are as yet unformed.

In embryos of about 10 mm the various components of the peripheral nervous system already are laid down and may be recognized in a transverse section of any typical body segment (Fig. 3-7). The central processes of the spinal ganglion cells form the *dorsal* roots; the *ventral root* is composed of axons from cells in the anterior gray of the spinal cord (mantle layer). Distal to the ganglion, the ventral root unites with the peripheral processes of the spinal ganglion cells to form a mixed *spinal nerve* (Figs. 3-7 and 7-1). Each spinal nerve containing afferent and efferent fibers, divides into a *dorsal* and a *ventral ramus* and also sends a fiber bundle known as the *ramus communicans* to the vertebral sympathetic chain. The dorsal ramus supplies the muscles and skin of the

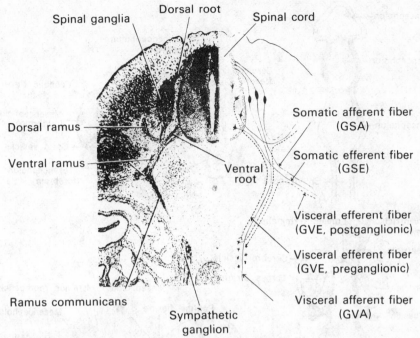

Fig. 3-7. Transverse section of 14 mm pig embryo. The functional categories of spinal nerve fibers are indicated on the right. Bielschowsky's silver stain. Photograph.

back; the larger ventral ramus goes to the ventrolateral parts of the body wall. Four functional types of peripheral nerve fibers may be distinguished: *general somatic afferent* (GSA), *general visceral afferent* (GVA), *general somatic efferent* (GSE) and *general visceral efferent* (GVE). All of these functional types of fibers are found in both dorsal and ventral rami. The somatic efferent or "motor" fibers arise from large cells in the anterior gray matter, leave the spinal cord through the ventral roots and go directly to the skeletal voluntary muscles of the body wall. The somatic afferent or "sensory" fibers are the peripheral processes of spinal ganglion cells, which terminate as receptors in the skin and deeper portions of the body wall. The central processes enter the cord as dorsal root fibers (Fig. 9-22).

The efferent innervation of visceral structures is different from that of the somatic muscles, for two neurons always are involved in the conduction of impulses from the central nervous system to the effector organs (Figs. 3-7 and 8-2). The *preganglionic visceral efferent* fibers are ax-

ons of spinal cord neurons which pass through the ventral root and ramus communicans to terminate in a vertebral or prevertebral sympathetic ganglion. The axons of sympathetic cells form the *postganglionic visceral efferent* fibers, which course through the ramus communicans in the reverse direction, join the main branches of the spinal nerve and are distributed to the smooth muscle and glandular epithelium of the body (Figs. 8-1 and 8-2). In the adult the ramus communicans consists of white and gray portions. The former contains the *myelinated* preganglionic fibers, the latter the *unmyelinated* postganglionic fibers.

Finally, *visceral afferent fibers* convey impulses from the thoracic and abdominal viscera. Like the somatic afferent fibers, their cell bodies are in the spinal ganglia and their central processes enter the spinal cord via the dorsal root (Fig. 9-22).

BRAIN

As soon as the anterior neuropore is closed, the rostral cavity of the neural tube shows three dilatations or brain vesicles.

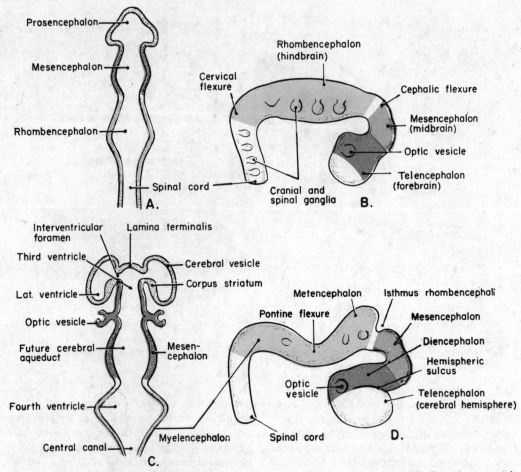

FIG. 3-8. Diagrams of the developing brain vesicles and ventricular system. *A* and *B*, Three brain vesicle stage of a 4-week embryo. *C* and *D*, Five brain vesicle stage of a 6-week human embryo. The prosencephalon, telencephalon and spinal cord are *stippled*. The diencephalon is shown in *dark red*, while the mesencephalon is *blue*. The derivatives of the rhombencephalon (pons and medulla) are in *light red* and the isthmus is *white* (modified from Hochstetter, '19, and Langman, '69).

These three early subdivisions are the *prosencephalon* or forebrain, the *mesencephalon* or midbrain and the *rhombencephalon* or hindbrain (Fig. 3-8A). The constricted region between the mesencephalon and rhombencephalon is known as the isthmus. The brain vesicles maintain many of the fundamental morphological features seen in more caudal parts of the embryonic neural tube, in that each has roof and floor plates and alar and basal plates. Although the walls of these vesicles are thin, the sulcus limitans is present at the junction of alar and basal plates in caudal brain vesicles (rhombencephalon

and mesencephalon). The large dilated cavities within each brain vesicle are the forerunners of the ventricular system, although they are destined to undergo extensive alterations in size, shape and extent as a consequence of cell proliferation, growth and various brain flexures. These ventricular cavities are continuous with the central canal of the spinal cord. The lateral margins of the prosencephalon develop shallow depressions, the optic sulci, which subsequently becomes evaginated to form the optic vesicle (Fig. 3-8B and C). Each optic vesicle becomes modified to form an *optic cup* which is joined to the

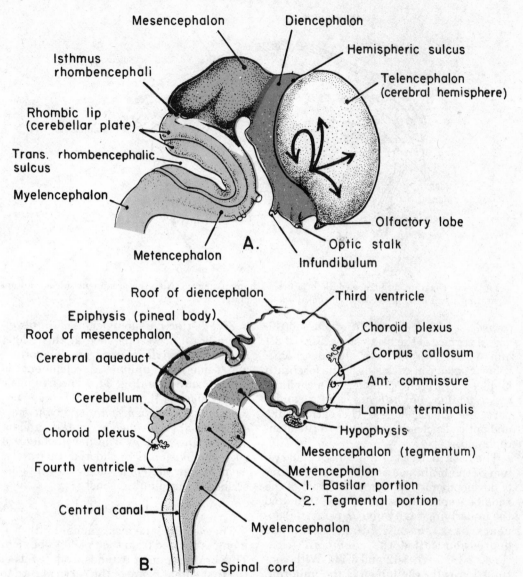

FIG. 3-9. Diagrams of the developing brain vesicles and ventricular system. *A*, Lateral view of cerebral vesicle and developing brain stem in human embryo of 8 weeks. *Arrows* indicate directions of growth and expansion of cerebral hemisphere. *B*, Sagittal section through the brain stem of a 12-week human fetus. The telencephalon is *stippled*, the diencephalon is *dark red* and the mesencephalon is *blue*. Rhombencephalic derivatives (metencephalon and myelencephalon) are *light red*, while the isthmus is *white* (modified from Hochstetter, '19).

prosencephalon by a hollow optic stalk.

Two prominent brain flexures appear at an early embryonic stage. The *cervical flexure* develops at the junction of rhombencephalon and spinal cord, with its concavity directed ventrally. A second ventral flexure, the *cephalic flexure*, occurs at the junction of mesencephalon and rhomben- cephalon (Fig. 3-9*B* and *D*). Rapid changes in the brain occur in the 4th and 5th week of development. In the 6th week a third impressive flexure with a dorsal concavity develops in the rhombencephalon and divides it into two segments, the *metence- phalon* and the *myelencephalon*. This prominent *pontine flexure* creates the

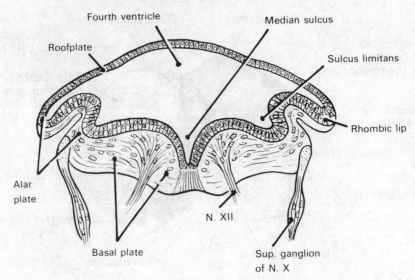

Fig. 3-10. Diagram through medulla of a 5-week human embryo. Note the prominent sulcus limitans separating structures derived from the basal and alar plates.

transverse rhombencephalic sulcus on the dorsal surface of the brain stem (Figs. 3-8*D* and 3-9*A*). A relatively shallow hemispheric sulcus on each side of the forebrain divides the prosencephalon into a cephalic *telencephalon*, or *endbrain*, and a caudal part, the *diencephalon*. The optic stalks and optic vesicles are attached to the diencephalon.

The basic pattern of the ventricular system of the brain is evident in early stages of development (Fig. 3-9*B*). The roof of the rhombencephalon is extremely thin and the underlying cavity (*fourth ventricle*) appears as a shallow, diamond-shaped depression called the *rhomboid fossa* (Figs. 2-18, 3-9*B*, 3-12 and 3-14). With continued growth, the lumen of the midbrain will become narrowed to form the *cerebral aqueduct*. Medial growth and expansion of the diencephalon also reduce the lumen of this segment of the brain to a thin vertical cleft, the *third ventricle*. A large opening (*interventricular foramen*) behind the lamina terminalis provides continuity between the third ventricle and the cavity of the laterally expanding cerebral hemisphere. The primitive *lateral ventricle* within each cerebral hemisphere will become altered extensively by subsequent development (Figs. 3-8 and 3-13).

Five distinctive subdivisions of the developing brain are established at this stage, and each subdivision undergoes elaborate, and sometimes unique, development as growth continues (Fig. 3-9). The five basic subdivisions of the brain are: (1) *the telencephalon*, (2) *the diencephalon*, (3) *the mesencephalon*, (4) *the metencephalon*, and (5) *the myelencephalon*. The development of each subdivision is considered separately, even though the embryological events described occur simultaneously.

Myelencephalon

The *medulla*, the most caudal brain segment, is derived from the myelencephalon. This brain segment extends from levels of the first spinal nerve of the cervical cord to the beginning of the pontine flexure (Fig. 3-9). As the future medulla oblongata, it differs from the spinal cord in that the walls are shifted laterally at higher levels by the expanding fourth ventricle. As a result the alar plate lies lateral to the basal plate. The sulcus limitans continues to mark the boundary between these two plates in both gross and microscopic specimens (Figs. 2-18, 3-10 and 11-16). Derivatives of the basal plate form the motor nuclei of cranial nerves, and come to occupy positions in the floor of the fourth

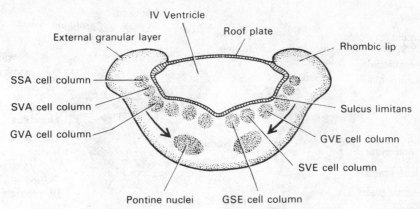

FIG. 3-11. Schematic drawing of a transverse section through the caudal metencephalon showing the cell columns of the cranial nerve nuclei with respect to the sulcus limitans. The rhombic lip lies dorsal to the sulcus limitans. The pontine nuclei originate from the alar plate and migrate ventrally (arrows). Cells of the external granular layer of the cerebellum migrate inward and ultimately form the granular layer of the cerebellar cortex (modified from Langman, '69).

ventricle medial to the sulcus limitans (Fig. 3-10). The most medial cell column gives rise to general somatic efferent (GSE) fibers that form cranial N. XII. Intermediate cell columns are associated with special visceral efferent (SVE) fibers, issuing from the nucleus ambiguus, that form components of cranial nerves IX, X and XI (Fig. 11-16). General visceral efferent (GVE) cell columns, also medial to the sulcus limitans, and represented by the dorsal motor nucleus of the vagus nerve (N. X) and inferior salivatory nucleus (N. IX), give rise to preganglionic parasympathetic fibers that are widely distributed.

Derivatives of the alar plate form sensory relay nuclei lateral to the sulcus limitans. The most lateral of these nuclei are the auditory and vestibular (special somatic afferent (SSA) cranial nerve components), and those of the trigeminal complex (general somatic afferent (GSA)). General and special visceral afferent (GVA and SVA) cell columns, represented by the solitary nuclei, lie medial to the above group (Fig. 3-11). The most medial and caudal cell groups of the alar lamina differentiate into the nuclei gracilis and cuneatus (general somatic afferent, GSA). Some cells derived from the alar lamina migrate ventrally to form portions of the *inferior olivary complex*, the largest cerebellar relay nucleus of the medulla (Fig. 11-13).

Fibers forming the medullary pyramids are cortically derived, late in appearance and occupy ventromedial regions near the midline.

In the region of the fourth ventricle, the roof plate consists of a single layer of ependymal cells covered by a thin layer of pia mater. These two layers form the tela choroidea, and prolongations project into the ventricle in the region of the transverse rhombencephalic sulcus to form the choroid plexus (Fig. 5-16). Openings in the roof plate appear (4 to 5 months) which establish continuity between the fourth ventricle and the subarachnoid space surrounding the brain stem. Two lateral apertures (foramina of Luschka) connect the lateral recesses of the fourth ventricle with the pontine cistern (Figs. 1-10 and 1-11). A single median aperture (foramen of Magendie) in the lower roof connects the fourth ventricle with the cerebellomedullary cistern.

Metencephalon

This rostral portion of the hindbrain, extending from the pontine flexure to the rhombencephalic isthmus, develops into two elaborate and distinctive components of the neuraxis. Both the pons and cerebellum are derived from the metencephalon (Figs. 3-11 and 3-12).

The *pons* consists of two parts: (1) a phy-

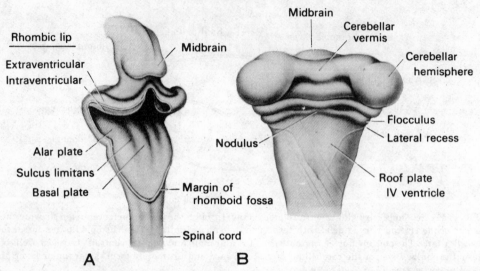

FIG. 3-12. Drawings of the developing cerebellum and hindbrain. *A*, Posterior oblique view of human embryo at 6 weeks. *B*, Posterior view of human fetus at 4 months' gestation (after Prentiss and Arey, '20).

logenetically older *dorsal portion*, lying in the floor of the fourth ventricle, referred to as the pontine tegmentum, and (2) a more recently acquired *ventral portion*, which cortical efferent fibers partially terminate in, and also traverse, in their passage to more caudal regions. The pontine tegmentum is derived from the basal plate (Fig. 3-11). A medial general somatic efferent (GSE) cell column gives rise to fibers of the abducens nerve (N. VI). An intermediate and interrupted cell column of typical motor neurons gives rise to special visceral efferent (SVE) fibers that form cranial nerves V and VII, and respectively innervate the musculature of the first and second branchial arches. General visceral efferent (GVE) cells contained in the superior salivatory nucleus supply preganglionic parasympathetic innervation for the submandibular, sublingual and lacrimal glands. Cells of the basal plate also contribute to the pontine reticular formation (Fig. 3-11).

Ventromedial portions of the alar plate form cell groups similar to those described for the medulla (Langman, '69). These cell groups are concerned with: (1) the vestibulocochlear nerve (SSA), (2) the trigeminal nuclear complex (GSA), and (3) the solitary nucleus (SVA and GVA). The *pontine*

nuclei which form massive cell collections in the newer ventral portion of the pons originate from the alar plate of both the metencephalon and myelencephalon (Fig. 3-11). Corticofugal fibers which develop later end, in part, upon these nuclei. The pontine nuclei give rise to a massive collection of fibers which cross the midline and enter the opposite cerebellar hemisphere; fibers in this bundle form the *middle cerebellar peduncle* (Figs. 2-19 and 2-25).

The *cerebellum* is derived from the dorsolateral portions of the alar plates which bend posteriorly and medially to form the rhombic lips (Figs. 3-9 and 3-12). The rhombic lips are at first widely separated from each other, and each lip projects partly into the fourth ventricle (intraventricular portion) and partly on the surface of the metencephalon above the roof·plate. Further deepening of the transverse rhombencephalic sulcus at the pontine flexure causes the cerebellar rudiments of both sides to fuse in the midline caudal to the roof of the mesencephalon (Hamilton and Mossman, '72). Fusion of the rhombic lips forms the transverse *cerebellar plate*. At 3 months these cerebellar primordia have a dumbbell-shaped appearance (Fig. 3-12) in which the unpaired central part represents the *vermis* and the two large lateral knobs represent the *hemispheres*. Near the end of the 4th month fissures begin to develop on the cerebellar surface. The first fissure to appear is the *posterolateral* (prenodular) *fissure* which separates the *nodulus* from other parts of the vermis and the *flocculus* from the rest of the cerebellar hemisphere. The *flocculonodular lobe* (*archicerebellum*), phylogenetically the oldest part of the cerebellum, has the most extensive connections with the vestibular system (Dow and Moruzzi, '58; Brodal et al., '62; Larsell and Jansen, '72). The portion of the cerebellar plate between the posterolateral fissure and the isthmus represents the rudiment of the *corpus cerebelli*. The first fissure to become visible in the corpus cerebelli is the *primary fissure*. The primary fissure is the deepest of all cerebellar fissures, and it separates the anterior and posterior lobes (Figs. 2-26 and 14-1). All parts of the cerebellum rostral to the primary fissure constitute the *paleocerebellum* (anterior lobe) while the *neocerebellum* (posterior lobe) lies between the primary and posterolateral fissures. The neocerebellum is subsequently divided into lobules by three transverse fissures, the prepyramidal, the horizontal and the posterior superior.

Cerebellar primordia initially consist of the three layers (ependymal, mantle and margin) which characterize the primitive neural tube. With development neuroblasts migrate through the mantle and marginal layers to the surface where they form the *external granular layer* (Uzman, '60; Miale and Sidman, '61; Hanaway, '67). Cells of the external granular layer retain their ability to divide, thus forming a proliferative zone on the surface of the cerebellum. Cells of the external granular layer eventually migrate inward and ultimately form the innermost cellular layer of the cerebellar cortex, the *granular layer*. *Purkinje cells* and *Golgi type II cells* are formed relatively early; Purkinje cells, representing the principal discharge element of the cerebellar cortex, form a distinctive layer along the outer margin of the granular layer. Although cells of the transient external granular layer migrate inward,

their processes, the *parallel fibers*, remain in the *molecular layer* where synaptic contacts are established with Purkinje cell dendrites.

The *deep cerebellar nuclei* are considered to be derived from neuroblasts located close to the ventricular surface of the cerebellum. The largest and most lateral of these nuclei, the *dentate nucleus*, has a convoluted appearance (Fig. 14-12) which becomes evident during the 5th month (Larsell and Jansen, '72). The *roof nuclei* (the fastigial nuclei) develop near the midline and have profuse connections with the vestibular nuclei. In lower forms the *globose* and *emboliform nuclei* are not clearly separated and are referred to as the *interposed nuclei*. Cranial and caudal portions of the thin metencephalic roof plate persist in the adult as the superior and inferior medullary veli (Figs. 2-20 and 2-21).

Mesencephalon

The *mesencephalon* is the most primitive of the brain vesicles and ultimately forms the smallest, least differentiated division of the brain stem. The alar and basal plates are separated by a well defined sulcus limitans (Fig. 3-9). The cavity of this vesicle is greatly reduced during development and ultimately becomes the cerebral aqueduct. The portion of the midbrain ventral to the aqueduct consists of the *midbrain tegmentum*, dorsally, and the *crus cerebri* ventrally; these structures are separated by the *substantia nigra* (Fig. 13-1). The tegmentum is derived from the basal and floor plates. Motor neurons derived from the basal plates form the general somatic efferent (GSE) cell columns that compose the oculomotor complex (N. III) and what must be regarded as a caudal appendage to it, the trochlear nuclei (N. IV). These cranial nerves, and the abducens nerve, innervate the extraocular muscles derived from the preotic somites. A smaller lateral cell group from the basal plate migrates dorsal to the somatic cell columns of cranial nerve III to form the visceral nuclei (GVE) of this complex. The marginal layer of each basal plate eventually is invaded by massive collections of corticofugal fibers which form the crus cerebri. These are corticospinal, corticopontine and corticobulbar fibers largely destined for more caudal regions of the neuraxis.

The alar plates of the mesencephalon proliferate and produce two longitudinal eminences separated by a median depression dorsal to the aqueduct. These eminences form the *quadrigeminal plate* (Fig. 3-14); a later developing transverse depression divides each longitudinal eminence into a *superior* and *inferior colliculus* (Fig. 2-18). Neuroblasts forming the inferior colliculus produce a central homogeneous cell mass surrounded by a narrow cortical rim. The superior colliculus is a more complex stratified structure formed by waves of migrating neuroblasts. Its development resembles that of the cerebral cortex in that cell migrations follow an "inside-out" sequence (Fujita, '64), which means that cells forming the deeper layers appear first and those destined for the superficial layers must pass through the deep layers. The inferior colliculus serves as a major relay complex in the auditory system, while the superior colliculus serves as a subcortical integrative center for the visual system.

The *midbrain reticular formation* and that specialized portion of it known as the *red nucleus* are considered to be derived from the alar plate (Langman, '69; Hamilton and Mossman, '72). The formation of the *substantia nigra* appears poorly understood. Some authors (Langman, '69) consider it to be derived from cells of the alar plate, while others (Shaner, '32, '36; Cooper, '46) suggest that the substantia nigra arises relatively late from cells that migrate ventrally from the basal plate. Cells of the pars compacta of the substantia nigra do not contain melanin pigment at birth; appreciable pigmentation does not develop until the 4th or 5th year. In the rabbit neurons of the substantia nigra have been found to contain dopamine on the 19th day of gestation (Tennyson et al., '73).

Diencephalon

The prosencephalon which divides into the diencephalon and the telencephalon gives rise to the entire central nervous system rostral to the midbrain (Fig. 3-8).

The *diencephalon* develops from the thickened lateral walls of the caudal portion of the original prosencephalic vesicle, which is considered to be formed only by the alar plates. The prosencephalon is caudally continuous with the mesencephalon, and at an early embryonic stage optic cups, formed from the optic vesicles, are attached to the lateral walls of the diencephalon. The cavity of the prosencephalon becomes narrowed to form the third ventricle. The *posterior commissure* is considered to mark the caudal limit of the diencephalon (Fig. 2-9), while the *interventricular foramen* represents its boundary with the telencephalon (Fig. 3-13). The *lamina terminalis*, representing the membrane formed by the closure of the anterior neuropore, is a telencephalic derivative, but its ventral part forms a matrix in which the *optic chiasm* ultimately develops.

The roof plate of the diencephalon becomes very thin and rostral parts of it invaginate to form the *choroid plexus* of the third ventricle (Figs. 3-9 and 3-13). Caudal portions of the roof plate thicken medially and evaginate posteriorly to form the *pineal gland*. This gland, which develops about the 7th week, ultimately becomes solid and lies in the midline dorsal to the posterior commissure. The roof plate of the diencephalon may form another evagination in the region of the interventricular foramen, known as the *paraphysis*. This epithelial sac may persist into adult life as a paraphysial cyst and produce intermittent blockages in the flow of cerebrospinal fluid (Dandy, '33; Bull and Sutton, '49). Other epithalamic structures, considered to be derived from the roof plate, or adjacent parts of the alar plate, are the *habenular nuclei* and *habenular commissure* (Kuhlenbeck, '51). These structures lie dorsally, immediately rostral to the posterior commissure. The habenular nucleus, which receives fibers of the *stria medullaris* and gives rise to the *fasciculus retroflexus*, links the septal nuclei with the midbrain reticular formation.

The alar plates forming the lateral walls and floor of the prosencephalon develop distinct longitudinal sulci on the surfaces facing the lumen. This depression is the *hypothalamic sulcus* which serves to divide the major part of the diencephalon into the *thalamus* and *hypothalamus* (Fig. 3-13). Some authors have suggested that the hypothalamic sulcus may be the diencephalic equivalent of the sulcus limitans, but this seems unlikely since it does not mark the division of alar and basal plates, or the boundary between sensory and motor regions. Active proliferation and cell differentiation produces an expansion of thalamic regions dorsal to the hypothalamic sulcus which greatly narrows the third ventricle. The thalamic nuclear masses of each side approach the midline and fuse in an *interthalamic adhesion* in about 80% of human brains. Cell growth in the thalamus proceeds rapidly and results in the formation of thalamic nuclear groups, some of which are clearly separated by medullary laminae (Fig. 2-22). The *principal nuclear groups* of the thalamus are: (1) the anterior, (2) the medial, (3) the ventral, and (4) the dorsal. The *medial* and *lateral geniculate bodies* (metathalamus) represent a caudal extension of the ventral nuclear group which function in part as relay neurons. The dorsal nuclear group, in general, serves as association neurons. Thalamic nuclear groups, readily detectable in gross specimens, include the anterior, the medial, the geniculate bodies and the pulvinar.

The part of the alar plate inferior to the hypothalamic sulcus (Figs. 3-9 and 3-13) on both sides of the third ventricle forms the hypothalamus. Cells in this region differentiate into a number of separate nuclear groups which subserve visceral, endocrine and regulatory functions. The most prominent nuclear group forms the *mammillary body*, a rounded protruberance on the ventral surface of the hypothalamus (Figs. 2-5 and 2-6). A small evagination in the floor of the diencephalon caudal to the optic chiasm forms the primordium of the *infundibulum*, which gives rise to the *neurohypophysis*. The *anterior lobe* of the *hypophysis* forms from an ectodermal diverticulum of stomodeum known as *Rathke's pouch*, which superiorly comes in contact with the infundibulum; Rathke's pouch loses its pharyngeal attachment and differentiates into the anterior lobe of the hypophysis (Fig. 3-9).

Telencephalon

This most rostral segment of the developing brain is composed of the two evaginating *cerebral vesicles* and their median connection, the *lamina terminalis* (Figs. 3-8 and 3-9). Each cerebral vesicle is in wide communication with the third ventricle via the interventricular foramen (Fig. 3-13) and expands upward, forward and backward. Through this caudal expansion the telencephalic vesicles cover the diencephalon dorsally and laterally. The region where the cerebral vesicle is attached to the roof of the diencephalon becomes very thin. Here the single layer of ependymal cells and the vascular mesenchyme in the roof of the third ventricle become continuous with similar layers in the lateral ventricle that form the choroid plexus. The line of invagination which first appears at the level of the interventricular foramen is called the *choroidal fissure*. Thus the choroid plexus of the third and lateral ventricles is continuous through the interventricular foramina along the line of vesicle evagination, the choroid fissure. A small horizontal cleft persists between the cerebral vesicle and the diencephalon (Fig. 3-14). This narrow triangular space dorsal to the thalamus is lined with a double layer of pia mater and filled with loose mesenchyme (velum interpositum, Fig. 2-22). This space represents the most rostral extension of the *transverse cerebral fissure*. The small *asterisk* (*) in Figure 3-13A and B is located within the transverse cerebral fissure. The lower pial layer of this fissure, as observed in frontal section, forms the roof of the diencephalon and becomes invaginated as the choroid plexus of the third ventricle (Figs. 2-22 and 3-13). The adult cerebral hemisphere also is separated from the cerebellum by the transverse cerebral fissure. The tentorium cere-

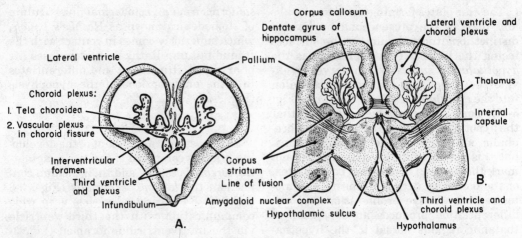

Fig. 3-13. Diagrams of frontal sections through diencephalon, ventricular system and choroid plexuses of the developing brain. *A*, Invagination of choroid plexuses into lateral and third ventricles. *B*, Choroid plexuses and secondary fusion of telencephalon with diencephalon. The transverse cerebral fissure is indicated in both *A* and *B* by an *asterisk* (*) (modified from Hamilton, Boyd and Mossman, '62).

belli occupies part of the transverse fissure and separates the inferior surfaces of the hemispheres from the superior surface of the cerebellum (Fig. 2-1).

Immediately above the choroid fissure the medial wall of the cerebral vesicle becomes thickened and forms the *hippocampal ridge* (Figs. 3-13 and 3-15). This ridge bulges into the lateral ventricle as a longitudinal elevation, the *hippocampal formation*. The hippocampal formation expands posteriorly and is carried downward into the temporal lobe. The medial surface of the hemisphere develops a corresponding groove, the *hippocampal fissure*, which runs parallel to the choroid fissure throughout its extent. The hippocampal formation and the dentate gyrus together constitute the *archipallium*, phylogenetically the oldest cortex.

The walls of the primitive telencephalic vesicle consist of ependymal, mantle and marginal layers and represent only the alar plates. The mantle layer ventrolaterally undergoes relatively rapid thickening as a consequence of cell proliferation and creates a cell mass that protrudes into the lumen of the vesicle. This thickened basal region is known as the *striatal portion* because it ultimately gives rise to the *corpus striatum* (Fig. 3-13). The thinner, more dorsal wall of the brain vesicle is

referred to as the *suprastriatal portion*. The suprastriatal portion is the primordium of the *cerebral cortex*.

Corpus Striatum and Internal Capsule. The thickened basal striatal region appears in the telencephalon at the level of the interventricular foramen (Fig. 3-13) (Hamilton and Mossman, '72). With the expansion of the cerebral hemispheres back over the diencephalon, part of the striatal ridge is carried in the wall of the lateral ventricle dorsal to the lateral border of the thalamus and down into the roof of the inferior horn of the lateral ventricle. Large numbers of developing corticofugal and corticopedal fibers projecting from, and to, the developing cerebral cortex incompletely divide the corpus striatum into a dorsomedial portion which bulges into the lateral ventricle and a ventrolateral portion medial to the insular region. The paraventricular striatal tissue medial to these fibers forms the *caudate nucleus* which throughout most of its extent is closely related to the lateral ventricle (Fig. 2-22). The portion of the corpus striatum lateral to these cortical fiber systems, which collectively form the *internal capsule*, constitutes the *lentiform nucleus* (Fig. 3-13). The lentiform nucleus is divided into two parts: (1) a larger lateral part known as the *putamen*, and (2) a

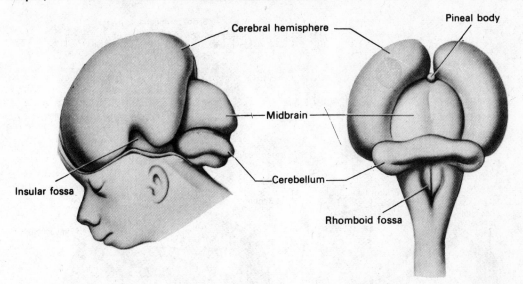

FIG. 3-14. Drawings of the cerebral vesicle and brain stem in the 12-week human fetus. *A*, Lateral view; *B*, Posterior view.

smaller inner part, the *globus pallidus*. Although the basal ganglia are classically regarded as subcortical telencephalic nuclei, some authors (Kuhlenbeck, '48; Kuhlenbeck and Haymaker, '49; Richter, '65) consider parts, or all, of the globus pallidus to be derived from portions of the hypothalamus. The *subthalamic nucleus*, a small nucleus with connections mainly with the globus pallidus, also is considered a hypothalamic derivative. The internal capsule, formed by fibers projecting to and from the cerebral cortex, has a complex development (Hewitt, '61), but ultimately forms two major limbs: (1) an *anterior limb* which partially separates the head of the caudate nucleus and the putamen, and (2) a larger *posterior limb* between the thalamus and the globus pallidus (Figs. 2-9 and 2-10).

The *cerebral hemispheres* grow and expand rapidly, first forward to form the frontal lobe area, then laterally and upward to form the future parietal lobe (*arrows* in Figs. 3-9 and 3-14). Posterior and inferior expansions soon produce the occipital and temporal lobes. The expansions of the cerebral hemispheres cover the diencephalon and posterior surface of the midbrain. The anterior, posterior and inferior expansions

during development explain the curved shape and the relations of several internal telencephalic structures in the adult brain (e.g., lateral ventricle, choroid plexus, caudate nucleus and fornix). The cortex covering the lenticular nucleus remains as a fixed area, the insula (Fig. 3-16). This region becomes buried in the floor of the lateral sulcus by the subsequent overgrowth of adjacent lobes (Fig. 3-15).

Cerebral Cortex. The early evolution of the forebrain is similar in all mammals, and has been reviewed (Åström, '67; Bernhard et al., '67; Stensaas, '68; Humphrey, '68; Ravic and Yakovlev, '68). The suprastriatal portion of the early telencephalic vesicle appears to be composed of three concentric zones during its smooth-surfaced (lissencephalic) stage. A *germinal* or *matrix zone* surrounds the lateral ventricle. Most of the cells of this zone migrate outwards to become nerve and glial cells upon maturation. However, some cells remain in this zone to form the internal limiting membrane, ependyma and the subependymal glial layer. The pale *intermediate zone* becomes the white matter of the cerebral hemispheres. It has many radiating fibers and is traversed by neuroblasts and glioblasts migrating from

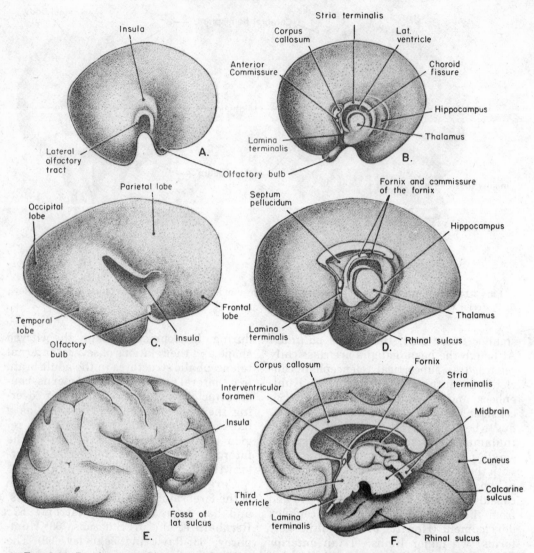

Fig. 3-15. Development of human cerebral hemisphere. *A* and *B*, Lateral and medial surfaces of the hemisphere in a fetus of 3 months. *C* and *D*, Lateral and medial surfaces of the hemisphere in a fetus at beginning of the 5th month. *E* and *F*, Lateral and medial surfaces of the hemisphere at the end of the 7th month (modified from Keibel and Mall, '12).

the matrix zone to the more superficial layer. An outer *cortical zone* or *plate* represents the prospective neopallium (isocortex). This zone has two distinct layers. The deeper pyramidal layer has many cells and will form layers II to VI of the adult six-layered cortex (Fig. 19-1). The marginal layer is composed mostly of fibers and becomes the molecular (plexiform) or most superficial layer (I). In areas of the olfactory cortex (allocortex) the six layers are not present. In these regions the migrant

neuroblasts and glioblasts enter the cortical zone and form a thin nuclear layer close to the surface.

There is evidence that the neuroblasts invade the cortical zone to form a primitive pyramidal layer before the glial cells arrive (Lorente de Nó, '33). It also has been shown that cells formed at the same time remain in the same part of the pyramidal layer; and that newly formed cells migrate beyond those already present (Angevine and Sidman, '61). Hence, cells in the

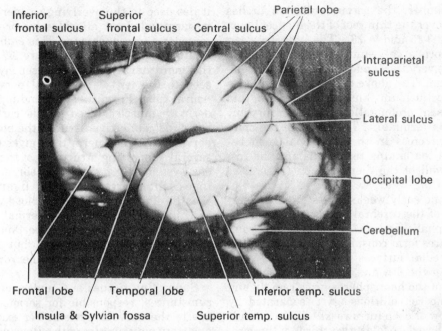

Inferior frontal sulcus   Superior frontal sulcus   Central sulcus   Parietal lobe

Intraparietal sulcus

Lateral sulcus

Occipital lobe

Cerebellum

Frontal lobe   Temporal lobe   Inferior temp. sulcus

Insula & Sylvian fossa   Superior temp. sulcus

FIG. 3-16. Lateral view of the brain of a 7-month human fetus. Note the primitive sulcal pattern and the exposure of the insular cortex. Photograph.

deeper strata of the pyramidal layer were formed earlier and are older than more superficially located cells. In man the cortical zone becomes highly cellular due to massive neuroblast migrations in the 12th week. At birth the human neopallium has assumed a stratified appearance as a result of neuron differentiation and laminae formation by the incoming and outgoing nerve fibers.

Although the hippocampal formation appears early in development (see page 66), its constituent cells are not organized into the characteristic adult arrangement until late embryonic life (Angevine, '65; Hamilton and Mossman, '72). The superior and rostral portions of the hippocampal formation undergo regressive changes in association with development of the corpus callosum, but these parts persist in the adult as the indusium griseum or supracallosal gyrus (Figs. 2-7 and 18-6).

Commissures. The medially placed *lamina terminalis* represents the cephalic end of the early neural tube and extends from the roof plate of the diencephalon to the optic chiasm (Figs. 3-9 and 3-15). This primitive midline telencephalic structure

thus provides the only bridge whereby nerve fibers can pass from one cerebral hemisphere to the other. The first fibers to cross between the two hemispheres (*commissural fibers*) are within the *anterior commissure*. This structure appears in the lower portion of the lamina terminalis by the 3rd month. It connects the olfactory bulb and portions of the temporal lobe of one side with the same structures of the opposite hemisphere (Figs. 18-3 and 18-7). The small *commissure of the fornix* is the second to appear in the lamina terminalis close to the roof of the diencephalon (Fig. 3-15D). Its fibers connect portions of the hippocampal formation with each other.

The largest and most important commissure to cross in the lamina is the *corpus callosum*. The first of these commissural fibers, connecting nonolfactory cortical areas of the two hemispheres, appears as a small bundle rostral to the commissure of the fornix. The size of the corpus callosum parallels the rapid growth and expansion of the neopallium. It first extends anteriorly to connect the frontal lobes and then enlarges posteriorly as the parietal lobes develop. As the constituent fibers increase in number, the corpus callosum arches back over the thin roof of the diencephalon (Figs. 3-15 and A-29). The area between the corpus callosum and the fornix becomes very thin and forms the septum pellucidum. The above commissures and septum pellucidum thus develop within, and represent prolongations of, the embryonic lamina terminalis. The fibers of the *optic chiasm* cross in the junctional zone between the lamina terminalis and the rostral wall of the diencephalon (Figs. 2-21 and 3-15).

In the early weeks of gestation the surfaces of the cerebral hemispheres are lissencephalic (smooth). The developing commissures form conspicuous bundles on the cut medial surfaces (Figs. 3-13 and 3-15). During the 6th and 7th months, the surfaces of the hemispheres grow rapidly and develop convolutions (*gyri*) separated by shallow or deep furrows (*sulci*). As a result of such surface folds, two-thirds of the cerebral cortex becomes buried in the walls and floor of the sulci when the brain attains its adult size. Fetal sulci appear in an orderly sequence; the phylogenetically older sulci appear first, and more recently acquired sulci appear later (Figs. 3-15*E*, 3-15*F* and 3-16). The principal sulci and gyri that form the characteristic pattern of the human cerebral cortex all can be identified in the full-term infant.

After the neural tube has been formed, it lies deep to the overlying ectoderm and is surrounded on all sides by primitive mesoderm (mesenchyme). This embryonic relationship is shown in Figure 3-7. Here the more darkly stained mesenchyme is seen to the left of the spinal nerve and neural tube. From the surrounding mesoderm the muscles, blood vessels, cartilage, bone and connective tissue of the body are derived. The mesoderm thus gives rise to several supporting structures of the nervous system (e.g., skull, vertebrae, meninges, intervertebral discs, ligaments, sheaths of peripheral nerves, blood vessels and microglia). These mesodermal structures are of paramount importance, for they provide not only support, but protection and nourishment, to the nervous system.

Supporting tissues are, under some circumstances, responsible for serious damage to the nervous system. For example, an artery may rupture with extensive hemorrhage, or the lumen of a vessel may be occluded suddenly and produce anoxia in the area of its neural distribution. Tumors commonly arise from the meninges, from the connective tissue sheaths along peripheral nerves or from glioblasts. An intervertebral disc may rupture posteriorly into the vertebral canal and compress the spinal cord or spinal nerves; also fractures of the skull and vertebrae often compress the underlying brain or spinal cord.

CHAPTER 4

The Neuron

The *neuron doctrine*, popularized by Waldeyer (1891), had its foundation in the extensive studies of Cajal ('09–'11), which were based upon the Golgi method (1882–1885, 1898a). This doctrine states that the individual nerve cell (i.e., neuron) constitutes the genetic, anatomic, trophic and functional unit of the nervous system. All neural pathways, circuits and reflex arcs are composed of individual neurons arranged in simple or complex patterns.

Each neuron consists of a cell body (i.e., perikaryon) from which one or more processes extend for variable distances. The most striking feature of the neuron is the presence of protoplasmic processes, some of which extend for long distances. The neuron is defined as a nerve cell and all processes which arise from it. A variety of staining technics have revealed the principal features of the neuron and the manner in which individual neurons are inter-related. The electron microscope and cytochemical technics have provided new insight into the fine structure and the functional roles of specific organelles. Recent data, acquired with these sophisticated technics, all support the neuron doctrine.

NEUROANATOMICAL METHODS

Although unstained fresh nerve tissue, or nerve tissue grown in tissue culture, may be studied with the phase microscope, the customary method is to use stained preparations. It is essential that fresh nerve tissue be fixed in a solution which kills bacteria, inactivates autolytic enzymes and produces minimal shrinkage, swelling or distortion. Appropriate fixatives also make components of the nerve cell receptive to suitable dyes or permeable to colloidal solutions. The most common fixatives for neural tissue are formalin and alcohols. These fixatives often are used in conjunction with a variety of chemicals, such as chloral hydrate, ammonia, pyridine, glacial acetic acid and mercuric chloride. In experimental studies in animals excellent fixation of neural tissue is achieved by perfusion technics, but this is not possible in man. Since several hours usually intervene between death and autopsy, it is rarely possible to obtain perfectly fixed human neural tissue. Appropriate fixation renders many components of the nerve cell, such as chromatin, receptive to suitable dyes (i.e., cresyl violet; Fig. 4-1E) or neurofilaments more permeable to colloidal silver solutions (Fig. 4-1A, B and C).

Formalin fixation followed by a mordanting in potassium dichromate preserves the normal lipids of myelin, and enhances the appearance of the myelin sheaths when stained with hematoxylin (e.g., Weigert method, Fig. 9-16). Primary fixation in potassium dichromate, followed by an osmic acid solution, selectively stains the fatty acids of degenerating myelin black, while the normal myelin remains a yellow-brown color (Marchi method, Fig. 10-5). When the initial fixative contains solvents (e.g., alcohol, ether, chloroform), lipids of myelin are removed and only a clear space remains (Fig. 4-2A and B). If such solvents are avoided the lipids of the normal myelin sheath are readily stained by osmic acid (Fig. 4-2C, D and E) and Luxol Fast Blue (Fig. 4-2F and H).

Nerve tissue has a strong affinity for weak silver solutions (i.e., argyrophilia). Blocks of nerve tissue are impregnated with silver salts for several days, and then placed in suitable reducing solutions. This action results in the deposition of silver particles within the nerve cell and its processes. The reduced silver particles in non-neural tissue are removed by subsequent solutions, so that the neurons and their processes appear golden brown or black against a light yellow background. The Cajal ('28) and Ranson ('14) technics both permit bulk staining of tissue blocks and are used to elucidate the structural features of the central and peripheral nervous system. Figures 4-1C and 4-2B show sympathetic ganglion cells and axons of a peripheral nerve stained by the Cajal silver nitrate method.

Other methods have been developed which permit the staining of mounted sections. In the Bodian ('36, '37) method the slides are placed in a silver protein solution (protargol) with metallic copper and incubated at 37°F. Again, the silver is reduced as in the bulk method. The silvered sections are then passed through a solution of gold chloride. Since gold has a higher atomic number and atomic weight than silver, the gold replaces the silver particles in the nerve tissues of the section. The sections then are developed in oxalic acid, and the non-neural gold particles are removed. Nerve cells, their nuclei and processes are all beautifully visualized by this method as shown in Figures 4-1A and B and 4-2A. The Holmes' ('43) silver technic is another useful silver modification giving consistently excellent results (see Fig. 4-2F and H).

For many years gold chloride was used to demonstrate the motor nerve endings in skeletal muscle, and the myenteric plexus of the intestine. Garven's modification ('25) of Ranvier's gold chloride method is still a useful procedure for the successful demonstration of motor nerve endings in teased muscle fiber preparations (Fig. 4-2G). One of the most valuable methods, the Nauta and Gygax ('51, '54) technic, results in a selective silver impregnation of degenerated axons. This staining method usually is done on frozen sections. Staining of normal nerve fibers and endings is suppressed and these have a golden yellow appearance (Figs. 9-24 and 9-25). Thick, as well as thin, degenerating axons of injured neurons appear as discontinuous black droplets or beaded segments arranged in an orderly linear fashion (degeneration "en passage"). Arborizing degenerating axons, observed in close proximity to nerve cells, represent "terminal" fiber degeneration. The Nauta procedure has been evaluated in detail by Eager and Barnett ('66). Selective staining of the terminal end feet of nerve processes (synaptic knobs, bouton termineaux) upon the dendrite or cell body of another neuron also is accomplished by the use of modified silver methods (Fig. 4-23). The technics of Barr ('39), Glees ('46), Rasmussen ('57), Fink and Heimer ('67) and Wiitanen ('69) have all been used in numerous studies to localize terminal fibers of pathways within the central nervous system (Fig 4-1F).

The Golgi silver technics are one of the oldest and most widely used methods for studying neurons and neuroglia (Golgi, 1882–1885). These technics produce a black deposit which literally "coats the surface" of the cell bodies and processes of many neurons. Although only a fraction of the total number of neurons and neuroglia are stained black, these often are revealed in great detail against a nearly colorless background (Fig. 4-1D). In addition to neurons and neuroglia the blood vessels also may be stained (Fig. 1-15). The method is empirical and the results are uncertain, but magnificent neuronal and neuroglial details are revealed in successful preparations (Figs. 5-2 and 14-7).

The illustrations of nerve tissue shown in Figures 4-1 and 4-2 represent a few of the basic methods used to study the neuron. A wide spectrum of additional technics are now in use, based upon recent advancements in the fields of neurochemistry, autoradiography, fluorescent and elec-

Fig. 4.1 (*on next page*)

Fig. 4-1. Shape, size and appearance of nerve cells stained by different technics. All photographs are ×370 except *D* which is ×125. *A*, Unipolar neurons of dorsal root ganglion. Three larger cells contain melanin granules. Silver protargol technic. *B*, Multipolar neuron of reticular formation. An area of cytoplasmic lipofuscin pigment appears between the nucleus and axon (*a*) of the large cell. Silver protargol technic. *C*, Multipolar neurons of sympathetic ganglion with interlacing of dendrites and small nerve fibers. Cajal silver nitrate technic. *D*, Purkinje cell of cerebellar cortex whose dendritic branches are studded with small gemmules. Adjacent blood vessels (*bv*) are identified in this preparation. Golgi technic. *E*, Cytoplasmic chromatin and nuclear appearances of normal (above) and injured (below) anterior horn cells of spinal cord. The small eccentric nucleus and depleted chromatin pattern (chromatolysis) resulted from earlier axonal destruction. Luxol Fast Blue-cresyl violet technic. *F*, Terminal degeneration in the ventral lateral nucleus of the thalamus following a localized lesion in the medial segment of the globus pallidus. Degenerated pallidothalamic fibers appear as black beaded strands and dots near the soma and dendrites of thalamic neurons. Wiitanen ('69) silver technic.

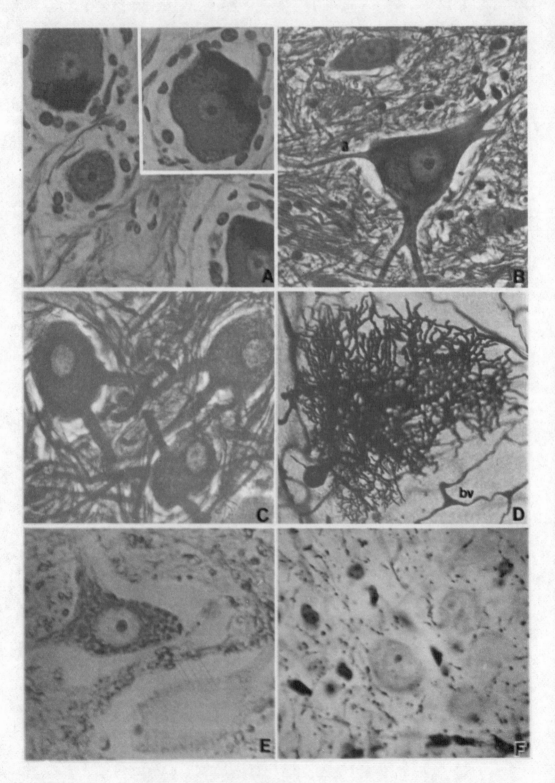

Fig. 4.1

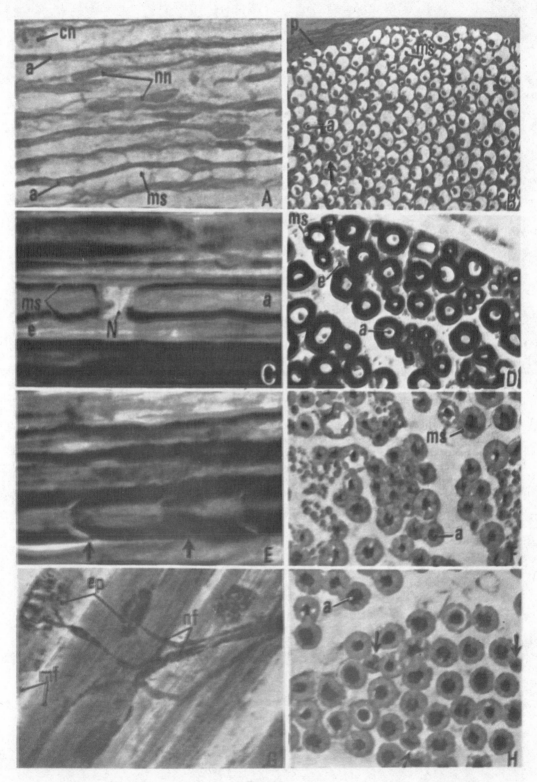

Fig. 4.2

FIG. 4.2 (on previous page)

FIG. 4-2. Size and appearance of nerve fibers stained by different technics. A, Longitudinal section of femoral nerve stained with silver protargol. Axons (a), Schwann cell (nn) and connective tissue (cn) nuclei are identified. The myelin sheath (ms) is dissolved and remains as a clear space in such silver preparations. ×370. B, Cross section of sciatic nerve stained with silver nitrate. Axons (a), myelin space (ms) and connective tissue of perineurium (p) are identified. Small black dots between larger fibers are axons of nonmyelinated fibers (arrow). ×130. C, Longitudinal section of myelinated nerve fiber and node of Ranvier (N) stained with osmic acid and light green. Myelin sheath (ms) stains black, axon (a) is unstained and connective tissue of endoneurium (e) is green. ×370. D, Cross section of lumbar nerve in cauda equina with osmic acid and light green. Endoneurium (e) derived from pia mater is green and myelin (ms) is black, while axons (a) are unstained. ×270. E, Longitudinal section of two myelinated nerve fibers with osmic acid and light green. Lower fiber with thicker myelin sheath exhibits Schmidt-Lantermann clefts (arrows). ×370. F, Cross section of intradural dorsal root sensory fibers with combined Holmes' silver and Luxol Blue technics. Axons (a) appear dark brown, and myelin sheath (ms) is blue. Note variation in size of myelinated and nonmyelinated axons. ×270. G, Longitudinal section of nerve fibers (nf) terminating as motor end plates (ep) on extrafusal skeletal muscle fibers (mf). Gold chloride technic. ×145. H, Cross section of intradural ventral root motor fibers stained as in F above. Larger fibers (a) terminate as motor end plates on extrafusal muscle fibers, while smaller γ efferent axons (arrows) end on intrafusal muscle fibers of neuromuscular spindle. ×270.

tron microscopy. Important contributions have been made with each of these different methods. Additional basic information and procedural steps in the more commonly used neurological stains can be found in text references edited by Windle ('57), Baker ('60), Ambrogi ('60), McManus and Mowry ('60), Jones ('61), Gasser ('61), Humason ('61), Culling ('63) and Adams et al. ('65).

FUNCTIONAL CONCEPT OF NEURONS

A generalized concept of neuron structure based upon the site of impulse origin, rather than the location of the cell body, has been proposed by Bodian ('62). The term "*dendritic zone*" is used to denote the receptor membrane of a neuron (Fig. 4-3) which may be cytoplasmic extensions (i.e., dendrites), portions of the cell soma or specialized receptors which act as transducers. The cell body (perikaryon) remains the focal point of embryonic outgrowth of dendrites and axon and of axonal regeneration; and it also maintains the trophic aspects of neuronal activity. The position of the perikaryon is irrelevant as far as the major electrochemical functions of the neuron are concerned. Its position is related to the outgrowth of processes and to metabolic maintenance rather than to the polarized conduction of the neuron.

This functional concept recognizes the site of impulse origin as the pivotal position in the neuron. This site may not necessarily be a fixed point in a particular neuron. Furthermore all surfaces bearing synapses (dendrites, cell body and axon) are related to response-generating functions. In these functional terms, the axon may be said to arise from any response-generating structure, such as a dendrite, the cell body or a receptor terminal. The functional role of the axon is to conduct signals away from the response-generating region. Impulse origin, or the physiological action potential ("spike"), occurs at or near the origin of the axon and conducts the nerve impulse away from the "dendritic zone." Axons are ensheathed by neuroglial or Schwann cells. Both axon diameter and sheath differentiation are related to the rate of impulse conduction. The branched

and variously differentiated terminals of axons are called "*telodendria*." They may show membrane and cytoplasmic differentiation related to synaptic transmission or neurosecretory activity (Fig. 8-8). Mitochondrial concentrations, synaptic vesicles or secretory granules are commonly present in their bulblike terminals which release chemical compounds known as neurotransmitters. The telodendria transmit electrical or chemical signals capable of producing generator potentials in the dendritic zones of other neurons and in muscle, or they can induce stimulatory effects in innervated glands. The terms axon, dendrite and cell body, used in this text, are in accordance with functional concepts described above.

VARIETIES OF NEURONS

Neurons show wide variations in size and an infinite variety in the arrangement of their processes. However, nerve cells subserving a similar function or located in a given region of the nervous system often resemble each other structurally (Figs. 4-1, 4-4, 4-5 and 4-6). Thus the *bipolar* neurons are sensory in function and subserve impulses generated by olfactory, visual, vestibular and auditory receptor endings (Fig. 4-6A). The T-shaped *unipolar neurons* are characteristic of the spinal ganglia and mesencephalic nucleus of the trigeminal nerve (Figs. 4-1A and 4-6B, C and D).

Such sensory neurons convey nerve impulses from a variety of specialized and nonspecialized receptors. *Multipolar neurons* transmit both sensory and motor nerve impulses, and are characteristic of the brain, spinal cord and peripheral autonomic nervous system (Figs. 4-1B through F, 4-4 and 4-6). The primary, secondary and tertiary dendritic branches of some multipolar neurons may be elaborate and enormously increase its synaptic surface (Figs. 4-4 and 4-5). A Purkinje cell of the cerebellar cortex serves as an illustrative example. Such dendrites are wide at the base, and taper rapidly. The primary, secondary and tertiary branches have a smooth surface, while the more distal dendritic branches are beset with great num-

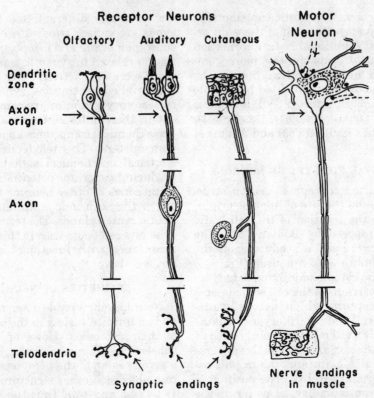

Fig. 4-3. Diagram of three sensory neurons and a motor neuron based on the site of impulse origin rather than location of the cell body. Dendritic zone is concerned with the generator potential in a receptor, as well as excitatory or inhibitory input of synaptic endings (*dotted lines* on motor neuron) of another nerve cell. The axon and its telodendria are related to conduction and synaptic transmission of the generated nerve impulse. The perikaryon of a neuron is the trophic center primarily concerned with the outgrowth and maintenance of processes, and their metabolic functions other than membrane activity. Note that the cell body may be located either in the dendritic zone or the region of the axon (after Bodian, '62).

bers of fine spines or *gemmules* (Fig. 4-5). Fox and Barnard ('57) reported the length of the spiny terminals of a single Purkinje cell to be 40,700 μ. The dendritic branchlets with their 61,000 spines have a combined synaptic surface area of 222,000 μ^2. These estimates of the spiny branchlets are now believed to be too conservative, and probably should be doubled (Fox et al., '67).

Arborizations of neurons in other parts of the CNS are less extensive, yet they reveal a characteristic pattern of branching. For example, nerve cells of the inferior olivary nuclear complex in the medulla (Fig. 4-4A) have radiating dendrites with curly branches, whereas neurons of the thalamus (Fig. 4-4K) have long radiating dendrites with numerous branches.

The cells of the *substantia gelatinosa* of the spinal cord, best seen in stained longitudinal sections, demonstrate only a few large dendrites that issue chiefly from one side of the cell (Fig. 4-4G). Smaller branches of these dendrites form a compact zone of fine parallel fibers.

It is instructive to compare the profuse dendritic branches of the central sensory and integrating neurons (Fig. 4-4A·, B, D, E and G through K) with the robust dendrites of motor neurons (Figs. 4-4C, F and L, and 4-6M, N and O). This comparison is even more striking if one contrasts the two principal cell types of the cerebellar and cerebral cortex (Fig. 4-5). The brushlike spread of dendrites of the Purkinje cell is similar to that of other central integrating neurons (Fig. 4-4A, I, J and K); yet each

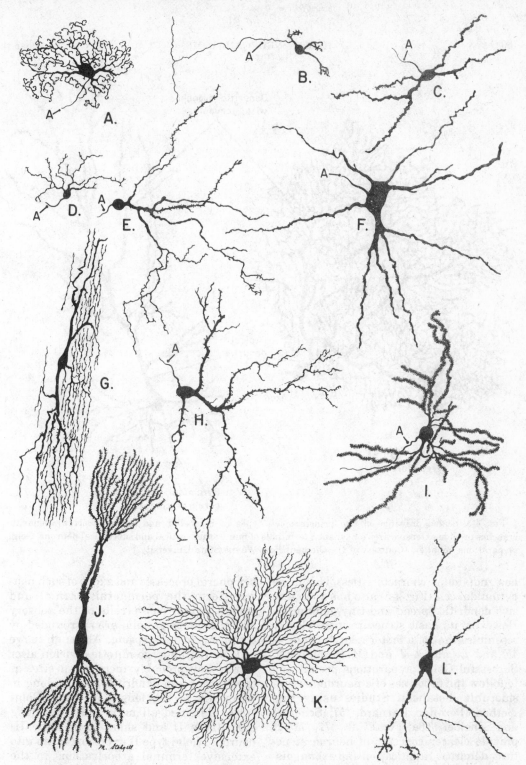

FIG. 4-4. Scaled drawings of some characteristic neurons whose axons (A) and dendrites remain within the central nervous system. *A*, Neuron of inferior olivary nucleus. *B*, granule cell of cerebellar cortex. *C*, small cell of reticular formation. *D*, small gelatinosa cell of spinal trigeminal nucleus. *E*, ovoid cell, nucleus of tractus solitarius. *F*, large cell of reticular formation. *G*, spindle-shaped cell, substantia gelatinosa of spinal cord. *H*, large cell of spinal trigeminal nucleus. *I*, spiny striatal neuron, putamen. *J*, double pyramidal cell, Ammon's horn of hippocampal cortex. *K*, cell from thalamic nucleus. *L*, cell from globus pallidus. Golgi preparations, monkey. (Courtesy of Dr. Clement Fox, Wayne State University.)

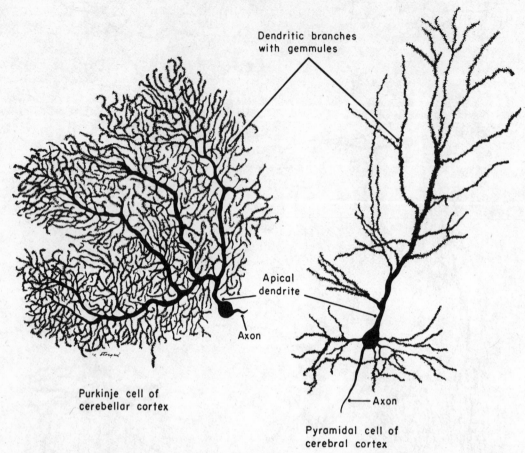

Fig. 4-5. Scaled drawings of two principal cell types in cerebellar and cerebral cortex. Dendritic branches provide extensive area for synaptic terminals of many other cortical and subcortical neurons. Golgi preparations, monkey. (Courtesy of Dr. Clement Fox, Wayne State University.)

has individual characteristics. The large pyramidal cell (Fig. 4-5) also has an extensive dendritic spread and tiny gemmules. However, its basic structure more closely resembles that of a motor neuron (Figs. 4-4F and L, and 4-6I and M through O). Successful Golgi preparations permit one to follow the processes of a neuron for considerable distances. Studies using this method (Fox and Barnard, '57; Scheibel and Scheibel, '58a; Fox et al., '71, '71/72) provide clearer concepts of neuron structure, dendritic ramification and axonal distribution within the cerebellar cortex, and brain stem reticular formation.

The somatic and visceral neurons of the central and peripheral nervous systems of man can be compared in Figure 4-6. The peripheral processes and axons of such neurons form the peripheral, cranial and spinal nerves. Nerve cells of the sensory and autonomic ganglia are surrounded by a thin nucleated capsule. Although nerve cells do not undergo mitotic division after birth, they probably increase in size, as their axons and dendrites grow in length. According to the length of axon, Golgi (1894) classified all nerve cells into long axon (type I) and short axon (type II) neurons. Golgi type II axons break up into extensive terminal arborizations in the immediate vicinity of the cell body.

The length of some nerve axons is quite remarkable. Giant pyramidal cells of the cerebral cortex may send axons to the caudal tip of the spinal cord, i.e., from the top

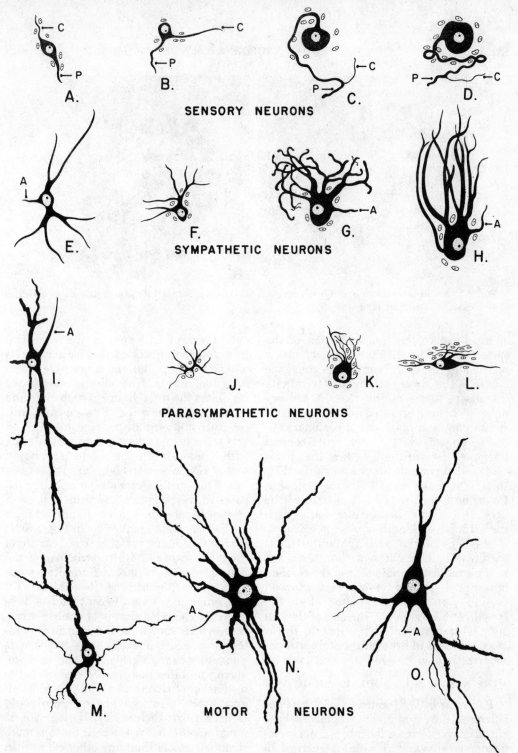

SENSORY NEURONS

SYMPATHETIC NEURONS

PARASYMPATHETIC NEURONS

MOTOR NEURONS

FIG. 4-6. Scaled drawings of representative neurons whose axons (A) are distributed in the peripheral nervous system of man. Capsular nuclei are shown about all ganglion cells. The central (C) and peripheral (P) processes of the sensory neurons are identified. *A*, Bipolar neuron, nodose ganglion (newborn). *B*, Pseudounipolar neuron, nodose ganglion (newborn). *C*, Unipolar neuron, dorsal root ganglion (newborn). *D*, Unipolar neuron, trigeminal ganglion. *E*, Multipolar neurons of intermediolateral nucleus of spinal cord. *F*, Superior cervical ganglion (newborn). *G* and *H*, Stellate ganglion. *I*, Dorsal motor nucleus N. X. *J*, Ciliary ganglion (newborn). *K*, Intracardiac ganglion. *L*, Myenteric ganglion. *M*, Nucleus ambiguus. *N*, Motor nucleus N. XII. *O*, Anterior horn cell.

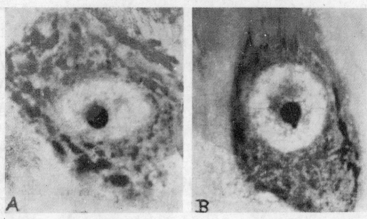

FIG. 4-7. Nucleolar satellite in motor cell of spinal cord (*A*) and Betz cell of motor cortex (*B*). Female cat. Cresyl violet. ×1200 (Barr et al., '50).

of the head to the lumbar region of the spinal cord (Fig. 10-13). Axons of motor neurons in the spinal cord may extend the length of the lower extremity to terminate in muscle fibers of the toes. A sensory unipolar neuron situated in the first sacral spinal ganglion may send a peripheral fiber to one of the toes, while its central fiber may ascend the length of the spinal cord and terminate in the medulla (Fig. 10-1). The total length of such a neuron would be from the toe to the nape of the neck. In a giraffe, such a fiber would reach the astounding length of over 15 feet.

The size of the perikaryon fluctuates within wide limits, from a diameter of 4 μ in the smallest granule cells of the cerebellum (Fig. 4-4*B*) and cerebral cortex to well over 100 μ in the largest motor cells of the spinal cord. In general, the size of the cell body is proportional to the length, thickness, richness of branchings and terminal arborizations of its dendrites and axon.

THE NERVE CELL BODY (PERIKARYON)

The neuron body consists of a nucleus surrounded by a mass of cytoplasm whose surface layer forms a delicate plasma membrane. It appears as a fine structure in stained sections when viewed with the light microscope (Figs. 4-1 and 4-7). As observed with the electron microscope, the plasma membrane (*PM* in Fig. 4-8) has a three-layered appearance similar to that of most tissue cells. It delimits sharply the

cytoplasm of the neuron (neuroplasm) from adjacent processes of other nerve cells and from neuroglial and connective tissue cells and fibers. The plasma membrane regulates the interchange of materials and ions between the cell and its environment, for it is differentially permeable, i.e., it acts selectively to permit the accumulation within the cell of some solutes and not of others (DeRobertis et al., '65; Robertson, '66). This surface membrane also participates in the reception and transmission of electrical potentials (nerve impulses) from one nerve cell to another (*sy* in Fig. 4-8). It is true that much remains to be learned of the significance and ultrastructure of the neuron plasma membrane and its associated subsurface cisterns (Rosenbluth, '62) and synaptic vesicles. Recent studies have provided clearer concepts of neuron structure, which show that the neuron is similar to an enormous glandlike cell that is constantly changing, synthesizing and producing proteins and lipoproteins with the mediation of ribonucleic acid (RNA) as an activator and governing molecule (Waelsch, '57; Richter, '57; Hydén, '60). It is significant that nerve cells contain more ribonucleic acid than any other cells, with the possible exception of the pancreatic cells in some animals (Brattgård et al., '58). All the ingredients and fluids for the synthesis of protein are dependent upon the integrity of the plasma membrane.

The cytoplasm of a neuron in a routinely

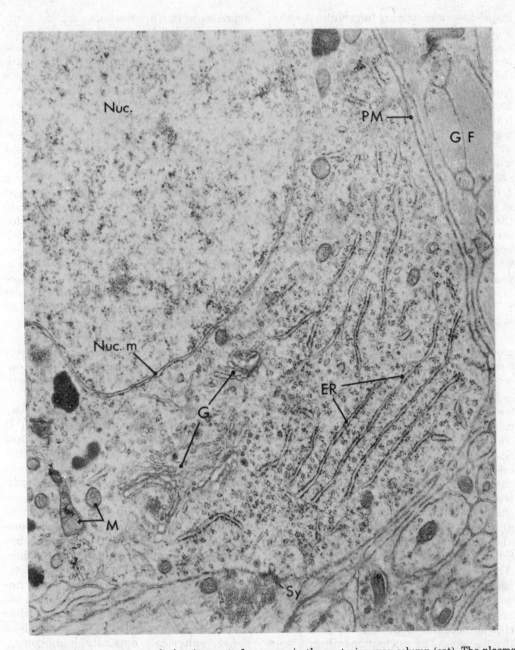

FIG. 4-8. Electron micrograph showing part of a neuron in the posterior gray column (cat). The plasma membrane (*PM*) separates cytoplasmic structures from glial fibers (*GF*) and a synapse (*sy*) which are identified in the adjacent neuropil. Part of the pale nucleus (*Nuc.*) and the nuclear membrane (*Nuc. m*) appear to the upper left. The cytoplasm demonstrates pouches and vesicles of the Golgi complex (*G*), mitochondria (*M*) and an array of individual ribonucleoprotein particles. Some appear as clumps or rosettes, while some ribosomes are attached to the outer surface membranes. The parallel stacks of cisternae of the granular endoplasmic reticulum (*ER*) are characteristic of Nissl bodies. Osmium fixation. ×75,000. (Courtesy of H. J. Ralston III.)

stained section appears basophilic and has a large, pale nucleus with a prominent nucleolus. After appropriate staining procedures, one also can demonstrate within the cytoplasm of nerve cells neurofibrils, chromophil substance (Nissl bodies), Golgi apparatus, mitochondria, at times a central body, and various inclusions such as pigment, fat and lipids. Neurofibrils are uniquely characteristic of nerve cells, whereas the other cytoplasmic constituents are observed in other tissue cells. The cytoplasm extends throughout the confines of the cell and all of its processes and, in the axon, is often called axoplasm. As observed by light microscopy, the cytoplasm appears open and somewhat dispersed, whereas it has a compact and crowded appearance in electron micrographs (Fig. 4-8). Many of the neuronal structures seen by light microscopy require specific stains (e.g., neurofibrils, mitochondria, Golgi apparatus, Nissl bodies and lipids), while most of these constituents are visualized simultaneously with the electron microscope.

Nucleus. This spherical structure varies in size from 3 to 18 μ, is generally proportional to cell size and is usually centrally located. A striking exception is the eccentric position of the nucleus in the cells of the nucleus dorsalis (of Clarke) in the spinal cord (Fig. 9-13). The nucleus often is displaced to one side of the cell in the neurons of the pelvic autonomic ganglia. Bi- and trinucleated neurons may also be observed in these same ganglia. Small aggregates of desoxyribonucleic acid (DNA) are scattered in a somewhat homogeneous nucleoplasm and account for the pale appearance of the nucleus (Figs. 4-1 and 4-8). Usually one deeply staining nucleolus occupies a prominent position in the nucleus. The nuclear membrane seen with the light microscope appears sharp and continuous, while electron micrographs reveal it as a double-layered membrane, periodically interrupted by nuclear pores (*Nuc. m.* in Fig. 4-8). The nuclei of Purkinje cells have a nuclear membrane that is wrinkled or puckered on the side facing the origin of the dendritic tree (Palay and Chan-Palay, '74). This irregular depression in the nucleus, stuffed with granular endoplasmic reticulum (Fig. 4-9), has been called the nuclear cap region. This region appears to contain more nuclear pores (650 Å in diameter) than smooth portions of the nuclear membrane. For a more detailed description of nuclear ultrastructure, the student is referred to the studies of Wischnitzer ('60), Hay and Revel ('63), Peters et al. ('70) and Palay and Chan-Palay ('74).

Nucleolus. This basophilic structure contains a large amount of RNA as well as a diffuse coating of DNA. It is known to have positive histochemical reactions for several enzyme systems associated with respiration, energy production and the synthesizing functions of the cell. It is particularly related to the production of nucleic acid and protein in nerve cells. In most electron micrographs the nucleolus shows no limiting membrane and the structure has a dense granular appearance. A "nucleolar satellite" 1 μ or less in diameter may be found closely apposed to the nucleus in nerve cells from female specimens (Barr et al., '50) as shown in Figure 4-7.

Chromophil Substance. There are two main types of nucleic acid in the cell: (1) ribonucleic acid [the sugar of the nucleotide is ribose (pentose)], and (2) desoxyribonucleic acid [the sugar is desoxyribose (desoxypentose)]. Cytochemical methods indicate that nucleoproteins of the desoxyribose type are found chiefly in the chromatin, which forms the spireme and chromosomes in mitosis and, during the intermitotic period, is partly represented by chromatin bodies known as karyosomes. Desoxyribonucleic acid also is found in the nucleolar satellite and in small quantities within the mitochondria. On the other hand, the true nucleolus is as a rule a dense, spherical, optically homogenous body that is rich in ribonucleic acid. Similar ribonucleoproteins are found in the cytoplasm, and there is good evidence for the assumption that the nucleolus plays an important part in cytoplasmic protein formation (Caspersson, '50).

In preparations stained with basic aniline dyes, the *chromophil substance* appears in the form of deeply staining granules or clumps of granules known as *Nissl (tigroid) bodies* (Fig. 4-1*E*). They are found in the cell bodies and dendrites of all large and many of the smaller cells, but are absent in the axon and in the axon hillock from which that process arises. They are most abundant and sharply defined in the larger cells, whose clear vesicular nucleus contains practically no basichromatin (Figs. 4-1 and 4-7).

The Nissl bodies are larger in motor than in sensory cells, and attempts have been made to distinguish the many neuron types by the size, shape, distribution and staining capacity of the chromophil granules.

Nissl bodies were presumed to result from protein precipitation during fixation. However, recent evidence has demonstrated their presence in living cells. In ganglion cells which have been centrifuged with tremendous force, the Nissl bodies become concentrated in the centrifugal pole of the cell without losing their individual discreteness (Beams and King, '35). Bensley and Gersh ('33), using the freeze-dry technic which eliminates many of the artifacts caused by commonly used fixation methods, have obtained Nissl pictures quite similar to those found in the usual histological preparations. Beams and King conclude that "Nissl bodies react like definite masses of greater density embedded in lighter substance." Deitch and Murray ('56) demonstrated an exact correspondence between the cytoplasmic masses seen by phase contrast microscopy in tissue culture cells of living chick ganglion cells and in the same cells fixed in 1% buffered osmium tetroxide. They believed the masses to be chromophilic material.

Confusion surrounding the Nissl bodies was resolved by the electron microscopy study of Palay and Palade ('55), in which the Nissl material was identified as masses of granular endoplasmic reticulum. Clusters of punctate ribonucleic acid granules, 10 to 30 mμ in diameter, were oriented upon and between the cisterns, tubules and vesicles to form a series of flattened, anastomosing, parallel-arranged sheets or membranes (Figs. 4-8 and 4-10). Dispersed ribonucleic acid granules

also can be observed along isolated cisternae within the neuron cytoplasm. With ultraviolet microscopy and ribonuclease, it has also been shown that ribonucleoprotein is one of the main constituents of the Nissl substance. Treatment of sections with the enzyme ribonuclease results in the loss of stainability with basic dyes, although the Nissl bodies remain intact.

Available evidence indicates that the Nissl bodies are part of a mechanism for the synthesis of cytoplasmic proteins. This mechanism serves to replace the protein constantly consumed during normal physiological activity and to restore the total cell mass when the neuron is suddenly deprived of a large amount of its protoplasm, as in axon amputation (Francoeur and Olszewski, '68). Following section of the axon, alterations in the discrete structure of the Nissl bodies can be demonstrated when stained by basic dyes and viewed with light microscopy (Fig. 4-1*E*). Nissl bodies in the cytoplasm about the nucleus appear dispersed or dissolved, a phenomenon termed *chromatolysis* (see page 107).

Neurofibrils. The neurofibrils are found in *all* nerve cells. As demonstrated by the reduced silver methods, they are delicate, homogeneous threads which are continuous throughout the cell body and its processes (Fig. 4-1*B* and *C*). In the cell body they cross and interlace. In processes they run parallel to each other and are more closely grouped, especially in the axon, which practically constitutes a cable of densely packed neurofibrils (Fig. 4-11). Neurofibrils have been described in the living nerve fibers of several invertebrates and in the living nerve cells of tissue culture (Weiss and Wang, '36; Geiger, '58).

The question whether neurofibrils exist as such in the living cell remained unsolved by the use of the conventional histological methods. Palay and Palade ('55) found nothing in their electron microscopy study comparable in size to the neurofibrillae observed by light microscopy. Similar negative results were obtained in other electron microscopy studies of both the developing and the adult nerve cell bodies and their processes (Palay, '56; Tennyson,

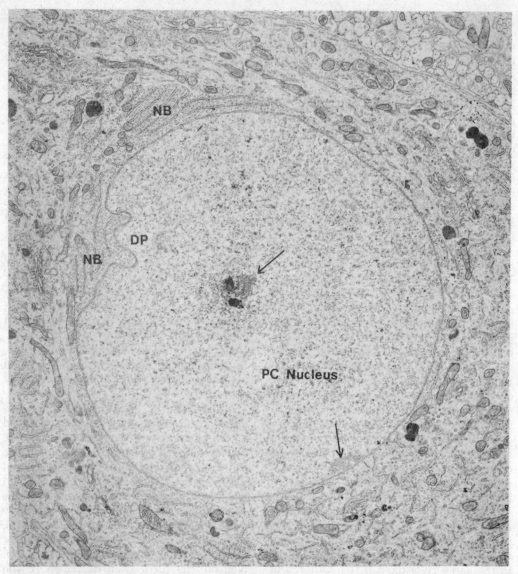

FIG. 4-9. Electron micrograph of a Purkinje cell nucleus of the rat. The nuclear chromatin is thinly and uniformly distributed throughout the nucleus, except for two sites indicated by *arrows*. The dendritic pole (*DP*) of the nucleus is wrinkled and capped by a small Nissl body (*NB*). ×14,000. (Courtesy of Drs. Sanford L. Palay and Victoria Chan-Palay, Harvard Medical School; Palay and Chan-Palay, '74.)

'62; Rhodin, '63). Recent investigators have observed fibrillar material in the axon, dendrites and perikaryon formed by long tubular elements 200 to 300 Å in diameter (Peters and Vaughn, '67). Such *neurotubules* have a smooth contour and are of variable length. In the axoplasm of peripheral and central nerves one usually can see neurotubules, as well as strands of canaliculi, vesicles of endoplasmic reticulum and a few ribosomes (Fig. 4-17). In addition to neurotubules there are finer axial components called *neurofilaments* which are about 100 Å in diameter. It seems generally accepted that the neurotubules and neurofilaments observed in electron microscopy become aggregated during fixation and form the neurofibrils observed

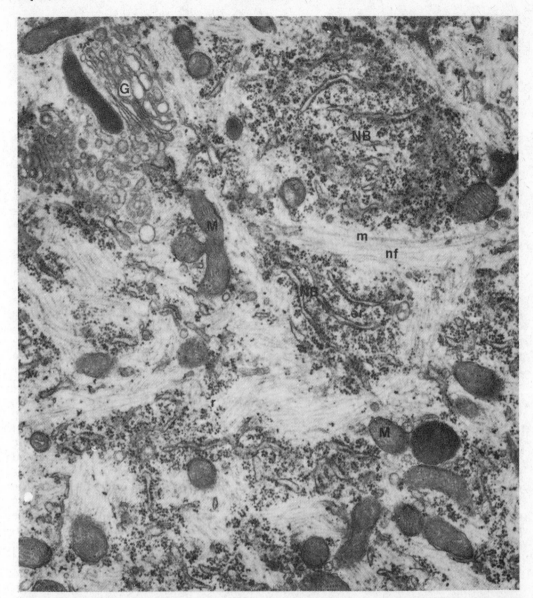

FIG. 4-10. Electron micrograph of the cytoplasm of a rat dorsal root ganglion cell. The cytoplasm contains well-defined Nissl bodies (*NB*) separated by spaces containing microtubules (*m*) and neurofilaments (*nf*). Some ribosomes in the Nissl bodies are arranged in rows attached to the outer surfaces of cisternae of the granular endoplasmic reticulum (*er*), while others lie free (*r*) in the cytoplasmic matrix. Free ribosomes appear in rosettes of six or more members. *G* in the upper left indicates part of the Golgi apparatus. ×46,000. (Courtesy of Drs. Henry De F. Webster and Sanford L. Palay; Peters et al., '70.)

with the light microscope (Gray and Guillery, '66; Peters et al., '70). It is interesting to note that microtubules predominate in dendrites, whereas neurofilaments are rare in the initial axon segment but become more common in the distal myeli-

nated segments of axons (Peters, '68). Nerve conduction takes place at the surface membrane of the axon, and neurotubules seem to have no role in this process. Whether the neurotubules are involved in axon growth, the transport of essential en-

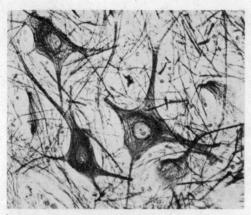

Fig. 4-11. Large motor neurons from infant spinal cord showing neurofibrillar structures. Portions of dendrites and axons of other neurons fill the field. Cajal silver method. Photograph.

zymes or the formation of protein and synaptic vesicles remains unresolved. The demonstration of electron-dense intraluminal granules in neurotubules of both central and peripheral nerves (Rodriguez-Echandîa et al., '68) suggests a relationship to axoplasmic flow (Weiss and Hiscoe, '48; Droz and Leblond, '62; Francoeur and Olszewski, '68).

Mitochondria. Granular or filamentous mitochondria are scattered throughout the entire cell body, dendrites and axon (Figs. 4-8, 4-12 and 4-21). These organelles occur even in the smallest ramifications and terminals of the neuron and are prominent electron microscopic features wherever intense metabolic activity occurs, such as at synapses and at sensory and motor endings (Palay and Palade, '55; Hartmann, '56; Dempsey, '56). These widely distributed cytoplasmic organelles are involved in glycolysis, biosynthesis and cell respiration, but their most important function is to serve as a source of energy for the cell. During cell respiration the enzymatic breakdown of carbohydrates and amino acids yields CO_2, water and energy. The energy, bound in adenosine triphosphate (ATP), is utilized in the transport of ions across cell membranes and protein synthesis (Waelsch, '57). The mitochondria (M in Figs. 4-8, 4-9, 4-10, 4-21 and 4-24) are recognized easily in most electron micrographs. The growing tips of dendrites often exhibit

varicosities or swellings which are filled with mitochondria (Sotelo and Palay, '68). Mitochondria in these varicosities are long and slender and are arranged either parallel to the long axis of the dendrite or form gentle swirls (Fig. 4-12). Their accumulation and breakdown at the nodes of Ranvier have been observed during the early stages of Wallerian degeneration (Webster, '62).

Centrosome. A microcentrum often is demonstrated in neuroblasts. It consists of one or two granules surrounded by a clear cytoplasmic area. In some instances, fine wavy fibrils may radiate from the clear area of cytoplasm. The significance of the centrosome is puzzling, for adult neurons are incapable of cell division. However, Murray and Stout ('47) and Murray ('57) have demonstrated that adult human sympathetic ganglia could survive, migrate and occasionally divide mitotically in tissue culture. Similar cultures of adult neurons of the human cerebral cortex have been observed to divide and survive after six subcultures for periods of 8 to 13 months (Geiger, '58).

Golgi Apparatus. The reticular Golgi complex is highly developed in nerve cells. With special silver-osmium stains the Golgi apparatus appears as a tangled skein of tortuous anastomosing strands and small vacuoles disposed around the nucleus. Some of the tortuous strands may extend into the larger dendrites, but none enter the axon. In other cells it may consist of disconnected granules or threads, and in some small cells it may be reduced to a single granule (Golgi body). The apparatus accurately reflects altered physiological and pathological conditions of the cell even more sensitively than the chromophilic substance. In the cell body of a neuron whose axon has been cut, the substance of the apparatus becomes dispersed toward the periphery, and subsequently is fragmented and dissolved. These phenomena have been termed "retispersion" and "retisolution," respectively (Penfield, '20).

The appearance of the Golgi apparatus as observed with the light microscope is quite different from that demonstrated in electron micrographs (G in Fig. 4-8). In

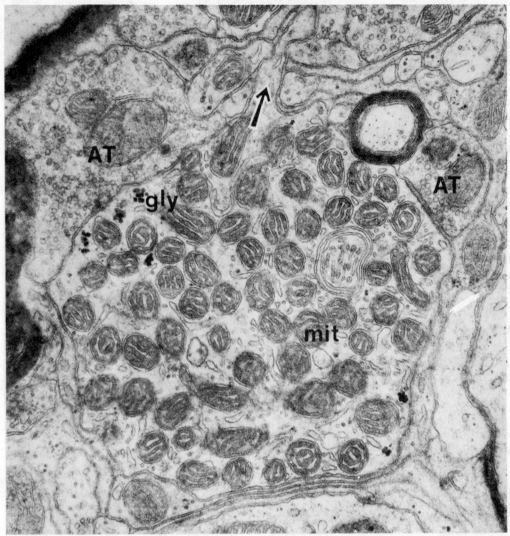

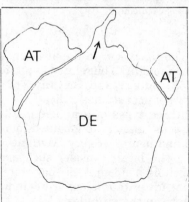

Fig. 4-12. Electron micrograph of a dendritic expansion (*DE*) filled with mitochondria (*mit*) and glycogen (*gly*) granules. This growing dendritic tip shows a filopodia-like expansion (*arrow*) and has two axonal terminals (*AT*) synapsing upon its surface. Dendritic profiles of this type are abundant in the dorsal part of the lateral vestibular nucleus in the rat. ×39,000. (Courtesy of Dr. C. Sotelo, Laboratoire d'Histologie Normale et Pathologique du Systeme Nerveux, Paris; Sotelo and Palay, '68.)

electron micrographs the Golgi apparatus appears as stacks of closely packed agranular membraneous cisternae associated with vacuoles and vesicles. Their close packing and the absence of ribosomes, either free or attached, distinguish the Golgi apparatus from the agranular endoplasmic reticulum and the Nissl substance (Peters et al., '70). Although the specific function of the Golgi apparatus is not fully understood, it appears to play a role in concentrating and packaging protein-rich materials. Recent evidence indicates that it is in the region of the Golgi apparatus that sugars are added to protein. It is possible that different cisternae within the Golgi complex may perform different functions. The innermost Golgi cisternae contain acid phosphatase and the "alveolate vesicles" of this region are full of hydrolytic enzymes (Friend and Farquhar, '67; Peters et al., '70). Thus the Golgi apparatus may be associated with the production of lysosomes, which contain hydrolases that break down protein, carbohydrates and nucleic acids (Holtzman et al., '67).

Inclusions. In addition to the organelles described above some nerve cells demonstrate dense cytoplasmic bodies and pigment granules. Most of the larger adult nerve cells contain a yellowish pigment known as *lipochrome* or *lipofuscin*. Lipofuscin generally is considered to be a wear and tear pigment, since the amount found within nerve cells increases with age. It appears in the form of granules which are usually aggregated in a dense mass in some part of the cell body (Fig. 4-1*B*). Occasionally they may be dispersed throughout the cell. They are insoluble in the usual lipoid solvents, are blackened by osmic acid and stained with Scharlach R. The cells of the newborn do not contain the pigment. It appears about the 6th year in in the spinal ganglia, a few years later in the spinal cord and after the 20th year in the cerebral cortex. It increases in amount with advancing years, and during senescence it may occupy a large part of the cytoplasm of some neurons (Truex, '40). Both histochemical and ultrastructural evidence suggests that lipofuscin granules are a form of lysosome (Essner and Novi-

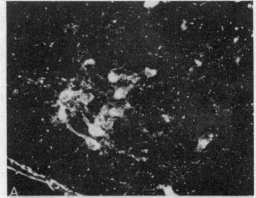
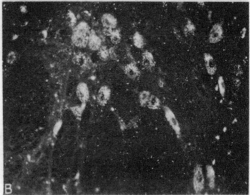

Fig. 4-13. Neurons containing biogenic amines in the squirrel monkey as demonstrated by fluorescence microscopy. *A*, Catecholamine-containing neurons located dorsolateral to the lateral reticular nucleus of the medulla. The background shows fine, beadlike varicosities containing catecholamines. ×400. *B*, Indoleamine-containing neurons in the dorsal nucleus of the raphe of the mesencephalon. ×400. (Courtesy of Dr. David Felten, Indiana University School of Medicine.)

koff, '60). The lipofuscin in the autonomic ganglia was thought to be related to ceroid (Sulkin, '53; Sulkin and Srivany, '60). Other histochemical studies indicate there are really three types of granules in the autonomic cells, namely, pigmented, nonpigmented and neurosecretory (Mytilineou et al., '63). The latter consider such material to include a lipoprotein that stores a neurotransmitter (norepinephrine) in an inactive state on the granules.

Granules of a blackish pigment known as *melanin* are found in the substantia nigra, locus ceruleus (nucleus pigmentosus) and certain pigmented cells scattered through the brain stem. It also is found in spinal and sympathetic ganglion cells (Fig. 4-1A). Melanin appears at the end of the 1st year and increases in amount until puberty, after which it apparently remains constant through senescence. Incubation of brain tissue in tritiated norepinephrine followed by radioautography reveals a heavy binding of norepinephrine at the surface membranes of pigmented cells of the substantia nigra, locus ceruleus and the dorsal motor nucleus of the vagus nerve (Ishii and Friede, '68). They suggested such binding was due to synaptic endings, and it may be related to the amount of catecholamines at the surface of the pigmented neurons.

Neurosecretion. One of the characteristics of all nerve cells is that they synthesize their own proteins. Synaptic neurosecretion of acetylcholine and norepinephrine in some neurons has been known for many years. Sensitive histochemical methods are available, at both the light and electron microscopic levels, for visualizing the intraneuronal distribution of a group of biogenic monoamines suspected of acting as neurotransmitters or modulators (Hökfelt and Ljungdahl, '72). These biogenic monoamines include dopamine, norepinephrine and 5-hydroxytryptamine which can be mapped with the Falck-Hillarp fluorescence method (Falck, '62). This method provides an estimate of the intraneuronal amine levels and reveals an uneven distribution; the cell body contains low to medium concentrations, while such concentrations are low in the axon, except for the terminal axonal enlargement (i.e., nerve endings) where amine levels are high (Fig. 4-13). Comparisons of norepinephrine neurons in the central and peripheral nervous system indicate that fluorescence is localized mainly in the perinuclear region and roughly corresponds to the position of the Golgi apparatus; in peripheral neurons the most intense fluorescence is seen in peripheral regions of the cytoplasm. At the ultrastructural level the distribution of granular vesicles closely parallels the distribution of fluorescence (Hökfelt and Van Orden, '72). Both small and large granular vesicles are present in

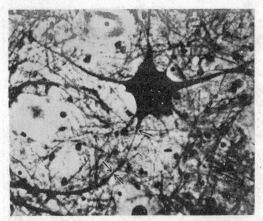

FIG. 4-14. Large motor neuron in the anterior gray horn of infant's spinal cord revealing several dendrites and the origin of the axon. The axon arises from the lower side of the cell body, tapers to thin thread for a short distance and thickens at the point where the myelin sheath develops. Small neuroglial nuclei are stained black. Modified Weigert's stain. Photograph.

monoamine neurons and some evidence suggests that the large granular vesicles contain large amounts of dopamine-β-hydroxylase and chromogranin A, and comparatively small amounts of norepinephrine. Small granular vesicles are thought to contain these substances in reverse proportions. Certain amino acids are suspected to be neurotransmitters. Those suspected of serving this function are gamma (γ) amino butyric acid (GABA), glycine and glutamate, but no histochemical methods are available by which they can be visualized in the light or electron microscope. Thus, in a sense all neurons may be considered as secretory cells.

In addition to the above examples, investigators have demonstrated the existence of certain glandlike neurons in both the invertebrate and vertebrate nervous systems (Speidel, '19; Scharrer and Scharrer, '40, '45; Palay, 45; Scharrer, '65). The hypothalamo-hypophyseal system of the vertebrate brain is the classical example of this neuroendocrine mechanism. These inter-relationships have been reviewed by Ortmann ('60), Bern and Knowles ('66) and Gabe ('66); see Chapter 16. Neurosecretory neurons constitute a link in the chain that unites the neural and endocrine systems.

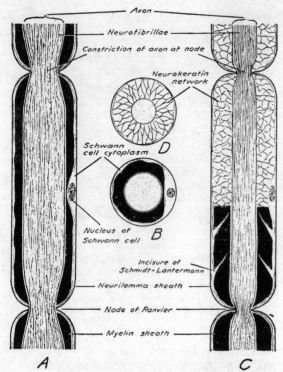

FIG. 4-15. *A* and *B*, Schematic drawings of peripheral myelin sheaths based on de Renyi's studies of living nerve fibers. *C* and *D* show them as seen in many fixed preparations. The cross membrane is not shown. (Copenhaver, '64.)

They represent the final pathway for conveying neural impulses to the endocrine system.

Neurosecretory neurons are "specialized" in a sense, yet they have retained all of the light and electron microscope characteristics of ordinary neurons. They demonstrate all of the cytoplasmic organelles discussed above including filaments, tubules and the proximodistal transport of axoplasm. However, the neurofilaments appear to be different in nature along the axon and in its preterminal region. The neurotubules may be 300 to 500 Å in diameter, and the axons also may demonstrate multilamellate bodies (Bern and Knowles, '66). Some neurosecretory neurons can conduct impulses and have an action potential of long duration (Bern and Yagi, '65). However, these elongated neurons have unusually electron-dense material associated with the Golgi membranes, and a prominent endoplasmic reticulum. It is presumed that "raw" protein material is synthesized by the endoplasmic reticulum which then passes it to the Golgi apparatus where it is packaged (proteinaceous neurosecretory material or NSM). Dense-core granules pass from the perikarya distally along the axon and may be concentrated in the preterminal regions of the fibers. Large masses of secretory material (Herring bodies) are observed along the course of these axons. The axon terminals containing neurosecretory granules are unique in that they abut upon a perivascular space rather than another neuron or effector cell. Their secretory product is released into the perivascular space, transported into the lumen of the vessel and carried via the blood to appropriate organs whose activity it can modify (Peters et al., '70). Experimental evidence suggests that the neurosecretory material produced by the supraoptic and paraventricular hypothalamic nuclei (Fig. 16-9) contains vasopressin and oxytocin (Bargmann, '66; Sloper, '66).

Inclusions of secretory material can be visualized by several histochemical stains and viewed with the light microscope (e.g., chromhematoxylin-phloxine stain). However, the refined cytological criteria established by electron microscopy provide the most meaningful features for identifying neurosecretory neurons. The supraoptic and paraventricular hypothalamic nuclei (Figs. 16-2, 16-4 and A-22) are the best known neurosecretory neurons in the human brain.

In mammals there is another neurosecretory system in the hypothalamus represented by the arcuate nucleus and the median eminence. Nerve fibers originating from the arcuate nucleus course into the median eminence and terminate in relationship to the perivascular spaces, as described for the supraopticohypophysial neurosecretory system (Figs. 16-1 and 16-9). Granule-containing vesicles in these nerve endings are smaller and of at least two types. The median eminence is considered to be involved in the elaboration and control of various releasing factors which regulate the adenohypophysis. Some of the

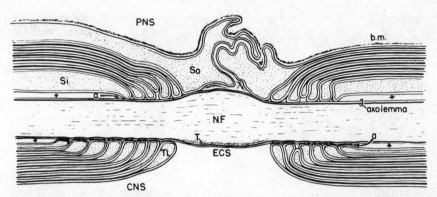

FIG. 4-16. Nodal regions from PNS (*above*) and CNS (*below*). In the PNS the Schwann cell provides both an inner collar (*Si*) and an outer collar (*So*) of cytoplasm in relation to the compact myelin. The outer collar (*So*) is extended into the nodal region as a series of loosely interdigitating processes. Terminating loops of the compact myelin come into close apposition to the axolemma in region near the node, apparently providing some barrier (*arrow at a*) for movement of material into or out of the periaxonal space (marked by *). The Schwann cell is covered externally by a basement membrane. In the CNS the myelin ends similarly in terminal loops (*tl*) near the node, and there are periodic thickenings of the axolemma where the glial membrane is applied in the paranodal region. These may serve as diffusion barriers and thus confine the material in the periaxonal space (marked *) so that movement in the direction of the arrow at "a" would be restrained. At many CNS nodes there is considerable extracellular space (*ECS*). Compare with CNS node shown in Figure 4-17. (Courtesy of Dr. R. P. Bunge, '68, and the American Physiological Society.)

small clear vesicles containing dense granules resemble those found in adrenergic nerve terminals.

THE NERVE FIBER

The axon is a slender, usually long process which arises from a conical mass of specialized protoplasm known as the implantation cone or axon hillock. It is distinguished from the cell body and dendrites by the complete absence of Nissl bodies, which also are lacking in the axon hillock. In smaller neurons an axon hillock is not easily identified in light microscopic preparations. The reason suggested by electron microscopy is that in these small cells there is little difference between the cytoplasm of the axon hillock and that of the neuronal cell body (Peters et al., '68). As the axon hillock narrows into the initial axonal segment, there is a gradual diminution in the number of ribosomes, but no abrupt change as suggested by light microscopic descriptions. Beyond the initial segment the axon contains mitochondria, neurofilaments, microtubules, agranular endoplasmic reticulum, vesicles and multivesicular bodies; no granular endoplasmic reticulum or ribosomes are present. Distally

each axon breaks up into simple or extensive terminal arborizations, the telodendria. The later may be synaptic endings on other neurons (e.g., sensory neurons), or effector endings in muscle and glands (Figs. 4-2G, 4-3 and 5 in Fig. 9-22).

In the central nervous system, the axons may be *myelinated* or *unmyelinated*. The former possess a sheath of myelin for at least a portion of their course. The oligodendrocyte forms and maintains the myelin sheath within the brain and spinal cord. In the unmyelinated fibers, the sheath is lacking. In the peripheral nervous system both myelinated and unmyelinated fibers have, in addition, an outer delicate nucleated membrane, the *sheath of Schwann*.

The *peripheral myelinated fiber* is structurally the most differentiated, consisting of axon (axis cylinder), myelin and sheath of Schwann. The myelin sheath is not continuous, but is interrupted at fairly regular intervals; the parts of the fiber free from myelin appear as constrictions known as the *nodes of Ranvier* (Figs. 4-2C and 4-15). In the fresh condition the semifluid axon is broad and homogeneous in appearance, and it occasionally shows

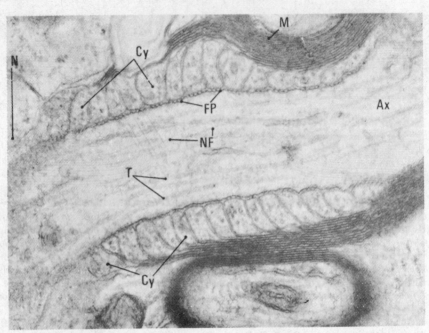

FIG. 4-17. Electron micrograph of node of Ranvier on nerve fiber of spinal cord (cat). The oligoglial cytoplasm (*CY*) forms loops of myelin (*M*) around the axon (*Ax*) at the node (*N*). Fusion points (*FP*) between the myelin and axon membranes are shown also. Neurotubules (*T*) and neurofilaments (*NF*) are identified in the axoplasm. Osmium fixation. ×70,000. (Courtesy of H. J. Ralston III.)

faint longitudinal striations. In silver stained preparations, it consists of closely packed, parallel-running neurofibrils imbedded in a scanty amount of homogeneous axoplasm (Fig. 4-2*A*). In most fixatives the axon usually shrinks to a thin axial thread. With special methods of fixation and tissue embedding its normal size may be more nearly approximated.

Between the axon and myelin sheath there is a delicate layer or membrane known as the axolemma (Fig. 4-16). Although difficult to demonstrate histologically, the membrane may be seen in ultraviolet photographs of the living nerve fiber, since the axolemma shows a much greater ultraviolet absorption than the axon or the myelin sheath. The axolemma is part of the neuron plasma membrane, and possesses a similar structure and specialized properties. It can be identified easily in high magnification electron micrographs as a delicate membrane surrounding the axon (Figs. 4-16 and 4-17).

Myelin. The myelin sheath is acquired a short distance from the cell body (Fig. 4-

14). The proximal portion of the axon is as a rule unmyelinated. The sheath is of varying thickness and is composed of a semifluid, doubly refracting substance known as *myelin,* which in the fresh state has a glistening white appearance. Physical technics have provided data concerning the orderly arrangement of lipoproteins that form myelin (Schmitt et al., '41; Sjöstrand, '63). Studies based upon polarized light, X-ray diffraction and electron microscopy have yielded a high degree of correlation and indicate that the myelin sheath is composed of concentric layers in which protein and lipid alternate. Lipid molecules are radially oriented in their layers while protein molecules are arranged tangentially. Myelin is composed of a fundamental, radially arranged repeating unit membrane with a spacing of 170 to 185 Å. The repeating unit membrane is composed of two subunits each consisting of a bimolecular lipid leaflet sandwiched between monolayers of protein. Each of these subunits corresponds to a single layer of plasma membrane de-

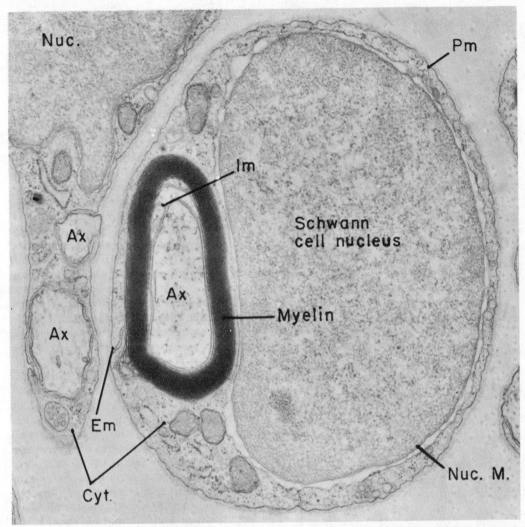

FIG. 4-18. Electron micrograph of a small myelinated nerve fiber from rat dorsal root ganglion matured in tissue culture. The infolding plasma membrane (*PM*) of the Schwann cell forms an external mesaxon (*Em*) continuous with the outermost lamella of the myelin sheath. An internal mesaxon (*Im*) surrounds the axon (*Ax*) and is continuous with the most internal lamella of the myelin sheath. Note the small amount of Schwann cell cytoplasm (*Cyt.*) between the nuclear (*Nuc. M.*) and plasma membranes. At the left are two unmyelinated axons associated with another Schwann cell. Osmium tetroxide fixation, Epon. Lead citrate stain. ×27,000. (Courtesy of Drs. M. B. Bunge and R. P. Bunge, Washington University School of Medicine, St. Louis.)

rived from the myelin-forming cell (Figs. 4-18 and 4-21).

With the limited magnification of light microscopy, it was presumed that peripheral myelinated nerves were enclosed by two separate layers, the myelin and Schwann cell sheaths. The histological appearances of myelinated nerves in cross section, when stained by the osmic acid and silver nitrate methods, are shown in Figure 4-2*B* and *D*. Electron microscopy studies have revealed that myelin was formed primarily by a double-layered infolding of the Schwann cell membrane, which became wrapped spirally around the axon in concentric layers (Geren, '54;

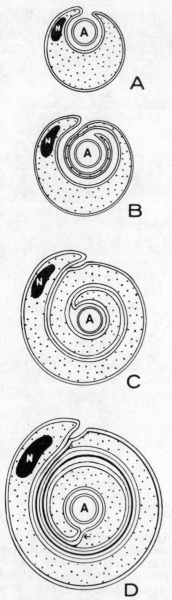

FIG. 4-19. Diagram of stages in the development of the myelin sheath about an axon (A). Cytoplasm of the Schwann cell is stippled and its nucleus is indicated (N). As additional layers of cell cytoplasm become wrapped around the axon (B and C), the cytoplasm is reduced in amount and the double-layered plasma membranes come into apposition (D). The outer membrane unit of the Schwann cell will become the future *intraperiod line* of myelin. The dark line (*major dense line*) represents the apposition of the inner (cytoplasmic) surface of the unit membrane as shown in D. The internal mesaxon is also indicated (*arrow in D*).

Robertson, '55, '58).

Four stages in the "jelly-roll theory" of myelin formation are depicted in Figure 4-19. In the peripheral nervous system the myelin sheath represents concentric layers of the Schwann cell, while the oligodendrocyte assumes the role of myelin formation within the central nervous system (Bunge, '68). In the latter case one oligodendrocyte may form a myelin layer on more than one axon (Fig. 5-9). It will be noted that the inner surfaces of the plasma membranes come into apposition and fuse to form *major dense lines* which are approximately 30 Å thick. Between each major dense line is a less dense *intraperiod line* formed by the union of the outer surfaces of the plasma membranes (Fig. 4-19). This fusion of membranes, accompanied by a reduction in cell cytoplasm, results in the repeating series of light and dark lines observed in electron micrographs (Figs. 4-18 and 4-21). Cytoplasmic remnants of the Schwann cell infolding may at times be identified at the axon-myelin junction (S in Fig. 4-21A). The primary infolding of the Schwann cell membrane often is present as an *internal mesaxon* (Im in Fig. 4-18). Continuity between the most superficial lamellae of the myelin sheath and the Schwann cell plasma membrane forms the *external mesaxon* (Em in Fig. 4-18).

These intimate relations of Schwann cell and myelin are further amplified by the tissue culture observations of Chu ('54), Peterson and Murray ('55) and Ross et al. ('62). They found that myelination began in isolated segments near the Schwann cell nucleus and extended along the fiber to a node of Ranvier. Remyelination of experimentally injured axons of the cat spinal cord appears to resemble the mechanism of myelination observed along peripheral nerves and in tissue culture (Bunge et al., '61).

Nodes of Ranvier. The myelin sheath is interrupted by constrictions at varying intervals on both central and peripheral axons. These areas can be identified in both the light and electron microscopes as regions where the myelin sheath is deficient (Figs. 4-2C and 4-17). At the nodal gap of peripheral nerves the axolemma is

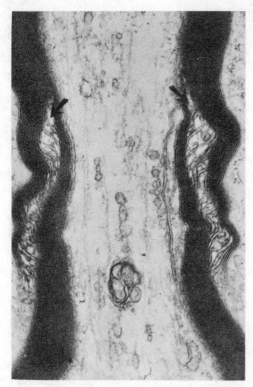

Fig. 4-20. Electron micrograph of a Schmidt-Lantermann cleft (*arrows*). Clear areas consist of Schwann cell cytoplasm. (Courtesy of Dr. R. P. Bunge, '67, and Rockefeller University Press.)

ensheathed by a fine basement membrane and small finger-like processes of the Schwann cell (Rhodin, '63). As shown in Figure 4-16 there are some characteristic differences between the nodes of central and peripheral axons. The internodal distance and nodal gap are both shorter on central axons. Such nodes also lack both interdigitating glial processes and a basement membrane. Thus nodes of Ranvier in the central nervous system have a greater extracellular space in the nodal region. The blunt spiral ends of the glial processes appear to fuse with the axolemma adjacent to a central node as shown in Figures 4-16 and 4-17. Paranodal terminations of myelin loops, on each side of the node, provide close apposition of plasma membranes rather than complete obliteration of the extracellular space about the axon (* in Fig. 4-16). Electron microscopy has provided essential information on the fine

structure of the node, and the following studies should be consulted for additional details (Uzman and Nogueira-Graf, '57; Robertson, '59; Peters, '60, '66; Metuzals, '65; Bunge, '68; Peters et al., '70). The length of the internodal segment varies considerably and is proportional to the diameter of the fiber, the thinner fibers having the shorter internodes. In the peroneal nerve of the rabbit the internodes on fibers 3 to 18 μ in diameter range from 400 to 1500 μ (Vizoso and Young, '48), and these figures probably pertain for other mammals and man.

At each node of Ranvier the axon is slightly constricted and is traversed by a delicate cross membrane or "Quermembran" which delimits adjacent internodal segments of the axon (Muralt, '46). Muralt has shown that the cross membrane is demonstrable in the living nerve fiber when viewed in polarized light. To date cross membranes have not been identified in electron micrographs. It will be observed later in the study of physiology that nerve impulses seem to travel by *saltatory transmission*. The flow of electric current, when recorded from a nerve, seems to skip along the nerve fiber from node to node at a rapid rate. An action current generated at one node thus acts as a stimulating current to the next node. Mitochondria tend to accumulate in the nodal areas of axons and suggest heightened metabolic activity at such sites. Collateral branches usually take origin from a parent axon at the nodal gap.

Schmidt-Lantermann Clefts. The myelin sheath of each internode is divided at intervals into conical segments by oblique, funnel-shaped clefts, which extend to the axon (Fig. 4-2*E*). These are best seen in preparations treated with osmic acid but also are visible in the living fiber, when it is viewed in polarized light. Several cone-shaped indentations may occur in a myelin segment between two nodes, while the myelin sheaths of adjacent axons may be devoid of such clefts for long distances. Although long regarded as artifacts, the clefts have been observed in electron microscopic studies as shearing defects in the lamellae of the myelin sheath (Robertson,

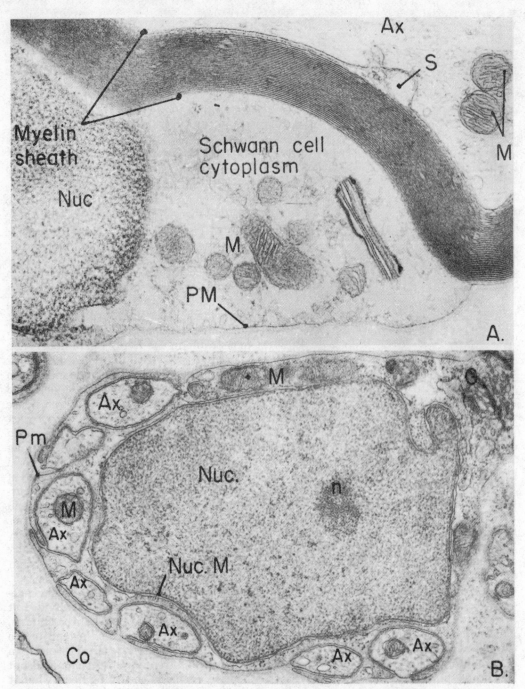

FIG. 4-21. *A*, Electron micrograph showing part of a myelinated nerve fiber in cross section. The Schwann cell cytoplasm and axoplasm (*Ax*) both contain mitochondria (*M*). Note the alternation of dense lamellae with less dense intermediate layers in the myelin sheath. This sheath is composed of thinned out Schwann cell cytoplasm wrapped concentrically around the axon (*Ax*). The innermost layer of the myelin sheath displays a local swelling (*S*). The plasma membrane (*PM*) of the Schwann cell envelops the entire structural complex. Mouse sciatic nerve. ×39,000. *B*, Electron micrograph showing the relationship of several unmyelinated axons (*Ax*) to the plasma membrane (*Pm*) of a Schwann cell. The nuclear membrane (*Nuc. M*), nucleus (*Nuc.*) and nucleolus (*n*) are identified. Mitochondria (*M*) and the Golgi complex (*G*) can be seen within the cytoplasm, while fine collagen fibrils (*Co*) surround the Schwann cell. Mouse sciatic nerve. Phosphate-buffered osmium tetroxide, Epon. Lead tartrate. ×26,000. (Preparations by Dr. J. Rhodin, School of Medicine, University of Michigan, Ann Arbor.)

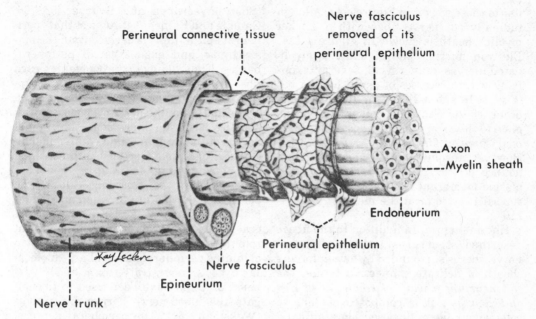

Perineural connective tissue

Nerve fasciculus
removed of its
perineural epithelium

Axon

Myelin sheath

Endoneurium

Perineural epithelium

Nerve fasciculus

Epineurium

Nerve trunk

FIG. 4-22. Diagram of the connective tissue sheaths about a peripheral nerve. Squamous cells of the perineural epithelium may function as a metabolic and blood-nerve diffusion barrier in the peripheral nerve. (Courtesy of Drs. T. R. Shanthaveerappa and G. H. Bourne, Emory University.)

'58; Rhodin, '63; Bunge et al., '67). Such clefts were shown to be areas of local separation of the spirally wrapped myelin lamellae which are nevertheless continuous across the incisure (Fig. 4-20). The light appearing regions between the lamellae consist of Schwann cell cytoplasm. In other preparations, the myelin sheath may exhibit a delicate trabecular reticulum, the *neurokeratin network* (Fig. 4-15). The network probably represents a precipitated protein residue of the myelin sheath rather than a true cytoplasmic reticulum. The myelin sheath ends at or near the point where the terminal arborizations are given off. No structure similar to the Schmidt-Lantermann clefts has been identified in myelin sheaths in the central nervous system.

Sheath of Schwann. This sheath of flattened cells forms the myelin of larger fibers. It also provides a thin attenuated cytoplasmic investment on nonmyelinated fibers of the cranial and spinal nerves (Figs. 4-18 and 4-21). Schwann cells, like the neurons, are of ectodermal origin (neural crest and neural tube). Each

Schwann cell has a flat, oval nucleus surrounded by a thin rim of cytoplasm which contains a Golgi complex and mitochondria (Fig. 4-18). The Schwann cells of both myelinated and nonmyelinated nerve fibers are surrounded by a typical basement membrane approximately 250 Å in thickness (*bm* in Fig. 4-16). This is separated from the plasma membrane of the Schwann cell by an interval of 250 Å. Ultrastructural studies indicate that the Schwann cell plasma membrane, with its surrounding basement membrane, represents the older term *"neurolemma sheath"* observed in light microscopy (Causey, '60; Thomas, '63). Nathaniel and Pease ('63a) regard only the granular basement membrane surrounding the Schwann cell as equivalent to the neurolemma.

One Schwann cell may have extensive cytoplasmic processes as it presides over, and maintains the integrity of, the segment of myelin between two nodes of Ranvier. If an ultrathin section were cut through a small myelinated nerve fiber to include the nucleus of a Schwann cell, it would reveal ultrastructural relations sim-

ilar to those shown in Figure 4-18. A longitudinally cut nerve fiber with a thicker
myelin sheath is shown in Figure 4-21A.
Electron micrographs of adult unmyelinated nerves may reveal several axons
lying within recesses of one Schwann cell
(Figs. 4-18 and 4-21B). The plasma membrane of the Schwann cell is closely applied to the axon except for a small periaxonal space of 150 to 200 Å (Bunge, '68).
However, at some point around the circum-
ference of each unmyelinated axon, the
plasma membrane is reflected and extends
superficially to form the mesaxon (Fig. 4-
21B).

Endoneurium. In addition to the above
described structures, each peripheral
nerve fiber is surrounded by a re-enforcing
sheath of delicate connective tissue, the
*endoneurium (sheath of Henle, or of Key
and Retzius)*. It is composed of delicate
collagenous fibers disposed longitudinally
for the most part, a homogeneous ground
substance and an occasional flattened fibroblast. A close contact between the endoneurial collagen and the basement membrane of Schwann cells is an inevitable
consequence of the ensheathing of nerve
fibers in collagen. Actual "collagen pock-
ets" surrounded by Schwann cells have
been observed along nonmyelinated axons. Thin bundles of collagen usually can
be observed within the typical basement
membrane surrounding a Schwann cell
(Gamble, '64). The endoneurium is continuous with the more abundant connective
tissue of the perineurium, which envelops
both small and large bundles of fibers
within a peripheral nerve trunk (Figs.
4-2B and 4-22).

Perineurium. The outermost layers of
the perineurium are composed of dense concentric layers of mostly longitudinally arranged strands of collagen. A few fibroblasts and macrophages also are present
among the strands. Perineural tissue is
somewhat unique in that it consists of fibroblasts and smooth lamellae that resemble mesothelium (Denny-Brown, '46). The
deeper concentric layers of flattened cells
have prominent basement membranes, often with closed contacts. The flattened
cells also have a slightly granular cytoplasm with scattered mitochondria and
rough-walled vesicles. Some investigators

(Shanthaveerappa and Bourne, '62, '66;
Gamble and Eames, '64) suggest that "perineural epithelium" is derived from the pia-
arachnoid and ensheaths all peripheral
nerves. They believe it accompanies each
fiber to its termination and forms the capsule of its end organ (Figs. 4-22 and 6-10).
Their concept of the derivation of cells is in
keeping with the knowledge that spinal
nerves of the human cauda equina demonstrate a pial sleeve or ensheathment and
endoneurium (Fig. 4-2F and H). Evidence
suggests that the squamous cells of the
perineural epithelium function as a metabolic and diffusion barrier in the peripheral nerve. It also may play an important
role in the degeneration and regeneration
of injured peripheral nerves. Large molecular dyes, silver nitrate, toxin and ^{131}I labeled proteins have been used to investi-
gate the blood-nerve barrier in animals
(Waksman, '61). The peripheral nerve of
the rabbit has an effective nerve barrier,
interpreted as due to the vascular endothelium rather than the mesothelial cells that
accompany the endoneurial connective tissue.

Epineurium. This dense, collagenous
layer forms an external connective tissue
ensheathment for all peripheral nerve
trunks (Fig. 4-22). It is continuous centrally with the dura mater of cranial and
spinal nerves. Its fibrous nature reinforces
the toughness of peripheral nerve trunks.
The collagen strands are disposed mainly
longitudinally, and the component fibers
have diameters between 700 and 850 Å.
A few elastic fibers and fibroblasts with
elongated processes are scattered throughout the epineurium. Axial arteries to peripheral nerves are derived from the large
arteries adjacent to nerve trunks. Arteries
that provide nourishment to a peripheral
nerve penetrate the epineurium and give
off several branches. The smaller arterioles pursue proximal or distal courses
within the perineurium of the nerve
trunk. Most of the capillaries supplying
the peripheral nerve fibers are located in
the endoneurium.

UNMYELINATED PERIPHERAL NERVE
FIBERS (FIBERS OF REMAK)

These slender axons are enveloped by
the thin Schwann cell sheath, its base-

ment membrane and fine strands of collagen (Figs. 4-18 and 4-21B). The critical point for fiber myelination of an axon in tissue culture is reported to be a diameter of 1 μ (Bunge et al., '67). Axons of thicker diameters always are invested with a myelin sheath. The peripheral axons of most postganglionic sympathetic neurons and many cells of the spinal ganglia are unmyelinated (Elfvin, '58). Numerous unmyelinated fibers also are found in the gray and white matter of the spinal cord and brain. Here they appear as fine naked axons embedded in glial cell processes with relationships similar to that of the Schwann cells on the peripheral unmyelinated fibers (Luse, '56, '56a; Bunge et al., '61).

Fiber Size. Myelinated fibers vary greatly in size. The fine fibers have a diameter from 1 to 4 μ; those of medium size from 5 to 10 μ; and the largest from 11 to 20 μ (Fig. 4-2).

Collaterals or branches are given off by most fibers of the central nervous system. They are usually of finer caliber than the parent stem, extend at right angles and often arise from the proximal unmyelinated part of the axon. In the myelinated portion they are given off at the nodes of Ranvier and become myelinated themselves. In the peripheral nervous system, the fibers of somatic motor neurons, which supply skeletal muscle, branch repeatedly at acute angles before reaching the muscle (Fig. 4-2G). Within the latter the branching may be very extensive, and a single nerve fiber may furnish motor terminals to many muscle fibers. Sensory fibers probably branch in a similar manner since their terminal arborizations extend over a considerable area. A single myelinated fiber may supply sensory endings to more than 300 hair follicle groups (Weddell, '41). The term "sensory unit" has been suggested for the sensory fiber and all its terminals.

Myelinated fibers conduct more rapidly than unmyelinated ones. Speed of conduction is proportional to the diameter of the fiber and, more especially, to the thickness of the myelin sheath. The myelin sheath may be regarded as insulation, while the extracellular space at the nodes of Ranvier and the periaxonal space provide ready avenues for ionic diffusion. This morphological substrate is required for the rapid reversibility of the excitation processes in order to account for the rapid conduction and relative indefatigability of the myelinated fiber.

Physical and Physiological Grouping of Nerve Fibers. When a wave of excitation, the *nerve impulse,* passes along a nerve fiber, it is accompanied by an electrical change known as the *action potential,* which can be recorded on a cathode ray oscillograph. The electrical record of an impulse consists of a strong negative deflection of short duration, the *spike potential,* which is usually followed by two longer but much weaker deviations known as the *negative* and *positive afterpotentials.* Since the traveling electric change and the impulse are inseparable from each other, a study of the electrical phenomena during excitation furnishes accurate information regarding the speed and frequency of the nerve impulse. The speed with which the spike potential travels over the nerve fiber constitutes the *conduction velocity* of the nerve impulse, and the number of successive potentials traversing the fiber are regarded as representing the frequency of the impulses.

Erlanger and Gasser ('37) demonstrated that different fibers in a nerve trunk conduct at varying velocities. The speed of conduction is proportional to the diameter of the fiber and of the myelin sheath. Each nerve has a characteristic pattern of velocities corresponding to an analogous pattern of fiber diameters in the nerve trunk. As a result of extensive physiological investigations supported by histological studies, nerve fibers have been grouped into four main classes, the A, B, C and γ fibers, whose potentials are known as the A, B, C and γ waves. Both A and B groups include several subdivisions. Criteria for the classification are fiber diameter, conduction velocity and nature of the electrical record (Bishop et al., '33; Heinbecker et al., '36; Gasser and Grundfest, '39; Grundfest, '39, '40; Lloyd, '43; Quensel, '44; Patton, '61a).

The A fibers are myelinated, range in diameter from 1 to 20 μ and conduct at rates of 5 to 120 meters/sec. The more finely myelinated B fibers have a diameter up to

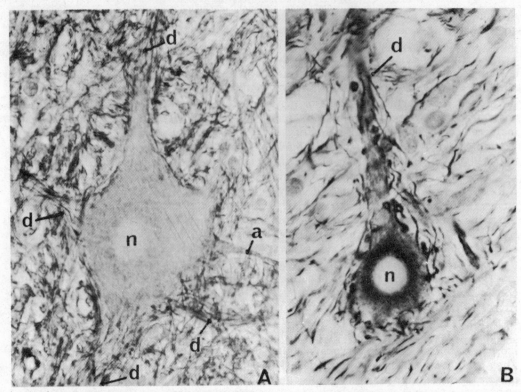

FIG. 4-23. Synaptic endings on human CNS neurons after silver impregnation and observed by light microscopy. Note numerous terminal boutons on the dendrites (*d*, axodendritic synapses) and some of the cell body (axosomatic synapses). The axon (*a*) and nucleus (*n*) are identified in *A*, which is a photograph of 650× magnification. The smaller neuron shown in *B* is magnified 920×.

3 μ and a conduction rate of about 3 to 15 meters/sec., although a higher velocity has been observed in some fibers of this group. The C fibers are unmyelinated and conduct very slowly, about 0.6 to 2 meters/sec. There is a certain amount of overlapping, so that a fiber of 2 μ could belong to either the A or B group, but certain features of the electrical record permit a definite classification. Thus the duration of the spike potential is always much longer in B fibers than in any A fiber, and the B fibers lack a negative afterpotential.

Studies on various types of nerves (muscular, cutaneous and autonomic) indicate a general functional grouping of the three fiber types. This grouping must not be regarded as rigid, since many fibers serving the same function may have widely different calibers. The A fibers include several subdivisions. The largest and most rapidly

conducting fibers (conduction velocity 60 to 120 meters/sec. in man) transmit motor impulses to skeletal muscles, while other A fibers convey afferent impulses from stretch receptors in muscle. The rest of the A fibers, varying considerably in diameter and speed of conduction, carry afferent impulses from cutaneous receptors. Fibers of intermediate size are related to touch and pressure. The finest fibers are believed to transmit impulses associated with pain, and perhaps some of these fibers conduct thermal and tactile impulses.

The B fibers are associated mainly with visceral innervation and are both efferent and afferent. All the preganglionic autonomic fibers belong to this group, as well as the postganglionic fibers from the ciliary ganglion, which are partly or wholly myelinated. The more rapidly conducting B fibers transmit afferent impulses from viscera. The unmyelinated C fibers comprise the efferent postganglionic autonomic fibers and afferent fibers which are believed to conduct impulses of poorly localized pain from the viscera and the periphery.

THE SYNAPSE

The simplest segmental reflex requires at least two neurons (Fig. 9-23). A wave of excitation, the nerve impulse, is set up in a peripheral sensory nerve ending and passes centrally along the axon of a ganglion cell into the spinal cord. There it activates a motor neuron, whose impulse travels along the motor fiber and causes a group of muscle fibers to contract (Fig. 9-22). Even more simple reactions have, as a rule, a third or *central* neuron interposed between the afferent and efferent cells (Fig. 9-23). In the more complicated neural circuits the number of such intercalated central neurons may be multiplied. All neural pathways therefore consist of chains of neurons so related to each other as to make possible the physiological continuity of nerve impulse conduction over the complete circuit. The point of junction of neurons, i.e., where the axonal arborizations of one neuron come in contact with the cell body or dendrites of another, is known as the *synapse*. The synapse is not a site of cytoplasmic confluence between neurons, but an interface at which they are functionally related. Axons terminating upon the dendrite of another neuron form *axodendritic synapses*, whereas axons terminating upon the cell soma or perikaryon form *axosomatic synapses*. Less frequently axon terminals of one neuron may be located directly on other axonic terminals, or on the initial segment of the axon of another neuron (*axoaxonic synapses*). The term "synapse" may be expanded to include not only the functional contacts between two neurons, but also those between neurons and effector cells, such as muscle cells.

Synaptic junctions show many structural variations (Fig. 4-23). Most commonly, the axon terminals end in small bulblike expansions or *neuropodia* (*end feet, boutons terminaux*). Each neuropodium consists of a neurofibrillar loop imbedded in perifibrillar substance; sometimes there are simply small neurofibrillar rings. A large motor neuron in the spinal cord may receive several thousand such endings, most of them 1 to 2 μ in diameter. In another type of synapse, the delicate axon terminals do not form end feet but come in lengthwise apposition with the dendrites or cell body, often for considerable distances. The most striking examples are the climbing fibers of the cerebellum (Figs. 14-4 and 14-5). In some cases, unmyelinated axons run at right angles to the dendrites and apparently come in contact with the spiny excrescences or *gemmules* with which the dendrites are beset (Fig. 4-5). Thus one axon may convey impulses to many neurons, and conversely one neuron (e.g., anterior horn cell) may receive impulses from many neurons, some of which are widely separated in the neuraxis.

Numerous electron microscopy studies have shown that synapses of the vertebrate nervous system possess the following basic similarities: (1) discontinuity between the cytoplasm of the two apposed membranes of a synapse, (2) direct contact of the presynaptic (plasma membrane of an axon terminal) and subsynaptic membranes, which are separated by a minute synaptic cleft, usually 100 to 200 Å in width (Figs. 4-24 and 4-25), and (3) the presence of mitochondria, a tail of neurofilaments and numerous synaptic vesicles on the presynaptic side of the synapse (Palay, '56; de Robertis, '59, '66; Gray and Guillery, '61; McLennan, '63; Peters et al., '70). The vesicles of the presynaptic terminals contain chemicals by which transmission across the synaptic membrane or at the neuromuscular junction is effected (de Robertis and Bennett, '54; de Robertis et al., '62; Whittaker, '65; de Robertis, '66, '67). Synaptic vesicles are considered to contain quanta of acetylcholine or catecholamines which are released in large numbers when an impulse arrives at the synapse (Katz, '66). At the neuromuscular junction quanta of acetylcholine, released a few at a time during quiescence, are associated

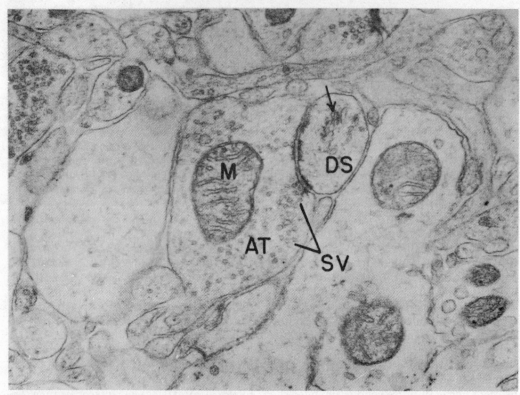

Fig. 4-24. Electron micrograph of an axodendritic synapse in the human cerebral cortex. The saclike enlargement comprising the axon terminal (AT) contains a mitochondrion (M) and numerous synaptic vesicles (SV). The axon terminal is indented by the dendritic spine (DS). Profiles of the spine apparatus (arrow) are seen above, while to the left the postsynaptic membrane of the dendritic spine is thickened in three places. Compare with synapse shown in Figure 4-23. Buffered osmium fixation, Epon. ×38,500. (Courtesy of Dr. J. Francis Hartmann, Presbyterian-St. Luke's Hospital, Chicago.)

with miniature end plate potentials. The "chemical synapse" involving the release of transmitter substance is the most common type of central nervous system synapse in mammals. In lower vertebrates (e.g., fish) "electrical synapses" function without a chemical transmitter; in these synapses there is a close contact between pre- and postsynaptic membranes.

The most commonly occurring synaptic vesicles are about 400 Å in diameter, are roughly spherical and have clear centers (Figs. 4-24 and 4-25). Vesicles of this type are found in axon terminals at neuromuscular junctions, throughout the central nervous system and in some sympathetic nerve endings. Circumstantial evidence suggests that these clear vesicles contain acetylcholine (Whittaker, '65; de Robertis,

'67). A slightly larger vesicle of about 500 Å in diameter containing a dense granule, 280 Å in diameter, is found in axon terminals of autonomic nerve fibers (Bloom and Barrnett, '66). Synaptic vesicles of this type are considered to be associated with catecholamines, especially norepinephrine. This type of synaptic vesicle appears in terminals of adrenergic nerve fibers, and may be seen in regions of the brain known to have a high amine content when tissue is fixed in potassium permanganate (Hökfelt, '67, '67a).

Many physiological peculiarities are associated with the synapse. While an activated nerve fiber conducts equally well in either direction (orthodromic and antidromic conduction), impulses are transmitted over the reflex arc, i.e., across the

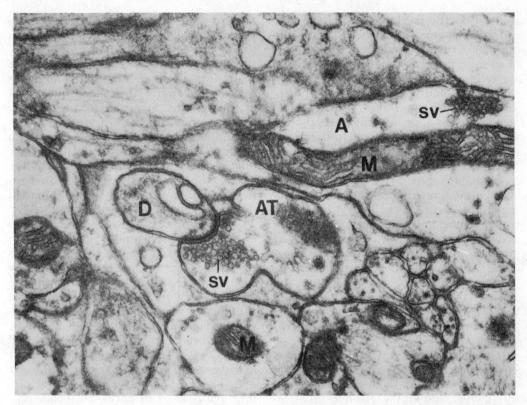

Fig. 4-25. Electron micrograph of an axodendritic synapse in monkey cerebellar cortex. Synaptic vesicles (*SV*) are present in the axon terminal (*AT*) and in the axon (*A*) in the upper right. Other organelles are: *D*, dendrite with spine apparatus, and *M*, mitochondria. ×48,000. (Courtesy of Dr. Ray C. Henrikson, College of Physicians and Surgeons, Columbia University.)

synapse, in one direction only. Thus the impulse travels from the axon of one neuron to the cell body, the dendrites or more rarely the axon of another, a phenomenon known as *dynamic polarization*. Hence synapses ensure that nerve fibers normally are used for one-way signal transmission. Some of the other ways in which conduction across the synapse differs from that in a nerve fiber may be briefly mentioned. Over a reflex arc (1) conduction is slower; (2) the response may persist after cessation of the stimulus (after-discharge); (3) the rhythm of stimulus and the rhythm of response correspond less closely; (4) repetition of a given stimulus may produce a response where a single stimulus will not (summation); (5) there is greater variability in the threshold value of a stimulus, i.e., the ease with which responses can be elicited; (6) there is much greater fatigabil-

ity; (7) there is greater dependence on oxygen supply and greater susceptibility to anesthetics and drugs; (8) there is a longer refractory period; and (9) there is re-enforcement or inhibition of one reflex by another.

Synapses control impulse traffic, the amount and pattern of information input, and consequently the behavior of a neuron or groups of neurons. Synapses are the units that provide mutual neuronal interdependence. Although each neuron in its entirety constitutes a "private line," there is no privacy in the central nervous system (Gelfan, '64). For additional details on the synaptic complex the reader is referred to the articles by Eccles ('59), Pappas ('66), DeRobertis ('66), Nathaniel and Nathaniel ('66), Katz ('66), Guillery ('67) and Peters et al. ('70).

Degeneration of Nerve Fibers. The

cell body is the trophic center of the neuron, and any process detached from it disintegrates. Crushing injuries or interruption of an axon produces detectable changes in the cell body (chromatolysis), as well as in the central and distal stumps of the injured fiber. When an axon is divided, degenerative changes of a traumatic character first affect the cut edges. In the proximal portion of the fiber, which is attached to the cell body, the degenerative changes (retrograde degeneration) extend only a short, although variable distance, depending on the nature of the injury. In a clean cut only one or two internodes may be involved. In more severe injuries, such as gunshot wounds or inflammatory processes, the retrograde degeneration may extend as much as 2 or 3 cm. However, the degeneration is soon succeeded by reparative processes leading to the formation of new axonal sprouts from the central stump.

In the distal portion, the axon and myelin sheath completely disintegrate, and degeneration occurs throughout the length of the fiber, including its terminal arborization. This process is known as *secondary* or *Wallerian degeneration*. The changes as a rule appear simultaneously along the length of the nerve fiber distal to the injury. Functional failure of the nerve also is abrupt down the length of the distal nerve trunk (Salafsky and Jasinski, '67; Novak and Salafsky, '67). In these studies muscle responses to distal nerve stimulation ceased 54 to 72 hr after sciatic nerve section, depending on whether nerve injury occurred in the thigh or at the level of the knee.

Axonal changes begin almost at once. Electron micrographs of the sciatic nerve following crush injury demonstrate that the initial change is an accumulation of mitochondria in the axoplasm at the nodes of Ranvier. This is followed by a breakdown of the axoplasm and mitochondria (Webster, '62). Twelve hours after injury the axon is swollen and irregular in shape. Within a few days it begins to break up into fragments. However, the breaking up process may continue for a considerable

time in some fibers, and fragments of degenerating axons have been found as late as 3 or 4 weeks after the injury. The synaptic terminals are affected similarly. The neurofibrils lose their staining capacity and assume an irregular shape; by the end of the 5th day many of the fibrils have become broken up to form granules. The myelin sheath likewise degenerates. Two or three days after section, constrictions appear which break the myelin into elongated ellipsoid segments, which in turn fragment into smaller ovoid or spherical droplets or granules (Figs. 4-26 and 4-27). The whole process resembles the breakup of a liquid column under surface tension and is ascribed to the fact that the fiber is no longer kept in a turgid condition by neuroplasmic pressure emanating from the cell body (Young, '49). It has been shown that under normal conditions there is a constant proximodistal axoplasmic flow from the cell body (Fig. 4-31) (Weiss and Hiscoe, '48). The autoradiographic studies of Droz and Leblond ('62) and Francoeur and Olszewski ('68) also indicate that protein synthesized in nerve cell bodies migrates distally along the axons. The phenomenon of axoplasmic transport makes it possible to trace axonal connections in the central nervous system by autoradiographic technics (Lasek, '70; Cowan et al., '72). Because the neuronal soma is the principal site of protein synthesis, the injection of tritiated amino acid precursors into the soma provides a label which is transported in the axon and accumulates in the axonal terminals.

The myelin changes, at first purely physical, are followed by chemical changes as well; the myelin breaks down into simpler intermediate substances, which react to the Marchi stain.

Ultrastructural studies provide information about the degenerative process. Nineteen hours after peripheral nerve injury there is a loosening of the myelin lamellae (Lee, '63). Myelin disintegration is evident at 4 days in Schwann cells and well advanced 96 hr after crushing dorsal roots of the cauda equina (Nathaniel and Pease, '63). These authors have elucidated the key roles of the Schwann cell and its basement membrane in both degeneration and regeneration. Schwann cells undergo hypertrophy, demonstrate unusual numbers of ribosomes, multiply in number, become mobile and form elaborate basement membranes. These cells are almost exclusively responsible for the removal of axon remnants and autodigestion of disintegrated myelin. There is no connective tissue response in the endoneurium, and leucocytes do not appear to participate in the phagocytosis of neuronal debris. The only endoneurial response is a slow accumulation, and slight increase, in the amount of collagen adjacent to the basement membranes. Newly formed and hypertrophied Schwann cells have extensive tapering and overlapping cytoplasmic processes, which in light microscopy formerly were interpreted as multinucleated syncytial cords (band fibers).

Nuclear division of the Schwann cells begins around the 4th day and continues actively to about the 25th, mitosis occurring over the whole length of the fiber. The increase in the number of nuclei is considerable, in some instances as much as 13 times the original population (Abercrombie and Johnson, '47).

During degeneration the Schwann cell plasma and basement membranes become separated from each other to markedly increase the extent and complexity of the extracellular spaces (Nathaniel and Pease, '63). The reactive Schwann cells form new elaborately folded and successive basement membranes one inside the other. These Schwann cells and basement membranes thus form numerous extracellular compartments or tubes surrounded by collagen of the endoneurium. Regenerating axonal sprouts from regions above the injury later enter these extracellular compartments or "tubes" between the basement membrane and Schwann cell. If no axonal sprouts enter the tube, it shrinks considerably and the walls thicken, due to the increase in the collagen content of the endoneurium.

Retrograde Degeneration. The neuronal body whose axon is injured likewise shows marked degenerative changes (Figs. 4-1E and 4-28). The cell body swells and becomes distended, the nucleus is displaced toward the periphery and the Nissl bodies undergo dissolution. Nissl body breakdown begins in the center of the cell and spreads outward (central chromatolysis). With light microscopy the fixed Nissl material appears to undergo lysis (Fig. 4-28). Cytochemical and electron microscopic studies indicate that there is little change in the total quantity of RNA in the perikaryon, and suggest that the cisternae and ribosomes are only dispersed and less concentrated. The fact that these cells imbibe water results in tremendous increases in cell volume. Ultrastructural changes also have been observed in many neuronal organelles (e.g., mitochondria, endoplasmic reticulum, Golgi apparatus, ribosomes and lysosomes) following nerve section or X-irradiation of ganglion cells in tissue culture (Masurovsky et al., '67; Holtzman et al., '67; Kirkpatrick, '68). Histochemical changes occur in a number of oxidative and hydrolytic enzymes within chromatolytic and regenerating neurons (Nandy, '68). Such changes reflect a reduction, or an increase, in glucose metabolism, a breakdown of Golgi bodies or increased RNA and nucleoprotein synthesis.

The extent and rapidity of these changes depend on the type of neuron involved, on the nature of the lesion and especially on the location of the injury. A lesion near the cell body produces a greater central effect than one more distantly placed. The effect depends upon the percentage of the neuron destroyed. If the lesion is near the cell body, the latter may ultimately die and the proximal portion of the nerve fiber attached to it degenerates. Chromatolysis in the cell body reaches its maximum 12 to 14 days following injury to the axon. This retrograde alteration of Nissl material (axon reaction) has been employed extensively in neuroanatomical research to locate the cells of origin of axons in central tracts, or in a peripheral nerve (Figs. 4-1E and 4-28).

Regeneration. If the neuron survives injury, *regeneration* takes place. Recovery

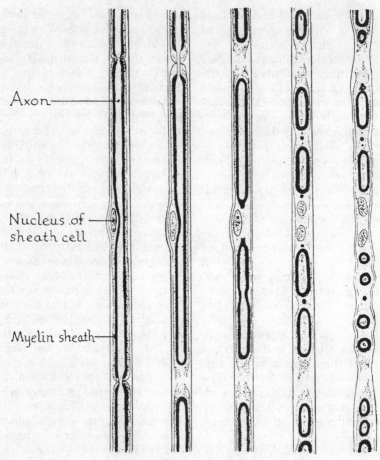

Axon

Nucleus of sheath cell

Myelin sheath

FIG. 4-26. Diagram showing breakup of myelin and axon during nerve degeneration. Note increase in sheath cell protoplasm and division of the nucleus (Young, '42).

in the cell body begins about the 3rd week and is characterized by the appearance of Nissl bodies around the nuclear membrane. The swelling of the perikaryon gradually subsides, the nucleus returns to its central position and the Nissl bodies are restored to their normal amount and distribution. Full recovery may take from 3 to 6 months, the time depending on the mass of axon to be reconstituted. While this is going on, regenerative processes appear in the axons of the central stump. As early as the 10th hr the axonal terminals begin to swell, owing to pressure emanating from the cell body. Each axon splits into numerous fine strands or fibers (Figs. 4-29 and 4-30) which traverse the scar formed at the site of the injury and reach the Schwann

tubes of the degenerating stump. Many of these fibers enter a single tube where they are disposed peripherally (Fig. 4-30). Later some of them move to a more central position and become completely surrounded by the plasma membrane of the sheath cells (Fig. 4-30). Along or within the bands, the regenerating axons grow distally for long distances to their peripheral destinations. Nathaniel and Pease ('63a) have found that regenerating axonal sprouts reach the extracellular spaces of the membrane envelope as early as 4 days after a lesion. Although many sprouts initially may occupy the spaces and gutters of the Schwann tube, only one persists and becomes remyelinated. This is usually the largest one (Fig. 4-30). The elimination of excess fibers

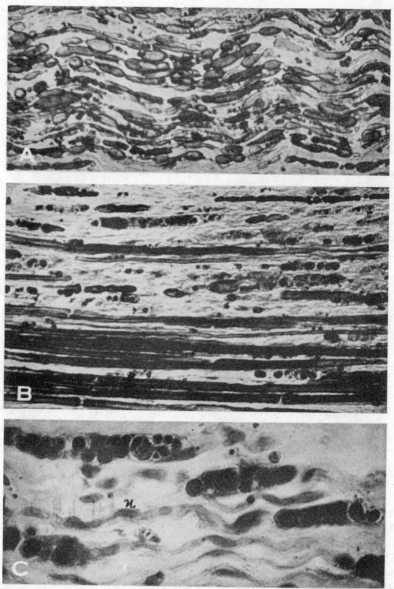

Fig. 4-27. *A*, Distal stump of a nerve cut 3 to 5 days previously. Osmic acid. *B*, Distal stump of a nerve partly cut 12 to 15 days previously. Osmic acid. Normal fibers and two nodes of Ranvier are shown at the bottom. *C*, Distal stump of a nerve cut 12 to 15 days previously. Osmic acid and iron hematoxylin. In addition to the clumps or islands of degenerating myelin, several band fibers and their nuclei (*n*) are shown. Photographs.

may take considerable time, and some of them still may be seen in tubes 3 or 4 months after section. The enlargement of one fiber and the elimination of the others occur only if the regenerating axons make sensory or motor contact with appropriate

receptor or effector endings in the periphery.

The thin regenerating axons, at first about 0.5 to 3 μ in diameter, gradually enlarge; the increase in diameter advances progressively down the tube, as if pro-

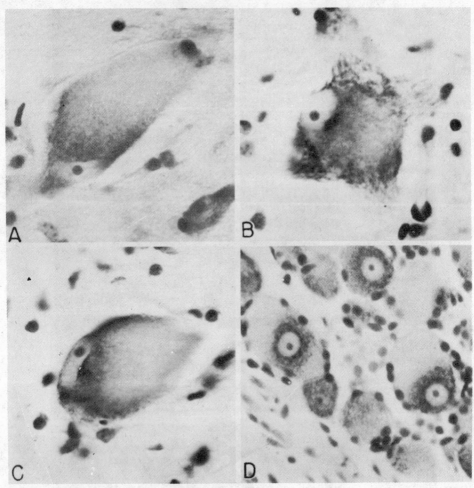

FIG. 4-28. Four examples of central chromatolysis in the monkey. *A* and *B*, Neurons in the brain stem reticular formation following section of the reticulospinal tracts. Cresyl violet. ×600; ×500. *C*, Retrograde cell change in lateral vestibular nucleus. Cresyl violet. ×500. *D*, Retrograde cell changes in the superior vagal ganglion. Cresyl violet. ×500.

pelled by some centrifugal force from the central stump. When the fiber reaches the periphery, growth in length ceases, but the increase in diameter continues until the original thickness is approximated. Myelination may occur as early as the 2nd or 3rd week in some fibers. It likewise advances in a proximodistal direction, and the process becomes somewhat slower in the more distal regions of the fiber. The myelin is at first laid down as a thin continuous sheath which subsequently becomes broken up into short internodal segments, about 150 to 700 μ in length. In fully regen-

erated nerve fibers, the internodes are shorter and more numerous, and there is no longer any definite relation between internodal length and diameter because fibers of varying thickness may possess similar internodal lengths. The time course of the events in degeneration and regeneration overlap each other. As noted above, regeneration of new axonal sprouts occurs before the disintegration of the axon and myelin sheath is completed in the distal segments of injured nerves. In a similar fashion regenerating axonal sprouts may traverse Schwann tubes

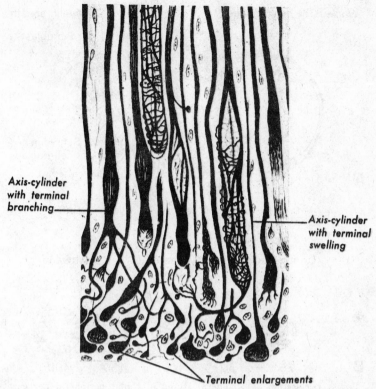

Axis-cylinder
with terminal
branching

Axis-cylinder
with terminal
swelling

Terminal enlargements

FIG. 4-29. Regenerating axons in the central stump of a cat's sciatic nerve 2¹/₂ days after section of the nerve (after Cajal, '09).

which still contain degeneration debris (Nathaniel and Pease,.'63a).

The growth processes observed during regeneration are remarkable. A slender axonal filament ultimately is transformed into a mature fiber whose volume in some instances may be several hundred times the volume of the original filament (Fig. 4-31, *B* through *E*). The manner in which this new axoplasm is formed has been investigated by Weiss and Hiscoe ('48) in a series of ingenious experiments. They fashioned small arterial rings which, when distended, could be slipped over the end of a cut nerve and placed in the desired position. The subsequent contraction of these rings produced localized constrictions with consequent reduction in the diameter of the individual fiber tubes (Fig. 4-31, *F* through *H*). The reduction in the lumen of the tube does not at first interfere with the advance of the slender regenerating axon,

which passes through the constricted zone and makes contact with the periphery. "But when the fiber, as it continues to enlarge, attains the dimensions of the constricted zone, a remarkable difference appears between those parts lying at the distal and at the proximal sides of the narrow neck. The distal segment ceases to grow and remains permanently undersized, while the proximal segment not only continues to enlarge, but near the entrance of the constricted zone, enlarges excessively." It was concluded that the axoplasm is exerting pressure in a distal direction and becomes dammed up where the channel narrows (Fig. 4-31*H*). The damming increases in intensity with time, and varies with the amount of constriction and the size of the fiber. Morphologically it is expressed in several ways, such as ballooning, beading, telescoping and coiling of the fibers. On release of the constriction, some

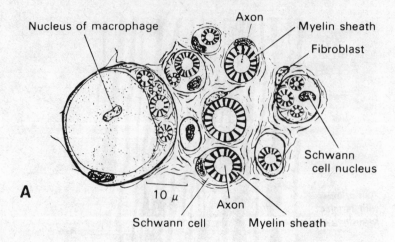

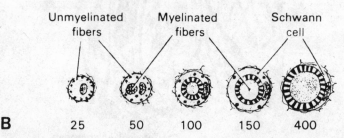

Fig. 4-30. *A*, Transverse section of peripheral stump of rabbit peripheral nerve severed 150 days previously. The stumps were left unsutured, but union was established by outgrowth. Most of the tubules contain one or more myelinated nerve fibers which are surrounded by protoplasm of the Schwann cells. *B*, Diagram of the progress of regeneration within the Schwann tubule distal to a good nerve suture at different time intervals (days). At 25 days there are many fibers near the edge of the tube; at 50 days one or two fibers are enlarged and surrounded by Schwann cell cytoplasm; at 100 days one large myelinated fiber occupies the center of the tube, while other smaller fibers are peripheral. At approximately 400 days, excess fibers disappear and a single large fiber attains its normal diameter (Young, '49).

of the dammed axoplasm flows into the distal portion, which consequently increases in thickness (Fig. 4-31*I*). The authors concluded that the formation of new axoplasm, i.e., growth in volume, occurs only in the cell body and that this axoplasm maintains a constant proximodistal motion that causes the elongation and enlargement of the regenerating fiber.

A knowledge of the mode of nerve regeneration is important as a basis for surgical treatment. If a nerve is severed, it is desirable to surgically approximate the cut ends promptly. If some time has elapsed since the injury, it is necessary to resect surrounding scar tissue and the neuroma on the proximal nerve stump before the nerve can be sutured. This subject is discussed further on page 188.

Fiber degeneration in the CNS is similar to that observed in the peripheral nerves. However, the degeneration proceeds at a slower pace, and the removal of neural debris by glial cells takes a longer time. It is known that the large fibers of the corticospinal tract and optic nerve degenerate faster than the fibers of small size (Van Crevel and Verhaart, '63, '63a). Such studies indicate that fibers of equal size tend to possess equal resistance to secondary degeneration. The large fibers degenerate faster, but are resorbed more slowly. Hence the debris of total degeneration in the central nervous system (CNS) is in evidence for several months.

Regeneration within the central nervous system of mammals has been studied with both anatomical and physiological

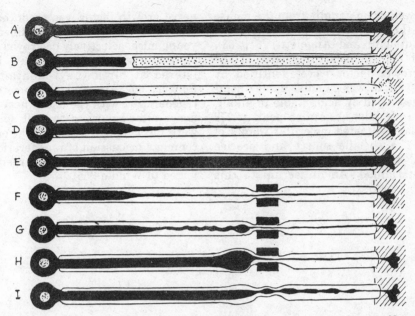

FIG. 4-31. Diagram of stages of nerve regeneration with and without constriction. *A*, Normal fiber; *B* through *E*, ordinary regeneration after simple crushing; *F* through *H*, regeneration after constriction; *I*, after release of constriction (Weiss and Hiscoe, '48).

technics (Sugar and Gerard, '40; Brown and McCouch, '47; Windle and Chambers, '50; Scott and Clemente, '52; Freeman, '52; Campbell et al., '57, '58). Such studies indicate that the central axons of injured nerve cells make abortive attempts to regenerate across an experimental gap in the spinal cord. Factors that influence and often hamper central regeneration are similar to those influencing regeneration in the peripheral nervous system (e.g., length of gap between severed stumps, hemorrhage and scar formation). Central regeneration is further thwarted by the absence of sheath cells to guide the regenerating axonal sprouts. Sugar and Gerard ('40) found evidence of functional regeneration in adult rats whose thoracic cords had been transected with care to prevent injury to the blood supply. No significant return of function has been noted in the higher mammals following complete transection of the spinal cord.

It has been shown that remyelination of experimentally injured axons of the spinal cord can take place in the cat (Bunge et al., '61). Just what effects the described "nerve growth factor" may have upon cen-

tral nervous system fiber regeneration is a moot question. Over the years various chemical compounds have been used in an attempt to stimulate the growth of the neurons and their processes. Bueker ('48) noted that a fragment of mouse sarcoma 180 implanted in the body wall of a 3-day chick embryo became invaded by sensory nerve fibers from the adjacent spinal ganglia. After 4 or 5 days the ganglia appeared to be considerably enlarged. This overall increase resulted from both the number and the size of the sensory neurons, while motor neurons remained unaffected. These observations were confirmed by Levi-Montalcini and Hamburger ('51), who also noted that the sympathetic nervous system contributed more fibers to the tumor graft than did sensory ganglia. Tissue cultures of chick spinal and sympathetic ganglia, when confronted with explants of a tumor at a distance of a few millimeters, produced an exceedingly dense outgrowth of fibers on the side of the ganglia facing the tumor (Levi-Montalcini et al., '54). An extract prepared from the mouse salivary glands also promoted exuberant nerve growth *in vitro* on chick ganglia, as well as on ganglia from the mouse and rat (Levi-Montalcini and Cohen, '60; Levi-Montalcini and Angeletti, '61, '63). Some of the chemical properties of the nerve growth factor were identified by Cohen ('60). It was nondialyzable, heat-labile, destroyed by acid, stable to alkali, had an ultraviolet absorption peak at 279 mμ and an estimated molecular weight of 44,000. The specific source and precise chemical structure of the protein have not been determined. An antiserum to this nerve growth factor was produced in rabbits. The antiserum, when injected into young mice, selectively destroyed the sympathetic chain ganglia, especially if administered at birth (Levi-Montalcini and Booker, '60). Attempts to promote neuron regeneration with the use of nerve growth factor after injury to the cat spinal cord were inconclusive (Scott, '63). For a more complete discussion of regeneration in the central nervous system, the reader is referred to Windle ('55).

CHAPTER 5

Neuroglia, Ependyma and Choroid Plexus

NEUROGLIA

The non-neural elements which form the interstitial tissue of the nervous system are known as neuroglia (i.e., "nerve glue," Virchow, 1860). Early investigators recognized that neuroglia separated neural elements from blood vessels and regarded neuroglia as an interstitial material in which characteristic stellate and spindle-shaped cells were suspended. Although peripheral nerves have a connective tissue supporting framework, this is lacking in the central nervous system. In the brain and spinal cord connective tissue is limited to membranes which surround and envelop them (i.e., the meninges) and small extensions of these membranes which accompany blood vessels that penetrate neural tissue. The meninges form a container in which the brain and spinal cord are "floated" in the cerebrospinal fluid. The structural features of neuroglia are difficult to demonstrate except by complex selective staining methods. In ordinary preparations stained with basophilic dyes usually only the nuclei are seen. Sections impregnated by the metallic technics of Golgi (1882–1885), Cajal ('13, '16) and Rió Hortega ('19, '21) reveal the different cell types, their processes and their relationships to neurons and blood vessels (Figs. 5-1, 5-2, 5-3, 5-4 and 5-7). The morphological characteristics of neuroglia as observed in the light microscope have been reviewed by Penfield ('32), Rió Hortega ('32), Glees ('55), Scheibel and Scheibel ('58), Windle ('58) and Polak ('65). Although metallic impregnation technics are capricious, studies based on these methods were used to identify neuroglial cell types in electron microscopic preparations. The superiority of electron microscopic studies is due to the fact that all elements of nervous tissue can be observed simultaneously, and tremendous magnifications permit clear delineation of membrane relationships. Electron microscopic studies indicate that the interstitial material of the central nervous system is composed only of neuroglia (Peters et al., '70). Thus the central nervous system is composed almost entirely of two elements, neurons and neuroglia, which are separated from each other by a capillary film of extracellular fluid contained in a space 100 to 200 Å in width (Palay and Palade, '55; Dempsey and Luse, '58).

There is some uncertainty as to the nature and physical magnitude of the *extracellular space* of the central nervous system. Electron microscopic studies indicate that neurons and neuroglia are tightly packed in the central nervous system with spaces no greater than 200 Å wide between individual cells. Estimates of the extracellular space on this basis suggest

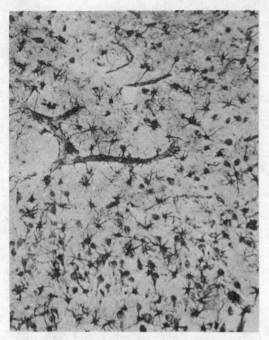

FIG. 5-1. Photomicrograph of astrocytes showing their radially arranged processes and "end feet." Cajal gold-sublimate method. ×150. (Courtesy of Dr. David Bodian, '67, and The Rockefeller University Press.)

the 200 Å extracellular space (Terry, '68). It is apparent that cerebral edema is not a uniform reaction in neural tissue.

In mammals neuroglial cells greatly outnumber nerve cells and they may comprise almost half of the total volume of the human brain. Their counterparts also are a constant feature of the peripheral nervous system. Similar supportive cells are present in all vertebrate nervous systems and in some invertebrate nervous tissue as well (Coggeshall and Fawcett, '64; Bullock and Horridge, '65). The stability of this class of cells phylogenetically suggests that their functional role must be of great importance. Glial cells of the mammalian brain are difficult to study because of their inaccessibility. For this reason information has been sought concerning neuroglia in invertebrates and lower vertebrates (Kuffler and Potter, '64; Kuffler et al., '66; Rosenbluth, '68) and in tissue culture studies (Pomerat, '58; Murray, '58, '65).

Although numerous hypotheses have been advanced concerning the functions of neuroglial cells, most of these are unconfirmed. Among the most widely accepted functions of neuroglia is the role of oligodendrocytes and the Schwann cells in the formation of myelin sheath (Bunge, '68). It has been suggested that neuroglia play an important role in isolating functionally distinct groups of neuronal elements which prevent axon terminals from influencing neighboring and unrelated receptive neuronal surfaces (Peters and Palay, '65; Palay, '66). Neuroglia may also participate actively in maintaining ionic homeostasis and thereby influence the composition of the surrounding extracellular fluid (Rosenbluth, '68). It appears fairly well established that astrocytes play a role in the repair of injuries in the brain and by proliferation can wall off damaged areas (Schultz and Pease, '59; Maxwell and Kruger, '65). A possible role of neuroglia in neuronal metabolism has been suggested because glial cells in invertebrates contain large quantities of glycogen and some lipid (Rosenbluth, '68). Although direct transfer of substrates from glia to neurons remains to be demonstrated, certain glia appear to constitute a reservoir of carbohydrate and lipid. In mammalian glia relatively little

that it occupies about 5% of the volume of the tissue (Horstmann and Meves, '59) which is small compared with other tissues. Measurements of the extracellular space based upon equilibration with sucrose suggest a volume of 10 to 15% (Davson and Bradbury, '65), but some results are misleading because of the blood-brain and blood-CSF barriers. Information concerning the volume, the nature of the fluid filling the extracellular space and the possibilities for controlling both its composition and volume is of great practical significance in relation to cerebral edema. It has been suggested that in a physiological sense, glial tissue, partly or completely, constitutes the cerebral extracellular space (Bakay, '65). Electron microscopic investigations suggest that experimental and clinical edema in the gray matter of the brain may be due to swelling of glial cells, particularly astrocytes (De Robertis, '65). In the white matter where edema is more severe, the enlargement is primarily in the extracellular region with marked widening of

Protoplasmic astrocytes of gray matter

Fibrous astrocytes of white matter

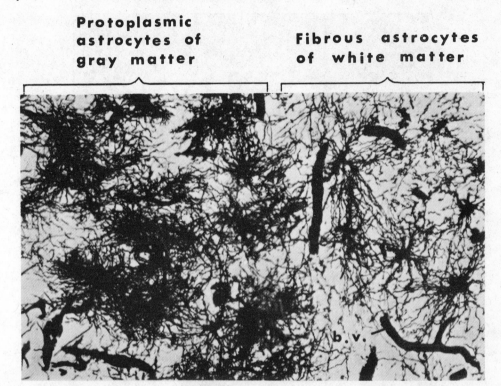

FIG. 5-2. Distribution and appearance of astrocytes in gray and white matter of human spinal cord. Smaller nerve cell bodies often are obscured by profuse branches of protoplasmic astrocytes. Blood vessels (b.v.) also are stained in such preparations and receive vascular end feet from adjacent astrocytes. Golgi stain. Photograph. ×175.

glycogen is present, but there is a correlation between glia and the length of axons in the central nervous system, which suggests that glia may be involved in the transfer of nutrients to neurons or the removal of metabolites from their environment. It seems certain that neuroglia constitute part of a local homeostatic system which serves to provide an optimal milieu in which neurons can carry out their specialized functions.

Two categories of supporting cells are recognized in the central nervous system, macroglia and microglia (Fig. 5-3). The *macroglia*, astrocytes and oligodendrocytes, are derived from ectoderm, have only one type of cytoplasmic process, do not generate action potentials (Kuffler et al., '66) and have not been observed to provide or receive synapses. Unlike neurons, neuroglia retain the ability to divide throughout life. Proliferation of macroglia occurs particularly in response to injury in

the nervous system (Schultz and Pease, '59). *Microglia* are considered to be of mesodermal origin and enter the embryonic brain and spinal cord when these developing structures are penetrated by blood vessels (Fig. 5-3). No morphological classification of neuroglia is entirely satisfactory, for there may be many intermediate forms between oligodendrocytes and astrocytes (Glees, '55; Luse, '56, '58; Schultz et al., '57; Ramon-Moliner, '58; Robertson and Vogel, '62), and some authors do not consider microglia to be true neuroglial cells (see Peters et al., '70). In the broadest sense neuroglia, often referred to simply as glia, should include the ependyma, the neurilemma cells (Schwann cells) and the satellite cells of peripheral sensory ganglia in addition to the macroglia and microglia. Ependymal, neurilemma and satellite cells are all derived from ectoderm; neurilemma and satellite cells are derivatives of the neural crest (Fig. 3-2).

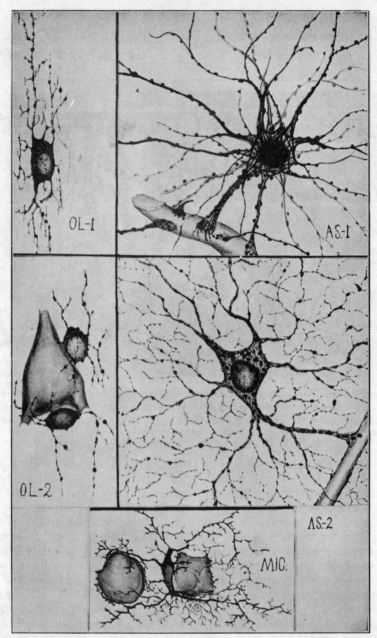

Fig. 5-3. Various types of neuroglia cells. *AS-1*, Fibrous astrocyte with one or two processes forming foot plates against a neighboring blood vessel; *AS-2*, protoplasmic astrocyte with foot plate containing gliosomes (dark granules) in its body and processes; *MIC*, microglia cell whose delicate spiny processes embrace the bodies of two neurons; *OL-1*, oligodendrocyte in the white matter (interfascicular form); *OL-2*, two oligodendrocytes lying against a nerve cell (perineuronal satellites) Penfield, '32).

Astrocytes. These cells are the largest, most numerous and most elaborate of all the glial elements. Astrocytes are recognized by their stellate-shaped cells and their many processes which extend into the surrounding neuropil (Figs. 5-1 and 5-2). Some of the long, branched processes from each cell form expansions that are applied to the surface of blood vessels, where they form the so-called "end feet" or

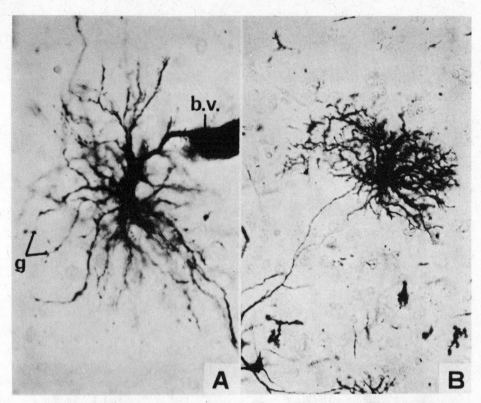

FIG. 5-4. Fibrous (*A*) and protoplasmic (*B*) astrocytes in white matter of adult cerebral cortex. Note numerous gliosomes (*g*) in the processes of the fibrous astrocyte and vascular end foot on blood vessel (*b.v.*). Golgi stain. Photograph. ×550.

"sucker processes." Processes of astrocytes extending to the surface of the central nervous system form similar expansions that constitute the superficial glial membrane beneath the pia mater (Fig. 1-9). Each neuron has a specific relationship with the astrocytic processes in its vicinity, ranging from complete encapsulation to none at all (Palay, '66). They form most of the "packing tissue" of the neuropil of the nervous system (Fig. 5-2), and reduce the extracellular space to a series of irregular and interlacing small clefts. With the Golgi stain these glial cells show a delicate but pervasive framework in which the neural elements appear to be suspended (Fig. 5-2). In sharp contrast to this somewhat rigid configuration, astrocytes in tissue culture show flowing veil-like expansions in all directions, and migrate with a slow, gliding motion (Murray, '65).

Two main types of astrocytes can be distinguished in both light and electron mi-

croscopy. The *fibrous astrocyte* (spider cell) is characterized by its thin, less branched processes which radiate from the cell body for considerable distances. These glial elements often are interposed between neurons and adjacent blood vessels and have prominent perivascular "end feet" (Figs. 5-3 and 5-4). Fibrous astrocytes are most numerous in the white matter (Fig. 5-2). With appropriate stains the cell body and processes are seen to contain many delicate fibrils. Each intracellular gliofilament is 60 Å in width and of indeterminate length. Such filaments correspond to the thicker fibrils observed in muscle and epithelial cells (i.e., myofibrils and tonofibrils). In the larger processes they are arranged in straight parallel bundles and can be followed for considerable distances. Such gliofibrils also are present in the protoplasmic astrocytes to be described below. Another feature common to both types of astrocytes are small granular swellings

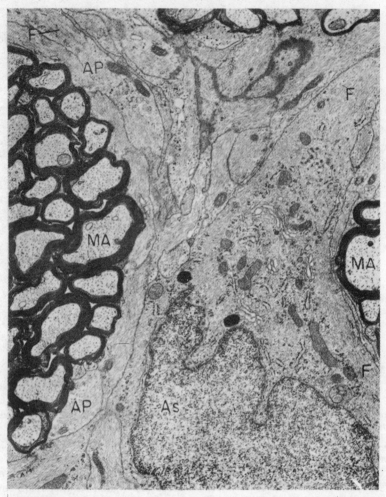

Fig. 5-5. An electron micrograph of a fibrous astrocyte (As) from normal, adult rat optic nerve. The astrocytic cell body contains numerous filaments (F) as do the astrocytic processes (AP) which subdivide the myelinated axons (MA) of the optic nerve into bundles. ×12,000. (Courtesy of Dr. James E. Vaughn, City of Hope Medical Center, Duarte, California.)

along the processes called *gliosomes* (Figs. 5-3 and *g* in 5-4). They occur in the cell body as well, and in electron micrographs they are seen to be clumps of mitochondria which contain a more dense matrix material.

The *protoplasmic astrocytes* (mossy cells) are most numerous and easy to identify in the gray matter (Fig. 5-2). They have numerous freely branching processes, perivascular "end feet," and often are observed in close proximity to neuronal perikarya and dendrites. If fibrous and protoplasmic astrocytes are examined in Golgi preparations (Fig. 5-4) one can

find sharp distinctive cells in each category. In the same sections one also can observe a host of intermediate and transitional cells that defy a precise morphological classification. Electron micrographs suggest the reason: they may represent different forms of the same cell (Maxwell and Kruger, '65; Peters et al., '70). Variations in cell type may in part be a reflection of the cytoarchitectural differences that exist between the gray and white matter of the brain and spinal cord. Electron microscopic features common to both types of astrocytes (Fig. 5-5) are the usual cytoplasmic organelles (dense mitochondria,

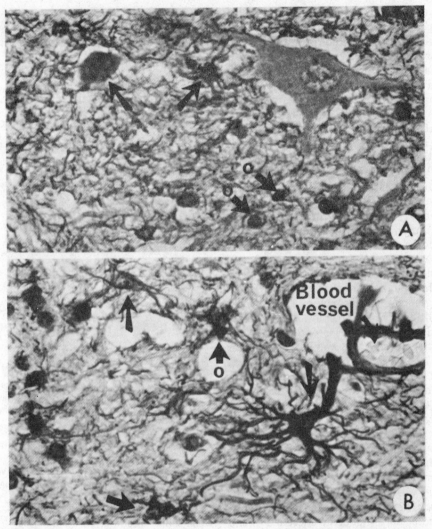

F IG. 5-6. Reactive astrocytes in gray matter of adult human cord 4 weeks after spinal stereotaxic lesion. *A,* Anterior horn cell with adjacent oligodendrocytes (*o*) and swollen astrocytes (*arrows*). *B,* A prominent and bizarre astrocyte with enlarged vascular end foot; several smaller astrocytes with gliofibrils are indicated by *arrows.* The cell body of an oligodendrocyte (*o*) is identified for comparison of relative sizes. Both photographs are of Holzer stain sections. ×550.

scanty granular and agranular endoplasmic reticulum, gliofilaments and an abundant watery cytoplasm). The nucleus is finely granular and only moderately dense, and nuclear pores have been identified (Palay, '58; Maxwell and Kruger, '65). Fine structural characteristics which identify the astrocyte alone were described by the latter authors. These include a watery cytoplasm that contains gliofilaments, and dense glycogen granules 150 to 400 Å in diameter.

Astrocytes, the major guardians of the extracellular space of the central nervous system, play an active role in ionic flow and the regulation of normal neuron metabolism. They demonstrate a wide variety of enzymes which suggests they may be involved in transport mechanisms between the blood and brain (Adams, '65). For example, stimulation of neurons for short periods leads to an increase in RNA, protein and respiratory enzyme activity, whereas there is a concomitant decrease in these units in the surrounding glial cells. Prolonged stimulation on the other hand decreases the RNA and protein of both neurons and glia. Friede ('62) has suggested a predominantly glycolytic role for the astrocyte which is subject to an adaptive change after a variety of injuries. Early accumulation of cytoplasmic glycogen granules in astrocytes has been demonstrated as a very prompt response to alpha (α) particle irradiation (Klatzo et al., '61; Maxwell and Kruger, '65). It is not surprising that the astrocytes show changes in response to a variety of brain injuries (application of solid carbon dioxide, damage to vascular endothelium, ischemia, irradiation, edema, etc.). They react to injury by undergoing swelling or hypertrophy and are said to be *"reactive astrocytes"* (Fig. 5-6). Such cells exhibit markedly increased staining of their perikarya by the periodic acid-Schiff method for certain oxidative enzymes. In the light microscope the reactive astrocytes persist for many weeks after injury. They can be identified by their increased size, prominent cytoplasmic gliofibrils and enlarged vascular "end feet" (Fig. 5-6). Ultrastructural study after α-irradiation has confirmed many of the previously suggested astrocytic alterations (Maxwell and Kruger, '65a). These authors observed a marked increase in the cytoplasmic glycogen granules within 24 hr. This was accompanied by a great increase in the number of dense mitochondria, and a more moderate increase in the Golgi membrane system. After 7 days the cytoplasm was expanded in volume, and the vascular "end feet" were enlarged with even greater amounts of glycogen. The peak in glycogen content occurred at the time when neuronal degeneration was first evident. Such glycogen accumulations in the astrocyte processes were useful markers which pinpointed the zone of maximal ionization. Some reactive astrocytes contained multiple nucleoli, but there was no evidence of mitotic division or that swollen astrocytes were engaged in phagocytosis of extracellular debris (Fig. 5-6). The processes of the astrocytes, filled with gliofibrils and diminished quantities of glycogen and mitochondria, were the major elements in the scar of a fully

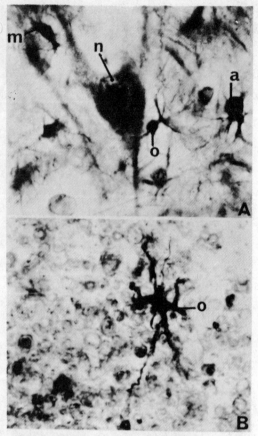

FIG. 5-7. Oligodendrocytes of human spinal cord. *A*, Newborn gray matter to demonstrate relative size of a neuron cell body (*n*), perineuronal (satellite) oligodendrocyte (*o*), astrocyte (*a*) and microglial cell (*m*). Cajal gold sublimate stain. ×565. *B*, Posterior white column of adult cord with oligodendrocyte (*o*). Golgi stain. ×550.

developed laminar lesion. Astrocytes play a similar role in the formation of "glial scars" in man. Whether an actual increase in the number of astrocytes (astrocytosis, hyperplasia) follows central nervous system injury remains unresolved.

Oligodendrocytes. The term oligodendroglia was introduced to describe small neuroglial cells with relatively few processes (Rió Hortega, '21a). The delicate slender processes radiate only a short distance from a spherical or pear-shaped cell body (Figs. 5-3 and 5-7). In sections stained with basic dyes the nuclei of oligodendrocytes are smaller, more regular and more chromophilic than astrocytic nuclei. These glial

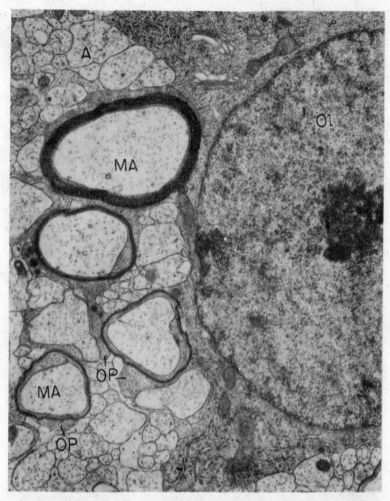

·FIG. 5-8. An electron micrograph of a myelin-forming oligodendrocyte (*Ol*) in a 6-day postnatal rat. Specimen is taken in the ventrolateral funiculus of the spinal cord near unmyelinated axons (*A*) and axons (*MA*) exhibiting different stages of myelination. Oligodendrocytic processes (*OP*) are closely associated with several newly formed myelin sheaths. ×16,000. (Courtesy of Dr. James E. Vaughn, City of Hope Medical Center, Duarte, California.)

cells differ from astrocytes in that: (1) their nuclei are smaller, rounder and more dense, (2) the cell body is smaller and gives rise to fewer processes, and (3) their cytoplasm is more dense, containing chiefly ribosomes, mitochondria and microtubules. The dense chromatin of the nucleus has light patches adjacent to numerous nuclear pores, while the cytoplasm has a crowded appearance, due to large quantities of free ribosomes and rough-surfaced endoplasmic reticulum. Other distinguishing features of their cytoplasm are prominent microtubules, dark and light multivesicular bodies and granular inclusions.

The cytoplasm has mitochondria and a Golgi apparatus, but contains neither fibrils nor glycogen granules (Mugnaini and Walberg, '64; Kruger and Maxwell, '66; Bunge, '68). The plasma membrane of the oligodendrocyte makes close contacts with adjacent myelin sheaths and the processes of adjacent glial cells (Fig. 5-8).

Three principal types of oligodendroglia can be identified by their location and relationships. *Perineuronal satellite cells* are closely apposed to neuron perikarya or their dendrites in the gray matter. This type is the most easily identified in adult material (*OL-2* in Fig. 5-3 and Fig. 5-7).

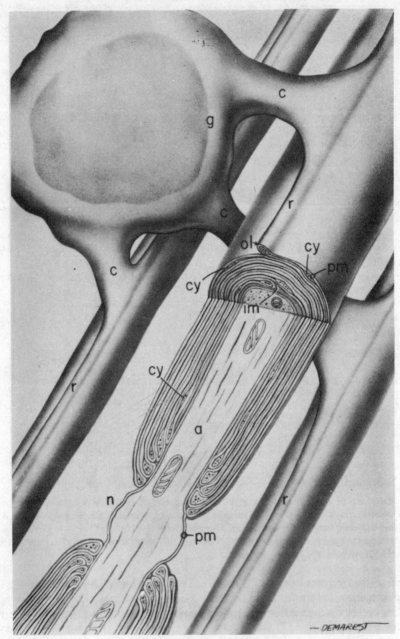

FIG. 5-9. Diagram of the relationship of the oligodendrocyte to the central myelin sheath. The trilaminar plasma membrane (*pm*) is designated by two lines, separated by a space, except in the mitochondrion, where it is represented by a single line. The inner mesaxon (*im*), formed as a glial process, completes the initial turn around the axon (*a*) and starts a second turn; it is retained after myelin formation is complete. Some cytoplasm of the glial process is trapped occasionally at *cy*. A bit of glial cytoplasm also is retained on the fully formed sheath exterior. In transverse sections, this cytoplasm is confined to a loop (*ol*), but along the internode length it forms a ridge (*r*) continuous with the glial cell body (*g*) at *c*. Viewed transversely, the sheath components form a spiral with only the innermost and outermost layers ending in loops. In the longitudinal plane, every myelin unit terminates in a separate loop near a node (*n*). Glial cytoplasm is retained within these loops. (Courtesy of Dr. R. P. Bunge, *Bailey's Textbook of Histology*, '71, and The Williams & Wilkins Company.)

Interfascicular cells occur in the white matter and often appear in rows between the myelinated fibers (*OL-1* in Fig. 5-3). The interfascicular oligodendrocytes are numerous in the white matter of the fetus and newborn. However, they rapidly diminish in number as myelination progresses. After the myelin sheath is formed, only the nucleus remains, so that in adult material their processes rarely are observed (Fig. 5-7B). The third type, *perivascular cells,* are observed less frequently. Oligodendrocytes whose delicate processes terminate as end feet upon adjacent blood vessels have been demonstrated by several authors (Cammermeyer, '66; Luse, '68).

It is suggested that oligodendrocytes act as: (1) an intermediary in neuronal metabolism, (2) a drainage cell, (3) a massaging device for various tissue elements, (4) an energizer to neurons, and lastly, (5) a cell forming the myelin sheath. There is little substantiating evidence for most of these presumed functions. The role of the oligodendrocyte in the myelination and remyelination after injury of central axons, however, does have supporting evidence. The fine structural continuity of the plasma membrane with the myelin sheath (Fig. 5-9), and their active participation in remyelination has been reported in detail (Bunge et al., '61; Bunge, '68). These cells are present in great numbers prior to myelin formation, and at this time there is a marked increase in glial enzyme activity (Friede, '61). In view of their cytoplasmic structure and role in myelin formation, these cells may be responsible for the high oxygen consumption so essential to the maintenance of myelin integrity (Blunt et al., '67). Astrocytes, as well, may participate in the latter function. It should be noted that in mammals the oligodendroglia react to injury by acute swelling, marked increases in a variety of osmiophilic organelles and increased acid phosphatase activity (Maxwell and Kruger, '66). Their study suggested a lysosomal intracellular breakdown of debris rather than phagocytosis by invading microgliocytes.

Microglia. Microglia were recognized as a distinctive glial element by Rió Hortega ('19, '32) when he introduced his silver carbonate staining method (Fig. 5-3). These cells are small in comparison to astrocytes, have elongated or triangular nuclei which stain deeply with basic dyes and have wavy, branching processes that give off spinelike projections. Microglia are found in both white and gray matter, but are more abundant in gray matter (Figs. 5-10 and 5-11). These cells, presumed to be of mesodermal origin, enter the nervous system as perivascular mesenchymal cells, and there is a suggestion that such cells may be preferentially situated near blood vessels. Approximately 10% of glial cells are classified as microglia in light microscopic preparations of the cerebral cortex (Brownson, '56).

Although microglial cells appear inactive in normal adult brain tissue, inflammatory or degenerative processes activate these cells which undergo rapid proliferation and migrate toward the site of injury. Histiocytes from the meninges and blood vessel walls behave similarly. Both types of cells become macrophages and phagocytize debris.

Small numbers of microglia in white matter have processes that wind along or follow myelinated fibers with a remarkable tortuosity (Cammermeyer, '65, '66). A microglia cell has an irregular perikaryon and a few thick processes which often appear to take off from each pole of the cell body. These large antler-like processes divide after variable distances into many smaller branches. Each branch then pursues an irregular and tortuous course either to adjacent neurons, or less often, to a blood vessel wall. The nucleus is ovoid or elongated, which aids in distinguishing the microglia from the oligodendrocyte. The cytoplasm is pervaded by myriads of minute vacuoles, which often gives the cell, or some of its processes, a sievelike appearance (Fig. 5-10A).

In spite of many descriptions of microglia in the light microscopic literature, this cell has not been identified in electron microscopic preparations (Peters et al., '70). Criteria for identification of microglial cells initially were arrived at by a process of elimination (Schultz et al., '57; Farquhar and Hartmann, '57; Mugnaini and Walberg, '64; Herndon, '64). The cell thought to correspond with the microglia

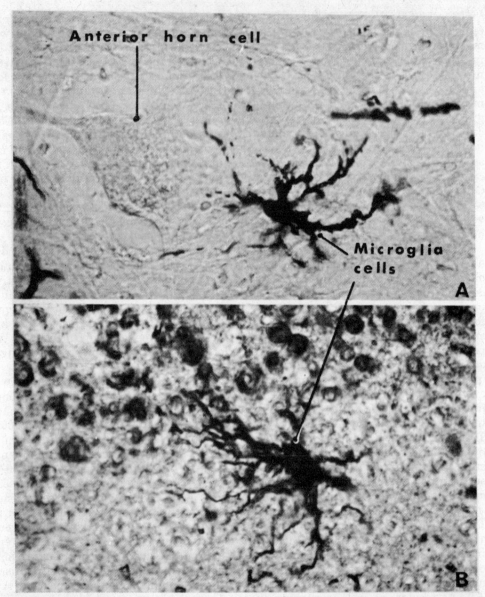

FIG. 5-10. Microglial cells in gray and white matter of adult human cord 3 weeks after a spinal stereotaxic lesion. *A,* Note thickened and stubby processes extending toward an adjacent anterior horn cell. *B,* Note knobby angular processes of microglial cell extending into the dark zone of degenerating fibers above. Golgi stain. Photographs. ×555.

was small with a dark nucleus, dark cytoplasm and compact organelles. Improved methods for fixing and handling central nervous tissue suggest that the crenated dark cells thought to be microglia were damaged cells. Explanations advanced for the failure to identify the microglia in the electron microscope suggest that: (1) oligo-dendrocytes and microglia may represent the same cell at the electron microscopic level, and (2) macrophages may be derived from pericytes of small vessels, rather than from neuroglial elements in the neuropil.

Microglia have long been considered the scavengers of the nervous system (i.e., the reticuloendothelial component of the nerv-

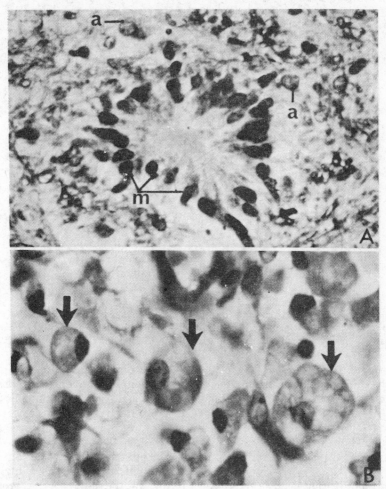

Fig. 5-11. *A*, Carousel formed by numerous microgliocytes (*m*) about a degenerating anterior horn cell 4 weeks after injury of its axon. Two astrocyte nuclei also are identified (*a*). Adult human cord. Luxol Fast Blue-cresyl violet stain. ×555. *B*, Three stages (*arrows*) in the formation of a microglial phagocyte (*gitter cell*). White matter of adult human cord, 4 weeks after a stereotaxic lesion. Luxol Fast Blue-cresyl violet stain. ×655.

ous system). They were presumed to be pleomorphic cells capable of: (1) metamorphosis into a macrophage, (2) undergoing mitotic division and migrating at will through the already formed neuropil, and (3) autolyzing or phagocytizing as a microglia cell (Rió-Hortega, '32; Penfield, '32).

Great numbers of discretely arranged microglial cells have been observed in the regions of experimental injury and edema (Rubinstein et al., '62). Such cellular mobilizations occur as early as 24 hr after cold injury (−50°C) and persist for days. Schultz and Pease ('59) observed a similar accumulation of microglial elements in the

acute phase 24 hr after stab wounds of the cerebral cortex. The microglia underwent a remarkable transformation within this period; they exhibited a rounded appearance as the cytoplasmic volume increased and became less dense so that the nuclei became more prominent. In about 1 week these changes culminated in the formation of typical macrophages with pale cytoplasm and no definite processes. An enlarged macrophage in the central nervous system with a foamy cytoplasmic appearance and ingested material is called a "gitter cell" (Fig. 5-11). As the cytoplasm of the macrophages became packed with in-

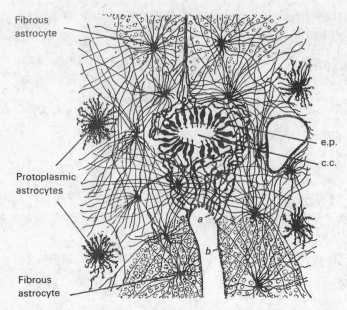

Fibrous astrocyte

Protoplasmic astrocytes

Fibrous astrocyte

e.p.

c.c.

a

b

FIG. 5-12. Ependyma and neuroglia in the central portion of the spinal cord of an infant 8 days old. Golgi impregnation. *a*, Terminal foot plate of ependymal cell; *b*, terminal foot plate of fibrous astrocyte; *c.c.*, central canal; *e.p.*, ependymal cell (after Cajal, '09).

gested material the nucleus was often pushed to the cell periphery. Such phagocytosed particles included myelin and lipoid droplets. Gitter cells dominated their lesions for the 1st week, then decreased in number until 90 days, at which time only an occasional phagocyte was seen (Fig. 5-11).

A similar mobilization is observed in the human nervous system after neuron injury (Fig. 5-11*A*). Three stages in the formation of a gitter cell are indicated by arrows in Figure 5-11*B*. These large vacuolated macrophages may assume a gigantic size and a bloated appearance. When suitable fat stains are used (e.g., osmic acid, oil red O, Sudan black, Sudan III or IV) the vacuolated gitter cells display an unusual number of fat droplets of varying size. There is much speculation, but little evidence concerning the origin of these macrophages. Some investigators consider them to be transformed microglial cells; others believe them to be transformed monocytes, or undifferentiated cells of the perivascular mesenchyme. Maxwell and Kruger ('65a) have presented the strongest evidence to date. They observed a fine structure correlation between the vascular peri-

cyte, the microglia and the gitter cells. They believe the only cerebral element which displays macrophage activity is derived from the vascular pericyte.

EPENDYMA

The ependyma lines the central canal of the spinal cord and the ventricles of the brain. In the embryo the processes traverse the entire thickness of the neural tube to become attached to the pia mater and superficial glial membrane (external limiting membrane) by terminal expansions. Most of the processes retract, so that at birth these processes reach only the pia where the neural wall is thin, as in the basal plate region (Fig. 5-12). In fetal life the ependyma consists of several layers of nuclei, and one can see the large pale nuclei of the germinal cells (*arrow* in Fig. 5-13*A*). Mitotic figures also are easy to identify (*). Cilia are observed in only the embryological stages of man, but persist in some adult animals, such as the rabbit and dog (Figs. 5-13*C* and 5-14). In the human adult the single layer of ependymal cells is cuboidal, while their retracted processes are entwined in the packed astrocytic processes of the *subependymal* (*SE* in Fig. 5-

13) or internal limiting *glial membrane*. There are few places in the nervous system where typical astrocytes and their processes are as concentrated as in this subependymal limiting membrane. During development, the pia-arachnoid pushes a layer of ependymal cells ahead of it, and invaginates into each of the primitive brain ventricles to form the tufted choroid plexuses (Figs. 3-9 and 3-13). The points of attachment, composed of pia mater and the cuboid ependymal cells, form the *tela choroidea* of the fourth, third and lateral ventricles (Fig. 5-16). These points of junction or reflection can be observed in gross brain specimens after the choroid plexus has been removed. The macroscopic torn edge of the ependyma is referred to as the *tenia choroidea* (Fig. 2-22). At the embryonal transition point between the lamina terminalis and tela choroidea of the third ventricle (rostral wall in midline) in mammals one often finds a peculiar mass called the *subfornical organ*. It is located a slight distance above the anterior commissure and medial preoptic area, between the diverging anterior columns of the fornix. This peculiar admixture of tall, modified ependymal cells, glialike cells, nerve cells, fibers and sinusoids appears to be a phylogenetically old structure of unknown function. Akert et al. ('61) have identified this organ in several mammals, and believed it was related to the septal nuclei. Others have ascribed a secretory function or role in the regulation of water balance to this unique cell cluster. Another lamina of ependymal cells is located below the posterior commissure at the junction of the diencephalon and midbrain (Fig. 13-9). This group of cells forms the *subcommissural organ* which is discussed in Chapter 13 (page 376).

Electron micrographs (Fig. 5-14) reveal that the ependymal cell cytoplasm contains small slender mitochondria, vesicles of ergastoplasm, an agranular reticulum, a Golgi complex and compact bundles of fine filaments 90 to 95 Å in diameter, which may be protein (Palay '58; Tennyson and Pappas, '65). Histochemically, the ependymal epithelium exhibits high oxidative activity as reflected by its enzyme content (i.e., acid and alkaline diphosphatase,

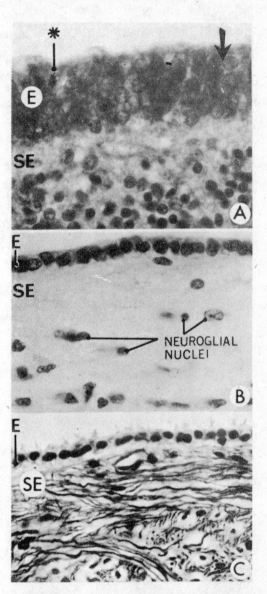

Fig. 5-13. Ependyma of human and rabbit brains. *A,* Ependymal cells *(E)* and subependymal glial membrane *(SE)* in a human fetus of 80 mm crown-rump (C-R) length. Mitotic figure (*) and pale germinal cell nuclei *(arrow)* are indicated. Luxol Fast Blue-cresyl violet stain. *B,* Ependymal cells lining adult human third ventricle. Luxol Fast Blue-cresyl violet stain. *C,* Ciliated ependymal cells lining adult rabbit fourth ventricle. Bodian stain. All photographs. ×655.

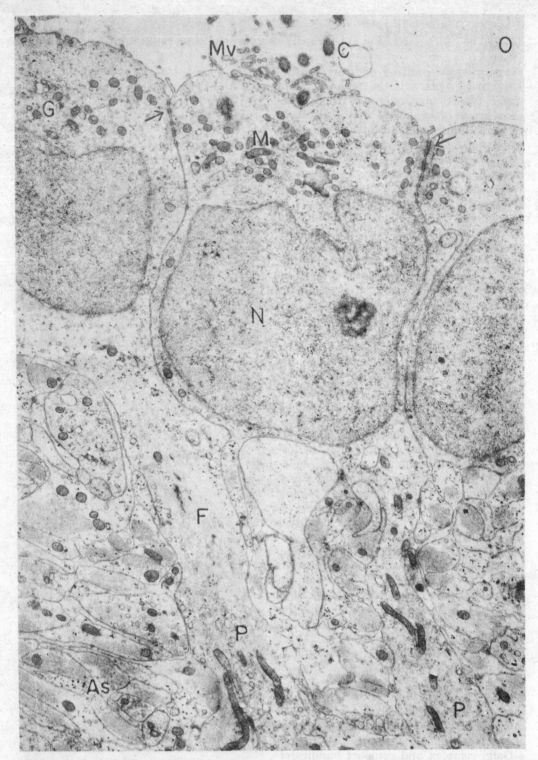

Fig. 5-14. Ependymal cells with long basal processes (P) line the aqueduct of the dog. The apical surface may exhibit short microvilli (Mv) and cilia (C), or may be relatively smooth. Rows of desmosomal-like plaques (*arrows*) join adjacent cells apically. Most of the mitochondria (M) in the cells are scattered randomly, but they are also aligned in rows close to the junctions. The Golgi complex (G) is usually in a supranuclear position. The nucleus (N) may be ovoid or indented and sometimes a nucleolus is seen. Fine filaments (F), similar to those found in the subependymal astrocytic processes (As), are present in the ependymal processes. ×7,800. (Courtesy of Dr. Virginia Tennyson, College of Physicians and Surgeons, Columbia University.)

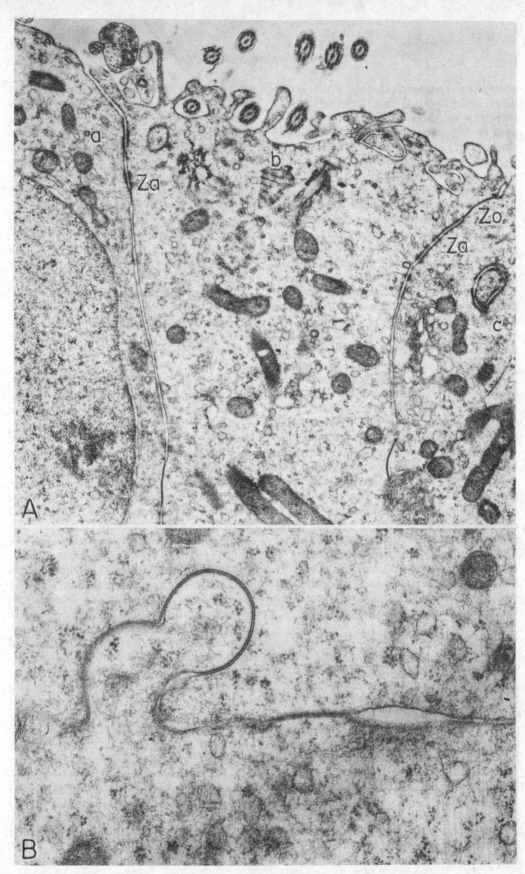

Fig. 5-15 (Legend on Next Page)

131

adenosine triphosphatase). Both structural and chemical reactions reflect the secretory and absorptive functions attributed to the ependymal cells and choroid epithelium (Adams, '65).

It will be recalled that the surface layer of ependymal cells and subjacent astrocytes (i.e., subependymal glial membrane) constitute a brain-cerebrospinal fluid barrier (Fig. 1-16). The lateral cell surfaces of ependymal cells are comparatively simple without elaborate folds or interdigitations. Near the apices of contiguous cells, the apposed surface membranes contribute to the formation of complex intercellular junctions which in light microscopy have been called terminal bars. Electron microscopic studies of the ependyma in the rat brain indicate that the lateral portions of the plasmalemma of contiguous cells are fused at discrete sites to form five-layered junctions, referred to as *zonulae occludens;* which obliterate the intercellular space (Brightman and Palay, '63). These fusions occur at some distance below the free surface (Fig. 5-15). Another type of intercellular junction, the *zonula adhaerens,* occurs near the apices of contiguous cells. Segments of the plasmalemma comprising this junction are characterized by their increased density, and the interspace of the junction contains filamentous material. This structural arrangement appears to form the brain-cerebrospinal fluid barrier, but it is still uncertain whether the ependymal zonula occludens completely seals the intercellular space from the ventricle.

CHOROID EPITHELIUM

The choroid plexuses are formed as a result of the invagination of the ependymal roof plate into the ventricular cavities by the blood vessels of the pia mater (page 65). In human embryos the primordia of all the choroid plexuses develop during the 2nd month of gestation. A mesenchymal invagination into the thin roof area of the fourth ventricle appears first at 6 weeks. The primordia of the telencephalic choroid plexuses become visible in the 7th week, followed in the 8th week by an invagination into the roof of the third ventricle. It is not surprising that extensive structural alterations in shape and microscopic appearances accompany the different stages of choroid plexus development. Four stages were delimited and described in detail by Shuangshoti and Netsky ('66). For our purposes, it will suffice to note that each primordium enlarges, becomes lobulated, and each lobule later demonstrates frondlike expansions (Fig. 5-16). In still later stages many villi develop on the surface. The entire lobulated, vascularized mass remains attached by a broad stalk at the point of the original invagination. The covering cells are at first pseudostratified tall epithelial cells 50 to 60 μ in thickness with a brush border on the luminal surface. At 11 weeks the choroid plexus fills 75% of the lateral ventricle, and the covering tall columnar cells have an abundance of cytoplasmic glycogen (Fig. 5-17). At this stage the mesenchyme of the underlying connective stroma becomes extremely loose and accumulates a large amount of mucin. In the interval between 15 and 17 weeks of gestation the entire plexus gradually decreases in size and the primary villi are better developed. The epithelium changes from low columnar to cuboidal and measures 15x15 μ. The loose underlying mesenchyme decreases in amount, while distinct connective tissue fibers (mostly collagen) make their appearance in the stroma. Between 29 weeks and full term the large cuboidal cells are replaced by smaller ones which are 10x10 μ. The cytoplasm loses its glycogen, while meningocytes, foamy cells and fat-laden macrophages are scattered through the stroma. Once removed, the glycogen never reappears as a normal constituent of the adult choroid epithelium. Such disappear-

FIG. 5-15. *A,* The apical cytoplasm of three contiguous ependymal cells (*a, b* and *c*). The luminal surfaces of cells are joined by the *zonula occludens* (*zo*) which is directly continuous with a *zonula adhaerens* (*za*). ×21,000. In *B,* a *zonula occludens* forms a dovetail type junction between the base of two ependymal cells. The interval between the two dense, parallel membranes can be compared with the usual intercellular space at the right. ×49,000. (Courtesy of Drs. M. W. Brightman and S. L. Palay, '63, and The Rockefeller University Press.)

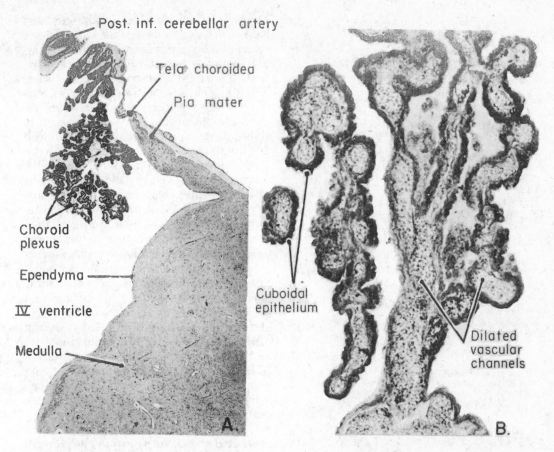

Post. inf. cerebellar artery

Tela choroidea

Pia mater

Choroid plexus

Ependyma

IV ventricle

Medulla

Cuboidal epithelium

Dilated vascular channels

A.

B.

FIG. 5-16. Photographs of human choroid plexus. *A*, Low magnification to show topography and relations of the plexus in the fourth ventricle. *B*, Higher magnification to demonstrate the epithelium and vascularity of two choroid villi.

ance of glycogen after birth, or at the beginning of aerobic oxidation, suggests that the developing nervous tissue uses energy which is released by the anaerobic metabolism of glycogen. Epithelial indentations lining the interlobular clefts may become buried in the stroma during early development and form the choroid cysts observed in the adult human brain (Shuangshoti and Netsky, '66). They appear red due to the blood in the stromal vessels, and the fine leaflike projections endow the choroid plexus with a shaggy surface appearance. Hardened bodies composed of concentric rings of calcium carbonate, calcium and magnesium phosphate also occur in the adult choroid plexus (psammoma bodies). They are generally spherical and originate

around a group of degenerated cells (Schaltenbrand, '55). Psammomatous bodies are usually of small diameter (0.01 to 0.15 mm) and appear to increase in number with age. Studies of morphological and histochemical alterations of the choroid plexus with age indicate that the height of the cuboidal epithelium gradually decreases, proliferated cells eventually desquamate and cytoplasmic vacuoles increase in number (Shuangshoti and Netsky, '70). It seems likely that lipid in the cytoplasm of desquamated choroidal epithelial cells may be one source of lipids in the cerebrospinal fluid.

The histological appearance of the adult choroid epithelial cells after routine staining is shown in Figures 5-16 and 5-17*B*.

They are low cuboidal cells with round and basally located nuclei. The bases of the cells are moderately smooth, while the lateral boundaries interdigitate with adjacent cells and demonstrate terminal bars. Small inpocketings can be seen on all surfaces of the cell (*pinocytosis*) and are regarded as a mechanism whereby surface solutes can be taken into the cell (cell drinking). An occasional cilium may occur on the apical surface of adult choroid cells. Each cell is bounded by a dense continuous cell membrane. On the ventricular surface, each cell is thrown into elaborate, finger-like extensions 80 to 90 mμ in diameter which contain cytoplasmic cores (striated or brush border of light microscopy; *microvilli* in electron micrographs). Microvilli in this instance are a structural device to increase the cell surface and thereby enhance its secretory and possibly absorptive functions (Fig. 5-18). Electron microscopic studies on the developing choroid plexus of the rabbit suggest such a "dual secretory-absorptive" role (Tennyson and Pappas, '61, '64, '68; Tennyson, '71). Their ultrastructural observations also confirm and greatly extend the embryological data of light microscopy which were presented above. As shown in one electron micrograph (Fig. 5-18) the adult choroidal cell contains numerous mitochondria, a Golgi complex, cisternal and tubular elements of the endoplasmic reticulum, numerous small vesicles, dense bodies with a heterogeneous content and occasional cilia. These investigators also called attention to the "pores" present in the capillar-

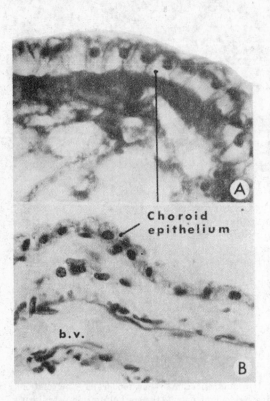

Choroid
epithelium

b.v.

FIG. 5-17. Choroid epithelium of man. *A*, Tall columnar choroid cells in a human fetus of 100 mm C-R length. Holmes' silver with hematoxylin counterstain. *B*, Cuboidal choroid cells of adult brain. A subjacent blood vessel (*b.v.*) is identified. Luxol Fast Blue-cresyl violet stain. Both photographs. ×655.

FIG. 5-18. *A*, Adult rabbit choroid plexus of the fourth ventricle. The cuboidal epithelial cells have a large nucleus (*N*). An occasional cilium (*C*) and polypoid microvilli (*Mv*) line the ventricular surface. Apically, a tight junction seals adjacent cells (*arrow*); near their base, elaborate infoldings (*I*) of the cell surfaces occur. A paranuclear Golgi complex (*G*), numerous mitochondria (*M*), heterogenous dense bodies (*B*) and vesicles are present in the cytoplasm. A basement membrane (*double arrows*) separates the choroidal epithelial cells from the connective tissue which contains collagen (*c*), processes of fibroblasts and other interstitial cells and blood vessels (*bv*). The thin wall of this choroidal capillary is typical. ×8,000. *B*, The thin capillary wall is interrupted by "pores," which exhibit a diaphragm (*arrows*) between the lumen (*bv*) and the interstitial space. A basement membrane (*bm*) coats the surface of the capillary. Fibroblast (*F*). ×66,000. (Courtesy of Dr. Virginia Tennyson, College of Physicians and Surgeons, Columbia University.)

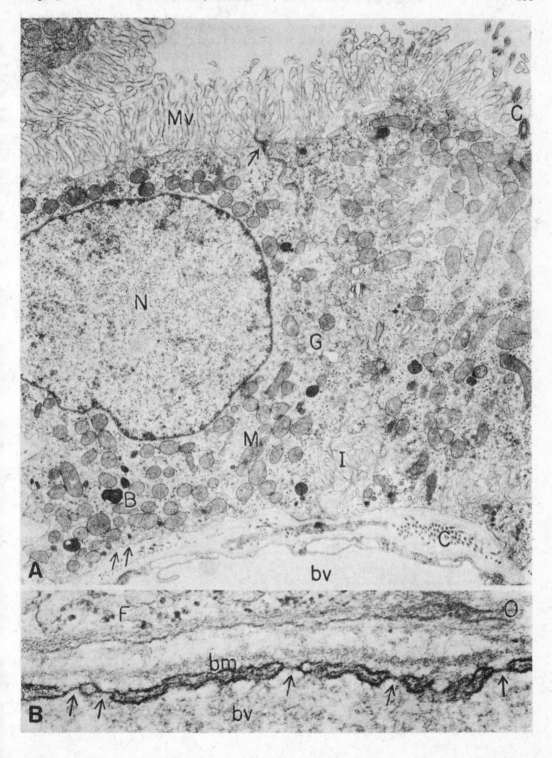

ies of the newborn and adult choroid plexus. However, they found no evidence that thorium dioxide, when injected intravenously, traversed these pores to attain a location within the connective tissue stroma. The authors interpreted such evidence as indicating the existence of a blood-cerebrospinal fluid barrier for this substance in the newborn rabbit. Histochemical demonstration of phosphatase activity in choroid cells, particularly the intracellular location of adenosine triphosphatase and acid phosphatase, should be noted. These hydrolytic enzymes play key roles in metabolically active cells; adenosine triphosphatase participates in the ionic transport at membrane surfaces, and in oxidative phosphorylation within mitochondria. Acid phosphatase is an important constituent of the lysosomes (dense bodies of electron micrographs) which gives rise to pinocytotic vacuoles and appears to play an important part in transcellular transport and digestion, as well as phagocytosis, necrosis and autolysis (Adams, '65). Additional information concerning structure and function of the choroid plexus is available in recent reviews (Dohrmann, '70; Cserr, '71).

It should be recalled that the vascular endothelium, choroidal epithelium and their basement membranes act as an effective barrier which prevents large molecular substances from entering the cerebrospinal fluid (e.g., tagged serum proteins, inulin and fluorescent dyes). However, such substances when injected into the ventricles can slowly pass through the ependyma and subependymal glia to enter the extracellular space of the brain which is guarded by astrocytes (Fig. 1-16). Thus all the neuroglial elements must be considered not only as an impressive structural skeleton, but also as dynamic units that regulate the chemical milieu of nerve cells and probably their metabolism.

CHAPTER 6

Receptors and Effectors

All information we have concerning the world about us is conveyed to the brain by an elaborate sensory system. This input, initiated from the external world, reaches the central nervous system via first order sensory nerve fibers. Sensory receptors and sensory endings act as transducers which change physical and chemical stimuli in our environment into nerve impulses which the brain can read. A *sensory unit* consists of a single peripheral neuron, located in a spinal or cranial nerve ganglion, its peripheral and central ramifications, and, in certain instances, the nonneural transducer cells with which the peripheral nerve fiber may be associated. Information conveyed centrally by sensory units provides an ongoing, constantly changing total picture of the external environment and the stimuli which it presents. From this massive barrage of sensory impulses generated in many different types of receptors and nerve endings, the central nervous system derives precise information concerning the quality, the intensity, the locus and the spatial and temporal patterns of stimuli that elicit sensations. Stimuli in our environment elicit sensory experiences that, within certain limits, can be recognized, described and classified. Each more or less unique sensory experience is referred to as a *sensory modality*. Sensations of color compose a single modality, as do those of tones. General somatic sensibility consists of several sensory modalities which differ in quality and can be distinguished readily as touch-pressure, pain, warmth, cold and sense of position or movement of limbs at joints. Certain substances can be readily differentiated by the way they taste, and the capacity of man and animals to distinguish and discriminate a great diversity of odors is well known. The spatial position of a tactile stimulus can be located with considerable accuracy, especially in certain surfaces of the body, such as the hand or face. Certain forms of sensation arising in abdominal and thoracic viscera are poorly localized, difficult for the patient to describe and sometimes referred to false locations.

A *peripheral receptive field* is the spatial area within which a stimulus of appropriate quality and strength will cause the discharge of an afferent impulse. The receptive field may represent an area of skin in which a mechanical stimulus will excite cutaneous receptors, the angle of joint rotation necessary to excite sensory units, or an area of the visual field in which a light stimulus will evoke discharges in retinal units or the optic nerve. Within a peripheral receptive field the threshold for adequate stimulation varies in that it is usually lowest in the central region where the density of receptor elements is highest. Peripheral branches of one sensory unit often overlap those of adjacent sensory units, and peripheral receptive fields on the body surface vary greatly in size. Cutaneous receptive fields on the digits of the hand are small in comparison to those on proximal portions of the limbs and on the trunk, but the central representation of these densely innervated areas in the cerebral cortex is massive.

Muller's "doctrine of specific energies," interpreted in modern physiological terms, states that different sets of nerve fibers, when activated, elicit different sensations by virtue of their unique central connections (Mountcastle, '74). A particular sensory nerve fiber provokes an identical sensation regardless of how it is excited, that is, by a natural adequate stimulus or by an artificial stimulus. Within a receptive surface, such as the skin, different sets of nerve endings and receptors are distributed in an interdigitated mosaic. Why a particular set of nerve fibers that terminates in an area common to other receptive elements responds selectively to a stimulus of a particular quality is unknown. The modalities and qualities of sensation seem to depend upon the temporal and spatial patterns of activation, the specificity of the sensory endings and the central connections (Davis, '61).

The four elemental qualities of cutaneous sensibility are not distributed uniformly over an area of skin. Within a cutaneous area there is a local differential sensitivity to touch, warmth, cold and pain (Blix, 1884). Each spot receives terminal branches from several afferent nerve fibers and a single nerve fiber may innervate several sensory spots. Regardless of how a particular spot is excited, only one elementary sensory experience is evoked, if the excitation is local. Variations of the elementary sensory experience can be produced by temporal and quantitative variations of the stimulus. The wide variety of complex sensory experiences are thought to be synthesized in the central nervous system from the combinations of activities evoked in afferent nerve fibers, each of which when acting alone is associated with a sensory quality of some purity (Mountcastle, '74).

The manner in which receptors behave in response to a continuing stimulus varies. Some receptors discharge only at the onset of a steady stimulus; these receptors are called *quick adapting*. Other receptors respond to a continuing stimulus with a high frequency discharge for its full duration; these receptors are called *slow adapting*.

RECEPTORS

Classification

No single classification of receptors has evolved which can adequately correlate the principles of structural organization, distribution and function. The three simple categories suggested by Miller et al. ('58, '60) are the least elaborate and restrictive. They suggested that the entire body is served by a basic triad of sensory nerve endings which are either "free," "expanded-tip" or "encapsulated." Such designations are applicable to the endings in glabrous skin and the subpapillary dermis. These terms also apply to the endings observed in fascia, tendons, ligaments, periosteum and synovial membranes (Figs. 6-1 and 6-3). However, difficulty is encountered with such categories in hairy skin and muscle spindle receptors where free nerve and expanded-tip endings are also encapsulated.

Sherrington ('06) classified all receptors into three main groups: *exteroceptors, proprioceptors* and *interoceptors* (Fig. 9-22). Exteroceptors on the external body surface receive impressions from the outside which may, or may not, result in somatic movements. They include touch, light pressure, pain and temperature, smell, sight and hearing. Some of these are *contact receptors;* others, such as smell, sight, hearing and aspects of thermal sense, are activated by distant stimuli and are known as *teloreceptors*.

The conscious proprioceptors, which receive stimuli from the deeper portions of the body wall, especially from the joints, joint capsules, ligaments and fascia, give rise to position sense and the sense of movement (i.e., kinesthesis). They are primarily concerned with the regulation of movement in response to exteroceptive stimuli. These receptors provide sensory information which is utilized in the cerebral cortex to synthesize a conscious awareness of bodily muscle activity and joint movements (*kinesthetic sense*). Most of the receptors related to the knee and temporomandibular joints are diffuse unencapsulated nerve terminals (Gardner, '44; Keller and Moffett, '68). Other specialized receptors (spindles) in skeletal muscle and tendon are activated by muscle contraction and stretch. Their encoded signals regulate muscular activities, either at spinal cord levels (e.g., myotatic, flexor and extensor reflexes), or they reflexly regulate muscle

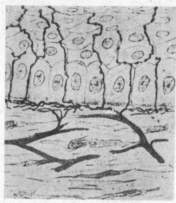

FIG. 6-1. Sensory nerve terminations in corneal epithelium (Cajal, '11).

tone and coordination of muscle activities (i.e., synergy) via projections to specific parts of the cerebellum. Muscle spindles and Golgi tendon organs are somatic receptors, but they contribute no sensory information which enters the conscious sphere; these receptors play no direct role in conscious kinesthetic sense. Nerve endings in skin, joints, fascia, muscle and tendons all transmit afferent nerve impulses from the soma or body wall. Hence exteroceptors, conscious proprioceptors and stretch receptors in muscles and tendons are grouped together as somatic receptors.

The interoceptors (visceroceptors) are the visceral sense organs that receive and transmit poorly localized sensory impulses related to digestion, excretion, circulation and respiration, which are primarily under the control of the autonomic system. They give rise to sensations of taste and visceral pain, to the more obscure forms of visceral sensibility such as hunger, thirst and sexual feelings, and to the general feelings of well-being or of malaise. Smell, although not interoceptive, has close visceral affiliations and may be considered partly visceral.

Sensibility may also be divided into *superficial* and *deep*. The former obviously coincides with exteroceptive sense, and the latter comprises both interoceptive and proprioceptive sense, including deep pressure. A special form of sensation is the ability to recognize the vibrations of a tuning fork applied to bone or skin. This is known as *vibratory* sense, a form of mechanoreceptive sensibility dependent for its unique qualities upon the temporal pattern of the neural inputs. The perception of vibratory sense appears dependent upon two sets of primary afferents, one innervating the skin and one innervating deep tissue (Mountcastle et al., '67). Cutaneous afferents probably convey impulses from Meissner's corpuscles, and deep afferents probably end in Pacinian corpuscles.

In an analysis of clinical problems related to sensation, Head ('05, '20) proposed that there are two different kinds of sensation subserved by dual sensory mechanisms at the periphery. This dual innervation was postulated to consist of a *protopathic* system and an *epicritic* system. Protopathic sensation was considered to be mediated by a primitive system subserving pain and extreme temperature differences which yield ungraded, diffuse impressions of a marked affective character. Epicritic sensation was thought to be mediated by a phylogenetically more advanced system sensitive to smaller temperature changes and concerned with the discriminative aspects of tactile sensation (i.e., precise localization and stimulus intensity). The concept of a duality of cutaneous sensations has been severely criticized (Walshe, '42), but considerable uncertainty still exists with respect to the classification of some sensations which have a psychophysical basis. It seems likely that the protopathic system may be anatomically related to free nerve endings (Rose and Mountcastle, '59), which raises the question whether such endings mediate sensations other than pain. Affective sensations are related primarily to reactions indirectly involving bodily welfare, and neuronal activities at thalamic levels may play an important role in this form of sensation. Thus, affective sensations often are regarded as *vital* or *thalamic*. Discriminative sensibility forms the basis for cognitive and complex associative reactions which involve the cerebral cortex; this form of sensation is regarded as *gnostic* or *cortical*. In a general way, pain, thermal, visceral sensibility and certain aspects of touch are predominantly affective, while tactile sense, kinesthesis and teleceptive sensibilities are predominantly discriminative.

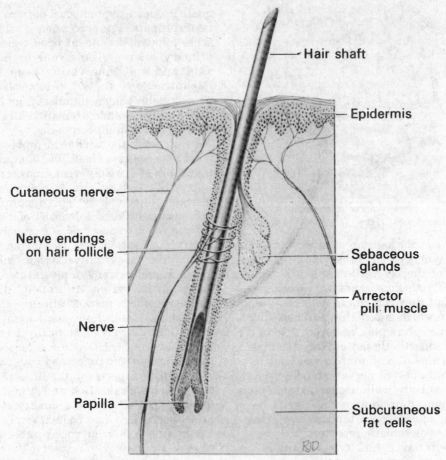

Hair shaft

Epidermis

Cutaneous nerve

Nerve endings
on hair follicle

Sebaceous
glands

Arrector
pili muscle

Nerve

Papilla

Subcutaneous
fat cells

RJD

FIG. 6-2. Nerves and nerve endings in skin and hair follicle.

Physiologically receptors can be classified in terms of the form of energy to which they respond at the lowest stimulus intensity. *Mechanoreceptors,* responding to mechanical forces, include those that subserve touch-pressure in the skin, and position sense and kinesthesis (joints and joint capsules), as well as stretch receptors in muscle, visceral pressure receptors and hair cells in the cochlea. *Thermoreceptors,* responding separately and differentially to warmth and cold, are distributed in spotlike fashion in the skin and vary greatly in their density in different parts of the body. *Photoreceptors* subserving vision respond to light, and *chemoreceptors* initiate impulses concerned with taste and olfaction.

Pain receptors are collectively referred to as *nociceptors* since pain can be produced by different forms of energy (electrical, mechanical, chemical or thermal).

Pain, frequently a frightening sensory experience, is associated with noxious stimuli that injure or threaten to destroy tissue. Because almost all descriptions of pain come from studies in man, many distinctive forms are recognized. Descriptions of particular kinds of pain guide the astute physician in his search to determine the nature and extent of the underlying pathological process. Two aspects of pain are recognized: (1) the distinct sensation, and (2) the psychological reaction to pain which depends upon many variables. Certain stimuli which commonly produce pain evoke other kinds of sensory experience at weaker intensities. Melzack and Wall ('65) have proposed a gate control theory of pain which suggests that pain perception and reactions to pain are triggered after the cutaneous sensory input has been modulated by both sensory feedback mecha-

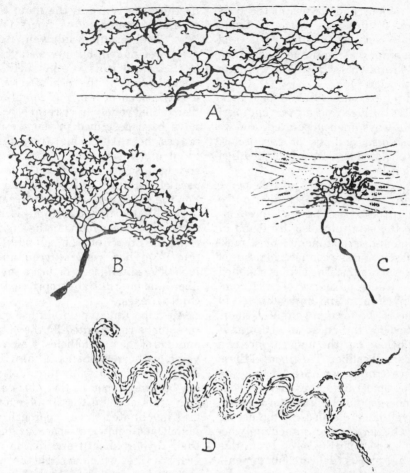

Fig. 6-3. Afferent nerve endings in various visceral structures. *A*, On a large pancreatic blood vessel (after De Castro, '23); *B*, in endocardium of dog (after Smirnow, 1895); *C*, in bronchial musculature of child (after Larsell and Dow, '33); *D*, in longitudinal muscle coat of stomach of cat (after Carpenter, '18).

nisms and the influences of the central nervous system.

Receptors may be regarded as miniature transducers capable of responding readily to appropriate forms of energy (adequate stimulus). An appropriate external stimulus applied to a receptor gives rise to a graded electrical response, known as a "receptor potential." The term "generator potential" is used to define the electrical potential that triggers the "all or none" response in the initial segment of the sensory nerve fiber. If the receptor potential is generated in the first sensory neuron, then it is also the generator potential (Gray, '59; Davis, '61). Such physiological events have been demonstrated best in the Pacinian corpuscle (Loewenstein and Altamirano-Orrego, '58; Loewenstein, '59, '60, '71).

Receptor endings have numerous mitochondria, microvesicles, neurofilaments and even acetylcholinesterase in the case of nerve endings related to hairs. Other receptors are associated with supportive cells that demonstrate a variety of enzyme activities. Free nerve endings appear to be the receptors in fetal life, whereas encapsulated endings appear after birth (Cauna and Mannan, '61). Throughout life receptors show a continuous cycle of breakdown, renewal and reorganization (Cauna, '65). This observation accounts for the variable appearance of Pacinian and Meissner's corpuscles in older individuals.

Different regions and tissues of the body have marked differences in the type and number of receptors. Detailed reviews of cutaneous innervation have been published by Granit ('55), Gray ('59), Quilliam ('66) and Sinclair ('67).

Two main types of receptors appear to be justified: (1) the *free* and *diffuse endings*, which are always unencapsulated, and (2) the *encapsulated* endings or corpuscles, which are enclosed in a capsule of modified supporting cells.

Free Nerve Endings. The free nerve endings are the most widely distributed receptors in the body. They are most numerous in the skin, but also are found in the mucous and serous membranes, muscle, deep fascia and the connective tissue of many visceral organs. The skin is supplied by many cutaneous nerve trunks composed of myelinated and unmyelinated fibers. Some of the large myelinated fibers are destined for the encapsulated organs described below, but the majority are of a relatively small caliber. The fibers of these small nerve trunks separate as they approach the epidermis, lose their myelin sheath, undergo branching and form extensive unmyelinated plexuses in the deeper portion of the dermis and immediately beneath the epidermis (Fig. 6-2). From this subepithelial plexus, delicate fibers penetrate the epithelium, divide repeatedly and form an end arborization of delicate terminal fibrils which wind vertically through the epidermis and end in small knoblike thickenings, upon the surface of the epithelial cells (Figs. 6-1 and 6-2). In the cornea, which has no horny layer, these intraepithelial endings may reach the surface, but in the skin they do not extend beyond the germinative layer. Intraepithelial endings also are found in mucous membranes lined by stratified epithelium, such as the esophagus and bladder. Similar endings may be seen in simple columnar epithelium as well.

Other nerve fibers form unmyelinated arborizations or terminal nets in the connective tissue of the dermis. There is some evidence that the intraepithelial endings are derived from fine myelinated fibers, while the subepidermal arborizations and plexiform nets are in the main terminals of unmyelinated nerve fibers (Woollard, '35). Such terminal unmyelinated fibers are never naked, but are always invested by Schwann cells (Cauna, '66). Diffuse nerve endings in the form of nerve nets, or arborizations of varying complexity, are distributed widely in visceral organs. They have been described in the serous membranes, heart, bronchial tree, alimentary canal and blood vessels (Fig. 6-3). Such endings also are found in the choroid plexuses of the brain and in skeletal muscle. For the most part, they are terminals of unmyelinated fibers. Complicated arborizations have been found in the smooth muscle of the bronchi by Larsell and Dow ('33) (Fig. 6-3). These visceral receptors are endings of medium-sized or large myelinated fibers and may initiate proprioceptive bronchial reflexes.

An important type of diffuse cutaneous receptor is represented by the *peritrichial* endings of the hair follicles, which are activated by the movements of hairs (Fig. 6-2). They vary considerably in complexity and are best developed in the vibrissae of certain mammals. In the simpler forms several myelinated fibers approach the hair follicle just below its sebaceous gland, lose their myelin sheath and divide into several branches which encircle the outer root sheath (Fig. 6-2). From these branches numerous fine fibers run for a short distance upward and downward in the outer root sheath and terminate in flattened or bulbous endings. The smallest hair follicles have at least two stem nerve fibers which form an outer circular plexus and an inner palisading one formed by the longitudinally directed fibers. Larger follicles are supplied by 6 to 10 fibers, while the largest receive between 20 and 30. In the rabbit each myelinated fiber sends branches to 4 to 120 hairs, and an average of 4 different dorsal root fibers supply each hair (Weddell et al., '55). Only free epidermal and dermal endings, and the fibers associated with hair follicles, are found in truly hairy skin.

Besides the intraepithelial endings described above, which end among or upon ordinary epithelial cells, the deeper por-

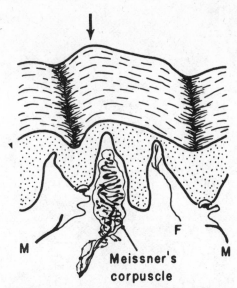

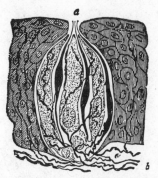

Fig. 6-5. Taste bud from circumvallate papilla of tongue. *a*, Taste pore; *b*, nerve fiber entering taste bud and ending upon neuroepithelial cells. On either side are some free intraepithelial endings (Merkel, 1875).

Fig. 6-4. Diagram of the papillary ridge in glabrous skin showing Meissner's corpuscle in a dermal papilla and Merkel's discs (*M*) on the deep edges of the sweat ridges. A free nerve ending (*F*) is shown in adjacent papilla. *Arrow* indicates direction of most effective epidermal stimulation to elicit touch and tactile two point discrimination (modified after Cauna, '65).

tion of the germinative layer contains somewhat more specialized endings known as the *tactile discs* of Merkel (Fig. 6-4). Each consists of a concave neurofibrillar disc or meniscus closely applied to a single epithelial cell of modified structure. A single epidermal nerve fiber may, by repeated branching, give rise to a number of such discs. These simple endings lie along the deeper sweat ridges between dermal papillae (Fig. 6-4). They are numerous at birth but gradually diminish with age. With the electron microscope the Merkel cell of man and the opossum can be distinguished from epidermal cells (Munger, '65, '66). The Merkel cell has a lobulated nucleus and a massive accumulation of secretory granules (glycoprotein) in the cytoplasm that is apposed to the neurite. Cauna ('65) believes them to be touch receptors which respond to the lever movement that results from deformation of the surface epidermis. In areas of transition to glabrous skin there is a gradual increase in the number of Merkel's discs and Meissner's corpuscles. In glabrous skin, such as

the volar surface of the finger, the epidermis and dermal papillae contain a profuse array of free nerve endings, Merkel's discs and the encapsulated Meissner's corpuscle (Fig. 6-4). The subpapillary dermis under such skin contains a wide variety of endings including the end bulbs of Ruffini, and Krause and Pacinian corpuscles.

The tendency toward modification of epithelial cells receiving sensory nerve endings is exemplified in various *neuroepithelial* cells which have special forms and show staining affinities similar to nerve cells. The specific cells of the taste buds (Fig. 6-5), olfactory mucosa and hair cells in the sensory epithelia of the cochlear and vestibular apparatus are examples of such neuroepithelial cells. Such supportive cells, as well as those forming the lamellae of encapsulated endings, have surrounding basement membranes. It remains to be determined whether they are modified epithelial or transformed Schwann cells.

Diffuse Endings. The deep somatic structures of the human body have unencapsulated sensory endings that are more profuse than those observed in visceral structures (Fig. 6-3). Elaborate nerve endings have been demonstrated by Ralston et al. ('60) in the tendons, ligaments, joint capsules, deep fascia and periosteum of man (Fig. 6-6). Ruffini (1894) originally described an encapsulated fusiform end organ in the skin and adipose tissue. Although long considered as a corpuscle, its morphology is vague and most investiga-

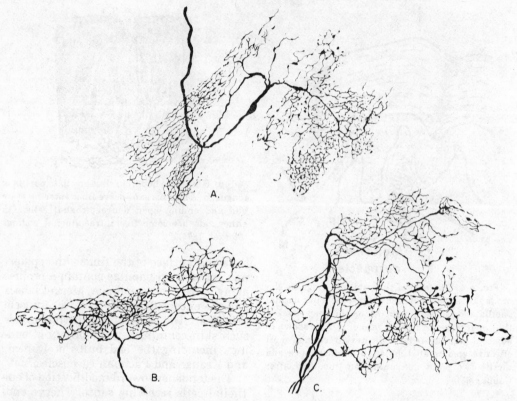

FIG. 6-6. Unencapsulated somatic nerve endings in deep somatic tissues of man. *A*, Patellar ligament; *B*, capsule of knee joint; *C*, periosteum of femur (after Ralston et al., '60).

tors have failed to verify its abundant distribution in man. It may well represent a variation of the diffuse, expanded-tip, unencapsulated endings described by Miller et al. ('60). Encoded messages from these diffuse unencapsulated receptors appear to be an important component of impulses carried by the axons of the posterior white columns. Proprioceptive nerve impulses from these deep receptors play an important role centrally in that they make us aware of the numerous localized body changes that occur during locomotion, standing or sitting.

Encapsulated Endings. These include the *tactile corpuscles of Meissner*, the *end bulbs*, the *Pacinian corpuscles*, the *Golgi-Mazzoni corpuscles*, the *neuromuscular spindles* and the *neurotendinous organs of Golgi*.

The *tactile corpuscles of Meissner* are elongated ovoid bodies, 90 to 120 μ in length, found in the dermal papillae, close to the epidermis (Figs. 6-4 and 6-7). Each corpuscle is surrounded by a thin, nucleated connective tissue sheath, while the interior consists of many flattened epithelioid cells whose nuclei are placed transversely to the long axis of the corpuscle. From one to four myelinated nerve fibers supply each corpuscle. As each fiber enters, its connective tissue sheath becomes continuous with the fibrous capsule. The myelin sheath disappears and the naked axon winds spirally among the epithelioid cells, giving off numerous branches which likewise spiral, show numerous varicosities and end in flattened neurofibrillar expansions. Besides the myelinated fibers, the corpuscles also may receive one or more fine unmyelinated fibers. Meissner corpuscles occur mainly in the hairless portion of the skin and are most numerous on the volar surface of the fingers, toes, hands and feet. They are found in lesser numbers in the lips, eyelids, tip of the tongue and

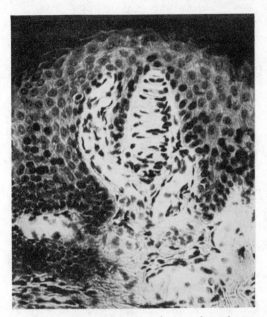

FIG. 6-7. Meissner's corpuscle in a dermal papilla of human finger tip. Photograph.

volar surface of the forearm. It is now apparent that Meissner's corpuscles are formed in excess of adult requirements, and those that survive possess a capacity for continuous growth and reorganization (Miller et al., '60; Cauna, '65). In young persons nearly every dermal papilla contains a small Meissner corpuscle, 25 μ in length. In older individuals, only a few papillae contain corpuscles which are larger and of more irregular arrangement. These endings always are associated with the papillary ridge which plays an essential role in their stimulation. Their relationship is designed so that the nerve endings are stimulated effectively through one surface elevation of the epidermis, which is in line with the long axis of the corpuscle (*arrow* in Fig. 6-4). This arrangement makes the Meissner corpuscle particularly suitable for tactile two-point discrimination (Cauna, '65).

The *end bulbs* resemble the tactile corpuscles in structure and are spherical or ovoid bodies which vary greatly in dimension. The simplest and smallest ones are found in the conjunctiva (Oppenheimer et al., '58); the largest in the connective tissue of the external genitalia, where they are known as *genital corpuscles*. In its

simplest form (Fig. 6-8A), the end bulb consists of a nucleated capsule enclosing a soft gelatinous core in which nuclei may often be seen. One or more myelinated fibers lose their myelin on entering the capsule and give off numerous lateral branches which form a complicated terminal arborization. Some end bulbs may be compound. End bulbs of various forms have a wide distribution, being found in the conjunctiva, mouth, tongue, epiglottis, nasal cavity, peritoneum (and other serous membranes), lower end of rectum and external genitalia, especially the glans penis and clitoris. They also are found in tendons, ligaments, synovial membranes and in the connective tissue of nerve trunks.

The *Pacinian corpuscles (Vater-Pacini)* are the largest and most widely distributed of the encapsulated receptors (Figs. 6-9 and 6-10). They are laminated, elliptical structures of whitish color, and each is supplied by a large myelinated fiber. They differ from the other encapsulated organs mainly in the greater development of their perineural capsule. This capsule is formed by a large number of concentric lamellae; each lamella of the outer bulb consists of a single continuous layer of flattened cells, and is supported by fine collagen fibrils of the interlamellar spaces. The interlamellar spaces contain a network of fine fibers, blood vessels and some free cells in a semifluid substance. Blood vessels accompany the nerve fiber to the capsule but ramify only in the outer bulb. At birth the Schwann cell and myelin sheaths are lost as the large nerve fiber enters the inner bulb. However, the capsule continues to grow and enlarge, so that in the human adult both the Schwann cell and myelin elements can at times be identified within the inner bulb (Cauna and Mannan, '58, '59). No fine nerves enter the inner bulb with the large fiber. Cauna and Mannan found that the average length of the corpuscle at birth was from 500 to 700 μ. The size increases gradually throughout life to become 3 to 4 mm in length. In persons over 70 years of age the corpuscles are less numerous, show regressive changes and are smaller and more irregular. Cauna and Mannan conclude that the Pacinian corpuscle may be a receptor mechanism

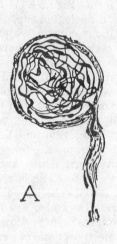

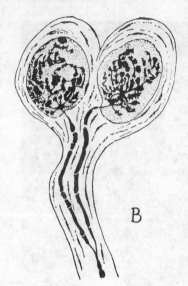

A

B

Fig. 6-8. *A*, End bulb of Krause from conjunctiva (Dogiel, 1891). *B*, Compound corpuscle of Golgi-Mazzoni from the subcutaneous tissue of the finger tip (Ruffini, 1894).

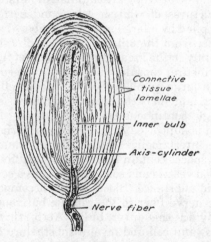

Connective
tissue
lamellae

Inner bulb

Axis-cylinder

Nerve fiber

Fig. 6-9. Human Pacinian corpuscle (after Cajal, '11).

for signalling changes in local blood supply rather than changes in pressure. The entire length of the unmyelinated fiber within the corpuscle is sensitive to deformation, and can initiate "all or none" responses (Ozeki and Sato, '64, '65). They removed the surrounding capsule and found the mechanoreceptor function was still intact. These authors concluded that the short-lasting receptor potential, obtained from intact corpuscles, must be attributed to the mechanical filtering proper-

ties of the lamellae. In addition to pressure the Pacinian corpuscle deep in the limbs may be sensitive to vibratory stimuli. The corpuscles are found in subcutaneous tissue, especially of the hand and foot, in the peritoneum, pleura, mesenteries, penis, clitoris, urethra, nipple, mammary glands and pancreas and in the walls of many viscera. They are especially numerous in the periosteum, ligaments and joint capsules, and they also occur in muscular septa and occasionally in the muscle itself.

Related to the Pacinian corpuscles are the lamellated *corpuscles of Golgi-Mazzoni*, found in the subcutaneous tissue of the fingers and on the surface of tendons (Fig. 6-8*B*). They are ovoid bodies with lamellated capsules of varying thickness and a central core of granular protoplasm in which the single myelinated fiber forms a rich arborization with varicosities and terminal expansions.

Stretch Receptors. Among the most highly specialized encapsulated end organs are the stretch receptors, represented by the neuromuscular spindles and neurotendinous organs.

The *neuromuscular spindles* (muscle spindles) are fusiform in shape and widely scattered in the fleshy bellies of skeletal muscles. Each spindle consists of from 2 to

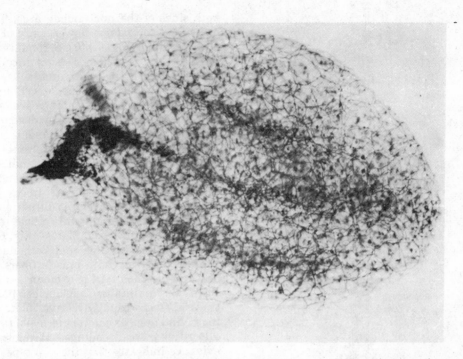

Fig. 6-10. Whole mount of Pacinian corpuscle. Note nuclei of sheets of squamous cells laid one on top of the other, and their continuity with perineural epithelium covering the entering nerve which supplies the corpuscle. Silver nitrate and cresyl violet stain. ×90. (Courtesy of Drs. Shanthaveerappa and Bourne, '66, and the Wistar Press.)

10 slender striated muscle fibers, enclosed within a thin connective tissue capsule, and attached at both ends to the epimysium or ordinary striated muscle (Fig. 6-11). These slender muscle fibers, innervated by γ fibers (3 to 7 μ), are known as *intrafusal fibers,* and they are tiny compared with the *extrafusal fibers* that produce contractile tension within a muscle.

Intrafusal muscle fibers are of two distinct sizes: one is of smaller diameter (10 to 12 μ), is shorter in length (3 to 4 mm) and has a single chain of central nuclei; the second or larger spindle fibers are about 25 μ in diameter, are 7 to 8 mm in length and in the equatorial region are enlarged to accommodate an area of numerous small nuclei ("nuclear bag" of Barker, '48). The small intrafusal fibers are known as "nuclear chain fibers," and the larger ones are designated "nuclear bag fibers" (Boyd, '62, 62a; Barker and Cope, '62). The ends of the nuclear chain fibers are attached to the polar parts of the longer nuclear bag fi-

bers. There are usually two of the longer fibers and five of the smaller fibers in each spindle, but these numbers are variable. A nuclear bag fiber with its capsule and associated sensory and motor nerve endings is shown in Figures 6-11 and 6-12. Two or more myelinated afferent fibers enter each spindle. A thick primary afferent fiber forms a spiral, branching and reticulated ending within the nuclear bag area (primary, annulospiral or nuclear bag ending). Silver-stained primary and secondary sensory endings on intrafusal muscle fibers are shown in Figure 6-13. The primary receptor has a low threshold to stretching of the muscle or its tendon, and also discharges a volley of impulses when the intrafusal fiber contracts as a result of stimulation by a γ efferent motor end plate (Fig. 6-11). The neuromuscular spindle is arranged parallel to the extrafusal or contractile fibers of the muscle; hence tension on the spindle is relaxed and afferent volleys from the annulospiral endings cease

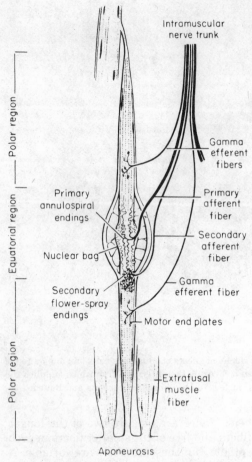

Intramuscular nerve trunk

Polar region

Equatorial region

Polar region

Gamma efferent fibers

Primary annulospiral endings

Primary afferent fiber

Secondary afferent fiber

Nuclear bag

Gamma efferent fiber

Secondary flower-spray endings

Motor end plates

Extrafusal muscle fiber

Aponeurosis

FIG. 6-11. Diagram of a nuclear bag intrafusal muscle fiber within a neuromuscular spindle. The intrinsic sensory and motor nerve endings on the spindle fiber are identified, and the polar and equatorial regions are indicated on the left. Normally there are 2 to 10 small and large intrafusal fibers within each neuromuscular spindle (after Barker, '48).

during active muscle contraction (i.e., the spindle is unloaded, and its receptors are silent). The primary afferent fibers (*Ia* in Fig. 6-12*A*) are 8 to 12 μ in diameter, have fast conduction velocities and their central processes within the spinal cord participate in the monosynaptic stretch (myotatic) reflex that regulates muscle tone (Figs. 9-26 and 9-27).

The myelinated secondary afferent fibers (*II* in Fig. 6-13*B*), with diameters of 6 to 9 μ, also enter the spindle to form small rings, coils and spraylike varicosities on

both sides of the nuclear bag area. These are called secondary, flower-spray or myotube endings (Fig. 6-13*B*). Secondary endings are the principal sensory terminals associated with nuclear chain fibers (Boyd, '62, '62a; Barker and Cope, '62). Both the primary and secondary endings are terminals of sensory fibers, for they degenerate after section of appropriate dorsal roots.

Small fusimotor fibers (γ efferents), 3 to 7 μ in diameter, enter each spindle and terminate. Two kinds of γ fiber endings upon the intrafusal muscle fibers have been described. Some end as diffuse, multiterminal "trail fibers," while others terminate in miniature "end plates" (Fig. 6-14). Barker ('67) maintains that both nuclear bag and nuclear chain muscle fibers usually receive each type of γ motor endings. Boyd ('62) maintains that nuclear bag intrafusal fibers usually receive "plate endings," and nuclear chain muscle fibers usually receive "trail endings." Physiological evidence indicates that the two types of γ axon terminations subserve different spindle functions, and thereby alter the nerve impulses that are generated subsequently by primary and secondary afferent endings of the neuromuscular spindle. Mixed B fibers have been described that innervate both intrafusal and extrafusal muscle fibers (Bessou et al., '63; Adal and Barker, '65).

As noted above, the contraction of intrafusal muscle fibers by γ efferent nerves induces discharges in the afferent nerves from the spindle. The fusimotor fibers thus reset the spindle mechanism and thereby regulate the sensitivity of the receptor. Contraction of the spindle fibers contributes nothing *per se* to the contractile tension of the muscle (Patton, '61). In addition, the neuromuscular spindles receive a variable number of fine unmyelinated fibers which appear to be vasomotor to the small vessels within the spindle. Other fine nerve fibers ramify in the capsule and probably mediate pain impulses.

The recorded dimensions of human muscle spindles vary enormously, the extremes for length being 0.05 and 13 mm. The usual length is 2 to 4 mm. Spindles have been found in practically all muscles but they are most numerous in the muscles of the extremities. They are especially abundant in the small muscles of the hand and foot. Fewer muscle spindles are present in the extraocular muscles (Cooper and Daniel, '49; Merrilles et al., '50; Cooper et al., '55; Greene and Jampel, '66). Cells in part of the trigeminal ganglion convey afferent impulses from muscle spindles in the extraocular muscles (Manni et al., '66).

Information conveyed centrally from the neuromuscular spindles play a major role in the reflex regulation of muscle tonus. Ascending impulses from these receptors are conveyed via relay nuclei in the spinal cord and medulla mainly to the cerebellum and are not concerned with conscious sensory experience. Responses of primary and secondary endings to mechanical stimuli differ in that the primary ending is more sensitive to the dynamic component of the stimulus. Thus, primary endings measure both velocity of stretching and length, while secondary endings measure mainly length. Collaterals from these sensory fibers have monosynaptic junctions with alpha (α) motor neurons (Figs. 9-22, 9-25 and 9-27). More than one internuncial neuron is interposed between these collaterals and the γ efferent neurons as shown in Figure 9-22. If the primary fiber (Ia) from the annulospiral ending is stimulated, there is a central delay of 2 msec before the efferent fiber response is recorded. Hence the annulospiral collaterals use central internuncial neurons to influence γ efferent neurons, and such connections are polysynaptic (Matthews, '64).

Neurotendinous organs (Golgi tendon organs, GTO) are encapsulated spindle-shaped receptors found at the junction of muscle and tendon, and occasionally in muscular septa and sheaths. Golgi tendon organs have been demonstrated in practically all muscles. The capsule of the Golgi tendon organ is approximately 8 to 10 times longer than it is wide and consists of several concentric lamellae that form cytoplasmic sheets closely applied to each other (Merrillees, '62). Cells of one lamella extensively overlap adjacent cells in the same concentric lamella. The outer lamina appears as typical squamous epithelium

without fenestrations, and the extensive overlap of neighboring cell processes suggests that intracapsular fluids are not easily exchanged with extracapsular fluids. The cells which form the capsule of the Golgi tendon organ resemble those of the perineural epithelial sheath surrounding nerve trunks, and the capsule is regarded as a direct continuation of the perineural sheath.

The GTO capsule exhibits four morphologically distinct levels (Schoultz and Swett, '72). At the proximal opening several loosely organized cellular lamellae surround entering muscle fibers. A slight distance below the capsule opening is the proximal collar, where collagen bundles of the muscle fibers are tightly enveloped by capsule cells so as to provide an effective seal between intracapsular and extracapsular fluids (Fig. 6-15). Distally there also is a capsular collar from which collagen bundles leave their capsular investments in a staggered fashion to join the central tendon. The receptor body, occupying nearly 80% of the length of the GTO, lies between the proximal and distal collars. The capsule wall of the receptor body is uninterrupted except for an opening near the midpoint through which the primary afferent fiber (Ib) enters the lumen of the capsule. The lumen of the receptor body is divided by thin cytoplasmic processes into longitudinally oriented compartments which in cross section have a honeycombed appearance. Cells and their processes which partition the lumen have been termed septal cells. These cells resemble fibroblasts and probably originate from lamellae of the capsule wall. In the greater part of the receptor body compartments contain a mixed assortment of collagen fibrils from muscle fibers (Fig. 6-16). A large number of collagen fibrils appear to terminate within the capsule lumen in an undetermined manner.

The primary afferent fiber (Ib) enters the capsule lumen in the equatorial region of the receptor body and divides into major ascending and descending branches. Unmyelinated collaterals from the major branches project radially through openings between septal cells to penetrate pe-

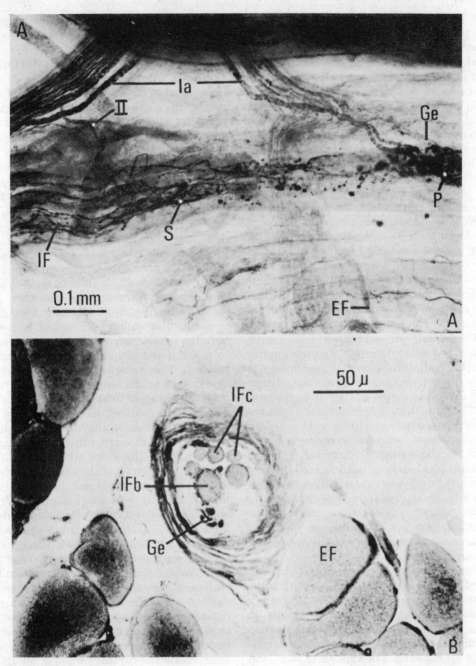

FIG. 6-12. Human intercostal neuromuscular spindle. *A*, Longitudinal squashed preparation showing sensory and motor neural elements related to the intrafusal muscle fibers (*IF*). Compare diameters of sensory fibers (*Ia*) related to primary (*P*, annulospiral) ending, sensory fiber (*II*) of secondary (*S*, flower-spray) ending, and γ efferent (*Ge*) fiber. An adjacent extrafusal muscle fiber (*EF*) and artery (*A*) are identified. *B*, Cross section of muscle spindle demonstrating its multilayered capsule and the diameters of the nuclear bag (*IFb*) and nuclear chain (*IFc*) intrafusal fibers. Gamma efferent axons (*Ge*) and extrafusal muscle fibers are identified. Modified De Castro silver stain. (Courtesy of Dr. W. R. Kennedy, University of Minnesota.)

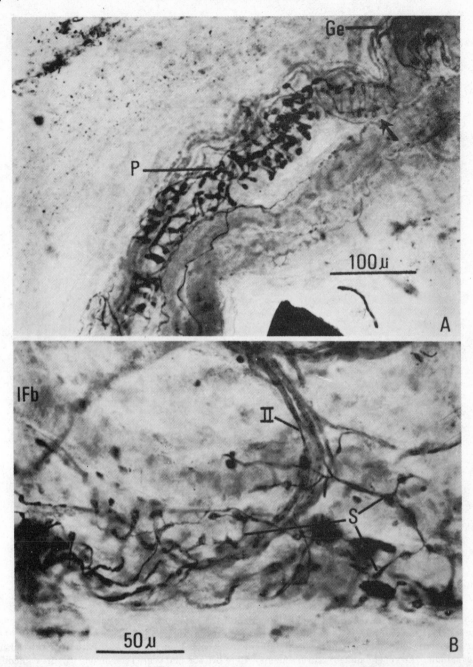

FIG. 6-13. Human intercostal neuromuscular spindles with two types of sensory endings. *A*, Primary (*P*, annulospiral) ending on each intrafusal muscle fiber has a thick axon with many side branches and terminal enlargements. The slender coil (*arrow*) is not seen on all primary endings. Adjacent γ efferent axons (*Ge*) are identified. *B*, Secondary (*S*, flower-spray) endings found on both bag and chain intrafusal muscle fibers (*IFb*). Architecture is similar to that of primary ending except for the slender, delicate nature of the branches. The axon related to this secondary ending is identified (*II*). Modified De Castro silver stain. (Courtesy of Dr. W. R. Kennedy, University of Minnesota.)

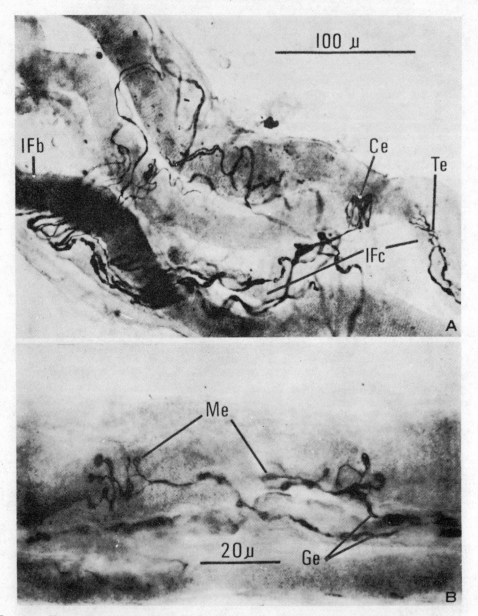

FIG. 6-14. Human intercostal neuromuscular spindle. *A*, γ efferent axons near sensory area that demonstrate trail (*Te*) and coiled (*Ce*) endings. In other sections these axons and endings are found on bag (*IFb*) and chain (*IFc*) intrafusal muscle fibers. *B*, γ efferent (*Ge*) motor end plates (*Me*) found toward capsular pole of spindle. Pairs of end plates occur frequently. Here two end plates are seen on one bag fiber. Modified De Castro silver stain. (Courtesy of Dr. W. R. Kennedy, University of Minnesota.)

ripherally located compartments containing longitudinal collagen bundles derived from muscle fibers. Preterminal nerve fibers branch extensively and spiral around discrete collagen bundles. Attempted se-

rial reconstructions of the GTO indicate that collagen bundles spiral about one another like the strands of a rope and often split to entrap smaller nerve fibers and terminals (Fig. 6-16). Evidence suggests

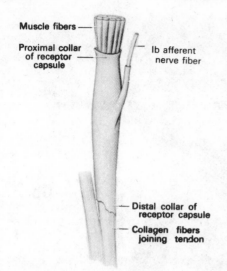

Muscle fibers

Proximal collar
of receptor
capsule

Ib afferent
nerve fiber

Distal collar of
receptor capsule

Collagen fibers
joining tendon

Fig. 6-15. Schematic diagram of a Golgi tendon organ. Muscle fibers converge as they enter the proximal opening of receptor capsule, below which is a slight constriction known as the proximal collar. Ib afferent fiber emerges from the central region of the receptor capsule in a connective tissue sleeve. Near the distal collar of the capsule collagen bundles emerge, and at staggered levels join the fibrils of the central tendon (modified from Schoultz and Swett, '72).

that the mechanical component of the transducer process must involve physical distortion of the axonal membranes during an increase in tensile forces along the collagen strands. It has been suggested that contraction, or passive muscle stretch, would tighten the braided strands of collagen in the GTO, reduce the size of the septal spaces and pinch nerves laced between them (Schoultz and Swett, '72).

The afferent nerve fibers from tendon organ receptors are large fibers of about 12 μ diameter. Golgi tendon organs are relatively insensitive to passive stretch because they lie in series with the contractile muscle that absorbs most of the stretch and prevents elongation of the tendon. Muscle contraction causes the tendon organs to discharge proportional to the tension developed. Contractions which shorten the muscle without developing much tension produce only weak excitation of the tendon organ. If the contraction shortens the muscle, lengthens the tendon

and develops tension, the tendon organs fire vigorously (Fig. 9-26) (Henneman, '68). If the stimulus is appropriate, the tendon organ is an extremely sensitive receptor. Contractions produced by stimulation of an isolated motor unit can easily cause individual tendon organs lying in series with it to discharge (Houk and Henneman, '67).

Afferent nerve fibers from the muscle spindle (primary) and the Golgi tendon organ are large and conduct impulses centrally at rapid rates. In order to distinguish between these two subgroups, the annulospiral afferent nerves are designated as Group Ia, while the tendon organ afferents are referred to as Ib nerve fibers. Stretch receptors in muscle do not furnish information which enters the conscious sphere concerning the position of a limb or joint. These receptors function in the automatic control of muscle tone.

Besides the neuromuscular and neurotendinous organs, muscle and tendon have a variety of other sensory structures: free nerve endings, end bulbs and Pacinian corpuscles. The latter are especially numerous in tendons.

Relation of Receptors to Sensory Modalities

It is generally maintained, although not proven, that each type of receptor is activated by only one kind of physical or chemical change and hence is associated with only one kind of sensory modality. The problem of relating the various receptors to specific sensory modalities has been exceedingly difficult and many important details remain unknown (Sinclair, '67).

It seems probable that painful impulses are received by the diffuse, cutaneous end arborizations. Not only would their universal presence and unspecialized terminals indicate this, but also their sole presence in places where stimuli give rise only to pain (e.g., the tympanic membrane of the ear, the cornea of the eye and the pulp of the teeth). Evidence suggests that the intraepithelial endings derived from fine myelinated fibers are related to sharply local-

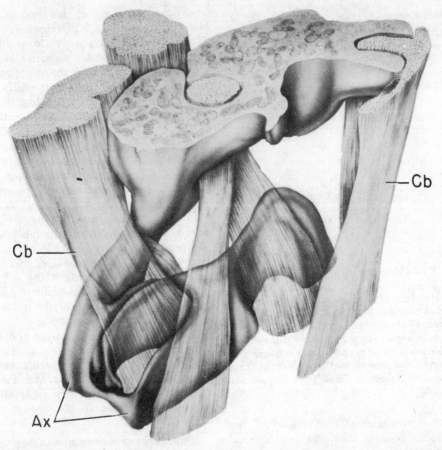

Fig. 6-16. Three-dimensional reconstruction of relationships between axonal branches (*Ax*) and longitudinally oriented collagen bundles (*Cb*) in a septal cell compartment of a Golgi tendon organ (*GTO*). The spiraling axon threads its way through the collagen bundles. Most collagen bundles do not run a straight parallel course through the GTO lumen, but twist like the strands of a braided rope. Increasing tensile forces on the collagen strands cause them to straighten and twist which results in pinching of the axonal branches trapped between them. (Courtesy of Drs. T. W. Schoultz and J. E. Swett, '72, Universities of Arkansas and Colorado, and Chapman and Hall, London.)

ized pain, while poorly localized pain is represented by the subepidermal terminations of unmyelinated fibers (Woollard, '35). It is probable, however, that the intraepithelial fibers also mediate a form of tactile sensibility (Waterston, '33).

Touch is represented by the endings in hair follicles, Meissner's corpuscles, and probably by tactile discs and some other intraepithelial endings. The peritrichial endings, stimulated by movements of the hair, give rise to a sensibility quite delicate and discriminative, yet having a marked affective tone. Shaving greatly reduces the sensibility to touch. On the hairless parts of the body tactile stimuli are received primarily by the corpuscles of Meissner, which are probably the chief sense organs of discriminative touch.

The receptors for temperature are not well known, but they are probably end bulbs of various kinds. Possibly some are diffuse endings. It is known that the margin of the cornea is sensitive only to cold and pain, and is provided only with diffuse endings and end bulbs of Krause. Hence the latter and similar subcutaneous end bulbs are believed to be receptors for cold. In the same way, the diffuse unencapsulated nerve endings are believed to be related to warmth.

The different parts of the body surface

vary considerably as to their capacity for affective and discriminative sensibility. The skin of the hand and fingers is particularly sensitive, and provides a variety of exteroceptive impulses that are integrated in the cerebral cortex. In other regions such as the back, abdomen and especially the genitalia, affective sensibility predominates, to the partial exclusion of discriminative aspects of sensation.

The Pacinian corpuscles, found in both deep subcutaneous and visceral structures, appear physiologically to be pressure transducers, but there is no evidence that they subserve steady pressure, or that pressure sensitivity is particularly acute in regions where Pacinian corpuscles are found. The rapidly adapting nature of the Pacinian corpuscle suggests that it may be particularly sensitive to vibration. This receptor may play a role in the threshold detection of tactile stimuli, despite its deep position, because it has a lower threshold for short mechanical stimuli than more superficial intracutaneous receptors (Lindblom and Lund, '66).

The proprioceptive stimuli of position and movement are initiated by the constant or varying tension states of the skeletal muscles, and their tendons, and by the movements of the joints. The changes in tension and pressure are received by the Pacinian and unencapsulated corpuscles found in the joint capsules, ligaments and periosteum (Fig. 6-6). Such afferent inputs are transmitted to cortical levels where they are utilized in the formulation of kinesthetic sense (conscious proprioception or kinesthesis). On the other hand, proprioceptive impulses from neuromuscular and tendon spindles are used for regulation of the spinal myotatic reflex, or via cerebellar pathways to regulate muscle tonus and synergy (i.e., such sensory inputs are for subcortical reflex control of skeletal muscle). The subcortical regulation of muscle tone and posture thus provides a background of muscle tone upon which discrete cortical (voluntary) activity, such as locomotion and fine finger movements, is based.

There is much that is still obscure about visceral sensibility. It is known that the viscera are insensitive to many mechanical and chemical stimuli, yet they may be the source of intense pain as well as of the organic sensations of hunger, thirst and so on. Visceral pain is due mainly to either distension or spasm of the muscle coats. Hence the intramuscular diffuse nerve endings appear to be the receptors for these stimuli (Fig. 6-3). The blood vessels also may give rise to painful sensation, which is likewise due to muscular spasms in their walls and to the resulting stimulation of similar diffuse endings. The totality of stimuli, constantly initiated by these diffuse visceral receptors during normal and abnormal function, probably gives rise to the general affective sensibility of internal well-being or of malaise.

Referred Pain. One peculiarity of visceral pain is that painful visceral stimuli are often "felt" in the corresponding somatic segment, or segments, of the external body wall, a phenomenon known as "referred pain." Centrally the receptive nuclei for somatic and visceral pain impulses are associated closely within the dorsal gray column of the spinal cord. For this reason, referred pain is most likely due to central mechanisms within the spinal cord, although the precise neurons involved have not been ascertained. A common explanation is that the constant bombardment of pain impulses, from a diseased viscus, lowers the threshold of stimulation of adjacent central (somatic) relay neurons. Normally these relay neurons are concerned with somatic sensations and not with transmission of visceral pain. As a result, normal incoming somatic sensory impulses that terminate in this "sensitized" neuron pool are relayed to higher centers, where they are misinterpreted as painful stimuli coming from body surfaces.

Sinclair et al. ('48) have suggested that the production of referred pain may be due to the branching of the sensory fibers which conduct painful impulses. One limb of a branched axon goes to the visceral site where the disturbance originates, while others go to the peripheral soma to which the pain is referred.

Pain referred to the skin from a viscus tends to be "felt" in a relatively small circumscribed area, usually, but not always, within the compass of the dermatome of the same spinal segment that supplies the viscus. This pain rarely occupies the whole, or even the major part, of the corresponding dermatome. In the reference zone there may be changes in the quality of sensation in response to stimuli and alterations of threshold (Sinclair, '67). Pain is the only sensory modality commonly referred in this manner. Thus, referred pain has a dermatomal distribution corresponding to the spinal nerves. The following are some classical examples of a diseased viscus that causes pain to be referred to the overlying soma and corresponding dermatomes: diaphragm referred to dermatome C4; heart referred to dermatomes C8 to T8; bladder referred to dermatomes T1 to 10; stomach referred to dermatomes T6 to 9; intestine referred to dermatomes T7 to 10; testes, prostate and uterus referred to dermatomes T10 to 12; kidneys referred to dermatomes T11 to L1; and rectum referred to dermatomes S2 to 4 (Figs. 7-1, 7-11 and 7-12).

EFFECTORS

The endings of the peripheral fibers in the effector organs of the body fall into two groups: somatic efferent and visceral efferent. The somatic efferent terminations represent the motor terminals of myelinated axons whose cell bodies are located in the anterior horn of the spinal cord. These fibers go directly to the skeletal muscles. The visceral endings are terminals of unmyelinated fibers which arise from cells of the various autonomic ganglia. These fibers supply the heart (cardiomotor), visceral muscle (visceromotor), blood vessels (vasomotor), hair (pilomotor), salivary and digestive glands (secretory) and sweat glands (sudomotor).

Somatic Effectors. The somatic efferent fibers terminate upon the skeletal muscle fibers in small, flattened oval expansions, the *motor end plates* or myoneural junction (Figs. 4-2G and 6-14). Motor end plates are located in narrow zones in a given muscle. Each end plate always lies in the midportion of the fiber it supplies. Larger muscle fibers have larger end

plates, and in the rabbit and monkey the diameters of end plates differ in "red" and "white" muscle fibers (Coers and Woolf, '59). For example, in red extrafusal fibers the end plates are significantly larger. These muscle fibers are known to be slow reacting and capable of sustained contraction. According to Coers ('55) the mean diameter of adult human limb motor end plates is 32.2 μ. In man most of the end plates have a length of 40 to 60 μ. The myelinated fibers, in their course to the muscle, repeatedly divide, and branch even more extensively as they spread out within the fleshy belly of the muscle. In this manner a single motor nerve fiber provides end plates to a variable number of the large extrafusal muscle fibers (Fig. 4-2G). Each terminal nerve branch loses its myelin sheath as it approaches the sarcolemma of a muscle fiber, while the Schwann cell sheath continues to invest even the smallest terminals. Electron microscopy has confirmed and elucidated many of the structural features of the motor end plate (Reger, '55, '57; Robertson, '56, '60; Couteaux, '58, Zacks, '64). The axoplasm of the small nerve branches contains numerous mitochondria, vesicles, round and oval profiles, small granular elements and tubular-appearing components of the endoplasmic reticulum. Such nerve terminals do not lie within the sarcoplasm of the muscle fiber, as believed previously, but occupy troughs which are hollowed out by infoldings of the sarcolemma (Fig. 6-17). The floor of the trough is usually corrugated by numerous secondary invaginations of the sarcoplasm (junctional folds). The entire depressed area is called a "synaptic gutter." Within the gutter the axon membrane and sarcolemma remain as discrete structures separated by a gap, or synaptic cleft. The whole ending is covered over by Schwann cell cytoplasm. The membranes of the Schwann cell, axon and sarcolemma are all separated from each other by a thin layer of moderately electron dense material (gap substance) which also extends out into the extracellular space around the entire ending.

The synaptic vesicles within the axon terminals of the end plate are presumed to represent the storage form of acetylcholine

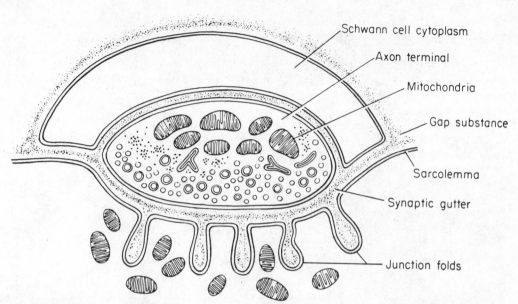

Schwann cell cytoplasm

Axon terminal

Mitochondria

Gap substance

Sarcolemma

Synaptic gutter

Junction folds

FIG. 6-17. Diagram of motor ending on a skeletal muscle fiber as seen in transverse section by electron microscopy. The mitochondria are presumed to play an active role in the synthesis of acetylcholine, whereas the numerous smaller vesicles shown in this diagram may represent a bound state of acetylcholine. Small clusters of dark granules also are found in the axon terminal. Note the separation of axon, Schwann cell and muscle membranes by gap substance. (Modified from Robertson, '56, '60; and from Couteaux, '58.)

(Fig. 6-17). With the arrival of a nerve impulse, numerous quanta of acetylcholine (ACH) are released through the presynaptic membrane into the synaptic gutter. The liberated acetylcholine is absorbed at selective postsynaptic receptor sites, and alters the permeability of the postsynaptic (sarcolemmal) membrane of the muscle fiber. Depolarization and a muscle action potential result from this series of events. That acetylcholine is the chemical transmitter at motor end plates is supported by several pieces of evidence. Acetylcholine occurs widely in the human nervous system, and is released during nerve stimulation. The enzyme acetylcholinesterase is present in the subneural complex of the motor end plate, and rapidly inactivates released acetylcholine. A large number of microscopic histochemical technics have been used to localize the enzymes of the motor end plate in man and numerous animals. These have been reviewed extensively by McLennan ('63) and Zacks ('64). If an inadequate amount of acetylcholine is produced (or it is destroyed too rapidly by acetylcholinesterase), muscle contraction is altered and the involved muscles are prone to early fatigue (e.g., myasthenia gravis). If the en-

zyme acetylcholinesterase is inactivated by anticholinesterase medication (e.g., by neostigmine), the endogenous acetylcholine is preserved at the end plate for longer periods. This rationale when applied to patients with myasthenia gravis often results in a dramatic recovery of muscle strength, and the ability of a muscle to respond to repetitive nerve stimulation.

The axon of one motor neuron supplies a variable number of skeletal muscle fibers. In the larger back muscles (e.g., sacrospinalis, gluteus maximus), a single anterior horn cell may provide motor end plates to over 100 muscle fibers. Each motor neuron to a muscle of the thumb, or an extrinsic eye muscle, may supply only a few skeletal muscle fibers. Namba et al. ('68) have described two kinds of motor endings in the extraocular muscles of man. The superior rectus muscle had both *en plaque* and *en grappe* endings. The levator palpebrae had only *en plaque* terminals with a mean diameter of 27 μ. As many as 12 *en grappe* endings were found on superior rectus fibers 10 to 20 μ thick. *En grappe* endings had a mean diameter of only 9.6 μ. All the skeletal muscle fibers supplied by one motor neuron and its axon constitute a *motor*

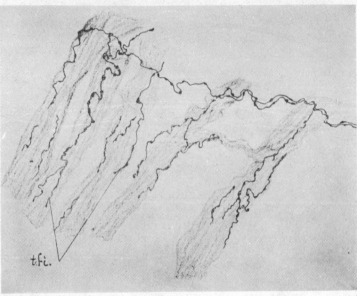

FIG. 6-18. Motor nerve terminations in the smooth muscle bands of a bronchus. Rabbit. *tfi*, Terminal fibrils (Larsell and Dow, '33).

unit. A muscle with many motor units for a given number of muscle fibers is capable of more precise movements than a muscle with a few motor units for the same number of muscle fibers. It also follows that only a few anterior horn cells and motor units are required to maintain reflex muscle tone during periods of rest or sleep. However, many or all motor units may be called into operation when demands are made upon the muscle for maximal contraction.

Visceral Effectors. The unmyelinated autonomic fibers which supply visceral muscle either end in simple arborizations, or first form extensive intramuscular plexuses from which the terminals arise. The terminal fibrils wind between the smooth muscle cells and end in small neurofibrillar thickenings, or delicate loops on the surface of the muscle fibers (Fig. 6-18). Similar terminals arise from delicate plexuses which surround the tubules or acini of glands, pass between the cells and terminate upon the plasma membrane of the glandular cells. Terminal endings occupy small troughs in the plasma membranes of both cardiac and smooth muscle fibers, sometimes for long distances. However, no end plates, or specialized endings, have been observed on the terminals of visceral

motor fibers by either light or electron microscopy. Groups of tiny axons surrounded by Schwann cell cytoplasm do come into intimate contact with single smooth muscle cells of the small intestine (multiaxonal junctions). In the large intestine (toad) single axons diverge from nerve bundles and come to lie, free of the Schwann sheath, in shallow grooves in the muscle cell. It is likely that one muscle cell has several widely separated single axon junctions (Rogers and Burnstock, '66). Axon terminals have either a predominance of granular or agranular vesicles and numerous mitochondria. A plethora of fine nerve fibers and plexuses have been demonstrated about blood vessels and in a variety of tissues by the fluorescence technic developed by Falck et al. ('62). This technic reveals an exquisite array of adrenergic nerve fibers and their terminals and has been used to study the course and relations of adrenergic nerve fibers to the smooth muscle within several organs (Fig. 8-7). The meticulous studies of Thaemert ('66, '66a) are equally informative. He has made three-dimensional montages from serial section electron micrographs to demonstrate the intricate nerve-muscle fiber relationships in both smooth and cardiac muscle.

CHAPTER 7

Segmental and Peripheral Innervation

Although the spinal cord is a long cylindrical, unsegmented structure, the 31 pairs of spinal nerves associated with localized regions produce an external segmentation. On the basis of this external segmentation the spinal cord is considered to consist of 31 segments, each of which receives and furnishes paired dorsal and ventral root filaments (Fig. 9-1). The spinal segments are divided in the following manner: 8 cervical, 12 thoracic, 5 lumbar, 5 sacral and 1 coccygeal. Thus there are 31 pairs of segmentally arranged spinal nerves which receive and distribute fibers to various parts of the body. Spinal nerves emerge from the vertebral canal via the intervertebral foramina. The first cervical nerve emerges between the atlas and the occiput (Fig. 1-4). The eighth cervical nerve emerges from the intervertebral foramen between C7 and T1; all more caudal spinal nerves emerge from the intervertebral foramina beneath the vertebrae of their same number (Fig. 9-3).

Spinal Nerve. Each spinal nerve arises from a region of the spinal cord by two roots, a dorsal afferent root and a ventral efferent one. The two roots traverse the dural sac, penetrate the dura and reach the intervertebral foramen, where the dorsal root swells into the spinal ganglion that contains the cells of origin of the affer-

ent fibers (Figs. 4-1A and 7-1). Distal to the ganglion, the dorsal and ventral roots unite and emerge from the intervertebral foramen as a *mixed spinal nerve* or *common nerve trunk,* containing both afferent and efferent fibers. The dorsal roots are, as a rule, thicker than the ventral ones and vary with the size of their respective ganglia. The first cervical and the first coccygeal nerves represent exceptions in that the dorsal root fibers frequently are absent.

Each dorsal root is composed of myelinated and unmyelinated nerve fibers which vary in size from 0.5 to 20 μ. They are the processes of the large, medium-sized, or small dorsal root ganglion cells. The larger myelinated fibers (10 to 20 μ) convey sensory impulses to the spinal cord from elaborate receptors located in the dermis, subcutaneous connective tissue, muscles, tendons, joint capsules, ligaments, periosteum and deep fasciae. Large afferent fibers conduct rapidly (5 to 120 m/sec) and, by virtue of their several physiological properties, are classified as the *A fiber* component of peripheral nerves. Smaller myelinated nerve fibers in dorsal roots (0.5 to 10 μ) convey sensory information to the cord from less specialized receptors, and from free nerve endings in the skin, viscera, muscles and connective tissues of the body.

159

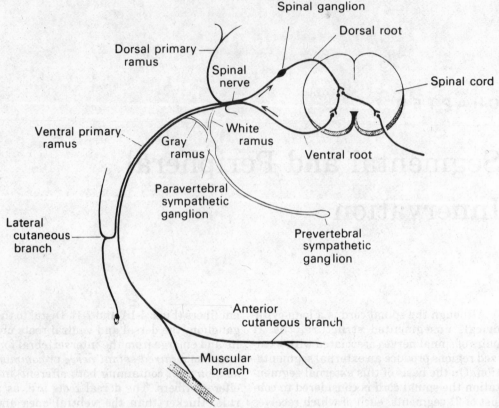

FIG. 7-1. Schematic diagram of a typical thoracic spinal nerve and its branches.

Small, unmyelinated, slow-conducting sensory fibers of the dorsal roots are classified physiologically as *C fibers*. The diameter spectra of the fibers within a dorsal root are shown in Figure 7-6.

The ventral root of a spinal nerve is composed of myelinated axons that vary in diameter from 3 to 13 μ. The vast majority are the axons (9 to 13 μ) of large anterior horn cells (GSE, general somatic efferent) of the spinal cord (Figs. 7-6B and 9-22). They conduct rapidly and have functional properties similar to the large sensory A fibers of the dorsal root. Each large A(α) fiber in the ventral root enters a peripheral nerve and supplies motor impulses to a variable number of *extrafusal muscle fibers* (Fig. 4-2G). Smaller myelinated fibers, 3 to 6 μ in diameter, form a second component of the ventral root (γ efferent fibers). These finer axons arise from smaller multipolar neurons scattered among the larger cells of the anterior gray horn (Figs. 9-21 and 9-22). Such small motor axons of ventral roots and motor nerves are designated as "gamma efferents," and they innervate the *intrafusal fibers* of the neuromuscular spindle (Figs. 6-11 and 9-22). A third fiber component is found only in the ventral roots of spinal nerves T1 to L2 (Fig. 8-1). Such myelinated fibers range from 3 to 10 μ in diameter and are the preganglionic axons of visceral motor neurons (GVE, general visceral efferent) located in the intermediolateral cell column of the spinal cord. These preganglionic visceral efferent fibers leave the ventral root to enter the ganglia of the sympathetic trunk through a white communicating ramus (Figs. 8-1, 8-2 and 9-22). The preganglionic visceral components of the ventral spinal roots conduct more slowly (3 to 15 m/sec); they are concerned with visceral reflexes and are designated as *B fibers*.

Similar preganglionic visceral efferent fibers (parasympathetic) are found in the ventral roots of sacral nerves 2, 3 and 4 (Fig. 8-1).

Spinal Ganglia. The spinal and autonomic ganglia are part of the peripheral nervous system. Almost all of the afferent fibers, both somatic and visceral, have their cell bodies in the spinal ganglia. These aggregations of unipolar nerve cells form spindle-shaped swellings on the dorsal roots (Figs. 1-4, 1-5, 7-1 and 9-1). Each ganglion is surrounded by a connective tissue capsule that is continuous with the epineurium of the spinal nerves. Cells of the spinal ganglia have a peripheral location beneath the capsule, and bundles of nerve fibers entering and leaving the ganglia form a central core (Fig. 7-2). In the trigeminal ganglion the cells and fibers are more loosely arranged. In spinal ganglia the interneural spaces contain large and small axons, satellite cells, Schwann cells and blood vessels.

The unipolar neurons are ovoid or spherical in shape, and often have indentations on their surface contour (Fig. 4-1A). Their cell diameters range from 20 to over 100 μ. Sensory ganglion cells grown in tissue culture and studied by electron microscopy have all the cytoplasmic organelles possessed by other neurons (Tennyson, '65; Bunge et al., '67; Pineda et al., '67). However, these sensory neurons have less prominent Nissl bodies, and scattered cytoplasmic chromatin; the axon often is coiled to form a "glomerulus" within its capsule, and each cell has a variable number of satellite cells. On the basis of their staining properties two types of ganglion cells have been described in the light microscope. The larger cells are lighter, while smaller cells often appear dark (obscure cells; Fig. 7-3). Rapidly preserved tissue fails to demonstrate these two cell types, suggesting that such staining variations may reflect differences in cell metabolism at the moment of fixation (Pineda et al., '67). Bunge et al. ('67) observed light and dark cells in tissue culture and believed this appearance depended on the amount of cytoplasmic neurofilaments. Angular and indented surface margins of the peri-

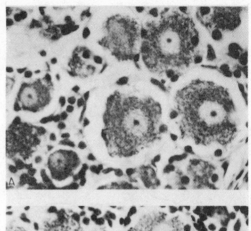
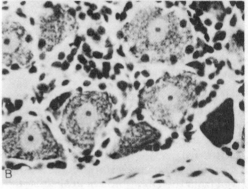

FIG. 7-2. Photomicrographs of normal cells in lumbar spinal ganglion (A) and the superior glossopharyngeal ganglion (B) of the monkey. Note variations in ganglion cell size and small dark nuclei of the capsule cells (Carmel and Stein, '69). Cresyl violet stain. ×500.

karyon represent interdigitations with the processes of surrounding satellite cells. Such ultrastructural extensions of the perikaryon explain the surface spines and excrescences that have been observed in Golgi, silver and methylene blue preparations. These typical, and often bizarre, sensory neurons commonly are observed in ganglia from older individuals (Fig. 7-4). The numerous processes may divide repeatedly or terminate as elaborate end bulbs within the capsule. Sensory neurons with such supernumerary processes have been mistaken by some as multipolar (motor) neurons. However, no one has yet reported vesicle-containing axon terminals or morphological evidence of synaptic contacts within the spinal or trigeminal ganglia. A more detailed study of the sensory ganglia

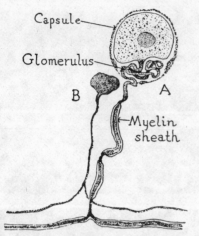

Capsule

Glomerulus

B

A

Myelin
sheath

FIG. 7-3. Two cells from vagus ganglion of cat. A, Large clear cell; B, small "obscure" cell with deeply staining cytoplasm. Ehrlich's methylene blue. (After Cajal, '11.)

and neuronal variations that accompany senescense have been presented by Warrington and Griffith ('04), Dogiel ('08), Ranson ('12), Truex ('40, '41) and Sosa and De-Zorilla ('66).

Satellite cells (capsular nuclei) are derived from the embryonic neural crest and, in the adult, form a concentric layer which closely invests the perikaryon and its unmyelinated axonic coils (Wyburn, '58). The round or elongated nuclei of the satellite cells are more dense than the adjacent perikaryon, and are identified easily with the light microscope (Figs. 4-1A, 7-2 and 7-4). They have ultrastructural features that distinguish them from Schwann cells. Satellite cells display plasma membrane redundancy in the form of folds on the surface that faces the neuron. Such folds and processes may form several layers and interdigitate with the surface evaginations of the perikaryon. The outer surface of the satellite cell is invested with a basal lamina which is continuous with that investing the myelin at the first internode (Pineda et al., '67). The capsule of satellite cells separates the perikarya from adjacent ganglionic capillaries, and must be involved in fluid transport mechanisms. They can increase in number after birth, and may play a role in the metabolism of the ganglion cells.

Studies of cell changes in sensory ganglia, spinal and cranial, in the monkey

indicate that: (1) section of the nerves proximal to the ganglia produces no cellular changes but causes centrally projecting fibers to degenerate, and (2) section of sensory nerves distal to the ganglia produces profuse chromatolytic changes in cells of all sizes and types within the ganglia (Fig. 7-5), but no central degeneration (Carmel and Stein, '69). Severance of nerve fibers distal to sensory ganglia appears to eliminate peripheral neurotrophic influences necessary for the growth and maintenance of the ganglion cell. The integrity of this influence is sufficient to sustain sensory ganglion cells after their central processes have been sectioned.

The Mixed Nerve. After union of the dorsal and ventral roots, the common nerve trunk divides into four branches or rami: dorsal ramus, ventral ramus, meningeal ramus and ramus communicans (Figs. 3-7 and 7-1). The dorsal rami supply the muscles and skin of the back; the larger ventral rami innervate the ventrolateral portion of the body wall and all the extremities. The ramus communicans connects the common spinal trunk with the sympathetic ganglia and consists of white and gray portions (Fig. 8-2). The former contains the myelinated preganglionic fibers passing from the spinal cord to the sympathetic ganglion, while the gray rami contain the unmyelinated postganglionic fibers which rejoin the ventral rami to be distributed to the body wall. The white rami also contain afferent fibers from the viscera whose cell bodies are situated in the spinal ganglia (Fig. 9-22).

The meningeal branch is a small nerve trunk which usually arises as several twigs from both the common trunk and the ramus communicans (Fig. 7-1). It re-enters the intervertebral foramen to supply the meninges, blood vessels and vertebral column.

The dorsal and ventral rami divide into superficial (cutaneous) and deep (muscular) peripheral nerves. These nerve trunks branch repeatedly and become progressively smaller as they extend peripherally. Ultimately these branches break up into individual nerve fibers which terminate in receptors or effectors. The cutaneous nerves are composed mainly of sensory fi-

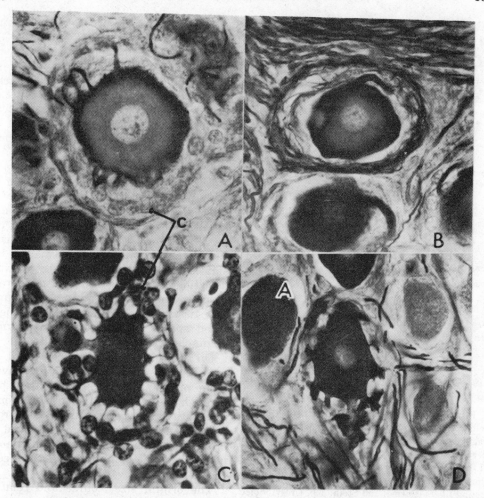

Fig. 7-4. Atypical sensory neurons of adult human trigeminal ganglion. *A*, Fenestrated cell with three looped processes on surface of perikaryon. Satellite and capsular nuclei are identified (*c*). *B*, Pericellular plexus of nerve fibers surrounding unipolar ganglion cell. *C*, Frayed cell (of Cajal) with multiple short processes, most of which terminate in the surrounding capsule. Counterstained with hematoxylin to demonstrate capsular nuclei (*c*). *D*, Erethized or irritated cell (of DeCastro). Note thick, palm-leaf expansions or supernumerary processes that issue from perikaryon and axon. Types shown in *A*, *C* and *D* are often observed in sensory ganglia of older individuals (Truex, '40). Cajal silver stain. All photographs. ×650.

bers of various size, but they also contain efferent vasomotor, pilomotor and secretory fibers for the blood vessels, hair and glands of the skin. In muscle nerves there also is a mixture of sensory and motor fibers. Both somatic α and γ efferent fibers go to the skeletal muscle fibers, while numerous large (A) and small afferent fibers pass centrally from receptors in the neuromuscular spindles and tendon organs. Small pain afferents and postganglionic vasomotor (C) fibers to the blood vessels also are found in the nerves that enter each muscle. Thus in each peripheral nerve there are fibers of various categories: myelinated and unmyelinated, large and small, visceral and somatic, sensory and motor.

While each spinal nerve supplies its own body segment, there is considerable intermixture and "anastomosis" of adjacent nerve trunks. The dorsal rami remain relatively distinct, although interconnections between rami of adjacent segments are common in the cervical and sacral regions (Pearson et al., '66). The ventral primary

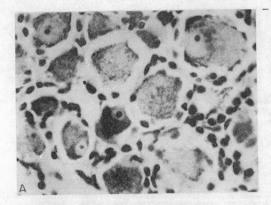

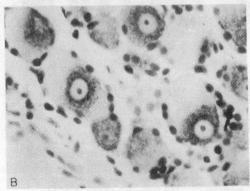

FIG. 7-5. Photomicrographs of chromatolytic cells in lumbar spinal ganglion (A) and the superior vagal ganglion (B) of the monkey after section of the nerve fibers distal to the ganglia. Although lesions of this type produce classic retrograde cell changes, they produce no degeneration in the centrally projecting fibers (Carmel and Stein, '69). Cresyl violet stain. ×500.

rami, however, form more extensive connections. With the exception of the thoracic nerves, which retain their segmental distribution, the cervical and lumbosacral ventral rami branch and anastomose to form the cervical, brachial and lumbosacral plexuses (Figs. 7-14, 7-15, 7-19 and 7-20). In these plexuses a regrouping of fibers occurs, so that each of the peripheral nerves which arises from the plexus contains contributions from two, three or even four ventral rami. The peripheral nerves are therefore "mixed" in a double sense; they consist not only of afferent and efferent fibers, but also of fibers which come from several spinal cord segments.

Connective Tissue Sheaths. Morphologically each peripheral nerve consists of parallel-running nerve fibers invested by a

thick sheath of rather loose connective tissue, the *epineurium* (Figs. 4-22 and 7-7). From this sheath septa extend into the interior and divide the fibers into bundles or *fascicles* of varying size, each of which is surrounded by a fairly distinct perifascicular sheath or *perineurium*. These fascicles do not run like isolated cables but repeatedly divide and join adjacent fascicles in an interchange of fibers (Fig. 7-7). As a result, the fascicular arrangement at different levels varies greatly in portions of the same nerve.

From the perineurium delicate strands invade the bundle as intrafascicular connective tissue or *endoneurium*. This tissue separates the fibers into smaller and smaller bundles and ultimately invests each fiber as a delicate tubular membrane. In the epineurial and perineurial connective tissue blood vessels and endothelial lined spaces communicate with lymph channels within smaller fascicles.

On emerging from the spinal cord, the dorsal and ventral roots receive an investment of connective tissue as they pass through the pia. This tissue is reinforced by additional connective tissue as the roots pass through the arachnoid and dura, the latter becoming continuous with the epineurium of the spinal nerve (root sleeve, Fig. 9-2).

The origin, size, course and relationships of spinal nerves to their respective vertebrae are of great clinical significance. These features of spinal nerves are described in Chapter 9 (page 213) and illustrated in Figures 9-1 and 9-3.

SEGMENTAL INNERVATION

The external segmentation of the spinal cord produced by the spinal nerves corresponds to the general metamerism of the body. Each pair of spinal nerves innervates symmetrically arranged paired somites (metamere). The embryonic somites formed from paraxial mesoderm differentiate into: (1) a *myotome,* which gives rise to muscle, and (2) a *sclerotome,* concerned with the development of the axial skeleton. Efferent fibers in the ventral roots innervate somatic musculature (myotomes) and some ventral roots contain pregang-

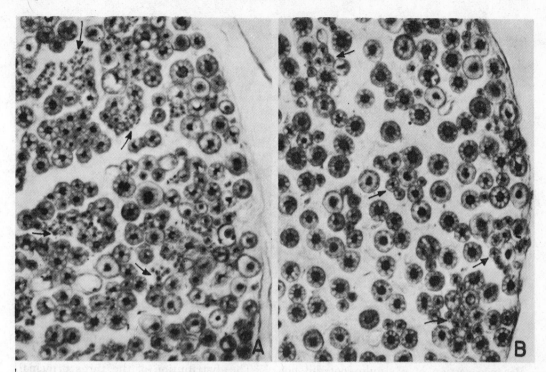

FIG. 7-6. Nerve fibers of dorsal and ventral roots. *A*, Cross section of L4 dorsal root within the dura mater. *Arrows* indicate groups of unmyelinated C fibers. *B*, Cross section of L4 ventral root within the dura mater. *Arrows* indicate axons of smaller γ efferent neurons to spindle muscle fibers. Larger α axons supply groups of skeletal muscle fibers. Holmes' silver-Luxol Fast Blue stain. Photograph. ×275.

lionic autonomic fibers which pass to autonomic ganglia which in turn give rise to postganglionic fibers that innervate blood vessels, visceral muscle and glandular epithelium. The dorsal roots contain all afferent fibers, somatic and visceral (Fig. 9-22). The cutaneous area supplied by fibers from a single dorsal root and its ganglion is called a *dermatome* (Figs. 7-9, 7-11, 7-12 and 7-13).

In the adult, the correspondence between neural and body metameres is recognized readily in the trunk region, where each spinal nerve supplies the musculature and cutaneous area of its own segment. In this region the dermatomes follow one another consecutively, each forming a band encircling the body from the midposterior to the midanterior line (Figs. 7-11 and 7-12). In the extremities, the dermatomes have a more complex arrangement. During development, the metameres migrate distally into the limb buds and arrange themselves parallel to the long axis of the future limb (Fig. 7-8). In each extremity consecutive segments which have migrated peripherally are arranged about an axial line (Fig. 7-9). As a consequence of limb development, the fourth cervical dermatome comes to lie adjacent to the second thoracic dermatome, and the dermatomes of C5 through T1 lie in the upper extremity (Figs. 7-8, 7-9, 7-11 and 7-12). For similar reasons, the dermatomes of L2 and S3 are adjacent posteriorly (Fig. 7-9). The intervening segments have migrated peripherally to form the more distal dermatomes of the lower extremity. This migration of metameres in the formation of limbs and the rotation of the lower extremity appears to explain the more complex arrangement of dermatomes in the extremities (Fig. 7-8). In each extremity, there is thus formed an axial line along which are placed a number of consecutive segments which have wandered out from the axial portions.

Sherrington (1893) demonstrated experi-

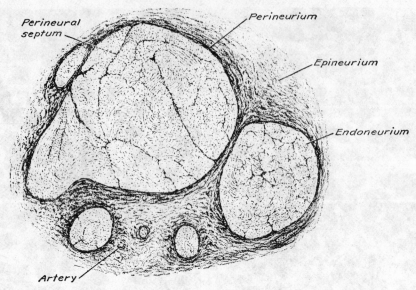

Fig. 7-7. Cross section of sciatic nerve of monkey (Copenhaver, '64).

mentally in the monkey the cutaneous areas supplied by the various dorsal roots. Because section of a single root did not produce a detectable anesthesia anywhere, he selected a specific root for study and cut two or three adjacent roots above and below. He found that each dermatome overlapped the sensory cutaneous areas of adjacent roots, being coinnervated by the one above and the one below (Fig. 7-10); hence at least three contiguous dorsal roots had to be sectioned to produce a region of complete anesthesia. Findings similar to those of Sherrington were obtained by irritating single roots or ganglia with strychnine and noting the resulting hypersensitive areas (Dusser de Barenne, '24).

Dermatomes in man were first outlined by mapping the areas of cutaneous eruption and hyperalgesia occurring in association with herpes zoster (shingles), a virus which often affects a single spinal ganglion (Head, '20). Foerster ('33, '36) furnished a remarkably complete map of human dermatomes based upon surgical section of various dorsal roots for the alleviation of spastic conditions, and cases of root injury due to tumors or other causes. His dermatomal maps correspond closely to those of Head ('20) and show the same overlap described by Sherrington (1893) in monkeys. Most dermatomes are supplied by fibers of three, occasionally even four, dorsal roots.

The distribution of the three principal divisions of the trigeminal nerve and the cervical spinal nerves innervating cutaneous regions of the head and neck are shown in Figure 7-13. The only spinal root whose section produces an area of complete anesthesia is C2. Neither C3 nor branches of the trigeminal nerve supply cutaneous regions in the back of the head. There also is virtually no overlap in the areas supplied by the three divisions of the trigeminal nerve. This is in sharp contrast to the overlap demonstrated for spinal dermatomes. In spinal dermatomes the overlap is greater for tactile sense than for pain and thermal sense. The distribution of the human dermatomes is shown in Figures 7-11 and 7-12.

The segmental innervation of the skeletal musculature (myotomes) has been worked out in man and animals by: (1) selective stimulation of the ventral roots (Wichmann, '00; Brendler, '68); (2) study of the pathological changes which occur in the anterior horn cells when a ventral root or motor nerve is cut (Figs. 4-1E, 9-1, 9-21 and 9-22); or (3) study of secondary degeneration of peripheral nerve fibers to muscle after central and peripheral lesions. As in the dermatomes, the majority of the

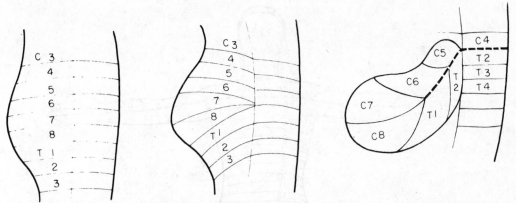

Fig. 7-8. Diagram of various stages in the development of the limb bud for the upper extremity. Dermatomes C5, C6 and C7 occupy the preaxial part of the limb bud, while dermatomes C8, T1 and T2 are postaxial. The axial line is indicated by a *dashed line* (modified from Haymaker and Woodhall, '45).

muscles, especially those of the extremities, are innervated by two or three, and occasionally even four, ventral roots. Hence injury to a single ventral root may only weaken a muscle or have no apparent effect. Only the very short muscles of the trunk and spinal column and a few others, such as the abductor pollicis, are formed from single myotomes and retain a mono-segmental innervation. The peripheral projection of individual spinal cord segments to a specific muscle thus provides a clue to the myotomic origin of skeletal muscle. The segmental motor supply to the major trunk and extremity muscles is shown graphically in Figures 7-16, 7-17 and 7-18. Because this information is essential to a full appreciation of muscle physiology, these figures are included for reference.

Following is a list of some of the important reflex and visceral activities with the locations in the spinal cord of the anterior horn cells that carry them out.

Movements of the head (by muscles of neck), C1 to C4.

Movements of diaphragm (phrenic center), C3 to C5.

Movements of upper extremity, C5 to T1.

Biceps tendon reflex (flexion of forearm on percussion of biceps tendon), C5 and C6.

Triceps tendon reflex (extension of forearm on percussion of triceps tendon), C6 to C8.

Radial periosteal reflex (flexion of forearm on percussion of distal end of radius), C7 and C8.

Wrist tendon reflexes (flexion of fingers on percussion of wrist tendons), C8 to T1.

Movements of trunk, T1 to T12.

Abdominal superficial reflexes (ipsilateral contraction of subjacent abdominal muscles on stroking skin of upper, middle and lower abdomen); upper (epigastric), T6 and T7; middle, T8 and T9; lower, T10 and T12.

Movements of lower extremity, L1 to S2.

Cremasteric superficial reflex (elevation of scrotum on stroking skin on the inner aspect of the thigh), T12 to L2.

Genital center for ejaculation, L1 and L2 (smooth muscle); S3 and S4 (skeletal muscles).

Vesical center for retention of urine, T12 to L2.

Patellar tendon reflex or knee jerk (extension of leg on percussion of patellar ligament), L2 to L4.

Gluteal superficial reflex (contraction of glutei on stroking skin over glutei), L4 to S1.

Plantar superficial reflex (flexion of toes on stroking sole of foot), L5 to S2.

Achilles tendon reflex or ankle jerk (plantar flexion of foot on percussion of Achilles tendon), L5 to S2.

Genital center of erection, S2 to S4.

Vesical center for evacuation of bladder, S3 to S5.

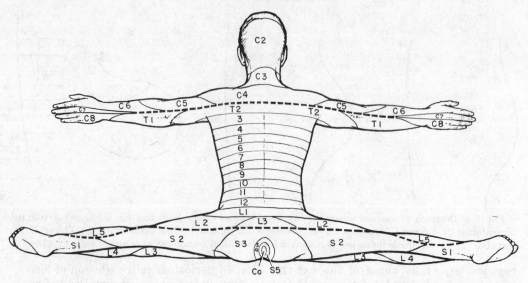

Fig. 7-9. Diagram illustrating the position of the posterior (*dashed lines*) and anterior (*solid line*) axial lines. In the upper extremity the axial lines extend down the middle of the corresponding surfaces of the limb. In the lower extremity the posterior axial line courses down the more lateral part of the leg to the region of the ankle; the anterior axial line begins in the pubic region and winds around the inner aspect of the thigh to reach the posterior surface of the thigh. The pattern of dermatomes is shown with respect to the axial lines (modified from Haymaker and Woodhall, '45).

Bulbocavernosus reflex (contraction of bulbocavernosus muscle on pinching penis), S3 to S4.

Anal reflex (contraction of external rectal sphincter on stroking perianal region), S4, S5 and coccygeal.

PERIPHERAL INNERVATION

In a general way each spinal nerve supplies its own body segment, but there is considerable intermixing and anastomosing of adjacent nerve trunks before they reach their peripheral termination. The primary dorsal rami remain relatively distinct, although interconnections are common in the cervical and sacral regions (Pearson et al., '66). The ventral rami form more elaborate connections. Except for the thoracic nerves, which largely retain their segmental distribution, the cervical and lumbosacral rami innervating the extremities anastomose and branch to form extensive plexuses in which a radical regrouping of fibers occurs. Each of the peripheral nerves arising from these plexuses contains fibers contributed by two, three, four or even five ventral rami. As a result the cutaneous areas (dermatomes) supplied by the peripheral nerves do not correspond with the cutaneous areas supplied by the individual dorsal roots. The peripheral and dermatomal distributions of sensory nerve fibers are contrasted in the anterior and posterior body views shown in Figures 7-11 and 7-12. Similarly, several ventral roots may contribute fibers to a single muscle, and conversely several muscles may receive fibers from a single ventral root. A knowledge of the cutaneous and muscular distribution of the peripheral nerves is of importance to the neurologist in determining the segmental level of peripheral nerve injuries; hence the more important morphological features are presented briefly. A more complete account will be found in textbooks of anatomy and clinical neurology.

Dorsal Rami

The dorsal rami of the spinal nerves innervate the intrinsic dorsal muscles of the back and neck, and the overlying skin from vertex to coccyx (Figs. 7-1 and 7-12). These muscles constitute the extensors of the vertebral column. In the middle of the back the cutaneous area roughly corresponds to that of the underlying muscles, but in the upper and lower portions of the

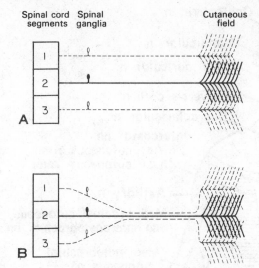

Spinal cord Spinal   Cutaneous
segments   ganglia   field

FIG. 7-10. Schematic diagram illustrating the overlap of cutaneous fields of segmental innervation. In *A*, three intercostal nerves are shown. In *B*, the analogous arrangement is shown for a peripheral nerve in an extremity. Because of the extensive overlaps, section of one spinal dorsal root produces little or no change in cutaneous sensibility (modified from Haymaker and Woodhall, '45).

trunk it widens laterally to reach the acromial region above and the region of the great trochanter below. With certain exceptions the dorsal rami have a typical segmental distribution, the field of each overlapping with that of the adjacent segments above and below (Fig. 7-10). Each ramus usually divides into a medial and a lateral branch, both of which may contain sensory and motor fibers, although the lateral branches of the cervical rami are purely motor. Deviations are found in the upper two cervical nerves (Fig. 7-13) and in the lumbosacral rami. The first or *suboccipital* nerve is purely motor and terminates in the short posterior muscles of the head (rectus capitis and obliquus capitis). The main branch of the second cervical ramus, known as the *greater occipital* nerve, ascends to the region of the superior nuchal line, where it becomes subcutaneous, and supplies the scalp on the back of the head to the vertex, occasionally extending as far as the coronal suture (Figs. 7-12 and 7-13). This nerve is joined by a filament from the third cervical ramus. The lateral branches of the upper three lumbar and upper three sacral rami send

cutaneous twigs which supply the upper part of the gluteal area, extending laterally to the region of the great trochanter. These branches are known as the *superior* (lumbar) and *medial* (sacral) *clunial nerves* (Fig. 7-12).

Ventral Rami

The ventral rami of the spinal nerves supply the ventrolateral muscles and the skin of the trunk, as well as the extremities (Figs. 7-1 and 7-9). With the exception of most thoracic nerves, the ventral rami of adjacent nerves unite and anastomose to form the cervical, brachial and lumbosacral plexuses.

Cervical Plexus

The cervical plexus is formed from the ventral rami of the four upper cervical nerves. It furnishes cutaneous nerves for the ventrolateral portions of the neck and shoulder and for the lateral portions of the back of the head. The muscular branches supply the deep cervical muscles of the spinal column, the infrahyoid muscles and the diaphragm. They also contribute to the innervation of the trapezius (nerves C1 to 4) and sternocleidomastoid muscles, which are chiefly supplied by the accessory nerve (N. XI).

The *lesser occipital nerve* (C2 and C3) is distributed to the upper pole of the pinna and to the lateral area on the back of the head, overlapping only slightly the field of the greater occipital nerve (Figs. 7-12 and 7-13). The *great auricular nerve* (C2 and C3) supplies the larger, lower portion of the pinna and the skin over the angle of the mandible. The *transverse colli* (C2 and C3) innervates the ventral and lateral parts of the neck from chin to sternum (supra- and infrahyoid region). The *supraclavicular nerves* (C3 and C4), which have a variable number of branches, are distributed to the shoulder, the most lateral regions of the neck and the upper part of the breast, where their end branches overlap those of the second intercostal nerve (Figs. 7-11, 7-12 and 7-13).

The chief muscular nerve is the *phrenic,* which supplies the diaphragm and is derived mainly from C4, but receives smaller contributions from C3 or C5, or from both (Fig. 7-15). It frequently receives an anas-

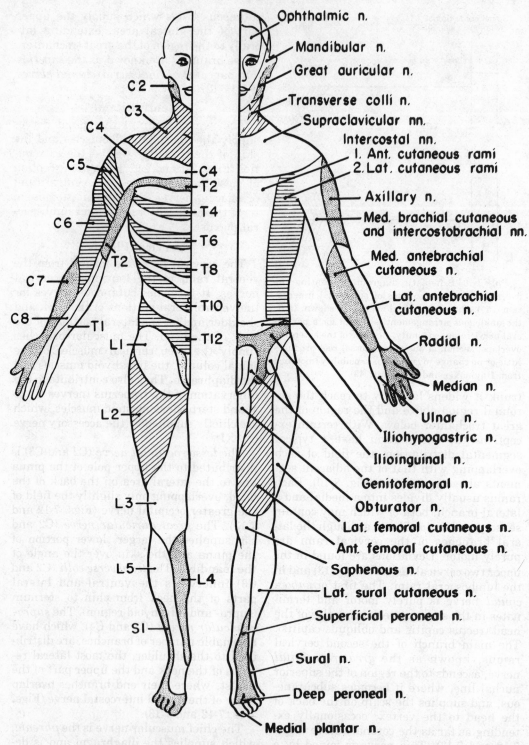

C2
C3
C4
C5
C6
C7
C8
T1
L1
L2
L3
L5
L4
S1

C4
T2
T4
T6
T8
T10
T12
T2

Ophthalmic n.

Mandibular n.

Great auricular n.

Transverse colli n.

Supraclavicular nn.

Intercostal nn.
1. Ant. cutaneous rami
2. Lat. cutaneous rami

Axillary n.

Med. brachial cutaneous
and intercostobrachial nn.

Med. antebrachial
cutaneous n.

Lat. antebrachial
cutaneous n.

Radial n.

Median n.

Ulnar n.

Iliohypogastric n.

Ilioinguinal n.

Genitofemoral n.

Obturator n.

Lat. femoral cutaneous n.

Ant. femoral cutaneous n.

Saphenous n.

Lat. sural cutaneous n.

Superficial peroneal n.

Sural n.

Deep peroneal n.

Medial plantar n.

FIG. 7-11. Anterior view of dermatomes (*left*) and cutaneous areas supplied by individual peripheral nerves (*right*).

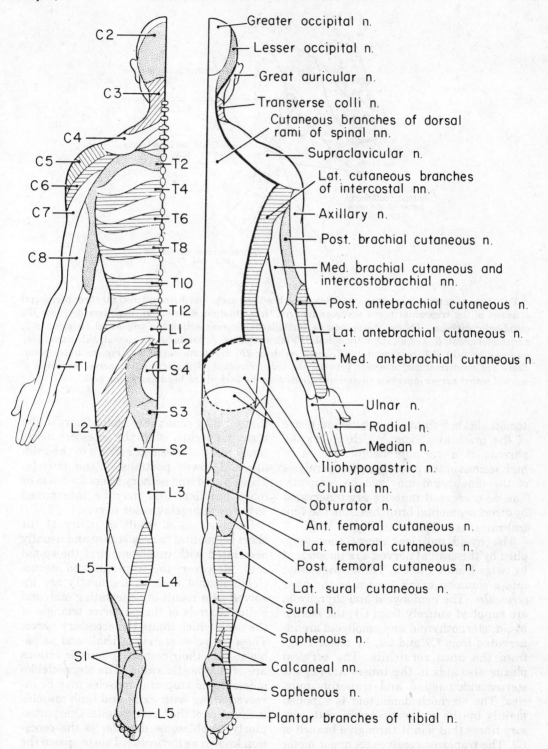

FIG. 7-12. Posterior view of dermatomes (*left*) and cutaneous areas supplied by individual peripheral nerves (*right*).

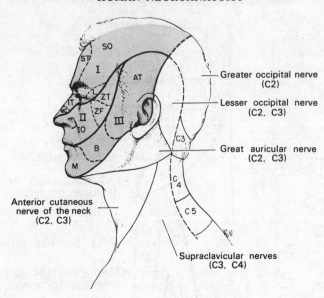

FIG. 7-13. Diagram of the cutaneous fields of the head and neck. The distribution of the three peripheral divisions of the trigeminal nerve are shown in *red* (I, ophthalmic division; II, maxillary division; III, mandibular division). Abbreviations indicate the following nerves within the trigeminal divisions: *AT*, auriculotemporal; *B*, buccal; *IO*, infraorbital; *IT*, infratrochlear; *L*, lacrimal; *M*, mental; *NC*, nasociliary (external branch); *SO*, supraorbital; *ST*, supratrochlear; *ZF*, zygomaticofacial; *ZT*, zygomaticotemporal. There are no dermatomal overlaps between the three divisions of the trigeminal nerve. Branches of cervical spinal nerves innervate cutaneous regions over the back of the head and in the neck.

tomotic branch from the subclavian nerve of the brachial plexus, which enters the phrenic at a variable height. Hence in high lesions of the phrenic nerve, paralysis of the diaphragm may not be complete. The deep cervical muscles are innervated by direct segmental branches from the ventral rami, as indicated in Figure 7-16.

The hyoid muscles, except those supplied by the cranial nerves, are innervated by twigs from C1 to C3. These twigs unite into a common trunk known as the *ansa cervicalis*. The geniohyoid and thyrohyoid are supplied entirely from C1; the sternohyoid, sternothyroid and omohyoid are innervated from C2 and C3, by motor twigs from the ansa cervicalis. The cervical plexus also aids in the innervation of the sternocleidomastoid and trapezius muscles. The sternocleidomastoid is supplied mainly by the accessory nerve, with sensory fibers that join it through a branch of C2. The trapezius receives its major motor contributions from the accessory nerve, and additional motor fibers from C2, C3 and C4. Brendler ('68) also demonstrated

that C1 may contribute motor fibers to the upper trapezius, while the accessory nerve sends most of the motor fibers to the middle and lower portions of the muscle. These motor and sensory fibers form one or more bundles, and may be intermixed with the supraclavicular nerves.

Paralysis as a result of injury of the short segmental nerves is rare and usually associated with involvement of the spinal cord. However, the trapezius and sternocleidomastoid muscles frequently are involved as a result of penetrating stab and bullet wounds of the posterior triangle of the neck which injure the accessory nerve. These muscles are superficial, and palpable so that their respective muscle actions are of diagnostic value. The sternocleidomastoid and trapezius muscles may be involved along with axial and limb muscles in diseases of the basal ganglia. One particularly troublesome disorder is the condition known as *torticollis*. Due to spasm the contracted sternocleidomastoid muscle stands out as a large cord, and the head usually is involuntarily rotated toward the opposite side. This awkward position may be maintained for long periods. Spasmodic torticollis may be associated with neuroses. In the latter cases it is often difficult to distinguish between a functional disorder and organic disease. Emotional stress usually aggravates these involuntary muscle movements.

Brachial Plexus

The nerves supplying the upper extremity and forming the brachial plexus are derived as a rule from the ventral rami of the four lower cervical and the first thoracic nerves, with a small contribution from the fourth cervical nerve (Figs. 7-14 and 7-15). Considerable variations are not uncommon. If the contribution from the fourth cervical nerve is strong and that of the first thoracic negligible, the plexus is referred to as the *prefixed* type. It is called *postfixed* when the fourth cervical does not participate at all, but the first thoracic makes a strong contribution and the second thoracic sends a branch. Between these extremes there are many intermediate conditions, depending on the stronger or weaker participation of the fourth cervical, on the one hand, and the second thoracic, on the other. These variations are dependent on embryological factors. The limb buds of both arms and legs may vary in longitudinal extent and especially in their relative position to the neuraxis. The more cephalic the position of the limbs, the more cephalic will be the nerves contributing to the plexus, and vice versa.

The ventral rami supplying the plexus give rise to three *primary trunks:* C5 and C6 unite to form the *superior trunk;* C8 and T1 form the *inferior trunk;* and C7 is continued as the *middle trunk* (Fig. 7-14). Each trunk splits into a posterior and an anterior division. The posterior divisions of all three trunks fuse to form the *posterior cord,* situated behind the axillary artery. The anterior divisions of the superior and middle trunk form the *lateral cord,* while the anterior division of the inferior trunks is continued as the *medial cord* (Fig. 7-14).

Many of the nerves supplying the shoulder muscles are given off directly from the ventral rami, or from the primary trunks and their branches before these unite to form the secondary cords. Thus the *dorsal scapular* nerve supplying the rhomboids arises from the dorsal surface of C5, and the *long thoracic* nerve to the serratus anterior arises from the dorsal surface of C5, C6 and C7. From the superior trunk the *suprascapular* nerve (C4, C5 and C6) for the supraspinatus and infraspinatus emerges dorsally, and the small nerve to the subclavius (C5 and C6) arises ventrally. The roots of the *medial and lateral pectoral* nerves (C5 to T1), which innervate the pectoralis major and minor, arise in part from the ventral surface of the superior and medial trunks, and in part from the medial cord (Fig. 7-15).

The three large peripheral nerves of the forearm (radial, median and ulnar) are formed in the following manner. The posterior cord, which receives contributions from all the plexus nerves, gives off the *thoracodorsal* (C6 to C8) and the *subscapular* nerves (C5 to C8), the former supplying the latissimus dorsi, the latter innervating the teres major and subscapularis (Fig. 7-15). Then the posterior cord splits into its two terminal branches, the larger *radial* nerve and the smaller *axillary* nerve. The lateral and medial cords each split into two branches, thus forming four nerves (Fig. 7-14). The two middle branches, one from the lateral cord and one from the medial cord, unite to form the *median* nerve. The outer branch, derived from the lateral cord, becomes the *musculocutaneous nerve.* The large innermost branch, derived from the medial cord, gives off the purely sensory *medial brachial cutaneous* and *medial antebrachial cutaneous* nerves, and its continuation becomes the *ulnar nerve* (Fig. 7-15).

A brief reference to embryology aids in explaining the formation of the plexus. During early development the primitive muscle mass of the limb is split into posterior and anterior layers, which are separated by the anlage of the humerus. The primary ventral nerve rami invading the limb split into posterior and anterior branches to supply corresponding muscles and the overlying skin. Within the primitive musculature, many simple muscles fuse to form larger and more complex ones

MAIN BRANCHES	CORDS	DIVISIONS	TRUNKS	VENTRAL RAMI

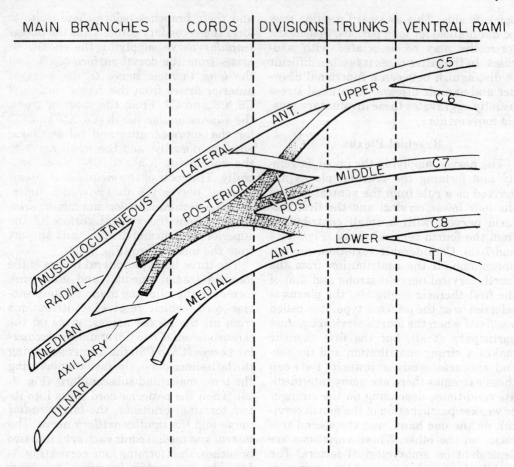

FIG. 7-14. Schematic drawing of the formation of the brachial plexus, indicating ventral rami, trunks, divisions, cords and main branches. The posterior divisions and the posterior cord are *shaded*.

and become supplied by two or more spinal nerves; as a result, the nerve fibers and plexuses interlace (Fig. 7-15). Such fusion usually occurs within either the posterior or the anterior musculature, and the muscles are innervated, respectively, by posterior or anterior divisions of the nerves. However, at the cephalic (preaxial) and the caudal (postaxial) borders of the limb, some muscles may be derived from both the posterior and the anterior musculature. These are supplied by fibers from both posterior and anterior nerves. A well known example is the brachialis muscle, which receives branches from the radial and musculocutaneous nerves. Thus the plexus primitively shows a division into posterior and anterior plates. The posterior plate innervates the posterior or extensor half of the arm and the posterior shoulder muscles; the anterior plate supplies the volar or flexor half and the anterior muscles of the shoulder. The nerves arising from the posterior plate are the dorsal scapular, long thoracic, suprascapular, subscapular, thoracodorsal, axillary and radial (*black* in Fig. 7-15). Those from the anterior plate include the subclavius, pectoral, musculocutaneous, median and ulnar, as well as the purely sensory medial brachial and medial antebrachial cutaneous nerves.

A summary of the peripheral distribution of the principal nerves of the upper extremity follows. The cutaneous areas of each nerve are shown in Figures 7-11 and 7-12. In their peripheral courses, some of the nerves of both the upper and lower extremity are particularly prone to trauma, or entrapment by fibrous tissue

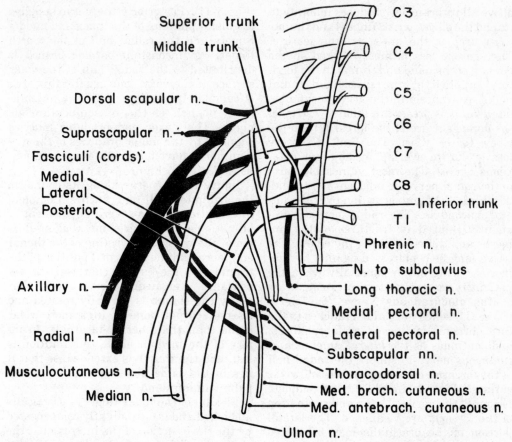

Superior trunk
Middle trunk

Dorsal scapular n.
Suprascapular n.
Fasciculi (cords):
Medial
Lateral
Posterior

Axillary n.

Radial n.

Musculocutaneous n.
Median n.

C3
C4
C5
C6
C7
C8
Inferior trunk
TI
Phrenic n.
N. to subclavius
Long thoracic n.
Medial pectoral n.
Lateral pectoral n.
Subscapular nn.
Thoracodorsal n.
Med. brach. cutaneous n.
Med. antebrach. cutaneous n.
Ulnar n.

Fig. 7-15. Diagram of the brachial plexus. The posterior divisions, posterior cords and peripheral nerves formed from the posterior divisions are shown in *black*. Cords and peripheral nerves formed from the anterior divisions of the ventral primary rami are in *white*.

related to either muscles, tendons, ligaments or fascia (Kopell and Thompson, '63). Sensory and motor symptoms that accompany such neuropathies depend on whether the nerves are primarily motor or sensory.

Axillary Nerve. This nerve innervates the deltoid and teres minor muscles and sends the *lateral brachial cutaneous* nerve to the skin of the upper outer surface of the arm, mainly in the deltoid region. After complete section of the axillary nerve, the deltoid muscle is paralyzed and abduction without external rotation is practically impossible. In time deltoid atrophy leads to loss of the round contour normally present at the shoulder. The sensory loss is less extensive, owing to the overlap of neighboring cutaneous nerves.

Radial Nerve. This nerve (C5 and T1)

supplies motor branches to the triceps muscle and all of the extensor muscles of the elbow, hands and fingers, and to the brachioradialis, supinator and abductor pollicis longus muscles. In addition, it usually sends a twig to the brachialis. Its cutaneous branches, distributed to the posterior surface of the extremity, are the *posterior brachial cutaneous nerve* to the arm, the *posterior antebrachial cutaneous* to the forearm and the *superficial radial nerve* which innervates the radial half of the dorsum of the hand and fingers as far as the distal interphalangeal joints (Fig. 7-12). The segmental innervation of the muscles supplied by the radial nerve is indicated in Figure 7-17.

Injuries of the radial nerve give variable symptoms which depend upon the location of the lesion. Complete section of the nerve above all its branches produces inability to extend the elbow, wrist, fingers and thumb; wrist drop is the most striking feature. The sensory loss is most marked on the dorsum of the hand and thumb in the territory supplied by the superficial radial nerve. Anesthesia in the arm is negligible but usually is present in a narrow strip on the dorsal surface of the forearm from the elbow to the wrist. The limited sensory loss is due to overlap by adjacent cutaneous nerves. The most vulnerable parts of the radial nerve lie adjacent to the middle third of the humerus and over the lateral epicondyle. The radial nerve is frequently injured in fractures of the humerus and those involving the elbow. The nerve may be compressed against the humerus during sleep, expecially when the patient is anesthetized or intoxicated.

Musculocutaneous Nerve. This nerve (C5 to C7) sends muscular branches to the coracobrachialis, biceps and brachialis, and continues as the *lateral antebrachial cutaneous* nerve to supply the radial half of the forearm, on both posterior and volar surfaces (Figs. 7-11 and 7-12). In complete lesions of the nerve, flexion and supination of the forearm are weakened. The lateral portion of the brachialis may be spared since it receives, as a rule, a branch from the radial nerve, and in addition flexion can still be produced by the brachioradialis. The sensory loss is variable in extent. It is poorly defined posteriorly, owing to overlap with the posterior antebrachial cutaneous nerve (a branch of the radial nerve). On the volar side, it is more extensive and more nearly approximates the territory supplied by the nerve.

Median Nerve. This nerve (C6 to T1, and sometimes C5) supplies all the muscles on the volar surface of the forearm except the flexor carpi ulnaris and the ulnar head of the flexor digitorum profundis. In the hand its branches innervate the outer lumbricals (I and II) and the muscles of the thenar eminence, except for the adductor pollicis and deep head of the flexor pollicis brevis. The sensory innervation is limited to the hand; it comprises the volar surface of the thumb, index and middle fingers; the radial half of the fourth finger; and corresponding portions of the palm

(Fig. 7-11). Posteriorly the nerve supplies the distal phalanx of the index and middle fingers and the radial half of the fourth finger. An inconstant *palmar* branch is distributed to the radial half of the volar surface of the wrist, but usually this area is completely overlapped by the antebrachial branch of the musculocutaneous nerve. The flexor and pronator muscles supplied by the motor branches of the median nerve have a segmental innervation, as indicated in Figure 7-17.

Injury to the nerve along its course in the arm affects all its branches. Complete interruption causes severe impairment of pronation of the forearm and weakens flexion at the wrist. The wasting of the thenar eminence and the abnormal position of the thumb give the hand a characteristic appearance after median nerve injury. Normally the thumb is partially rotated and its metacarpal bone is in a more volar plane than the other metacarpals. In injury of the median nerve this rotation is lost, and the thumb is extended, so that it lies in the same plane as the rest of the palm (simian hand).

Flexion of the index finger is practically abolished and is only slightly compensated by the flexor action of the interossei at the metacarpophalangeal joint. The middle finger is more variably affected. In the thumb, flexion of the terminal phalanx is completely lost, as are abduction and opposition. Makeshift movements of opposition, without abduction and rotation, can still be affected by the abductor pollicis and the deep head of the flexor brevis (pseudo-opposition). The motor defects are brought out readily in attempts to make a fist. The fourth and fifth fingers flex, but the thumb and index finger, and to a variable degree the middle finger, remain partially extended.

Sensory loss following a lesion of the median nerve is somewhat variable; usually it is less extensive than the area supplied by the nerve (Figs. 7-11 and 7-12), and it is most constant on the volar surface of the index and middle finger. Loss of appreciation of light touch generally is more constant and extensive than appreciation of pin-prick, and extends from the radial border of the thumb to the base of the thenar eminence and across the palm to include the palmar aspect of the ring finger on the radial side. On the dorsum of the hand it includes the radial side of the terminal two-thirds of the ring finger and the middle and index fingers as far proximal as the middle of the proximal phalanges. Deep sensibility usually is lost in the terminal phalanges of the index and middle fingers. The median nerve is prone to injury in deep cuts at the wrist and to entrapment as it passes beneath the transverse carpal ligament with the flexor tendons (carpal tunnel syndrome). Nerve compression may follow fractures (carpal and distal radial bones) or occur without external stress. Injuries here, as well as lesions of the nerve anywhere along its course, may be accompanied by secondary autonomic system overactivity. Following partial or incomplete median nerve regeneration an intense, persistent "burning pain" may be found over one or more points in the distal course of the nerve (*causalgia*). The median nerve is the most common site of causalgia.

Ulnar Nerve. This nerve (C8 and T1) supplies the flexor carpi ulnaris and the ulnar head of the flexor digitorum profundis muscles in the forearm. In the hand, it innervates the adductor pollicis, the deep head of the flexor pollicis brevis, the interossei, the two inner lumbricals and the muscles of the hypothenar eminence. It gives off three cutaneous branches. The *palmar cutaneous* branch supplies the ulnar half of the volar surface of the wrist, an area extensively overlapped by the medial antebrachial cutaneous nerve (Fig. 7-11). The posterior branch goes to the ulnar half of the dorsum of the hand and all of the little finger, and to the proximal phalanx of the ulnar half of the ring finger. The *superficial volar* branch supplies the volar surface of the fifth, and the ulnar half of the fourth fingers, and the corresponding ulnar portion of the palm (hypothenar region) (Figs. 7-11 and 7-12). The segmental innervation of muscles supplied by the ulnar nerve is indicated in Figure 7-17.

As in the case of the median nerve, injury to the ulnar nerve in the arm region affects its whole distribution. Flexion of the wrist is weakened, as are flexion of the fourth and fifth fingers and adduction of the thumb. There is marked wasting of the hypothenar and interossei muscles. The paralysis of these small muscles is particularly disturbing, for it makes execution of the finger movements required for writing, sewing and other skilled activities exceedingly difficult. The interossei flex the basal phalanges and extend the middle and distal ones. Hence paralysis of the interossei results in: (1) overextension of the basal phalanges by the extensor digitorum communis, and (2) flexion of the middle and distal phalanges by the flexor digitorum sublimis (claw hand).

Sensory disturbances are variable and depend upon the level of nerve injury. Total anesthesia as a rule is limited to the little finger and the hypothenar region. The ulnar nerve is prone to trauma as it crosses the medial epicondyle of the humerus, and to entrapment as it passes from the wrist to the hand.

Medial Antebrachial Cutaneous Nerve. This nerve (C8 and T1) supplies the medial half of the forearm, on both posterior and volar surfaces (Figs. 7-11 and 7-12). The extent of the sensory deficits caused by injury to this nerve varies in individual cases. On the volar side it often reaches to the middle of the arm. On the posterior surface the sensory deficit is somewhat smaller than the area of supply shown in Figure 7-12.

Medial Brachial Cutaneous Nerve. This nerve (T1) usually is associated with the *intercostobrachial* nerve derived from the second and often from the third thoracic (intercostal) nerves. These two nerves supply the axillary region and the inner surface of the arm, the area being considerably larger on the volar surface than on the posterior surface (Figs. 7-11 and 7-12). The area is overlapped extensively by adjacent cutaneous nerves. Injury to one of the nerves produces negligible symptoms. In injuries of both, the anesthesia is limited to the axillary region and medial surface of the upper arm.

Injuries of the Brachial Plexus

The motor and sensory deficits of plexus lesions vary considerably, depending on

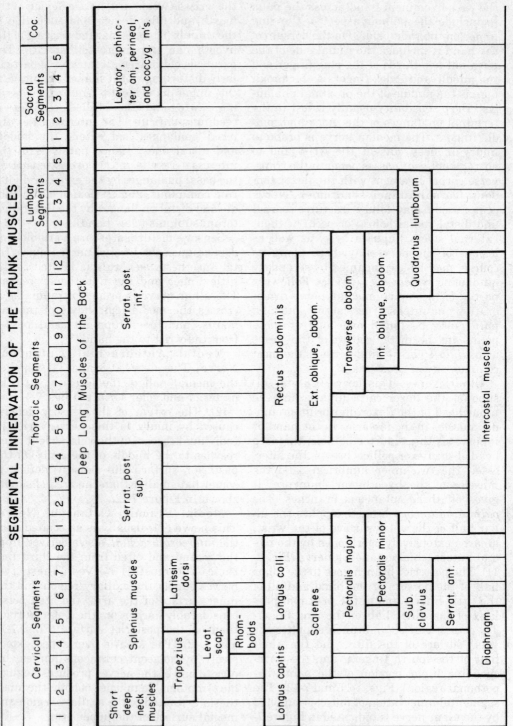

Fig. 7-16. Segments of spinal cord that contribute somatic motor nerve fibers to individual trunk muscles (after Haymaker, '56).

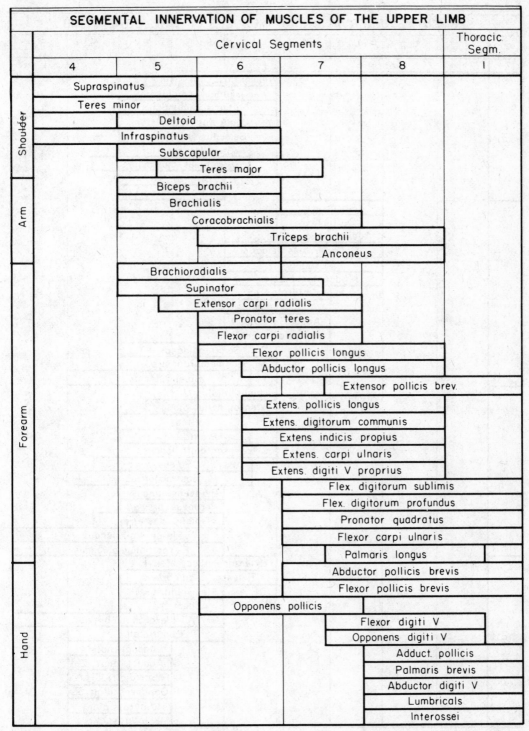

FIG. 7-17. Segments of spinal cord that contribute somatic motor nerve fibers to the individual muscles of shoulder and upper extremity (after Haymaker, '56).

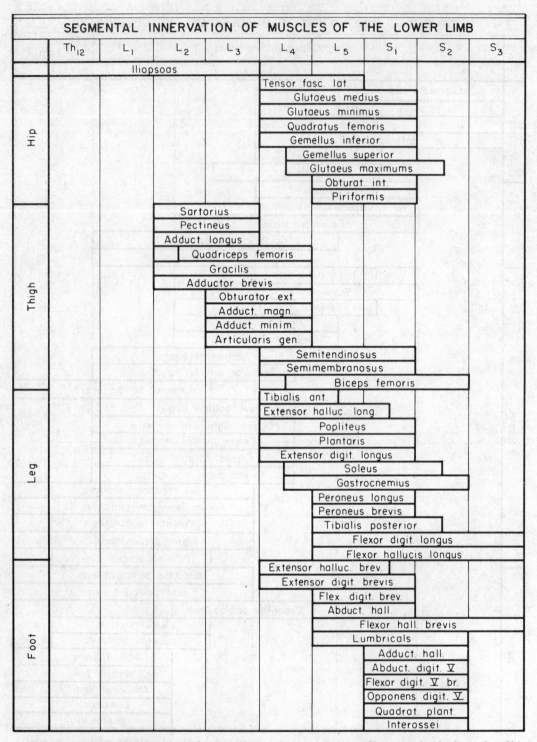

FIG. 7-18. Segments of spinal cord that contribute somatic motor nerve fibers to individual muscles of hip and lower extremity (after Haymaker, '56).

the extent of the injury, and on whether the primary trunks, divisions or cords are involved. In injury of the trunks the symptoms are segmental in character, and two main syndromes may be recognized. One syndrome affects the upper trunk and the other the lower trunk. The upper trunk syndrome (Duchenne-Erb) involves the muscles supplied by C5 and C6, namely the deltoid, biceps, brachialis, brachioradialis, supinator, teres major, teres minor, supraspinatus and infraspinatus. In this syndrome there is difficulty in elevation and external rotation of the arm, accompanied by a severe loss of flexion and supination of the forearm. Owing to the overlap of adjacent roots, the sensory deficit is as a rule limited to the deltoid region and lateral aspect of the arm.

The lower trunk syndrome (Klumpke or Duchenne-Aran) is relatively rare and affects primarily the small muscles of the hand innervated by C8 and T1 (Fig. 7-17). The palmaris longus and the long digital flexors usually are involved; hence the chief disabilities are in the finger and wrist movements. The sensory loss is along the medial aspects of the arm, forearm and hand. If preganglionic sympathetic fibers of the first thoracic root are included in the injury, there is drooping of the eyelid, diminution in the size of the pupil and narrowing of the palpebral fissure (Horner's syndrome, see page 210 and Fig. 10-26).

Injuries of the cords of the brachial plexus produce symptoms similar to those of peripheral nerves, except that several peripheral nerves are affected at the same time. Thus a lesion of the posterior cord involves the radial and axillary nerves and often the thoracodorsal and subscapular nerves (Fig. 7-15). Interruption of the lateral cord affects the musculocutaneous and the lateral portion of the median nerve. Injury to the medial cord involves the ulnar and the medial portion of the median nerve, as well as the medial brachial and antebrachial cutaneous nerves.

Lumbosacral Plexus

The plexus innervating the lower extremity is as a rule formed by the primary ventral rami of L1 to S2 and the larger portion of S3; frequently there is a small contributing branch from T12 (Figs. 7-19 and 7-20). As in the case of the brachial plexus, there may be anatomical variations. The plexus is *prefixed* when it is supplied by T12 to S2, and *postfixed* when it is formed from roots L2 to S4. There are also many intermediate forms, but the maximum shift in either direction rarely exceeds the extent of a single spinal nerve. These conditions are determined by the individual variations in the position of the limb buds during development. According to Foerster ('29) prefixed lumbosacral plexuses are rare. The lumbosacral plexus, excluding the pudendal and coccygeal portions, which are not distributed to the leg, is conveniently subdivided into an upper *lumbar* and a lower *sacral* plexus.

The *lumbar plexus* is formed by L1, L2, L3, the larger part of L4 and usually a communicating branch from T12 (Fig. 7-19). The larger *sacral plexus* is supplied by the smaller portion of L4 (furcal nerve), which joins L5 to form the large lumbosacral trunk, and by S1, S2 and the greater portion of S3 (Fig. 7-20). Except for the uppermost portion supplied mainly by L1, where the conditions are somewhat obscure, both plexuses show an organization into posterior and anterior divisions. The arrangement is simpler than in the brachial plexus. The undivided lumbosacral primary rami do not form interlacing trunks but split directly into posterior and anterior divisions related, respectively, to the primitive posterior and anterior musculature of the leg. The peripheral nerves to the extremity are formed by the union of a variable number of either posterior or anterior divisions (Figs. 7-19 and 7-20). In the lumbar plexus, the anterior divisions give rise to the *iliohypogastric* (anterior branch), *ilioinguinal, genitofemoral* and *obturator nerves;* and the posterior divisions give rise to the *iliohypogastric* (posterior branch), *iliopsoas, femoral* and *lateral femoral cutaneous nerves.* In the sacral plexus, the anterior divisions furnish the *tibial nerve* and the nerves to the hamstring, quadratus femoris, obturator internus and gemelli muscles; the posterior divi-

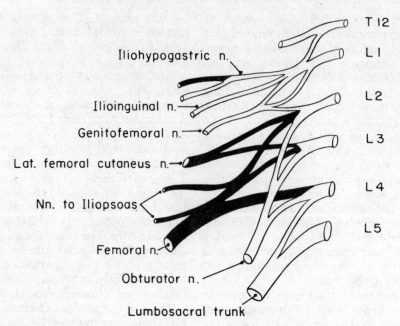

FIG. 7-19. Diagram of lumbar plexus. Peripheral nerves formed by anterior divisions of ventral primary rami are *white;* nerves formed by posterior divisions of ventral primary rami are *black*.

sions form the *common peroneal* and the *superior* and *inferior gluteal nerves.* The *posterior femoral cutaneous nerve,* which supplies the back of the thigh, receives fibers from both posterior and anterior divisions. As in the case of the arm, muscles derived from both the posterior and the anterior primitive musculature are innervated by both posterior and anterior divisions. Thus the biceps femoris receives branches from the tibial, as well as peroneal portions of the sciatic nerve.

Following is a summary of the peripheral distribution of the principal nerves of the lower extremity. The cutaneous areas supplied by these nerves are shown in Figures 7-11 and 7-12.

Obturator Nerve. The obturator nerve (L2 to L4) supplies the adductor muscles of the thigh and the gracilis muscle; it sends an inconstant branch to the pectineus, which more often is innervated by the femoral nerve. Its cutaneous branch is distributed to the inner surface of the thigh (Figs. 7-11 and 7-12), the area being extensively overlapped by adjacent cutaneous nerves. The segmental innervation of the muscles

supplied by the obturator nerve is indicated in Figure 7-18.

In injury of this nerve, adduction of the thigh is weakened severely but not lost, since the adductor magnus also receives some fibers from the sciatic nerve. The sensory defects usually involve only a small triangular area of the anatomical field. The obturator nerve is vulnerable to entrapment by the obturator membrane as it passes through the obturator canal.

Femoral Nerve. The femoral nerve (L2 to L4) sends motor branches to the extensors of the leg, the iliopsoas, the sartorius and also the pectineus. Occasionally a branch may go to the adductor longus. The cutaneous branches are the *anterior femoral cutaneous* nerves for the thigh and the *saphenous* nerve for the leg and foot (Figs. 7-11 and 7-12). The former supply the anterior and anteromedial surface of the thigh, comprising a relatively large autonomous sensory field. The saphenous nerve sends an infrapatellar branch to the skin in front of the kneecap and then is distributed to the medial side of the leg; the lowermost branches are distributed from the medial

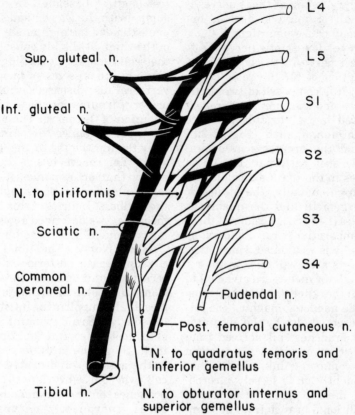

Sup. gluteal n.

Inf. gluteal n.

N. to piriformis

Sciatic n.

Common peroneal n.

Tibial n.

L 4

L 5

S I

S 2

S 3

S 4

Pudendal n.

Post. femoral cutaneous n.

N. to quadratus femoris and inferior gemellus

N. to obturator internus and superior gemellus

FIG. 7-20. Diagram of lumbosacral plexus. Peripheral nerves formed by anterior divisions of ventral primary rami are *white;* nerves formed by posterior divisions of ventral primary rami are *black.*

margin of the foot to the proximal phalanx of the great toe.

The segmental innervation of the quadriceps femoris, iliopsoas, sartorius and pectineus is shown in Figure 7-18.

Injury of the femoral nerve causes inability to extend the leg. If the lesion is high enough to involve the iliopsoas, flexion of the thigh at the hip is severely impaired. Sensory disturbances are manifested throughout the field of supply, and there are relatively large areas of total anesthesia. If the thigh nerves alone are involved the anesthesia is most extensive on the anterior surface of the thigh above the knee. In isolated lesions of the saphenous nerve, the anesthetic field extends on the inner surface of the leg from below the knee to the medial margin of the foot. The femoral nerve may become involved sec-

ondary to an abscess in the psoas muscle. The terminal sensory branch of the femoral (saphenous nerve) is subject to entrapment as it leaves the subsartorial canal.

Lateral Femoral Cutaneous Nerve. The lateral femoral cutaneous nerve (L2 and L3) supplies the lateral half of the thigh, from the lateral buttock region to the knee (Figs. 7-11 and 7-12). In spite of overlap by adjacent cutaneous nerves, injury of this nerve produces a considerable area of anesthesia on the lateral aspect of the thigh.

The cutaneous areas supplied by the *iliohypogastric* (L1), *ilioinguinal* (L1) and *genitofemoral* (L1 and L2) nerves are shown in Figures 7-11 and 7-12. The iliohypogastric and ilioinguinal nerves also send motor fibers to the internal oblique and transverse abdominal muscles. Sensory loss due to injury to one of these nerves is relatively small or may be absent, but such lesions may cause neuralgia.

Sciatic Nerve. The sciatic nerve (L4 to S3), the largest nerve in the body, is the chief continuation of all the roots of the sacral plexus. It is composed of two parts, the *tibial nerve* and the *common peroneal nerve,* enclosed for a variable distance within a common sheath (Fig. 7-20). Emerging from the greater sciatic foramen, or while still within it, the nerve sends branches to the main external rotators of the thigh, namely, the obturator internus, the gemelli and the quadratus femoris muscles (L4 to S1). Lesions of these nerves are comparatively rare, and external rotation only is weakened, since other external rotators are available. In the region of the thigh, branches are given off to the flexors of the knee (hamstring muscles) and to the adductor magnus, the latter being innervated also by the obturator nerve. These branches, all derived from the tibial portion of the sciatic, often spring from a common trunk, which either runs independently or is loosely incorporated in the medial side of the sciatic nerve. An additional branch from the common peroneal nerve supplies the short head of the biceps femoris muscle. In injuries of the hamstring nerves flexion of the knee is impaired severely, but weak flexion still may be produced by the action of the gracilis and sartorius muscle.

The sciatic nerve splits into its two terminal nerves at varying levels in the thigh. The muscular branches of the common trunk provide motor and sensory fibers to the quadratus femoris, the obturator internus, the gemelli, the semitendinosus, the semimembranosus and the biceps femoris.

Normal peripheral nerve can be damaged by excessive stretch, as may occur in the roots and cords of the brachial plexus following undue angulation of the head and shoulder, or arm traction, during delivery. Reaction to stretch in a diseased nerve with a long course such as the sciatic, often produces pain, and paresthesias. One of the best known nerve stretching mechanisms is the straight leg-raising test (sign of Lasègue). In a person lying supine with the legs extended, elevation of one extended (straightened) leg by flexion of the thigh at the hip causes stretching of the sciatic nerve. Stretching of the sciatic nerve in the presence of meningitis, intervertebral disc disease, peripheral neuritis or nerve trauma, produces pain in the distribution of the nerve. The patient usually attempts to relieve the pain by automatically flexing the leg at the knee (Kernig's sign). This nerve has a prominent axial artery that accompanies it, as well as a large number of postganglionic sympathetic fibers. Injuries of this nerve, like the median nerve described above, are particularly prone to be followed by causalgia.

Tibial Nerve. The tibial nerve (L4 to S3) supplies the posterior calf muscles concerned with: (1) plantar flexion and inversion of the foot, and (2) plantar flexion of the toes. It also supplies the intrinsic muscles of the sole, which aid in maintaining the arch of the foot. One cutaneous branch given off in the thigh, the *sural* nerve, is distributed to the posterior and medial surface of the calf, where it is overlapped extensively by branches of the saphenous and lateral sural (peroneal) nerves. Terminal branches of the sural nerve (*lateral calcaneal*) supply the outer margin of the heel and a triangular area on the outer surface of the foot which extends to the lower portion of the Achilles tendon (Fig. 7-12). Other cutaneous branches of the tibial nerve (*medial calcaneal* and *plantar*) supply the back and medial margin of the heel, the plantar surface of the foot and toes and the dorsal phalanges (Figs. 7-11 and 7-12). The terminal branches of the tibial nerve are the *medial* and *lateral plantar* nerves. The segmental innervation of the calf and plantar muscles supplied by the tibial nerve is indicated in Figure 7-18.

Complete interruption of the tibial nerve above all its branches abolishes plantar flexion of the foot and toes and severely impairs inversion of the foot. Atrophy of the plantar muscles increases the concavity of the plantar arch (pes cavus). Sensory disturbances are negligible in the calf region, in which only a narrow strip may show reduced sensitivity. Total anesthesia is found on the sole of the foot, the plantar surface of the toes, the heel, and often in a triangular area on the outer surface of the foot. This nerve is vulnerable to fractures and dislocations of the medial melleolus, calcaneus and astragalus bones. It also can be compressed as it passes through the osseofibrous canal with three tendons, deep to the flexor retinaculum or deltoid ligament (tarsal tunnel syndrome).

Common Peroneal Nerve. The common peroneal nerve (L4 to S2) supplies the lateral and anterior muscles of the leg and the dorsal muscles of the foot, effecting dorsal flexion and eversion of the foot and dorsal flexion of the toes. The chief cutaneous nerves are the *lateral sural cutaneous* and the *superficial peroneal nerve* (Fig. 7-11). The former, given off in the thigh, is distributed to the outer side of the leg from the knee region to nearly the outer margin of the sole, where it invades the territories of the superficial peroneal and sural nerves. The superficial peroneal nerve supplies the dorsum of the foot and toes to the distal phalanges and a portion of the anterior surface of the leg. A small cutaneous branch of the deep peroneal nerve is distributed to the cleft between the adjacent surfaces of the great and second toe (Fig. 7-11). The common peroneal nerve divides into its superficial and deep branches as it passes to the lateral side of the neck of the fibula under cover of the peroneus longus muscle. The segmental innervation of the peronei, tibialis anterior and extensor muscles on the dorsum of the foot is indicated in Figure 7-18.

Complete section of the peroneal nerve causes paralysis of dorsal flexion and eversion of the foot and paralysis of dorsal flexion (extension) of the toes. The most striking feature is inability to elevate the foot and toes (foot drop). If the condition is prolonged, shortening of the Achilles tendon will produce a permanent plantar hyperflexion and the foot will assume an equinovarus deformity. Sensory defects will be found on the dorsum of the foot, the outer part of the leg, and the skin between the great and second toe. The extent of the sensory loss is much smaller than the ana-

tomical field, since cutaneous areas on both, foot and leg, are overlapped extensively by the adjacent cutaneous nerves. The common peroneal nerve is subject to injury both by compression and fracture at the neck of the fibula. A terminal branch of the deep peroneal nerve is frequently injured as it crosses the dorsum of the foot. The terminal sensory fibers of the superficial peroneal nerve may become entrapped as they pierce the deep fascia at the distal and lateral part of the leg.

Gluteal Nerves. The *superior gluteal nerve* (L4 to S1) supplies the gluteus medius, gluteus minimus and tensor fasciae latae muscles, which abduct the hip and rotate it internally. These movements are impaired by injury to the nerve.

The *inferior gluteal nerve* (L5 to S2) is distributed to the gluteus maximus, the strongest extensor of the hip. Injury causes wasting of the buttock. There is difficulty in rising from a sitting position, walking uphill or climbing stairs, where powerful contraction of the muscle is required for raising the body.

Posterior Femoral Cutaneous Nerve. The posterior femoral cutaneous nerve (S1 to S3) gives off several branches (*inferior clunial*) which supply the lower portions of the buttocks. These nerves overlap branches of the lumbar and sacral dorsal rami (superior and medial clunial nerves) (Fig. 7-12). Another small branch (*perineal*) goes to the lower innermost part of the buttock, the dorsal surface of the scrotum (or labia majora) and reaches the inner surface of the thigh. The main nerve supplies the posterior aspect of the thigh, often extending below the knee and widely overlapping the territories of adjacent nerves. Injuries produce a relatively broad strip of anesthesia on the posterior surface of the thigh from the buttocks to the knee.

FUNCTIONAL CONSIDERATIONS

The origin, size, course and relations of the spinal nerves to their respective vertebrae are important factors (Figs. 9-1, 9-2 and 9-3). Meninges, intervertebral discs, size of the intervertebral foramina and vertebral mobility often can be correlated anatomically with a variety of spinal nerve root syndromes (Davis, '57). For example, degenerated or ruptured intervertebral discs may lead to compression of spinal nerve roots as they approach the intervertebral foramen, or the foramina may be narrowed due to osteoarthritis. Effects of stress and strain on the erect spine appear first at the weakest points. Here motion occurs and the mechanical impacts of postural strain and trauma usually are recorded (i.e., cervical and lumbar regions). Dorsal roots, except for C1, are nearly three times larger than ventral roots. However, the spinal roots vary in size in different regions. The largest are those that participate in the formation of the nerve plexuses that supply the limbs. The sixth cervical is the largest of the cervical nerves and from this point upward the roots diminish in size. Root size in relation to bony foramina have some interesting correlations with attendant liability to mechanical irritation or compression. Cervical roots occupy only one-fourth of their respective intervertebral foramen. In contrast, from the first lumbar nerve downward the size of the nerve increases in relation to the size of the foramen. The first to third lumbar nerves never completely fill the foramina, and the fourth root rarely does, whereas the fifth lumbar nerve root frequently fills the intervertebral foramen. This suggests a possible explanation for the high incidence of compression of the fibers of the fifth lumbar nerve root.

Nerve compression by disease or injury can result in a variety of root symptoms, usually associated with pain of short duration. Pain often dominates the clinical picture. If the ventral roots are involved, muscle spasm, weakness and vasomotor disturbances may accompany the pain. A knowledge of the radicular (segmental) distribution of the spinal nerves is helpful in evaluating root lesions which may lie in and around the vertebra of a given region.

Injury to the spinal nerves or their peripheral branches causes disturbances of both sensation and movement. Section of a dorsal root rarely produces a loss of sensation (anesthesia), although it may impair reflexes (hyporeflexia) initiated by appropriate stimuli in the areas supplied by that root. Owing to the overlapping distribution of fibers of adjacent roots, anesthesia will not be detectable unless several contiguous roots are cut (Fig. 7-10). The hyporeflexia involves superficial and deep reflexes and it is associated with a diminution of tone (hypotonia) in the affected muscles.

The various activities of the central nervous system can be expressed only by impulses which impinge (i.e., synapse) upon neurons, somatic and visceral, whose axons pass peripherally to effector organs. The large α motor neurons of the anterior horn of the spinal cord give rise to axons which emerge via the ventral root and innervate striated muscle. The α motor neurons and their axons constitute anatomical and physiological units, referred to as the final common pathway or the *lower motor neuron* (Sherrington, '06). The concept of the lower motor neuron is not limited to the spinal cord, even though it is frequently used in that context. Cells of the motor cranial nerve nuclei (nerves III, IV, V, VI, VII, IX, X, XI and XII) which innervate the muscles of the head and neck, also must be classified as lower motor neurons. Lesions selectively involving the lower motor neuron in the spinal cord, in the ventral root or in a peripheral nerve, produce weakness or paralysis, loss of muscle tone, loss of reflex activity and atrophy. All of these changes are confined to the affected muscles (Carpenter, '71). Atrophy as a consequence of a lower motor neuron lesion develops gradually and in time is obvious on inspection.

Since the anterior horn cells that innervate a single muscle extend longitudinally through several spinal segments, and since several such cell columns exist at each spinal level, a lesion confined to one spinal segment will cause weakness, but not complete paralysis, in all muscles innervated by this segment. Complete paralysis will occur only when the lesion involves the column of cells in several spinal segments that innervate a particular muscle, or the ventral root fibers that arise from these cells. Because most appendicular muscles are innervated by fibers arising from parts of three spinal segments

(Figs. 7-16, 7-17 and 7-18), complete paralysis of a muscle implies a central lesion involving anterior horn cells in several spinal segments, or a lesion involving ventral root fibers from several spinal segments (Figs. 9-21 and 9-22). Since neighboring cell columns are likely to be affected at each level, such lesions usually produce paralysis in muscle groups rather than individual muscles.

The denervated muscle also shows certain changes in its reaction to electrical stimulation. Healthy muscle responds to stimulation by both the faradic (interrupted) and galvanic (continuous) current. In faradic stimulation, the response lasts as long as the stimulus is applied. In galvanic stimulation the response occurs only on closing or opening the circuit. Normally it is the application of the negative pole or cathode which produces the strongest contraction on closing the current. In the complete *reaction of degeneration*, which appears 10 to 14 days after nerve injury, the muscle no longer responds to stimulation of its motor nerve. However, the muscle still responds to direct stimulation with slow wavelike contractions, but it is the positive pole or anode which induces the strongest response on closing the circuit.

If preganglionic visceral fibers also are involved, as in the case of the thoracic and upper lumbar roots, there are sudomotor, vasomotor, and atrophic disturbances expressed by dryness and smoothness of the skin.

It becomes necessary to distinguish the deficits which occur as a consequence of lesions in spinal segments from those that occur in spinal roots, mixed spinal nerves and peripheral nerves. A lesion in ventral root fibers usually produces the same motor deficits as those resulting from destruction of anterior horn cells. However, at certain levels (i.e., thoracolumbar and sacral), section of ventral root fibers produces additional autonomic deficits which may not accompany lesions of the anterior horn cells. Section of a single ventral root, for example C5, would produce weakness in the supraspinatus, infraspinatus subscapularis, biceps brachii and brachioradialis, but not complete paralysis of any of these muscles. This pattern of distribution is unique to the C5 ventral root and different from that of any single peripheral nerve.

Lesions of mixed spinal nerves produce motor and sensory deficits that correspond to those of combined dorsal and ventral root lesions. While the motor deficits correspond almost exactly to those seen with pure lesions of the ventral root, sensory deficits follow a dermatomal distribution and tend to be less extensive because of the overlapping innervation characteristic of dermatomes. If only one mixed spinal nerve were injured, for example C5, the motor weakness would be the same as described above, but no sensory loss would be detectable. Involvement of several contiguous mixed spinal nerves would produce marked weakness or paralysis in the muscles innervated by those spinal segments and detectable sensory loss in at least one dermatome.

The above findings are in sharp contrast to the motor and sensory deficits associated with peripheral nerve lesions. With a peripheral nerve lesion the muscle paralysis and the sensory loss correspond to the peripheral distribution of the particular nerve.

In certain diseases of the lower motor neuron, the muscles exhibit small, localized spontaneous contractions known as *fasciculations*. These muscle twitches, visible under the skin, represent the discharge of squads of muscle fibers innervated by nerve fibers arising from lower motor neurons. Fasciculations occur asynchronously in different parts of various muscles and are thought to be triggered by motor unit discharges that occur within the cell body of the motor neuron. Fasciculations commonly are seen in amyotrophic lateral sclerosis (Fig. 10-24), occasionally in acute inflammatory lesions of peripheral nerves and generally do not occur when the anterior horn cells are rapidly destroyed (i.e., acute poliomyelitis). The term *fibrillations*, frequently misused as the equivalent of the term fasciculations, refers to small (10 to 20 μV) potentials of 1 or 2 msec duration that occur irregularly and asynchronously in electromyograms of denervated muscle. These spontaneous discharges cannot be observed under the skin and produce no detectable shortening of muscles. These potentials represent the spontaneous activation of individual muscle fibers.

Regeneration of Injured Peripheral Nerves. Our knowledge of the processes of degeneration and regeneraton has been greatly increased in recent years by investigations on mammalian nerves under various experimental conditions. Valuable information was obtained by clinical and surgical studies of the peripheral nerve injuries during the war. Seddon ('43) distinguishes three types of nerve injury: (1) complete anatomical division; (2) crush or compression injuries in which the continuity of the nerve fibers is broken but the sheaths and supporting tissue remain intact; and (3) temporary impairment or nerve block. Nerve section nearly always demands surgical intervention to re-establish continuity. The recovery is more or less successful, but never complete, since many of the regenerating fibers fail to reach their respective end organs. After nerve crush there also is complete degeneration of the severed nerve fibers. Both nerve section and nerve crush are followed by loss of sensation and movement; wasting of muscles and reaction of degeneration. However, the damaged nerve fibers and their sheaths are in close anatomical contiguity after nerve crush, and subsequent regeneration usually leads to more complete recovery. In mild compression or block, there are varying degrees of paralysis, but electrical exitability remains normal. Because the nerve fibers are not severed, there is no peripheral degeneration. Recovery is more rapid; it begins in a few weeks and usually is completed within 2 or 3 months. These three types of nerve injury may appear as separate entities or in various combinations. Since the clinical symptoms after nerve section and crush are the same until regeneration is completed, surgical exploration usually is indicated to determine the nature of the injury (Stookey and Scarff, '43).

In a simple crush, although the continuity of the axons is interrupted, the endoneurium and other supporting tissues remain essentially intact. As a result, regenerating nerve fibers from the central stump can grow distally, traverse the minimal scar tissue between the severed axonal ends and enter appropriate Schwann cell tubes of the distal stump. After complete anatomical severance, the conditions are quite different at the site of injury. The cut ends are separated by a gap of variable extent which becomes filled with connective tissue and sheath cells, so that a scar of union is formed between the stumps. Hemorrhage and the vascular mesenchyme contribute cells to the scar tissue. These cellular elements in the lesion area seriously impede the growth of fine sprouts of regenerating axons from the proximal stump of the nerve. An enlarged heterogeneous mass at the cut end of a previously injured nerve is known as a *traumatic neuroma* (amputation or pseudoneuroma). It consists of Schwann cells, connective tissue cells and fibers, macrophages and an abundance of tangled aberrant nerve fibers. Such a skein of "lost" nerve fibers in scar tissue can be a most serious complication following peripheral nerve section or injury. Many of these fibers are "functional" processes of dorsal root ganglion cells, and these tangled ends still can transmit nerve impulses into the spinal cord. Such neuroma explains why a patient may have localized "phantom pain" and/or paresthesias in a previously amputated hand or foot.

The behavior of the Schwann cells after anatomical severance is especially significant. About the 4th day, they become elongated and migrate out of the stumps into the scar, coming mainly from the peripheral stump but, to a lesser extent, also from the central one. These cells arrange themselves end to end, and form strands which traverse the fibrous tissue of the scar and establish continuity between the intact axons and the degenerating tubes of the peripheral stump. In some animals, under suitable conditions, gaps of 2 cm have been naturally bridged in this manner. In man gaps of several millimeters may be similarly bridged. Under most circumstances, however, the mass of scar tissue is too extensive to be handled by the sheath cells themselves, and surgical intervention is required. Scar tissue must be removed from both ends of the severed nerve, and these ends must be approximated and maintained by epineural sutures. The central axonal tips swell and produce a number of fine branches which enter the injured area by the 3rd day. At first they appear free in the connective tissue. Soon they apply themselves to the surface of the sheath cell strands and are led to the peripheral stump, where many of the branches enter the old Schwann cell tubes (Figs. 4-29 and 4-30). However, the number of fibers entering the distal tubes is always smaller after section of the nerve than after crush. Moreover, many nerve fibers enter tubes which are structurally unsuitable for full functional maturation. Once the fibers have entered the distal tubes, the processes of growth and maturation are the same as after crush. These are described in Chapter 4.

The rate of nerve regeneration has been studied by a number of investigators. After primary suture of the peroneal nerve in the rabbit, it takes about 7 days for the growing axon tips of the central stump to traverse the scar of the gap and reach the peripheral stump (Gutmann et al., '42; Gutmann and Young, '44; Sunderland, '52). After crush the "scar" delay was about 5 days. Then the fastest axonal tips grew at the rate of 3.5 mm a day after suture, and 4.4 mm after a crush. Most of the axons grow distally at 3 mm a day after the peroneal nerve is crushed, and 2 mm a day after nerve section and suture. When the fine regenerated axons attain the periphery they increase in diameter and most of them ultimately become remyelinated. If a sufficient number of such fibers reach and successfully re-establish contact with appropriate sensory and motor end organs, there will be an eventual return of function. The total latent period in the rabbit between nerve regeneration and functional recovery was 20 days following nerve crush and 36 days after nerve suture.

In the longer nerves of man the process is slower, although a rate of 4.4 mm a day for growing axons was found after a crush of one of the digital nerves (Bowden and Gutmann, '44). The rate of functional regeneration falls off with the distance traversed, since increase in diameter and myelination occurs more slowly in the distal portions of the fiber. A justifiable assumption for axonal growth in man under ideal conditions is about 3 mm/day. The average latent period until functional maturity after distal nerve injuries is 20 days after crush and 50 days after suture.

Regeneration can occur when two stumps are sutured after being left apart for a considerable period of time. However, it is generally agreed that functional recoveries after long-delayed sutures usually are unsatisfactory. The difficulties occasioned by long delay are due to a number of factors which interfere with the regenerative processes, and these effects become progressively more serious. Some of the factors may be briefly mentioned. After a long delay, the distal stump atrophies and the outgrowth of sheath cells is reduced or ceases. Hence good apposition of the cut nerve ends is difficult, and many axons fail to reach the degenerated atrophic Schwann cell tubes of the distal stump. The tubes themselves are greatly shrunken and receive fewer fibers, so that the chances for appropriate peripheral connections are reduced. Myelinization is delayed and increase in diameter of the nerve fiber is restricted by the thickened endoneurium, which forms a large portion of the tube. Of special importance is the progressive atrophy of the muscles and end organs. In early stages, where the motor end plates remain intact and connected with the Schwann cell tubes, new fibers can enter directly and restore the original pattern. In later stages these channels become occluded and the end organs may completely disintegrate. The regenerating fibers often fail to enter the old sensory and motor endings or their previous locations. These fibers wander along the muscle fibers, ultimately forming new motor end plates of a more primitive character, whose distribution is irregular and different from the original pattern of innervation. All studies favor early nerve suture, perhaps 3 or 4 weeks after injury. At this time sheath cell activity is at its height and the somewhat thickened perineurium permits easier surgical apposition of the injured nerve stumps (Young, '49). Delays of 6 months or more before suture may seriously interfere with the reparative processes but failure is not necessarily encountered in all cases. Good recovery is possible after long-delayed suture if enough axons reach appropriate Schwann cell tubes and the muscles are maintained in good condition by appropriate therapy. Sunderland ('50) has reported good restoration of function in human hand and finger muscles which had been denervated for 12 months.

CHAPTER 8

The Autonomic Nervous System

Portions of the central and peripheral nervous system concerned primarily with the regulation and control of visceral functions are termed collectively the *visceral, vegetative* or *autonomic nervous system* (Fig. 8-1). Visceral reactions and functions are initiated mainly by internal changes that activate visceroceptors. Visceral motor responses in smooth muscle and glands are to a large extent involuntary and unconscious. Such visceral reactions as do reach conscious levels are vague, poorly localized and predominantly of an effective character. Tactile sensibility is practically absent, and temperature sense is appreciated only in certain places, such as the esophagus, stomach, colon and rectum. On the other hand, distention or spasms of the muscular walls of hollow viscera or blood vessels may produce severe distress or acute pain.

As defined by Langley ('21) the *autonomic system* was purely a visceral motor system consisting of "visceral efferent cells and fibers that pass to tissues other than the skeletal muscle." This rigid definition limited the term autonomic to a two neuron visceral efferent system, and excluded visceral afferent fibers. Yet sensory fibers accompany most visceral motor fibers and form the afferent links of most visceral reflex arcs. Visceral afferent fibers have their cells of origin in the spinal and specific cranial nerve ganglia (Figs. 8-2 and 9-22). They, like the higher brain centers, play a constant and dynamic role in the regulation of autonomic activities. In recent years the above limited concept has been liberalized to make the term "autonomic" more synonymous with "visceral," and to include both peripheral and central neural structures (Hess, '48). It behooves all concerned with visceral function to remember that central neurons and visceral afferent neurons are vital and integral parts of the autonomic system, regardless of arbitrary definitions. In similar fashion no attempt should be made to sharply delineate the nervous system into somatic and visceral portions. This is a convenient physiological subdivision, but the two are merely different parts of a single integrated neural mechanism. The higher brain centers regulate both somatic and visceral functions, and throughout most neural levels there is intermingling and association of visceral and somatic neurons. Moreover, visceral reflexes may be initiated by impulses passing through somatic afferent fibers from any receptor, and conversely visceral changes may give rise to somatic activities. Through some mechanism, as yet unexplained, stimulation of peripheral visceral efferent neurons also can alter the activity of somatic sensory receptors.

Interposed in the efferent peripheral pathway between the central nervous sys-

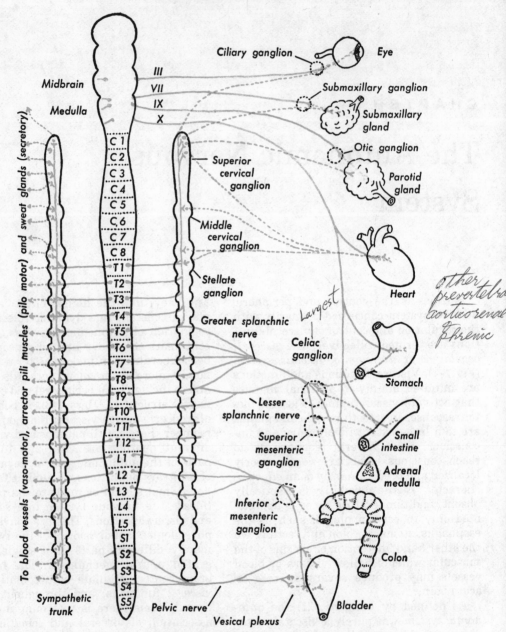

FIG. 8-1. Schematic diagram showing general arrangement of the autonomic system. The sympathetic components are shown in *red*; while the parasympathetic components are in *blue*. *Solid lines* represent preganglionic fibers; *broken lines* indicate postganglionic fibers. For clearness the sympathetic fibers to the blood vessels, hair and sweat glands are shown separately in figure 8-2.

tem and the visceral structures are aggregations of nerve cells known as the *autonomic ganglia*. The cells of these peripheral ganglia are in synaptic relation with fibers from the spinal cord or brain stem, and they send out axons which terminate in the visceral effectors: smooth muscle, heart muscle and glandular epithelium.

Pre- and Postganglionic Neurons. Thus unlike skeletal muscle, which is directly innervated by axons of centrally located neurons, the transmission of im-

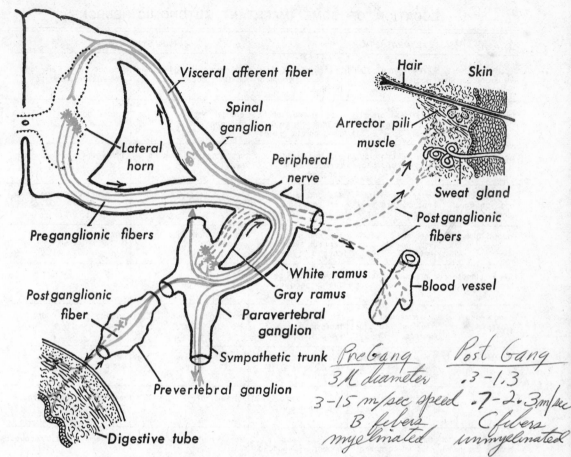

FIG. 8-2. Diagram of neural reflex arcs of the sympathetic system.

pulses from the central nervous system to the viscera always involves two different neurons (Figs. 8-1 and 8-3). The first neuron, situated in the brain stem or spinal cord, sends a thinly myelinated *preganglionic* fiber to an autonomic ganglion, where it synapses with one or more *postganglionic* cells. Preganglionic fibers of the cranial and spinal nerves are approximately 3 μ in diameter, have slow conduction velocities (i.e., 3 to 15 m/sec) and are designated as the B fibers of peripheral nerves (Patton, '61). The usually unmyelinated axons of autonomic ganglion cells then pass as *postganglionic* fibers to visceral effectors (Fig. 9-22). Postganglionic autonomic axons have smaller diameters (0.3 to 1.3 μ), possess slower conduction velocities (0.7 to 2.3 m/sec) and are usually classified as the C fibers of peripheral nerves. Therefore even the simplest visceral reflex arc will involve at least three neurons: (1) visceral afferent, (2) preganglionic visceral efferent, and (3) postganglionic visceral efferent (Figs. 8-2 and 9-22).

The autonomic ganglia, which have a wide distribution in the visceral periphery, may be classified in three groups: (1) the *paravertebral*, (2) the *prevertebral* (*collateral*), and (3) the *terminal*. The paravertebral ganglia are arranged in a segmental fashion along the anterolateral surface of the vertebral column and are connected with each other by longitudinal fibers to form the two *sympathetic trunks* or ganglionated cords (Fig. 8-1). The prevertebral ganglia are irregular aggregations of cells found in the mesenteric neural plexuses surrounding the abdominal aorta and its larger visceral branches. The terminal ganglia are parasympathetic and are located within, or close to, the structures

LOCATION OF SOME IMPORTANT AUTONOMIC NEURONS

Structure Supplied	SYMPATHETIC		PARASYMPATHETIC	
	Preganglionic Cell Bodies in CNS Nuclei	Postganglionic Cell Bodies in Peripheral Ganglia	Preganglionic Cell Bodies in CNS Nuclei	Postganglionic Cell Bodies in Peripheral Ganglia
Iris of eye	intermediolateral nuc. in cord segments C8-T2 (3)	sup. cervical ganglion and scattered along carotid plexus	Edinger-Westphal nuc. of midbrain	ciliary ganglion
Lacrimal gland	intermediolateral nuc. in cord segments T1-2	sup. and middle cervical symp. ganglia	sup. salivatory nuc. in pons	pterygopalatine ganglion
Submandibular and sublingual glands	intermediolateral nuc. in cord segments T1-3(4)	sup. and middle cervical symp. ganglia	sup. salivatory nuc. in pons	submandibular ganglion
Parotid gland	intermediolateral nuc. in cord segments T1-3(4)	sup. and middle cervical symp. ganglia	inf. salivatory nuc. in medulla	otic ganglion
Sweat glands of head and neck	intermediolateral nuc. in cord segments T1-3	3 cervical sympathetic ganglia		
Lungs and bronchi	intermediolateral nuc. in cord segments T1-5	inf. cervical and thoracic (T1-5) symp. ganglia	dorsal motor nuc. N. X	ganglia of pulmonary plexi
Heart	intermediolateral nuc. in cord segments T1-5(6,7)	3 cervical and thoracic (T1-6) symp. ganglia	dorsal motor nuc. N. X	intra-cardiac ganglia of atria
Esophagus	intermediolateral nuc. in cord segments T1-6	thoracic symp. T(1-3) 4-6 ganglia	dorsal motor nuc. N. X	myenteric and submucous plexi
Stomach, small intestine; ascending and transverse colon	intermediolateral nuc. in cord segments T5-11	celiac and sup. mesenteric ganglia	dorsal motor nuc. N. X	myenteric and submucous plexi
Descending colon and rectum	intermediolateral nuc. in cord segments T12-L3	lumbar and inf. mesenteric symp. ganglia	autonomic nuc. of intermediate gray in cord segment S2-4	ganglia of hemorrhoidal myenteric and submucous plexi
Sex organs	intermediolateral nuc. in cord segments T10-L2	lumbar, sacral and inf. mesenteric symp. ganglia	autonomic nuc. of intermediate gray in cord segments S2-4	ganglia along branches of aorta and int. iliac arteries (e.g. ovarian, uterine)
Urinary bladder	intermediolateral nuc. in cord segments T12-L2	lumbar and inf. mesenteric symp. ganglia	autonomic nuc. of intermediate gray in cord segments S2-4	ganglia along vesical branches of int. iliac artery
Sweat glands and blood vessels of lower extremity	intermediolateral nuc. in cord segments L1-2	lumbar and sacral symp. ganglia		

FIG. 8-3. Location of preganglionic and postganglionic autonomic neurons to important visceral structures.

they innervate. These ganglia show extreme variations in size and compactness of organization. Some are organized into distinct anatomically encapsulated structures, as in the case of the sympathetic trunks and the autonomic ganglia of the head. Others form extensive plexuses of nerve cells and fibers, as in the intramural intestinal plexuses. Small ganglionic masses or scattered cell groups are found within, or near, the walls of visceral structures (e.g., heart, bronchi, pancreas and urinary bladder).

The outflow of preganglionic fibers from

the central nervous system, which establishes synaptic connections with peripheral autonomic ganglia, arises from three well defined regions. The *cranial outflow* arises from visceral cell groups of the brain stem associated with the oculomotor, facial, glossopharyngeal and vagus nerves and emerges from the brain stem in association with these cranial nerves (*blue* in Fig. 8-1). Preganglionic fibers arising from these nuclei are parasympathetic and terminate either in cranial autonomic ganglia (i.e., ciliary, pterygopalatine, submandibular or otic), or in terminal ganglia within the walls of thoracic or abdominal viscera (e.g., heart, lungs, esophagus and stomach). The *thoracolumbar outflow* arises from cells of the intermediolateral cell column in all thoracic and the upper two or three lumbar spinal segments. The peripheral processes of these cells give rise to preganglionic sympathetic fibers which emerge from the spinal cord via the ventral roots of the thoracic and upper lumbar spinal nerves (*red* in Fig. 8-1). Peripherally these fibers leave the mixed spinal nerve as the *white rami communicantes*, enter the sympathetic trunk and terminate upon cells in the paravertebral and prevertebral ganglia (Fig. 8-2). Although the thoracolumbar outflow arises from a cell column in a restricted region of the spinal cord (i.e., T1 to L3), it represents the total sympathetic output for the entire body. This is possible because some preganglionic sympathetic fibers ascend and descend in the sympathetic trunk for considerable distances before terminating upon postganglionic neurons. The *sacral outflow* arises from preganglionic visceral neurons in the second, third and fourth sacral segments of the spinal cord. These preganglionic parasympathetic fibers emerge from sacral spinal segments via their corresponding ventral roots and pass to terminal ganglia within the walls of pelvic viscera (*blue* in Fig. 8-1).

Although preganglionic neurons are located in three distinct regions of the central nervous system, only two main divisions of the autonomic nervous system are recognized: (1) the *sympathetic* or *thoracolumbar system*, and (2) the *parasympathetic* or *craniosacral system* (Figs. 8-1 and

8-2). In spite of the restricted central origins of preganglionic sympathetic and parasympathetic fibers, most viscera receive a double autonomic innervation. Peripherally fibers of the two divisions of the autonomic nervous system often are intermingled, but they retain their functional independence, which usually is antagonistic but closely integrated. The thoracolumbar outflow provides sympathetic innervation for all visceral structures of the body via synaptic articulations with postganglionic sympathetic neurons in peripheral autonomic ganglia. The cranial portion of the parasympathetic system supplies specific visceral structures in the head via postganglionic parasympathetic fibers from autonomic ganglia, and thoracic and abdominal viscera via the vagus nerve and postganglionic fibers from terminal ganglia. Pelvic viscera are innervated by the parasympathetic sacral outflow and postganglionic fibers from terminal ganglia.

The Sympathetic System. The sympathetic trunks are two ganglionated cords symmetrically placed along the anterolateral aspects of the vertebral column that extend from the base of the skull to the coccyx. The cervical portion contains three ganglia formed by the fusion of the original eight segmental ganglia. The *superior cervical ganglion*, the largest of the paravertebral ganglia, is situated near the second and third cervical vertebrae. The small *middle cervical ganglion* (often absent), when present, lies near the sixth cervical vertebra. The *inferior cervical ganglion* lies at the lower border of the seventh cervical vertebra, behind the subclavian artery. This ganglion frequently fuses with the first thoracic ganglion to form the *stellate ganglion* (Fig. 8-1). In the thoracic, lumbar and sacral regions, the ganglia are segmentally arranged. There are 11 or 12 thoracic, 3 or 4 lumbar and 4 or 5 sacral ganglia. In the sacral portion, the two trunks gradually approach each other and fuse at the coccyx in the unpaired coccygeal ganglion.

The prevertebral ganglia are irregular ganglionic masses surrounding the visceral branches of the aorta. The largest prevertebral ganglia are the paired celiac ganglia embedded in a mass of connective tissue and nerve fibers. Other prevertebral ganglia are the aorticorenal, the phrenic and the superior and inferior mesenteric. These ganglia are closely interconnected by numerous nerve fibers (Fig. 8-1) and will be described in relation to the celiac and subsidiary plexuses.

The sympathetic ganglia receive preganglionic fibers from the spinal cord through the ventral roots of all the thoracic and the upper two lumbar nerves (Sheehan, '41, '41a; Pick and Sheehan, '46). These fibers leave the ventral roots, pass through the white rami communicantes and enter the sympathetic trunk, where they have two general destinations: (1) the paravertebral ganglia, or (2) the prevertebral ganglia. Those that terminate in the paravertebral sympathetic ganglia either end in the first one entered, or pass up or down in the sympathetic trunk giving off collaterals, and finally terminate in ganglia above or below the level of their entrance (Fig. 8-1). The preganglionic fibers from the upper five thoracic nerves pass mainly upward and, in the cat, T1 contributes the smallest number of ascending fibers in the cervical sympathetic trunk (Foley and Schnitzlein, '57). Those from the middle thoracic segments (T7 to T10) pass up or down, while those of the lowest thoracic and lumbar segments pass only downward. The preganglionic fibers that terminate in the prevertebral ganglia do not synapse in the paravertebral ganglia, but merely pass through them and emerge as the splanchnic nerves (Figs. 8-1 and 8-2). While the sympathetic pathway from the spinal cord to the viscera always involves two neurons, there are never more than two. Thus, synapses between pre- and postganglionic neurons occur either in the paravertebral or prevertebral ganglia, but not in both.

While the white rami communicantes are limited to the thoracic and upper lumbar nerves, each spinal nerve receives a *gray ramus communicans* from the sympathetic trunk (Fig. 8-2). The gray ramus consists of unmyelinated postganglionic fibers which innervate the blood vessels, arrector pili muscles and glands of the body wall.

The cervical sympathetic ganglia receive ascending preganglionic fibers from the white rami of the upper thoracic nerves, most of which go to the superior cervical ganglion.

The *superior cervical ganglion* gives rise to postganglionic fibers distributed as gray rami to: (1) the lower four cranial nerves, (2) the upper three or four cervical nerves, (3) the pharynx, (4) the external and internal carotid arteries, and (5) the superior cervical cardiac nerve. Postganglionic sympathetic fibers passing to the external and internal carotid arteries form plexuses about these vessels and their branches (Mitchell, '53). From these vascular plexuses the postganglionic fibers pass through cranial autonomic ganglia to join branches of the cranial nerves. Such sympathetic postganglionic fibers supply the dilator muscle of the iris, the smooth muscle portion of the levator palpebrae, the orbital muscle of Müller, the blood vessels, sweat glands, hair of the head and face and the lacrimal and salivary glands (Fig. 8-3). The superior cervical cardiac nerve passes to the cardiac plexus.

The *middle cervical ganglion*, when present, supplies gray rami to cervical nerves C5 and C6, and sometimes also to C4 and C7. When this ganglion is absent these spinal nerves receive gray rami from the sympathetic trunk.

The *inferior cervical ganglion* furnishes gray rami to spinal nerves C7, C8 and T1 (Fig. 8-3). Thus a single ganglion may supply two or more of the lower cervical nerves, and a single nerve may be supplied by two ganglia. Potts ('24) has found that the lower four cervical nerves may each receive three gray rami derived from the sympathetic trunk and from the middle and inferior cervical ganglia. In addition, the middle and inferior cervical ganglia give off, respectively, the middle and inferior cardiac nerves, which take part in the formation of the cardiac plexus (Fig. 8-1).

The thoracic, lumbar and sacral ganglia furnish gray rami to the remaining spinal nerves. Delicate branches from the upper four or five thoracic ganglia go to the cardiac plexuses as the thoracic cardiac nerves. Other fibers from the inferior cervical ganglion reach the pulmonary plexuses to innervate the bronchial musculature and blood vessels of the lungs (Fig. 8-3). Shorter mediastinal branches from both the thoracic and lumbar ganglia form plexuses around the thoracic and abdominal aorta. In addition to these, there are two, sometimes three, important branches known as the *splanchnic nerves* which arise from the thoracic portion of the sympathetic trunk, pierce the diaphragm and terminate in the prevertebral ganglia of the mesenteric plexuses (Fig. 8-1). Although the splanchnic nerves appear to be branches of thoracic ganglia, they represent axons of preganglionic neurons which merely pass through paravertebral ganglia and the sympathetic trunk en route to the celiac and mesenteric ganglia. Thus the splanchnic nerves correspond to white rami communicantes. The *greater splanchnic nerve* arises by roots from the fifth to the ninth thoracic ganglia and goes to the celiac plexus. The *lesser splanchnic nerve* usually arises by two roots from the tenth and eleventh ganglia, and either unites with the greater splanchnic, or continues as an independent nerve to that portion of the celiac plexus which surrounds the roots of the renal arteries and terminates in the aorticorenal ganglion (Mitchell, '53). The *smallest splanchnic nerve*, when present, arises from the last thoracic ganglion and goes to the renal plexus. Often this nerve is represented by a branch from the lesser splanchnic nerve.

The *celiac plexus*, the largest of all autonomic plexuses, surrounds the celiac and superior mesenteric arteries. This asymmetrical paired plexus extends cranially to the diaphragm, caudally to the renal arteries and laterally to the suprarenal bodies. It becomes continuous below with the abdominal aortic plexuses. From the main plexus paired and unpaired subsidiary plexuses are given off which accompany the branches of the celiac and superior mesenteric arteries as well as other branches of the abdominal aorta. The paired plexuses include the phrenic, suprarenal and spermatic (or ovarian); the gastric, hepatic, splenic and superior mesenteric plexuses are unpaired. Within the celiac plexus are found two relatively large ganglionic masses, the *celiac ganglia*, lying on either side of the celiac artery and connected with each other by delicate fiber strands. Occasionally the two may be so close as to form a single unpaired ganglion encircling the artery. Other ganglionic masses found in the plexus include the paired aorticorenal ganglia and the *superior mesenteric ganglion* lying near the roots of their respective arteries. All these ganglia receive preganglionic fibers from the splanchnic nerves.

Caudally the celiac plexus becomes continuous with the abdominal aortic plexuses lying on either side of the aorta. From these plexuses nerve strands pass to the root of the inferior mesenteric artery and form the inferior mesenteric plexus, which surrounds that artery and its branches. Within this plexus and lying close to the root of the artery is another prevertebral ganglionic mass, the *inferior mesenteric ganglion* (Figs. 8-1 and 8-11). Further caudally, the abdominal aortic plexuses are continued into the unpaired *hypogastric* or *pelvic plexus*, which also receives strands from the inferior mesenteric plexus. On entering the pelvis the plexus breaks up into a number of subsidiary plexuses adjacent to the rectum, bladder and accessory genital organs (Figs. 8-9 and 8-11). The preganglionic fibers supplying the pelvic organs come from the white rami of the two upper lumbar nerves and from the lowest thoracic nerve. They pass through the corresponding ganglia of the sympathetic trunk, and terminate in the inferior mesenteric ganglion (Fig. 8-1). The cells of this ganglion then send their postganglionic axons by way of the inferior mesenteric and hypogastric plexuses to the pelvic viscera (Fig. 8-11).

The Parasympathetic System. The preganglionic fibers of the craniosacral division form synaptic relations with postganglionic neurons in cranial autonomic, or terminal ganglia. In the *cranial* region four such ganglia are related topographically to the branches of the trigeminal nerve (Fig. 8-1). The *ciliary ganglion* lying against the lateral surface of the optic nerve receives preganglionic fibers from the visceral nuclei of the oculomotor nerve (III) and sends postganglionic fibers (short ciliary nerves) to the sphincter of the iris and the smooth muscle of the ciliary body. The *pterygopalatine ganglion*, in the pterygopalatine fossa, and the *submandibular ganglion*, lying over the submandibular gland, receive fibers from the superior salivatory nucleus via the intermediate portion of the facial nerve (VII) (Figs. 8-1 and 12-15). The preganglionic fibers pass by way of the major petrosal nerve to the pterygopalatine ganglion, and by way of the chorda tympani nerve to the submandibular ganglion. The latter usually is broken up into submandibular and sublingual portions. The pterygopalatine ganglion sends postganglionic fibers to the lacrimal glands and to the blood vessels and glands of the mucous membranes of the nose and palate. Postganglionic fibers from the submandibular ganglion go to the submandibular and sublingual salivary glands and also to the mucous membranes of the floor of the mouth. The *otic ganglion* is situated mesially to the mandibular nerve as it leaves the oval foramen. It receives preganglionic fibers from the inferior salivatory nucleus of the glossopharyngeal nerve (IX) by way of the minor petrosal nerve and sends postganglionic fibers to the parotid gland (Fig. 8-1). All of these cranial autonomic ganglia receive nerve filaments from the superior cervical ganglion, passing by way of the internal and external carotid plexuses. These filaments do not synapse with the ganglionic cells, but merely pass through the cranial parasympathetic ganglia to furnish sympathetic innervation to blood vessels, smooth muscle and glands.

The largest source of preganglionic parasympathetic fibers is the dorsal motor nucleus of the vagus nerve (X), which supplies practically all the thoracic and abdominal viscera except those in the pelvic region (Figs. 8-1 and 8-3). In the thorax, these preganglionic fibers enter the pulmonary, cardiac and esophageal plexuses to be distributed to the terminal (intrinsic) ganglia of the heart and bronchial musculature. Short postganglionic fibers then go to the heart and bronchial muscle. In the

abdomen, the parasympathetic fibers of the vagus nerve go to the stomach, and pass through the celiac and its subsidiary plexuses, to end in the terminal ganglia of the intestine, liver, pancreas and probably the kidneys. In the alimentary canal these terminal ganglia form the extensive ganglionated plexuses of Auerbach (myenteric) and of Meissner (submucosal). They extend the whole length of the digestive tube from the upper portion of the esophagus to the internal anal sphincter. These plexuses are composed of numerous small aggregations of ganglion cells intimately connected to each other by delicate transverse and longitudinal fiber bundles. From intramural neurons short postganglionic fibers terminate in the smooth muscle and glandular epithelium and serve motor and secretory functions. The alimentary innervation of the vagus extends as far as the descending colon (Figs. 8-1 and 8-3).

The *sacral* preganglionic parasympathetic fibers exit from the spinal cord via the second, third and fourth sacral nerves which form the *pelvic nerve* (N. erigentes) and go to the terminal ganglia of the pelvic plexuses, as well as to the myenteric and submucosal plexuses of the descending colon and rectum (Fig. 8-1). Postganglionic fibers from terminal ganglia supply the urinary bladder, descending colon, rectum and accessory reproductive organs. The sacral autonomic fibers innervate viscera not supplied by the vagus (Figs. 8-3 and 8-11).

The enteric plexuses differ from the other autonomic plexuses in one important respect. They contain some intrinsic mechanism for local reflex action, since coordinated peristalsis occurs on stimulation of the gut after section of all the nerves which connect these plexuses with the central nervous system. The nature of this reflex mechanism is not fully understood.

It is evident from the above that all the autonomic plexuses consist of complicated intermixtures of sympathetic and parasympathetic fibers which are difficult to distinguish morphologically. It should be emphasized again that the sympathetic preganglionic fibers are interrupted in the paravertebral and prevertebral ganglia, while

perikarya

the parasympathetic preganglionic fibers pass by way of the plexuses to the terminal ganglia.

Visceral Afferent Fibers. There are numerous receptors in the viscera whose afferent fibers, myelinated or unmyelinated, travel centrally by way of the autonomic nerves, both sympathetic and parasympathetic. The largest myelinated fibers come principally from Pacinian corpuscles, while the smaller myelinated and the unmyelinated ones come from the more numerous diffuse visceral receptors (Fig. 6-3). Sensory fibers from the thoracic, abdominal and pelvic viscera traverse sympathetic and splanchnic nerves to reach the sympathetic trunk. They pass uninterruptedly through the trunk and white communicating rami to their perikarya of origin in the dorsal root ganglia (Figs. 8-2, 8-11 and 9-22). The parasympathetic nerves likewise contain many visceral afferent fibers. The visceral afferent fibers of the vagus nerve, whose cell bodies are in the inferior (nodose) ganglion, are distributed peripherally to the heart, lungs and other viscera. Similar fibers from the bladder, rectum and accessory genital organs pass by way of the pelvic nerves and enter the spinal cord through the second, third and fourth sacral dorsal roots (Fig. 8-11). Their cell bodies are located in corresponding sacral spinal ganglia. Visceral sensory fibers from the bladder also enter the spinal cord through the lower thoracic and lumbar spinal nerves (Fig. 8-11). The sacral visceral afferent fibers, which convey impulses from stretch receptors in the wall of the urinary bladder, play a dominant role both in reflex control and the mediation of vesical pain impulses. These afferents accompany the sacral parasympathetic outflow and convey the sensory impulses that signal bladder distension. The sensation of a distended bladder is abolished by anesthetic block of the pelvic nerves, resection of these nerves or the cutting of dorsal roots S2, S3 and S4. Visceral afferents from the bladder and adjacent viscera which ascend to the lumbar and lower thoracic dorsal root ganglia appear to play a minor role in the regulation of the bladder. Resection of the presacral nerve and hypo-

gastric plexus in man produces little or no alteration of vesical function.

The afferent visceral fibers are important in the initiation of various visceral and viscerosomatic reflexes mediated through the spinal cord and brain stem. Many of these reactions remain at a subconscious level, but afferent impulses also give rise to visceral pain or distress, nausea, hunger and other poorly localized visceral sensations. It is the constant stream of afferent visceral impulses that is responsible for the general feeling of internal well being, or of malaise.

Visceral pain from most abdominal and pelvic organs is carried chiefly by the sympathetic nerves. Vagal sensory fibers are concerned with specific visceromotor, vasomotor and secretory reflexes, most of which do not reach consciousness. It should be recalled that pain carried by visceral afferent fibers from diseased or inflamed organs may be "referred" to skin areas supplied by somatic afferent fibers of the same segment (see page 155). The sense of taste is mediated by afferent fibers of the vagus, glossopharyngeal and facial nerves, while impulses giving rise to the sensation of hunger probably are carried by the vagus. *implies immature form*

Structure of Autonomic Ganglia. The *see p 57* autonomic ganglia are aggregations of multipolar neurons of varying size and shape, each surrounded by a connective tissue capsule. Trabeculae extending from the capsule form an internal framework which contains numerous, often pigmented perikarya, between which are irregular plexuses of myelinated and unmyelinated fibers (Figs. 4-1C and 8-4). Besides these ganglia, isolated autonomic cells or nonencapsulated aggregations of such cells are found widely distributed throughout the viscera.

The diameter of autonomic cells ranges from 20 to 60 μ, and the number and length of their branching dendrites is exceedingly variable. There may be as few as 3 or 4 on some perikarya, and as many as 20 on others. The cells have a clear ovoid and often eccentric nucleus, delicate neurofibrils and fine chromophilic bodies. Binucleated or even multinucleated cells are not uncommon. Most of the cells are surrounded by cellular capsules similar to those surrounding spinal ganglion cells (Figs. 4-6 and 7-2). Electron microscopic studies of autonomic ganglion cells reveal large pigmented granules, numerous small dense bodies and the usual perikaryonal components. Neuronal processes are readily identified as they emerge from cells or, when viewed without this continuity, by the striking number of synaptic and presynaptic junctions with which they are studded (Pick, '70). Processes filled with Nissl substance, mitochondria, large inclusion bodies and pigment particles usually are considered to be dendrites. Neuronal processes containing only neurofilaments and some smooth vesicles are regarded as axons, but the distinction between dendrites and axons on the basis of the presence or absence of Nissl substance is not easy to make. Furthermore there are no reliable morphological criteria for distinguishing between cells and fibers belonging to the sympathetic and parasympathetic systems.

Some of the cells have short dendrites which ramify within the capsules. These are numerous in the autonomic ganglia of man (Fig. 8-4). Others have long, slender dendrites which pierce the capsule and run for varying distances in the intercellular plexuses. Some cells possess both short and long processes. The intracapsular dendrites may arborize symmetrically on all sides of the cell or they may form interlocking dendritic processes between two or more cells, enclosed within a single capsule (Fig. 8-5A). Such cells probably receive common terminal arborizations of preganglionic fibers. The extracapsular dendrites have similar terminal arborizations at varying distances from the cell body.

Preganglionic fibers end in synaptic relation with the perikarya and dendrites of many postganglionic cells (Fig. 8-5B). They branch repeatedly within the ganglion and form pericellular arborizations; some of the terminals end by neurofibrillar rings or loops on the cell body. More common are the axodendritic synapses where the preganglionic fibers end in diffuse arborizations about the intracapsular and extracapsular dendrites. Although the synaptic arrangements within autonomic ganglia are not fully known, there are suggestions that these ganglia are not simple relays transmitting impulses between preganglionic and postganglionic neurons (Hillarp, '60). Because small cells interpreted as internuncial neurons have been described (Williams, '67), questions are raised as to the possible role of interneurons.

If the superior cervical ganglion (Fig. 8-1) is isolated by section of all incoming preganglionic fibers, the postganglionic perikarya do not degenerate. The isolated postganglionic perikarya may decrease slightly in diameter and show alterations of Nissl substance, endoplasmic reticulum and mitochondria, but they survive, i.e., the perikarya do not demonstrate transneuronal degeneration (Hamlyn, '54; Barton and Causey, '58). However, following section of postganglionic axons of the cervical and ciliary ganglia, the perikarya show central chromatolysis and changes in their electrophysiological properties (Warwick, '54; Barton and Causey, '58; Hunt and Riker, '66).

The capsule cells of the autonomic ganglia are known to contain a variety of enzymes (Truex, '51; Adams, '65). They have been considered as homologous to the oligodendrocytes by Schwyn ('67); to satellite and Schwann cells of dorsal root ganglia by Barton and Causey ('58); or as connective tissue fibroblasts and interstitial cells. These supportive cells show a marked hyperplasia following stimulation of the preganglionic fibers for periods of 105 to 180 min (Schwyn, '67). This author believes the capsule cells participate in neuronal metabolism and DNA turnover during periods of increased metabolism and synaptic activity.

Chemical Mediation at Synapse. The investigations of Dale ('14), Loewi ('21, '45), Cannon ('29) and many others have demonstrated that autonomic effects are mediated by chemical substances, known as *neurohumoral transmitters*, liberated at preganglionic and postganglionic nerve terminals. The neurohumoral transmitter of all preganglionic autonomic fibers, of all postganglionic parasympathetic fibers and

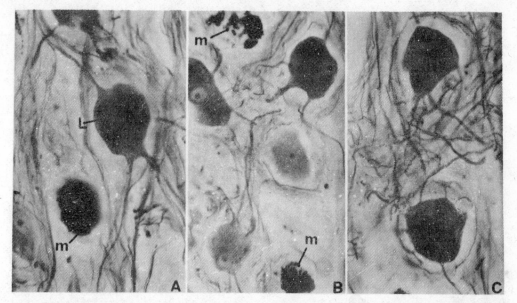

FIG. 8-4. Adult human sympathetic neurons. Note interdigitating dendrites that often form a pericellular plexus. Perikarya show some eccentric nuclei, melanin granules (*m*) and lipofuscin (*L*). The nuclei of the capsule cells are not stained. Cajal silver stain. ×490.

of postganglionic sympathetic nerve fibers innervating sweat glands is acetylcholine. Acetylcholine also is the transmitter at somatic motor nerve terminals in skeletal muscle, and numerous investigations suggest that acetylcholine is involved in synaptic transmission in the central nervous system, although it is not the universal central transmitter. An impulse transmitted to an autonomic ganglion; or a somatic neuromuscular junction, causes the synchronous release of several hundred quanta of acetylcholine stored in synaptic vesicles at axonal terminals. The transmitter diffuses across the synaptic cleft (200 Å) and combines with receptors on the postjunctional membrane, which may result in a localized depolarization and propagation of an impulse. Nerves which liberate acetylcholine as the neurohumoral transmitter at their terminals are called *cholingeric fibers*. At cholinergic junctions impulse transmission liberates a specialized enzyme, *acetylcholinesterase*, which readily hydrolyzes free acetylcholine to choline and acetic acid. Thus, acetylcholinesterase serves to terminate the transmitter action of acetylcholine at postsynaptic sites and at effector junctions. Nerve impulses conveyed by cholinergic fibers pro-

duce rapid, localized responses of short duration in postjunctional effectors. Since acetylcholine serves as the neurohumoral transmitter at various peripheral junctions, postjunctional cholinergic receptors are assumed to share certain common features. Because individual drugs vary in respect to their potency at different cholinoceptive sites, various receptors must have distinctive, as well as common, features. Drugs which combine with a cholinergic receptor produce either: (1) the same effect as acetylcholine (i.e., cholinomimetic effect), or (2) no apparent effect, because occupation of the receptor site prevents the action of acetylcholine (i.e., cholinergic blockade). Cholinomimetic responses of drugs at autonomic effector cells are referred to as *muscarinic effects*. Drugs which produce responses in sequence are said to produce *nicotinic effects*, because nicotine in low doses stimulates, while higher doses paralyze autonomic ganglia. Atropine selectively blocks all muscarinic responses to acetylcholine and related cholinomimetic drugs. Nicotinic receptors in autonomic ganglia and skeletal muscle are not identical in that tetraethylammonium and hexamethonium selectively block ganglionic transmission, and *d*-tubocurarine

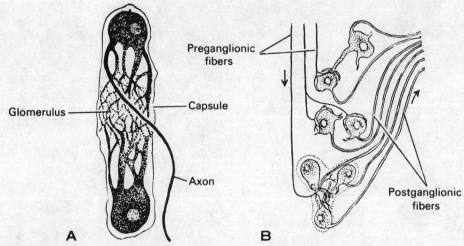

Fig. 8-5. *A*, Glomerulus formed by dendrites of two sympathetic ganglion cells (after Cajal, '11). *B*, Diagram of the relationships between preganglionic fibers and sympathetic ganglion cells. One preganglionic fiber may come into synaptic relationships with several sympathetic cells (after Ranson and Billingsley, '18).

blocks transmission at both the somatic motor end plates and at autonomic ganglia, although its action at the motor end plate predominates. Cholinergic neurons of the central nervous system also exhibit either nicotinic or muscarinic responses.

Drugs which inhibit or inactivate acetylcholinesterase cause acetylcholine to accumulate at cholinergic sites and produce effects equivalent to continuous stimulation of cholinergic fibers. Physostigmine (eserine), neostigmine and edrophonium (tensilon) are "reversible" anticholinesterase drugs useful in treating myasthenia gravis, glaucoma and atony of smooth muscle. "Irreversible" anticholinesterase compounds form the basis for "nerve gases" which are among the most potent synthetic toxic agents known (Koelle, '70).

The majority of postganglionic sympathetic nerves release norepinephrine as the transmitter substance and probably should be classified as *noradrenergic*, although the older term, *adrenergic*, is more widely used (Cannon and Rosenblueth, '33, '37; McLennan, '63; von Euler, '56, '61; Norberg, '67). The widespread distribution of sympathetic nerves and the demonstration of monoaminergic neurons in the central nervous system suggest that monoaminergic mechanisms are of immense importance. The fundamental discovery (Falck

et al., '62) that certain monoamines and precursors could be made intensely fluorescent by formaldehyde gas led to the application of this principle to tissue sections (Falck, '62; Falck and Torp, '62). This method permits anatomical localization of monoamines and investigations of problems related to the synthesis, storage, release and metabolism of the amines in neurons and their terminals (Figs. 4-13, 8-6, 8-7, 12-26 and 13-18). Fluorescence histochemical observations indicate that in postganglionic sympathetic nerves, norepinephrine is present not only in synaptic terminals, but in the entire sympathetic neuron (von Euler, '56, '61; Falck, '62; Norberg, '67). Norepinephrine, as found by the fluorescence method, appears to be especially intense in enlargements of the nerve terminals referred to as varicosities. Terminal varicosities form a ground plexus in close contact with effector cells, and according to Hillarp ('59) the transmitter is released along the entire length of the terminals (Fig. 8-7). Evidence indicates that the norepinephrine content of the terminals can be depleted by electrical stimulation (Malmfors, '64; Norberg, '67). Thus there is little doubt that the varicosities are specialized structures involved in the storage and release of the transmitter. Histochemical studies have shown

α = excite   β = inhibit
EXCEPT —1) β in heart = excite; 2) α & β in GI tct are inhibitory and additive

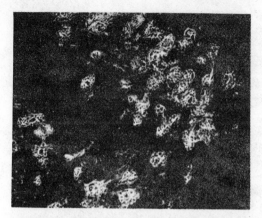

FIG. 8-6. Catecholamine-containing neurons surrounding the mesencephalic tract of the trigeminal nucleus in the squirrel monkey as demonstrated by fluorescent histochemical technics. In some cells the fluorescent material can be seen in cell processes. ×400. (Courtesy of Dr. David Felten, School of Medicine, Indiana University.)

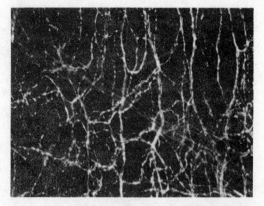

FIG. 8-7. Normal rat iris. Strands of the adrenergic ground plexus over the dilator muscle are demonstrated by fluorescent histochemical technics. Several nerve terminals demonstrate pronounced varicosities. ×250. (Courtesy of Dr. Torbjörn Malmfors, Karolinska Institutet, Sweden.)

that the transmitter is stored in special granules within the adrenergic neurons and electron microscopic observations indicate that the storage granules and "densecored" vesicles (Figs. 8-7 and 8-8) are identical (Wolfe et al., '62; von Euler, '66; Hökfelt, '66). All parts of the sympathetic adrenergic neuron contain norepinephrine, but the terminals contain the highest concentrations (von Euler, '56). Recent evidence indicates that transmitter granules in adrenergic neurons are formed in the cell body, transported peripherally in the axon and stored in terminal varicosities (Dahlström, '65; Norberg, '67).

In the adrenal medulla the release of acetylcholine by preganglionic sympathetic fibers and its combination with receptors on chromaffin cells is followed by the liberation of epinephrine into the extracellular fluid which ultimately enters the circulation. Osmophilic granules have been isolated from the adrenal medulla which contain high concentrations of catecholamines and collectively represent a major storage depot of epinephrine.

The adrenergic neuron also contains mechanisms for the inactivation of the transmitter substance, but these are not as rapid and efficient as those involved in the breakdown of acetylcholine. Monoamine oxidase (MAO) is an intraneuronal en-

zyme considered to be involved in regulating the amine level within the neuron (Carlsson, '65). The adrenergic transmitter released at synaptic junctions is inactivated by several mechanisms: (1) diffusion, (2) the enzyme catechol-o-methyltransferase (COMT) which occurs extraneuronally, and (3) binding to extraneuronal sites not involved in nerve conduction. The inactivating mechanism of greatest physiological importance is the reuptake of transmitter substance by adrenergic terminals. This uptake occurs at the neuronal cell membrane by an active mechanism called the membrane pump (Carlsson, '65; Norberg, '67). The membrane pump in the nerve terminals has the ability to concentrate the amine more than 1,000 times.

Smooth muscle can be either excited or inhibited by norepinephrine, epinephrine and other catecholamines, depending upon the site and the concentration. Norepinephrine excites smooth muscle, isoproterenol inhibits smooth muscle and epinephrine can both excite and inhibit. Ahlquist ('48) postulated two types of adrenergic receptors: (1) α receptors associated with excitatory responses and (2) β receptors associated with inhibition. There are two major exceptions to the above: (1) stimulation of β receptors in cardiac muscle produces excitatory effects, and (2) stimulation of

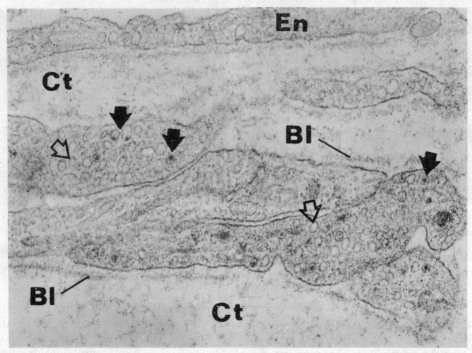

Fig. 8-8. Electron micrograph of a sympathetic nerve terminating in the pericapillary connective tissue (*Ct*) of a rat pineal gland. The axons, close to their terminals, lack a Schwann cell investment and are covered only by a basal lamina (*Bl*). Agranular vesicles (*open arrows*) and granular vesicles (*solid arrows*), which contain a biogenic amine, are numerous. *En* identifies the capillary endothelial cell. ×50,000. (Courtesy of Dr. W. Bondareff, School of Medicine, Northwestern University.)

either α or β receptors in the gastrointestinal tract produces inhibitory responses that are additive. Synthetic compounds which structurally resemble naturally occurring catecholamines can combine with α or β receptors and produce sympathomimetic effects. The term *adrenergic blocking agent* is used for compounds that selectively inhibit certain responses to adrenergic nerves, epinephrine and sympathomimetic amines. Since adrenergic blocking agents are selective and specific for either α or β receptors, two distinctive classes of agents are recognized (Nickerson, '70).

Acetylcholine, norepinephrine and certain other catecholamines probably serve as transmitters at certain sites within the central nervous system. *Dopamine,* an intermediary compound in the synthesis of norepinephrine, appears to be the predominant transmitter of impulses from the substantia nigra to the striatum (Fig. 13-18) (Fuxe and Andén, '66; Hökfelt and Ungerstedt, '69). Serotonin (5-hydroxytrypt-amine), found particularly in the raphe nuclei of the brain stem (Ungerstedt, '71), also is considered to be a synaptic transmitter, but its precise role is obscure (Fig. 4-13*B*). There is some evidence that it may be involved in mechanisms that induce sleep (Jouvet, '68). The locus ceruleus, a pigmented structure in the upper pons, is composed of neurons containing norepinephrine which give rise to ascending monosynaptic pathways widely distributed in the cerebral cortex, the cerebellar cortex and diencephalic structures (Figs. 8-6 and 12-26) (Olson and Fuxe, '71; Ungerstedt, '71). Norepinephrine neurons in the locus ceruleus may exert activating influences upon all cortices. The monoamine pathways in the central nervous system are much more extensive than indicated here and have been mapped in some animals (Ungerstedt, '71; Felten et al., '74). Furthermore all three monoamine systems mentioned here (dopamine, serotonin and norepinephrine) have networks or terminals in the hypothalamus and are considered to be involved in neuroendocrine functions (Fuxe and Hökfelt, '70). An increasing number of studies suggest that γ-aminobutyric acid (GABA) may serve as an inhibitory neurotransmitter in the central nervous system, but no histochemical methods exist by which it can be visualized directly in tissue (Hökfelt and Ljungdahl, '72).

Figure 8-8 shows autonomic axon terminals in the rat pineal body which contain biogenic amines. Available evidence indicates that the dense or granulated vesicles of the pineal body contain an adrenergic transmitter, whereas the clear, or nongranulated, vesicles are storage sites of acetylcholine and other transmitter substances (see De Robertis et al., '65).

The terms "adrenergic" and "cholinergic" do not correspond completely with "sympathetic" and "parasympathetic," respectively. Thus the postganglionic fibers to the sweat glands (sudomotor fibers), although anatomically part of the sympathetic system, are cholinergic. Moreover they react to certain drugs, such as pilocarpine and atropine, in the same way as parasympathetic fibers. It should be recalled that the upper and lower extremities have no parasympathetic nerve fibers. In these regions the sympathetic postganglionic fibers are of two distinct types: most are adrenergic, but those to the sweat glands are cholinergic (Figs. 8-9 and 8-10). There are other instances of mixed autonomic nerves. For example, the splanchnic nerves contain both adrenergic and cholinergic fibers. The latter are destined for the adrenal medulla, where acetylcholine is the transmitter substance. Overactivity of both adrenergic and cholinergic fibers is indicative of either autonomic imbalance, irritating lesions or abnormal regeneration along the course of the fibers. These may be expressed as excessive or abnormal sweating and salivation, alterations in gastrointestinal motility or increased peripheral vasoconstriction as in hypertension. Appropriate drugs can either enhance or inhibit impulses at the sympathetic and parasympathetic ganglionic synapses, or block the membrane receptor sites upon which the neurotransmitter substances produce their effects (e.g., muscle, heart, glands, blood vessels).

Denervation Sensitization. It was noted above that the postganglionic perikarya and their processes persist following section of the appropriate preganglionic fibers. It is known that section of the preganglionic fibers results in increased sensitivity of the isolated neurons and the tissues they supply to circulating adrenaline. The exact way in which the neuroeffector mechanism is altered remains unknown. However, it was observed that complete section of the postganglionic fibers to an organ or region resulted in far greater sensitization to adrenaline than that which followed complete preganglionic nerve section. Hampel ('35) observed the qualitative responses of the nictitating membrane of the cat to adrenaline on successive days after denervation. He found that the response reached a maximum about 8 days after preganglionic denervation. Postganglionic denervation resulted in sensitization responses that were twice as great as those that followed preganglionic section. Similar responses are observed in most other tissues supplied by the adrenergic fibers. Increased sensitivity has been observed as well in structures supplied by the cholinergic fibers (e.g., lacrimal, sweat and salivary glands). The latter become sensitive to acetylcholine, which is equally true of denervated skeletal muscle. This peculiar phenomenon often is referred to as Cannon's ('39) law of denervation: "When in a series of efferent neurons a unit is destroyed, an increased irritability to chemical agents develops in the isolated structure or structures. The effect being maximal in the part directly denervated." Such denervation accounts for the increased sensitization of the superior cervical ganglion cells to acetylcholine which occurs after severance of its preganglionic fibers.

The paralysis after denervation of smooth muscle is very different from that seen in skeletal muscle where there is a persisting flaccid paralysis. Restoration of smooth muscle tone is due in part to the sensitization of the neuroeffector mechanism to circulating epinephrine. The anatomical arrangement of the preganglionic

IMPORTANT FUNCTIONS OF SOME AUTONOMIC PATHWAYS

FUNCTION	SYMPATHETIC	PARASYMPATHETIC
Iris	dilates the pupil (mydriasis)	constricts the pupil (miosis)
Lacrimal gland	little or no effect on secretion	stimulates secretion
Salivary glands	secretion reduced in amount and viscid	secretion increased in amount and watery
Sweat glands of head, neck, trunk, and extremities	stimulates secretion (cholinergic fibers) nerve fibers	little or no effect on secretion
Bronchi	dilates lumen	constricts lumen
Heart	accelerates rate, augments ventricular contraction	decreases heart rate
GI motility and secretion	inhibits	stimulates
GI sphincters	constricts	relaxes
Sex organs	contraction of ductus deferens, seminal vesicle, prostatic and uterine musculature; vasoconstriction	vasodilation and erection
Urinary bladder	little or no effect on bladder	contracts bladder wall, promotes emptying
Adrenal medulla	stimulates secretion (cholinergic nerve fibers)	little or no effect
Blood vessels of trunk and extremities	constricts	no effect

FIG. 8-9. Sympathetic and parasympathetic actions upon visceral structures.

and postganglionic sympathetic vasoconstrictor fibers to the hand and foot serves as an excellent example to illustrate this point (Fig. 8-10). In Reynaud's disease the small arteries and arterioles of the upper extremities, usually the hands, undergo episodic vasoconstriction in response to cold. As a result, the extremity demonstrates pallor and reactive hyperemia (i.e., an increased amount of blood in a part, or congestion). In chronic cases trophic changes develop with atrophy of the skin and subcutaneous tissues. Long-standing cases may develop skin ulceration or even ischemic gangrene. Removal of the inferior cervical, first and second thoracic sympathetic ganglia eliminates the vasoconstriction but destroys both the preganglionic as well as the postganglionic fibers to the forearm and hand (Fig. 8-10A). The smooth muscle of the arteries and arterioles will, in time, regain some vascular tone since the smooth muscle is also highly sensitized by removal of the postganglionic cells and fibers. Better results usually are obtained in the foot following removal of

the second and third lumbar sympathetic ganglia (Fig. 8-10B). Here the partial sympathectomy interrupts the preganglionic outflow. However, it leaves intact the postganglionic cells and fibers in the lower lumbar and sacral ganglia which reach the foot through the sciatic nerve and its branches. Thus the vessels of the leg and foot regions are less sensitized to neurohumeral catecholamines.

Central Autonomic Pathways. Visceral structures innervated by the autonomic nervous system normally maintain a constant internal environment within the organism (homeostasis). Preganglionic neurons within the central nervous system (Figs. 8-1 and 8-3) are maintained in a continuous, but quantitatively variable, state of activity by a multitude of segmental and suprasegmental mechanisms. Regulation from higher levels is not accomplished by one or even two neuron pathways. This regulation appears to be mediated by a series of synaptic relays between several interposed neurons located at successively lower levels of the brain stem (i.e., it is a somewhat diffuse multisynaptic descending system).

The hypothalamus commonly is regarded as the principal locus of central autonomic integration (see page 478). Simply stated, the most voluminous afferent connections of the hypothalamus originate from the hippocampal formation, the amygdaloid nuclear complex and the olfactory cortex, and indirectly from cortical regions which form portions of the limbic lobe (Raisman, '66; Nauta, '72). Many of these structures are involved in neural circuitry that begins in the septal region and extends in a paramedian zone through the preoptic region and hypothalamus into the rostral mesencephalon (Fig. 16-5). In this view the hypothalamus is the central part of a continuum which suggests the term "septo-hypothalamo-mesencephalic continuum" (Nauta, '72). There are a great number of reciprocal connections between structures within this subcortical continuum and phylogenetically older derivatives of the forebrain. There are no direct descending connections from the hypothalamus that extend beyond the mesencephalic tegmentum (Guillery, '57; Raisman, '66). Mesencephalic structures receive an input from the hypothalamus via: (1) a descending component of the medial forebrain bundle, (2) the mammillary bodies (mammillotegmental tract), and (3) descending projections in the periventricular gray (Fig. 16-7). It seems certain that hypothalamic impulses conveyed to the mesencephalon are transmitted to more caudal parts of the neuraxis via numerous synaptic relays within the brain stem reticular formation, although these pathways must be exceedingly complex (Nauta, '72). It is presumed that reticular neurons convey impulses to visceral motor nuclei in the brain stem and spinal cord.

In the midbrain and upper pons, these descending tracts are located dorsally and medially near the central gray matter and floor of the fourth ventricle (Smith and Clarke, '64; Wolf and Sutin, '66; Cheatham and Matzke, '66; Bradley and Conway, '66). In man and most mammals that have been studied, the fibers descending into the upper midbrain stream through the prerubral field and region above the red nucleus. Stereotaxic surgery for dyskinesia in this area of the human brain has resulted in widespread autonomic deficits (Carmel, '68). These deficits included ptosis (drooping) of the eyelid, miosis (constriction) of the pupil and a loss of sweating (hemianhydrosis) on the same side (ipsilateral) of the body as the lesion. In man these descending fibers are uncrossed below the level of the red nucleus. These fibers are located more laterally in the pontine tegmentum and reticular formation of the medulla. Through this descending fiber system, the hypothalamus and other suprasegmental structures contribute to the regulation of a variety of visceral reflex activities (e.g., blood pressure, body temperature, sweating, secretion, eye, vesicle, rectal and sexual reflexes). Lesions of these descending central tracts can result in a complete loss, or altered control, of visceral activities at lower segmental levels. For example, lesions in the lateral reticular formation of the medulla interrupt the fibers regulating sympathetic control of the smooth muscle of the eye and may result in a Horner's syndrome (see page 210).

A most unusual clinical entity (Riley et al., '49; Riley, '52, '57; Riley and Moore, '66) serves as an excellent example of the disseminated and abnormal functional activities of these descending autonomic fibers. The authors originally postulated a central, possibly congenital, diencephalic origin to account for these symptoms in children of Jewish extraction: deficiency of lacrimation; transient and extreme elevation in blood pressure induced by mild anxiety; excessive sweating and drooling of saliva; and the occurrence of sharply demarcated, bilateral and symmetrical erethymatous blotches on the skin (*familial dysautonomia* or *Riley-Day syndrome*). Subsequent study has revealed other disturbances that support a diagnosis of this syndrome. These include postural hypotension, feeding difficulties from birth onward, a relative indifference to pain, erratic control of body temperature, emotional lability, absent corneal reflexes and corneal anesthesia, absent deep tendon reflexes,

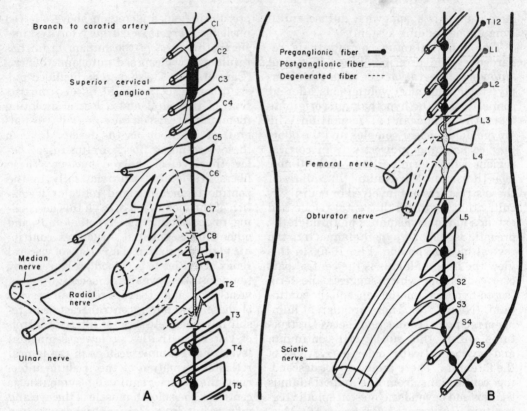

Fig. 8-10. Anatomical course of preganglionic and postganglionic sympathetic vasoconstrictor fibers to the upper and lower extremities. *A*, After cervicothoracic ganglionectomy (inferior cervical, T1 and T2, *stippled*) all of the postganglionic fibers to the hand degenerate. *B*, Resection of sympathetic ganglia L2 and L3 (*stippled*) interrupts only descending preganglionic fibers to lower lumbar and sacral sympathetic ganglia. Postganglionic fibers to the sciatic nerve and foot region do not degenerate (modified from White et al., '36).

abnormal pupillary response to methacholine and an abnormal intradermal response to histamine. Hypotonus, poor motor coordination and developmental retardation may accompany the above findings. The precise pathological causes remain unknown, but lesions have been found in the thalamus, reticular formation of pons and medulla, spinal cord, sympathetic ganglia and the myenteric plexus (Riley and Moore, '66).

Bilateral lesions of the lateral white funiculi may result in altered sweating in regions supplied by the cord segments below the level of such lesions. Control of the bladder and rectum also may be lost. After spinal cord transection the autonomic reflexes are at first depressed (spinal shock), temperature regulation and sweating are absent and blood pressure falls profoundly. Weeks later, after spinal shock has waned, segmental reflexes caudal to the lesion reappear. Somatic segmental reflexes in time become exaggerated, but visceral reflexes usually are sluggish.

FUNCTIONAL CONSIDERATIONS

Gaskell ('16) has pointed out that when a visceral structure is innervated by both sympathetic and parasympathetic fibers, the effects of the two are as a rule antagonistic. The sympathetic neurons dilate the pupil, accelerate the heart, inhibit intestinal movements and contract the vesical and rectal sphincters. The parasympathetic neurons constrict the pupil, slow the heart, further peristaltic movement and relax the above named sphincters (Fig. 8-

9). The apparently haphazard effects on smooth and cardiac muscle produced by each autonomic division in different organs (contraction in one, inhibition in another) are more readily explained when the *overall* activities of the two systems are taken into consideration. The parasympathetic deals primarily with anabolic activities concerned with the restoration and conservation of bodily energy and the resting of vital organs. In the words of Cannon ('29), "a glance at these various functions of the cranial division reveals at once that they serve for bodily conservation; by narrowing the pupil they shield the retina from excessive light; by slowing the heart rate they give the cardiac muscle longer periods for rest and invigoration; and by providing for the flow of saliva and gastric juice, and by supplying the necessary muscular tone for the contraction of the alimentary canal, they prove fundamentally essential to the processes of proper digestion and absorption, by which energy-yielding material is taken into the body and stored. To the cranial division belongs the great service of building up reserves and fortifying the body against times of need and stress." The sacral division supplements the cranial by ridding the body of intestinal and urinary wastes.

On the other hand, stimulation of the sympathetic component equips the body for the intense muscular action required in offense and defense. It is a mechanism that quickly mobilizes the existing reserves of the body during emergencies or emotional crises. The pupils dilate, respiration is deepened and the rate and force of the cardiac contractions are increased. The blood vessels of the viscera and the skin are constricted, the blood pressure is raised and an ample blood supply is made available to the skeletal muscles, lungs heart and brain. The peaceful activities are slowed or stopped; blood is drained from the huge intestinal reservoir, peristalsis and alimentary secretion are inhibited and the urinary and rectal outlets are blocked by contraction of their sphincters.

The two systems are reciprocal, and their dual activities are integrated into coordinated responses ensuring the maintenance of an adequate internal environment to meet the demands of any given situation. The parasympathetic activities are initiated primarily by internal changes in the viscera themselves. The sympathetic system is in considerable part activated by exteroceptive impulses that pass over somatic afferent fibers and are initiated by favorable or unfavorable changes in the external environment.

The preganglionic fibers of the sympathetic system arise from a continuous cell column in the spinal cord, and a single fiber may form synaptic relations with many cells in different paravertebral or prevertebral ganglia (Fig. 8-5*B*). Both types of ganglia are placed at considerable distances from the organs innervated, and from them postganglionic fibers are distributed to extensive visceral areas (Figs. 8-1 and 8-11). Such a mechanism permits a wide radiation of impulses. The norepinephrine released at most sympathetic terminals further enhances the widespread and prolonged effects of sympathetic stimulation. Thus, stimulation of a thoracic ventral root, or white ramus, causes piloerection and vasoconstriction in five, six or even more segmental skin areas.

In the parasympathetic system the preganglionic neurons are represented by more isolated cell groups whose fibers pass out in separate nerves and go directly to the terminal ganglia within or near the organs. Each preganglionic parasympathetic fiber enters into synaptic relations with fewer postganglionic neurons than is the case in the sympathetic division. Thus in the superior cervical ganglion of the cat, the ratio of preganglionic fibers to postganglionic neurons is about 1:15 or more, while in the ciliary ganglion the ratio is only 1:2 (Wolf, '41). Parasympathetic action is more discrete and is limited to the portion stimulated. The liberation and rapid hydrolysis of acetylcholine by the parasympathetic postganglionic fibers is compatible with such localized autonomic responses. Thus stimulation of the glossopharyngeal nerve increases parotid gland secretion, while stimulation of the oculomotor nerve constricts the pupil, in each case without the appearance of other parasympathetic effects.

The functions of the two subdivisions of

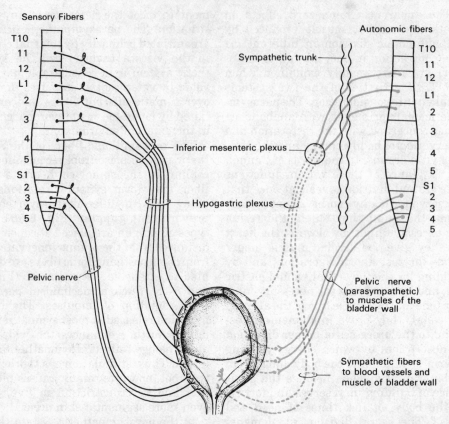

FIG. 8-11. Diagram of the sensory and autonomic innervation of the urinary bladder. Preganglionic parasympathetic visceral motor (*blue*) fibers from S2, S3 and S4 pass to terminal ganglia which give rise to postganglionic fibers that induce contractions of the detrusor muscle. Afferent impulses from stretch receptors (*black*) in the bladder wall enter upper lumbar and lower thoracic spinal segments via the hypogastric plexus, and S2, S3 and S4 spinal segments via the pelvic nerve. Descending sympathetic fibers (*red*) in the hypogastric plexus play no essential role in micturition. Somatic motor fibers from S2, S3 and S4 spinal segments (not shown) innervate the external vesicle sphincter. Relaxation of the external sphincter and contraction of the detrusor muscle are essential for micturition.

the autonomic system are most easily understood by contrasting the individual structures innervated and noting the reciprocal actions of their dual nerve supply (Fig. 8-9). The autonomic fibers to the eye provide an excellent example of this dual innervation. The sympathetic division stimulates the smooth muscle fibers of the dilator muscle of the iris, the tarsal muscle and the orbital muscle (of Müller). The tarsal muscle extends from the levator palpebrae muscle to the tarsal plate of the upper lid and aids in full elevation of the upper eyelid. The orbital muscle, at least in lower forms, keeps the ocular bulb forward in the bony orbit. Lesions in either the central or peripheral sympathetic path-

ways to the eye produce a triad of symptoms known as *Horner's syndrome*. As a result of sympathetic injury, the parasympathetic innervation is unopposed, and results in constriction of the ipsilateral pupil (miosis), dropping of the upper eyelid (pseudoptosis) and an apparent sinking in of the eyeball (enophthalmos). Vasodilation and dryness of the skin of the face also may be evident. Sympathetic fibers destined for the eye follow the internal carotid artery, while those to sweat glands on the face course along the branches of the external carotid artery. This dichotomy of postganglionic fibers from the cervical ganglia explains the altered patterns of autonomic function that can occur after injuries in the face, deep neck or within the skull. There may be loss of sweating on the face with preservation of sympathetic innervation to the eye or vice versa. Lesions of the cervical sympathetic trunk, inferior cervical ganglion or ventral roots of the upper thoracic nerves interrupt the fibers before they divide to follow separate courses.

Parasympathetic fibers to the eye stimulate the sphincter muscle of the iris and bring about constriction of the pupil. These axons also stimulate the ciliary muscle. Contraction of the circular fibers of the ciliary muscle causes relaxation of the ciliary zonule and thereby decreases the tension of the lens capsule. As a result of such parasympathetic activity, the pupil is constricted and the convexity of the lens is increased for near vision (accommodation).

Innervation of the salivary glands was long believed due solely to secretory fibers in the cranial parasympathetic nerves (Fig. 8-9). Many differences have been found between the several glands of the different species studied, but both parts of the autonomic system send secretory fibers to the salivary glands. Sympathetic fibers provide for vasoconstriction of blood vessels, contraction of the myoepithelial cells of the ducts and secretory fibers to the demilune gland cells (Babkin, '50). Stimulation of the human sympathetic trunk in the neck, or the injection of adrenaline into the salivary duct, evokes a flow of saliva from the submandibular, but not from the parotid gland. The secretory response to sympathetic stimulation is of short duration when compared to the long acting response that follows parasympathetic stimulation (Emmelin and Stromblad, '54). Parasympathetic fibers in cranial nerves VII and IX provide for vasodilation of the blood vessels and secretory fibers to the alveolar and acinar cells of the parotid, submandibular, sublingual and retrolingual glands. The vagus nerve contains secretory fibers to the glands of the trachea and upper digestive tract. For additional details on the innervation of the salivary glands the reader is referred to the extensive reviews by Babkin ('50), Lundberg ('58), Burgen and Emmelin ('61) and Emmelin ('67).

The innervation of the urinary bladder and the control of micturition represent a complex and specific autonomic function of great practical importance (Fig. 8-11). The smooth muscle of the urinary bladder exhibits two types of activity: (1) intermittent contractions which occur as the organ adapts its capacity to an increasing volume, and (2) sustained contractions associated with relaxation of the external sphincter which occur during micturition.

Visceral motor fibers of S2, S3 and S4 leave the sacral nerves, and as the *pelvic nerve,* course to the lateral wall of the bladder where the fibers terminate in small vesical ganglia. Short postganglionic parasympathetic fibers to the bladder musculature induce contraction of the detrusor smooth muscle (Fig. 8-11). Somatic motor fibers from sacral spinal segments 2, 3 and 4 become incorporated in the *pudendal* (pudic) *nerve,* and via a branch of that nerve, the perineal nerve, innervate the external vesicle sphincter. Relaxation of the external sphincter (somatic nerves) and contraction of the bladder wall (sacral visceral motor) are the two events essential for micturition. The descending sympathetic fibers in the hypogastric plexus play no essential motor role in the process of urination. They are concerned with the innervation of the vesical trigone and lower ureter, vasomotor control and the mechanism of ejaculation.

Afferent impulses responsible for the detrusor reflex arise from stretch receptors in the bladder wall and enter the spinal cord via the pelvic nerves (Talaat, '27; Root, '69). If the bladder is greatly distended, afferent impulses pass via the hypogastric nerves and plexus to reach their perikarya (spinal ganglia) and spinal segments T10 to L2 (Fig. 8-11). When the intravesical pressure attains a certain value, the detrusor muscle contracts, the external sphincter relaxes and the bladder is effectively emptied. *Vesical afferents* ascending in the hypogastric nerves serve as a sensory input to the "vesical center for retention of urine" located in cord segments T12 to L2. It should be recalled that the desire to urinate is dependent upon intravesical pressure rather than fluid-volume content. The vesical capacity and frequency of urination vary with age and are influenced by reflex, psychic and local irritative factors. In children 8 to 10 years of age the initial desire to void occurs with an intravesical pressure of 9 to 11 cm of water (bladder volume 80 to 100 ml of urine). In adults with a fluid capacity of 140 to 180 ml, an intravesical pressure of 15 to 16 cm of water induces the desire to void (Campbell, '57). The most essential sensory fibers from the bladder return to the spinal cord via the pelvic nerve and dorsal roots S2, S3 and S4. These afferents participate in reflexes that are integrated with the "vesical center for bladder evacuation" located in cord segments S3 to S5. The sacral afferent impulses to the spinal cord apparently reach conscious level through the long pathways which are poorly defined. It has been suggested that these pathways lie in the dorsal half of the lateral funiculus (Barrington, '21; McMichael, '45; Root, '69). Facilitating and inhibiting suprasegmental influences upon spinal mechanisms concerned with micturition suggest that regions in the pontine and midbrain tegmentum are involved (Tang and Ruch, '56). In addition the cerebral cortex appears to exert some control over bladder function. Clinical studies indicate that portions of the superior frontal gyrus on the medial surface of the hemisphere may be specially concerned with control of micturition and defecation (Andrew and Nathan, '64). Lesions in this region, involving one or both frontal lobes, may cause urgency, frequency of micturition or incontinence. Such lesions also are associated with lack of awareness of all vesical events including the sensation of the desire to micturate and the sensation that micturition is imminent. Disturbances of bladder function associated with spinal cord injury are described on page 279.

A familiarity with the information in Figure 8-9 proves most useful in evaluating the overall functional status of the autonomic nervous system. Vital body processes such as circulation, secretion, digestion and excretion are essentially autonomic reflex responses. The autonomic nervous system also participates in many somatic-visceral and visceral-somatic reflexes which involve either cranial or spinal nerves (e.g., respiration, pupillary, lacrimal, palatal, pharyngeal, sneeze, cough, swallowing, vomiting, carotid sinus, vasomotor, sudomotor, pilomotor, vesicle, genital and emotional reflexes). Some of these reflexes will be presented as individual nerves are discussed. Metabolic or mechanical irritations of autonomic nerve fibers in the periphery may cause exaggerations of some of the sympathetic and parasympathetic functions included in Figure 8-9. Partial or complete lesions of autonomic fibers may occur in either the central or the peripheral nervous system (Fig. 10-26). An appreciation of the nuclei, fiber pathways and resulting reflex deficits from injuries can be useful as a diagnostic aid in exploring the diffuse distribution of the autonomic system. In the periphery the postganglionic sympathetic fibers that rejoin spinal nerves (Fig. 8-2) have a distribution which compares closely to that of the sensory dermatomes (Richter and Woodruff, '45; DeJong, '58). Hence changes in cutaneous sudomotor and vasomotor reflexes, changes in skin temperature and increased skin resistance to passage of a minute electric current implicate the involvement of sympathetic nerve fibers. A knowledge of dermatomal and peripheral nerve distributions (Figs. 7-11, 7-12, 7-16, 7-17 and 7-18), correlated with the segmental nuclear origins of autonomic neurons (Figs. 8-1 and 8-3), often can provide additional evidence to substantiate both the location and level of a nerve injury.

CHAPTER 9

Spinal Cord: Gross Anatomy and Internal Structure

The spinal cord is the least modified portion of the embryonic neural tube and the only part of the adult nervous system in which the primitive segmental arrangement clearly is preserved.

GROSS ANATOMY

The spinal cord is a long, cylindrical structure, invested by meninges, which lies in the vertebral canal. It extends from the foramen magnum (Fig. 1-4), where it is continuous with the medulla, to the lower border of the first lumbar vertebra (Fig. 1-6). The spinal cord has two enlargements, cervical and lumbar, each associated with nerve roots which innervate, respectively, the upper and lower extremities (Fig. 9-1). Caudal to the lumbar enlargement, the spinal cord has a conical termination, the *conus medullaris* (Figs. 1-6 and 9-1). A condensation of pia mater, extending caudally from the conus medullaris, forms the *filum terminale*; the latter structure penetrates the dural tube at levels of the second sacral vertebra, becomes invested by dura and continues as the coccygeal ligament to the posterior surface of the coccyx (Fig. 1-6).

While the spinal cord is a continuous unsegmented structure, the 31 pairs of spinal nerves associated with localized regions produce an external segmentation (Fig. 9-1). On the basis of this external segmentation, the spinal cord is considered to consist of 31 segments, each of which receives and furnishes paired dorsal and ventral root filaments (Fig. 9-2). The spinal segments are divided in the following manner: 8 cervical, 12 thoracic, 5 lumbar, 5 sacral and 1 coccygeal. Up to the 3rd month of fetal life the spinal cord occupies the entire length of the vertebral canal, but after that time the differential rate of growth of the vertebral column exceeds that of the spinal cord. At birth the conus medullaris is located near the L3 vertebra; in the adult it is between the L1 and L2 vertebrae, and occupies only the upper two-thirds of the vertebral canal (Fig. 9-3). The sites of emergence of the spinal nerve do not change, but there is a lengthening of root filaments between the intervertebral foramina and the spinal cord; this is most marked for the lumbar and sacral spinal roots. These roots descend for a considerable distance within the dural sac before reaching their respective intervertebral foramina. The large number of lumbosacral roots surrounding the filum terminale is known as the *cauda equina* (Fig. 1-6). Spinal nerves emerge from the vertebral canal via the intervertebral foramina. The first cervical nerve emerges between the atlas and the occiput (Fig. 1-4). The eighth cervical root emerges from the intervertebral foramen between C7 and T1; all

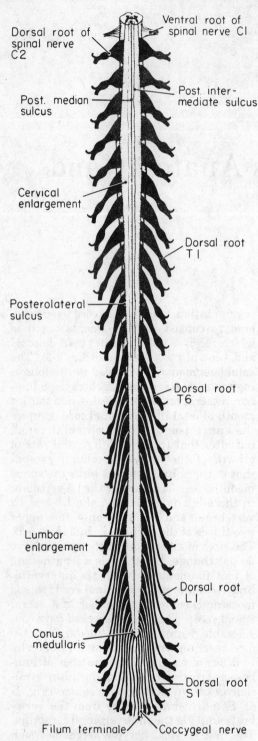

FIG. 9-1. Posterior view of spinal cord showing attached dorsal root filaments and spinal ganglia. *Letters* and *numbers* indicate corresponding spinal nerves.

more caudal spinal nerves emerge from the intervertebral foramina beneath the vertebrae of their same number (Fig. 9-3). Dorsal root fibers usually are absent in the first cervical and the coccygeal roots, and there are no corresponding dermatomes for these segments. (Figs. 7-11, 7-12 and 7-13).

The spinal cord, like all of the central nervous system, is derived from the embryonic neural tube. The central canal, lined by ependymal cells, represents the vestigial lumen (Fig. 9-4).

The length of the spinal cord from its junction with the medulla to the tip of the conus medullaris is about 45 cm in the male and 43 cm in the female. In contrast, the length of the vertebral column is about 70 cm. Its weight is about 35 g. In the midthoracic region, the transverse and sagittal diameters are about 10 mm and 8 mm, respectively; in the cervical enlargement (sixth cervical), 13 to 14 mm and 9 mm; in the lumbar enlargement (third lumbar), about 12 mm and 8.5 mm (see Fig. 9-5).

General Topography. When freed from its meninges, the surface of the cord shows a number of longitudinal furrows (Figs. 9-1, 9-2, 9-6 and 9-7). On the anterior surface is the deep *anterior median fissure*, which penetrates into the cord for a depth of some 3 mm, and into which extends a fold of the epipia containing blood vessels. On the posterior surface is the shallow *posterior median sulcus*. This sulcus is continuous with a delicate glial partition, the *posterior median septum*, which extends into the cord to a depth of 5 mm and reaches the deep-lying gray. More laterally are the *posterolateral* and *anterolateral sulci*. The former is a fairly distinct furrow into which the filaments of the dorsal roots enter (Figs. 9-1, 9-2 and 9-8). The anterolateral sulcus marks the exit of the ventral root fibers and is hardly distinguishable, since the ventral roots emerge in groups of irregular filaments occupying an area of about 2 mm in transverse diameter. In the cervical and upper thoracic cord another furrow, the *posterior intermediate sulcus*, extends internally between the median and posterolateral sulci (Fig. 9-6). The anterior median fissure and posterior median septum divide the cord into two incompletely

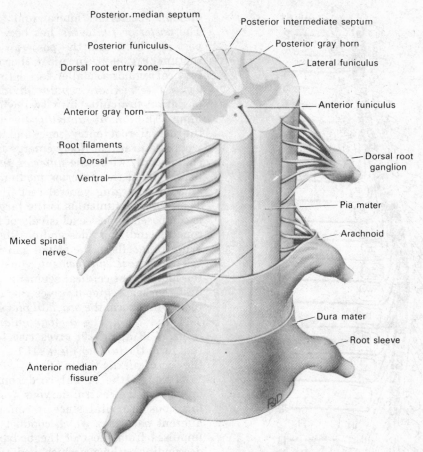

Posterior median septum

Posterior intermediate septum

Posterior funiculus

Posterior gray horn

Dorsal root entry zone

Lateral funiculus

Anterior gray horn

Anterior funiculus

Root filaments

Dorsal

Ventral

Dorsal root ganglion

Pia mater

Arachnoid

Mixed spinal nerve

Dura mater

Root sleeve

Anterior median fissure

FIG. 9-2. Drawing of the spinal cord, nerve roots and meninges. The blood supply and venous drainage of the spinal cord are shown in Figures 20-1 and 20-2.

separated halves connected by a narrow median bridge, or commissure, composed of gray and white matter.

In transverse section the spinal cord consists of: (1) a butterfly-shaped central gray substance composed of collections of cell bodies and their processes, and (2) a surrounding mantle of white matter composed of bundles of myelinated fibers, most of which are either ascending or descending (Figs. 9-2 and 9-7). The symmetrical butterfly-shaped gray consists of cell columns which extend the length of the spinal cord and vary in configuration at different levels (Figs. 9-5 and 9-6). Each half of the spinal cord has a *posterior gray column* or *horn* which extends posterolaterally almost to the surface. An *anterior gray column* or *horn* extends anteriorly but does not reach the surface. In thoracic spinal segments a small, pointed *lateral*

horn is evident near the base of the anterior horn (Fig. 9-7). A *gray commissure*, connecting the gray substance of the two sides, encompasses the central canal. Surrounding the central canal is a light granular area composed mainly of neuroglia, known as the central gelatinous substance (substantia gliosa). Anterior to the anterior gray commissure is a bundle of transverse fibers, the *anterior white commissure*, composed of crossing fibers arising from nerve cells in the gray substance (Fig. 9-7).

Ascending and descending fibers occupying particular regions of the white matter of the spinal cord are organized into more or less distinct bundles (Figs. 9-6 and 9-10). Fiber bundles having the same, or similar, origin, course and termination are known as *tracts* or *fasciculi*. The white matter of the spinal cord is divided into three paired

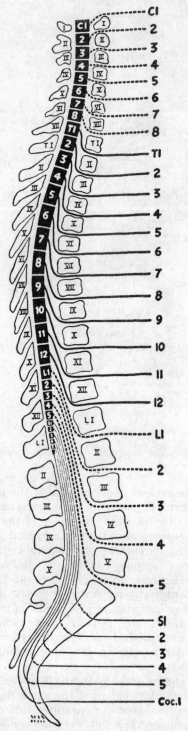

FIG. 9-3. Diagram of the position of the spinal cord segments with reference to the bodies and spinous processes of the vertebrae (Haymaker and Woodhall, '45).

funiculi: posterior, lateral and anterior. The *posterior funiculus* lies between the posterior horn and the posterior median septum (Fig. 9-2). In upper thoracic and cervical regions a smaller, less definite *posterior intermediate septum* divides each posterior funiculus into two white columns. The *lateral funiculus* lies between the dorsal root entry zone and the site where ventral root fibers emerge from the spinal cord, while the *anterior funiculus* lies between the anterior median fissure and the emerging ventral root filaments. The posterior funiculus is the largest and is composed almost exclusively of long ascending and short descending fibers that arise from cells in the spinal ganglia.

The *cervical enlargement,* consisting of the four lowest cervical segments and the first thoracic segment, gives rise to nerve roots which form the *brachial plexus* (Figs. 7-14 and 7-15). The *lumbar enlargement* (Figs. 7-19 and 7-20) gives rise to fibers that form the *lumbar plexus* (L1 to L4) and the *sacral plexus* (L4 to S2).

Although the spinal cord constitutes only 2% of the central nervous system, its functions are vital since it contains: (1) afferent pathways which conduct sensory impulses from most of the body, (2) the descending pathways which mediate voluntary motor function, and (3) fiber systems and neurons which provide autonomic control for most of the viscera. The blood supply of the spinal cord is described in detail in Chapter 20.

INTERNAL STRUCTURE

The microscopical appearance of the adult spinal cord is vastly altered from the three-layered embryonic neural tube (Fig. 3-3). The incoming and outgoing processes of ganglion cells and intrinsic neurons produce marked changes in the embryonic marginal and mantle layers. The embryonic layers become longitudinal columns of gray and white matter in the adult spinal cord, each having microscopical landmarks and subdivisions (Figs. 9-2 and 9-6). Individual segments of the spinal cord show variations at different levels, for there is great variation in the size and number of fibers in the individual spinal nerves (Fig. 9-1).

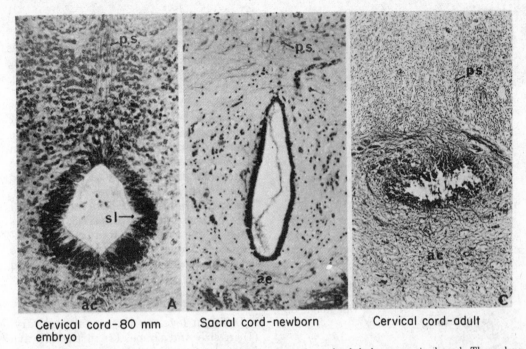

Cervical cord–80 mm   Sacral cord–newborn   Cervical cord–adult
embryo

FIG. 9-4. Ependymal cells and central canal of embryonic and adult human spinal cord. The sulcus limitans (*sl* in *A*) becomes lost in the adult. Processes of the ependymal cells entering the posterior median septum (*ps*) can be seen and the fibers of the anterior white commissure are identified (*ac*). *A*, Holmes silver stain, ×263; *B*, Luxol Fast Blue-cresyl violet, ×112; *C*, Holmes silver-cresyl violet, ×108.

Gray and White Substance

The gray and white matter are composed of neural elements supported by an interstitial neuroglial framework. The mesodermal structures comprise the blood vessels and their contents. The larger vessels are accompanied by prolongations of pial connective tissue. The gray matter contains the nerve cells, dendrites and portions of myelinated and unmyelinated nerve fibers. These fibers are axons of nerve cells located in the gray matter which pass into the white matter, or portions of the axons in the white matter which enter the gray to terminate. The preponderance of neurons, neuroglia and capillaries imparts a firm consistency to the H-shaped gray substance (Fig. 9-7). This density is enhanced further by the multitude of fine glial processes, fibrils, synaptic terminals and dendrites, which collectively form an intricate meshwork, or *neuropil*, that invests the neurons. In sections prepared with either hematoxylin and eosin or Nissl stains, the gray substance has a highly cellular appearance, whereas the fibrous elements of the neuropil are unstained (Fig. 9-9). In such sections one sees only the neuronal perikarya, glial and endothelial nuclei. The enormous dendritic plexus of the neurons and their synaptic endings remain unstained (Fig. 4-23). Lorente de Nó ('53) has estimated that the soma of the perikaryon forms only 6% of the surface of a neuron. Hence the unstained neuropil of the gray matter in Figure 9-9 is where most dendritic plexuses are located. The central canal, surrounded by ependymal cells, is located in the cross bar of the H-shaped gray matter (Figs. 9-4 and 9-7). A sharply delineated central canal is seen only in fetal and newborn spinal cords. In the adult the ependymal lining often is discontinuous and the lumen may contain debris, round cells, macrophages and neuroglial processes (Fig. 9-4C). Surrounding the central canal are clumps of fibrous astrocytes which are otherwise scarce in the gray matter (Figs. 5-2 and 5-12). The two slender bands of gray matter above and below

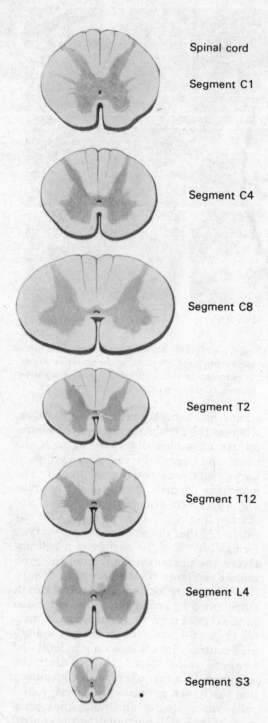

Spinal cord

Segment C1

Segment C4

Segment C8

Segment T2

Segment T12

Segment L4

Segment S3

FIG. 9-5. Diagram of selected spinal cord segments at different levels showing the variations in size, shape and topography of gray and white matter.

the central canal form the posterior and anterior gray commissures.

The white matter contains few neurons or dendrites, but is composed of ascending and descending myelinated and unmyelinated nerve fibers. The longitudinally arranged fiber bundles and their supportive neuroglial cells surround the gray matter as the posterior, lateral and anterior white funiculi. Numerous myelinated axons can be observed entering or leaving the white funiculi as dark fibers in sections stained by the Weigert method (Figs. 9-7 and 9-19). The structure and distribution of the glial cells are presented in Chapter 5. The processes of the astrocytes form a *superficial glial membrane* which is adherent to the deep surface of the pia mater (Figs. 1-8 and 1-9).

Spinal Cord Levels

Different levels of the spinal cord vary: (1) in size and shape, (2) in the relative amounts of gray and white matter, and (3) in the disposition and configuration of the gray matter (Fig. 9-5). Cervical spinal segments contain the largest number of fibers in the white matter because: (1) descending fiber systems have not yet contributed fibers to lower segmental levels, and (2) ascending fiber systems, augmented at each successively rostral segment, reach their maximum. The gray columns are maximal in the cervical and lumbar enlargements which are associated with the larger nerves that innervate the extremities. Lumbosacral segments contain large amounts of gray matter, relative to both the size of the cord segments and the amount of white matter.

Cervical Segments. These segments are characterized by their relatively large size, relatively large amounts of white matter and an oval shape (Figs. 9-5 and 9-8). The transverse diameter exceeds the anteroposterior diameter at nearly all levels. On each side the posterior funiculus is divided by a prominent posterior intermediate septum into a *fasciculus gracilis* (medial) and a *fasciculus cuneatus* (lateral).

In the lower cervical segments (C5 and below) related to the brachial plexus, the posterior horns are enlarged, and well de-

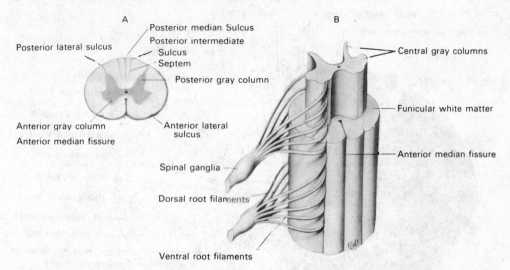

A

Posterior median Sulcus

Posterior intermediate
Sulcus

Posterior lateral sulcus

Septem

Posterior gray column

B

Central gray columns

Funicular white matter

Anterior gray column

Anterior lateral
sulcus

Anterior median fissure

Spinal ganglia

Dorsal root filaments

Anterior median fissure

Ventral root filaments

FIG. 9-6. *A*, External and internal topography of cervical spinal cord. *B*, Diagram showing internal arrangement of gray and white matter of the spinal cord.

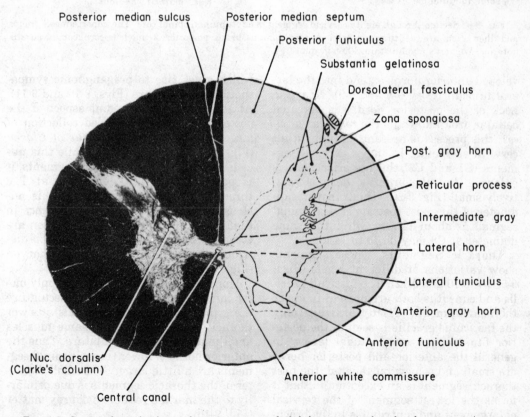

Posterior median sulcus   Posterior median septum

Posterior funiculus

Substantia gelatinosa

Dorsolateral fasciculus

Zona spongiosa

Post. gray horn

Reticular process

Intermediate gray

Lateral horn

Lateral funiculus

Anterior gray horn

Anterior funiculus

Anterior white commissure

Nuc. dorsalis
(Clarke's column)

Central canal

FIG. 9-7. Section through a lower thoracic segment of adult human spinal cord to demonstrate important subdivisions of the gray and white matter. Photograph of Weigert's myelin stain on *left* and schematic drawing on *right*. Area surrounding the gray matter, and limited peripherally by the *dotted line*, is composed of shorter ascending and descending fibers of the fasciculus proprius system.

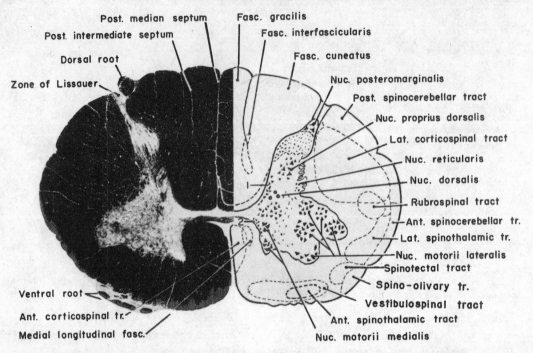

FIG. 9-8. Section through eighth cervical segment of adult human spinal cord. The important cell groups and fiber tracts are identified. *1*, Nucleus cornucommissuralis posterior; *2*, nucleus cornucommissuralis anterior. Weigert's myelin stain. Photograph.

veloped anterior horns extend into the lateral funiculi (Figs. 9-8 and 9-9). Near the neck of the posterior horn is a serrated cellular area known as the *reticular process*; this process is present throughout all cervical segments. In upper cervical segments (C1 and C2) the posterior horn is enlarged, but the anterior horn is relatively small (Fig. 9-20). The transverse diameter of the most rostral cervical spinal segment is about 12 mm, while this same diameter at C8 may be 13 to 14 mm.

Thoracic Segments. These segments show variations at different levels (Figs. 9-5, 9-7, 9-10 and 9-12). The fasciculi gracilis and cuneatus both are present in upper thoracic segments (T1 to T6), while only the fasciculus gracilis is seen in the posterior funiculus at more caudal levels. In general the anterior and posterior horns are small and somewhat tapered; the first thoracic segment is an exception in that it forms the lowest segment of the cervical enlargement and contributes to the brachial plexus. A prominent, but small, lateral horn is present at all thoracic levels and contains the intermediolateral cell column

which gives rise to preganglionic sympathetic efferent fibers (Figs. 9-10 and 9-11). At the base of the medial aspect of the posterior horn is a rounded collection of large cells, the *dorsal nucleus of Clarke* (Figs. 9-10, 9-11 and 9-12). While this nucleus is present in all thoracic segments, it is particularly well developed at T10 through T12. The large cells of this nucleus have a characteristic appearance in that their large vesicular nuclei often are eccentric, and chromophilic material is distributed peripherally in the perikaryon (Fig. 9-13).

Upper thoracic spinal nerves supply motor innervation only to axial musculature (i.e., the back and intercostals). Lower thoracic nerves supply the same muscles and the abdominal musculature. Thus the anterior horns of lower thoracic spinal segments are a little larger. The small diameter of the thoracic segments is due primarily to the marked reduction of gray matter (Fig. 9-10).

Lumbar Segments. These segments are nearly circular in transverse section, have massive anterior and posterior horns and

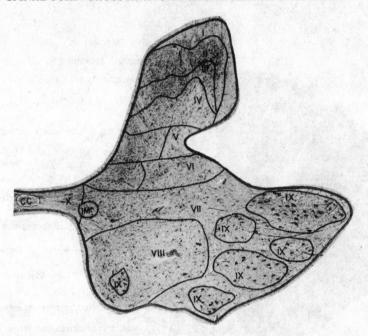

FIG. 9-9. Structural lamination indicated on thick section of human cord segment C6. The central canal (*cc*) and intermediomedial nucleus (*IM*) are identified. Compare with Figure 9-8. Thionin stain. Photograph. ×9.

contain relatively and absolutely less white matter than cervical segments (Figs. 9-5, 9-14 and 9-15). The fasciculi gracilis which compose the posterior funiculus are not as broad as at higher levels, especially near the gray commissure, and have a highly characteristic configuration (Fig. 9-14). The well developed anterior horns have a blunt process that extends into the lateral funiculi; motor cells in this process in segments L3 through L5 innervate large muscle groups in the lower extremities. Upper lumbar levels (L1 and L2) resemble lower thoracic spinal segments (Figs. 9-7 and 9-12). The dorsal nucleus of Clarke in upper lumbar segments (L1, L2 and L3) is especially well developed, and its presence facilitates identification of these levels. The transition between T12 and L1 is subtle, and these levels are difficult to identify precisely.

Sacral Segments. These segments are characterized by their small size, relatively large amounts of gray matter, relatively small amounts of white matter and a short, thick gray commissure (Figs. 9-5, 9-16 and 9-17). The anterior and posterior horns are large and thick, but the anterior horn is not bayed out laterally as in lumbar spinal segments. In caudal sequence sacral segments conspicuously diminish in overall diameter but retain relatively large proportions of gray matter. The substantia gelatinosa is particularly well developed in sacral segments, and this accounts for the thickened posterior gray column (Figs. 9-16 and 9-17).

Nuclei and Cell Groups

The butterfly-shaped gray matter of the spinal cord contains an enormous number of neurons of varying size and structure. Basically these cells can be classified as *root cells* and *column cells*. Root cells lie in the anterior and lateral horns and give rise to axons which exit via the ventral root to innervate somatic or visceral effectors. Processes of column cells are confined to the central nervous system. Although these neurons can be subdivided into *central, internuncial, commissural* and *association neurons,* a relatively large number give rise to fibers which enter the white matter. These fibers bifurcate, ascend and descend for variable distances and form part of an intersegmental fiber system.

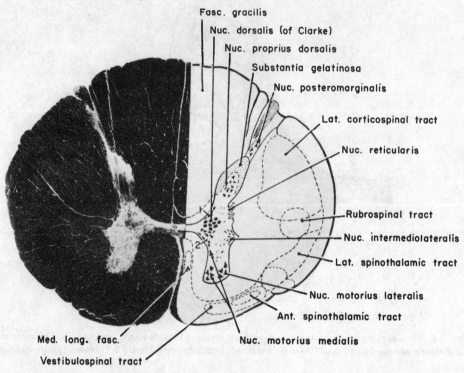

Fasc. gracilis
Nuc. dorsalis (of Clarke)
Nuc. proprius dorsalis
Substantia gelatinosa
Nuc. posteromarginalis
Lat. corticospinal tract
Nuc. reticularis
Rubrospinal tract
Nuc. intermediolateralis
Lat. spinothalamic tract
Nuc. motorius lateralis
Ant. spinothalamic tract
Med. long. fasc.
Nuc. motorius medialis
Vestibulospinal tract

FIG. 9-10. Section through fifth thoracic segment of adult human spinal cord. Important cell groups and fiber tracts are identified. *1*, Nucleus cornucommissuralis posterior; *2*, nucleus cornucommissuralis anterior. Weigert's myelin stain. Photograph.

Some of these fibers have long processes which ascend to higher levels of the neuraxis and transmit impulses related to specific sensory receptors. Nerve cells are organized in the gray matter into more or less definite groups which extend longitudinally and are referred to as cell columns or nuclei. In the neuroanatomical sense, a nucleus consists of a collection of cells with common cytological characteristics, which give rise to fibers that follow a common path, have a common termination and subserve the same function. Most of our information concerning the structural organization of the central nervous system is centered around this simple concept.

The spinal gray also contains Golgi type II cells whose short unmyelinated axons do not reach the white matter, but terminate in the gray close to their origin. Some Golgi type II cells may be commissural in that their axons cross to the gray of the opposite side, while others ascend or descend variable distances as intersegmental fibers.

Nuclear groups as well as their dendritic patterns are observed best in longitudinal sections of the cord following thionin and Golgi staining procedures. However, this plane of section is difficult for the beginning student to interpret. Transverse sections cut at 80 to 100 μ and stained with thionin, or cresyl violet, provide a more complete picture of neuronal groupings as shown in Figures 9-9, 9-11, 9-15 and 9-17. Such nuclear groups are most prominent in the human newborn; they are less sharply defined in the adult cord, particularly in thin sections. Thicker sections demonstrate more perikarya, but certain cellular details are lost or compromised.

Cytoarchitectural Lamination

For many years innumerable and often conflicting terms were used to locate and describe the nuclear grouping of cells in the spinal cord. Some were based on cell size and appearance (e.g., substantia gelatinosa), and others were subdivided on the basis of their location in the gray matter

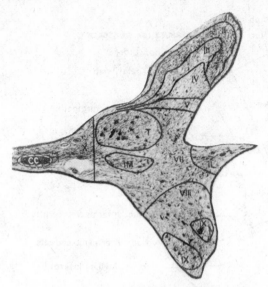

(e.g., motor nuclei of the anterior horn). Although eponyms have been used widely, some believed the only logical terminology should be based on a synaptological principle (i.e., to class the neurons according to their synaptic connections). In a series of illuminating papers Rexed ('52, '54, '64) described an architectural organization of neurons in the cat spinal cord that has proven valuable. His several zones have been corroborated and used by other investigators to describe terminal degeneration in this experimental animal. It is generally accepted that a similar lamination or zoning of the gray matter exists in all higher mammals. Examination of the spinal cord segments in the newborn and many adult human spinal cords revealed the presence of laminae comparable to those described by Rexed in the cat (Truex and Taylor, '68). This lamination of cell groups in the spinal cord resolved much of the confusion in terminology, and has become a widely used method for localizing axonal degeneration in the mammalian spinal cord. These studies of the *cytoarchitectonic organization* of the spinal cord recognize nine distinct cellular laminae in

most regions, which are represented by Roman numerals and an area X (Fig. 9-18). Area X, the central gray substance, surrounding the central gray, is present in all segments and appears fairly uniform throughout the spinal cord.

Thick frozen sections of the human spinal cord from different segmental levels are shown in Figures 9-9, 9-11, 9-15 and 9-17. They are stained to demonstrate neurons, and the boundaries of Rexed's laminae are indicated in each figure. For ease of comparison combined Weigert-Nissl stained nuclear groups are illustrated at levels near those of the laminae. There are differences in laminar configuration at various segmental levels of the spinal cord. The laminae constitute regions with characteristic properties, but their boundaries are zones of transition, where changes may occur either gradually or abruptly. Only the principal features of individual lamina are included in this brief presentation. Some of the laminae correspond to recognized cell columns and nuclei, while others are regional admixtures of cells (Fig. 9-18).

Lamina I is a thin veil of scattered gray substance that caps the surface of the posterior horn and bends around its margins. It has a spongy appearance and is penetrated by many small and large fiber bundles (Figs. 9-14, 9-15 and 9-18). It contains small, medium and large cells, but these are not numerous. The cytoplasm of these cells is rich in granular endoplasmic reticulum and other organelles (Ralston, '68, '68a). This lamina contains a complex array of nonmyelinated axons, small dendrites and synaptic knobs. Only a few dorsal root fibers establish synapses within this lamina. This lamina corresponds to the *posteromarginal nucleus* and in light microscopic preparations is best identified in sections through the lumbar enlargement (Figs. 9-14 and 9-16).

Lamina II consists of tightly packed small cells and corresponds to the substantia gelatinosa of the earlier literature. Neurons are spindle-shaped with little cytoplasm and few cytoplasmic organelles. It is traversed by many strands of large fibers from the posterior funiculus (Fig. 9-19), but has few synaptic endings of dorsal root

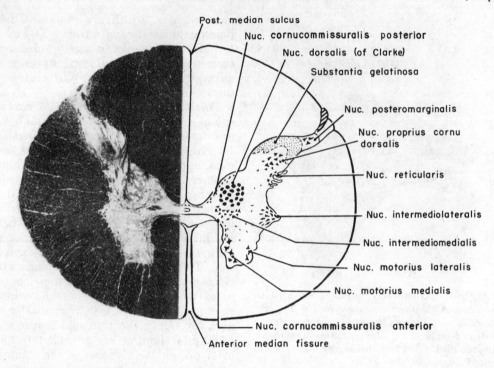

Post. median sulcus
Nuc. cornucommissuralis posterior
Nuc. dorsalis (of Clarke)
Substantia gelatinosa
Nuc. posteromarginalis
Nuc. proprius cornu dorsalis
Nuc. reticularis
Nuc. intermediolateralis
Nuc. intermediomedialis
Nuc. motorius lateralis
Nuc. motorius medialis
Nuc. cornucommissuralis anterior
Anterior median fissure

FIG. 9-12. Section through the twelfth thoracic segment of the adult human spinal cord. Important cell groups are identified on the right. Weigert's myelin stain. Photograph.

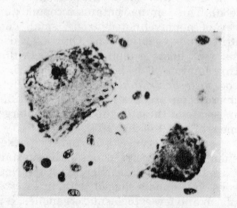

FIG. 9-13. Two cells from nucleus dorsalis (Clarke's column) of human spinal cord. Nissl stain. Photograph.

fibers (Ralston, '68a). The entire lamina has a very low population of glial cells and fibers.

Lamina III forms a band across the posterior horn and consists of less densely packed larger neurons. It has a lighter appearance, and the zone has less breadth in man than in the cat. This zone is rich in myelinated axons, and cells in this layer receive the greatest number of axodendritic synapses from entering dorsal root fibers (Ralston, '68a).

Lamina IV is the broadest of the first four layers, and its borders are sometimes diffuse (Figs. 9-9, 9-11, 9-15, 9-17 and 9-18). Small to large-sized cells of variable shapes scattered throughout this zone give it a heterogeneous, less compact appearance. Axodendritic and axosomatic synapses of dorsal root fibers are found commonly on the large and medium-sized cells of this layer. Cells in laminae III and IV correspond to the *proper sensory nucleus* (nucleus proprius cornu dorsalis) of the older terminology (Figs. 9-10, 9-12, 9-14 and 9-16).

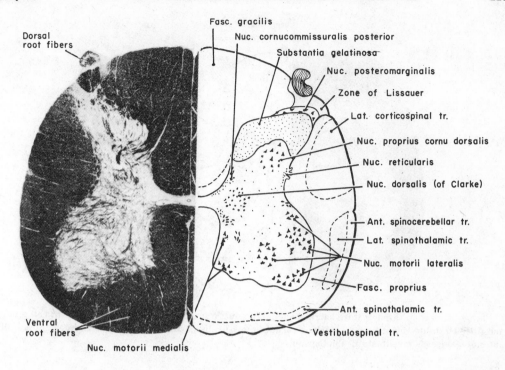

FIG. 9-14. Section through the fourth lumbar segment of adult human spinal cord. The important cell groups and fiber tracts are identified. Weigert's myelin stain. Photograph.

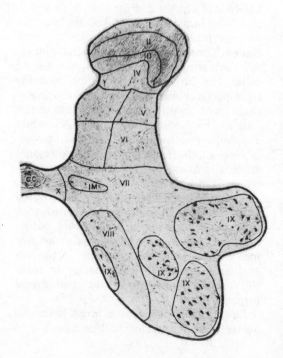

Lamina V is a broad zone extending across the neck of the posterior horn, which is divided into medial and lateral subdivisions, except in the thoracic region (Fig. 9-11). Many fiber bundles pass through the lateral zone, giving it a reticulated appearance. The lateral part of lamina V (Rexed, '52) is the reticular nucleus, which is particularly prominent at cervical levels (Figs. 9-8 and 9-10). It has large perikarya with coarse Nissl bodies. The medial zone extends to the posterior funiculus and has fewer, smaller perikarya with small amounts of Nissl substance. Dorsal root fibers as well as descending suprasegmental fiber systems (e.g., corticospinal

FIG. 9-15. Structural lamination indicated on thick section of human cord segment L5. The central canal (*cc*) and intermediomedial nucleus (*IM*) are identified. Compare with Figure 9-14. Thionin stain. Photograph. ×7.5.

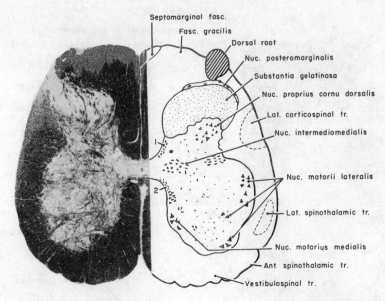

Septomarginal fasc.
Fasc. gracilis
Dorsal root
Nuc. posteromarginalis
Substantia gelatinosa
Nuc. proprius cornu dorsalis
Lat. corticospinal tr.
Nuc. intermediomedialis
Nuc. motorii lateralis
Lat. spinothalamic tr.
Nuc. motorius medialis
Ant. spinothalamic tr.
Vestibulospinal tr.

FIG. 9-16. Section through third sacral segment of adult human spinal cord. The important cell groups and fiber tracts are identified. *1*, Nucleus cornucommissuralis posterior; *2*, nucleus cornucommissuralis anterior. Weigert's myelin stain. Photograph.

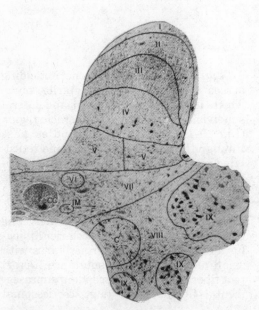

FIG. 9-17. Structural lamination indicated on thick section of human cord segment S4. Structures identified are the commissural nucleus (*C*), central canal (*cc*) and the intermediomedial nucleus (*IM*). Compare with Figure 9-16. Thionin stain. Photograph. ×15.

and rubrospinal) synapse upon neurons in this lamina (Fig. 9-20).

Lamina VI is a broad layer at the base of the posterior horn which is best developed in the cord enlargements and is absent between T4 and L2 (Figs. 9-9, 9-15 and 9-18). Like lamina V, it is divided into medial and lateral regions. The smaller, more compact, medial region contains numerous dark-staining medium and small-sized cells. The larger lateral region contains triangular or star-shaped neurons. Many dorsal root group I muscle afferents terminate in the medial zone of layer VI, while descending pathways are known to project to cells in the lateral zone. Physiological studies indicate functional differences between laminae in the dorsal horn (Wall, '67). Cutaneous afferents are distributed more dorsally than those concerned with proprioceptive sense or kinesthesis, but no lamina can be related to particular sensory modalities. Some axons of cells in the lateral zone leave the gray matter to enter the fasciculus proprius system and lateral funiculus.

Lamina VII occupies a large heterogeneous region anterior to laminae V and

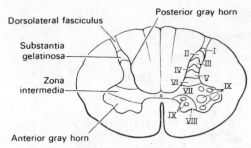

FIG. 9-18. Schematic drawing through the eighth cervical spinal segment with the laminae of Rexed ('52, '54) on the *right* and more general divisions of the spinal gray indicated on the *left* (Carpenter, '71; courtesy of The W. B. Saunders Company).

VI, extending across the spinal gray on each side. This region, also known as the *zona intermedia* (intermediate gray), has boundaries which vary at different spinal levels (Fig. 9-7). In the cervical and lumbosacral enlargements lamina VII extends laterally and ventrally into the anterior horn (Fig. 9-18). Lamina VII contains a large number of internuncial neurons at all levels, but in particular regions well defined cell columns are readily recognized. These well defined cell columns are the dorsal nucleus, the intermediolateral nucleus and the intermediomedial nucleus.

The *dorsal nucleus of Clarke* forms a prominent round or oval cell column in the medial part of lamina VII that extends throughout thoracic and upper lumbar segments (Figs. 9-7, 9-10, 9-11 and 9-12). The large multipolar or oval cells of this nucleus have coarse Nissl granules and eccentric nuclei (Fig. 9-13). This nucleus achieves its greatest size in lower thoracic and upper lumbar segments. Collaterals of dorsal root afferents establish secure synapses upon cells of this nucleus at their levels of entrance and at adjoining levels which exhibit extensive overlap. The large cells of the dorsal nucleus give rise to the uncrossed posterior spinocerebellar tract.

The *intermediolateral nucleus* consists of a cell column which occupies the apical region of the lateral horn in thoracic and upper lumbar segments (T1 through L2 or L3). Cells of this nucleus are spindle-shaped or ovoid with vesicular nuclei and fine Nissl granules (Figs. 9-10, 9-11 and 9-

12). These cells, considerably smaller than somatic motor neurons, give rise to preganglionic sympathetic fibers that exit via the ventral root and reach various sympathetic ganglia via the white rami communicantes. *Sacral autonomic nuclei* occupy a corresponding position in the lateral part of lamina VII of segments S2, S3 and S4 (Schnitzlein et al., '63), even though no lateral horn is present (Fig. 9-16). Cells of these nuclei resemble those of the intermediolateral cell column, but give rise to preganglionic parasympathetic fibers that exit via the sacral ventral roots to form the "pelvic nerves." The fibers synapse upon postganglionic neurons in, or near, the walls of pelvic viscera; postganglionic fibers in turn innervate the pelvic viscera (Fig. 8-11).

The *intermediomedial nucleus,* unlike other cell columns described in lamina VII, extends virtually the entire length of the spinal cord (Figs. 9-9, 9-11, 9-12, 9-15 and 9-17). This nucleus consists of a group of small and medium-sized cells with a triangular shape that lie in the most medial part of lamina VII, lateral to the central canal. The nucleus consistently receives a small number of fibers from the dorsal root at all levels (Shriver et al., '68; Carpenter et al., '68). It has been suggested that the intermediomedial nucleus may receive visceral afferent fibers and serve as an intermediary relay in transmis-

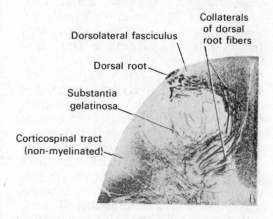

FIG. 9-19. Portion of transverse section of the lumbar spinal cord in an infant showing entrance of dorsal root fibers and collaterals. Weigert's myelin stain. Photograph.

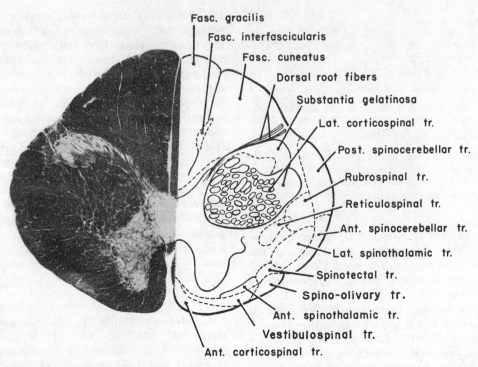

Fasc. gracilis
Fasc. interfascicularis
Fasc. cuneatus
Dorsal root fibers
Substantia gelatinosa
Lat. corticospinal tr.
Post. spinocerebellar tr.
Rubrospinal tr.
Reticulospinal tr.
Ant. spinocerebellar tr.
Lat. spinothalamic tr.
Spinotectal tr.
Spino-olivary tr.
Ant. spinothalamic tr.
Vestibulospinal tr.
Ant. corticospinal tr.

FIG. 9-20. Section through upper portion of first cervical segment of adult human spinal cord. Some of the important fiber tracts are identified. Weigert's myelin stain. Photograph.

sion of impulses to visceral motor neurons (Petras and Cummings, '72).

Lamina VIII includes a zone at the base of the anterior horn, but its size and shape differ at various cord levels. In the cord enlargements, this lamina occupies only the medial part of the anterior horn (Figs. 9-9, 9-15 and 9-18); at other levels it extends across the base of the anterior horn ventral to lamina VII (Fig. 9-11). Cells of this lamina vary greatly in size but are mostly triangular and stellate-shaped. The cells have relatively large amounts of cytoplasm and contain large Nissl granules. Axons of some medially located neurons are considered to cross the midline in the anterior white commissure. This lamina constitutes an entity of importance since certain descending fiber systems terminate upon cells in this region. Descending spinal tracts terminating, in part, within lamina VIII include the vestibulospinal, the medial longitudinal fasciculus, the pontine reticulospinal and the tectospinal (Figs. 9-20 and 10-21).

Lamina IX consists of several distinct groups of somatic motor neurons (Figs. 9-8, 9-9, 9-10, 9-11, 9-14, 9-15, 9-16 and 9-17). Anterior horn cells of this lamina are large multipolar neurons (30 to 70 μ in diameter) regarded as the prototype of motor neurons. These cells have large central vesicular nuclei, coarse Nissl bodies, multiple dendrites and large axons which form the ventral root. Somatic efferent neurons are largest in size and number in the cervical and lumbar enlargements where the cell groups spread both laterally and dorsally (Figs. 9-8 and 9-14).

The lateral nuclear masses are always sharply delimited. Within each nuclear group one can see also both large and small perikarya that are rich in Nissl bodies. The medial nuclear masses are often less sharply defined and share a diffuse border with lamina VIII (Figs. 9-11 and 9-15).

The large somatic motor cells of the anterior horn which innervate striate muscle are referred to as alpha (α) motor neurons.

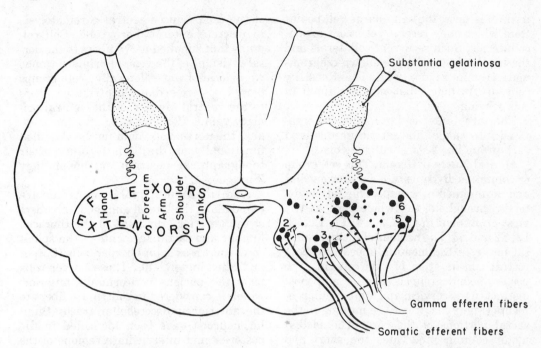

FIG. 9-21. Diagram of motor nuclei in anterior gray horn of lower cervical segment of spinal cord. On the *left* is shown the general location of anterior horn cells that send motor axons to specific muscle groups of the upper extremity. Motor nuclei indicated on the *right* are: *1*, posteromedial; *2*, anteromedial; *3*, anterior; *4*, central; *5*, anterolateral; *6*, posterolateral; *7*, retroposterolateral. Smaller anterior horn cells send axons (γ efferents) to supply small muscle fibers of neuromuscular spindle (Fig. 9-27). Note the collaterals from somatic efferent axons that return to gray matter and synapse on small medially placed "Renshaw cells." Smaller cells appearing as the *dotted zone* in the intermediate gray indicate the area of the internuncial neuron pool.

Scattered among these large motor cells are a number of smaller neurons (gamma (γ) neurons) which give rise to efferent fibers; these emerge via the ventral root and supply the contractile elements of the muscle spindle (i.e., intrafusal muscle fibers). Gamma efferent fibers play an essential role in the maintenance of muscle tone and bring the muscle spindle under control of spinal and supraspinal influences (Fig. 9-27).

Many of the motor nuclei have been subdivided and named on the basis of their location in the gray matter (Fig. 9-21). As shown in Figure 9-21, there is a topographical distribution of perikarya whose axons supply the different muscle groups of the extremity.

Somatic Efferent Neurons

These neurons contribute axons to the respective ventral roots of the spinal nerves and are organized into named nuclear groups which may vary from segment to segment (Figs. 9-8, 9-10, 9-14 and 9-16). These large multipolar neurons have 3 to 20 dendrites and axons with diameters of 10 to 13 μ. Each cell has a large central vesicular nucleus and coarse Nissl bodies in the cytoplasm (Figs. 4-1E and 4-7A). These somatic efferent neurons are largest in the lumbar and cervical enlargements and smaller in the thoracic segments of the spinal cord (Fig. 9-11). Scattered among the large anterior horn cells are γ neurons which give rise to γ efferent fibers (Fig. 9-27). Other small medially placed neurons in the anterior gray horn have been identified physiologically, but not anatomically. These small neurons (Renshaw, '40, '41, '46) presumably receive synaptic terminals from the recurrent axonal collaterals of α motor neurons. Axons of "Renshaw cells" probably end as synaptic terminals upon the same large cell bodies from which they receive recurrent axonal collaterals. Such recurrent collaterals and the involved neurons are shown diagrammatically in Figure 9-21. The Renshaw cells are included (but not identified) in this schema.

The large anterior horn cells are organized into medial and lateral groups, and each group has several subdivisions.

Medial Nuclear Group. This cell group or column is divisible into a posteromedial and anteromedial group. The latter extends throughout the whole cord and is most prominent in C1, C2, C4, T1, T2, L3, L4, S2 and S3. The nucleus of the hypoglossal nerve in the medulla appears to be a rostral continuation of this column. The posteromedial group is smaller and most distinct in the cervical and lumbar enlargements (Fig. 9-21). It may be missing in the sacral portions of the cord. The medial motor column innervates the short and long muscles attached to the axial skeleton.

Lateral Nuclear Group. This motor cell group innervates the rest of the body musculature. In the thoracic segments, it is small and undivided and innervates the intercostal and other anterolateral trunk muscles (Fig. 9-10). In the cervical and lumbar enlargements, it is enlarged and a number of subgroups may be distinguished. The group is especially prominent in those segments which participate in the innervation of the most distal portions of the extremities. Here may be distinguished anterolateral, posterolateral, anterior, central and retroposterolateral groups (Figs. 9-14 and 9-21). The exact innervation of individual muscles in the extremities by each of these groups has not been completely worked out, but in general the more distal muscles are supplied by the more lateral cell groups. Passing from the most mesial part of the anterior horn to its lateral periphery, the successive innervation is spine, trunk, shoulder and hip girdle, upper leg and arm, and lower leg and arm. The retroposterolateral group supplies the muscles of the hand and foot. Experimental denervation studies in animals have produced variable results. Section of specific peripheral motor nerves

of the cat produced central chromatolysis in discrete anterior horn cells. Cell columns that supplied nerve fibers to the dorsal divisions of the ventral primary ramus were located anterolaterally; cell groups placed posteromedially contributed fibers to the ventral division of the ventral primary ramus (Romanes, '51). In the monkey, the nerve cells could not be classified functionally on the basis of either their topographical position or morphology (Sprague, '51).

Additional multipolar neurons are found along the lateral and medial borders of the anterior gray horn in the thoracic, lumbar and sacral segments of the spinal cord, known as spinal border cells (Cooper and Sherrington, '40). These border cells form the nucleus pericornualis anterior, which is considered to contribute fibers to the anterior spinocerebellar tracts. Similar neurons have been identified in the posterior and intermediate regions of the anterior gray horn of the monkey (Sprague, '51).

Visceral Efferent Neurons

Axons of these neurons pass by way of the ventral roots and white rami communicantes to the various sympathetic ganglia. They are small ovoid or spindle-shaped cells with thin, short dendrites, vesicular nuclei and fine chromophilic bodies (Figs. 4-6 and 9-11). They range in size from 12 to 45 μ, and may be divided into two groups.

Intermediolateral Nucleus *(Figs. 9-10 and 9-11).* This nucleus consists of several adjacent cell columns. The most lateral apical cell group constitutes the lateral horn. The nucleus begins in the lower portion of C8 and extends caudally through L2 or L3. Axons of neurons in the intermediolateral nucleus leave the cord in the ventral roots of spinal nerves T1 and L3 (Poliak, '24; Bok, '28) to terminate in the ganglionated sympathetic chain, or in more peripheral ganglia along the aorta (Figs. 8-1 and 9-22). Each preganglionic axon has synaptic endings upon the dendrites and cell bodies of many postganglionic neurons in outlying sympathetic ganglia.

Sacral Autonomic Nuclei. Scattered small neurons are found along the lateral surface at the base of the anterior gray horn in sacral segments S2, S3 and S4 (Fig. 9-16). Such cells bear a striking resemblance to those found in the intermediolateral nucleus. Axons of these scattered cells leave the cord in the corresponding ventral roots as preganglionic (sacral) parasympathetic fibers. These fibers in turn have multiple synapses with many postganglionic cells located in or near the wall of the pelvic viscera (Fig. 8-1).

Posterior Horn Neurons

These cells and their processes are confined entirely to the central nervous system. In the posterior and intermediate gray especially, they receive the collaterals or direct terminations of dorsal root fibers. In turn, they send their axons either directly to anterior horn cells of the same segments or to the white matter, where, by bifurcating, they become ascending and descending longitudinal fibers, forming intersegmental tracts of varying length (Fig. 9-23). The cells vary in size, form and internal structure. Some are organized into definite cell groups that are easily distinguished in transverse sections; others are scattered irregularly in the gray matter.

The *nucleus posteromarginalis (nucleus magnocellularis pericornualis, marginal cells)* forms a thin layer of cells covering the tip of the posterior horn and situated in lamina I (Figs. 9-10, 9-14 and 9-16). They are large, tangentially arranged stellate or spindle-shaped cells reaching a diameter of over 50 μ. Their axons pass into the lateral white funiculus and bifurcate into ascending and descending fibers, probably forming intersegmental pathways. These cells are found throughout the cord, but are most numerous in the lumbosacral segments.

Beneath the marginal cells is the *substantia gelatinosa* (lamina II) which forms the outer caplike portion of the head of the posterior horn. It extends the whole length of the cord and is largest in the lumbosacral and first cervical segments (Figs. 9-17 and 9-20). Its variations in size are to some extent related to the size of the dorsal root. The nucleus is composed of rows of small ovoid or polygonal cells with deeply staining nuclei about 6 and 20 μ in diameter

(Fig. 4-4G). Some unmyelinated or finely myelinated axons end in the substantia gelatinosa. The large number and small size of the cells suggest that they give rise to short, principally intrasegmental fibers. The nucleus constitutes the chief associative center of the posterior horn for incoming impulses.

The head and cervix of the posterior horn is occupied by the *nucleus proprius cornu posterior (nucleus centrodorsalis, nucleus magnocellularis centralis).* This nucleus corresponds to laminae III and IV as seen in Figures 9-9 to 9-16. Some are spindle-shaped cells of more than medium size; others are large polygonal cells with numerous dendrites that approach the size of a motor anterior horn cell. This rather poorly defined cell column is found in all segments, the cells being most numerous in the lumbosacral cord. Lateral to this nucleus, the small- and medium-sized cells found in the reticular process (lamina V) have been termed the *nucleus reticularis* (Figs. 9-8 and 9-14).

The *nucleus dorsalis (nucleus thoracicus, column of Clarke, nucleus magnocellularis basalis, nucleus spinocerebellaris)* is a striking cell column in the medial portion of the base of the posterior horn. The nucleus begins to be well defined in C8 and extends through the thoracic and upper lumbar segments, being most prominent in T10, T12 and L1 (Figs. 9-11 and 9-12). Below L3 it becomes indistinguishable, although occasional cells are found.

In the intermediate gray a rather diffusely organized cell group constitutes the *nucleus intermediomedialis,* as contrasted with the intermediolateral nucleus. The small- and medium-sized cells, 10 to 24 μ in size, are found in varying numbers throughout the spinal cord (Fig. 9-12).

Two less definite cell columns extending the length of the cord are the *nuclei cornucommissurales posterior* and *anterior* (Fig. 9-16). The former, in section, is a thin cell strip occupying the medial margin of the posterior horn and extending along the border of the posterior gray commissure. It lies over the column of Clarke where the latter is present. The anterior is a similar cell group along the medial surface of the anterior horn and anterior gray commis-

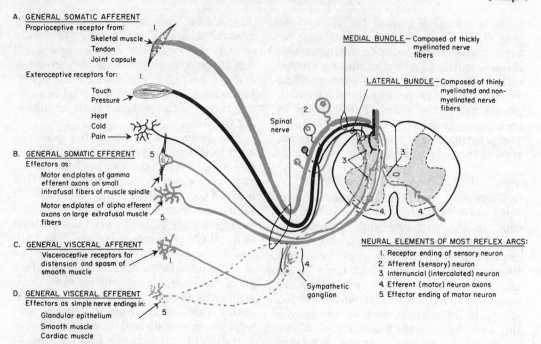

Fig. 9-22. Diagram of functional components of a thoracic spinal nerve, and the arrangement of dorsal root fibers as they enter the spinal cord. Skeletal muscle afferent and efferent fibers are indicated in *red*. Visceral afferent and efferent fibers are shown in *blue*. An afferent fiber from a Pacinian corpuscle (*black*) and a thin pain fiber (*black*) also are shown. *Numbers* in the diagram correspond to neural elements that form reflex arcs.

sure. These nuclei consist of small- and medium-sized spindle-shaped cells whose axons probably form intersegmental tracts in the posterior and anterior white funiculi, respectively.

ARRANGEMENT OF ENTERING AFFERENT FIBERS

Central processes of cells in the spinal ganglia enter the dorsolateral aspect of the spinal cord in small fascicles over a considerable distance (Fig. 9-2). The dorsal roots break up into a number of filaments, or rootlets, which enter the spinal cord in a linear manner. Peripheral processes of these cells conveying impulses centrally from various somatic and visceral receptors have been described as forming two bundles (Ranson, '14). Thick myelinated fibers of the *medial bundle* are described as representing the central processes of spinal ganglion cells conveying impulses from large encapsulated somatic receptors, such as neuromuscular spindles, neurotendinous organs, Pacinian corpuscles and

Meissner's corpuscles (Fig. 9-22). The smaller, less conspicuous *lateral bundle*, composed of thinly myelinated fibers, is described as representing the central processes of smaller ganglion cells related to free nerve endings, tactile, thermal and other somatic and visceral receptors. Evidence based upon Golgi studies has shown that thinly myelinated fibers from the dorsal root actually pass both medially and laterally to the posterior horn (Szentágothai, '64). Upon entering the spinal cord, central processes of each spinal ganglion cell divide into ascending and descending branches (Ranson, '13), which in turn give rise to numerous collaterals (Fig. 9-23). Most of the collateral branches are given off in the segment of entry, where they either relay impulses to second order neurons, or participate in intrasegmental reflexes (Fig. 9-23). Primary ascending and descending branches extending into adjacent spinal cord segments, together with their collaterals, constitute the anatomical basis of intersegmental reflexes, and the

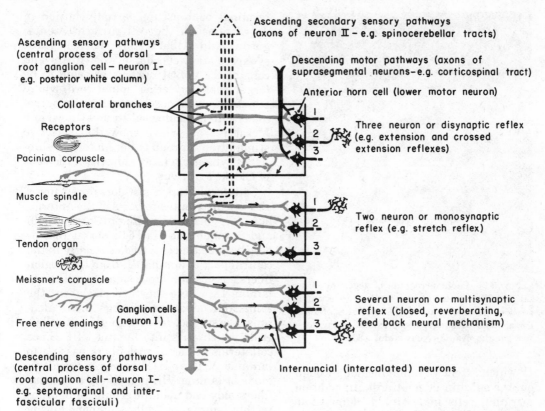

FIG. 9-23. Diagram of major branches and collaterals of dorsal root ganglion cells within three spinal cord segments. On the *left* are various receptors that generate impulses in response to different kinds of stimuli. Impulses from muscle spindles initiate the myotatic or stretch reflex involving two neurons (monosynaptic reflex). Impulses from the tendon organ initiate disynaptic reflex circuits involving inhibitory mechanisms. Other reflex circuits may involve many neurons (multisynaptic). Also indicated are ascending and descending branches of dorsal root fibers in the posterior white column (see Fig. 10-1) and collateral pathways that project fibers to the cerebellum (see Fig. 10-10).

relay of impulses to secondary sensory pathways (Figs. 9-22 and 9-23). The longer ascending primary branches of the medial bundle enter the ipsilateral posterior funiculus, and many of these ascend without synapse as far as the medulla. Some of the fine, thinly myelinated fibers of the lateral bundle of the dorsal root, conveying impulses of pain, thermal and light tactile sense, enter the medial part of the *zone of Lissauer (fasciculus dorsolateralis)* (Figs. 9-7, 9-8 and 9-14). The central course and branches of one dorsal root ganglion cell may be far more extensive than shown schematically in Figures 9-22 and 9-23.

The zone of Lissauer (fasciculus dorsolateralis) is composed of: (1) fine myelinated and unmyelinated dorsal root fibers which enter medial parts, and (2) a far larger

number of endogenous propriospinal fibers which interconnect different levels of the substantia gelatinosa (Ranson, '14; Earle, '52; Szentágothai, '64). In Golgi preparations axons of cells in laminae I, II and III can be followed into lateral parts of the zone of Lissauer. The number of dorsal root fiber collaterals terminating in the substantia gelatinosa is small, although this structure is traversed by fiber bundles passing to laminae III and IV (Szentágothai, '64; Ralston, '65; Stein and Carpenter, '65; Shriver et al., '68; Carpenter et al., '68). It seems likely that afferent impulses excite the substantia gelatinosa polysynaptically via interneurons in deeper portions of the posterior horn. This view is suggested by the rich dendritic arborizations of the large cells of lamina

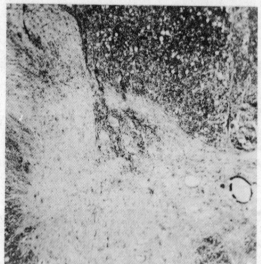

FIG. 9-24. Photomicrograph of degenerated dorsal root fibers in the rhesus monkey projecting directly to the dorsal nucleus of Clarke at L2. Lumbar dorsal roots were sectioned proximal to the dorsal root ganglia. Nauta-Gygax stain. ×80.

IV which extend in radial fashion throughout the substantia gelatinosa. In addition, marginal cells in lamina I, supplied by small dorsal root fibers, also may send axons into the substantia gelatinosa. Studies of the fine structure of the substantia gelatinosa (Ralston, '65) reveal extensive axo-dendritic and axo-axonal contacts, but infrequent axo-somatic contacts.

One of the principal sites of termination of large myelinated dorsal root fibers is the dorsal nucleus of Clarke (Fig. 9-24). Clarke's nucleus receives fibers from all ipsilateral spinal roots except the upper cervical roots (Grant and Rexed, '58; Shriver et al., '68). Studies of dorsal root afferents to Clarke's nucleus (Liu, '56; Grant and Rexed, '58) indicate: (1) the greatest number of fibers come from dorsal roots of the hindlimb, (2) there is considerable overlap of different dorsal root fibers distributed to the nucleus, and (3) fibers enter the nucleus via both ascending and descending collateral branches of the dorsal root. Synapses of dorsal root afferents upon the cells of Clarke's nucleus appear unique in that terminal fibers have long parallel contact with the dendrites of Clarke's neurons, and unusually large

terminal boutons are partially buried in depressions on the cell surface (Szentágothai and Albert, '55). These "giant synapses" between dorsal root fibers and cells of the dorsal nucleus are said to be larger than any other spinal cord synapses. Anatomical observations are in agreement with physiological studies (Lloyd and McIntyre, '50) which show that selective stimulation of group I afferent fibers establishes synaptic relationships with the cells of Clarke's nucleus.

Collateral branches of dorsal root fibers also are distributed to parts of the anterior horn (Fig. 9-25). According to Sprague ('58) and Sprague and Ha ('64), dorsal root fibers become concentrated especially in the central part of lamina VI; from this region fibers pass in numerous small bundles into lamina IX where they arborize about the soma and dendrites of large motor neurons. Dorsal root fibers also give off collaterals which pass into lamina VIII. Since collaterals of dorsal root fibers passing to laminae VIII and IX traverse broad regions of lamina VII, it is likely that some fibers may end upon internuncial neurons in this lamina, as well as on dendrites of motor nuclei which extend beyond the limits of Rexed's lamina IX. Dorsal root fibers

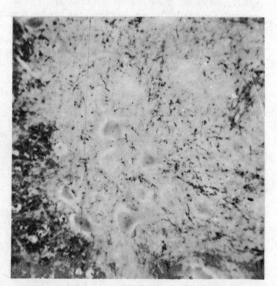

FIG. 9-25. Photomicrograph of terminal degeneration projecting around anterior horn cells at C6 in the rhesus monkey. Cervical dorsal roots were sectioned in this animal. Nauta-Gygax stain. ×220.

from group Ia afferent fibers projecting to lamina IX are involved in the monosynaptic myotatic reflex (Figs. 9-26 and 9-27). Group Ib and group II afferent fibers also generate synaptic potentials in central parts of laminae V, VI and VII (Sprague and Ha, '64).

Spinal Reflexes

The five essential elements required for most spinal reflexes are: (1) peripheral receptors, (2) sensory neurons, (3) internuncial neurons, (4) motor neurons, and (5) terminal effectors. The *myotatic* or *stretch reflex* is a monosynaptic reflex dependent upon two neurons. Stretch-sensitive proprioceptive endings located in muscle (muscle spindle) and tendon (Golgi tendon organ) are the receptors stimulated by a sudden brisk stretch of muscle. The *muscle spindle*, consisting of bundles of specialized slender muscle fibers (intrafusal fibers) surrounded by a connective tissue capsule, is attached to the endomysium of extrafusal muscle fibers (Fig. 6-11). Stretching of the noncontractile nuclear bag region (equatorial region) of the muscle spindle constitutes the mechanical stimulus required to fire the annulospiral or primary afferent fiber (group Ia) of this receptor. Gamma efferent fibers from the smaller anterior horn cells terminating in the polar (contractile) portions of the muscle spindle (intrafusal muscle fibers) bring this receptor under the control of spinal and supraspinal influences. *Golgi tendon organs* are found in tendons close to their muscular attachments (Figs. 6-15 and 6-16). As first pointed out by Fulton and PiﾒSuñer ('27-'28), the muscle spindle is arranged in "parallel" with extrafusal fibers, so that stretching of a muscle causes the spindle to discharge, while contraction of the extrafusal fibers tends to "unload" the spindle. The Golgi tendon organ is in "series" with extrafusal muscle fibers and thus can be caused to discharge by either a stretch or a contraction of the muscle (Fig. 9-26). Current physiological belief, based largely upon indirect evidence, indicates that the low threshold muscle spindles are the prime receptors involved in the stretch reflex. However, γ efferent fibers to the muscle spindle can exert potent influences

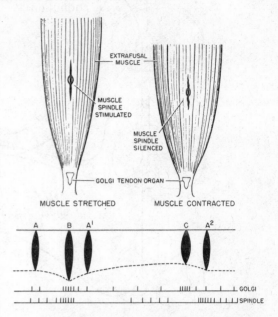

FIG. 9-26. Diagram showing the anatomical and functional relationships of the muscle spindle and the Golgi tendon organ to extrafusal muscle fibers. The muscle spindles are arranged in "parallel" with the extrafusal muscle fibers, so that stretching the muscle causes the spindles to discharge. Contraction of the muscle tends to "unload" or "silence" the muscle spindles. The Golgi tendon organs are arranged in "series" with respect to the extrafusal muscle fibers. Thus the Golgi tendon organs can be discharged either by a stretch of the tendon or a contraction of the muscle. The threshold of the Golgi tendon organ is relatively higher than that of the muscle spindle. The *lower diagram* summarizes the functional characteristics of the muscle spindle and Golgi tendon in relation to changes in muscle length. At A, the muscle is shown at its resting length, and the slow spontaneous discharge of the tendon organ and muscle spindle is indicated. At B, the muscle is stretched and both receptors discharge, although the adaptation of the muscle spindle is more rapid. At A^1, the muscle resumes its original length and tension, and there is a temporary reduction in the frequency of spontaneous firing of the muscle spindle. At C, where the muscle is contracted and shortened, the muscle spindle is silenced, but the rate of discharge of the tendon organ is increased. At A^2, the muscle is stretched out to its resting length, and the muscle spindles are therefore discharged, while the tendon organs are silenced by the drop in tension (Granit, '55).

upon the activity of this receptor. The myotatic reflex can be elicited in almost any muscle by sharply tapping either the mus-

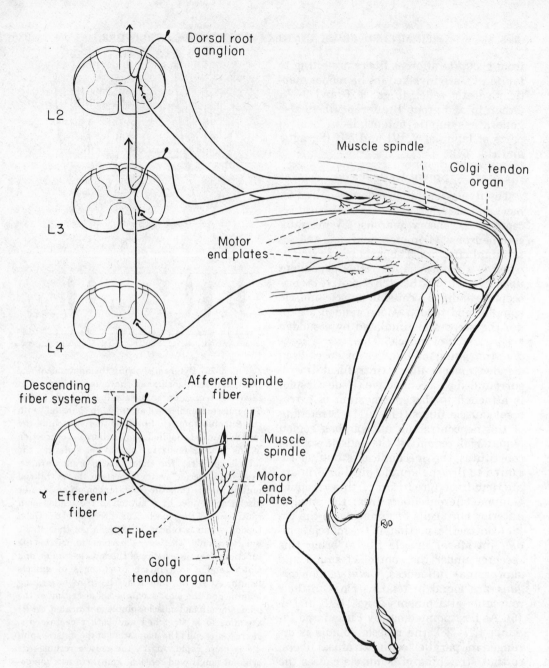

Fig. 9-27. Schematic diagram of patellar tendon reflex. Motor and sensory fibers of the femoral nerve associated with spinal segments L2, L3 and L4 mediate this myotatic reflex. The principal receptors are the muscle spindles, which respond to a brisk stretching of the muscle effected usually by tapping the patellar tendon. Afferent fibers from muscle spindles are shown entering only the L3 spinal segment, while afferent fibers from the Golgi tendon organ are shown entering only the L2 spinal segment. In this monosynaptic reflex, afferent fibers entering spinal segments L2, L3 and L4 and efferent fibers issuing from the anterior horn cells of these levels complete the reflex arc. Motor fibers shown leaving the L4 spinal segment and passing to the hamstring muscles demonstrate the pathway by which inhibitory influences are exerted upon an antagonistic muscle group during the reflex. The *small diagram below* illustrates the γ loop. Gamma efferent fibers pass to the polar portions of the muscle spindle. Contractions of the intrafusal fibers in the polar parts of the spindle stretch the nuclear bag region and thus cause an afferent impulse to be conducted centrally. The afferent fibers from the spindle synapse upon an α motor neuron, whose peripheral processes pass to extrafusal muscle fibers, thus completing the loop. Both α and γ motor neurons can be influenced by descending fiber systems from supraspinal levels. These are indicated separately.

cle, or its tendon, in such a way as to produce a brief sudden stretch of the muscle. Thus, striking the tendon of the quadriceps femoris muscle provokes a forceful contraction of the stretched muscle and a quick extension of the leg at the knee (Fig. 9-27). In this example, both the sensory and motor nerve fibers leave and enter the quadriceps muscle as constituents of the femoral nerve. It will be recalled that parts of two, three or more myotomes are incorporated in each muscle, and that two, three or more spinal nerves and cord segments provide sensory and motor fibers. The femoral nerve is composed of sensory and motor fibers from spinal nerves L2, L3 and L4. Thus, the synapses between these sensory and motor fibers must be within spinal cord segments L2, L3 and L4. The myotatic reflex is clinically useful in determining the levels of motor integrity of the nervous system, and also may reveal evidence of release of higher control.

Afferent fibers from Golgi tendon organs (group Ib) have disynaptic inhibitory influ-ences upon α motor neurons (Fig. 9-27). Although Golgi tendon organs have a higher threshold than the muscle spindles, afferent discharge of Ib fibers can exert inhibitory influences upon α motor neurons which reduce muscle tone. Unlike the muscle spindle, the Golgi tendon organ does not receive efferent fibers from the central nervous system.

As shown in this schema, other spinal reflexes have one or more internuncial neurons interposed between sensory and motor neurons (2 and 3 in Fig. 9-23), and some of these may form complex circuits. An anterior horn cell (lower motor neuron) thus may be facilitated, or inhibited, by the sum total of all the impulses that play upon it through literally thousands of synaptic terminals. Such synaptic endings may be terminals of incoming sensory fibers, internuncial neurons or several of the descending motor pathways arising from higher levels of the neuraxis. This is the basic organization of the spinal cord segment and its attached spinal nerves.

CHAPTER 10

Tracts of the Spinal Cord

The ascending and descending fibers of the spinal cord are organized into more or less distinct bundles which occupy particular areas in the white matter. Fiber bundles having the same origin, course and termination are known as tracts or fasciculi. It is customary to divide the white matter of the spinal cord into three funiculi: posterior, lateral and anterior (Figs. 9-2 and 9-6). Thus a funiculus may contain several fasciculi, but owing to the overlapping and intermingling of fibers, these may not be demarcated sharply. In general, long tracts tend to be located peripherally, while shorter tracts tend to be situated medially.

LONG ASCENDING SPINAL TRACTS

Although dorsal root afferent fibers entering the spinal cord convey impulses from all general types of somatic and visceral receptors, the impulses conveyed rostrally in the spinal cord are segregated so that impulses concerned with pain, thermal sense, touch and kinesthesis (sense of movement and joint position) from various body segments ascend together in more or less specific tracts, sometimes widely separated from each other. Ascending tracts not only convey impulses concerned with specific sensory modalities that reach consciousness, but they also transmit impulses from stretch receptors and tactile receptors that project to the cerebellum which are not concerned with conscious sensory perception. Ascending impulses

projected to the cerebellum are considered to be concerned with the regulation of muscle tone and with the coordination of motor function.

Posterior White Columns (*Fasciculus gracilis and fasciculus cuneatus*). Since the posterior funiculus is composed predominantly of dorsal root fibers, both the ascending and descending courses of these fibers will be described (Fig. 9-23).

A large proportion of heavily myelinated fibers of the dorsal root enter the posterior funiculus medial to the posterior horn, where they bifurcate into long ascending and short descending branches. Ascending fibers from lower levels gradually are shifted medially and posteriorly as they continue upward in the posterior funiculus of the spinal cord. Longer ascending fibers are displaced medially by shorter ascending dorsal root fibers entering the spinal cord at successively higher levels. This arrangement of ascending fibers in the posterior columns produces a crude overlapping laminar arrangement in which the longer sacral fibers are most medial, the shorter cervical fibers are most lateral, and lumbar and thoracic fibers occupy intermediate positions (Figs. 10-1 and 10-2). The number of ascending fibers derived from a particular dorsal root bears a relationship to the size of the root. Dorsal roots of the cervical and lumbar enlargements contribute the largest number of fibers.

In the cervical and upper thoracic re-

238

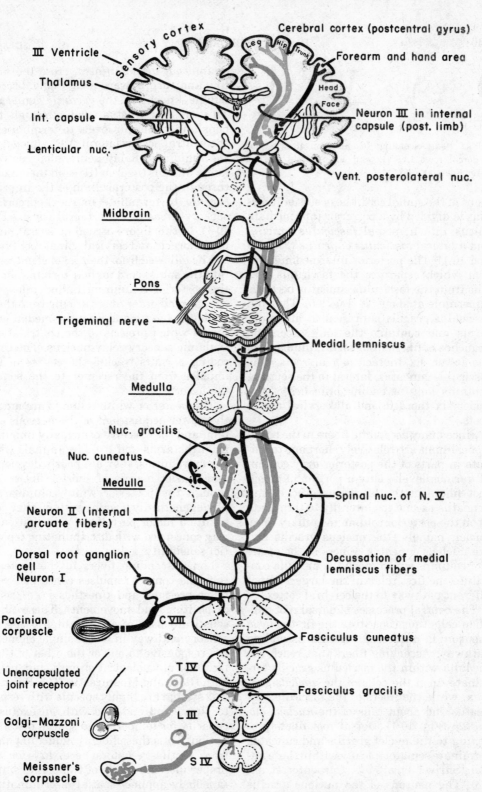

Fig. 10-1. Diagram of the formation and course of the posterior white columns and the medial lemniscus. Fibers in the posterior white columns in the spinal cord are uncrossed, while all fibers of the medial lemniscus are crossed. Impulses mediated by this pathway concern discriminative tactile sense (touch and pressure) and kinesthetic sense (i.e., sense of position and movement). *Letters* and *numbers* indicate segmental levels of the spinal cord.

239

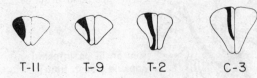

Fig. 10-2. Ascending degeneration after section of dorsal roots L1, T12 and T11. Marchi method (after Foerster, '36).

gions of the spinal cord, the posterior funiculus is divided by a posterior intermediate sulcus into a medial *fasciculus gracilis* and a lateral *fasciculus cuneatus* (Fig. 9-8 and 10-1). The posterior intermediate septum which separates the fasciculus gracilis from the fasciculus cuneatus becomes discernible at about T6 (Fig. 9-5). Thus the fasciculus gracilis is present at all spinal levels and contains the long ascending branches of fibers from sacral, lumbar and the lower six thoracic dorsal roots. The fasciculus cuneatus, lateral to the septum, contains long ascending branches of the upper six thoracic and all cervical dorsal roots.

Since many ascending fibers in the posterior columns are relatively short and terminate in parts of the posterior gray column at various levels, only a portion of dorsal root fibers in the fasciculus gracilis and cuneatus ascend ipsilaterally to terminate upon the posterior column medullary relay nuclei, namely, the nucleus gracilis and the nucleus cuneatus. Fibers in the posterior columns which reach the medulla constitute the first relay in the largest spinal afferent pathway to the cerebral cortex.

The central processes of dorsal root ganglion cells thus constitute the first neuron (neuron I, uncrossed) of this ascending pathway. Ascending fibers that reach the medulla within the fasciculus gracilis terminate upon the cells of the *nucleus gracilis*, while the fibers of the fasciculus cuneatus end about cells of the *nucleus cuneatus* (Fig. 10-1). Dorsal root fibers projecting to the nuclei gracilis and cuneatus terminate somatotopically within these nuclei (Shriver et al., '68; Carpenter et al., '68). The neurons of the nucleus gracilis and cuneatus constitute the second neuron (neuron II) in this afferent system. The axons of neuron II sweep ventromedially

as *internal arcuate fibers*, cross the midline and turn upward as a single discrete bundle known as the *medial lemniscus*. This crossed tract ascends through the pons and midbrain levels to terminate in the ventral posterolateral (VPL) nucleus of the thalamus. Relay neurons of this thalamic nucleus (neuron III) send their axons through the posterior limb of the internal capsule to terminate in the appropriate sensory areas of the cerebral cortex (Fig. 10-1). In this figure ascending sacral, lumbar, thoracic and cervical spinal root fibers can be followed from their level of entrance into the spinal cord to their termination in the posterior column medullary relay nuclei. Second order fibers arising from these nuclei decussate and form the medial lemniscus which projects to the contralateral thalamic sensory relay nucleus. The color coding permits tracing the course of the impulse from the receptor to the somesthetic cortex.

The posterior white columns are among the newer acquisitions of the nervous system, and they receive principally impulses from the arms and legs. In animals without extremities, they are poorly developed and consist mainly of shorter fibers. Although the posterior white columns are phylogenetically a young system, they constitute a major part of the principal pathway concerned with discriminating (epicritic) sensibility.

Long ascending fibers in the posterior columns convey impulses concerned with touch-pressure and kinesthesis (i.e., sense of position and movement). These fibers constitute part of a large highly specific sensory pathway in which single elements are responsive to one or the other of these forms of physiological stimuli, but not to both (Rose and Mountcastle, '59). Fibers of this system are highly specific with respect to place, and endowed with an exquisite capacity for temporal and spatial discrimination. Thus these fibers conduct impulses from tactile receptors necessary for the proper discrimination of two points simultaneously applied (spatial discrimination) and for exact tactile localization. Rapid successive stimuli, produced by applying a tuning fork to a bony prominence or skin, result in a sense of vibration. "Vibratory sense" is not a specific sensory modality, but a temporal modulation of tactile sense (Calne and Pallis, '66). The end organs involved in perception of vibratory sense probably are Pacinian corpuscles found in subcutaneous connective tissue and in periosteum. Impulses conveying this form of temporally modulated tactile sense are considered to ascend in both the posterior and lateral columns of the spinal cord (Calne and Pallis, '66). The ascending impulses in the posterior columns conducted from receptors on joint surfaces and in joint capsules, which are excited by movement, are of great importance because they convey information concerning the position of different parts of the body (kinesthesis).

The posterior columns also contain group Ia muscle spindle afferents. Most of these fibers ascend for variable distances, leave the posterior columns and terminate upon portions of the dorsal nucleus of Clarke. An important exception exists with respect to group Ia fibers from cervical and upper thoracic segments (Shriver et al., '68). These fibers ascend in the fasciculus cuneatus to low medullary levels and terminate somatotopically in different portions of the *accessory cuneate nucleus*. The accessory cuneate nucleus has cells which resemble those of Clarke's nucleus and, like that nucleus, projects fibers to the cerebellum (Figs. 10-10, 11-9 and 11-12).

The *descending branches of the dorsal root fibers* vary in length, and become displaced medially and somewhat posteriorly as they pass to lower segments of the spinal cord. They are relatively shorter fibers, but some may descend a distance of ten or more segments. In the cervical, and most of the thoracic, spinal cord they form a small plug-shaped bundle, the *fasciculus interfascicularis* or *comma tract of Schultze*, lying in the middle of the posterior funiculus (Figs. 9-8 and 10-21). In the lumbar region they descend near the middle of the posterior septum in the *septomarginal fasciculus* (*oval area of Flechsig*), which in the sacral cord occupies a small triangle near the posteromedian periphery (*triangle of Phillippe-Gombault*) (Fig. 9-

16). Besides the descending root fibers, the above named fascicles also contain descending fibers from cells of the posterior horn.

Lesions of the posterior columns naturally abolish or diminish discriminating tactile and kinesthetic sense and the symptoms appear on the same side as the lesion. Mere contact and pressure appear normal; but tactile localization is poor, and two-point discrimination and vibratory sense are lost or diminished. There is loss of appreciation of differences in weight and inability to identify objects placed in the hand by feeling them. These symptoms are most acute on the fingers and more acute on the extremities than on the trunk. Position and movement sense is severely affected, especially in the distal parts of the extremities. Small passive movements are not recognized as movements at all, but as touch or pressure. Even in long excursions the direction and extent of the movement may not be perceived. Loss of position sense greatly impairs the performance of voluntary motor function. This sensory loss causes movements to be clumsy, uncertain and poorly coordinated (posterior column ataxia).

Since a fiber severed from its cell of origin degenerates, injury to the ascending fibers of the posterior white column will produce microscopic evidences of fiber degeneration. These large myelinated fibers frequently are involved totally, or in part, by toxins, or by demyelinating or metabolic diseases. Sections prepared by the Weigert method yield a "negative picture of myelin degeneration" after injury, for only the normal intact fibers are stained (Figs. 10-3 and 10-4). A knowledge of tract formation (Fig. 10-1) enables one to distinguish which region of the spinal cord has been injured sometime prior to death. The series shown in Figure 10-3 was made following injury in the lumbosacral region, and the antemortem neurological signs and symptoms involved the lower extremities and pelvis. Note the decrease of ascending degeneration in the fasciculus gracilis as it ascends to the second cervical segment. Also observe the progressive increase of normal fibers that have entered

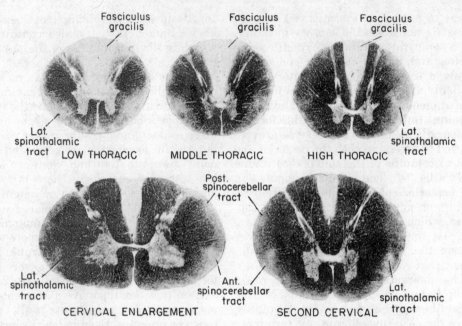

Fig. 10-3. Transverse sections of human spinal cord crushed some time previously in the lumbosacral region. In the posterior columns the progressive diminution of the degenerated area is due to passage into the gray matter of short and medium length ascending branches of lumbosacral dorsal root fibers. The progressive increase in normal fibers adjacent to the posterior horns is due to the addition of ascending branches of dorsal root fibers entering above the level of the injury. Weigert's myelin stain.

the spinal cord above the level of the injury. Contrast the appearance of the second cervical segments shown in Figures 10-3 and 10-4. The antemortem posterior column symptoms were far more extensive in the patient with a cervical cord crush (Fig. 10-4). Here all ascending posterior column fibers were interrupted bilaterally, including part of the sensory fibers from the brachial plexus. Note that only a few normal upper cervical root fibers have entered the fasciculus cuneatus above the level of injury.

Sections of the cord prepared by the Marchi method demonstrate a "positive picture of fiber degeneration" (Figs. 10-2 and 10-5). In such preparations the degenerated myelin sheaths stain as fine brown or black granules. The ascending degeneration, after destroying only the dorsal roots of L1, T12 and T11, is shown in Figure 10-2. In such an injury outside the spinal cord, normal sacral and lumbar fibers remain and are visible in the most medial part of the fasciculus gracilis. The fasciculus cuneatus is completely normal. A section of the

cervical cord after lumbar injury (Fig. 10-5) shows that degeneration is limited to the most medial fibers within the fasciculus gracilis.

The Marchi method yields important information concerning the course of large well myelinated tracts, but it does not provide information concerning the terminations of degenerated fibers. Great care must be used in interpreting Marchi preparations, for this method often produces deceiving artifacts (Smith, '51, '56).

Evidence of degeneration in the posterior columns also can be detected in Nissl stained sections after a considerable period of time. Relatively dense gliosis is present in the areas of degenerated fibers (Fig. 10-6).

Anterior Spinothalamic Tract. For many years it has been assumed that the spinothalamic tracts arose primarily from the large cells of the proper sensory nucleus (i.e., nucleus centrodorsalis, laminae III and IV of Rexed, '52) of the dorsal horn (Fig. 9-18); axons of these cells were considered to cross obliquely in the anterior

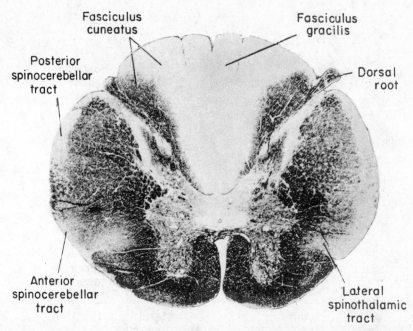

Fasciculus
cuneatus

Fasciculus
gracilis

Posterior
spinocerebellar
tract

Dorsal
root

Anterior
spinocerebellar
tract

Lateral
spinothalamic
tract

FIG. 10-4. Section through second cervical segment of a human spinal cord which had been crushed some time previously in the lower cervical region. Owing to the high level of the injury, practically all the fibers of the spinocerebellar and spinothalamic tracts have undergone degeneration. Also degenerated are all ascending branches of dorsal root fibers in the posterior white column, except those of dorsal root fibers which have entered above the upper level of the lesion (about C6). Weigert's myelin stain. Photograph.

white commissure and ascend contralaterally as part of the spinothalamic system. Studies of Golgi stained preparations have failed to reveal any fibers arising from cells of lamina III and IV that could be followed into the anterior white commissure (Pearsons, '52; Szentágothai, '64). Thus it seems unlikely that spinothalamic fibers arise directly from the proper sensory nucleus. Available evidence suggests that fibers crossing in the anterior white commissure and entering the spinothalamic system arise mainly from laminae VI, VII and perhaps from parts of lamina VIII (Szentágothai, '64). The manner in which cells of the proper sensory nucleus make contact with the cells of origin of the spinothalamic system is unknown.

In spite of these gaps in our knowledge, it seems well established that spinothalamic fibers cross in the anterior white commissure, and that the decussation takes place through several spinal segments. Fibers ascending contralaterally in the anterior and anterolateral funiculi form the anterior spinothalamic tract

(Figs. 10-5 and 10-7). Fibers of the anterior spinothalamic tract are somatotopically arranged so that those originating from the most caudal segments of the spinal cord are situated laterally with respect to those from more rostral spinal segments. A small number of uncrossed fibers may ascend in the anterior spinothalamic tract; these are not indicated in Figure 10-7.

Fibers of the anterior spinothalamic tract usually are described as ascending without interruption to thalamic levels. As this tract ascends in the brain stem a conspicuous reduction in the number of fibers is evident. In the medulla the tract is located dorsolaterally to the inferior olivary nucleus, where it appears to join the lateral spinothalamic tract. At medullary levels some fibers of this tract, or collaterals, project into the brain stem reticular formation, while others terminate about cells of the lateral reticular nucleus of the medulla, a cerebellar relay nucleus. Fibers projected to these locations explain the reduction in size of this tract in the lower brain stem. At levels through the upper

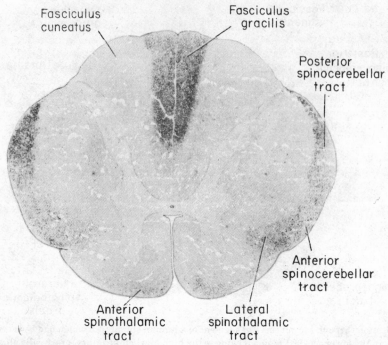

FIG. 10-5. Section through second cervical segment of a human spinal cord which had been crushed several weeks previously in the upper lumbar region. The ascending degenerating fibers are seen as *black granules*. Marchi stain. Photograph.

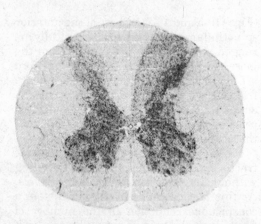

FIG. 10-6. Photomicrograph of the fifth cervical spinal segment in a rhesus monkey following multiple cervical dorsal rhizotomies on the right and section of the C5 dorsal root on the left. Intense gliosis sharply outlines the fasciculus cuneatus on the right, while more restricted gliosis on the left occupies the area of degenerated C5 dorsal root fibers. Nissl stain. ×10.

pons and midbrain, the tract becomes closely associated with the medial lemniscus. Fibers of this ascending sensory system terminate upon cells of the ventral posterolateral (VPL) nucleus of the thala-

mus. From this thalamic nucleus impulses are relayed to the cerebral cortex.

The anterior spinothalamic tract transmits impulses associated with what is called "light touch" to higher levels of the neuraxis. Light touch is the sensation provoked by stroking an area of skin devoid of hair (glabrous skin) with a feather or wisp of cotton. This sensation supplements deep touch (pressure) and discriminative tactile sense conveyed in the posterior white columns. Because tactile sensation is transmitted centrally by both the posterior white columns and the anterior spinothalamic tracts, clinically this sensory modality is of limited value in localizing injuries of the spinal cord. Injury to the anterior spinothalamic tract in the spinal cord produces little, if any, disturbance in tactile sensibility. The pleasant or unpleasant character of certain sensations, however, is considered to be related to conduction in the anterolateral funiculi. Bilateral destruction of these columns may cause complete loss of such affective qualities as itching, tickling and libidinous feeling (Foerster and Gagel, '32).

Lateral Spinothalamic Tract. Closely related to the anterior spinothalamic tract is the lateral spinothalamic tract. It is treated separately in view of its tremendous clinical importance. Its component fibers are more concentrated than those in the anterior spinothalamic tract, and it contains more numerous long fibers that go directly to the thalamus. The receptors of pain and thermal sense represent peripheral endings of the small- and medium-sized dorsal root ganglion cells, whose thin central processes enter the zone of Lissauer (Fig. 10-8). Statements made in regard to the cells of origin of the anterior spinothalamic tract apply also to the lateral spinothalamic tract. Thus it seems likely that cells of laminae VI, VII and perhaps VIII give rise to axons that cross in the anterior white commissure and ascend in the opposite lateral funiculus, as the lateral spinothalamic tract. Fibers of this tract cross obliquely to the opposite side within the segment of entry, although some may ascend one segment before crossing. Fibers of this tract are medial to those of the anterior spinocerebellar tract (Figs. 10-5 and 10-21).

The fibers show an anteromedial segmental arrangement in the lateral spinothalamic tract. The most lateral and posterior fibers represent the lowest portion of the body, whereas the more medial and anterior fibers are related to the upper extremity and neck (Fig. 10-8). As shown on the left of level C8, there is also a lamination of the sensory modalities within this tract; fibers concerned with thermal sense are posterior while fibers associated with pain are located more anteriorly. Injuries of this compact pathway ordinarily affect both pain and thermal sense. At higher levels this tract sends numerous collaterals into the brain stem reticular formation.

Detailed studies of anterolateral cordotomy in the monkey (Bowsher, '57, '61; Mehler et al., '60) indicate that the thalamic projections of the spinothalamic system are more complex than classic studies suggest. Unilateral anterolateral cordotomy produces thalamic degeneration: (1) predominantly ipsilaterally in the ventral posterolateral (VPL) nucleus, and (2) bilat-

erally in certain intralaminar nuclei and in a posterior thalamic zone (near the magnocellular part of the medial geniculate body). These anatomical observations, confirmed by physiological studies (Poggio and Mountcastle, '60; Whitlock and Perl, '61; Perl and Whitlock, '61), indicate that in the ventral posterolateral nucleus: (1) the body surface is represented in a distorted, but orderly topographical manner, (2) cells of this nucleus are related to small specific receptive fields contralaterally, and (3) most cells are not activated by noxious stimuli. In the posterior thalamic zone there is a crude topographical representation; cells in this region are activated from large receptive fields, both ipsilaterally and contralaterally, and respond readily to noxious stimuli.

Unilateral section of this tract produces a complete loss of pain and thermal sense (analgesia and thermoanesthesia) on the opposite side of the body. This contralateral sensory loss extends to a level one segment below that of the lesion, owing to the oblique crossing of fibers (Fig. 10-23). The anesthesia involves the superficial and deep portions of the body wall, but not the viscera, which appear to be represented bilaterally. The anogenital region is not markedly affected with unilateral lesions. After a variable period there is often some return of pain sensibility, due perhaps to the presence of uncrossed spinothalamic fibers. Such pain impulses also may ascend by shorter relays along spinospinal and spinoreticular pathways. A return of thermal sense also may be encountered.

In certain instances bilateral surgical section of the lateral spinothalamic tracts (cordotomy) is performed on selected patients to relieve pain and produce a complete and more enduring sensory loss. The spinothalamic and trigeminothalamic pathways both may be destroyed by one laterally placed lesion in the medulla or midbrain, where these two tracts occupy a superficial position (Figs. 10-8 and 12-22). Interruption of both tracts at midbrain levels results in a loss of pain and thermal sense over the face, neck, trunk and extremities on the opposite side of the body.

Nathan and Smith ('51) have presented

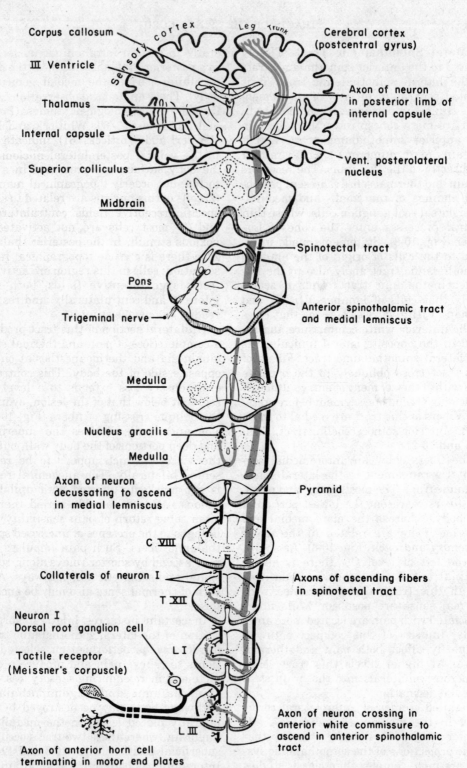

Corpus callosum
Ⅲ Ventricle
Thalamus
Internal capsule
Superior colliculus

Sensory cortex
Leg Trunk
Cerebral cortex
(postcentral gyrus)

Axon of neuron
in posterior limb of
internal capsule

Vent. posterolateral
nucleus

Midbrain

Spinotectal tract

Pons

Trigeminal nerve

Anterior spinothalamic tract
and medial lemniscus

Medulla

Medulla

Nucleus gracilis

Axon of neuron
decussating to ascend
in medial lemniscus

Pyramid

C Ⅷ

Collaterals of neuron I

Axons of ascending fibers
in spinotectal tract

T Ⅻ

Neuron I
Dorsal root ganglion cell

Tactile receptor
(Meissner's corpuscle)

L I

Axon of neuron crossing in
anterior white commissure to
ascend in anterior spinothalamic
tract

L Ⅲ

Axon of anterior horn cell
terminating in motor end plates

FIG. 10-7. Diagram of the anterior spinothalamic and spinotectal tracts. Although the precise cells of origin of these tracts are not known, spinothalamic fibers are considered to arise mainly from cells in laminae VI, VII and VIII of Rexed. The anterior spinothalamic tract conveys impulses of light touch. The spinotectal tract projects to the deep layers of the superior colliculus and lateral regions of the central gray. *Letters* and *numbers* indicate segmental spinal levels.

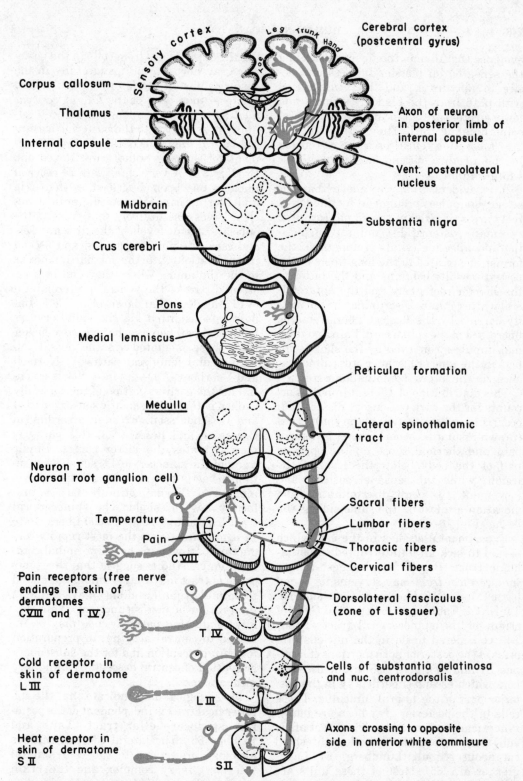

FIG. 10-8. Diagram of the lateral spinothalamic tract. The location of the cells or origin of the lateral spinothalamic tract appears to be in laminae VI, VII and VIII of Rexed. Fibers of this tract usually cross to the opposite side within one segment. Fibers of the lateral spinothalamic tract have a more complex termination in the thalamus than indicated here. The lateral spinothalamic tract conveys impulses of pain and thermal sense and has a somatotopic lamination. *Letters* and *numbers* indicate segmental spinal levels.

evidence that in man the fibers subserving the sensation of bladder fullness and desire to micturate, and fibers associated with pain from the bladder, urethra and lower ureter, are all located in the lateral spinothalamic tract. They believe that fibers mediating touch, pressure or tension in the urethra ascend in the posterior white column.

It is evident from the above that the sensory impulses brought in by the dorsal roots are organized in the spinal cord into two main systems: discriminative (epicritic) and affective (vital, protopathic); the former are related to the long fibers of the posterior white columns and the latter to the shorter root fibers and the anterolateral white column. Discriminative sensibility carried by the longest fibers remains uncrossed in the spinal cord. Pain and thermal impulses conveyed by the shortest fibers in the zone of Lissauer cross almost at once via the lateral spinothalamic tract.

This distribution of afferent impulses accounts for the curious sensory dissociation occurring in hemisection of the spinal cord (Brown-Séquard), where there is loss of pain and thermal sense on the opposite half of the body below the level of the lesion, while the sense of position and movement, two-point discrimination and vibration are lost on the same side as the lesion (Fig. 10-23).

Experimental studies in the cat, which is said to lack an uninterrupted spinothalamic tract (Busch, '61), suggest that a *spinocervical tract* may serve as its homologue (Morin, '55; Morin and Catalano, '55; Taub, '64; Taub and Bishop, '65). Cells of origin of the spinocervical tract (Taub, '64), considered to lie in the nucleus proprius of the posterior horn (portions of laminae III and IV), give rise to uncrossed fibers which ascend superficially in the posterior part of the lateral funiculus. These cells in the posterior gray horn are monosynaptically activated by dorsal root afferents that respond chiefly to low threshold cutaneous stimuli (Lundberg, '64; Landgren et al., '65). Most of these units are activated by tactile stimuli from relatively restricted receptive fields, but additional activation results from pressure and pinch-

ing the skin. Axons from cells in the posterior gray horn ascend ipsilaterally in the posterior part of the lateral funiculus and synapse upon cells of the *lateral cervical nucleus* (Fig. 10-9), a longitudinal cell column anterolateral to the posterior horn in the lateral funiculus of the C1 and C2 segments of the cat's spinal cord (Rexed and Brodal, '51). A very small lateral cervical nucleus has been described in man (Ha and Morin, '64). The lateral cervical nucleus gives rise to fibers that cross to the opposite side at levels of the first and second cervical spinal segments, and ascend in association with the medial lemniscus to the thalamus, where they end in a restricted part of the ventral posterolateral (VPL) nucleus (Landgren et al., '65). Impulses transmitted via the spinocervicallemniscal pathway reach the cortex earlier than those mediated via the dorsal column-medial lemniscal pathway (Norrsell and Voorhoeve, '62). Its integrity is essential for the earliest portion of the cortically evoked potential in somatic sensory areas I and II (Andersson, '62), and according to Oscarsson and Rosén ('66), this pathway also activates the motor cortex. Single units of the spinocervical tract show spontaneous activity and respond to hair movement and thermal stimuli with a uniformly low threshold. The spinocervical tract, containing 2000 to 3000 fibers, 10 to 14 μ in diameter, is the most rapidly conducting pathway in the feline spinal cord. Anatomical studies suggest that the spinocervical tract may convey impulses related to painful stimuli and also plays a role in integration of motor functions. This rapidly conducting pathway also may be involved in central alerting, in preparation for pain perception and for the subsequent activation of central descending inhibitory mechanisms.

Physiological data indicate that the spinocervical tract is independent of the posterior spinocerebellar tract (Taub and Bishop, '65). The lateral cervical nucleus also has projections to the contralateral inferior olivary complex and the brain stem reticular formation (Morin, '55; Morin and Catalano, '55; DiBiagio and Grundfest, '56), and it receives a cutaneous

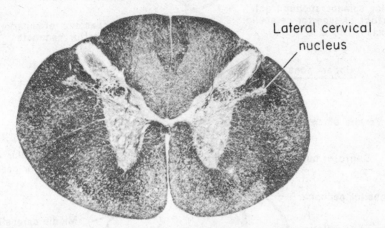

Lateral cervical
nucleus

Fig. 10-9. Transverse section of the first cervical spinal segment in the cat showing the lateral cervical nucleus. Cells of this nucleus receive fibers of the spinocervical tract, considered as the feline equivalent of the spinothalamic tract. Fibers arising from cells in the lateral cervical nucleus cross in the upper cervical spinal segments and ascend in association with the medial lemniscus to the thalamus. Weil stain. ×16.

trigeminal projection (Wall and Taub, '62).

Spinotectal Tract. The cells of origin of the small spinotectal tract, like those of the spinothalamic system, are not known. Fibers of this crossed tract, located in the anterolateral part of the spinal cord (Figs. 10-7 and 10-21), ascend in the spinal cord and brain stem in close association with the spinothalamic system (Poirier and Bertrand, '55). At midbrain levels fibers of the spinotectal tract project medially into the deep layers of the superior colliculus and to lateral regions of the central gray substance. While the functional significance of the spinotectal tract is largely conjecture, certain evidence suggests that it may be part of a multisynaptic pathway transmitting nociceptive impulses (Mehler et al., '60). This view is supported by observations (Magoun et al., '37; Spiegel et al., '54) of behavioral reactions which suggest painful sensations as a consequence of stimulation of the superior colliculus and periaqueductal gray.

Posterior Spinocerebellar Tract. This prominent uncrossed ascending tract, situated along the posterolateral periphery of the spinal cord (Figs. 10-4, 10-5, 10-10 and 10-21), arises from the large cells of Clarke's column (dorsal nucleus) which extend from the third lumbar (L3) to the eight cervical (C8) segment. Afferent fibers reach the nuclei via the dorsal roots (Fig. 9-24). The cells of Clarke's nucleus give rise to large fibers which pass laterally in the ipsilateral white matter and ascend the entire length of the spinal cord. In the medulla fibers of this tract become incorporated in the inferior cerebellar peduncle (Figs. 2-19 and 2-25), enter the cerebellum and terminate in both cephalic and caudal portions of the vermis. The tract first appears in the upper lumbar cord (L3) and increases in size until the upper limit of Clarke's nucleus is reached (C8). Since the column of Clarke is not present in lower lumbar and sacral spinal segments, impulses entering via these caudal dorsal roots, and destined for the cerebellum, are first conveyed rostrally in the fasciculus gracilis by ascending branches of dorsal root fibers; at higher levels where Clarke's column is present, these fibers leave the fasciculus gracilis and enter the dorsal nucleus (Figs. 9-19 and 10-10).

Experimental evidence (Liu, '56; Grant and Rexed, '58; Shriver et al., '68; Carpenter et al., '68) indicates that Clarke's nucleus receives both ascending and descending collaterals of dorsal root fibers, and a single dorsal root may supply afferent fibers to Clarke's nucleus in as many as six or seven spinal segments. Thus there is extensive overlapping of afferent fibers of certain dorsal roots in their termination in Clarke's nucleus. Clarke's nucleus re-

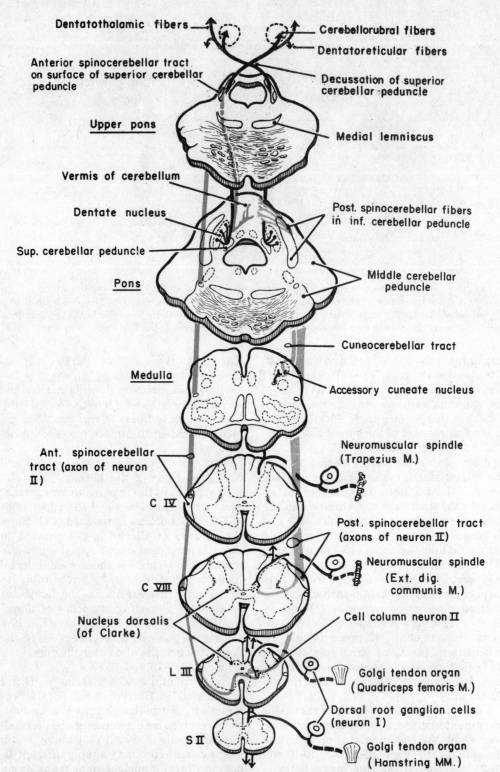

FIG. 10-10. Diagram of the anterior (*red*) and posterior (*blue*) spinocerebellar tracts and the cuneocerebellar tract (*blue*). Impulses conveyed by the posterior spinocerebellar tract arise from muscle spindles and Golgi tendon organs. Crossed fibers of the anterior spinocerebellar tract are considered to arise from cells in parts of laminae V, VI and VII of Rexed, and are activated by impulses from Golgi tendon organs. The cuneocerebellar tract, arising from cells of the accessory cuneate nucleus in the medulla, is considered the upper limb equivalent of the posterior spinocerebellar tract. The rostral spinocerebellar tract, considered the upper limb equivalent of the anterior spinocerebellar tract in the cat, is not shown. *Letters* and *numbers* indicate segmental spinal levels.

ceives afferent fibers via dorsal roots from all parts of the body except the head and neck (C1 to C4 dorsal roots), but functionally this nucleus appears related primarily to the hindlimb and caudal part of the body.

Fibers of the posterior spinocerebellar tract have conduction velocities ranging from 30 to 110 m/sec (Lloyd and McIntyre, '50; Oscarsson, '65). Fibers of this tract terminate ipsilaterally in the cerebellar vermal cortex (Grant, '62). Cerebellar areas of fiber termination in the anterior lobe correspond to Larsell's lobules I to IV (Fig. 14-1), while those in posterior areas end mainly in parts of the pyramis and paramedian lobule. According to physiological studies (Snider and Stowell, '44, Carrea and Grundfest, '54; Combs, '56) these cerebellar cortical areas represent mainly the hindlimb.

This uncrossed pathway from periphery to cerebellum is composed of two neurons, the spinal ganglion cells and the cells of Clarke's column (dorsal nucleus) (Fig. 10-10). Degeneration studies in man have emphasized that the anterior and posterior spinocerebellar tracts are difficult to delimit as they form the margins of the lateral funiculus in the spinal cord. Many fibers of the anterior spinocerebellar tract move posteriorly as they ascend and become incorporated within the posterior spinocerebellar tract (Smith, '57).

Impulses relayed to the cerebellum via the posterior spinocerebellar tract arise from stimulation of stretch receptors in muscle, the muscle spindles and the Golgi tendon organs. Neurons of Clarke's column receive monosynaptic excitation by group Ia and Ib afferent fibers via the dorsal root ganglion, and often there is additional excitation from group II muscle spindle afferents (Oscarsson, '65). There is no evidence that the posterior spinocerebellar tract is activated by stimulation of low threshold joint receptors. The synaptic linkage between group I afferents and the dorsal nucleus allows transmission of impulses at high frequencies, and little spatial summation is required for eliciting a discharge in the posterior spinocerebellar tract. The majority of neurons in Clarke's column are activated by either Ia or Ib afferents, but some neurons apparently receive excitation from both types of afferents. The occasional convergence of Ia and Ib excitation is said to be of little functional significance. Certain exteroceptive impulses also are transmitted by the posterior spinocerebellar tract (Oscarsson, '65). These exteroceptive impulses are related to touch and pressure receptors in the skin, and slowly adapting pressure receptors in foot pads.

Thus the posterior spinocerebellar tract relays impulses from stretch receptors, touch receptors and pressure receptors directly from spinal levels to particular parts of the cerebellum. The tract is somatotopically organized in its course and termination, and transmission is little influenced by supraspinal mechanisms. Present information suggests that impulses conveyed by this tract are utilized in the fine coordination of posture and movement of individual limb muscles.

Anterior Spinocerebellar Tract. Situated along the lateral periphery of the spinal cord anterior to the posterior spinocerebellar tract, and posterior to the site of emergence of ventral root fibers (Figs. 10-4, 10-5 and 10-10), is the anterior spinocerebellar tract. Medial to this tract is the lateral spinothalamic tract. The tract makes its first appearance in the lower lumbar spinal cord. In upper cervical spinal segments some fibers of the tract become incorporated within the posterior spinocerebellar tract (Smith, '57). In the human brain stem the anterior spinocerebellar tract appears quite small.

Fibers of the anterior spinocerebellar tract were considered by Cooper and Sherrington ('40) to arise in lumbar spinal segments from cells in the periphery of the anterior horn, known as "spinal border cells" or the *nucleus pericornualis anterior*. Investigations by Hubbard and Oscarsson ('62) in the cat indicate that cells of origin of this tract occupy the lateral part of the base and neck of the posterior horn and the lateral part of the intermediate zone (i.e., parts of laminae V, VI and VII of Rexed). These cells form a column extending caudally as far as sacral segments

(Grant '62), or coccygeal segments (Ha and Liu, '68). The investigations of Ha and Liu ('68) indicate that the cells of origin of the anterior spinocerebellar tract are widely distributed in the dorsolateral part of the anterior gray. While some of these cells are "spinal border cells," they do not form the principal part of the cell column. Morphologically these neurons are almost impossible to distinguish from motor neurons in Nissl preparations of normal spinal cord. In the cat, cells of this scattered cell column extend rostrally to the L1 segment; there is no "forelimb" component. Fibers of the anterior spinocerebellar tract are less numerous than those of the posterior spinocerebellar tract, are composed of uniformly large fibers (11 to 20 μ), have conduction velocities of 70 to 120 m/sec and virtually all are crossed.

This pathway to the cerebellum is composed of two neurons: neuron I in the dorsal root ganglia, and neuron II in the cell column at the base of the anterior and posterior horns in lumbar and sacral spinal segments. Fibers of neuron II cross in the spinal cord, and ascend through the spinal cord, medulla and pons. At upper pontine levels the tract enters the cerebellum by coursing along the dorsal surface of the superior cerebellar peduncle (Figs. 10-10 and 14-18). Although physiological studies (Carrea and Grundfest, '54; Combs, '56) indicate that fibers of this ascending system cross initially at spinal levels and recross again within the cerebellum, anatomical studies in man indicate that only a small number of these fibers cross in the cerebellum (Smith, '61). Experimental studies (Lundberg and Oscarsson, '62; Grant, '62; Oscarsson, '65) show that the majority of fibers of this tract in the cat terminate contralaterally; about 10% end ipsilaterally and about 15%, after branching, end both ipsilaterally and contralaterally. Within the cerebellar cortex, fibers of this tract have a rostrocaudal distribution similar to that of the posterior spinocerebellar tract, except that the main area of termination is in the anterior lobe (lobules I to IV) (Grant, '62; Oscarsson and Uddenberg, '64).

Cells which give rise to the anterior spinocerebellar tract receive monosynaptic excitation from ipsilateral group Ib afferents, and polysynaptic excitation and inhibition from ipsilateral and contralateral flexor reflex afferents (Oscarsson, '65). Fibers of this tract are activated by afferent impulses from Golgi tendon organs with receptive fields which often include one synergic muscle group at each joint of the ipsilateral limb. It is presumed that the fibers of this system convey information concerning movement or posture of the whole limb rather than information about movements in individual muscles. The significance of polysynaptic excitation and inhibition received via flexor reflex afferents remains obscure. Transmission of impulses in the anterior spinocerebellar tract is said to be controlled by supraspinal systems that might allow selection of information from either tendon organ afferents or flexor reflex afferents.

The effects of injury to these spinocerebellar tracts in the spinal cord are difficult to judge, since other tracts usually are involved simultaneously. Injury to the cerebellum itself results in reduced muscle tone and in an incoordination of muscular action producing disturbances of posture and movement (cerebellar ataxia or asynergia). There is no loss of proprioceptive sense as a consequence of these lesions since impulses projected to the cerebellum do not enter the conscious sphere.

Cuneocerebellar Tract. Since the column of Clarke is not present above C8, large fibers of cervical spinal nerves entering above this level ascend ipsilaterally in the fasciculus cuneatus. Fibers conveying impulses from group Ia muscle afferents and some cutaneous afferents pass to the *accessory cuneate nucleus*, a group of large cells in the dorsolateral part of the medulla with cytological features similar to those of the dorsal nucleus of Clarke (Figs. 10-10 and 11-9). The accessory cuneate nucleus in the monkey receives afferents via the dorsal roots from T7 to C1 (Shriver et al., '68) which terminate in an overlapping systematic fashion (Fig. 11-12). Cells of the accessory cuneate nucleus give rise to the cuneocerebellar tract, the upper limb equivalent of the posterior spinocerebellar tract. Fibers of this tract, posterior external arcuate fibers, enter the cerebellum as a component of the inferior cerebellar peduncle and terminate in the ipsilateral cerebellar cortex (lobule V). These cerebellar afferent fibers are distributed to the forelimb area of the intermediate zone in the anterior lobe and to forelimb areas of the pyramis and paramedian lobule (Fig. 14-1).

In the cat another spinocerebellar pathway, the *rostral spinocerebellar tract,* has been described (Oscarsson, '64, '65; Oscarsson and Uddenberg, '64) as the ipsilateral forelimb equivalent of the anterior spinocerebellar tract. The position of the cells of origin of this tract is unknown, but they are located rostral to the column of Clarke in the cervical spinal cord, and give rise to an uncrossed tract having an anterior position in the spinal cord which reaches the cerebellum via both the inferior and superior cerebellar peduncles. This tract resembles the anterior spinocerebellar tract which it partially overlaps, except that it is uncrossed; fibers of the tract are distributed mainly to ipsilateral parts of the anterior lobe (lobules I to V) of the cerebellum (Fig. 14-1).

Thus in addition to the posterior and anterior spinocerebellar tracts, related primarily to the hindlimbs and caudal parts of the body, there are two equivalent tracts, the cuneocerebellar and the rostral spinocerebellar, that relay sensory information from the forelimbs and rostral parts of the body (Oscarsson, '65). The posterior spinocerebellar and cuneocerebellar tracts are similar and convey information from muscle spindles, tendon organs (not demonstrated in cuneocerebellar tract) and touch and pressure receptors in the skin. The anterior spinocerebellar and rostral spinocerebellar tracts are similar in that they convey impulses from tendon organ afferents and flexor reflex afferents, both from wide receptive fields.

Spinoreticular Fibers. Impulses from the spinal cord also project to widespread regions of the brain stem reticular formation. Spinoreticular fibers originate from all spinal levels, presumably from cells located in the posterior horn (Brodal, '49;

Morin et al., '51; Mehler et al., '56; Rossi and Brodal, '57). These fibers ascend in the anterolateral funiculus, and those terminating in the medullary reticular formation are preponderantly uncrossed (Fig. 10-11). In the medulla these fibers terminate chiefly upon cells of the nucleus reticularis gigantocellularis and parts of the lateral reticular nucleus. The lateral reticular nucleus of the medulla (Fig. 11-8) is known to project to specific portions of the cerebellum, indicating that some fibers in this pathway may be concerned with the transmission of exteroceptive impulses to the cerebellum. Large cells of the nucleus reticularis gigantocellularis project to spinal levels as well as to more rostral regions of the brain stem. Spinoreticular fibers passing to pontine levels are distributed bilaterally and are less numerous than those terminating in the medulla. Most of these fibers end in the nucleus reticularis pontis caudalis (Brodal, '57). A small number of spinoreticular fibers have been found in the mesencephalic reticular formation (O'Leary et al., '58). Functionally, the spinoreticular fibers represent part of a phylogenetically old, polysynaptic system which plays a significant role in the maintenance of the state of consciousness and awareness. This complex, referred to as the ascending reticular system (Moruzzi and Magoun, '49), is considered in more detail in Chapter 13.

Other Ascending Fiber Systems in the Spinal Cord. In addition to the ascending fiber systems mentioned in preceding sections, several other ascending pathways have been described. While the existence of these anatomical pathways seems certain, relatively little is known of their functional significance.

A *spinocortical tract* has been described in man and experimental animals (Brodal and Walberg, '52; Nathan and Smith, '55a). Fibers of this tract arise from all levels of the spinal cord, but the contribution from the cervical region is greatest. Some of these ascending fibers appear to cross in the spinal cord, but the majority cross in the pyramidal decussation. In the brain stem these fibers follow the corticospinal tract in a reverse direction. Spino-

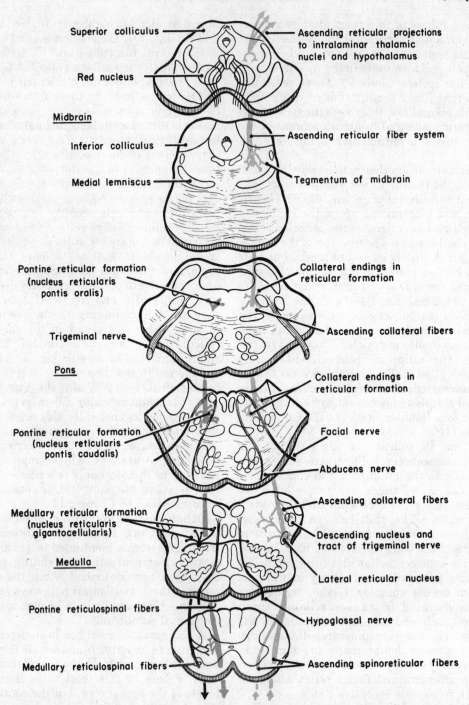

Fig. 10-11. Schematic diagram of ascending and descending reticular fiber systems. Ascending spinoreticular and collateral reticular projections are shown on the *right* (*blue*). This system gives off collateral fibers at various brain stem levels and is augmented by rostrally projecting reticular fibers. Pontine reticulospinal fibers (*red*) are uncrossed and originate largely from the nucleus reticularis pontis caudalis. Medullary reticulospinal fibers (*black*) are predominantly uncrossed and arise from the nucleus reticularis gigantocellularis. Fibers from these sources are not sharply segregated in the spinal cord. (Based upon Olszewski and Baxter, '54; Brodal, '57; and Nauta and Kuypers, '58).

cortical fibers have been traced through the internal capsule and into the lower layers of the cerebral cortex. Other ascending fiber systems described include the spino-olivary, spinovestibular and spinopontine.

Spino-olivary fibers originate from all levels of the spinal cord, ascend contralaterally mainly in the anterior funiculus and terminate mostly in specific parts of the dorsal and medial accessory olivary nuclei. Somewhat more than half of these fibers cross in the medulla. Since fibers from the inferior olivary nuclei project to the cerebellum, the spino-olivary fibers would seem to constitute a component of a spinocerebellar pathway which presents certain similarities to that of the posterior spinocerebellar tract (Brodal et al., '50). Spinoolivary fibers are activated by cutaneous afferents and probably by Golgi tendon organ afferents (Grant and Oscarsson, '66). Physiological studies suggest a dorsal spino-olivary tract, in addition to the ventral spino-olivary tract described above, in which impulses reach the accessory olivary nuclei via the posterior column nuclei (Oscarsson, '67).

Spinovestibular fibers project largely upon the dorsal part of the lateral vestibular nucleus. These fibers ascend ipsilaterally in the spinal cord from levels as far caudally as lumbar segments (Pompeiano and Brodal, '57). Fibers of this tract are partially intermingled with those of the posterior spinocerebellar tract.

Spinopontine fibers ascend with the spinocortical fibers previously described. These fibers, probably collaterals of the spinocortical tract, terminate upon pontine nuclei. It has been suggested that these fibers may be concerned with transmission of certain exteroceptive impulses to the cerebellum (Walberg and Brodal, '53).

LONG DESCENDING SPINAL TRACTS

The descending spinal tracts are concerned with somatic movement (motor function), visceral innervation, the modification of muscle tone, segmental reflexes and central transmission of sensory impulses. The largest and most important of these tracts arises from the cerebral cortex; all other descending spinal tracts arise from localized cell masses in the three lowest segments of the brain stem.

Corticospinal System. These tracts consist of all fibers which: (1) originate from cells within the cerebral cortex, (2) pass through the medullary pyramid, and (3) enter the spinal cord. They constitute the largest and most important descending fiber system in the human neuraxis. Each tract is composed of over 1,000,000 fibers of which some 700,000 are myelinated (Lassek and Rasmussen, '39; Lassek, '42, '54). Approximately 90% of these myelinated fibers have a diameter of 1 to 4 μ; most of the remaining myelinated fibers range in caliber from 5 to 10 μ, but include among them some 30,000 to 40,000 very large fibers having a thickness of 10 to 22 μ. Fibers of the corticospinal system arise almost exclusively from areas 4 (motor area), 6 (premotor area) and portions of the parietal lobe (Fig. 10-12). The largest fibers arise mainly from the giant pyramidal cells of Betz in the precentral gyrus (area 4 of Brodmann; Fig. 19-5), but some may arise from adjacent cortical areas. These corticofugal fibers converge in the corona radiata and pass downward through the internal capsule, crus cerebri, pons and medulla (Figs. 2-8, 10-12 and 10-13). As this large tract descends in the brain stem, it passes close to the emerging root fibers of cranial nerves III, VI and XII. *Corticobulbar fibers* conveying impulses to motor nuclei of the brain stem are closely associated with corticospinal fibers in the internal capsule and brain stem. The corticospinal tract comes to the surface in the medulla as the pyramid. At the junction of medulla and cord, the fibers undergo an incomplete decussation giving rise to three tracts: (1) a large *lateral corticospinal tract* (crossed), (2) an *anterior corticospinal tract* (uncrossed), and (3) a small *anterolateral corticospinal tract* (uncrossed and not illustrated in Fig. 10-13).

The majority of the fibers, 75 to 90%, cross in the pyramidal decussation and descend in the posterior part of the lateral funiculus as the lateral or crossed corticospinal tract, lying between the posterior spinocerebellar tract and the lateral fasciculus proprius (Figs. 10-14 and 10-15). In

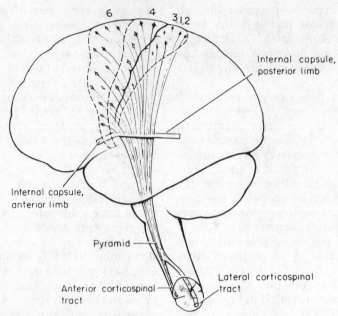

FIG. 10-12. Schematic diagram of the lateral and anterior corticospinal tracts indicating their regions of origin and course (Carpenter, '71; courtesy of The W. B. Saunders Company).

lower lumbar and sacral spinal segments, caudal to the posterior spinocerebellar tract fibers of the corticospinal tract reach the lateral surface of the spinal cord (Fig. 10-16). In the uppermost cervical segments some fibers of that tract occupy, for a short distance, an aberrant position external to the posterior spinocerebellar fibers. The tract extends to the most caudal part of the cord and progressively diminishes in size as more and more fibers leave to terminate in the gray matter.

A smaller portion of the pyramidal fibers descend uncrossed as the anterior or direct corticospinal tract (bundle of Türck), occupying an oval area adjacent to the anterior median fissure (Figs. 10-12, 10-13, 10-14 and 10-15). It normally extends only to the upper thoracic cord, and innervates primarily the muscles of the upper extremities and neck. This tract is found only in man and the higher apes and shows considerable variation, because the proportion of decussating fibers is not constant. In extreme cases the tract may be absent. In rare cases, the pyramidal fibers of one or both sides may not cross at all and may give rise to huge anterior corticospinal tracts (Verhaart and Kramer, '52).

Besides the two tracts discussed, there are other uncrossed corticospinal fibers which form the *anterolateral corticospinal tract* of Barnes ("Fibres pyramidales homolaterales superficielles" of Déjérine). This tract is composed of fine fibers which descend more anteriorly in the lateral funiculus.

Fibers of the crossed lateral corticospinal tract enter the gray matter laterally in the region of the intermediate zone. Silver impregnation studies (Nyberg-Hansen and Brodal, '63) in the cat show that entering fibers divide into dorsomedial and ventromedial components. Fibers of the dorsomedial component are distributed to laminae IV, V and part of VI, while the ventromedial component supplies fibers to lamina VI and the dorsal part of lamina VII. In the cat no degenerated fibers are found in lamina IX, where large motor neurons of the anterior horn are located. In the monkey Liu and Chambers ('64) describe corticospinal fibers passing into lamina VII and into the base of both the posterior and anterior horns. A few fibers of the lateral corticospinal tract have been described as crossing in the posterior and anterior gray commissures to end in the

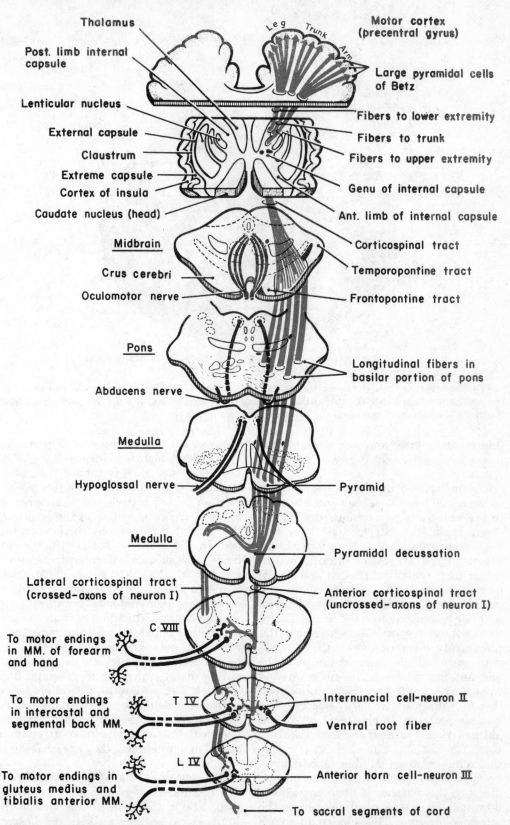

Thalamus

Post. limb internal capsule

Lenticular nucleus

External capsule

Claustrum

Extreme capsule

Cortex of insula

Caudate nucleus (head)

Leg Trunk Arm

Motor cortex (precentral gyrus)

Large pyramidal cells of Betz

Fibers to lower extremity

Fibers to trunk

Fibers to upper extremity

Genu of internal capsule

Ant. limb of internal capsule

Midbrain

Crus cerebri

Oculomotor nerve

Corticospinal tract

Temporopontine tract

Frontopontine tract

Pons

Abducens nerve

Longitudinal fibers in basilar portion of pons

Medulla

Hypoglossal nerve

Pyramid

Medulla

Pyramidal decussation

Lateral corticospinal tract (crossed-axons of neuron I)

Anterior corticospinal tract (uncrossed-axons of neuron I)

C VIII

To motor endings in MM. of forearm and hand

To motor endings in intercostal and segmental back MM.

T IV

Internuncial cell-neuron II

Ventral root fiber

L IV

To motor endings in gluteus medius and tibialis anterior MM.

Anterior horn cell-neuron III

To sacral segments of cord

FIG. 10-13. Diagram of lateral and anterior corticospinal tracts—the principal descending motor pathway concerned with skilled, voluntary motor activity. The locations of the corticobulbar tracts appear in each level of the brain stem as *black areas* (*right side*). *Letters* and *numbers* indicate corresponding segments of the spinal cord.

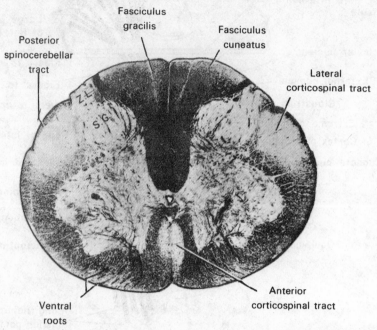

Fasciculus
gracilis

Fasciculus
cuneatus

Posterior
spinocerebellar
tract

Lateral
corticospinal tract

Z.L.

S.G.

Ventral
roots

Anterior
corticospinal tract

Fɪɢ. 10-14. Section through the cervical enlargement of spinal cord of 7- to 8-month human fetus. The corticospinal tracts are unmyelinated at this stage and hence are unstained. *S.G.*, Substantia gelatinosa; *S.L.*, zone of Lissauer. Weigert's myelin stain. Photograph.

intermediate gray and the dorsomedial and central parts of the contralateral anterior horn.

The majority of axons in the anterior corticospinal tract have been found to cross in the anterior white commissure and to terminate in the intermediate gray and the centromedial part of the anterior horn. Fibers of the uncrossed lateral corticospinal tract remain uncrossed and terminate in the base of the posterior horn, the intermediate gray and central parts of the anterior horn. According to Liu and Chambers ('64) corticospinal fibers arising in the precentral gyrus terminate in the intermediate gray and the base of the posterior and anterior horns, while fibers arising from the postcentral gyrus terminate primarily in the posterior horn, especially the nucleus proprius. In the monkey several authors (Hoff, '32a; Hoff and Hoff, '34; Kuypers, '60; Liu and Chambers, '64) report that some corticospinal fibers end in direct synaptic contact with anterior horn cells, although the majority of fibers are said to terminate on internuncial neurons in the intermediate zone. This species difference

between cat and monkey is supported by electrophysiological evidence (Lloyd, '41; Bernhard et al., '53; Bernhard and Bohm, '54; Hern and Phillips, '59; Hern et al., '60; Preston and Whitlock, '61; Landgren et al., '62) indicating monosynaptic activation of motor neurons by corticospinal fibers in the monkey, but not in the cat. Some physiological (Bernhard, '54; Preston and Whitlock, '60, '61) and anatomical (Kuypers, '60; Liu and Chambers, '64) studies suggest a somatotopical organization in the monkey in which fibers from the precentral gyrus pass to epi-axial motor neurons, but not axial motor neurons. The contralateral projection is to neurons innervating distal (chiefly) and proximal limb muscles. The ipsilateral cortical projection is to motor neurons innervating proximal limb muscles. Although some fibers from the postcentral gyrus pass directly to spinal motor neurons, they are far fewer in number.

It has been estimated that about 55% of all pyramidal fibers end in the cervical cord, 20% in the thoracic and 25% in the lumbosacral segments (Weil and Lassek,

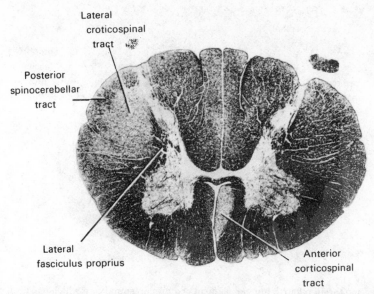

Lateral
croticospinal
tract

Posterior
spinocerebellar
tract

Lateral
fasciculus proprius

Anterior
corticospinal
tract

FIG. 10-15. Transverse section through cervical enlargement of spinal cord of a hemiplegic man. The lateral corticospinal tract of one side and the anterior corticospinal tract of the other side are degenerated and demyelinated. Weigert's myelin stain. Photograph.

'29). This would suggest that pyramidal control over the upper extremity is much greater than over the lower. Myelination of the corticospinal fibers begins near birth and is not completed until the end of the 2nd year.

The pyramidal tract conveys impulses to the spinal cord associated with volitional movements, especially isolated individual movements of the fingers and hand which form the basis for the acquisition of manual skills. Destruction of the tract produces a loss of voluntary movement that is most marked in the distal parts of the extremities. The proximal joints and grosser movement are less severely and permanently affected. At the onset of a vascular accident involving corticospinal fibers, there is a loss of tone in the affected muscles. But after a period of days, or sometimes weeks, the muscles gradually become resistant to passive movement (spasticity), and the deep tendon (myotatic) reflexes, especially in the leg, are increased in force and amplitude (hyper-reflexia). On the other hand, the superficial reflexes, such as the abdominals, cremasteric and normal plantar, are lost or diminished.

In individuals of advanced age there is a tendency for the superficial abdominal reflexes to be absent. These reflexes are absent more often in females than in males (Madonick, '57). Absence of the superficial abdominal reflexes is not in itself indicative of neurological disease. The abnormal plantar response, elicited by stroking the sole of the foot with a blunt instrument, is characterized by extension of the great toe and fanning of the other toes (*sign of Babinski*). The normal plantar response is a brisk flexion of all toes. The Babinski sign usually is indicative of injury to the corticospinal system, but it is not an infallible sign. The extensor toe response commonly can be elicited in the newborn infant, the sleeping or intoxicated adult or following a generalized seizure. It also may be absent in some patients with lesions of the corticospinal tract (Nathan and Smith, '55).

The cause of the spasticity usually occurring in human hemiplegia is still a subject of considerable controversy. Lesions of the pyramidal tract in cats and monkeys produce a hypotonic paralysis, or paresis of discrete movements, although in the chimpanzee the hypotonia is more obscure

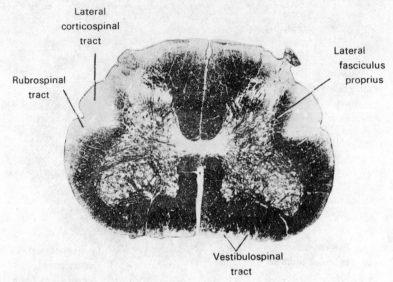

Fig. 10-16. Section through fourth lumbar segment of a human spinal cord which had been crushed some time previously in the lower cervical region. The degenerated long descending tracts are unstained. Note that the lateral corticospinal tract reaches the lateral periphery of the cord. Weigert's myelin stain. Photograph.

(Tower, '49). Similarly, Fulton and Kennard ('34) have reported that ablation of the motor area (area 4) in monkeys and chimpanzees produces a flaccid paralysis. When the motor area (area 4) and the premotor area (area 6) are both ablated, there is a slight increase in resistance to passive movements, but usually not of the degree that characterizes true clinical spasticity (see Chapter 19, page 583).

It must be remembered that the corticospinal tract is a complex fiber system arising from extensive cortical areas, and only part of it originates from the giant pyramidal cells of Betz in the precentral gyrus. These cells are relatively few in number, about 25,000 according to Campbell ('05), some 34,000 in the more careful count of Lassek ('40). They probably furnish the larger fibers, 10 to 22 μ in diameter, whose number has been estimated at about 40,-000 (Lassek and Rasmussen, '39). The more numerous finer fibers come in considerable part from other cortical regions. Thus there are at least two components in the pyramidal tract: a large-fibered component from the motor area, and a fine-fibered one mainly from other areas. Lesions of the entire pyramidal tract involve

both components; ablation of the motor area alone destroys only the large-fibered one (Häggqvist, '37). It is probable that fibers of the Betz cells are concerned with the finer isolated movements of the distal parts of the extremities, which are primarily affected in pyramidal lesions. The more numerous finer fibers may be related to grosser movement and tonic control, and injury to them may be the cause of the increase in muscle tone and the hyperactive deep tendon reflexes. These fibers which form an integral part of the pyramidal tract, its largest portion, descend uninterruptedly from the cerebral cortex through the medullary pyramids to the spinal cord. They come from cortical areas which also give rise to fibers which project to subcortical nuclei that in turn convey impulses to spinal levels.

The pyramidal cells and their axons constitute the "*upper motor neurons*" in contrast to the "*lower motor neurons*" (anterior horn cells), which directly innervate the skeletal muscle. The symptoms of a pyramidal lesion, loss of volitional movement, spasticity, increased deep tendon reflexes, loss of superficial reflexes and the sign of Babinski, therefore are designated as "upper motor neuron" type paralysis (spastic or supranuclear paralysis). In "lower motor neuron" paralysis, there is loss of all movement, reflex and voluntary, as well as loss of tone and atrophy of the affected muscles.

Paralysis of both arm and leg on one side is termed a *hemiplegia,* while paralysis of a single limb is called a *monoplegia. Diplegia* denotes the paralysis of two corresponding parts on opposite sides of the body, such as both arms. When both legs are paralyzed the term *paraplegia* is used. Paralysis of all four extremities is known as *tetraplegia* or *quadriplegia.*

All descending spinal tracts, other than the corticospinal, arise from nuclear masses in the brain stem. Three descending tracts arise from the midbrain. These are the tectospinal, interstitiospinal and rubrospinal tracts.

Tectospinal Tract. Fibers of this tract arise from neurons in the deeper layers of the superior colliculus, a complex neural structure which serves primarily as an optic relay center (Fig. 10-17). The tract is formed by fibers that sweep anteromedially about the periaqueductal gray and cross the midline anterior to the medial longitudinal fasiculus in the *dorsal tegmental decussation.* In the upper brain stem this tract descends near the median raphe anterior to the medial longitudinal fasciculus; at medullary levels tectospinal fibers become incorporated within the medial longitudinal fasciculus (Fig. 10-17). In the older literature tectospinal fibers are referred to as the predorsal bundle. In the spinal cord tectospinal fibers descend in the anterior part of the anterior funiculus near the anterior median fissure (Fig. 10-21). The majority of fibers terminate in the upper four cervical spinal segments, but a few reach lower cervical segments (Altman and Carpenter, '61; Nyberg-Hansen, '66; Petras, '67). Tectospinal fibers enter the ventromedial part of the anterior horn and radiate into laminae VIII, VII and parts of lamina VI (Nyberg-Hansen, '66). None of these fibers terminate directly upon large motor neurons. The functional significance of the tectospinal tract is not known, but it is presumed to mediate reflex postural movements in response to visual and perhaps auditory stimuli.

The superior colliculus also gives rise to fibers distributed bilaterally in the mesencephalic reticular formation and to medial regions of the contralateral pontine and medullary reticular formation (Altman and Carpenter, '61). These fibers are referred to as *tectobulbar fibers.*

Rubrospinal Tract. Fibers of the rubrospinal tract arise from cells of the red nucleus, a well-defined structure in the central part of the mesencephalic tegmentum (Figs. 10-17, 13-1 and 13-4). The red nucleus is a large, oval cell mass which in transverse sections has a circular appearance (Fig. 13-1). This nucleus is divided into a rostral parvocellular part and a caudal magnocellular part; the extent of these two divisions shows variations in size in different animals. In the monkey three distinctive types of neurons are found in the red nucleus: (1) large giant neurons with coarse, evenly distributed, Nissl granules which characterize the magnocellular part, (2) medium-sized triangular neurons with prominent nucleoli and a Nissl substance that does not form distinct granules, which characterize the parvocellular part, and (3) small neurons, found in both magnocellular and parvocellular parts, which are achromatic and have scant cytoplasm (King et al., '71). In the cat there is no adequate basis for distinguishing magnocellular and parvocellular portions of the red nucleus. In this animal the rubrospinal tract arises from cells of all sizes in the caudal three-fourths of the nucleus (Pompeiano and Brodal, '57a). In the monkey the rubrospinal tract arises largely from the magnocellular region which occupies the caudal third of the red nucleus (Keller and Hare, '34; Orioli and Mettler, '56; Poirier and Bouvier, '66; Kuypers and Lawrence, '67; Massion, '67).

Rubrospinal fibers are given off from the medial border of the red nucleus, cross the median raphe immediately in the ventral tegmental decussation and descend to spinal levels, where fibers lie anterior to, and partially intermingled with, fibers of the lateral corticospinal tract (Figs. 10-17 and 10-21). Fibers of the rubrospinal tract

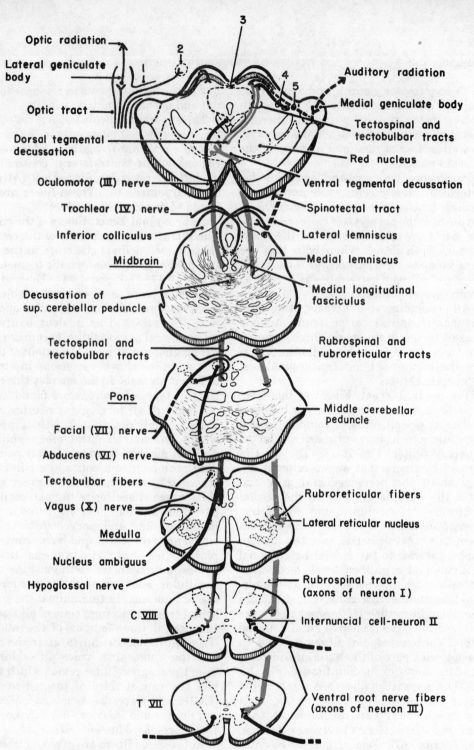

Optic radiation
Lateral geniculate body
Optic tract
Dorsal tegmental decussation
Oculomotor (III) nerve
Trochlear (IV) nerve
Inferior colliculus
Midbrain
Decussation of sup. cerebellar peduncle
Tectospinal and tectobulbar tracts
Pons
Facial (VII) nerve
Abducens (VI) nerve
Tectobulbar fibers
Vagus (X) nerve
Medulla
Nucleus ambiguus
Hypoglossal nerve
C VIII
T VII

Auditory radiation
Medial geniculate body
Tectospinal and tectobulbar tracts
Red nucleus
Ventral tegmental decussation
Spinotectal tract
Lateral lemniscus
Medial lemniscus
Medial longitudinal fasciculus
Rubrospinal and rubroreticular tracts
Middle cerebellar peduncle
Rubroreticular fibers
Lateral reticular nucleus
Rubrospinal tract (axons of neuron I)
Internuncial cell-neuron II
Ventral root nerve fibers (axons of neuron III)

FIG. 10-17. Diagram of the rubrospinal (*red*) and tectospinal (*blue*) tracts. Rubrospinal fibers arise somatotopically from the red nucleus, cross in the ventral tegmental decussation and descend to spinal levels where fibers terminate in parts of laminae V, VI and VII of Rexed. Crossed rubrobulbar fibers project to parts of the facial nucleus (not shown) and to the lateral reticular nucleus of the medulla (rubroreticular fibers). Uncrossed rubrobulbar fibers (not shown) descend in the central tegmental tract and terminate in the dorsal lamella of the ipsilateral principal olivary nucleus. Tectospinal fibers arise from deep layers of the superior colliculus, cross in the dorsal tegmental decussation and descend initially ventral to the medial longitudinal fasciculus. At medullary levels these fibers become incorporated in the medial longitudinal fasciculus. Fibers of the tectospinal tract descend only to lower cervical spinal segments. Numbered midbrain structures include: *1*, the brachium of the superior colliculus; *2*, the pretectal area; *3*, commissure of the superior colliculus; *4*, spinotectal tract; and *5*, collicular fibers from the lateral lemniscus.

262

arise somatotopically from the red nucleus (Pompeiano and Brodal, '57a). Fibers projecting to cervical spinal segments arise from dorsal and dorsomedial parts of the nucleus, while fibers passing to lumbosacral regions of the spinal cord arise from ventral and ventrolateral parts of the red nucleus. Thoracic spinal segments receive fibers that originate from intermediate regions of the nucleus. While the rubrospinal tract extends the length of the spinal cord in most mammals, it has not been demonstrated below thoracic spinal segments in man (Stern, '38). Conclusions that the rubrospinal tract in man is rudimentary are based partially on the fact that cells of the human red nucleus are small. It seems likely that many of the rubrospinal fibers in man are thin and poorly myelinated, thus making their identification difficult. In the cat cervical spinal segments receive the greatest number of rubrospinal fibers and thoracic segments receive a smaller number of fibers than do lumbar segments (Hinman and Carpenter, '59; Nyberg-Hansen and Brodal, '64). Fibers of this tract enter the spinal gray laterally and radiate in fan-shaped fashion into the lateral half of lamina V, lamina VI and dorsal and central parts of lamina VII (Nyberg-Hansen, '66). These fibers terminate on somata and dendrites of large and small cells within these laminae (Nyberg-Hansen and Brodal, '64).

In their descent through the brain stem, some collateral fibers of the rubrospinal tract are given off which project to the cerebellum (Courville and Brodal, '66), the facial nucleus (Courville, '66) and the lateral reticular nucleus of the medulla (Walberg, '58; Hinman and Carpenter, '59; Courville, '66). The parvocellular part of the red nucleus also gives rise to uncrossed rubral efferent fibers that project to dorsal parts of the principal inferior olivary nucleus (Poirier and Bouvier, '66); these fibers are referred to as uncrossed rubrobulbar fibers (Walberg, '56).

The red nucleus receives fibers from the cerebellum and the cerebral cortex. In the cat and monkey corticorubral fibers arise mainly from the "motor" cortex, descend ipsilaterally and terminate upon cells in all parts of the red nucleus (Rinvik and Walberg, '63; Kuypers and Lawrence, '67). Corticorubral fibers are somatotopically organized with respect to both origin and termination. The magnocellular part of the red nucleus receives cortical projections primarily from the precentral gyrus, while the parvocellular part receives fibers from the precentral gyrus, the rostrally adjacent frontal areas and the supplementary motor area (Kuypers and Lawrence, '67). Thus the synaptic linkage of corticorubral and rubrospinal fibers, both of which are somatotopically organized, constitutes a two-neuronal pathway from the motor cortex to spinal levels. Cells of the red nucleus projecting to the spinal cord are excited monosynaptically by corticorubral projections (Tsukahara et al., '67).

All parts of the red nucleus receive crossed cerebellar efferent fibers via the superior cerebellar peduncle. Fibers from the dentate nucleus project mainly to the rostral third of the red nucleus, while fibers from a part of the interposed nucleus (equivalent to the emboliform nucleus in man) pass to the caudal two-thirds of the nucleus (Courville, '66; Massion, '67). Rubral afferent fibers from part of the interposed nucleus (anterior part) are somatotopically organized.

Stimulation of the red nucleus (Pompeiano, '56, '57) in the cat produces flexion in either the forelimb or hindlimb on the opposite side, depending upon which part of the nucleus is stimulated. Flexion limited to a single limb is explained by the somatotopic organization of fibers in the rubrospinal tract. Microelectrode studies (Sasaki et al., '60; Hongo et al., '69) have demonstrated that stimulation of cells in the red nucleus produces excitatory postsynaptic potentials in contralateral flexor α motor neurons, and inhibitory postsynaptic potentials in extensor α motor neurons. A convergence of rubrospinal fibers and primary afferents also provides for excitatory actions upon spinal interneurons involved in reflex pathways (Hongo et al., '69a). The most important function of the rubrospinal tract is the control of muscle tone in flexor muscle groups (Massion, '67). The rubrospinal tract excites flexor motor neurons via polysynaptic pathways, and stimulation of the red nucleus during locomotion enhances flexor muscle activity during the swing phase (Orlovsky, '72a). Modulation of activity in rubrospinal neurons according to locomotor rhythm occurs only when the cerebellum is intact. The spinocerebellar pathways participate in this modulation in that they provide the main inputs into regions of the cerebellar cortex which are somatotopically linked with the interposed nuclei (within the cerebellum), which in turn project to the red nuclei. Since rubrospinal fibers do not end directly upon anterior horn cells, impulses conveyed by these fibers could be mediated in one of two ways: (1) by spinal interneurons which in turn facilitate flexor α motor neurons, or (2) by effects upon γ motor neurons which indirectly influence α motor neurons through the γ loop (Fig. 9-27).

The *interstitiospinal tract* is uncrossed and forms a component of the descending medial longitudinal fasciculus (MLF); it will be discussed with that composite bundle.

Two major descending spinal tracts arise from the pons. These are the vestibulospinal and pontine reticulospinal tracts. The pontine and medullary reticulospinal tracts will be discussed together.

Vestibulospinal Tract. The vestibular nuclei constitute a cytological complex in the floor of the fourth ventricle in both the pons and medulla. The four major nuclei of this complex receive afferent fibers from the vestibular nerve and the cerebellum which are distributed differentially (Fig. 10-18 and 12-14). The vestibulospinal tract, the principal descending spinal pathway from this complex, arises exclusively from the lateral vestibular nucleus. The *lateral vestibular nucleus* consists of a fairly discrete collection of giant cells in the lateral part of the complex near the level of entry of the vestibular nerve root. Practically all cells of the lateral vestibular nucleus contribute fibers to the formation of this tract which descends the length of the spinal cord in the anterior part of the lateral funiculus (Figs. 10-18 and 10-19).

The vestibulospinal tract, like the rubrospinal tract, is somatotopically organized

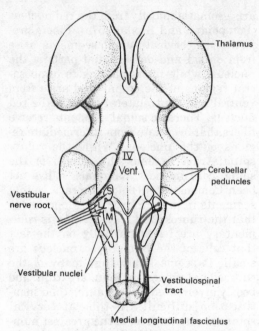

FIG. 10-18. Schematic diagram of the spinal projections from the vestibular nuclei. The vestibulospinal tract (*blue*) arises only from cells of the lateral vestibular nucleus. This tract is uncrossed, somatotopically organized and concerned with the facilitation of extensor muscle tone. Vestibular fibers descending in the medial longitudinal fasciculus (*red*) arise largely from the medial vestibular nucleus and are mainly uncrossed. *S* indicates superior vestibular nucleus; *L* indicates the lateral vestibular nucleus; and *I* and *M* indicate the inferior and medial vestibular nuclei.

(Pompeiano and Brodal, '57b). Cells in different portions of the lateral vestibular nucleus project fibers to specific parts of the spinal cord. The ventrorostral region of the nucleus projects fibers to cervical spinal segments, while cells in the dorsocaudal part of the nucleus pass to lumbosacral spinal segments. Fibers passing to thoracic spinal segments are derived from intermediate regions of the nucleus. While there is some overlap between regions sending fibers to particular spinal segments, the evidence for this somatotopical arrangement is definite. Fibers of the vestibulospinal tract descend the entire length of the spinal cord. Cervical and lumbar spinal segments receive the greatest number of vestibulospinal fibers; thoracic spinal segments receive fewer fibers. In

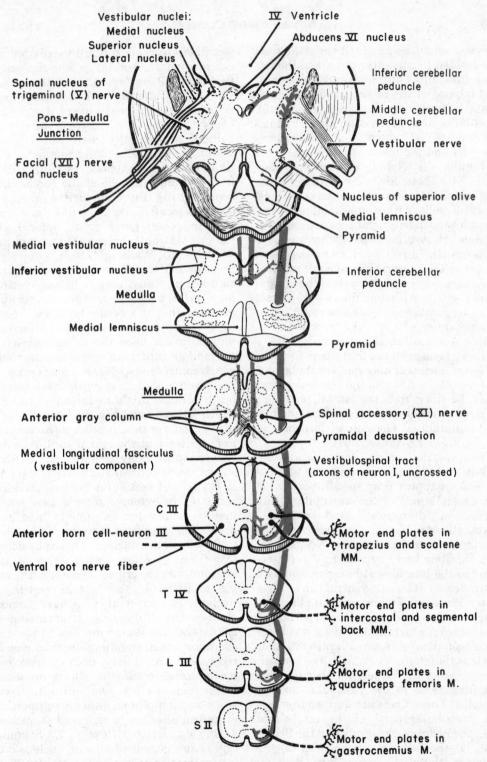

Vestibular nuclei:
Medial nucleus
Superior nucleus
Lateral nucleus

IV Ventricle

Abducens VI nucleus

Inferior cerebellar peduncle

Middle cerebellar peduncle

Vestibular nerve

Spinal nucleus of trigeminal (V) nerve

Pons-Medulla Junction

Facial (VII) nerve and nucleus

Nucleus of superior olive

Medial lemniscus

Pyramid

Medial vestibular nucleus

Inferior vestibular nucleus

Medulla

Inferior cerebellar peduncle

Medial lemniscus

Pyramid

Medulla

Anterior gray column

Spinal accessory (XI) nerve

Pyramidal decussation

Medial longitudinal fasciculus (vestibular component)

Vestibulospinal tract (axons of neuron I, uncrossed)

C III

Anterior horn cell-neuron III

Motor end plates in trapezius and scalene MM.

Ventral root nerve fiber

T IV

Motor end plates in intercostal and segmental back MM.

L III

Motor end plates in quadriceps femoris M.

S II

Motor end plates in gastrocnemius M.

FIG. 10-19. Diagram of the vestibulospinal tract (*blue*) and descending vestibular fibers in the medial longitudinal fasciculus (*red*). Fibers of the vestibulospinal tract have a somatotopic origin in the lateral vestibular nucleus, descend the length of the spinal cord and terminate predominantly in lamina VIII of Rexed. Descending vestibular fibers in the medial longitudinal fasciculus arise from the medial vestibular nucleus. In the lower brain stem these fibers are bilateral, but in the cervical spinal cord they are ipsilateral. *Letters* and *numbers* indicate segmental spinal levels.

265

cervical spinal segments fibers of the tract are located in the anterior part of the lateral funiculus, but in lumbosacral segments most of the fibers are found in the anterior funiculus (Figs. 9-8 and 10-16). Vestibulospinal fibers enter the gray matter and are distributed to all parts of lamina VIII and the medial and central parts of lamina VII (Nyberg-Hansen and Mascitti, '64). These fibers form axodendritic and axosomatic synaptic contacts with all types of cells within these laminae, although axodendritic synapses are most numerous. No vestibulospinal fibers appear to terminate directly on motor neurons, except in the thoracic spinal cord, where a few fibers may end upon cells of the anteromedial group. Although fibers in this tract in man probably are less numerous than in other mammals, it is still a tract of considerable size and functional significance.

There is no evidence that fibers from the inferior, medial or superior vestibular nuclei contribute fibers to the vestibulospinal tract. No fibers from the lateral vestibular nucleus reach the spinal cord via the medial longitudinal fasciculus (Carpenter et al., '60; Nyberg-Hansen, '64).

The vestibulospinal tract relays impulses to the spinal cord from the vestibular end organ and from specific portions of the cerebellum. Primary vestibular fibers terminate differentially and selectively upon cells in all four major divisions of the vestibular nuclear complex (Walberg et al., '58; Stein and Carpenter, '67). Projections to the lateral vestibular nucleus are restricted to its rostroventral part. Electron microscopic findings indicate that primary vestibular fibers end upon perikarya and spines of proximal and distal dendrites of cells of all sizes in the lateral vestibular nucleus (Mugnaini et al., '67). The cerebellum provides the largest number of afferent projections to the vestibular nuclear complex. These fibers are derived from: (1) the "vestibular part" of the cerebellum (i.e., the nodulus, the uvula and the flocculus), (2) the fastigial nuclei, and (3) the anterior lobe of the cerebellum (Walberg and Jansen, '61; Walberg et al., '62; Mugnaini and Walberg, '67; Walberg, '72). "Vestibular parts" of the cerebellum pro-

ject fibers to regions of all vestibular nuclei in a pattern similar to that of primary vestibular fibers, except that the projection to the lateral vestibular nucleus is scant. Fastigiovestibular fibers are crossed and uncrossed, topographically arranged and supply different regions within the lateral, medial and inferior vestibular nuclei. Cerebellovestibular fibers from the anterior lobe of the cerebellum, representing Purkinje cell axons, are somatotopically arranged and terminate only in dorsal parts of the lateral and inferior vestibular nuclei (Muganiani and Walberg, '67; Walberg, '72). It is apparent that vestibular influences upon the spinal cord are mediated largely by the vestibulospinal tract. There is considerable evidence that the vestibular nuclei, especially the lateral nucleus, exert a facilitatory influence upon the reflex activity of the spinal cord and spinal mechanisms which control muscle tone. This perhaps is best exemplified in experimental decerebrate animals by the reduction of rigidity which follows lesions in the lateral vestibular nucleus or interruption of the vestibulospinal tract in the spinal cord. Another experimental study (Pompeiano, '60) has shown that electrical stimulation of points in the lateral vestibular nucleus produces increases in extensor muscle tone which may be localized to forelimb or hindlimb, depending upon the position of the electrode within the nucleus. These physiological findings offer confirmation. of the anatomically described somatotopical origin of fibers in the lateral vestibular nucleus. Sasaki et al. ('62) have demonstrated that following stimulation of the lateral vestibular nucleus in the cat, excitatory postsynaptic potentials can be recorded intracellularly from extensor motor neurons, while the effects on flexor motor neurons are insignificant. Excitatory vestibulospinal influences upon extensor muscles can be observed at rest and during locomotion (Orlovsky, '72). Stimulation of the lateral vestibular nucleus during locomotion enhances the activity of extensor muscles during the stance phase of the step. Modulation of vestibulospinal neurons with locomotor rhythm occurs only when the cerebellum is intact. Anatomical data suggest that these facilitatory effects must be mediated via interneurons in laminae VII and VIII. The abundant fibers from the cerebellum which project in a specific manner to the vestibular nuclei suggest that significant cerebellar influences upon extensor muscle tone and posture also are mediated to spinal levels via the vestibulospinal tract.

Clinically, examples of impulses conveyed by the vestibulospinal tract are seen in the tendency to fall after being rapidly rotated, and in the "past-pointing" reaction. In the latter, after being rotated in a certain direction, vertical voluntary movements tend to deviate in the direction of prior rotation, and the person misses objects he endeavors to touch with his eyes closed.

Reticulospinal Tracts. Two relatively large regions of the brain stem reticular formation give rise to fibers that descend to spinal levels. One of these regions is in the pontine tegmentum, while the other lies in the medulla; hence it is proper to refer to these as the pontine and medullary reticulospinal tracts (Figs. 10-11 and 10-20).

The *pontine reticulospinal tract* arises from aggregations of cells in the medial pontine tegmentum referred to as the *nuclei reticularis pontis caudalis* and *oralis* (Olszewski and Baxter, '54; Brodal, '57; Torvik and Brodal, '57). The caudal pontine reticular nucleus begins in the caudal pontine tegmentum and extends rostrally to the level of the motor trigeminal nucleus. This nucleus contains a number of giant cells in addition to various types of smaller cells. The oral pontine reticular nucleus, present in more rostral parts of the medial pontine tegmentum, extends into the caudal mesencephalic reticular formation; giant cells are found only in the more caudal parts of this nucleus. Reticulospinal fibers arise from cells in all parts of the nucleus reticularis pontis caudalis but only from the caudal part of the nucleus reticularis pontis oralis. More than half of the large cells in the caudal pontine reticular nucleus project fibers to spinal levels (Torvik and Brodal, '57). The pon-tine reticulospinal tract is almost entirely ipsilateral and descends chiefly in the medial part of the anterior funiculus (Fig. 10-20). In the brain stem part of these fibers descend in close association with the medial longitudinal fasciculus. Pontine reticulospinal fibers are more numerous than those arising in the medulla, descend the entire length of the spinal cord and terminate in lamina VIII and adjacent parts of lamina VII (Fig. 10-20). A few pontine reticulospinal fibers cross at spinal levels in the anterior white commissure. The gray laminae that receive terminations of pontine reticulospinal fibers also contain terminals of vestibulospinal, tectospinal and interstitiospinal fibers. This spinal projection is not somatotopically organized.

The *medullary reticulospinal tract* arises from the medial two-thirds of the medullary reticular formation (Brodal, '57). The largest number of fibers arise from the *nucleus reticularis gigantocellularis*, lying dorsal to the inferior olivary complex and lateral to the paramedian region (Fig. 10-20). As the name of this nucleus implies, it is composed of characteristic large cells, but large cells are not as conspicuous in man as in lower animals. In addition, there are many medium-sized and small cells. Fibers of the medullary reticulospinal tract are mainly ipsilateral, but some crossed fibers are present. The latter cross at medullary levels. The medullary reticulospinal tract descends the length of the spinal cord in the anterior part of the lateral funiculus (Figs. 10-11 and 10-20). Reticulospinal fibers from the pons and medulla are not segregated sharply in the spinal cord. Fibers entering the spinal gray radiate into all parts of lamina VII and terminate mainly in central parts of this lamina (Fig. 10-20); other fibers enter lamina IX and appear to end in relationship to both large and small neurons (Nyberg-Hansen, '66). Medullary reticulospinal fibers terminate in parts of the gray spinal laminae that also receive fibers from the rubrospinal and corticospinal tracts. Reticulospinal fibers from both the pons and medulla terminate upon cells of all sizes and on both the somata

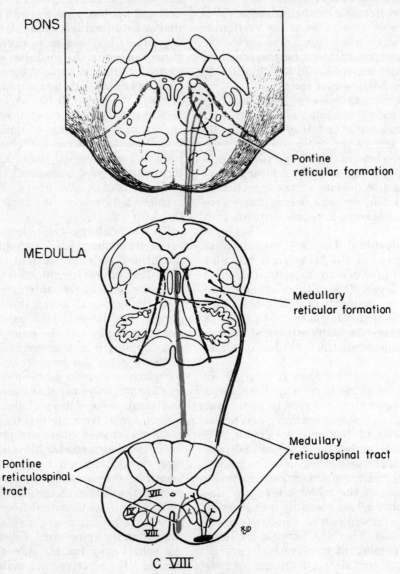

PONS

Pontine
reticular formation

MEDULLA

Medullary
reticular formation

Medullary
reticulospinal tract

Pontine
reticulospinal
tract

VII

IX

VIII

C VIII

FIG. 10-20. Diagram of the reticulospinal tracts indicating their regions of origin, course and terminations. Pontine reticulospinal fibers (*red*) terminate in lamina VIII and adjacent parts of lamina VII. Medullary reticulospinal fibers (*black*) terminate chiefly in lamina VII, but some end in lamina IX.

and dendrites. The above evidence suggests that impulses arising from the reticular formation which influence γ motor neurons probably are mediated largely by internuncial neurons in parts of laminae VII and VIII (Eldred et al., '53; Eldred and Fujimori, '58).

Although early experimental studies suggested that the reticulospinal tracts did not descend caudal to thoracic spinal segments, virtually all recent data indicate that these tracts descend the entire length of the spinal cord (Staal, '61; Nyberg-Hansen, '65, '66; Petras, '67). Information concerning the reticulospinal tracts in man is very meager (Nathan and Smith, '55a), and conclusive data are not available. Autonomic fibers from higher levels of the neuraxis probably descend in close association with both the reticulospinal and corticospinal tracts to end about visceral motor cells of the intermediate gray matter.

The brain stem reticular formation receives inputs from many sources, but direct corticoreticular projections seem especially important. Corticoreticular fibers arise from widespread areas of the cortex, although the greatest number originate from the "motor area." While these fibers arise from different cortical areas, they mainly terminate in two fairly restricted regions of the reticular formation, one in the pons and one in the medulla (Rossi and Brodal, '56). In the pons these fibers end mainly in the nucleus reticularis pontis oralis and in the rostral part of the caudal pontine reticular nucleus. In the medulla such fibers terminate in the nucleus reticularis gigantocellularis. Corticoreticular fibers are distributed bilaterally with some crossed preponderance. The regions of termination within the reticular formation correspond to those that give rise to the reticulospinal tracts. Thus the synaptic linkage of corticoreticular and reticulospinal fibers forms a pathway from the cortex to spinal levels. There is no evidence of a somatotopic arrangement within this system (Brodal, '57).

Experimental studies have demonstrated that stimulation of the brain stem reticular formation can: (1) facilitate or inhibit voluntary movement, cortically induced movement and reflex activity; (2) influence muscle tone; (3) affect inspiratory phases of respiration; (4) exert pressor or depressor effects on the circulatory system; and (5) exert depressant effects on the central transmission of sensory impulses. Areas of the medullary reticular formation from which medullary reticulospinal fibers arise appear to correspond closely with the regions from which inspiratory, inhibitory and depressor effects have been obtained (Pitts et al., '39; Pitts, '40; Amoroso et al., '54; Torvik and Brodal, '57). Areas of the brain stem reticular formation related to facilitatory influences, expiratory effects and pressor vasomotor phenomena are mainly rostral to the medulla and appear to extend beyond those regions which give rise to direct reticulospinal fibers (Brodal, '57). Thus some facilitatory influences from the upper brain stem reticular formation probably are not transmitted directly to spinal levels by reticulospinal pathways.

Recent studies have shown that the reticular formation can influence muscle tone by acting upon γ motor neurons which innervate the contractile portions of the muscle spindle (Eldred et al., '53; Granit, '55). Inhibitory effects on the muscle spindle are obtained most easily from the medullary reticular formation, while facilitatory effects are elicited from more rostral regions. It is probably by this means that the reticulospinal systems can modify tendon reflex activity. The reticular formation and its great functional significance will be considered in more detail in Chapter 13.

Medial Longitudinal Fasciculus (MLF). The posterior part of the anterior funiculus contains a composite bundle of descending fibers that originates from different nuclei at various brain stem levels and is collectively referred to as the *medial longitudinal fasciculus* (abbreviated MLF). Such descending fibers represent only a portion of the brain stem tract that is designated by the same name, but is composed of both ascending and descending fibers (Fig. 12-14). In the brain stem and spinal cord, fibers of this tract are

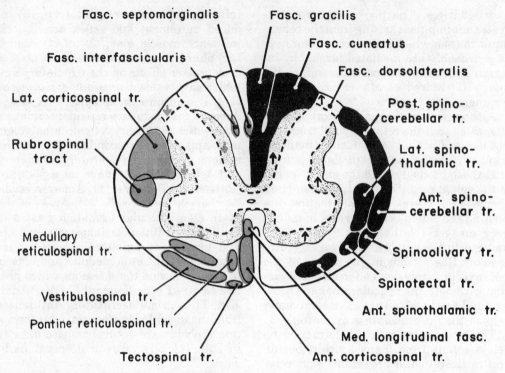

FIG. 10-21. Diagram of ascending (*black*) and descending (*red*) pathways of the spinal cord. The fasciculus proprius system (*stippled*) and dorsolateral fasciculus contain both ascending and descending nerve fibers.

always near the median raphe and immediately ventral to the cerebral aqueduct, fourth ventricle or central canal (Figs. 10-18 and 10-19). Descending fibers of the medial longitudinal fasciculus in the spinal cord originate from the medial vestibular nucleus, the reticular formation, the superior colliculus (tectospinal fibers) and the interstitial nucleus of Cajal (interstitiospinal fibers). Fibers of this bundle form a well-defined tract only in the upper cervical segments of the spinal cord (Figs. 10-18, 10-19 and 10-21). Below that level most fibers are difficult to follow, although fibers have been traced to sacral levels. Most of these fibers are believed to terminate among internuncial neurons in the most medial part of the anterior horn.

Vestibular fibers descending in the medial longitudinal fasciculus arise only from the medial vestibular nucleus (Fig. 10-18), are predominantly ipsilateral in the spinal cord and terminate in the dorsal part of lamina VIII and adjacent parts of lamina VII (Nyberg-Hansen, '64; McMasters et

al., '66). Physiological studies suggest that fibers from the medial vestibular nucleus convey monosynaptic inhibitory influences directly to upper cervical motor neurons (Wilson and Yoshida, '69). This unusual direct inhibitory pathway appears to play a role in the labyrinthine regulation of head positions. The largest component of descending fibers in the medial longitudinal fasciculus at spinal levels is the pontine reticulospinal tract; these fibers descend the length of the spinal cord and terminate mainly in lamina VIII and parts of VII (Fig. 10-20). Fibers of the interstitiospinal tract are uncrossed, descend in the most posterior part of the anterior funiculus near the anteromedian fissure and terminate in dorsal parts of lamina VIII and neighboring parts of lamina VII (Staal, '61; Nyberg-Hansen, '66). While most of the fibers of this tract are given off in upper portions of the spinal cord, some fibers project as far caudally as sacral levels.

Olivospinal Tract. This tract is considered to be a complex tract composed of fine fibers which stain lightly in Weigert preparations. This bundle, located on the anterior surface of the spinal cord at the zone of transition between the lateral and anterior funiculi, is partially traversed by ventral root fibers. While this tract has been described as containing descending fibers from the inferior olivary nucleus, the evidence is not conclusive. Some fibers from higher levels traversing this area have been considered as part of the anterolateral corticospinal tract (Barnes, '01; Déjérine, '01). Experimental studies indicate that this tract actually may contain primarily spino-olivary fibers ascending to the medial and dorsal accessory olivary nuclei (Brodal et al., '50).

Descending Autonomic Pathways. The descending tracts described in the preceding pages are parts of pathways by which impulses ultimately reach, or influence the activity of, voluntary striated muscles through the somatic anterior horn cells. The spinal cord also contains descending fibers which come in relation with the intermediolateral column and other preganglionic cell groups for the innervation of visceral structures (smooth muscle, heart muscle and glandular epithelium). The highest coordinating center of this pathway is the hypothalamus, which in turn is under the influence of visceral neurons within portions of the cerebral cortex. Other important autonomic centers lie in the tegmentum of the midbrain, pons and medulla. These descending paths are diffuse and probably are interrupted by relay neurons in the reticular formation. In the spinal cord these fibers descend mainly in the anterior and anterolateral portions of the white matter, in close relation to the lateral fasciculus proprius system and the reticulospinal tracts.

ASCENDING AND DESCENDING SPINAL TRACTS

A series of schematic diagrams have represented the ascending and descending tracts of the spinal cord described in this chapter. It should be emphasized that at different levels of the spinal cord these tracts occupy slightly different positions,

and that they show variations in size depending upon the particular level. Considerable intermingling and overlapping of fiber pathways are found at all spinal levels. Major ascending and descending spinal pathways are diagramed schematically in Figure 10-21.

FASCICULI PROPRII

The shorter fiber systems which form part of the intrinsic reflex mechanism of the spinal cord are as important as the long ascending and descending tracts. In its simplest form a spinal reflex arc may consist of only two neurons: an afferent peripheral neuron (spinal ganglion cell), and an efferent peripheral neuron (anterior horn cell) with a single synapse in the gray (Fig. 9-23). These monosynaptic reflexes are as a rule uncrossed and usually involve only one segment or closely adjacent ones (i.e., they are primarily segmental reflexes). This same reflex arc, which is dependent upon impulses from the muscle spindles, plays a vital role in the unconscious neural control of muscular contraction during movement and the maintenance of posture. It has been suggested (Merton, '53) that this reflex arc behaves as a servo-mechanism, or automatic control, which is activated by an "error signal" occurring in a closed loop and possessing power amplification. The closed loop consists of the muscle spindle, group Ia afferent fibers, the synapse with α motor neurons, and α fibers innervating extrafusal muscle (Fig. 9-27). The power amplification is provided by the contraction of extrafusal muscle. Thus contraction of the muscle opposes applied tension and tends to maintain the muscle at a constant length. The "error signal" may be considered to be the difference in the frequency of firing of the primary endings when the muscle is unloaded, and when it is loaded (Matthews, '64).

However, only part of the collaterals of dorsal root fibers terminate directly upon anterior horn cells (Hoff, '32; Foerster et al., '33; Sprague and Ha, '64). Hence in most reflex arcs there is at least one central or internuncial neuron interposed between the afferent and efferent neurons. These central cells then send their axons to the motor cells of the same segment, or to higher and lower segments, for the completion of various intersegmental arcs. Many of the fibers are axons of internuncial cells which ascend or descend in the white columns of the same side. Others come from commissural cells and pass to the white matter of the opposite side. All these ascending and descending fibers, crossed and uncrossed, which begin and end in the spinal cord and connect its various levels, constitute the *spinospinal* or *fundamental* columns (*fasciculi proprii*) of the spinal cord (Figs. 9-7 and 10-21). To this spinal reflex mechanism also belong the descending root fibers of the interfascicular and septomarginal bundles, which previously were described, and the collaterals and many terminals of ascending dorsal root fibers. Impulses entering the cord at any segment may travel along these fibers to higher or lower levels before connecting directly or through internuncial neurons with the anterior horn cells (Fig. 9-23).

The spinospinal fibers are found in all funiculi: posterior, anterior and lateral. They occupy the area adjacent to the gray matter, and between the gray matter and the more peripherally placed long tracts with which they intermingle. They are most numerous in the anterolateral white columns. In the posterior funiculus they form a narrow zone along the posterior commissure and adjacent portions of the posterior horn. In general, the shortest fibers lie nearest the gray and connect adjacent segments. The longer fibers lie more peripherally and continue up or down through several segments.

It must be kept in mind that under normal circumstances there are no *isolated* reflexes, and that every neural reaction involving any given arc always influences, and is influenced by, other parts of the nervous system. The primitive nervous system is organized for the production of generalized muscle movements and total response. Studies of fetal behavior suggest that local reflexes appear later (Herrick and Coghill, '15; Coghill, '29; Hooker, '44).

UPPER AND LOWER MOTOR NEURONS

One of the most important concepts in neurological diagnosis rests upon distin-guishing the abnormalities of motor function which result from pathological involvement of, or injury to, the upper or lower motor neuron. This relatively simple, yet frequently puzzling, distinction forms one of the cornerstones of clinical neurology. The ability to distinguish upper and lower motor neuron lesions constitutes the first step in attempting to localize the site of a neural lesion that manifests itself by disturbances of normal motor function. Once the site of the neural lesion has been established, the clinician can begin to consider the pathological processes which might be responsible (Carpenter, '71).

Anterior horn cells (α motor neurons) and their axons, which innervate striated muscle, constitute anatomical and physiological units referred to as the final common motor pathway, or the *lower motor neuron*. The concept of the lower motor neuron is not limited to the spinal cord, even though it is most frequently used in that context. Cells of the motor cranial nerve nuclei (nerves III, IV, V, VI, VII, IX, X, XI and XII), which provide innervation for muscles of the head and neck, also must be classified as lower motor neurons, even though these nuclei form discontinuous cell columns in the brain stem. The anterior horn cells are regarded as the prototype for all motor neurons.

The segmental input to the lower motor neuron is profuse, both direct and indirect, and largely, but not exclusively, ipsilateral. Muscle spindle afferents (group Ia) project directly to the lower motor neuron (Figs. 9-25 and 9-27), while afferents from most other receptors, including the Golgi tendon organ (Fig. 9-27), influence the lower motor neuron indirectly via internuncial neurons. Afferent inputs from stretch receptors (i.e., muscle spindle and Golgi tendon organ) activate ipsilateral cell groups in the spinal cord, while afferent impulses from other sensory receptors are distributed by multisynaptic circuits to both sides of the spinal cord. The lower motor neuron also is under powerful indirect suprasegmental control provided by impulses transmitted via descending spinal systems (Fig. 10-21).

Lesions selectively involving the lower motor neuron result in weakness or paralysis, loss of muscle tone, loss of reflex activity and atrophy. All of these changes are confined to the affected muscles. *Weakness* or *paralysis,* occurring in affected muscles, bears a direct relationship to the extent and severity of the lesion. Since the anterior horn cells that innervate a single muscle extend longitudinally through several spinal segments, and since several such cell columns exist at each spinal level, a lesion confined to one spinal segment will cause weakness, but not complete paralysis, in all muscles innervated by this segment. Complete paralysis will occur only when the lesion involves the column of cells in several spinal segments that innervate a particular muscle, or the ventral root fibers that arise from these cells. Because most of the appendicular muscles are innervated by fibers arising from parts of three spinal segments, complete paralysis of a muscle resulting from a central lesion in the anterior horn indicates involvement of several spinal segments. Furthermore, because neighboring cell columns are likely to be affected at each level, such a lesion usually produces paralysis in muscle groups, rather than in individual muscles.

Since the lower motor neuron consists of the anterior horn cells and their axons, which innervate striated muscle, it becomes necessary to distinguish the motor deficits that occur as a consequence of lesions in spinal segments from those which occur in ventral roots, spinal nerves and peripheral nerves. A lesion in ventral root fibers usually produces motor deficits similar to those resulting from destruction of anterior horn cells. At certain levels (i.e., thoracolumbar and sacral) section of the ventral root fibers would produce additional autonomic deficits which might not accompany anterior horn cell lesions at the same level (Fig. 10-22). Lesions of mixed spinal nerves produce motor and sensory deficits that correspond to those of combined dorsal and ventral root lesions. While the motor deficit corresponds almost exactly to that seen with pure lesions of the ventral root, sensory disturbances and loss follow a dermatomal distribution and tend to be less extensive because of overlapping innervation characteristic of dermatomes (Figs. 7-10, 7-11 and 7-12). With a

peripheral nerve lesion, the muscle paralysis and sensory loss correspond to the distribution of the particular nerve (Figs. 7-11 and 7-12).

Loss of muscle tone, *hypotonia,* is a characteristic and constant finding in lower motor neuron lesions. Flaccidity of the affected muscles is evidenced by greatly diminished resistance to passive movement. This reduction in muscle tone results from the withdrawal of streams of impulses transmitted to muscles that normally maintain a state of variable, but sometimes sustained, contraction in some of the muscle units.

Reflexes in the affected muscles are diminished or lost (areflexia) in lower motor neuron lesions because the reflex arc is interrupted (Fig. 9-27). In this type of lesion the effector mechanism is destroyed.

Although paralysis, hypotonia and areflexia occur almost immediately following a lower motor neuron lesion, atrophy or muscle wasting does not become evident for 2 or 3 weeks. The *atrophy* develops gradually and in time is obvious on inspection. Why muscles deprived of their innervation atrophy and degenerate is not adequately understood, and in a sense seems to contradict the neuron doctrine. It seems likely that the morphological and functional properties of muscle are dependent upon transmitter substances provided by the terminals of motor nerve fibers. Atrophy, of the type seen in lower motor neuron disease, does not result from depriving anterior horn cells of afferent impulses from either suprasegmental or segmental levels (Tower, '37).

In certain diseases of the lower motor neuron, the muscles exhibit small, localized spontaneous contractions known as *fasciculations*. These muscle twitches, visible through the skin, represent the discharge of squads of muscle fibers innervated by nerve fibers arising from a single lower motor neuron. Fasciculations occur asynchronously in different parts of various muscles and are thought to be due to a triggering of motor unit discharges that occur within the cell body of the motor neuron. Fasciculations of this type are interpreted as a disease process attacking the lower motor neurons in the anterior gray horn. Fasciculations commonly are

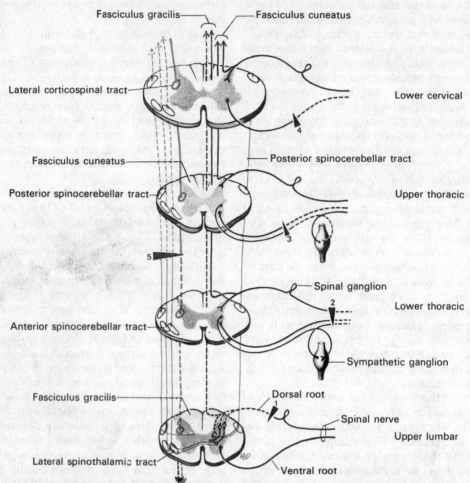

FIG. 10-22. Simplified schematic diagram of degeneration resulting from certain lesions of the spinal nerves, spinal roots and spinal cord. Sites of lesions are indicated by *small black triangles*. Dorsal and ventral root fibers, peripheral nerve fibers, fibers in the posterior white columns and certain short relays are in *black*; other ascending spinal tracts are in *blue*, and the corticospinal tract is in *red*. A lesion of the dorsal root, *1*, at upper lumbar levels produces degeneration in the posterior and anterior gray horns (not shown) and ascending degeneration in parts of the fasciculus gracilis (*dashed lines*). No degeneration is present in other ascending spinal tracts because degeneration does not pass beyond the synapse. A lesion of a spinal nerve as at *2* produces peripheral degeneration (*dashed lines*) in somatic motor, sensory and postganglionic sympathetic fibers. A lesion of the ventral root at site *3* produces degeneration in somatic motor and preganglionic sympathetic fibers. A lesion at *4* produces degeneration only in somatic motor fibers distal to the lesion. The lesion at *5* destroys the lateral funiculus and produces ascending degeneration in the posterior and anterior spinocerebellar tracts (*blue*) and in the spinothalamic tracts (only the lateral spinothalamic tract (*blue*) shown here) above the level of the lesion. This lesion also produces descending degeneration in the corticospinal tract (*red*) below the level of the lesion. Although other spinal tracts which would degenerate are not indicated, the same principle applies.

seen in amyotrophic lateral sclerosis, occasionally in acute inflammatory lesions of peripheral nerves and rarely occur when anterior horn cells are rapidly injured or destroyed (i.e., in acute poliomyelitis).

The term *fibrillation*, frequently misused as the equivalent of the term fasciculation, refers to the small (10 to 200 μV) potentials of 1 to 2 msec duration that occur irregularly and asynchronously in electromyograms of denervated muscle. These spontaneous discharges cannot be observed through the skin and produce no detectable shortening of muscles.

All of the descending fiber systems that can influence and modify the activity of the lower motor neuron constitute the *upper motor neuron* (Fig. 10-21). This is a more inclusive definition than that used by many clinicians who equate the upper motor neuron solely with the corticospinal system. The narrower concept has become a rule of thumb because of: (1) the overwhelming clinical importance of the corticospinal system, and (2) poorly defined information concerning the functional influences of descending nonpyramidal fiber systems. Recent anatomical and physiological data concerning descending nonpyramidal fiber systems make it necessary to modify this venerable rule of thumb and to consider the concept of the upper motor neuron in its broadest sense. Descending impulses, transmitted to spinal levels by a group of heterogenous tracts, are concerned mainly with: (1) mediation of somatic motor activity, (2) control of muscle tone, (3) maintenance of posture and equilibrium, (4) suprasegmental control of reflex activity, (5) inervation of visceral and autonomic structures, and (6) modification of sensory input.

Lesions involving the upper motor neuron, at a wide variety of locations and resulting from many different kinds of pathological processes, produce paralysis, alterations of muscle tone and alterations of reflex activity. Lesions destroying the upper motor neuron are rarely selective, usually incomplete and frequently involve adjacent pathways and nuclear structures. The degree of paresis or paralysis does not bear a direct relationship to the size of the lesion, or to the extent of involvment of the corticospinal tract (Lassek, '54). Destruction of the upper motor neuron may result from vascular disease, trauma, neoplasm and infectious and degenerative diseases. Unilateral lesions in the cerebral hemisphere and brain stem produce contralateral paralysis, usually hemiplegia. Spinal lesions, most commonly the result of trauma, are usually bilateral and cause a paraplegia.

Initially symptoms associated with upper motor neuron lesions are both focal and general in character. Generalized symptoms include headache, vomiting, convulsions and coma. Focal symptoms, such as paralysis, sensory loss or impairment of speech, are related to the site of the lesion and the structures involved. Immediately after a cerebral vascular lesion, the paralyzed limbs contralateral to the lesion usually are flaccid and the myotatic reflexes are depressed, or absent. After variable periods, the myotatic reflexes reappear in an exaggerated form in the paralyzed limbs. The superficial abdominal reflexes, elicited by stroking the skin over the abdomen, and the cremasteric reflexes in the male, disappear on the side of the paralysis. The plantar response, elicited by stroking the sole of the foot, becomes extensor. The latter response, known as the *sign of Babinski*, consists of extension of the great toe and fanning of the other toes. Although the sign of Babinski is of great clinical importance, the physiological mechanism underlying it is not understood.

After a variable period of time muscle tone gradually returns in the affected limb and ultimately exceeds that of the normal side. This exaggeration of muscle tone is referred to as *hypertonicity* or *spasticity*. The exaggeration of muscle tone is not exhibited by all muscles in the affected limbs. Spasticity involves the antigravity muscles. In the affected upper extremity spasticity is present particularly in the adductors and internal rotators of the shoulder, in the flexors of the elbow, wrist and digits and in the pronators of the forearm.

In the affected lower extremity spasticity develops in the adductors of the hip, the extensors of the hip and knee and in the plantar-flexors of foot and toes. *Spasticity* is relatively easy to describe but extremely difficult to define. Descriptively spasticity is characterized by: (1) increased resistance to passive movement, (2) extraordinarily hyperactive myotatic (deep tendon) reflexes that exhibit a low threshold, a large amplitude, an enlarged reflexogenous zone and have a briskness much greater than normal, and (3) the presence of clonus (Magoun and Rhines, '47). *Clonus* is a manifestation of the exaggerated stretch reflex in which the contractions of one muscle group are sufficient to stretch antagonistic muscle groups and initiate myotatic responses in that muscle group. Clonus has a tendency to perpetuate itself in a synchronized manner. In some instances the threshold for this extreme exaggeration of the myotatic reflex is so low that passively moving a limb may initiate it.

The paralysis, which may appear complete at the onset of the cerebral vascular accident, tends to become less severe in time. Even the weakness tends ultimately to involve one limb more than the other. The motor functions affected most are those associated with fine, skilled movements. Gross movements, and those which involve a whole limb, are least affected and show considerable restitution. Atrophy of the type seen with lower motor neuron lesions does not occur with upper motor neuron lesions. However, after a period of years some atrophy of disuse becomes evident.

Many hemiplegic patients recover considerable motor function in time. Those that become ambulatory have a characteristic gait. The paralyzed leg is circumducted at the hip *en bloc* and swung forward, because of the difficulty in flexing the knee. The foot is plantar-flexed and the toe of the shoe is dragged in a circular fashion. The arm on the affected side is flexed at the elbow and wrist, the forearm is pronated and the digits are flexed. The arm usually is held close to the body, but if the arm is swung at all in walking, it moves primarily at the shoulder. Upper motor neuron syndromes resulting from lesions in the brain stem produce disturbances of motor function similar to those described above, except that they frequently also involve cranial nerves.

LESIONS OF THE SPINAL CORD AND NERVE ROOTS

The origin, course and terminations of ascending and descending spinal pathways are among the best documented pathways in the central nervous system (Nathan and Smith, '55a; van Beusekom, '55; Brodal, '57; Brodal et al., '62; Massion, '67). However, considerable anatomical and physiological detail concerning small and diffuse pathways continues to be developed from: (1) experimental anatomical studies in animals using silver impregnation technics and methods dependent upon axoplasmic transport, (2) neurophysiological stimulation and recording under controlled conditions, and (3) detailed neuropathological studies in man.

The study of secondary or Wallerian degeneration has been expecially valuable in tracing fiber pathways (Fig. 10-22). When a nerve fiber is cut, not only does the part severed from the cell body undergo complete degeneration, but the cell body itself exhibits certain pathological changes, such as central chromatolysis, swelling and nuclear eccentricity. Thus, if the spinal cord is transected, all the ascending fibers will degenerate above the level of injury ("ascending" degeneration). Their cell bodies, located below the injury, may show these pathological changes (Figs. 4-1E and 4-28). Below the level of injury the descending fibers will degenerate ("descending" degeneration), since their cell bodies are above the cut. In the same way the central continuations of the dorsal root fibers may be determined by following their secondary degeneration in the spinal cord after section of the dorsal roots proximal to the spinal ganglia (Fig. 10-22). Although chromatolysis of spinal ganglion cells might be expected following surgical section of the dorsal root in this location, only very minimal cell changes are seen (Hare and Hinsey, '40). However, section of the mixed spinal nerve produces retrograde cell changes in the spinal ganglia (Fig. 7-5) and in some anterior horns (Carmel and Stein, '69). The location of the cell bodies whose axons form the ventral roots may be similarly determined by cutting the ventral root and ascertaining which cell bodies in the cord show retrograde changes (axon reaction). The Marchi method (Marchi and Algeri, 1885) which stains the degenerated myelin sheath may be useful in tracing the course of relatively large fiber bundles (Fig. 10-5). Silver impregnation technics (Figs. 4-1F, 9-24 and 9-25) provide more precise data concerning the course and termination of both myelinated and unmyelinated fibers (Nauta and Gygax, '51, '54; Glees and Nauta, '55; Fink and Heimer, '67; Wiitanen, '69; Heimer, '70).

Dorsal Root Lesions. It should be obvious that cutting a dorsal root of a spinal nerve (i.e., dorsal rhizotomy) will abolish all of its incoming sensory impulses as well as interrupt the afferent arms of some segmental reflexes (Fig. 10-22). Due to the overlap of dermatomes in the periphery, destruction of one dorsal root does not result in diminished cutaneous innervation (hypesthesia); three consecutive dorsal roots must be destroyed before there is complete *anesthesia* in a dermatome (Fig. 7-10). Muscle tone also is dependent upon the integrity of segmental reflexes, although two or more segments usually supply a single muscle. For example, total resection of dorsal root C5 will result in severe loss of muscle tone in the supraspinatus and rhomboid muscles (derived from cervical myotomes 4 and 5, mostly 5). Such a lesion also diminishes, but does not abolish, reflex tone in the deltoid, subscapularis, biceps brachii, brachialis and brachioradialis muscles (derived from cervical myotomes 5 and 6). However, if dorsal roots C5 and C6 are both destroyed, all proprioceptive sensory nerve fibers from these muscles are lost and there are no reflexes (*areflexia*).As a result the normal tone of these muscles is abolished completely (*atonia*). However, these muscles can still contract for their ventral root fibers remain intact.

The difference in the physiological deficits occurring with dorsal rhizotomies involving all roots to a limb and those sparing certain roots is impressive. Mott and Sherrington (1895) showed that complete deafferentation of an extremity resulted in virtual paralysis of the limb. Monkeys with such rhizotomies could not use the deafferented limb for walking, climbing or grasping. The motor deficits resulting from incomplete deafferentation of an extremity are quite different. If only one dorsal root distributing cutaneous afferents to any part of the hand or foot remained intact, little motor deficit resulted. These authors differentially sectioned certain dorsal roots and found that if cutaneous afferents alone were left intact, little impairment of function resulted. However, when muscle afferents were intact and cutaneous afferents were sectioned, the hand was virtually useless. From these studies, it was concluded that, "afferent impulses, both from the skin and from muscle, especially the former, as related to the palm or sole, are necessary for the carrying out of highest level movements." Subsequent investigations (Lassek, '53) indicate that preservation of the C7 dorsal root appears to be of the greatest significance for use of the upper extremity. According to Twitchell ('54) monkeys with incomplete deafferentation of the arm direct movement of the limb by contact alone. These observations serve to emphasize the important role that different sensory inputs play in the integration of motor function.

Ventral Root Lesions. Injury to the emerging ventral root of a spinal nerve produces deficits in segmental motor responses due to interruption of somatic efferent axons (Figs. 9-21, 9-22 and 10-22). If a thoracic or upper lumbar spinal nerve is injured, visceral efferent neurons (and reflexes) also would be involved (Figs. 8-1, 8-2, 9-22 and 10-22). Thus the destruction of the C8 spinal ventral root would partly paralyze the small muscles of the hand (via median and ulnar nerves), whereas a lesion of both ventral roots C8 and T1 would produce a complete flaccid paralysis and atrophy of these muscles (fig. 7-17). The inclusion of ventral root T1 in the injury would also interrupt most of the preganglionic visceral efferent fibers en route to the superior cervical sympathetic ganglion (Figs. 9-22 and 10-26). Loss of these visceral motor fibers to the smooth muscle of the eye and levator palpebrae muscle results in a triad of clinical symptoms known as Horner's syndrome (page 210). This syndrome usually is accompanied by altered sweating on the face. It should be noted that destruction of either the anterior horn cells (e.g., poliomyelitis), or their peripheral axons, results in a lower motor neuron lesion (Figs. 10-24 and 10-26), which deprives the appropriate muscles of the tonic influence of motor nerves.

If the mixed nerve is injured distal to the junction of the dorsal and ventral root (Fig. 10-22), the combined sensory and motor losses enumerated above will be present. It should be noted that if such combined nerve lesions are extensive, they may be followed by trophic changes in the skin (smoothness, dryness) and in capillary circulation (cyanosis). The trophic alterations presumably are due to the loss of peripheral vasomotor and afferent nerve fibers.

Spinal Cord Transection. Complete spinal cord transection immediately produces, below the level of the lesion, loss of all: (1) somatic sensation, (2) visceral sensation, (3) motor function, (4) muscle tone, and (5) reflex activity. This state, referred to as *spinal shock,* is characterized by complete lack of neural function in the isolated spinal cord caudal to the lesion. Spinal shock occurs in all animals and man following complete transection of the spinal cord and is considered to be due to the sudden and abrupt interruption of descending excitatory influences. The period of spinal shock varies in different animals but in man ranges from 1 to 6 weeks and averages about 3 weeks. During this time there is no evidence of neural activity below the level of the lesion. The termination of the period of spinal shock is heralded by the appearance of the Babinski sign. A fairly orderly sequence of events follows which vary in duration. The various phases involved in the recovery of function in the isolated human spinal cord have been carefully analyzed by Kuhn ('50). These phases in recovery of neural function are: (1) minimal reflex activity (3 to 6 weeks), (2) flexor spasms (6 to 16 weeks), (3) alternate flexor and extensor spasms (after 4 months), and (4) predominant extensor spasms (after 6 months). The phase of minimal reflex activity is characterized by weak flexor responses to nociceptive stimuli, which begin distally and later involve proximal muscle groups in the extremities. During this period the Babinski sign can be obtained bilaterally, but the muscles are flaccid and the deep tendon reflexes cannot be elicited.

The phase of flexor muscle spasms is characterized by increasing tone in the flexor muscles and by stronger flexor responses to nociceptive stimuli, which progressively involve more proximal muscle groups. It is during this phase that the so-called *triple flexion response* is first seen. This involves flexion of the lower extremity at the hip, knee and ankle in response to a relatively mild nociceptive stimulus. The most exaggerated form of this reaction is the *mass reflex,* in which a relatively mild, and sometimes nonspecific, stimulus results in powerful bilateral triple flexion responses. These responses are characterized by repeated discharge of motor units throughout the caudal part of the spinal cord. The mass reflex appears to be due to the spread of afferent impulses from one segment to the next and dispersion of impulses in such a manner as to cause motor units to continue to fire after the exciting stimulus has been withdrawn. The mass reflex is distressing to the patient because it is almost impossible to control. This reflex becomes less severe about 4 months after spinal transection when extensor muscle tone gradually begins to increase. During this phase both flexor and extensor muscle spasms occur, but within a relatively short time extensor muscle tone may be so great that the patient can momentarily support his weight in a standing position (Kuhn, '50).

Examination of the patient 1 year after complete spinal cord transection reveals the following: (1) complete paralysis below the level of the lesion, (2) loss of all sensation (somatic and visceral) below the lesion, (3) marked extensor muscle tone (spasticity) below the lesion (Guttmann, '46, '52), (4) hyperactive deep tendon (myotatic) reflexes below the lesion, (5) clonus in both lower extremities, and (6) bilateral Babinski signs. Paralysis of bowel and bladder, present from the time of spinal transection, constitutes one of the major problems, but with good nursing care, reflex emptying of bowel and bladder can be established. In many patients there is reflex spinal sweating in response to noxious stimuli. This type of sweating is not under thermoregulatory control. In the male there is also a disturbance of sexual activity.

Bladder and bowel functions are disturbed in all transections of the cord, for they are no longer under voluntary control. Interruption of descending autonomic fibers, particularly those *en route* to parasympathetic nuclei in the sacral cord (S2, S3, S4), leads to loss of rectal motility. There are reflex spasms of the external anal sphincters and fecal retention. Defecation occurs involuntarily after long intervals. If cord segments S2, S3 and S4 are destroyed, there is a permanent paralysis of the external sphincter and fecal incontinence (Fig. 8-11). When these sacral segments are involved, there is in addition paralytic incontinence, and usually bladder distention, impotence and perianal, or saddle, anesthesia. However, normal sensory and motor function is retained in the lower extremities (conus medullaris syndrome).

Bladder disturbances usually occur in three phases after cord transection. At the outset there is always *retention,* due to paralysis of the muscular bladder wall (detrusor muscle), and spasm of the vesicle sphincter. Two or 3 weeks later (range 2 days to 18 months) the second phase or *overflow incontinence* is observed. This phase consists of an intermittent dribbling of urine due to gradual hypertrophy of the detrusor smooth muscle. The muscle can overcome the resistance of the external sphincter for short periods of time. In most cases continued hypertrophy of the bladder

wall eventually permits the bladder to expel small amounts of urine automatically, providing bladder infections have not intervened. This is the third phase, known as *automatic micturition.* Such automaticity of the bladder is poor if lumbar spinal cord segments are involved, and absent (paralytic incontinence) when the sacral segments are destroyed.

In partial or incomplete transection of the spinal cord, some ascending or descending fibers escape injury. The sensory deficits may not correspond to the level of motor loss, and some voluntary function may return within 1 or 2 weeks. Vasomotor and visceral disturbances usually are less pronounced, and irritative sensory phenomena are more common (e.g., pains, paresthesias, hyperesthesias). Marked priapism is more likely to accompany an incomplete transection of the cord. Haymaker ('56) has stated that the only reliable criterion of total transection, in the early stages after spinal injury, is "a complete flaccid paraplegia with areflexia and complete sensory loss which lasts longer than 2 to 5 days."

Although complete transections of the spinal cord produce degeneration in ascending tracts above the level of the lesion (Fig. 10-3) and in descending tracts below the level of the lesion (Fig. 10-16), the lesion rarely is sharply localized, and considerable degeneration usually is present in nearly all systems in the immediate vicinity of the lesion.

Spinal Hemisection. Hemisection of the spinal cord is probably the most instructive spinal lesion for teaching purposes, in spite of the fact that precise lesions of this kind are encountered only rarely in clinical neurology. The signs and symptoms associated with hemisection of the spinal cord constitute the *Brown-Séquard* syndrome (Fig. 10-23). Neurological findings in the illustrated hemisection would include: (1) loss of sensory impulses transmitted by the posterior white columns from below the lesion on the same side; (2) an upper motor neuron lesion below the level of injury on the same side; (3) lower motor neuron symptoms and vasomotor paralysis in areas supplied by the in-

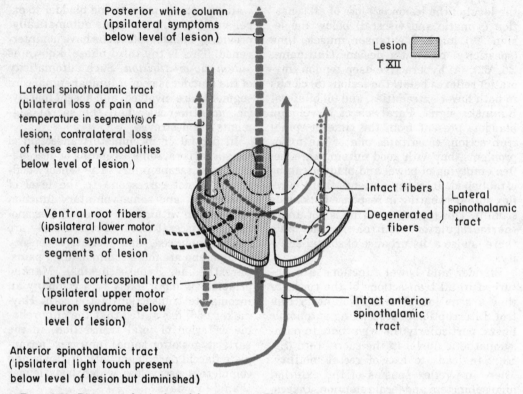

Posterior white column
(ipsilateral symptoms
below level of lesion)

Lateral spinothalamic tract
(bilateral loss of pain and
temperature in segment(s) of
lesion; contralateral loss
of these sensory modalities
below level of lesion)

Lesion
T XII

Intact fibers
Degenerated fibers
Lateral spinothalamic tract

Ventral root fibers
(ipsilateral lower motor
neuron syndrome in
segments of lesion

Lateral corticospinal tract
(ipsilateral upper motor
neuron syndrome below
level of lesion)

Intact anterior spinothalamic tract

Anterior spinothalamic tract
(ipsilateral light touch present
below level of lesion but diminished)

FIG. 10-23. Diagram of spinal cord hemisection. This lesion results in a Brown-Séquard syndrome. *Arrows* show direction of impulse conduction; *broken lines* indicate degenerated nerve fibers.

jured segments on the side of the lesion; (4) bilateral loss of pain and thermal sense within the area of the lesion; and (5) loss of pain and thermal sense below T12 on the opposite side of the body (i.e., lower extremity, genitals and perineum). With a lesion at the T12 spinal segment, sensory and pyramidal symptoms would be manifested through spinal nerves of the lumbar and sacral plexuses. The lower motor neuron damage at cord segment T12 would produce no atrophy in muscles of the lower extremity and the reflex arcs below the level of the lesion would remain intact.

Complete and incomplete transections of the human spinal cord may result from missile wounds or fracture-dislocation of vertebrae. Similar damage may follow ischemic necrosis due to occlusion or interruption of radicular arteries that supply the vulnerable upper thoracic segments (Fig. 20-1) of the spinal cord (Bolton, '39; Mettler, '48; Zülch, '54). Neoplasms also

may compress the spinal cord and secondarily compromise the blood supply. In such spinal cord lesions, the symptoms are severe and the complications are numerous, regardless of the level of injury.

In spinal hemisection the basic principle with respect to degeneration pertains, in that virtually all degeneration is on the side of the lesion; ascending tracts will degenerate above the level of the lesion, and descending tracts will degenerate below the level of the lesion (Fig. 10-23). However, if the lesion involves several spinal segments, a small amount of degeneration may be detected in the contralateral spinothalamic tracts (and anterior spinocerebellar tract if the lesion involves lumbar spinal segments).

Amyotrophic Lateral Sclerosis. This spinal cord disease involves both upper and lower motor neurons. It is a progressive degenerative disease of unknown etiology, occurring with greatest frequency in

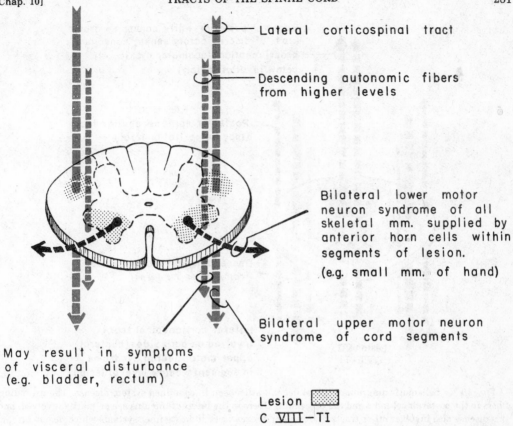

Lateral corticospinal tract

Descending autonomic fibers from higher levels

Bilateral lower motor neuron syndrome of all skeletal mm. supplied by anterior horn cells within segments of lesion.

(e.g. small mm. of hand)

Bilateral upper motor neuron syndrome of cord segments

May result in symptoms of visceral disturbance (e.g. bladder, rectum)

Lesion ▒▒

C Ⅷ–TI

FIG. 10-24. Diagram of the spinal cord lesion in amyotrophic lateral sclerosis. *Arrows* show direction of impulse conduction; *broken lines* indicate degenerated nerve fibers.

the fifth and sixth decades of life, characterized by degeneration of the corticospinal tracts and the anterior horn cells. When degeneration of anterior horn cells begins in the cervical region (Fig. 10-24), the disease manifests itself by progressive muscular atrophy in the upper extremities, usually in the small intrinsic hand muscles, and spastic weakness of the muscles of the trunk and lower extremities. Muscular weakness usually is symmetrical and becomes generalized in the terminal phases of the disease. Fasciculations (i.e., involuntary twitching of muscle fascicles) in affected muscles can be observed and felt by the patient and the examiner. Myotatic irritability of affected muscles persists until atrophy is complete. Late in the course of this progressive disease the above findings may be accompanied by functional disturbances of the bladder and

rectum due to injury of descending autonomic fibers en route to lumbar and sacral segments of the cord. Such fibers lie close to both the reticulospinal and corticospinal tracts and can be looked upon as "suprasegmental" to the visceral nuclei of the spinal cord.

Combined System Disease. The neurological manifestations of pernicious anemia result in degenerative changes in peripheral nerves and in the central nervous system. The anemia and the degenerative changes in the nervous system result from a deficiency of vitamin B_{12}. A defect in gastric secretion deprives these patients of an enzyme specifically required for absorption of vitamin B_{12}. Peripheral nerves and spinal tracts undergo varying degrees of degeneration. The degeneration in the spinal cord appears to affect especially the posterior white columns and the cortico-

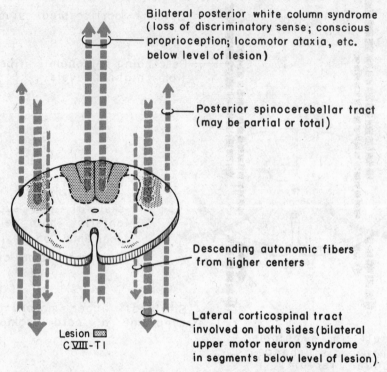

Bilateral posterior white column syndrome
(loss of discriminatory sense; conscious
proprioception; locomotor ataxia, etc.
below level of lesion)

Posterior spinocerebellar tract
(may be partial or total)

Descending autonomic fibers
from higher centers

Lateral corticospinal tract
involved on both sides (bilateral
upper motor neuron syndrome
in segments below level of lesion)

Lesion ▨
C VIII - T I

FIG. 10-25. Schematic diagram of spinal degeneration seen in combined system disease. The ascending fibers in the posterior columns and the descending fibers in the lateral funiculus are primarily involved, but this disease also involves other tracts. *Arrows* and *broken lines* indicate fiber systems which degenerate in this disease. The extent of degeneration in the posterior spinocerebellar tract is variable.

spinal tracts, but it is not confined to these systems (Fig. 10-25). Patients with this disease have both sensory and motor disturbances. The sensory disturbances include numbness and tingling, "pins and needles" sensation, loss of position sense and loss of vibratory sense. These sensory disturbances are greatest in distal portions of the extremities and tend to be symmetrical. There is little impairment of tactile, thermal or pain sense. Weakness in the lower extremities is common and the gait may be spastic and ataxic. The myotatic reflexes in the lower extremities usually are reduced while those in the upper extremity are normal. The sign of Babinski can be elicited bilaterally. Moderate muscular wasting usually occurs in the late stages of the disease.

Syringomyelia. This is a chronic disease characterized pathologically by long cavities, surrounded by glial elements, that develop in relationship to the central canal of the spinal cord. These cavities may extend into the medulla (syringobulbia). Syringomyelia probably is related embryologically to an abnormal closure of the central canal. Incomplete closure of the central canal may leave cavities around which a secondary gliosis develops. Characteristically syringomyelia involves the lower cervical and upper thoracic regions of the spinal cord. The affected region of the spinal cord is enlarged and transverse sections reveal a large irregular cavity containing a clear or yellow fluid.

The hallmark of this disease is an early impairment, or loss, of pain and thermal sense with preservation of tactile sense. This selective loss of pain and thermal sense, frequently noted first in the hands and forearms, results from interruption of decussating sensory fibers (i.e., spinothalamic tracts) in several consecutive segments. This kind of sensory loss is referred to as a "dissociated sensory" loss because

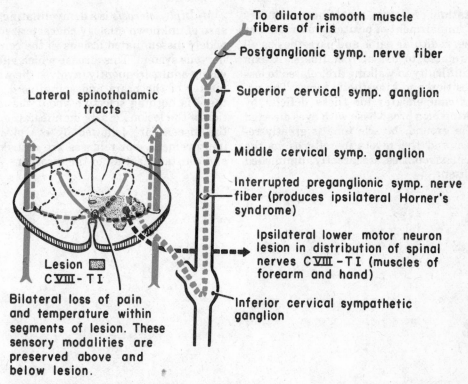

Fig. 10-26. Diagram of syringomyelia with lateral extension of the cavity into anterior gray horn of spinal cord. *Arrows* show direction of impulse conduction; *broken lines* indicate degenerated nerve fibers.

other forms of sensation are preserved. Later the cavity may enlarge in a lateral, posterior, cranial or caudal direction, and it may destroy adjacent fiber tracts or gray matter. An example of such a case is illustrated schematically in Figure 10-26. Here the lesion interrupts the crossing fibers of the lateral spinothalamic tract in cord segments C8 and T1. Injured axons distal to the point of the lesion are separated from their cells of origin and undergo degeneration (*broken lines* in Fig. 10-26). Destruction of these crossing fibers from both sides of the cord results in a bilateral loss of pain and thermal sense in the distribution of spinal nerves and dermatomes of C8 to T1. All pain and termperature fibers of T1 are destroyed, but some of the C8 fibers are spared inasmuch as a few fibers ascend and cross in the C7 cord segment. This type of lesion results in a "dissociated sensory" loss as described above. The remainder of the lateral spinothalamic tract contains normal fibers that have crossed in spinal cord segments either above or below

the area of the lesion. In this case, the lateral extension of the cavity also has destroyed the anterior gray horn and nerve fibers passing through it (Fig. 10-26). A patient with such a lesion would have symptoms and signs of a unilateral lower motor neuron lesion and a Horner's syndrome in addition to the classic sensory disturbances. These neurological findings aid in localizing the lesion to spinal segments C8 and T1.

Other Spinal Syndromes. There are many varieties of spinal cord lesions and syndromes in addition to those briefly described here. *Tabes dorsalis* (locomotor ataxia) is a central nervous system form of syphilis which produces degeneration in the central processes of dorsal root ganglion cells. This results in extensive demyelination and degeneration of fibers in the fasciculus gracilis. There is no unanimity of opinion as to why the degenerative lesions in tabes dorsalis have this selective character. The principal symptoms of tabes are attributable to degeneration and irritation of dorsal root fibers. Sensory loss, impairment of position and vibratory sense, radicular pains and paresthesias all are related to dorsal root fibers. Ataxia and difficulty in walking are related to loss of position and kinesthetic sense. The patient compensates for these deficits by walking on a broad base with eyes directed to the ground. Muscle tone is greatly reduced and the myotatic reflexes in the lower extremities are greatly diminished or absent.

Multiple sclerosis is a demyelinating disease of unknown etiology characterized by widely disseminated lesions in the central nervous system. This disease which affects young adults frequently involves the white matter of the brain and spinal cord, but there is nothing selective about the location of the lesions. Early manifestations of the disease are followed by conspicuous improvement, but relapses are a striking and constant feature of the disorder.

CHAPTER 11

The Medulla

The medulla (myelencephalon), the most caudal segment of the brain stem, represents a conical, expanded continuation of the upper cervical spinal cord. Externally the transition from spinal cord to lower medulla is gradual, without sharp demarcation. The caudal limit of the medulla is rostral to the highest rootlets of the first cervical spinal nerve at about the level of the foramen magnum. Above the level of transition, the medulla increases in size and its external features become distinctive. Changes in the external appearance of the medulla are due chiefly to structural rearrangement and development of structures peculiar to the medulla. The development of the fourth ventricle causes structures previously located posteriorly to be shifted posterolaterally, while the appearance of the pyramids on the anterior surface partially obliterates the anterior median fissure. The oval eminences posterolateral to the pyramids, produced by the inferior olivary nuclei, give the medulla above the zone of transition a characteristic configuration. The gross features of the brain stem are shown in anterior and posterior views in Figures 11-1 and 11-2.

While the spinal cord throughout most of its length presents a relatively uniform internal organization, graded sections through the medulla disclose numerous important changes from level to level. Among the principal changes taking place in the medulla are the following: (1) the development of the fourth ventricle, representing the rostral continuation of the central canal of the spinal cord, (2) the replacement of the butterfly-shaped central gray of the spinal cord by large cellular aggregations and interlacing fibers constituting the reticular formation, (3) the decussation of the medullary pyramids, (4) the termination of ascending first order fibers contained in the fasciculi gracilis and cuneatus upon their respective nuclei, and the formation of a composite second order lemniscal pathway, (5) the gradual replacement of spinal fibers in the zone of Lissauer by fibers of the spinal trigeminal tract, (6) the development of cranial nerve nuclei, their interconnecting fiber systems and their afferent and efferent root fibers, and (7) the appearance of groups of relay nuclei, most of which project fibers to the cerebellum.

In the floor of the fourth ventricle the sulcus limitans can be seen lateral to the median sulcus. This groove continues to demarcate afferent and efferent cell columns (Fig. 11-16) as it did in the developing spinal cord (Fig. 3-3A). The reticular formation, phylogenetically one of the oldest portions of the neuraxis, represents the core of the brain stem. Structurally, it is composed of complex collections of cells of different sizes, types and shapes forming both diffuse cellular aggregations and circumscribed nuclei (Figs. 11-8 and 11-9). Fibers entering, leaving and traversing the reticular core seemingly pass haphazardly in all directions. However, studies of Golgi-stained preparations of this region

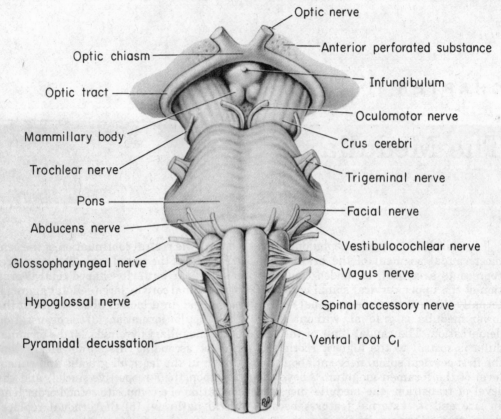

FIG. 11-1. Drawing of the anterior aspect of the medulla, pons and midbrain.

(Scheibel and Scheibel, '58) indicate that fibers and cellular groups are organized in specific patterns. The reticular formation of the medulla is continuous with that of the pons and higher levels of the brain stem. Figure 11-3 indicates the level and plane of section of most of the brain stem photomicrographs described in this and succeeding chapters.

SPINOMEDULLARY TRANSITION

At the junction of the spinal cord and medulla (Figs. 11-4 and A-1) transverse sections resemble those of the upper cervical spinal cord with certain modifications. The substantia gelatinosa has increased in size, and coarse descending myelinated fibers can be found in the zone of Lissauer. At this level the zone of Lissauer contains fine ascending root fibers from the uppermost cervical nerves and coarser descending fibers of the trigeminal nerve (N. V) which enter at pontine levels and descend

in the dorsolateral part of the brain stem. Some of these descending spinal trigeminal fibers can be found as low as the second cervical segment. The substantia gelatinosa becomes the spinal trigeminal nucleus at high cervical levels, and it retains the same relative position and size throughout the medulla. Descending trigeminal fibers terminate directly, or by collaterals, in parts of the spinal trigeminal nucleus.

A conspicuous increase in the gray surrounding the central canal is evident (Figs. 11-4 and 11-5). The lateral corticospinal tract has become clearly separated from the medial longitudinal fasciculus by its passage into the posterior part of the lateral funiculus. It is broken up into a number of obliquely or transversely cut bundles, between which are strands of gray matter. A few fibers of the spinal portion of the spinal accessory nerve can be seen arching posterolaterally to emerge

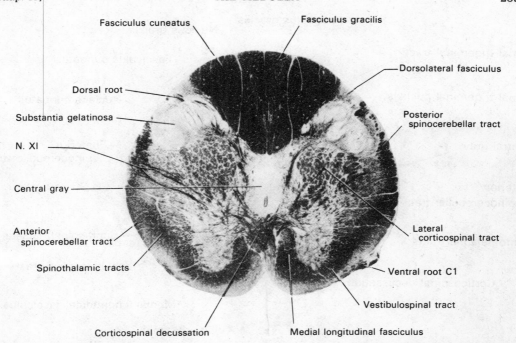

Fasciculus cuneatus

Fasciculus gracilis

Dorsolateral fasciculus

Dorsal root

Substantia gelatinosa

N. XI

Central gray

Posterior
spinocerebellar tract

Anterior
spinocerebellar tract

Spinothalamic tracts

Lateral
corticospinal tract

Ventral root C1

Vestibulospinal tract

Corticospinal decussation

Medial longitudinal fasciculus

FIG. 11-4. Transverse section through the junction of spinal cord and medulla. Some of the most caudal decussating fibers of the corticospinal tract can be seen passing into the posterior part of the lateral funiculus. The structure labeled substantia gelatinosa also contains cell groups of the spinal trigeminal nucleus. Weigert's myelin stain. Photograph.

Posterior Column Nuclei. In the posterior white columns nuclear masses have appeared in the fasciculi gracilis and cuneatus. These are the nuclei of the posterior funiculi, known respectively as the *nucleus gracilis* and *nucleus cuneatus*. The long ascending branches of the cells in the dorsal root ganglia, coursing in the posterior funiculus, terminate upon these nuclei (Figs. 9-23, 10-1 and 11-2). At these levels the fasciculus cuneatus is massive and only a small caudal part of the nucleus cuneatus protrudes into the ventral part of the fasciculus (Figs. 11-5 and 11-6). The nucleus gracilis is larger, occupies a more central position and is capped dorsally and laterally by fibers of the fasciculus gracilis. At progressively higher levels, increasing numbers of fibers terminate in these nuclei. The nuclei increase in size (Fig. 11-7) while the fasciculi correspondingly decrease (Fig. 11-8). At levels through the caudal part of the inferior olivary complex, the entire fasciculus gracilis and most of the fasciculus cuneatus have

been replaced by their respective nuclei (Figs. 11-8 and 11-9).

In animals three cytologically distinct regions of the nucleus gracilis have been recognized (Cajal, '09; Taber, '61; Kuypers and Tuerk, '64): (1) a reticular region rostral to the obex characterized by a loose organization of cells, (2) a "cell nest" region caudal to the obex characterized by cell clusters, and (3) a caudal region characterized by scattered cells occurring singly or in small clusters. Ascending dorsal root fibers project somatotopically to the nucleus gracilis (Ferraro and Barrera, '35; Walker and Weaver, '42; Hand, '66; Carpenter et al., '68). According to Hand ('66) lumbosacral dorsal root fibers exhibit a somatotopic lamination chiefly in the "cell nest" region, while terminations in the reticular region are diffuse with intersegmental overlap. Certain physiological studies in the cat suggest that neurons in the nucleus gracilis exhibit rostrocaudal differences with respect to: (1) the size of the peripheral receptive fields which supply

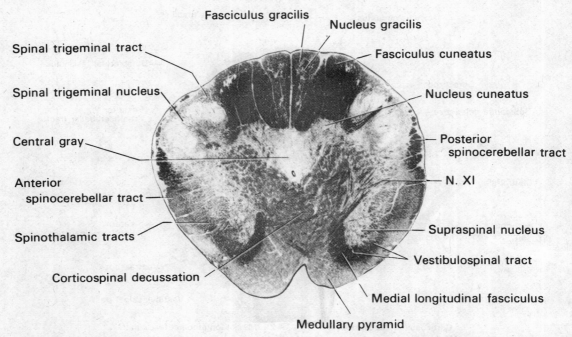

Fasciculus gracilis

Nucleus gracilis

Spinal trigeminal tract

Fasciculus cuneatus

Spinal trigeminal nucleus

Nucleus cuneatus

Central gray

Posterior spinocerebellar tract

Anterior spinocerebellar tract

N. XI

Spinothalamic tracts

Supraspinal nucleus

Vestibulospinal tract

Corticospinal decussation

Medial longitudinal fasciculus

Medullary pyramid

FIG. 11-5. Transverse section of the medulla through the decussation of the corticospinal tracts. Weigert's myelin stain. Photograph.

afferent input (Gordon and Paine, '60; McComas, '63), and (2) segregation of sensory modality (Kuhn, '49; Perl et al., '62; Gordon and Jukes, '64; Winter, '65). Rostral portions of the nucleus (i.e., reticular region) are said to be related to deep pressure and joint movement, while the "cell nest" and caudal regions of the nucleus are related to hair and skin receptors. Other physiological data (Kruger et al., '61), based upon single neuron analysis of posterior column nuclei, provide no evidence of rostrocaudal differentiation in terms of either somatotopy or modality segregation. The latter finding supports experimental studies (Mountcastle and Powell, '59; Poggio and Mountcastle, '60) which indicate that: (1) the somatotopic organization of the posterior columns and the medial lemniscus is maintained at the level of the posterior column nuclei, and (2) neural elements devoted to kinesthesis and tactile sense are intermingled in a single and mutual somatotopic pattern. Studies in the monkey indicate that lower thoracic, lumbar and sacrococcygeal dorsal roots project in overlapping somatotopic fashion throughout the rostrocaudal extent of the nucleus gracilis (Carpenter et al., '68). Zones of the nucleus gracilis receiving terminal dorsal root fibers are organized so that: (1) roots of the lumbar enlargement project to irregular-shaped areas in the central core of the nucleus, (2) lower thoracic and upper lumbar roots project in serial fashion to narrow, oblique laminae lateral to the core region, and (3) sacral and coccygeal dorsal roots project in serial fashion to crescent-shaped laminae in dorsomedial parts of the nucleus. The areas of the terminal projection zones in the nucleus gracilis are related to the size of the dorsal root and the number of ascending fibers they contribute to the fasciculus gracilis.

The nucleus cuneatus also exhibits regional differences in its cytoarchitecture (Meesen and Olszewski, '49; Olszewski and Baxter, '54). According to Kuypers and Tuerk ('64) dorsal areas of the cuneate nucleus contain clusters of round cells with bushy dendrites, while basal areas contain triangular, multipolar and fusiform cells with long, sparse dendrites.

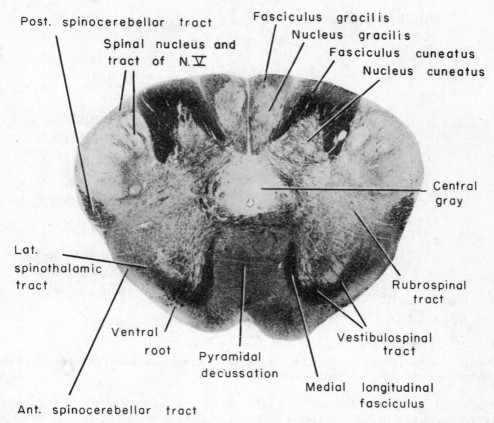

Post. spinocerebellar tract

Spinal nucleus and
tract of N. V

Fasciculus gracilis

Nucleus gracilis

Fasciculus cuneatus

Nucleus cuneatus

Central
gray

Lat.
spinothalamic
tract

Rubrospinal
tract

Ventral
root

Pyramidal
decussation

Vestibulospinal
tract

Medial longitudinal
fasciculus

Ant. spinocerebellar tract

FIG. 11-6. Transverse section of the medulla through the upper part of the corticospinal decussation. Weigert's myelin stain. Photograph.

These authors considered the round cell clusters to receive afferents principally from distal parts of the body and to be related to small cutaneous receptive fields. Triangular and multipolar cells were considered to receive afferents primarily from proximal parts of the limb and trunk, and were regarded as being related to larger cutaneous receptive fields. These studies suggested that dorsal root fibers have a dual termination with some fibers ending in cell clusters and others among basal triangular cells.

A systematic study of dorsal root projections to the cuneate nucleus in the monkey has shown that: (1) fibers from C1 through T1 terminate in both exclusive and overlapping zones, (2) fibers from C5 through C8 terminate in a central core region about which other dorsal root fibers terminate in oblique serial laminae, (3) rostral dorsal root fibers (C1 through C4) terminate in ventrolateral regions, and (4) caudal dorsal root fibers (T1 through T7) terminate in dorsomedial regions (Shriver et al., '68) (Figs. 11-10 and 11-11). Comparisons of the patterns of dorsal root terminations in the nuclei gracilis and cuneatus in the monkey (Carpenter et al., '68) suggest that in the nucleus gracilis: (1) overlapping terminations are more extensive and irregular than in the cuneate nucleus, and (2) there is less autonomous terminal representation of individual dorsal root fibers in the nucleus gracilis.

Decussation of the Medial Lemniscus. In transverse sections of the medulla above the corticospinal decussation (Figs. 11-8, 11-9 and A-3), the nucleus gracilis reaches its greatest extent, and practically all fibers of the fasciculus gracilis have terminated in portions of the nucleus. Al-

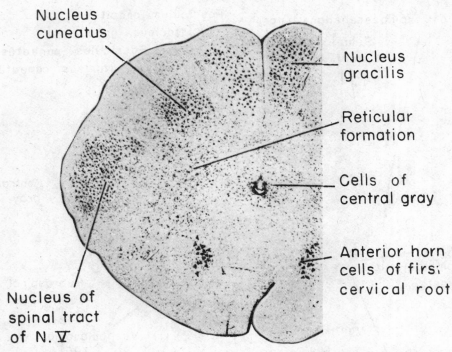

Nucleus
cuneatus

Nucleus
gracilis

Reticular
formation

Cells of
central gray

Anterior horn
cells of first
cervical root

Nucleus of
spinal tract
of N. Ⅴ

FIG. 11-7. Section through medulla of 1-month infant at about same level as in Figure 11-5. Cresyl violet. Photograph, with cell groups blocked in schematically.

though the nucleus cuneatus is much larger than shown in Figures 11-6 or 11-7, a considerable number of fibers of the fasciculus cuneatus remain dorsal to the nuclei. From the nuclei gracilis and cuneatus, myelinated fibers arise which sweep ventromedially around the central gray. These fibers, known as *internal arcuate fibers,* cross the median raphe and contralaterally form a well-defined ascending bundle, the *medial lemniscus.* This large ascending fiber bundle can be readily followed through the brain stem to its termination in the ventral posterolateral nucleus (VPL) of the thalamus (Fig. 10-1). The medial lemniscus constitutes the second neuron of the posterior column pathway conveying kinesthetic sense and discriminative tactile sense to higher levels of the neuraxis. The decussation of the medial lemniscus provides part of the anatomical basis for sensory representation of half of the body in the contralateral cerebral cortex. Consequently, injury to the medial lemniscus causes characteristic kines-

thetic and tactile deficits on the opposite side of the body.

Lateral to the cuneate nucleus is a group of large cells similar to those of the dorsal nucleus of Clarke, known as the *accessory cuneate* nucleus (Figs. 10-10, 11-8, 11-9, A-3 and A-4). This nucleus is considered to be the medullary equivalent of the dorsal nucleus (Sherrington, 1893a; Pass, '33; Brodal, '41). These nuclei share the following anatomical and functional features: (1) cells are morphologically similar with eccentric nuclei, (2) afferent fibers are derived from dorsal roots, (3) both nuclei give rise to uncrossed cerebellar afferent fibers, and (4) both nuclei relay impulses from muscle spindles, type II muscle afferents and cutaneous afferents (Oscarsson, '65). Although impulses from Golgi tendon organs are relayed via the dorsal nucleus, similar relays have not been established for the accessory cuneate nucleus. Ascending fibers conveyed by the fasciculus cuneatus and terminating in the accessory cuneate nucleus are derived from the same

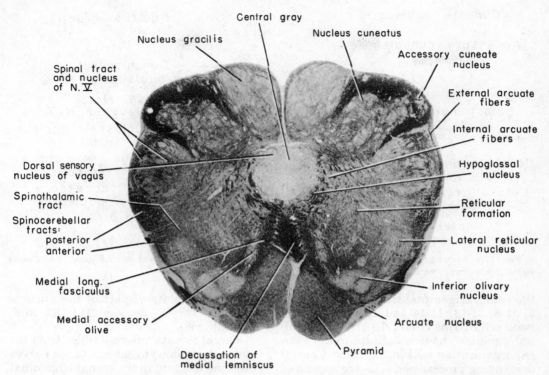

Central gray
Nucleus gracilis
Nucleus cuneatus
Accessory cuneate nucleus
Spinal tract and nucleus of N. V
External arcuate fibers
Internal arcuate fibers
Dorsal sensory nucleus of vagus
Hypoglossal nucleus
Spinothalamic tract
Reticular formation
Spinocerebellar tracts:
posterior
anterior
Lateral reticular nucleus
Medial long. fasciculus
Inferior olivary nucleus
Medial accessory olive
Arcuate nucleus
Decussation of medial lemniscus
Pyramid

FIG. 11-8. Transverse section of medulla through the decussation of the medial lemniscus. Weigert's myelin stain. Photograph.

dorsal root ganglia as those projecting to the cuneate nucleus, namely those of cervical and upper thoracic spinal segments. Dorsal root fibers, projecting to the accessory cuneate nucleus, terminate somatotopically (Liu, '56; Shriver et al., '68), in overlapping laminae. In the monkey (Shriver et al., '68) the pattern of termination of fibers from C1 through T1 dorsal roots in the accessory cuneate nucleus is similar to that of the cuneate nucleus in that fibers from: (1) C5 through C8 terminate in the central core region about which other dorsal root fibers terminate in oblique serial laminae, (2) rostral roots terminate in ventrolateral regions, while those from more caudal roots end in dorsomedial regions, and (3) all of these roots, except C1 and C2, terminate throughout the rostrocaudal extent of the nucleus (Figs. 11-10 and 11-12). Fibers from the above-mentioned dorsal roots terminating in the accessory cuneate nucleus end in both exclusive and overlapping zones; fi-

bers from one dorsal root partially overlap the territory of the next highest root. Upper thoracic dorsal root fibers (other than T1) exhibit greater overlap and terminate in smaller zones in the lateral part of the nucleus.

Although fibers from parts of the fasciculus cuneatus terminate upon cells of the accessory cuneate nucleus, these cells do not contribute fibers to the formation of the medial lemniscus. Cells of the accessory cuneate nucleus give rise to uncrossed *cuneocerebellar fibers* that at higher levels enter the cerebellum via the inferior cerebellar peduncle (Fig. 10-10). Fibers of the cuneocerebellar tract, conveying impulses from receptors in muscles of the upper extremity and neck, represent the upper limb equivalent of the posterior spinocerebellar tract.

Spinal Trigeminal Tract. Afferent trigeminal root fibers, which enter the brain stem at upper pontine levels, descend in the dorsolateral part of the brain stem as

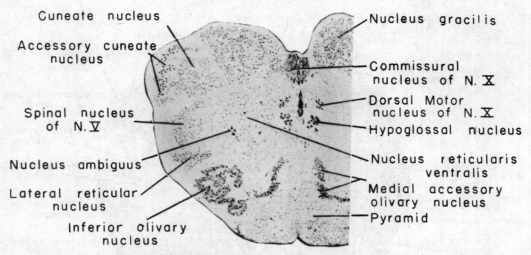

FIG. 11-9. Section through medulla of 1-month infant about the same level as in Figure 11-8. Cresyl violet. Photograph, with cell groups blocked in schematically.

the spinal trigeminal tract (Figs. 11-5, 11-6, 11-8, 11-13, 11-14 and 12-21). These fibers, originating from cells of the trigeminal ganglion, have a definite topographical organization within the tract. Central descending processes of cells are organized so that: (1) fibers of the mandibular division are most dorsal, (2) fibers of the ophthalmic division are most ventral, and (3) fibers of the maxillary division occupy an intermediate position. Clinicopathological studies (Taylor et al., '22; Smyth, '39; Falconer, '49) suggest that fibers of the separate divisions extend caudally for different distances, with those of the mandibular division terminating at medullary levels and those of the ophthalmic division terminating in upper cervical spinal segments. Experimental studies (Torvik, '56; Kruger and Michel, '62; Kerr, '63; Rhoton et al., '66) indicate that there is little difference in the caudal extent of fibers in the different trigeminal divisions, and that some fibers from all divisions extend into upper cervical spinal segments. As this tract descends it becomes progressively smaller as fibers leave the tract and terminate in the adjacent spinal trigeminal nucleus. In the rostral medulla a surprisingly large number of trigeminal fibers in the dorsal part of the spinal trigeminal tract project medially to terminate in a re-

stricted ventrolateral part of the nucleus solitarius (Torvik, '56; Kerr, '61, '63; Rhoton et al., '66).

General somatic afferent fibers from the vagus, glossopharyngeal and facial nerves enter and descend in the spinal trigeminal tract. Vagal and glossopharyngeal fibers descend in the dorsomedial part of the tract for a considerable distance and terminate in the magnocellular division of the caudal part of the spinal trigeminal nucleus (Torvik, '56; Kimmel et al., '61; Kerr, '62; Rhoton et al., '66). Only a modest number of facial nerve fibers enter the spinal trigeminal tract.

Spinal Trigeminal Nucleus. This nucleus, which lies along the medial border of the tract, extends from the level of entry of the trigeminal root in the pons to the second cervical spinal segment (Figs. 12-20, 12-21 and 12-22). Fibers from the spinal trigeminal tract terminate upon cells of the nucleus at various levels throughout its extent. Cytoarchitecturally the spinal trigeminal nucleus has been subdivided into three parts (Olszewski, '50): (1) an *oral part* extending caudally to the level of the rostral pole of the hypoglossal nucleus, (2) an *interpolar part* extending caudally to the level of the obex, and (3) a *caudal part* which begins at the level of the obex, closely resembles the posterior horn of the

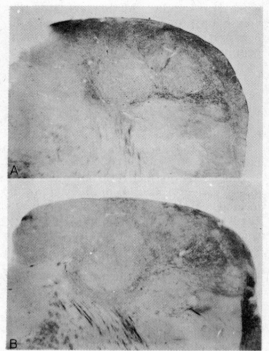

FIG. 11-10. Photomicrograph of terminal degeneration in the cuneate and accessory cuneate nuclei in the monkey following section of the fifth (A) and sixth (B) cervical dorsal roots. Compare localization of degeneration with that plotted in Figures 11-11 and 11-12. Nauta-Gygax stain. ×16.

spinal cord and extends caudally as far as the second cervical spinal segment. The inner, medial part of the caudal subdivision, containing irregularly arranged medium-sized cells of triangular or multipolar shape, constitutes the magnocellular (division) subnucleus. Fibers in different parts of the spinal trigeminal tract terminate within sharply circumscribed sectors of the spinal trigeminal nucleus. Fibers conveying impulses from the mandibular division terminate in dorsal parts of the nucleus, while fibers of the ophthalmic division terminate in ventral parts of the nucleus. A number of descending trigeminal fibers pass beyond the spinal trigeminal nucleus to terminate in dorsal parts of the reticular formation and portions of the solitary nucleus. Many neurons of the spinal trigeminal nucleus give rise to an extensive axonal plexus of small fiber bundles which lie adjacent to the nucleus.

These so-called "deep bundles" emit collaterals which effectively link different levels of the spinal trigeminal nucleus (Gobel and Purvis, '72).

Descending fibers in the spinal trigeminal tract convey impulses concerned with pain, thermal, and tactile sense from the face, forehead, and mucous membranes of the nose and mouth (Fig. 7-13). While other portions of the trigeminal complex are concerned with tactile sense, the spinal trigeminal tract and nucleus appear to be the only part of this complex uniquely concerned with the perception of pain and thermal sense. The most decisive evidence for this modality segregation is that medullary trigeminal tractotomy markedly reduces pain and thermal sense without impairing tactile sense (Sjöqvist, '38). Physiological studies (Kruger and Michel, '62a) indicate that it is extremely difficult to isolate or identify neurons in the spinal trigeminal nucleus concerned with transmission of impulses related to pain, while virtually all neurons in this nucleus can be excited by delicate tactile stimuli. It has been suggested that the representation of pain in the spinal trigeminal nucleus may involve tactile neurons excited by small fibers which are known to convey impulses related to painful sensations in certain circumstances.

From the spinal nucleus fibers arise which form the secondary trigeminal tracts. These fibers arise, a few at each level, and cross through the reticular formation to the opposite side. Most of these fibers ascend to thalamic levels in association with the contralateral medial lemniscus (Fig. 12-22); others appear to terminate upon cells of the reticular formation. These are trigeminothalamic fibers which constitute the second neuron in the sensory pathway from face to cortex. Other uncrossed fibers ascend and descend on the same side, forming reflex connections with the motor nuclei of the hypoglossal, vagus, facial and other cranial nerves (Figs. 12-20 and 12-22). A considerable number of trigeminocerebellar fibers arise from the spinal trigeminal nucleus and enter the cerebellum via the inferior cerebellar peduncle (Carpenter and Hanna, '61).

CUNEATE NUCLEUS

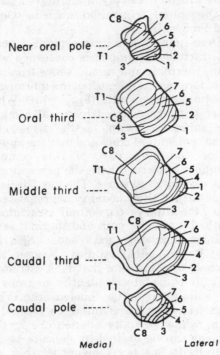

Fig. 11-11. Diagram of the somatotopic terminations of cervical and T1 dorsal root fibers in the cuneate nucleus in the monkey. The nucleus is shown in drawings of transverse sections from the right side. Thoracic dorsal root fibers T2 through T7 terminate in overlapping fashion along the dorsomedial margin of the nucleus (Shriver et al., '68).

Since the spinal trigeminal tract and nucleus are located close to the spinothalamic tract, injury to the dorsolateral region of the medulla produces the curious clinical picture of an alternating hemianalgesia and hemithermo-anesthesia of the face and body. There is loss or diminution of pain and thermal sense on the same side of the face, and on the opposite side of the body and neck (Fig. 12-22).

Reticular Formation. The reticular formation at the level of the decussation of the medial lemniscus occupies the region ventral to the posterior column nuclei and the spinal trigeminal complex and dorsolateral to the pyramid (Fig. 11-8). It contains numerous cells of various sizes arranged in more or less definite groups and is traversed by both longitudinal and transverse fiber bundles. At this level it is traversed by numerous internal arcuate fibers and smaller bundles of secondary trigeminal fibers. Cells in the above described region constitute the ventral reticular nucleus (Fig. 11-9). Peripheral to the reticular formation the long tracts retain their relative lateral and anterior positions. Fibers of the medial longitudinal fasciculus are dorsal to the pyramids and lateral to the decussation of the medial lemniscus.

One of the distinct reticular nuclei, the *lateral reticular nucleus of the medulla,* is located ventrolaterally (Fig. 11-8). This nucleus begins caudal to the inferior olivary complex and extends rostrally to midolivary levels (Figs. 11-9 and 11-13). In man this nucleus consists of a large ventral cell group dorsolateral to the inferior olive and a small subtrigeminal cell group beneath the spinal trigeminal nucleus (Walberg, '52). Neurons composing these nuclear groups project fibers to specific portions of the cerebellum via the ipsilateral inferior cerebellar peduncle. The lateral reticular nucleus of the medulla receives afferent fibers from the spinal cord via spinoreticular pathways and collaterals from the spinothalamic tracts. Crossed descending rubrobulbar fibers also terminate upon cells of this nucleus (Walberg, '58; Hinman and Carpenter, '59). Physiological data suggest that exteroceptive impulses may be conveyed to the cerebellum via the lateral reticular nucleus (Morin and Gardner, '53; Combs, '56).

On the anterior aspect of the pyramid is the *arcuate nucleus,* whose position varies somewhat in different levels (Figs. 11-8, 11-13, 11-14 and 11-15). In rostral portions of the medulla the nucleus enlarges considerably (nucleus precursorius pontis) and appears to become continuous with the nuclei of the pons. Afferent fibers to this nucleus are derived from the cerebral cortex, and its efferent fibers project as ventral external arcuate fibers to the cerebellum. Fibers from this small nucleus are thought to be crossed.

Aréa Postrema. Immediately rostral to the obex on each side of the fourth ventricle is the *area postrema* (Fig. 11-13), a slightly rounded eminence containing as-

ACCESSORY CUNEATE NUCLEUS

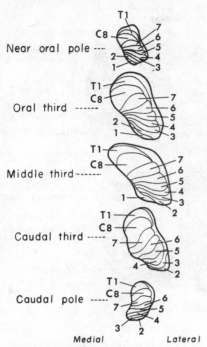

Near oral pole

Oral third

Middle third

Caudal third

Caudal pole

Medial   Lateral

FIG. 11-12. Diagram of the somatotopic termination of cervical and T1 dorsal root fibers in the accessory cuneate nucleus in the monkey. The nucleus is shown in drawings of transverse sections from the right side. Fibers from these roots partially overlap the terminal zone of the next higher root. Thoracic dorsal root fibers T2 through T7 terminate in overlapping fashion along the dorsolateral margin of the nucleus (Shriver et al., '68).

troblast-like cells, arterioles, sinusoids and probably some apolar or unipolar neurons (Cammermeyer, '47; Brizzee and Neal, '54). The area postrema in the dog has been demonstrated to function as an emetic chemoreceptor trigger zone that responds to apomorphine and intravenous digitalis glycosides (Borison and Wang, '49, '53). The area postrema receives fibers from the nucleus solitarius (Morest, '60) as well as some fibers ascending in the posterior and lateral columns of the spinal cord (Morest, '67). It is suggested that impulses transmitted by ascending spinal pathways from viscera may play a role in the physiology of vomiting. Axons from neurons in the area postrema have been traced into caudal parts of the medial nucleus solitarius (Morest, '67).

Cranial Nerve Nuclei. At these levels, the cranial nerve nuclei, other than the spinal trigeminal nucleus, include the hypoglossal (N. XII) and those of the vagus (N. X) nerve (Figs. 11-9, 11-13 and 11-14). The latter nuclei are in the gray surrounding the central canal. Anterolateral to the central canal are small collections of typical large motor neurons which constitute the caudal portions of the hypoglossal nucleus. Lateral to the central canal collections of smaller spindle-shaped cells form the dorsal motor nucleus of the vagus nerve. These cells give rise to preganglionic parasympathetic fibers. Dorsal to the central canal on each side of the median raphe is the commissural nucleus of the vagus nerve. The cells represent the most caudal extension of the medial portion of the nucleus solitarius; they receive visceral afferent fibers. The nucleus ambiguus lies in the reticular formation dorsal to the inferior olivary complex and medial to the lateral reticular nucleus (Figs. 11-9 and 11-13).

OLIVARY LEVELS OF THE MEDULLA

The most characteristic features of the medulla are present in transverse sections through the inferior olivary complex (Figs. 11-9, 11-13, 11-14, A-4 and A-5). The central canal has opened into the fourth ventricle, which widens progressively at higher levels. The tela choroidea and choroid plexus form a thin roof over the ventricle, while the floor of the fourth ventricle contains several rounded eminences formed by specific nuclear groups. The medial eminence, or *trigonum hypoglossi,* is produced by the nucleus of N. XII; the intermediate eminence, known as the *trigonum vagi,* overlies certain vagal nuclei; the lateral eminence in the fourth ventricle is the *area vestibularis,* which is occupied by the caudal poles of the medial and inferior vestibular nuclei (Figs. 11-2, 11-14 and 11-15).

Although the nucleus gracilis has disappeared at this level and the nucleus cuneatus is greatly reduced in size, internal arcuate fibers can be seen sweeping ventromedially through the reticular formation to enter the contralateral medial lemniscus. At this level the medial lemnisci oc-

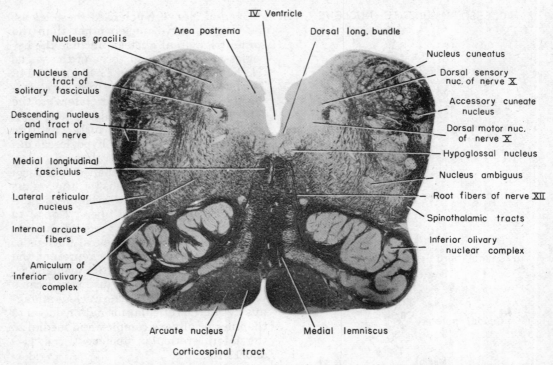

FIG. 11-13. Transverse section of the medulla through the caudal part of the fourth ventricle, the area postrema and the lower part of the inferior olivary nucleus. Weigert's myelin stain. Photograph.

cupy triangular areas on each side of the median raphe, bounded ventrally by the pyramids and laterally by the inferior olivary nuclei. Dorsal to the medial lemnisci on each side of the median raphe are the medial longitudinal fasciculi (Figs. 11-13 and 11-14). The spinal trigeminal nucleus and tract, somewhat inconspicuous in Weigert-stained sections, retain the same general position; the accessory cuneate nucleus is dorsal, and the fibers forming the inferior cerebellar peduncle are dorsolateral.

Inferior Olivary Nuclear Complex. The most characteristic and striking nuclear structure in the medulla is a convoluted gray band of cells known as the inferior olivary nuclear complex (Figs. 11-9, 11-13 and 11-14). This complex consists of: (1) the *principal inferior olivary nucleus*, appearing as a folded bag with the opening or hilus directed medially; (2) a *medial accessory olivary nucleus* along the lateral border of the medial lemniscus; and (3) a *dorsal accessory olivary nucleus*, dorsal to

the main nucleus (Bowman and Sladek, '73). These nuclei are composed of relatively small, round or pear-shaped cells with numerous short branching dendrites. Fibers emerging from the inferior olivary nucleus fill the interior of the bag-shaped nucleus, pass through the hilus, traverse the medial lemnisci and course both through and around the opposite inferior olivary nuclei. Contralaterally these fibers traverse the reticular formation and parts of the spinal trigeminal complex to enter the inferior cerebellar peduncle. The accessory olivary nuclei and the most medial part of the main olivary nucleus are phylogenetically the oldest and project their fibers largely to the cerebellar vermis. The larger convoluted lateral portion of the main nucleus projects its fibers to the opposite cerebellar hemisphere (neocerebellum). The olivocerebellar projection is remarkably specific, and all parts of the cerebellar cortex, as well as the deep cerebellar nuclei, receive olivary projections (Brodal, '40). Olivocerebellar fibers end as climbing

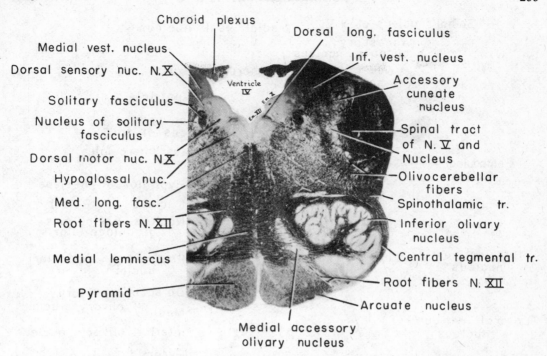

Choroid plexus

Medial vest. nucleus

Dorsal sensory nuc. N.X

Solitary fasciculus

Nucleus of solitary
fasciculus

Dorsal motor nuc. N X

Hypoglossal nuc.

Med. long. fasc.

Root fibers N. XII

Medial lemniscus

Pyramid

Dorsal long. fasciculus

Inf. vest. nucleus

Accessory
cuneate
nucleus

Spinal tract
of N. V and
Nucleus

Olivocerebellar
fibers

Spinothalamic tr.

Inferior olivary
nucleus

Central tegmental tr.

Root fibers N. XII

Arcuate nucleus

Medial accessory
olivary nucleus

Ventricle IV

FIG. 11-14. Transverse section of the medulla through the inferior olive complex rostral to that shown in Figure 11-13. *Em. X,* eminentia vagi; *Em. XII,* eminentia hypoglossi. Weigert's myelin stain. Photograph.

fibers (i.e., fibers which ascend Purkinje cell dendrites) in the cerebellar cortex (Hámori and Szentágothai, '66; Eccles et al., '67). As more and more olivocerebellar fibers are given off, the inferior cerebellar peduncle increases in size. While this peduncle is a composite bundle containing fibers from a large number of specific nuclei, olivocerebellar fibers constitute the largest component of this bundle (Figs. 11-21, 11-22 and 14-22).

The principal olivary nucleus is surrounded by a dense band of myelinated fibers, the *amiculum olivae,* composed largely of axons terminating in the nucleus. Descending fibers terminating upon cells of the inferior olivary complex arise from the cerebral cortex, the red nucleus and the periaqueductal gray of the mesencephalon (Mettler, '44; Walberg, '56, '74). Cortico-olivary fibers appear to arise from frontal, parietal, temporal and occipital cortex, descend in most of their course with corticospinal fibers and terminate bilaterally, primarily upon the ventral lamella of the principal olive. Rubro-olivary

fibers and fibers arising from the periaqueductal gray of the mesencephalon enter a composite bundle known as the central tegmental tract and descend (Figs. 11-25, 12-1 and 12-4). These uncrossed fibers terminate in different portions of the principal olive. Rubro-olivary fibers end in the dorsal lamella, while fibers from the periaqueductal gray terminate in the rostral parts of the principal and medial accessory olivary nuclei (Walberg, '74). Spino-olivary fibers, ascending in the anterior funiculus of the spinal cord, terminate largely on parts of the dorsal and medial accessory olivary nuclei; more than half of these fibers cross in the medulla. The inferior olivary nuclear complex is the largest of the medullary cerebellar relay nuclei.

The tracts ventrolateral to the reticular formation have been pushed dorsally by the olivary nuclei. The anterior spinocerebellar, rubrospinal and spinothalamic tracts occupy the lateral periphery between the inferior cerebellar peduncle and the olivary complex. Fibers of the vestibulospinal tract are scattered along the poste-

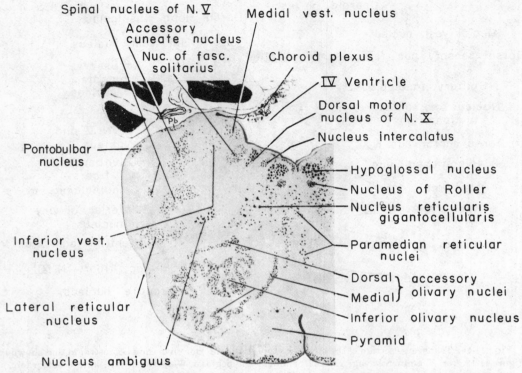

FIG. 11-15. Section through midolivary region of the medulla. Cresyl violet. Photograph, with schematic representation of main cell groups.

rior surface of the inferior olive. Posteriorly on each side of the medial raphe lie the medial longitudinal fasciculi, containing at this level predominately descending fiber bundles of mixed origin. Descending fibers in this tract are derived from certain vestibular nuclei, portions of the brain stem reticular formation and certain nuclei in the midbrain. The interstitial nucleus of Cajal (interstitiospinal tract) contributes a small number of fibers to the dorsomedial part of the medial longitudinal fasciculus. Tectospinal fibers from the superior colliculus form a loosely organized group of fibers in the ventral part of the bundle.

MEDULLARY RETICULAR FORMATION

The term "reticular formation" is a somewhat vague designation given a variety of special connotations; it originated to describe portions of the brain stem core characterized structurally by a wealth of cells of various sizes and types, arranged in diverse aggregations, and enmeshed in a complicated fiber network. In a sense, the reticular formation constitutes a matrix within which "specific" nuclei and tracts are embedded. Cajal ('11) considered reticular neurons to be composed largely of third order sensory neurons and, to a lesser extent, of second order motor neurons. Phylogenetically the reticular formation is very old. In primitive forms it may represent the largest part of the central nervous system. In higher vertebrates the reticular core of the brain stem constitutes a mass of considerable proportions, due in part to the process of encephalization. Although some authors have regarded the reticular formation as a diffusely organized brain stem component, anatomical studies (Brodal, '57) indicate that it is not diffusely organized, and that it can be subdivided into specific regions, possessing distinctive cytoarchitecture, fiber connections and intrinsic organization. In spite of this, these regions cannot be considered as entirely independent entities, since complex fiber connections provide innumerable possibilities for interaction between the various subdivisions.

Golgi-stained sections of the reticular formation have yielded important information concerning its intrinsic organization. Such studies (Scheibel and Scheibel, '58) indicate that almost all reticular axons project for some distance in both rostral and caudal directions. A large number of these emit branching collaterals along their course which terminate in a variety of different types of endings. The majority of primary bifurcating axons are oriented in the longitudinal axis of the brain stem, but project collateral branches in all directions. Many of these collateral fibers arborize extensively about cranial nerve nuclei, and in some instances they may end upon both motor and sensory nuclei.

Physiological data indicate that the reticular formation is predominantly a polysynaptic pathway involving chains of neurons which fire successively. The inability to demonstrate short-axoned, Golgi type II cells in the reticular formation in Golgi-stained material (Scheibel and Scheibel, '58) suggests that the polysynaptic transmission of impulses probably is due to lateral dispersion along collateral fibers. Impulses conducted rapidly in the reticular core (Adey et al., '57) appear to be transmitted by long projecting axons of reticular neurons. Thus the organizational pattern of the reticular formation suggests that a single reticular neuron may convey impulses both rostrally and caudally, may exert its influences both locally and at a distance and may participate in both rapid and slow conduction of impulses.

The reticular formation proper begins in the medulla a little above the corticospinal decussation (Figs. 11-7 and 11-8). One of the particularly discrete nuclei of the reticular formation, the *lateral reticular nucleus* of the medulla, has been described (Figs. 11-8 and 11-9). In sections through the lower medulla, the area dorsal to the caudal half of the inferior olivary nucleus and medial to the lateral reticular nucleus is the location of the *nucleus reticularis ventralis* (Fig. 11-9). At higher levels the

reticular area located medial and dorsal to the rostral half of the inferior olivary nucleus is occupied by the *nucleus reticularis gigantocellularis* (Olszewski and Baxter, '54; Figs. 11-15 and A-5). The latter nucleus is the rostal continuation of the nucleus reticularis ventralis. The nucleus reticularis gigantocellularis is a relatively large nuclear complex composed of characteristic large cells, as well as medium and small cells (Fig. 11-15). Giant cells in this nucleus are not as conspicuous in man as in lower forms. Descending fibers from this reticular nucleus form the medullary reticulospinal tract described earlier (Figs. 10-11 and 10-20).

At the midolivary levels of the medulla small groups of cells are situated near the midline, dorsal to the inferior olivary complex. These cells, which have been subdivided into a dorsal, a ventral and an accessory group, constitute the *paramedian reticular nuclei* (Fig. 11-15). Experimental studies (Brodal, '53) have shown that these reticular neurons project most of their fibers to the cerebellum.

The *nucleus reticularis parvicellularis* is a small-celled reticular nucleus situated dorsolaterally, medial to the spinal trigeminal nucleus and ventral to the vestibular area. This portion of the reticular formation has been referred to as the "sensory" part (Brodal, '57), since numerous studies have shown that collateral fibers from secondary sensory systems terminate in this region.

In essence the medullary reticular formation consists of three principal nuclear masses: (1) a *paramedian reticular nuclear group,* (2) a *central group* (i.e., the ventral reticular and gigantocellular reticular nuclei), and (3) a *lateral nuclear group* consisting of the lateral reticular and parvicellular reticular nuclei.

Afferent Fibers to the Medullary Reticular Formation. While the exact cells of origin of spinoreticular fibers have not been established, it is accepted generally that these fibers ascend almost exclusively in the anterolateral funiculus (Mehler et al., '56; Rossi and Brodal, '57). *Spinoreticular fibers* terminate largely in the caudal and lateral portions of the medullary reticular formation, including the caudal half of the nucleus reticularis gigantocellularis (Figs. 10-11 and 11-15). Although some fibers of this system project to more rostral regions of the brain stem reticular formation, fibers passing to the nucleus reticularis parvicellularis appear scanty.

A large number of spinothalamic fibers have been shown to terminate in a somatotopic fashion upon cells of the lateral reticular nucleus of the medulla (Brodal, '49). Since almost all cells of this nucleus give rise to fibers which pass to specific parts of the cerebellum, this nucleus is considered primarily as a reticular relay nucleus in a spinocerebellar pathway. Physiological data support the thesis that exteroceptive impulses may be relayed to the cerebellum via this route (Combs, '56).

Other important sources of afferents to the reticular formation are *collateral fibers* from second order sensory neurons, such as spinothalamic fibers, secondary auditory pathways, secondary fibers from the nucleus of the solitary fasciculus, secondary trigeminal pathways and secondary vestibular pathways. Collaterals from these diverse sources appear to terminate largely in the lateral region of the reticular formation, which has been referred to as the "sensory" part. It is notable that few, if any, collaterals from the medial lemniscus enter the brain stem reticular formation. Except for a modest number of primary trigeminal fibers (Torvik, '56; Carpenter and Hanna, '61), primary sensory fibers do not appear to terminate in the reticular formation.

Cerebelloreticular fibers in the medullary reticular formation terminate primarily in the region of the paramedian reticular nuclei. Fibers originating in the fastigial nuclei reach this region via the uncinate fasciculus (Thomas et al., '56; Carpenter et al., '58), while fibers from the dentate nucleus pass via the descending division of the superior cerebellar peduncle (Carpenter and Nova, '60; Brodal and Szikla, '72).

Corticoreticular fibers originate from widespread areas of the cerebral cortex, but the majority of these fibers arise from the sensorimotor areas (Rossi and Brodal,

'56). These fibers for the most part terminate in areas of the reticular formation which give rise to reticulospinal fibers, the *nucleus reticularis pontis oralis,* the *nucleus reticularis pontis caudalis* and the *nucleus reticularis gigantocellularis* (Figs. 10-11, 10-20 and 11-15). Corticoreticular fibers are both crossed and uncrossed.

According to Golgi studies of afferents to the brain stem reticular formation, most of the long ascending and descending fiber systems, making connections in various regions, emit collateral or terminal fibers in planes perpendicular to the long axis of the brain stem. As a consequence of this arrangement, impulses from a wide variety of sources converge upon the reticular nuclei. The area of maximal overlap of afferent fields occurs in the medullary reticular formation, which gives rise to the largest number of long ascending and descending axons.

Efferent Fibers from the Medullary Reticular Formation. Ascending reticular fibers from the medulla arise from cells dorsal to the rostral half of the inferior olive and are localized in the medial two-thirds of the reticular formation. While most of these fibers originate from the nucleus reticularis gigantocellularis, some may arise from the nuclei reticularis ventralis and lateralis. These fibers ascend mainly in the area of the central tegmental fasciculus and are for the most part uncrossed (Fig. 12-4). Degeneration studies (Nauta and Kuypers, '58) indicate that they terminate in parts of the intralaminar and reticular nuclei of the thalamus. This same area of the reticular formation also projects descending fibers to spinal levels (Torvik and Brodal, '57; Figs. 10-11 and 10-20).

Efferent fibers from the paramedian reticular nuclei and the lateral reticular nuclei project to specific portions of the cerebellum. Fibers arising in the paramedian reticular nuclei, preponderantly uncrossed, terminate largely in the vermis of the anterior lobe (Brodal, '53). Cerebellar areas receiving fibers from the lateral reticular nucleus include the ipsilateral vermis, hemisphere and the flocculonodular lobule.

The medullary reticular formation, exclusive of the cerebellar projecting nuclei, may be divided into medial and lateral regions. The medial two-thirds of the reticular formation gives rise to most of the long ascending and descending fiber systems. Cells in the lateral third project axons medially and dendrites laterally. Morphological data suggest that the lateral regions of the reticular formation may serve "receptive" and/or "associative" functions, while the medial regions, capable of transmitting impulses to both spinal and higher brain stem levels, may be primarily the "effector" area (Brodal, '57).

Ascending and Descending Tracts. Ascending fibers of the medial lemniscus occupy an "L"-shaped area on each side of the median raphe posterior to the pyramid and medial to the inferior olivary complex (Figs. 11-13, 11-14 and 11-21). The spinothalamic tracts, which can no longer be designated as anterior and lateral, have merged and form essentially a single entity in the retro-olivary area. These tracts appear considerably smaller than at spinal levels, because an appreciable number of fibers terminate in the lateral reticular nucleus, and a number of spinoreticular fibers, which at spinal levels ascend in close association with these tracts, have passed medially into the gigantocellular reticular nucleus. The posterior spinocerebellar tract moves posterior at medullary levels and becomes incorporated in the inferior cerebellar peduncle (Fig. 11-21). The anterior spinocerebellar tract maintains a retro-olivary position and ultimately enters the cerebellum by coursing along the superior surface of the superior cerebellar peduncle. About one-third of the fibers of the rostral spinocerebellar tract enter the cerebellum via the inferior cerebellar peduncle; all other fibers of this uncrossed tract enter the cerebellum in association with the superior cerebellar peduncle (Oscarsson, '65).

The medial longitudinal fasciculus (MLF) lies anterior to the hypoglossal nucleus adjacent to the median raphe (Figs. 11-13, 11-14 and 11-21). Rubrospinal fibers descend in a retro-olivary position close to the lateral reticular nucleus; some crossed descending rubral efferent fibers, terminating in this cerebellar relay nucleus, are properly called *rubrobulbar fibers*. Uncrossed rubrobulbar fibers, arising from rostral parts of the red nucleus, descend in the central tegmental tract and end upon cells in the dorsal lamella of the principal inferior olivary nucleus. At midmedullary levels fibers of the vestibulospinal tract, which arise only from the lateral vestibular nucleus, are scattered in an area posterior to the inferior olivary complex. At more caudal levels, these fibers form a more compact bundle in the retro-olivary region. The medullary reticulospinal tract is not evident at these levels, but it cells of origin, the gigantocellular reticular nucleus, are present posteromedial to the inferior olivary complex (Fig. 11-13). The spinal trigeminal tract and nucleus occupy the same location as at more caudal levels.

Inferior Cerebellar Peduncle. This peduncle is a composite group of tracts and fibers which assemble along the posterolateral border of the medulla and first form a distinct bundle at about midolivary levels (Fig. A-4). Throughout the upper medulla the addition of fibers increases the size of the structure until it forms a large, well-defined mass of myelinated fibers (Figs. 11-21, 11-22, 11-25 and A-5). Tracts and fibers forming this peduncle originate in the medulla and spinal cord. The posterior spinocerebellar tract moves dorsally and enters the inferior cerebellar peduncle directly. Approximately one-third of the fibers of the rostral spinocerebellar tract enter this cerebellar peduncle. Crossed olivocerebellar fibers, originating from all parts of the inferior olivary complex, constitute quantitatively the largest group of fibers that enter the inferior cerebellar peduncle (Figs. 11-21, 11-25 and 14-22). A number of medullary nuclei contribute a relatively small number of fibers to the inferior cerebellar peduncle. These nuclei include: (1) the lateral reticular nucleus of the medulla, (2) the accessory cuneate nucleus, (3) the paramedian reticular nuclei, (4) the arcuate nucleus, and (5) the perihypoglossal nuclei (i.e., the nucleus intercalatus, the nucleus of Roller and the nucleus prepositus) (Figs. 11-15 and 11-21). Fibers

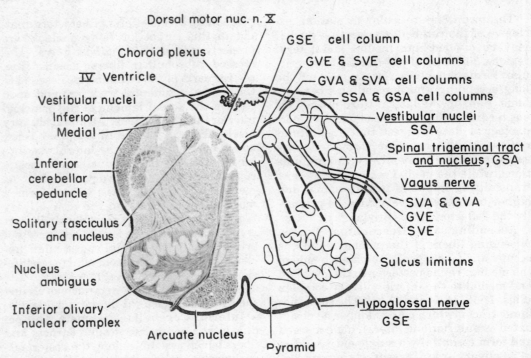

FIG. 11-16. Schematic transverse section of the medulla showing its basic features. Cell columns related to functional components of the cranial nerves are indicated on the *right*. Functional components of cranial nerves are both general and special. The vestibular nuclei shown at this level (and auditory nuclei at higher levels) form the special somatic afferent (SSA) cell columns. The spinal trigeminal nucleus forms the general somatic afferent (GSA) cell column and receives fibers from cranial nerves with this functional component (i.e., N. V, N. VII, N. IX, N. X). Functional components of the vagus nerve (except GSA) are shown in relation to particular nuclei. The hypoglossal nucleus (and the nuclei of N. VI, N. IV and N. III at higher brain stem levels) gives rise to general somatic efferent (GSE) fibers. *Heavy dashes* separate the nuclei of the various cell columns on the *right* side.

from the lateral reticular nucleus and the accessory cuneate nucleus are uncrossed, while those from the other nuclei are both crossed and uncrossed. At higher levels, the inferior cerebellar peduncle becomes covered laterally by fibers of the middle cerebellar peduncle (Figs. 11-25 and 12-2).

On the posterolateral aspect of the inferior cerebellar peduncle a small group of closely packed, medium-sized cells can be seen (Fig. 11-15). These cells constitute the caudal portion of the *pontobulbar nucleus*. At more rostral levels this cell column assumes a progressively more ventral position, until at the junction of pons and medulla it forms a fairly large cell mass ventral to the inferior cerebellar peduncle (Figs. 11-22 and 11-24). The cells of this

nucleus resemble those in the ventral portion of the pons and have been regarded as a caudal extension of the pontine nuclei.

CRANIAL NERVES OF THE MEDULLA

The schematic arrangement of the functional components of the cranial nerves of the medulla, and the cell columns to which they are related, is shown in Figure 11-16. This schema resembles that present in the spinal cord, although development of the fourth ventricle has shifted somatic and visceral afferent regions laterally. The functional components of a typical spinal nerve are four: (1) general somatic afferent (GSA), (2) general visceral afferent (GVA), (3) general somatic efferent (GSE), and (4) general visceral efferent (GVE). Functional components of the cranial nerves include the four types found in spinal nerves, plus three additional special categories: (1) special somatic afferent (SSA), (2) special visceral afferent (SVA), and (3) special visceral efferent (SVE). Somatic efferent fibers in both spinal and cranial nerves are regarded as a general component.

In the medulla, as in the spinal cord, the sulcus limitans divides afferent and efferent cell columns. Special somatic afferent (SSA) cranial nerves in the medulla are represented by the auditory and vestibular components of the vestibulocochlear nerve (VIII). General somatic afferent (GSA) fiber components of cranial nerves V, VII, IX and X descend in the spinal trigeminal tract. Fibers conveying taste (special visceral afferent, SVA) and general visceral afferent (GVA) impulses from components of cranial nerves VII, IX and X form a well-defined tract, the solitary fasciculus, which is embedded in the solitary nucleus (Figs. 11-13, 11-14, 11-17 and 11-18). The above cell columns lie posterolateral to an extension of the sulcus limitans (Fig. 11-16). Ventromedial to this hypothetically projected line are the efferent cell columns. The dorsal motor nucleus of the vagus nerve and the inferior salivatory nucleus of the glossopharyngeal nerve give rise to general visceral efferent (GVE) fibers. Cells of the nucleus ambiguus, located in the ventrolateral reticular formation posterior to the inferior olivary nuclear complex, give rise to special visceral efferent (SVE) fibers that pass peripherally as components of the XI, X and IX cranial nerves (Figs. 11-17 and 11-18). These fibers innervate muscles of the pharynx and larynx derived from the third and fourth branchial arches (i.e., branchiomeric muscles). Other motor nuclei, having similar locations in the pons, supply special visceral efferent fibers to muscles derived from the first and second branchial arches via cranial nerves V and VII (Figs. 11-17 and 11-18). The general visceral efferent (GVE) components (parasympathetic) forming parts of cranial nerves III, VII, IX and X are indicated in Figures 11-17 and 11-18. The hypoglossal nucleus located in

the floor of the fourth ventricle near the median raphe gives rise to general somatic efferent (GSE) fibers which innervate the muscles of the tongue. The general somatic efferent cranial nerve nuclei all lie near the median raphe and relatively close to the floor of the fourth ventricle or cerebral aqueduct. Other nuclei, at more rostral levels, belonging to this group are: the abducens, trochlear and oculomotor. Schematic diagrams showing these nuclei and their intramedullary course (Figs. 11-17 and 11-18) should help the student to understand the organization of the cranial nerves and their various components.

The Hypoglossal Nerve. The hypoglossal nerve is a motor nerve (GSE) innervating the somatic skeletal musculature of the tongue. It also appears to contain some afferent fibers, since the muscle spindles of the tongue degenerate following section of the nerve. These afferent fibers may be derived in part from inconstant ganglion cells found on the hypoglossal roots (Tarkhan and Abd-El-Malek, '50), but their principal source is still obscure. During fetal life the nerve apparently contains dorsal root fibers related to a small ganglion, but these disappear at a later period.

The nucleus of N. XII forms a column of typical multipolar motor cells about 18 mm long that occupies the central gray of the medial eminence. It begins caudal to the inferior olive and extends rostrally to the region of the striae medullares. Within the nucleus coarse myelinated fibers can be seen, which are the root fibers of the motor cells, and a network of finer fibers representing terminals of axons ending in the nucleus. The root fibers gather on the ventral surface of the nucleus, forming a series of rootlets which pass ventrally, lateral to the medial lemniscus, and emerge on the surface of the medulla between the pyramid and the inferior olivary complex (Figs. 11-1, 11-13, 11-14 and A-4).

The hypoglossal nuclei receive numerous fibers and collaterals from reticular neurons, which form delicate plexuses within and around the cells. Some of these fibers constitute the terminals of a "corticobulbar" fiber system effecting voluntary movements of the tongue. Fibers from the

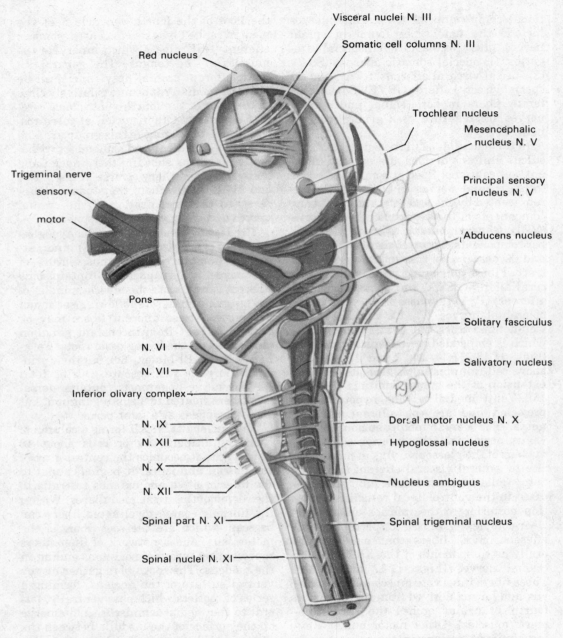

Visceral nuclei N. III

Somatic cell columns N. III

Red nucleus

Trochlear nucleus

Mesencephalic
nucleus N. V

Trigeminal nerve

sensory

Principal sensory
nucleus N. V

motor

Abducens nucleus

Pons

Solitary fasciculus

N. VI

N. VII

Salivatory nucleus

Inferior olivary complex

N. IX

Dorsal motor nucleus N. X

N. XII

Hypoglossal nucleus

N. X

N. XII

Nucleus ambiguus

Spinal part N. XI

Spinal trigeminal nucleus

Spinal nuclei N. XI

FIG. 11-17. Schematic diagram of the intramedullary course of the cranial nerves in a midsagittal view. The brain stem is represented as a hollow shell except for cranial nerve components. General somatic (GSE) and special visceral (SVE) efferent components of cranial nerves innervating striated muscles are shown in *red*. General visceral efferent (GVE) components of cranial nerves III, VII, IX and X, representing preganglionic parasympathetic fibers, are shown in *yellow*. General somatic (GSA), general visceral (GVA) and special visceral (SVA) afferent components of the cranial nerves are in *blue* (modified from Elze, '32).

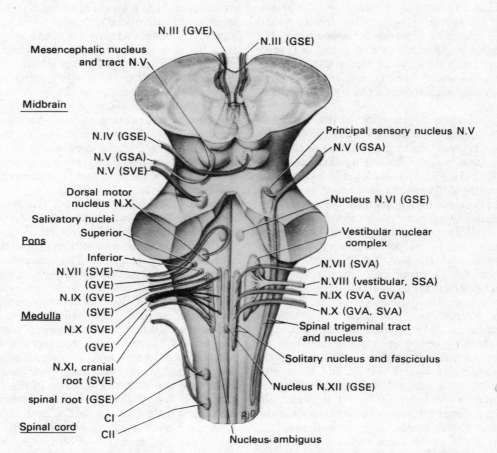

N.III (GVE)
N.III (GSE)
Mesencephalic nucleus
and tract N.V
Midbrain
N.IV (GSE)
N.V (GSA)
N.V (SVE)
Principal sensory nucleus N.V
N.V (GSA)
Dorsal motor
nucleus N.X
Salivatory nuclei
Superior
Pons
Inferior
N.VII (SVE)
(GVE)
N.IX (GVE)
Medulla   (SVE)
N.X (SVE)
(GVE)
N.XI, cranial
root (SVE)
spinal root (GSE)
CI
Spinal cord
CII
Nucleus ambiguus
Nucleus N.VI (GSE)
Vestibular nuclear
complex
N.VII (SVA)
N.VIII (vestibular, SSA)
N.IX (SVA, GVA)
N.X (GVA, SVA)
Spinal trigeminal tract
and nucleus
Solitary nucleus and fasciculus
Nucleus N.XII (GSE)

FIG. 11-18. Schematic representation of the infratentorial cranial nerves showing their nuclei of origin and termination, their intramedullary course and their functional components. The cochlear nerve and nuclei are not shown (see Fig. 12-10). General somatic afferent (GSA) components of the trigeminal nerve (N. V) are shown in *light blue*. General and special visceral afferent (GVA, SVA) components of the facial (N. VII), glossopharyngeal (N. IX) and vagus (N. X) nerves are shown in *dark blue*. The vestibular nerve which differentially distributes special somatic afferent (SSA) fibers to the vestibular nuclear complex is *white*. Similarities in the intramedullary course of fibers in the spinal trigeminal tract, the vestibular nerve root and the solitary fasciculus are evident on the *right*.

General somatic efferent (GSE) fibers from the oculomotor (N. III) and trochlear (N. IV) nuclei and those of the spinal root of the accessory nerve (N. XI) are *light red*. Only contributions from the first and second cervical segments to the spinal root of the accessory nerve are shown. Root fibers of the abducens (N. VI) and hypoglossal (N. XII) nuclei which exit ventrally and contain GSE fibers are not shown.

Special visceral efferent (SVE) fibers from the branchiomeric cranial nerves (N. V, N. VII, N. IX, N. X and N. XI) are shown in *light red*. General visceral efferent (GVE) fibers, representing preganglionic parasympathetic components, of the oculomotor (N. III), facial (N. VII), glossopharyngeal (N. IX) and vagus (N. X) nerves are in *dark red*.

reticular formation are crossed and uncrossed. Other fibers to these nuclei probably are secondary glossopharyngeal, vagal and trigeminal fibers which mediate reflex tongue movements in a response to stimuli from lingual, oral and pharyngeal mucous membranes. Fibers from visceral centers also may terminate in the hypoglossal nuclei.

Immediately posterior to the hypoglossal nucleus is a small bundle of fibers in the periventricular gray known as the *dorsal longitudinal fasciculus* (Schütz, 1891) (Figs. 11-13 and 11-14). This is a composite bundle of fibers consisting of ascending and descending components which are considered to be visceral in nature. While the prevailing conduction in this bundle appears to be in an ascending direction (Burgi and Bucher, '60; Nauta, '72), descending fibers arising from medial and periventricular hypothalamic cell groups have been identified (Krieg, '32; Ingram, '40; Nauta, '58), but these fibers do not extend caudally beyond the midbrain.

In the gray of the ventricular floor are several nuclear masses surrounding the hypoglossal nuclei whose functions and connections are not understood. The *nucleus intercalatus*, situated between the hypoglossal nucleus and dorsal motor nucleus of the vagus, is composed predominantly of small cells and a scattering of larger cells (Fig. 11-15). Rostral to the hypoglossal nucleus is the *nucleus prepositus* (Figs. 11-21 and 11-22), which extends from the oral pole of the hypoglossal nucleus almost to the abducens nucleus. It is composed of relatively large cells and a few smaller cells resembling those of the nucleus intercalatus, with which it is continuous at more caudal levels. The *nucleus of Roller*, composed of relatively large cells, lies ventral to the rostral pole of the hypoglossal nucleus and adjacent to its root fibers (Fig. 11-15). Collectively, the nucleus intercalatus, nucleus prepositus and nucleus of Roller constitute the so-called perihypoglossal nuclei.

Injury to the hypoglossal nerve produces a lower motor neuron paralysis of the ipsilateral half of the tongue with loss of movement, loss of tone and atrophy of the muscles. Since the genioglossus muscle effects protrusion of the tongue, the tongue, when protruded, will deviate to the side of the injury. The intrinsic muscles of the tongue alter the shape of the tongue; the extrinsic muscles alter its shape and position.

The juxtaposition of the emerging root fibers of N. XII and the corticospinal tract is the anatomical basis of the *inferior* or *hypoglossal alternating hemiplegia* resulting from ventral lesions of this area (Fig. 10-13). This syndrome consists of: (1) a lower motor neuron paralysis of the ipsilateral half of the tongue, and (2) a contralateral hemiplegia.

Spinal Accessory Nerve. The accessory nerve usually is divided into cranial and spinal portions which form, respectively, the internal and external branches of the nerve (Fig. 11-19). The *cranial root* of the nerve arises from neurons in the caudal pole of the nucleus ambiguus (SVE). Axons of these cells emerge from the lateral surface of the medulla caudal to the lowest filaments of the vagus nerve. The cranial fibers of the accessory nerve join the vagus nerve and, as motor fibers of the inferior (recurrent) laryngeal nerve, innervate the intrinsic muscles of the larynx. The *spinal portion* of the accessory nerve originates from a cell column in the anterior horn extending from the fifth (or sixth) cervical segment to about the middle of the pyramidal decussation. Caudally cells of this column occupy a lateral process of the anterior horn, but at higher levels they tend to assume a more central position. Root fibers from these cells arch posterolaterally to emerge from the lateral aspect of the spinal cord between the dorsal and ventral roots (Fig. 11-4). Rootlets of the spinal part of the accessory nerve unite to form a common trunk (external branch) which ascends in the spinal canal posterior to the denticulate ligaments, enters the skull through the foramen magnum and ultimately exits from the skull via the jugular foramen, together with the vagus and glossopharyngeal nerves (Fig. 11-19). The spinal nucleus of N. XI, like all motor nuclei, receives direct and indirect fiber projections from a variety of sources which mediate reflex activity related to cephalo-

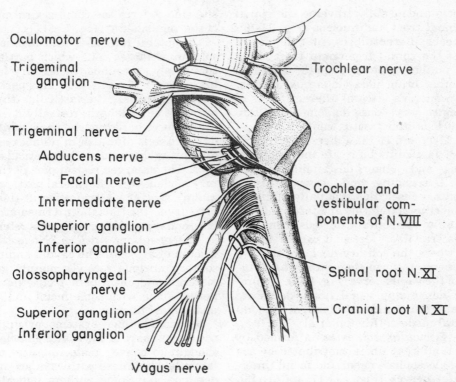

Oculomotor nerve

Trigeminal ganglion

Trochlear nerve

Trigeminal nerve

Abducens nerve

Facial nerve

Intermediate nerve

Superior ganglion

Inferior ganglion

Glossopharyngeal nerve

Superior ganglion

Inferior ganglion

Cochlear and vestibular components of N. VIII

Spinal root N. XI

Cranial root N. XI

Vagus nerve

Fig. 11-19. Semidiagrammatic sketch of brain stem and cranial nerves showing the peripheral ganglia.

gyric movements. The spinal portion of the accessory nerve supplies the sternocleidomastoid and upper parts of the trapezius muscles. Although contractions of the sternocleidomastoid muscle turn the head to the opposite side, unilateral lesions of N. XI usually do not produce any abnormality in the position of the head. Weakness in rotating the head to the opposite side can be detected on testing; when the neck is flexed, the chin tends to turn slightly to the paralyzed side. Paralysis of the upper part of the trapezius muscle is evidenced by: (1) downward and outward rotation of the upper part of the scapula, and (2) a moderate sagging of the shoulder on the affected side. Weakness of the upper part of the trapezius muscle also can be tested by having the patient shrug his shoulders against resistance.

The Vagus Nerve. This is a complex branchiomeric cranial nerve containing: (1) *general somatic afferent (GSA) fibers* distributed through the auricular branch

of the vagus to the skin in back of the ear and the posterior wall of the external auditory meatus, (2) *general visceral afferent (GVA) fibers* from the pharynx, larynx, trachea, esophagus and thoracic and abdominal viscera, (3) *special visceral afferent (SVA) fibers* from scattered taste buds in the region of the epiglottis, (4) *general visceral efferent (GVE; preganglionic) fibers* to terminal parasympathetic ganglia innervating the thoracic and abdominal viscera, and (5) *special visceral efferent (SVE; branchiomotor) fibers* to the voluntary striated muscles of the larynx and pharynx. General somatic afferent fibers of the vagus nerve arise from cells of the superior ganglion of the vagus nerve, located in, or immediately beneath, the jugular foramen (Fig. 11-19). Both general and special visceral afferent fibers of the vagus nerve arise from the larger inferior vagal ganglion (nodosal ganglion). Afferent vagal fibers enter the lateral surface of the medulla ventral to the inferior cerebellar peduncle and usually traverse the spinal trigeminal tract and nucleus (Fig. 11-16). Cutaneous afferent fibers enter the dorsal part of the spinal trigeminal tract along with similar general somatic afferents from other branchiomeric cranial nerves. More numerous visceral afferent fibers of the vagus nerve pass dorsomedially into the nucleus and tractus solitarius (Figs. 11-16, 11-17 and 11-18). Fibers entering the solitary fasciculus bifurcate into short ascending and longer descending components. Descending vagal components in the solitary fasciculus gradually diminish in number as collaterals and terminals are given off to the solitary nucleus. Some vagal visceral fibers descend caudal to the obex, where the solitary nuclei of the two sides merge to form the *commissural nucleus* of the vagus nerve (Fig. 11-9). A number of descending vagal fibers decussate and enter the contralateral half of the commissural nucleus (Rhoton et al., '66).

The *fasciculus solitarius* is formed by visceral afferent fibers contributed by the vagus, glossopharyngeal and facial (intermediate) nerves (Figs. 11-17 and 11-18). Fibers conveying taste from the anterior two-thirds of the tongue (chorda tympani) and from the posterior third of the tongue (glossopharyngeal nerve) enter rostral parts of the solitary fasciculus and mainly terminate in rostal parts of the solitary nucleus. Portions of the solitary fasciculus at the level of entry of the vagus nerve, and caudal to it, contain mainly general visceral afferent fibers, largely from the vagus nerve. The solitary fasciculus constitutes a composite descending bundle of visceral afferent fibers comparable to the spinal trigeminal tract which contains general somatic afferent fibers.

The *nucleus solitarius* can be divided into two parts: (1) a medial part, dorsolateral to the dorsal motor nucleus of the vagus, and (2) a lateral part, located along the lateral border of the solitary fasciculus (Figs. 11-14 and 11-20). Cells of the medial part extend rostrally slightly beyond the dorsal motor nucleus of the vagus (Fig. 11-20); this part of the nucleus extends caudal to the fourth ventricle and merges with the corresponding cell column on the opposite side to form the commissural nucleus of the vagus nerve (Fig. 11-9) (Torvik, '56).

The lateral part of the nucleus is a cell column of larger cells which partially or completely surrounds the solitary fasciculus (Figs. 11-14 and 11-20). This part of the nucleus parallels the fasciculus throughout most of its length; rostrally it extends to the lower border of the pons, while caudally its cells diminish in number and are difficult to distinguish from reticular neurons. The enlarged rostral part of the solitary nucleus (i.e., the lateral part) receives mainly special visceral afferent (taste) fibers from the facial (intermediate) and glossopharyngeal nerves and is referred to as the *gustatory nucleus* (Nageotte, '06; Rhoton et al., '66). The caudal and medial solitary nucleus receives mainly general visceral afferent fibers from the vagus nerve, along with some facial and glossopharyngeal fibers.

Secondary fiber systems arising from the lateral part of the solitary nucleus are thought to convey taste impulses to thalamic levels. These pathways are not understood, but some authors indicate that these fibers cross and ascend in conjunction with the contralateral medial lemniscus (Allen, '27). Some physiological evidence suggests that gustatory impulses are conveyed bilaterally to thalamic levels (Blomquist et al., '62). Caudal parts of the medial solitary nucleus do not project fibers to the thalamus (Morest, '67). These cells, which receive mainly nongustatory visceral afferents, project fibers into dorsal and lateral parts of the medullary reticular formation. These reticular projections from the solitary nucleus may be implicated in the central regulation of respiratory, cardiovascular and emetic functions.

Other secondary fibers from the sensory nuclei of N. X and N. IX go to various motor nuclei of the cranial and spinal nerves. As already stated, impulses pass to the hypoglossal and salivatory nuclei for lingual and secretory reflexes, either directly or through intercalated neurons. Impulses from the pharyngeal, respiratory and alimentary mucous membranes passing to the nucleus ambiguus probably are involved in pharyngeal and laryngeal re-

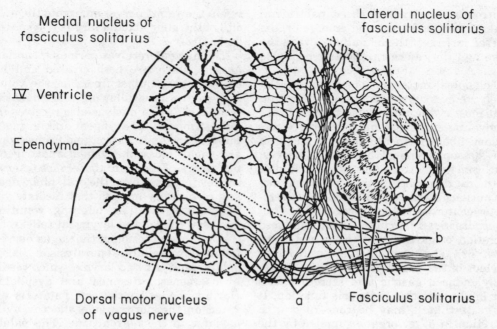

Medial nucleus of
fasciculus solitarius

Lateral nucleus of
fasciculus solitarius

IV Ventricle

Ependyma

Dorsal motor nucleus
of vagus nerve

a

Fasciculus solitarius

b

FIG. 11-20. The vagal nuclei in the floor of the fourth ventricle based upon a drawing of a Golgi preparation of newborn cat (Cajal, '09). Efferent (preganglionic) fibers from the dorsal motor nucleus of the vagus nerve are indicated by *a*, while *b* indicates fibers from the medial and lateral (sensory) nuclei of the fasciculus solitarius forming secondary vagoglossopharyngeal pathways. The medial nucleus of the fasciculus solitarius extends caudally to the fourth ventricle and merges with the corresponding cell group on the opposite side, forming the commissural nucleus of the vagus nerve (Fig. 11-9). The lateral nucleus of the fasciculus solitarius extends rostrally, increases in size and parallels the fasciculus solitarius throughout most of its length.

flexes. Additional impulses to the dorsal motor nucleus of N. X, the phrenic nucleus in the cervical spinal cord and the nuclei of the intercostal muscles in the thoracic cord are involved in coughing, vomiting and respiration. The connections with the spinal cord centers innervating the respiratory muscles probably are mediated by intercalated reticular neurons in the vicinity of the nucleus solitarius.

In the cat and the monkey the maintenance of rhythmic respiratory movements is mediated by diffusely arranged cell groups in the reticular formation dorsal to the olivary region, and longitudinally coextensive with the sensory and motor nuclei of the vagus nerve (Pitts, '46). The cells of this *"respiratory center"* not only are activated by vagal and other neural impulses, but also are affected directly by changes in their chemical environment (CO_2 accumulation, etc.). Ventral cell groups lying im-

mediately above the inferior olive are concerned with inspiratory movements, while more dorsal ones are concerned with expiration. The activities of the respiratory center are subject to regulation from higher neural levels in the brain stem and the cerebral cortex.

The *dorsal motor nucleus of the vagus nerve* occupies the medial portion of the trigonum vagi in the floor of the fourth ventricle (Figs. 11-13, 11-15 and 11-16). It is a column of cells extending both cranially and caudally a little beyond the hypoglossal nucleus. The nucleus is composed of relatively small, spindle-shaped cells among which are larger cells with coarser chromophilic bodies and scattered melanin pigment. The functional significance of the several cell types is not clear. Cells of this nucleus give rise to preganglionic parasympathetic fibers (GVE). The axons of the cells from the dorsal motor nucleus pass ventrolaterally, traverse the spinal trigeminal nucleus and tract and emerge on the lateral surface of the medulla between the olive and the inferior cerebellar peduncle (Figs. A-4 and A-5).

The dorsal motor nucleus contains relatively few myelinated fibers, indicating that most of the terminals entering it are unmyelinated. These are principally secondary fibers from the sensory nuclei of the glossopharyngeal and vagus nerves, and from visceral centers. Recent studies in the cat demonstrate that the dorsal motor nucleus is the vagal medullary secretomotor center, since destruction of this nucleus drastically reduces insulin-induced secretion of gastric acid (Kerr and Preshaw, '69). The fact that the dorsal motor nucleus of the vagus is responsible for vagally induced gastric acid secretion does not imply that this is its sole function. It suggests that it may be concerned with secretion in other organs supplied by the vagus nerve. Following destruction of the dorsal motor nucleus of the vagus, stimulation of the distal end of the transected vagus nerve has no visceral motor or cardioinhibitory effect (Kerr, '69; Kerr and Preshaw, '69).

The *nucleus ambiguus* is a column of cells in the reticular formation about half way between the spinal trigeminal nucleus and the inferior olivary complex (Figs. 11-9, 11-13, 11-15, 11-16, 11-17 and 11-18). This nucleus, extending from the level of the decussation of the medial lemniscus to levels through the rostral third of the inferior olivary complex, is composed of typical multipolar lower motor neurons. Fibers from the nucleus arch dorsally, join efferent fibers from the dorsal motor nucleus of the vagus nerve and emerge from the lateral surface of the medulla dorsal to the inferior olivary complex (Figs. 11-16, 11-17 and 11-18). Caudal parts of the nucleus ambiguus give rise to the cranial part of the spinal accessory nerve, while rostral parts of this cell column give rise to glossopharyngeal special visceral efferent fibers (which innervate the stylopharyngeus muscle). Special visceral efferent fibers of the vagus nerve (and those from the cranial part of the accessory nerve which rejoin the vagus nerve) innervate the muscles of the pharynx and larynx (Figs. 11-16 and 11-18).

The nucleus receives various terminals, among which are both crossed and uncrossed corticobulbar fibers for the voluntary control of swallowing and phonation (Fig. 11-23). The nucleus also receives impulses from the pharyngeal and laryngeal muscles for tonic control, and from secondary vagal, glossopharyngeal and trigeminal fibers. Fibers in these three nerves convey impulses from the oral, pharyngeal and respiratory mucosa that mediate various reflexes, such as coughing, vomiting, and pharyngeal and laryngeal reflexes.

A unilateral lesion of the vagus nerve is followed by ipsilateral paralysis of the soft palate, pharynx and larynx, which results in hoarseness, dyspnea and dysphagia. During phonation the soft palate is elevated on the normal side and the uvula deviates to the normal side. The palatal reflex is lost on the lesion side. Anesthesia of the pharynx and larynx results in an ipsilateral loss of the cough reflex. Destruction of visceral motor fibers of the vagus results in an ipsilateral loss of the carotid sinus reflex. As a rule visceral disturbances are not marked following a unilateral lesion of the vagus nerve. A unilateral lesion of the recurrent laryngeal nerve will result in hoarseness of the voice and coughing attacks which in time diminish and disappear. The abductor muscles of the larynx are affected first.

Bilateral lesions of the vagus nerves as a rule are fatal unless immediate precautions are instituted to prevent asphyxia, resulting from complete laryngeal paralysis. Paralysis and atonia of the esophagus and stomach induce pain and vomiting with the hazards of aspiration. These lesions also result in loss of vagal respiratory reflexes, dyspnea and cardiac acceleration. Bilateral lesions most frequently are due to pathology within the medulla.

The Glossopharyngeal Nerve. This nerve is related closely to the vagus nerve, having certain common intramedullary nuclei, and similar functional components. Fibers of this nerve enter and emerge from the medulla at levels rostral to the vagus

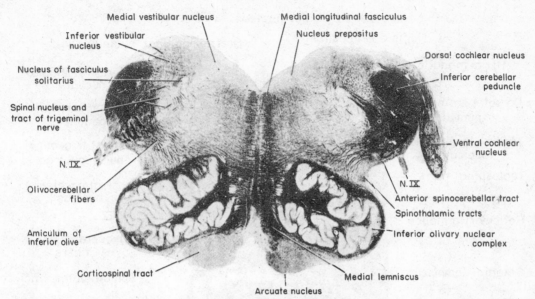

Medial vestibular nucleus

Inferior vestibular nucleus

Nucleus of fasciculus solitarius

Spinal nucleus and tract of trigeminal nerve

N. IX

Olivocerebellar fibers

Amiculum of inferior olive

Corticospinal tract

Arcuate nucleus

Medial longitudinal fasciculus

Nucleus prepositus

Dorsal cochlear nucleus

Inferior cerebellar peduncle

Ventral cochlear nucleus

N. IX

Anterior spinocerebellar tract

Spinothalamic tracts

Inferior olivary nuclear complex

Medial lemniscus

FIG. 11-21. Transverse section of medulla of 1-month infant through the cochlear nuclei and ninth nerve. Weigert's myelin stain. Photograph.

nerve, but like the vagus nerve, they traverse the spinal trigeminal tract and nucleus (Figs. 11-16, 11-21 and 11-22). The glossopharyngeal is a mixed branchiomeric cranial nerve with the following functional components: (1) *general visceral afferent (GVA) fibers*, (2) *special visceral afferent (SVA) fibers* (taste), (3) a few *general somatic afferent (GSA) fibers*, (4) *general visceral efferent (GVE) fibers*, and (5) a small number of *special visceral efferent (SVE) fibers*. Like the vagus nerve it has two peripheral ganglia, a small *superior ganglion* in the jugular foramen and a larger extracranial *inferior (petrosal) ganglion* (Fig. 11-19).

Primary sensory neurons mediating general somatic sense (GSA) from cutaneous areas back of the ear lie in the superior ganglion; central processes of these cells enter the spinal trigeminal tract and nucleus. Cell bodies of visceral afferent fibers lie in the inferior ganglion. General visceral afferent fibers convey impulses concerned with tactile sense, thermal sense and pain from the mucous membranes of the posterior third of the tongue, the tonsil, the posterior wall of the upper pharynx and the Eustachian tube. Special visceral afferent fibers convey taste sensation from

the posterior third of the tongue. Visceral afferent fibers enter the posterolateral part of the medulla and are distributed to rostral portions of the solitary fasciculus and its nucleus (Fig. 11-21). Rostral and lateral parts of the nucleus solitarius which receive fibers from the facial (intermediate) and glossopharyngeal nerves constitute what is called the "*gustatory nucleus*."

The *carotid sinus nerve* conveys impulses from the carotid sinus, a baroreceptor, located at the bifurcation of the common carotid artery. Increases in carotid arterial pressure excite carotid sinus baroreceptors, and impulses are conveyed centrally by the glossopharyngeal nerve. Collaterals of glossopharyngeal fibers project to the dorsal motor nucleus of the vagus nerve, excite these cells and bring about reductions in heart rate and arterial pressure via pre- and postganglionic vagal fibers that convey impulses to the sinoatrial and atrioventricular nodes, as well as to atrial heart muscle. The *carotid sinus reflex* involving glossopharyngeal visceral afferents and vagal general visceral efferents constitutes a mechanism for the regulation of arterial blood pressure.

General visceral efferent fibers, arising

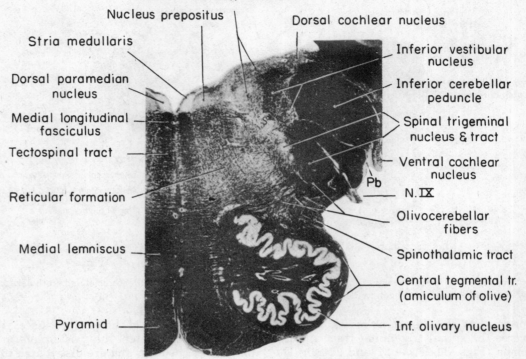

Medial vestibular nucleus

Nucleus prepositus

Stria medullaris

Dorsal cochlear nucleus

Dorsal paramedian nucleus

Inferior vestibular nucleus

Medial longitudinal fasciculus

Inferior cerebellar peduncle

Tectospinal tract

Spinal trigeminal nucleus & tract

Pb

Ventral cochlear nucleus

N. IX

Reticular formation

Olivocerebellar fibers

Medial lemniscus

Spinothalamic tract

Central tegmental tr. (amiculum of olive)

Pyramid

Inf. olivary nucleus

FIG. 11-22. Transverse section through the upper medulla at the level of the cochlear nuclei and the root fibers of the glossopharyngeal nerve. *S* indicates the lateral nucleus of the fasciculus solitarius; *Pb* indicates pontobulbar nucleus. Weigert's myelin stain. Photograph.

from the *inferior salivatory nucleus*, pass via the lesser petrosal nerve to the otic ganglion, situated below the foramen ovale and medial to the mandibular division of the trigeminal nerve. Postganglionic fibers originating from the cells of the otic ganglion convey parasympathetic secretory impulses to the parotid gland. Cells of the inferior salivatory nucleus are virtually impossible to distinguish from reticular neurons, but they are considered as a separate rostral cell group equivalent to the dorsal motor nucleus of the vagus.

Special visceral efferent fibers, as already described, arise from rostral portions of the nucleus ambiguus (Figs. 11-17 and 11-18). These fibers, small in number, innervate the stylopharyngeus muscle and perhaps portions of the superior pharyngeal constrictor muscle.

As the above description indicates, the glossopharyngeal nerve is predominantly

a sensory nerve, and a nerve contributing preganglionic parasympathetic fibers to the otic ganglion. Isolated lesions of the glossopharyngeal nerve are rare. Disturbances associated with lesions of the nerve include: (1) loss of the pharyngeal (gag) reflex, (2) loss of the carotid sinus reflex, and (3) loss of taste in the posterior third of the tongue. *Glossopharyngeal neuralgia* resembles trigeminal neuralgia in that the excruciating pain is paroxysmal and may be triggered by seemingly trivial stimuli such as coughing or swallowing. The pain associated with this syndrome radiates to regions behind the ear.

CORTICOBULBAR FIBERS

Corticofugal fibers projecting into the lower brain stem are referred to as *corticobulbar fibers*. These fibers arise mainly from the precentral and postcentral gyri, and are distributed to: (1) sensory relay nuclei, (2) parts of the reticular formation, and (3) certain motor cranial nerve nuclei in man and primates.

Sensory relay nuclei receiving corticobulbar fibers include the nuclei gracilis and cuneatus, the sensory trigeminal nuclei and the nucleus of the solitary fasciculus (Brodal et al., '56; Torvik, '56; Walberg, '57; Kuypers, '58, '58a, '58b, '58c, '60; Kuypers et al., '61; Kuypers and Tuerk, '64; Zimmerman et al., '64). Corticobulbar fibers to the posterior column nuclei leave the corticospinal tract and enter these nuclei, by either passing among the fibers of the medial lemniscus, or by traversing the reticular formation. After unilateral cortical lesions degenerated terminal fibers are distributed bilaterally to the posterior column nuclei, but are most numerous contralaterally. There are suggestions of somatotopic projections between portions of the precentral and postcentral gyri and the nuclei gracilis and cuneatus, but considerable overlap also is evident (Kuypers, '58b). According to Zimmerman et al. ('64), the projection from the primary somesthetic cortex in the rat is such that fibers from the forelimb cortical area pass to the nucleus cuneatus and those from the hindlimb area terminate in the nucleus gracilis. Studies of corticobulbar fibers projecting to the nuclei gracilis and cuneatus in the cat (Kuypers and Tuerk, '64) indicate that these fibers are distributed preferentially to portions of the nuclei containing loosely organized cells, and that few fibers from the cortex terminate in "cell nest" regions which receive ascending fibers from spinal dorsal roots. Fibers to all trigeminal sensory nuclei and the nucleus solitarius are derived from widespread cortical regions with the largest number arising from the frontoparietal region (Brodal et al., '56). Corticobulbar projections to trigeminal sensory nuclei appear to be nontopological (Zimmerman et al., '64), although Kuypers ('58b) suggests that in primates these fibers arise mainly from the postcentral gyrus. Corticofugal fibers to the nucleus solitarius terminate chiefly in its rostral part, near levels where facial and trigeminal afferents end.

Corticobulbar projections to the posterior column nuclei, and other sensory relay nuclei, underlie a physiological mechanism by which descending cortical impulses can influence the transmission of ascending sensory impulses at the second neuron level. Both excitatory and inhibitory influences upon these sensory relay nuclei can be produced following stimulation of the cerebral cortex (Hagbarth and Kerr, '54; Hernandez-Peon and Hagbarth, '55; Levitt et al., '60; Jabbur and Towe, '61; Gordon and Jukes, '64a). Experimental studies (Gordon and Jukes, '64, '64a) of descending cortical influences upon the nucleus gracilis suggest that excitatory and inhibitory influences are exerted differentially upon portions of the nucleus which are distinguishable on the basis of the size of the receptive field and sensory modality represented. Corticofugal inhibitory influences were found mainly in middle portions of the nucleus where individual cells responded to movement of hair, light touch to foot pads, pressure at the base of a claw or subcutaneous pressure. These cells exhibited small receptive fields and were inhibited by stimuli applied outside the physiological receptive field (i.e., surround inhibition). Corticofugal excitatory effects were found mainly on the rostral, and the deep part of the middle region of the nucleus where individual cells responded mainly to touch and pressure. These cells with rather large receptive fields did not show the phenomenon of surround inhibition.

Corticoreticular fibers projecting to the lower brain stem arise from broad areas of the cerebral cortex, but the largest number originates from the motor, premotor and somesthetic areas (Rossi and Brodal, '56a). These fibers descend with those of the corticospinal tract, but leave this bundle to enter the brain stem reticular formation. The largest number of these fibers terminate in two well circumscribed areas, one in the medulla and another in the pons. Terminations in the medulla are in the area of the nucleus reticularis gigantocellularis, while the pontine area of termination is mainly within the nucleus reticularis pontis oralis. Corticoreticular fibers are distributed bilaterally, but with a slight contralateral predominance (Zimmerman et al., '64). Some corticoreticular fibers also project to reticular cerebellar relay nuclei, such as the reticulotegmental nucleus in the pons, and the lateral reticular and paramedian reticular nuclei of the medulla. Regions of the reticular formation receiving corticofugal fibers give rise to: (1) long ascending and descending projections (Brodal and Rossi, '55; Torvik and Brodal, '57), (2) projections to the cerebellum (Brodal, '53; Combs, '56), and (3) abundant collateral fibers that project to cranial nerve nuclei (Scheibel and Scheibel, '58).

The *motor cranial nerve nuclei* innervating striated muscle receive impulses from the cerebral cortex via corticobulbar pathways. These fibers arise mainly from portions of the precentral gyrus, descend through the internal capsule and brain stem in association with the corticospinal tract (Figs. 2-8, 10-12 and 11-23) and constitute the upper motor neurons for the motor cranial nerve nuclei. Most fibers regarded as "corticobulbar" are distributed to neurons in the reticular formation which in turn relay impulses to the motor cranial nerve nuclei. In experimental studies (Walberg, '57a; Kuypers, '58; Zimmerman et al., '64) in the cat and rat, it has not been possible to trace terminal degeneration directly into any motor cranial nerve nucleus. These findings present a parallel to that accepted for the spinal cord, in that relatively few corticospinal fibers terminate directly upon anterior horn cells (Phalen and Davenport, '37; Szentágothai-Schimert, '41; Lloyd, '41). This indirect system is supplemented in man and primates by corticobulbar fibers that project directly to certain motor nuclei, namely, the trigeminal, the facial, the hypoglossal and the supraspinal (Kuypers, '58a). Fiber projections to the motor trigeminal and hypoglossal nuclei are bilateral and nearly equal (Fig. 11-23). Direct cortical projections to the facial nucleus are bilateral, but fibers passing to ventral cell groups, which innervate lower facial muscles, are most abundant contralaterally. These observations are in accord with clinical observations regarding one central type of

facial palsy to be discussed fully in the next chapter. Many of the direct corticobulbar fibers correspond to what early authors referred to as aberrant pyramidal bundles. An example of these obliquely running fascicles, frequently seen in the medulla and lower pons, is shown coursing into the pontine tegmentum in Figure 12-17. The more numerous corticoreticular fibers represent part of the phylogenetically older indirect corticobulbar pathway in which neurons of the reticular core serve as internuncials. Direct corticobulbar fibers found in man and primates represent a more recently developed parallel system.

Thus the supranuclear innervation of the motor cranial nerve nuclei is largely bilateral and more complex than that present at spinal levels. Bilateral projections are most evident to those nuclei innervating muscle groups which as a rule cannot be contracted voluntarily on one side (Fig. 11-23). These include the laryngeal, pharyngeal, palatal and upper facial muscles. This same principle applies to the muscles of mastication and the extraocular muscles. Because unilateral stimulation of the motor cortex produces isolated contraction of contralateral lower facial muscles, certain cell groups of the facial nucleus are considered to receive predominantly crossed corticobulbar fibers. The fact that unilateral stimulation of the motor cortex causes turning of the head to the opposite side has been interpreted as indicating that corticofugal fibers to nuclei innervating the sternocleidomastoid muscle probably are uncrossed, since contraction of this muscle turns the head to the opposite side. It seems likely that some uncrossed corticospinal fibers (Figs. 10-13 and 10-15) may project impulses to spinal accessory cell groups innervating this muscle and the upper part of the trapezius muscle, although direct fibers to these cells appear meager (Kuypers, '58a). Eye movements elicited by electrical stimulation of the cerebral cortex are always conjugate, indicating that the supranuclear innervation of the nuclei of the extraocular muscles is bilateral.

Because cortical control of motor cranial

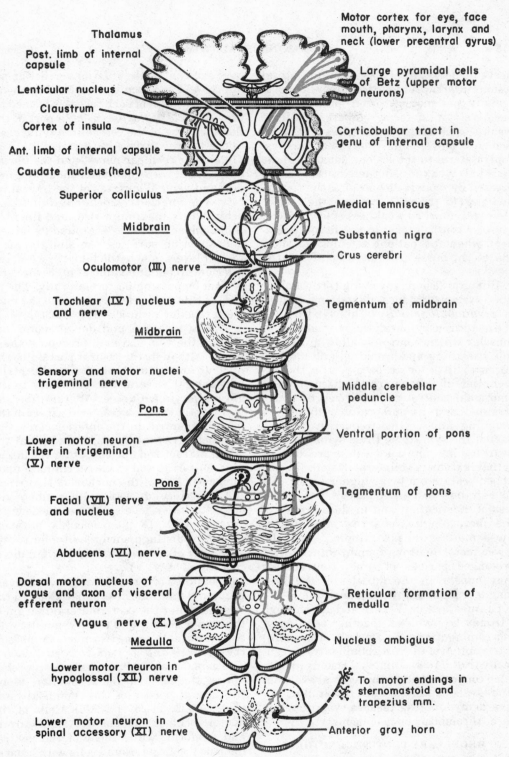

Thalamus

Post. limb of internal capsule

Lenticular nucleus

Claustrum

Cortex of insula

Ant. limb of internal capsule

Caudate nucleus (head)

Motor cortex for eye, face mouth, pharynx, larynx and neck (lower precentral gyrus)

Large pyramidal cells of Betz (upper motor neurons)

Corticobulbar tract in genu of internal capsule

Superior colliculus

Midbrain

Medial lemniscus

Substantia nigra

Crus cerebri

Oculomotor (III) nerve

Trochlear (IV) nucleus and nerve

Midbrain

Tegmentum of midbrain

Sensory and motor nuclei trigeminal nerve

Pons

Middle cerebellar peduncle

Lower motor neuron fiber in trigeminal (V) nerve

Ventral portion of pons

Pons

Facial (VII) nerve and nucleus

Tegmentum of pons

Abducens (VI) nerve

Dorsal motor nucleus of vagus and axon of visceral efferent neuron

Vagus nerve (X)

Medulla

Reticular formation of medulla

Nucleus ambiguus

Lower motor neuron in hypoglossal (XII) nerve

To motor endings in sternomastoid and trapezius mm.

Lower motor neuron in spinal accessory (XI) nerve

Anterior gray horn

FIG. 11-23. Diagram of "corticobulbar" pathways in the brain stem. Fibers of this upper motor neuron pathway to the motor cranial nerve nuclei arise in the cerebral cortex; pass caudally in the internal capsule, the crus cerebri and the ventral portion of the pons; and are distributed largely to neurons in the reticular formation bilaterally. Reticular neurons conveying the impulses to the motor cranial nerve nuclei correspond to the intercalated or internuncial neurons found at spinal levels. In man and primates this indirect system is paralleled by more recently developed direct corticobulbar fibers distributed to the motor nuclei of the trigeminal, facial and hypoglossal nerves (Kuypers, '58a).

nerve nuclei is largely bilateral, unilateral lesions interrupting corticobulbar fiber systems (upper motor neuron) produce comparatively mild forms of paresis. Slight weakness of tongue (genioglossus muscle) and jaw movements (pterygoid muscles) contralateral to the lesions usually can be detected. Weakness in these muscles is expressed by modest deviation of the tongue and jaw to the side opposite the lesion. However, marked weakness of lower facial muscles contralateral to the lesion is evident when the patient attempts to show the teeth, purse the lips or puff out the cheeks.

Bilateral lesions involving corticobulbar fiber systems produce a syndrome known as *pseudobulbar palsy*. This syndrome is characterized by paralysis or weakness of muscles which control swallowing, chewing, breathing and speaking, and may occur with little or no paralysis in the extremities, if lesions are localized. Loss of emotional control characterized by unrestrained and inappropriate outbursts of laughing and crying frequently form a part of the syndrome; these symptoms appear as the physiological expression of rather extensive bilateral lesions in the upper brain stem or at higher levels. Although there is marked paresis of the muscles of mastication and in the muscles of the face, tongue, pharynx and larynx, these muscles do not atrophy, since the lower motor neurons remain intact. After prolonged periods of time, contractures may appear in the muscles of the lips, tongue and palate (Haymaker, '56).

Cranial nerves V, VII and IX through XII may be involved, together or in varying combinations, as a result of bilateral interruption of the corticobulbar tracts centrally (Fig. 11-23). Bilateral lesions involving "corticobulbar pathways" above pontine levels usually are the result of extensive demyelinating disease, vascular disease, thrombosis or neoplasms.

MEDULLARY-PONTINE JUNCTION

The fourth ventricle reaches its maximum width at the level of the lateral recesses (Figs. 11-2, 11-24 and A–6). These lateral extensions of the fourth ventricle pass external to the inferior cerebellar peduncle and the cochlear nuclei (Fig. A–5). The lateral wall of each recess is formed by the *peduncle of the flocculus*, a part of the floccular lobe of the cerebellum lying close to the lateral surface of the medulla (Fig. 11-24). The cochlear nerve, and the *dorsal* and *ventral cochlear nuclei* lie on the medial and ventral surfaces of the lateral recess. The *inferior cerebellar peduncle* has achieved its maximum size, and fibers of the cochlear nerve curve around its lateral and superior surfaces. At slightly more rostral levels, above the lateral recess, the inferior cerebellar peduncle enters the cerebellum by passing posterolaterally. The fibers of this peduncle lie medial to the middle cerebellar peduncle (Fig. 11-25).

The hypoglossal and dorsal motor nucleus of the vagus are not present at these levels, although the rostral portion of the nucleus ambiguus is present and contributes special visceral efferent fibers to the glossopharyngeal nerve. Afferent fibers of N. IX enter the posterolateral aspect of the medulla ventral to the inferior cerebellar peduncle, traverse parts of the spinal trigeminal tract and nucleus, enter the fasciculus solitarius and in part terminate upon upper portions of the nucleus of that tract, the gustatory nucleus. Other fibers descend to lower levels. Above the level of entrance of N. IX the fasciculus solitarius cannot be distinguished readily, for it consists only of a small descending bundle of root fibers of N. VII.

Root fibers of the *cochlear* nerve, conveying impulses from the organ of Corti in the cochlea, enter the posterolateral margin of the upper medulla. Primary auditory fibers terminate upon two nuclear masses, the *ventral and dorsal cochlear nuclei*. The dorsal cochlear nucleus forms a prominence, the *tuberculum acusticum*, along the lateral border of the rhomboid fossa (Figs. 11-22, 11-25 and A-6). Cells of the dorsal cochlear nucleus are small, ovoid and fusiform, while those of the ventral nucleus are large, round cells with a dark-staining cytoplasm. Secondary auditory fibers arising from the dorsal and ventral cochlear nuclei become apparent at rostral brain stem levels.

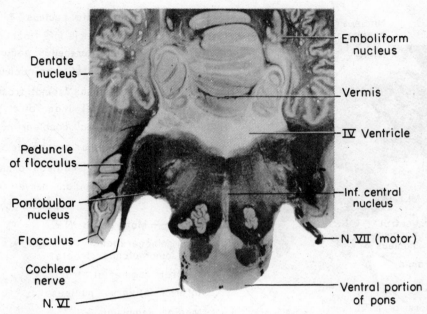

Dentate nucleus —

Peduncle of flocculus —

Pontobulbar nucleus —

Flocculus —

Cochlear nerve —

N. VI —

— Emboliform nucleus

— Vermis

— IV Ventricle

— Inf. central nucleus

— N. VII (motor)

— Ventral portion of pons

FIG. 11-24. Transverse section through the junction of medulla and pons in a 1-month infant. Portions of the cerebellum containing large parts of the intracerebellar nuclei are attached. Structures in and around the tegmentum are identified in Figure 11-25. Weigert's myelin stain. Photograph.

In the floor of the fourth ventricle the nucleus prepositus lies medially in the position previously occupied by the hypoglossal nucleus. Lateral to this nucleus are the vestibular nuclei (Figs. 11-21 and 11-25). At this level portions of the *medial* and *inferior vestibular nuclei* are seen. The inferior vestibular nucleus lies adjacent to the medial surface of the inferior cerebellar peduncle and is characterized by numerous, relatively coarse myelinated fiber bundles which course through it. These fibers, coursing in the longitudinal axis of the nucleus, are primary vestibular fibers and cerebellar efferent fibers which descend. The inferior vestibular nucleus has abundant reciprocal connections with vestibular portions of the cerebellum (Carpenter et al., '60).

The inferior olivary complex is still present, but is reduced in size (Fig. 11-24). The accessory olivary nuclei have disappeared. Anterior to the olivary complex the fibers of the pyramid are surrounded by pontine nuclei and some transverse fibers. The medial lemniscus and medial longitudinal fasciculus occupy the same positions as at more caudal levels, although

they are slightly separated from the corresponding tract on the opposite side by more fully developed nuclei in the median raphe. Other ascending and descending tracts maintain the same relative positions as at lower medullary levels.

The junction of medulla and pons (Figs. 11-24 and 11-25) is characterized by: (1) passage of the inferior cerebellar peduncle into the cerebellum, (2) reduction in size and, ultimately, disappearance of the inferior olivary complex, (3) gradual incorporation of the corticospinal tract within the ventral part of the pons, (4) enlargement of the reticular formation, and (5) appearance of cranial nerve nuclei and root fibers typical of this higher level.

Cranial nerves present at the junction of medulla and pons are the abducens, cochlear, vestibular and facial. The abducens nerve fibers emerge at the lower border of the pons lateral to the pyramids. All other cranial nerves at this level are grouped together at the *cerebellopontine angle*, formed by the junction of medulla, pons and cerebellum (Fig. 11-19). All of these nerves emerge from, or enter, the internal auditory meatus. The cochlear nerve is the

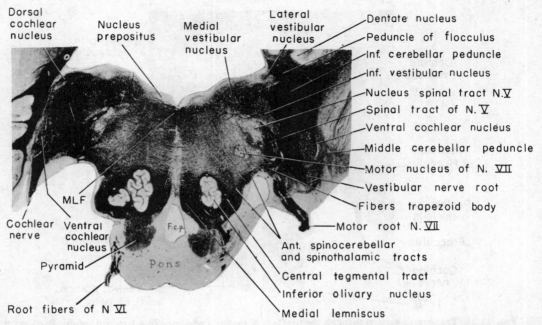

Dorsal cochlear nucleus

Nucleus prepositus

Medial vestibular nucleus

Lateral vestibular nucleus

Dentate nucleus

Peduncle of flocculus

Inf. cerebellar peduncle

Inf. vestibular nucleus

Nucleus spinal tract N.V

Spinal tract of N.V

Ventral cochlear nucleus

Middle cerebellar peduncle

Motor nucleus of N. VII

Vestibular nerve root

Fibers trapezoid body

Motor root N. VII

MLF

Cochlear nerve

Ventral cochlear nucleus

Pyramid

F.c.p.

Pons

Ant. spinocerebellar and spinothalamic tracts

Central tegmental tract

Inferior olivary nucleus

Root fibers of N VI

Medial lemniscus

FIG. 11-25. Transverse section of medulla of 1-month infant through caudal border of pons. *F.c.p.*, Foramen cecum posterior; *MLF*, medial longitudinal fasciculus. Weigert's myelin stain. Photograph.

most caudal and lateral, while the facial nerve is the most rostral and medial. The vestibular nerve lies between the cochlear and facial nerves. These cranial nerves will be described and discussed in the next chapter.

In the upper medulla the medial lemniscus reaches its full extent. It forms a vertical band of heavily myelinated fibers on either side of the raphe dorsal to the pyramids (Fig. 11-22). The formation and course of this tract are shown in Figure 10-1. The lateral and anterior spinothalamic tracts occupy a retro-olivary position (Fig. 11-22). Corticobulbar fibers leave the pyramids and pass dorsally into the reticular formation (Fig. 11-23); intercalated neurons lying in the reticular formation in turn project upon motor cranial nerve nuclei (Walberg, '57a).

The medial longitudinal fasciculus (abbreviated MLF), tectospinal and tectobulbar tracts occupy an area dorsal to the medial lemniscus on each side of the median raphe. The tracts are partially separated by lighter-stained areas representing the raphe nuclei. At somewhat higher

levels this position is occupied by the inferior central nucleus (Figs. 11-24 and 12-4). Other descending tracts, such as the rubrospinal and vestibulospinal, are difficult to distinguish in Weigert-stained material.

As the inferior cerebellar peduncle enters the medullary core of the cerebellum, it is covered externally by the fibers of the middle cerebellar peduncle, which arise from the ventral part of the pons. The development of the ventral portion of the pons envelops the medullary pyramids. The blind end of the anterior median fissure overhung by the pons is known as the *foramen cecum posterior* (Fig. 11-25). The attenuated rostral pole of the inferior olivary nucleus is flanked laterally by the fibers of the central tegmental tract and medially and ventrally by the medial lemniscus. The medial lemniscus gradually becomes flattened dorsoventrally and lies along the ventral border of the pontine tegmentum (Fig. 10-1). The light-staining area separating the medial lemnisci and the medial longitudinal fasciculi is occupied by the inferior central nucleus (nucleus of the raphe).

Experimentally, electrical stimulation of the lateral part of the medullary reticular formation and adjacent periventricular gray in lower animals (Wang, '55) produces elevation of arterial blood pressure and cardiac acceleration, probably as a consequence of activating sympathetic effectors. Descending pathways mediating these responses lie in the anterior and lateral funiculus of the spinal cord and are largely homolateral. Stimulations in the region of the obex, and in a wide area medial and ventral to the sympathetic area, produce a slowing of the heart rate. Part of this response appears to be vagal, but other evidence also suggests an inhibition of sympathetic neurons. Similar studies indicate that inspiratory and expiratory responses can be obtained from stimulations of circumscribed areas of the medulla (Ngai and Wang, '57).

Multiple medullary structures may be simultaneously involved by vascular lesions, neoplasms or other disease processes. Symptoms and signs resulting from such lesions bear a close correlation to the specific neural structures involved, and their nature depends in part upon whether the lesions are irritative or destructive. Although vascular lesions are subject to considerable variation in location and extent, the distribution of the principal blood vessels within the medulla shows some constant features (Figs. 20-13 and 20-14). Lesions involving structures in the dorsolateral part of the medulla (lateral medullary syndrome) are probably the most common at this level and give rise to a constellation of symptoms and signs that are readily recognizable (Currier et al., '61). While the classic feature of this syndrome is loss of pain and thermal sense in the ipsilateral half of the face and the contralateral half of the trunk and extremities, a variety of other severe symptoms occur. These include vertigo, nausea, vomiting, dysphonia, dysphagia, face and body pain, weakness of the face, disturbance of equilibrium and hiccup. In the past this syndrome has been attributed largely to occlusion or disease of a single vessel, the posterior inferior cerebellar artery (Figs. 20-1, 20-4 and 20-6), but current data (Baker, '61) indicate that involvement of the vertebral artery and its smaller penetrating branches plays an equally important role in the production of the syndrome. Particular attention should be given to the neuronal structures which lie within the area of distribution of both the posterior inferior cerebellar and vertebral arteries (Figs. 20-13 and 20-14).

CHAPTER 12

The Pons

The pons (metencephalon) represents the rostral part of the hindbrain. It consists of two distinctive parts: (1) a *dorsal portion*, the pontine tegmentum, and (2) a *ventral portion*, referred to as the pons proper (Fig. 12-1).

CAUDAL PONS

Dorsal Portion. The dorsal portion of the pons, known as the pontine tegmentum, is the rostral continuation of the medullary reticular formation. It contains cranial nerve nuclei, ascending and descending tracts and reticular nuclei (Fig. 12-1). Cranial nerve nuclei found in the pons are those of the V, VI, VII and VIII cranial nerves. The ascending tracts in this part of the brain stem are the same as those found in the medulla. The medial lemniscus occupies a different position than in the medulla and its configuration is changed. This large, flattened, elliptical bundle, present on each side of the median raphe, lies anteriorly, just above the ventral portion of the pons (Figs. 12-1 and 12-2). Crossing fibers of the trapezoid body traverse ventral parts of the bundle on each side. The medial longitudinal fasciculi (MLF) are situated dorsally on each side of the median raphe as in the medulla. The spinothalamic and anterior spinocerebellar tracts are difficult to distinguish but occupy positions in the anterolateral tegmentum. The spinal trigeminal tract and nucleus lie medial to the inferior cerebellar peduncle. The vestibular nuclei (i.e., medial and lateral) are present in the floor of the fourth ventricle, dorsal to the reticular formation (Fig. 12-2).

The pontine reticular formation is more extensive than the medullary reticular formation, but occupies a similar region. The medial two-thirds of the pontine reticular formation is represented by the pontine reticular nuclei (*nuclei reticularis pontis, pars caudalis* and *pars oralis;* Figs. 12-1 and 12-19) (Olszewski and Baxter, '54; Brodal, '57). The *pars caudalis* replaces the gigantocellular reticular nucleus of the medulla and extends rostrally to the level of the trigeminal motor nucleus (Fig. 12-3). The *pars oralis,* present in more rostral pontine levels, extends into the caudal mesencephalon (Fig. 12-19). The pontine reticular nuclei give rise to the pontine reticulospinal tract (Figs. 10-11 and 10-20). Lateral to the pars caudalis is a small-celled reticular nucleus (parvocellularis) similar to that described in the medulla. The median raphe contains the inferior central nucleus, and the subependymal area near the midline contains the nucleus of the *medial eminence* and the dorsal paramedian nucleus (Figs. 12-3 and 12-4).

The reticular formation posterolateral to the medial lemniscus contains a relatively large discrete bundle, the *central tegmental tract* (Figs. 12-1 and 12-4). This is a composite tract consisting of descending fibers from certain midbrain nuclei that project mainly to the inferior olivary complex, and ascending fibers from the lower

brain stem reticular formation that project
to certain thalamic nuclei.

In addition to the structures described,
the pontine tegmentum contains a number
of cranial nerve nuclei and nuclei related
to specific sensory systems. These include
the cochlear and vestibular components of
N. VIII, the motor and sensory components of the facial nerve, the abducens
nerve and large portions of the trigeminal
nuclear complex. Root fibers of the vestibulocochlear and facial nerves enter the caudal pons at the cerebellopontine angle
formed by the junction of the medulla,
pons and cerebellum (Fig. 11-19). Fibers of
the cochlear nerve root pass dorsally, lateral to the inferior cerebellar peduncle, to
terminate upon cells of both the dorsal and
ventral cochlear nuclei (Fig. 11-25). Vestibular root fibers, slightly medial and rostral
to those of the cochlear nerve, enter caudal
portions of the pons by passing between
the inferior cerebellar peduncle and the
spinal trigeminal tract (Figs. 12-2 and 12-
5). Primary vestibular fibers are distributed differentially within the vestibular
nuclear complex in the floor of the fourth
ventricle; a moderate number of vestibular
fibers project to specific parts of the cerebellum via the juxtarestiform body, a structure medial to the inferior cerebellar peduncle (Fig. 12-6). Ventral to the vestibular nerve are the intermediate and facial
nerves (Figs. 12-2 and 12-5). The intermediate nerve contains mainly special visceral
afferent (taste; SVA) and general visceral
efferent (parasympathetic; GVE) fibers.
The larger motor root of the facial nerve is
the most rostral and medial cranial nerve
in the cerebellopontine angle.

The *motor nucleus of N. VII* appears as
a pear-shaped gray mass in the lateral
part of the reticular formation immediately dorsal to the superior olive (Figs. 12-
1, 12-2 and 12-4). Within it may be seen the
usual plexus of fine terminals and the
coarser fibers which give origin to the facial root. The root fibers form a complicated intramedullary loop whose continuity cannot be seen in any one section (Figs.
12-1, 12-5, 12-6 and 12-7). Emerging as fine
bundles of fibers from the dorsal surface of
the nucleus, they pass dorsomedially to

the floor of the ventricle. There they form
a compact longitudinal bundle which ascends for a distance of about 2 mm, medial
to the abducens nucleus and dorsal to the
medial longitudinal fasciculus (Fig. 12-7).
At the cranial border of the abducens nucleus the bundle makes a sharp lateral
turn over the dorsal surface of the abducens nucleus, forming the *internal genu* of
the facial nerve (Fig. 12-15). Fibers of the
motor root of the facial nerve pass ventrolaterally, medial to the spinal trigeminal
complex, and emerge from the brain stem
near the caudal border of the pons (Fig. 11-
1).

The *abducens nucleus (N. VI)* is a
rounded gray cellular mass in the lateral
part of the medial eminence of the fourth
ventricle. Together with the genu of the
facial nerve, it forms the rounded prominence in the ventricular floor known as
the *colliculus facialis* (Figs. 12-1, 12-2, 12-3
and 12-7). Its root fibers exit from the medial surface of the abducens nucleus and
descend to emerge at the caudal border of
the pons (Figs. 11-1 and 12-1).

Ventral Portion. The ventral portion of
the pons is a massive structure consisting
of orderly arranged transverse and longitudinal fiber bundles between, and among,
which are large collections of pontine nuclei (Figs. 12-1, 12-3 and 12-4). Longitudinal fiber bundles coursing through the ventral portion of the pons are: (1) corticospinal, (2) corticobulbar, and (3) corticopontine (Figs. A-7, A-8 and A-9). The largest
groups of longitudinal fibers, the corticospinal tracts, traverse the pons, enter the
medullary pyramids, decussate incompletely and pass into the spinal cord (Figs.
10-13 and A-28). Corticobulbar fibers separate from the corticospinal tracts and enter
the reticular formation of the pontine tegmentum. Impulses pass to the motor cranial nerve nuclei directly and via intercalated neurons. While bundles of corticospinal fibers present a compact arrangement at rostral and caudal pontine levels,
in the middle regions of the pons these
bundles are broken up into a number of
small fascicles by transversely oriented
pontine fibers.

Other longitudinal fibers descending

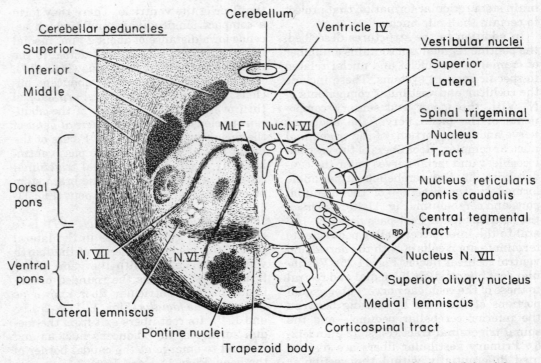

Fig. 12-1. Semidiagrammatic drawing of a transverse section of the pons at the level of the abducens nucleus. The dorsal portion of the pons, constituting the tegmentum, contains the reticular formation, cranial nerve nuclei and ascending and descending tracts. The ventral portion of the pons contains the pontine nuclei, massive bundles of corticofugal fibers and the transverse fibers of the pons which form the middle cerebellar peduncle.

from the cerebral cortex and terminating upon pontine nuclei are corticopontine fibers. These fibers arise from the cortex of the frontal (frontopontine), temporal (temporopontine), parietal (parietopontine) and occipital (occipitopontine) lobes, descend without crossing and end upon homolateral pontine nuclei. Corticopontine fibers from the primary sensorimotor cortex appear to be somatotopically organized and end upon circumscribed regions of the pontine nuclei (Brodal, '68). Each part of the cerebral cortex so far studied appears to give off fibers to several well defined areas within the pontine nuclei (Brodal, '72, '72a). The corticopontocerebellar pathway is quantitatively the most important route by which the cerebral cortex can influence the cerebellar cortex. These projection systems appear to be somatotopically organized in a precise manner. The corticopontine fibers are numerous in the upper portion of the pons, where they form bun-

dles difficult to distinguish from the pyramidal tracts (Figs. 12-18 and 12-23). Their number gradually diminishes as fibers terminate in the pontine nuclei. The corticopontine fibers and the transverse fibers to be described below do not become myelinated until some time after birth and are not distinguishable in brain sections of a 4-week infant stained by the Weigert technic (Fig. 12-2). They are shown in the adult pons in Figures 12-4, 12-7 and 12-23.

The transversely oriented fibers are axons of pontine nuclei (Fig. 12-3) which cross to the opposite side and form the massive *middle cerebellar peduncle*. These fibers pass dorsal and ventral to the corticospinal tract; the more dorsal fibers form the *deep layer,* while the more ventral ones constitute the *superficial layer* of the pons (Fig. A-26). Fibers of the middle cerebellar peduncle sweep dorsolaterally and somewhat caudally to enter the medullary core of the cerebellum superficial to

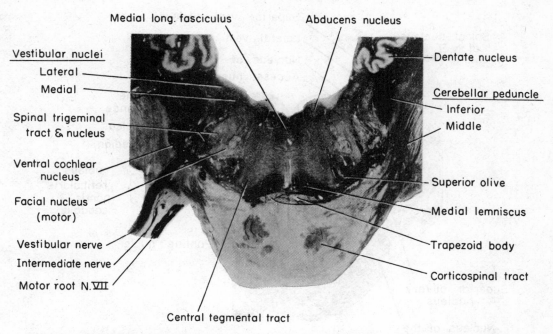

Medial long. fasciculus   Abducens nucleus

Vestibular nuclei
Lateral
Medial

Spinal trigeminal
tract & nucleus

Ventral cochlear
nucleus

Facial nucleus
(motor)

Vestibular nerve
Intermediate nerve
Motor root N. VII

Dentate nucleus

Cerebellar peduncle
Inferior
Middle

Superior olive

Medial lemniscus

Trapezoid body

Corticospinal tract

Central tegmental tract

FIG. 12-2. Slightly asymmetrical section of the pons of a 1-month infant. Root fibers of the vestibular and facial nerves are present on the left. Weigert's myelin stain. Photograph.

the inferior cerebellar peduncle. The ventral portion of the pons thus may be considered as a relay station in an extensive, phylogenetically new, two neuronal pathway from the cerebral cortex to the cerebellar cortex. The first neuron in the cerebral cortex projects an uncrossed corticopontine fiber to the pontine nuclei. The second pontine neuron sends a crossed pontocerebellar fiber to the cortex of the opposite cerebellar hemisphere via the middle cerebellar peduncle. In addition a small number of fibers from the superior colliculus (tectopontine fibers) descend ipsilaterally to terminate upon dorsolateral pontine nuclei (Altman and Carpenter, '61). These fibers and fibers from the pontine nuclei are considered to transmit optic impulses to restricted regions of the cerebellum.

The pontine nuclei are numerous, closely packed cellular aggregations situated between the transverse and longitudinal fibers (Fig. 12-3). In caudal regions the cells form a ring around the compact pyramidal tract, which more rostrally is broken up into smaller bundles by islands of pontine cells. In a general way the cells may be grouped into lateral, medial, dor-

sal and ventral nuclear masses (Fig. 12-7). In the lateral groups the polygonal cells are relatively large- or medium-sized; in the paramedian region they are smaller. Their dendrites ramify around adjacent cell bodies, and their axons, almost entirely crossed, form the middle cerebellar peduncle. Among these cells are found curiously shaped Golgi type II cells whose dendrites are beset with numerous hairlike processes, and whose short, branching axons terminate in the vicinity of the cell body.

Certain nuclei in the pontine tegmentum, like the reticulotegmental nucleus, project fibers into the ventral part of the pons which enter the cerebellum via the contralateral middle cerebellar peduncle (Figs. 12-19, 12-24, A-8 and A-9). The reticulotegmental nucleus is regarded by some as a tegmental extension of the pontine nuclei (Jacobson, '09).

VESTIBULOCOCHLEAR NERVE

The vestibulocochlear nerve (N. VIII) consists of two distinctive parts: (1) the cochlear part concerned with audition, and (2) the vestibular part conveying impulses

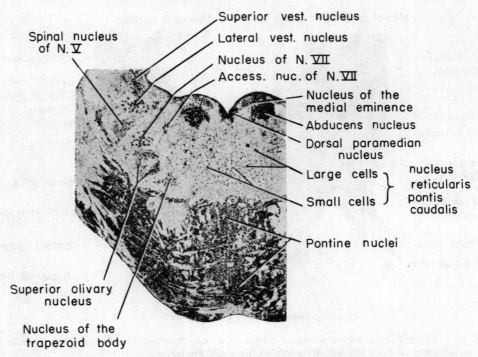

Spinal nucleus
of N. V

Superior vest. nucleus

Lateral vest. nucleus

Nucleus of N. VII

Access. nuc. of N. VII

Nucleus of the
medial eminence

Abducens nucleus

Dorsal paramedian
nucleus

Large cells ⎫ nucleus
          ⎬ reticularis
Small cells ⎭ pontis
             caudalis

Pontine nuclei

Superior olivary
nucleus

Nucleus of the
trapezoid body

FIG. 12-3. Section through pons and pontine tegmentum of 3-month infant at about same level as Figure 12-2. Cresyl violet. Photograph, with schematic representation of cell groups.

concerned with equilibrium and orientation in three-dimensional space. These two components of the vestibulocochlear nerve run together from the internal auditory meatus to the cerebellopontine angle, where they enter the brain stem (Figs. 11-1 and 11-19). Each of these nerves has distinctive central nuclei and connections.

The Cochlea. The cochlear portion of the labyrinth consists of a fluid-filled tube, coiled in a spiral of about two and a half turns, that serves as the auditory transducer (Fig. 12-8). The cochlea is partitioned by two membranes, the basilar membrane and vestibular (Reissner's) membrane, to form the scala vestibuli, the scala tympani and the cochlear duct (scala media). Energy from sound waves is transmitted to the base of the scala vestibuli (oval window) by the foot plate of the stapes. The round window is a flexible membrane at the base of the scala tympani. The cochlear duct contains the *organ of Corti;* the receptor organ consists of one row of inner hair cells and three rows of outer hair cells (Fig. 12-9). The tectorial

membrane, attached at one end to the spiral limbus, overlies the hair cells (Fig. 12-8). The basilar membrane is not under tension, but has a stiffness that varies 100-fold from one end to the other. This membrane is narrowest and stiffest at the base of the cochlea and widest and most pliable near the helicotrema (Goldstein, '68). Energy transmitted from fluid produces traveling waves in the basilar membrane that move from the base of the cochlea to the apex (Békésy, '60). Maximum displacement of the basilar membrane at different distances from the stapes can be correlated with specific sound frequencies. Displacement of the basilar membrane in response to an acoustic stimulus causes bending of hairs of the hair cells in contact with the tectorial membrane. The precise manner in which these forces produce excitation of primary auditory neurons is not known.

The Cochlear Nerve and Nuclei. The larger cochlear division of N. VIII enters the brain stem lateral and somewhat caudal to the vestibular division (Fig. 11-25). Its fibers originate in the *spiral ganglion,*

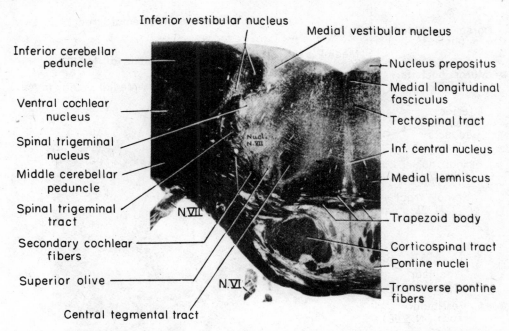

Inferior vestibular nucleus

Medial vestibular nucleus

Inferior cerebellar peduncle

Ventral cochlear nucleus

Spinal trigeminal nucleus

Middle cerebellar peduncle

Spinal trigeminal tract

Secondary cochlear fibers

Superior olive

Central tegmental tract

Nucleus prepositus

Medial longitudinal fasciculus

Tectospinal tract

Inf. central nucleus

Medial lemniscus

Trapezoid body

Corticospinal tract

Pontine nuclei

Transverse pontine fibers

N.VII

N.VI

FIG. 12-4. Transverse section of the adult pons at the level of emergence of the facial nerve root. Weigert's myelin stain. Photograph.

an aggregation of bipolar cells situated in the modiolus of the cochlea. The longer central processes of these cells form the cochlear nerve, while the short peripheral ones end in relation to the hair cells of the organ of Corti (Figs. 12-8 and 12-10). Fibers of the cochlear nerve terminate upon two nuclear masses, the *dorsal* and *ventral cochlear nuclei,* located on the lateral surface of the inferior cerebellar peduncle (Figs. 11-21, 11-25 and 12-10). Although the dorsal and ventral cochlear nuclei represent a more or less continuous cell mass dorsolateral and lateral to the inferior cerebellar peduncle, they have distinctive cells and cytoarchitectural organization. The dorsal cochlear nucleus forms an eminence on the most lateral portion of the ventricular floor known as the *acoustic tubercle* (Fig. 11-25). In most mammals this nucleus appears distinctly laminated in Nissl preparations (Powell and Erulkar, '62). Beneath the ependyma is a molecular layer of small round cells. Deep to this is a layer of spindle cells, two or three cells thick, regularly arranged with their long axes perpendicular to the surface. The innermost polymorphic layer is the thickest and

consists of sparsely distributed medium and relatively large pyramidal cells. In man the above described lamination is indistinct. Cells of the ventral cochlear nucleus are oval, or round, medium-sized cells with relatively large amounts of cytoplasm, fine evenly distributed Nissl substance and very short processes. There is no lamination as in the dorsal cochlear nucleus, but variations of cellular arrangement are present in different parts of the nucleus. Cells in medial portions of the nucleus are smaller, rounder, and more compactly arranged than in the lateral portion. In the cat the ventral cochlear nucleus has been divided into anterior and posterior parts on the basis of cellular arrangements (Rose et al., '59).

Primary Auditory Fibers. These fibers, representing the central processes of the spiral ganglion, enter the cochlear nuclei, bifurcate in an orderly sequence and are distributed to both dorsal and ventral cochlear nuclei (Lorente de Nóo, '33a). Experimental studies (Powell and Cowan, '62; Moskowitz and Liu, '72) indicate that after partial and complete lesions of the cochlea, degenerated fibers can be found in

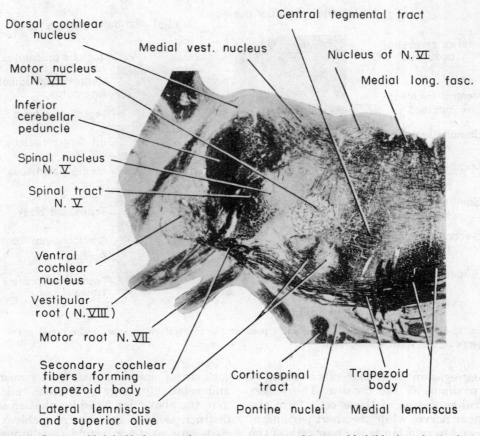

Dorsal cochlear nucleus

Central tegmental tract

Medial vest. nucleus

Nucleus of N. VI

Motor nucleus N. VII

Medial long. fasc.

Inferior cerebellar peduncle

Spinal nucleus N. V

Spinal tract N. V

Ventral cochlear nucleus

Vestibular root (N. VIII)

Motor root N. VII

Secondary cochlear fibers forming trapezoid body

Corticospinal tract

Trapezoid body

Lateral lemniscus and superior olive

Pontine nuclei

Medial lemniscus

FIG. 12-5. Section of left half of pons and pontine tegmentum of 3-year-old child whose brain showed a complete absence of the left cerebellar hemisphere and middle cerebellar peduncle. The origin of the trapezoid fibers from the ventral cochlear nucleus is clearly shown. Note also fibers of the dorsal acoustic stria passing into the tegmentum from the dorsal cochlear nucleus (Strong, '15). Weigert's myelin stain. Photograph.

both parts of the cochlear nuclear complex. Fibers to the dorsal cochlear nucleus terminate about cells in the deep polymorphic layer and on the deep dendrites of the spindle cells. In the ventral cochlear nucleus, cochlear fibers end in fine pericellular plexuses and boutons surrounding cell somata (Rasmussen, '57).

One of the characteristic features of the auditory system is the pattern of *tonotopic localization* evident at various levels. In the cochlea it has been shown that high tones are received in the basal coils, while the apical portion is sensitive to low frequencies (Crowe, '35; Tasaki, '54). Anatomical studies suggest that apical cochlear fibers terminate in ventral parts of the dorsal cochlear nucleus and in the ventral

nucleus, while fibers from basal portions of the cochlea end in the dorsal part of the dorsal cochlear nucleus (Lewy and Kobrak, '36). Physiological evidence (Rose et al., '59; Rose, '60), based upon microelectrode studies of frequency sensitive neurons in the cochlear nuclear complex, indicates that each major division possesses its own frequency sequence, and that each division seems to have a full tonal spectrum. In all three divisions of the cochlear complex in the cat (i.e., dorsal nucleus and anterior and posterior parts of the ventral nucleus) neurons responding to higher frequencies are dorsal, while those responding to lower frequencies are ventral. Thus there appears to be multiple tonotopic representation in the cochlear nuclear com-

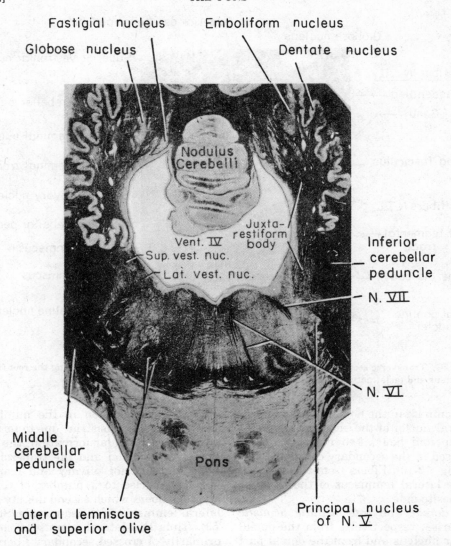

Fastigial nucleus   Emboliform nucleus

Globose nucleus   Dentate nucleus

Nodulus Cerebelli

Juxta-restiform body

Vent. IV

Sup. vest. nuc.

Lat. vest. nuc.

Inferior cerebellar peduncle

N. VII

N. VI

Middle cerebellar peduncle

Pons

Lateral lemniscus and superior olive

Principal nucleus of N. V

Fig. 12-6. Transverse section of the pons, pontine tegmentum and portions of the cerebellum at the level of the abducens nuclei. One-month infant. Weigert's myelin stain. Photograph.

plex which suggests that primary cochlear fibers bifurcate and terminate in an orderly dorsoventral sequence throughout the complex.

Auditory Pathways. Secondary auditory pathways in the brain stem are exceedingly complex and many details regarding their exact composition and course are uncertain. Most of the available information concerning these pathways is based upon studies in animals. Secondary auditory fibers arising from the dorsal and ventral cochlear nuclei are grouped into

three acoustic striae (Barnes et al., '43; Ades, '59). The *ventral acoustic stria* arises from the ventral cochlear nucleus (Strominger and Strominger, '71), and courses medially along the ventral border of the pontine tegmentum to form the trapezoid body (Figs. 12-5 and 12-10). Many of these fibers pass through or ventral to the medial lemniscus, cross the raphe and reach the dorsolateral border of the opposite *superior olive*, where they turn upward to form a longitudinal ascending bundle known as the *lateral lemniscus*. Other trapezoid fi-

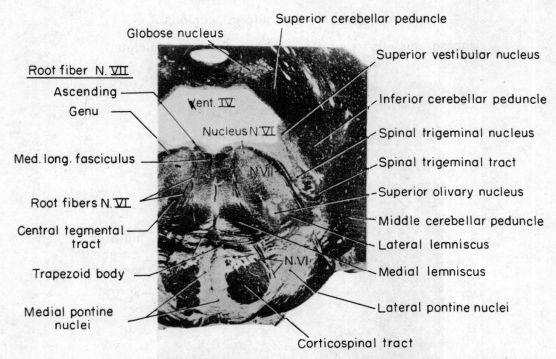

Globose nucleus

Superior cerebellar peduncle

Root fiber N. VII

Ascending

Genu

Med. long. fasciculus

Root fibers N. VII

Central tegmental tract

Trapezoid body

Medial pontine nuclei

Vent. IV

Nucleus N VI

N VII

N. VI

Superior vestibular nucleus

Inferior cerebellar peduncle

Spinal trigeminal nucleus

Spinal trigeminal tract

Superior olivary nucleus

Middle cerebellar peduncle

Lateral lemniscus

Medial lemniscus

Lateral pontine nuclei

Corticospinal tract

FIG. 12-7. Transverse section of the adult pons through the abducens nucleus showing the root fibers of the abducens and facial nerves. Weigert's myelin stain. Photograph.

bers terminate in the homolateral and contralateral nuclei of the superior olive and the trapezoid body, two nuclear masses interposed in the secondary cochlear pathway (Fig. 12-10). Fibers from these nuclei join the lateral lemniscus of the same or the opposite side.

The *dorsal* and *intermediate acoustic striae* arise, respectively, from the dorsal cochlear nucleus and from the dorsal part of the ventral cochlear nucleus. Both of these striae pass medially dorsal to the inferior cerebellar peduncle (Fig. 12-10). The dorsal stria crosses the median raphe ventral to the medial longitudinal fasciculus and fibers pass ventrally to join the lateral lemniscus of the opposite side. Fibers of the intermediate stria course medially through the reticular formation in an intermediate position, cross the midline and enter the contralateral lateral lemniscus. The dorsal stria is larger than the intermediate stria and the ventral stria is larger than the other two combined. In their passage through the tegmentum

there is a diminution in the number of fibers in the various striae due to terminations in the reticular formation, the superior olivary nuclei and the trapezoid nuclei. The superior olivary and trapezoid nuclei give rise to a number of tertiary auditory fibers which ascend mainly in the lateral lemniscus of the same side (Stotler, '53). Thus the lateral lemniscus consists primarily of crossed secondary fibers contributed by the three auditory striae and tertiary fibers from the superior olive and trapezoid nuclei. No direct fibers from the cochlear nuclei ascend in the ipsilateral lateral lemniscus (Barnes et al., '43). The number of ascending fibers in the lateral lemniscus is small compared with the total number of fibers arising from the dorsal and ventral cochlear nuclei.

The *trapezoid body* forms a conspicuous bundle of transverse fibers in the ventral part of the pontine tegmentum (Figs. 12-4, 12-5 and 12-7). These fibers arise principally from the ventral cochlear nucleus and, in a gentle arc, sweep medially toward the raphe. Most of these fibers cross to the opposite side, passing through or ventral to the medial lemniscus, and reach the ventrolateral portion of the tegmentum. Here they turn sharply in a longitudinal direction to form a new ascending fiber bundle, the lateral lemniscus (Fig. 12-10). The turn is made just dorsolateral to a nuclear mass known as the *superior olive* (Figs. 12-7 and A-27). This is a cellular column, about 4 mm long, extending from the level of the facial nucleus to the motor nucleus of the trigeminal nerve; it is in close contact ventrally with the lateral portion of the trapezoid body. It contains several distinct cell groups: an S-shaped principal nucleus composed of medium-sized polygonal cells, and a wedge-shaped medial accessory nucleus of closely packed somewhat larger fusiform cells (Figs. 12-3 and 12-4). The superior olive receives collaterals of secondary cochlear fibers and contributes fibers to the trapezoid body and lateral lemniscus. The medial accessory superior olivary nucleus receives afferents bilaterally from the anteroventral cochlear nuclei and gives rise to fibers that ascend in the ipsilateral lateral lemniscus (Stotler, '53; Osen, '69). From the dorsal surface of the medial accessory olivary nucleus a bundle of fibers, the *peduncle of the superior olive,* passes dorsomedially toward the abducens nucleus (Figs. 12-2 and A-7).

Other smaller cellular aggregations related to the trapezoid body are difficult to see in Weigert preparations (Fig. 12-5). They include the *trapezoid nucleus*, which is scattered among the trapezoid fibers medial to the superior olive, and the *internal* and *external preolivary nuclei*, which lie ventral to the superior olive. All these nuclei appear to be intercalated cell groups in the secondary auditory pathways (Fig. A-7).

The *lateral lemniscus*, the principal ascending auditory pathway in the brain stem, courses rostrally in the lateral part of the tegmentum. Initially this bundle lies lateral to the superior olivary complex (Figs. 12-7 and 12-10), but at isthmus levels its position is more dorsal (Fig. 12-23). Interposed in the course of the lateral

lemniscus in the upper portion of the pons are other more diffuse cellular aggregations which constitute the *nucleus of the lateral lemniscus* (Figs. 12-10 and 12-23). To these the lemniscus contributes some terminals, or at least collaterals, and probably receives additional fibers from them. The lateral lemniscus then reaches the midbrain, where most of the fibers terminate either directly, or by collaterals, in the inferior colliculus. Some fibers may reach the colliculus of the opposite side through the commissure of the inferior colliculi. The small number of remaining fibers in the lateral lemniscus may project directly to the medial geniculate body (Woollard and Harpman, '40). Thus fibers from the inferior colliculus, and possibly a few from the lateral lemniscus, constitute the *brachium of the inferior colliculus* (Fig. 12-10).

It is evident from the above that the auditory pathway receives contributions from a number of intercalated nuclear masses and has a more complex composition than sensory systems considered heretofore; it also has a considerable ipsilateral component consisting of ascending fibers arising mainly from the superior olivary complex. It is difficult to state the number of neurons involved in the auditory pathway from periphery to cortex, but the principal ones are: (1) cells of the spiral ganglion whose central processes form the cochlear nerve, (2) secondary fibers from the dorsal and ventral cochlear nuclei which form the three auditory striae and contribute primarily crossed fibers to the lateral lemniscus, (3) the nuclei of the superior olivary complex and the trapezoid body that contribute to the lateral lemnisci, (4) the nucleus of the lateral lemniscus which receives and contributes fibers to the bundle of the same name, (5) the inferior colliculus which receives fibers from the lateral lemniscus and projects via its brachium to the medial geniculate body, and (6) the medial geniculate body, which gives rise to geniculocortical fibers (auditory radiation) that project to the transverse temporal gyri of Heschl (Figs. 2-7 and 12-10). Whether the fibers contributed by all of these nuclei convey impulses

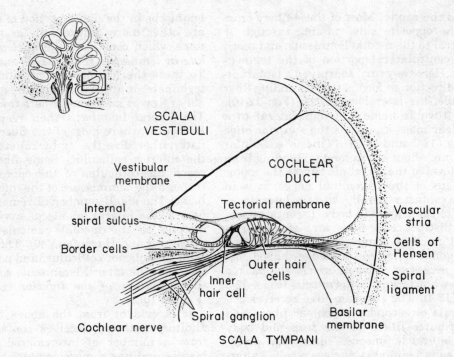

SCALA
VESTIBULI

Vestibular
membrane

COCHLEAR
DUCT

Internal
spiral sulcus

Tectorial membrane

Vascular
stria

Border cells

Cells of
Hensen

Outer hair
cells

Inner
hair cell

Spiral
ligament

Cochlear nerve

Spiral ganglion

Basilar
membrane

SCALA TYMPANI

Fig. 12-8. Drawing of a radial section through the cochlea showing the cochlear duct, the basilar membrane, the organ of Corti and the tectorial membrane. The small *diagram in the upper left* is an axial section of the cochlea. The *area enclosed in the rectangle* is reproduced in detail in the large drawing.

which ultimately reach the cerebral cortex remains undetermined. There is evidence (Winkler, '21) that some crossed fibers in the dorsal and intermediate acoustic striae may pass directly to the medial geniculate body. Most of the auditory impulses reaching the auditory cortex are conveyed by higher order neurons. Physiological studies indicate a definite tonotopic localization in the inferior colliculus (Rose et al., '63). Although there has been little evidence of a tonotopic organization in the medial geniculate body (Whitfield, '67), recent studies in the cat indicate a clear tonotopic organization (Aitkin and Webster, '71). In the medial geniculate body low frequencies are perceived laterally and high frequencies are represented medially in the principal division. Physiological data concerning the tonotopic representation of auditory impulses at the cortical level are discussed in Chapter 19.

Because of the large number of intercalated nuclei in the course of the auditory pathway (i.e., superior olive, trapezoid nu-

cleus, nucleus of the lateral lemniscus, inferior colliculus), the reflex cochlear connections are exceedingly complex. It seems likely that all of the relay nuclei along the auditory pathway are involved to some degree in reflex circuits by which various motor phenomena occur in response to cochlear stimulation. Experimental evidence suggests that a descending conduction system, from the auditory cortex to the cochlea (Rasmussen, '60), is associated with the classical ascending auditory system.

Efferent Cochlear Bundle. One of the most interesting cochlear reflex connections is the *olivocochlear bundle* or the *efferent cochlear bundle* described by Rasmussen ('46, '53). Crossed and uncrossed components of the olivocochlear bundle project from the brain stem to the cochlea in a number of vertebrates, including man, and form a pathway by which the central nervous system may influence its own sensory input (Rasmussen, '60; Gacek, '61). Electrical stimulation of the

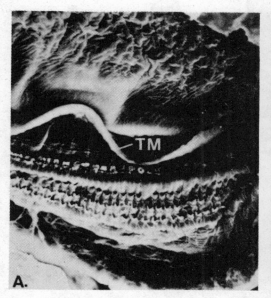 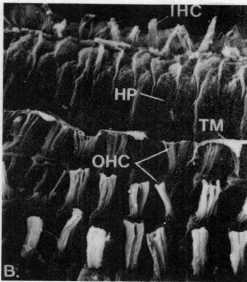

FIG. 12-9. Scanning electron micrographs of the cochlea of the rhesus monkey. *A*, View of the basal coil of the cochlea with the tectorial membrane (*TM*) reflected back. ×450. *B*, Surface view of the hair cells of the cochlea after removal of the tectorial membrane (*TM*), except for fragments attached to outer hair cells (*OHC*). *IHC*, inner hair cells; *HP*, head plate of inner pillar. ×2,100 (Rivera-Dominguez et al., '73).

crossed olivocochlear bundle in the cat results in a reduction of auditory nerve fiber responses to acoustic stimuli (Galambos, '56). Fibers of the crossed olivocochlear bundle in the cat arise from the region dorsal to the medial accessory superior olive (the medial periolivary nucleus), pass dorsally in the pontine tegmentum and cross the midline beneath the genu of the facial nerve (Fig. 12-11). Contralaterally these fibers emerge from the brain stem in association with the vestibular nerve. In the inner ear, fibers of this bundle pass via the vestibulocochlear anastomosis into the cochlear nerve and traverse the cochlear spirals before projecting into the organ of Corti (Rasmussen, '53). The uncrossed fibers of the olivocochlear bundle appear to arise from the region dorsal to the superior olive (the lateral periolivary nucleus) and join fibers of the crossed bundle in the ipsilateral vestibular nerve (Luk et al., '74). In the cat approximately 20% of the fibers in the olivocochlear bundle are uncrossed (Rasmussen, '60). Peripherally crossed and uncrossed fibers of the olivocochlear bundle make synaptic contact with the outer hair cells (Kimura and Wersäll, '62; Spoendlin and Gacek, '63;

Smith and Rasmussen, '63, '65). Certain efferent axons also enter the inner spiral bundle and appear to synapse with spiral ganglion fibers beneath the inner hair cells (Spoendlin, '66; Smith, '67). There are indications from electron micrographic studies that some fibers of the olivocochlear bundle are unmyelinated (Terayama and Yamamoto, '71). Recent studies of the origins of the crossed fibers of the olivocochlear bundle in the cat utilizing an acid phosphatase method suggest that these fibers arise from the dorsomedial periolivary nucleus, the ventral trapezoid nucleus and portions of the medial trapezoid nucleus (Luk et al., '74).

In addition to the efferent cochlear bundle, which represents essentially an inhibitory feedback system to the primary sensory receptor, other evidence (Rasmussen, '64) indicates that the cochlear nuclei receive descending efferent fibers from various relay nuclei in the auditory pathway. Structures giving rise to these fibers include the inferior colliculus, the nuclei of the lateral lemniscus and the principal superior olive. These descending pathways may inhibit impulses concerned with certain frequencies of the auditory spectrum

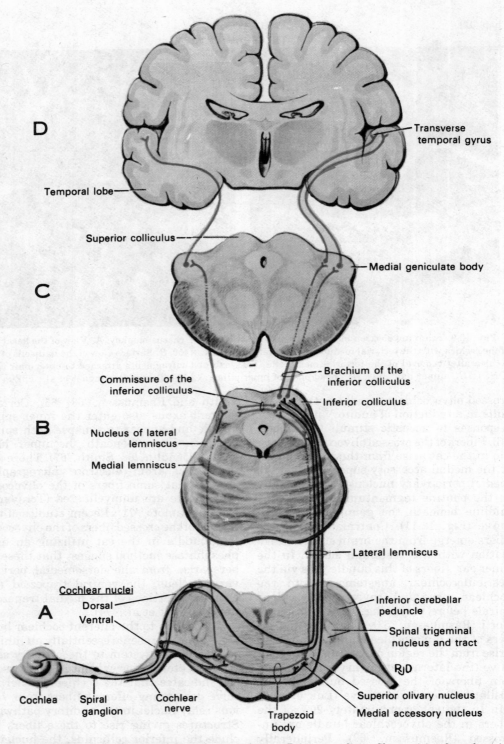

FIG. 12-10. Schematic diagram of the auditory pathways. Primary auditory fibers arising from the spiral ganglion are in *black*. Secondary auditory fibers arising from the dorsal and ventral cochlear nuclei and forming the acoustic striae are in *red*. Auditory fibers arising from relay nuclei are in *blue*. *A*, Medulla; *B*, level of inferior colliculus; *C*, level of superior colliculus; *D*, transverse section through the cerebral hemisphere. (From Carpenter, *Core Text of Neuroanatomy*, '72; courtesy of The Williams & Wilkins Company.)

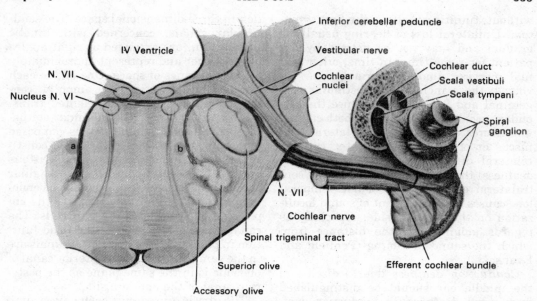

FIG. 12-11. Schematic drawing of efferent cochlear bundle in the cat. Crossed fibers of the olivocochlear bundle (*red, a*) arise dorsal to the accessory superior olivary nucleus, pass dorsomedially toward the floor of the fourth ventricle and cross to the opposite side. Uncrossed fibers of the olivocochlear bundle (*red, b*) arise dorsal to the superior olivary nucleus, join the crossed fibers and pass peripherally in association with the vestibular nerve. Peripherally efferent cochlear fibers join the cochlear nerve via the vestibulocochlear anastomosis and are distributed to the hair cells of the cochlea (modified from Rasmussen, '60).

and in this way result in a relative enhancement of those impulses not subject to inhibition. This phenomenon is referred to as auditory sharpening.

Additional secondary and higher order auditory fibers enter the brain stem reticular formation and may be involved in reflex closing of the eyes and turning of the head in response to a loud noise. Other acoustic reflex mechanisms involve middle ear muscles, such as the stapedius and tensor tympani, which serve as regulators of auditory input to the cochlea. Both of these reflex pathways involve neurons of the ventral cochlear nucleus, the trapezoid body and the medial superior olive (Borg, '73). In the reflex involving the stapedius muscle, fibers from the medial accessory superior olive project bilaterally to facial motor neurons. Contractions of the stapedius muscle serve to dampen the oscillations of the ear ossicles. In the reflex involving the tensor tympani muscle, fibers from the medial accessory superior olive project bilaterally to trigeminal motor neurons that innervate that muscle. The threshold for the tensor tympani reflex is

relatively high and its significance in man is obscure.

The nucleus of the lateral lemniscus gives rise to fibers which decussate and enter the inferior colliculus of the opposite side. The inferior colliculi are interconnected via commissural fibers and probably some fibers project to the superior colliculi. Recent physiological studies (Rose et al., '66) suggest that some neurons of the inferior colliculus are sensitive to interaural time relationships of binaurally applied stimuli, while others are sensitive to small interaural intensity differences. These data indicate that certain neurons in the inferior colliculus may be concerned with the localization of a sound source.

Lesions of the Auditory System. Destruction of the cochlear nerve, or of both cochlear nuclei, causes complete *deafness* on the same side. Among the more common disorders is the so-called acoustic neurinoma, a perineural fibroblastoma that probably arises from cells of the Schwann sheath. Although this benign tumor probably originates from the vestibular portion of the eighth nerve, loss of hearing with, or without, tinnitis usually is the first symptom. Unilateral loss of hearing usually is gradual and may not be noticed by the patient for some time. In time, other cranial nerves almost invariably are involved; these include the vestibular, trigeminal and facial nerves. Since the secondary cochlear pathways are both crossed and uncrossed, lesions of one lateral lemniscus or of the auditory cortex cause a bilateral diminution of hearing (partial deafness) that is most marked in the contralateral ear. Removal of one temporal lobe causes an impairment of sound localization on the opposite side, especially as regards judgment of the distance from which the sound is coming (Penfield and Evans, '32).

Conduction deafness due to disease of the middle ear should be distinguished from nerve deafness. In conduction deafness the ossicular chain fails to transmit vibrations from the tympanum to the oval window and to the scala vestibuli and scala media (i.e., cochlear duct; Fig. 12-8). When the ossicular chain is broken, vibrations of the tympanum pass via the air of the middle ear to the round window; this is inefficient because it lacks the impedence matching of the ossicular chain and most of the sound energy is lost. Hearing loss due to interruption of the ossicular chain ranges from 30 decibels for low tones to 65 decibels in the middle range. Fixation of the ossicular chain resulting from middle ear infections, or otosclerosis, is more common than interruptions of the ossicular chain. In *otosclerosis* even air conduction via the round window is impaired because this membrane is thickened. Early in the course of the disease patients with otosclerosis have either a loss of appreciation of low tones, or a mild loss in the entire auditory range. Later there is a marked perceptive deficit for high tones. Tinnitus, without vertigo, is common, and many patients hear better in the presence of loud noises (*paracusis*).

The Labyrinth. The vestibular portion of the inner ear consists of three *semicircular canals*, the *utricle* and the *saccule* (Fig. 12-12). Receptors in these structures are concerned with equilibrium, and orienta-

tion in three-dimensional space. The semicircular canals, concerned with kinetic equilibrium, are arranged at right angles to each other and represent approximately the three planes of space. One end of each canal has a dilatation, the ampulla, containing a ridge or crista oriented transversely to the canal. The columnar epithelium of the *crista ampullaris* is composed of neuroepithelial hair cells which constitute the vestibular receptor. Each crista is covered by a gelatinous cupula. Angular acceleration causes displacement of endolymphatic fluid and movement of the cupula which stimulates the hair cells. The canals on opposite sides of the head function in pairs (i.e., the horizontal canals are in the same plane and the anterior canal of one side is in the same plane as the posterior canal of the opposite side).

The utricle and saccule each have a similar patch of sensory epithelium, the *macula utriculi* and *macula sacculi*, but here the hair cells are in contact with a gelatinous covering containing small calcareous concretions or particles, the *otoliths*. The utricle and saccule together constitute the so-called "otolith organ."

The cristae of the semicircular canals are stimulated by rotatory movement (i.e., angular acceleration) which causes movement of endolymphatic fluid and deflection of hairs of the sensory epithelium. Endolymphatic flow is greatest in the pair of canals most nearly perpendicular to the axis of rotation. The utricular macula, concerned primarily with static equilibrium, responds to changes in gravitational forces, and to linear acceleration. Macular impulses convey information regarding the position of the head in space, the hair cells being stimulated by the otolithic particles, whose position varies under the influence of gravity. The functional role of the saccular macula in static equilibrium has not been resolved. Destruction of the sacculae does not produce detectable disturbance in the rabbit (Versteegh, '27) or in the frog (Tait and MacNally, '25). The experiments of Ashcroft and Hallpike ('34) demonstrated that the nerve from the saccular macula in the frog did not respond to tilting or rotation, but did respond accurately to vibration. These data have been interpreted as indicating that the saccule in man may be concerned with the reception of vibratory stimuli. Recent physiological studies of peripheral otolithic neurons in the monkey suggest that the saccule may have an equilibratory function (Fernandez et al., '72). Saccular neurons appear sensitive to dorsoventral accelerations, while utricular neurons are most sensitive to accelerations in a horizontal plane. Saccular afferents have a lower resting discharge and a lower sensitivity than utricular afferents.

Anatomical studies (Lorente de Nó, '33a; Stein and Carpenter, '67) show that the nerve fibers from the saccular macula do not join the cochlear nerve and that they are distributed to the vestibular nuclei in a manner similar to that of nerve fibers from the utricular macula and the semicircular canals.

The Vestibular Nerve and Nuclei. The maculae and cristae are innervated by cells of the vestibular ganglion (ganglion of Scarpa), an aggregation of bipolar cells located in the internal auditory meatus. The vestibular ganglion can be divided into superior and inferior vestibular ganglia which are connected by a narrow isthmus (Fig. 12-12). The shorter peripheral processes of these cells go to the receptor cells of the maculae and cristae; the longer central processes form the vestibular nerve. Cells of the superior vestibular ganglion innervate the cristae of the anterior and lateral semicircular canals and the macula of the utricle. Cells of the smaller inferior vestibular ganglion innervate the crista of the posterior semicircular canal and the macula of the saccule (Stein and Carpenter, '67; Carpenter et al., '72). The vestibular nerve enters the cerebellopontine angle medial to the cochlear nerve. Vestibular root fibers pass dorsally between the inferior cerebellar peduncle and the spinal trigeminal tract, and bifurcate into short ascending and long descending branches which are distributed to the vestibular nuclei (Figs. 11-18 and 12-13). Some primary vestibular fibers (i.e., root fibers) continue without interruption to particular parts of the cerebellum; these fibers

reach the ipsilateral half of the cerebellum via the juxtarestiform body (Fig. 12-6) and project mainly to the cortex of the nodulus, uvula and flocculus (Brodal and Høivik, '64; Carpenter et al., '72). The largest number of primary vestibular fibers terminate differentially in the four vestibular nuclei in the floor of the fourth ventricle (Fig. 12-14). The vestibular nuclei are the inferior, lateral, medial and superior. Because of the long rostrocaudal extent of the vestibular nuclei, usually only two nuclei can be seen in any one transverse section (Figs. 12-13, 12-14, A-4, A-5 and A-6).

The *inferior vestibular nucleus* begins caudally in the medulla medial to the accessory cuneate nucleus and extends rostrally medial to the inferior cerebellar peduncle to the point near the entrance of the vestibular nerve root (Fig. 12-4). Cytoarchitecturally the nucleus is composed of small- and medium-sized cells except in its most rostral part, where scattered large cells resemble those of the lateral vestibular nucleus. In the ventrolateral and caudal parts of the nucleus, a number of rather large cells form several densely packed groups. These cells (*group f* of Brodal and Pompeiano, '57) are of particular interest because they do not receive primary vestibular fibers and many of them project fibers to the cerebellum. In fiber-stained sections, the inferior vestibular nucleus is characterized by bundles of longitudinally oriented fibers, part of which are descending primary vestibular fibers. These descending fiber bundles facilitate the delineation of the inferior and medial vestibular nuclei (Figs. 11-22 and 12-4).

The *lateral vestibular nucleus* (Deiters' nucleus), located laterally in the ventricular floor at the level of entrance of the vestibular nerve, extends rostrally to the level of the abducens nucleus. This nucleus is characterized by multipolar giant cells with coarse Nissl granules. Although most of the cells of this nucleus are regarded as giant cells, considerable variations in cell size are found (Fig. 12-3). The nucleus also contains varying types of smaller cells. Cells of all sizes are intermingled throughout the nucleus except in a small dorsolateral protrusion that consists

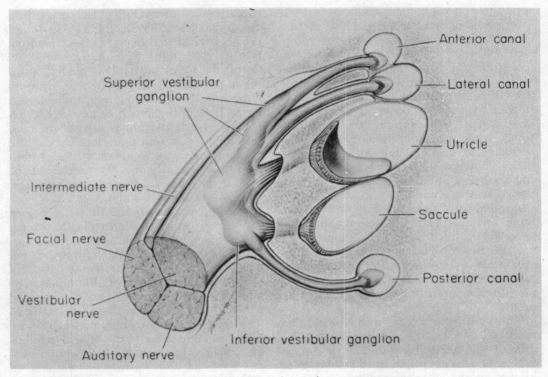

Fig. 12-12. Semischematic drawing of the vestibular ganglia and peripheral branches innervating anatomically distinctive portions of the labyrinth. Cells in the superior vestibular ganglion are arranged in a spiral fashion. Cells in the superior and distal portion of this ganglion innervate the cristae of the anterior and lateral semicircular canals. The broader proximal part of the superior vestibular ganglion contains cells which innervate the macula of the utricle. Cells of the inferior vestibular ganglion innervate the macula of the saccule and the crista of the posterior semicircular canal. The superior and inferior vestibular ganglia are joined by an isthmus of cells. The relationships between the facial, intermediate, vestibular and auditory nerves are shown on the left (Stein and Carpenter, '67).

only of medium-sized cells. There are some regional differences in the relative number and size of giant cells, which are most abundant in the caudal part of the nucleus.

The *medial vestibular nucleus* occupies the floor of the fourth ventricle medial to the inferior and lateral vestibular nuclei (Figs. 12-4 and 12-13). Its rostral and caudal boundaries are indistinct. Rostrally it fuses dorsolaterally with the superior vestibular nucleus.

Cells of the medial vestibular nucleus are small- and medium-sized, closely packed and fairly evenly distributed. Dorsolaterally some of the larger cells resemble those of the lateral vestibular nucleus, although none are true giant cells. The medial and inferior vestibular nuclei can

be distinguished readily at all levels in myelin-stained preparations because bundles of longitudinally coursing fibers are not present in the medial vestibular nucleus (Fig. 12-4).

The *superior vestibular nucleus* lies dorsal and mostly rostral to the lateral vestibular nucleus in the angle formed by the floor and the lateral wall of the fourth ventricle (Figs. 12-1 and 12-6). The superior cerebellar peduncle forms the dorsolateral border of the nucleus throughout most of its rostrocaudal extent. The mesencephalic and principal sensory nuclei of the trigeminal nerve are adjacent to the nucleus medially and ventrally, in its rostral two-thirds. The rostral pole of the nucleus is difficult to delimit. Cells of this nucleus are loosely scattered, medium- and small-

VESTIBULAR NUCLEI   VESTIBULAR GANGLIA

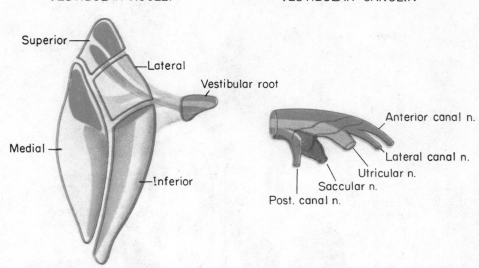

FIG. 12-13. Diagrammatic representation of the relationships between portions of the vestibular ganglia and central fibers projecting to parts of the vestibular nuclear complex. The vestibular ganglia are shown in a modified transverse plane, while the vestibular nerve root and the vestibular nuclear complex are drawn in a stylized fashion, as they would appear in horizontal sections of the brain stem. Only the principal central projections of distinctive parts of the vestibular ganglia are shown. Portions of the vestibular ganglia innervating the cristae of the semicircular canals (*red*) project primarily to the superior vestibular nucleus and rostral parts of the medial vestibular nucleus. Portions of the superior vestibular ganglion (*yellow*) innervating the macula of the utricle project central fibers primarily to parts of the inferior and medial vestibular nuclei. Fibers from portions of the inferior vestibular ganglion innervating the macula of the saccule (*blue*) project mainly to dorsolateral parts of the inferior vestibular nucleus. Some cells in the vestibular ganglia project fibers to parts of all vestibular nuclei, so that each part of the labyrinth has a unique as well as common projection, within the vestibular nuclear complex (Stein and Carpenter, '67).

sized, and round or spindle-shaped. Larger stellate cells in the central part of the nucleus form clusters.

Besides the main vestibular nuclei described above, there are several smaller accessory nuclei (Brodal and Pompeiano, '57), one of which consists of strands of cells between the root fibers of the vestibular nerve (interstitial nucleus of the vestibular nerve; Fig. 12-14).

Primary Vestibular Fibers. These fibers project to all four vestibular nuclei and the interstitial nucleus of the vestibular nerve, but their distribution is differential (Fig. 12-13). Upon entering the brain stem, primary vestibular fibers bifurcate into ascending and descending branches. Ascending branches supply the superior vestibular nucleus, rostral parts of the medial vestibular nucleus, and give off collaterals to the ventral part of the lateral ves-

tibular nucleus. Descending branches form the so-called descending root of the vestibular nerve, which provides fibers to the inferior vestibular nucleus and collaterals to the caudal parts of the medial vestibular nucleus (Stein and Carpenter, '67). Quantitatively the largest number of primary vestibular fibers pass to the inferior vestibular nucleus. Vestibular terminals are not distributed equally to all of the regions of the vestibular nuclei. Certain areas in each of the vestibular nuclei do not receive primary vestibular fibers (Walberg et al., '58). In the superior vestibular nucleus, primary vestibular fibers terminate mainly in the central regions of the nucleus. In the lateral vestibular nucleus, primary vestibular fibers are found only in the ventral parts of the nucleus. Electron microscopic findings confirm that these fibers establish synaptic contact primarily

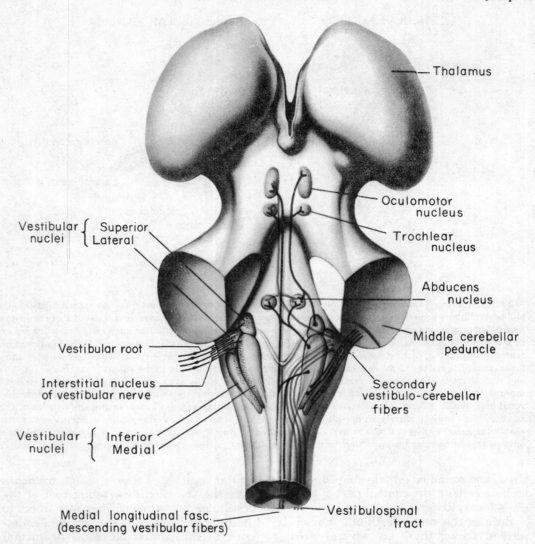

Thalamus

Oculomotor
nucleus

Trochlear
nucleus

Vestibular ⎰ Superior
nuclei ⎱ Lateral

Abducens
nucleus

Middle cerebellar
peduncle

Vestibular root

Secondary
vestibulo-cerebellar
fibers

Interstitial nucleus
of vestibular nerve

Vestibular ⎰ Inferior
nuclei ⎱ Medial

Medial longitudinal fasc.
(descending vestibular fibers)

Vestibulospinal
tract

FIG. 12-14. Schematic diagram of some of the principal fiber projections of the vestibular system. On the *left* the relationships and spatial disposition of the four main vestibular nuclei are indicated. Among the afferent root fibers are the cells of the interstitial nucleus of the vestibular nerve. *Dotted areas* in the vestibular nuclei represent the regions of the nuclear complex which receive the largest number of primary vestibular fibers. These areas are: (1) the ventral half of the lateral vestibular nucleus, (2) the lateral part of the medial vestibular nucleus, (3) the dorsomedial part of the inferior vestibular nucleus, and (4) the central part of the superior vestibular nucleus.

On the *right* the course of secondary vestibular fibers from individual nuclei is shown. Fibers from the superior vestibular nucleus (*red*) ascend ipsilaterally in the medial longitudinal fasciculus (MLF). Ascending fibers from the lateral vestibular nucleus (*blue*) appear to be largely crossed and ascend in the MLF. Descending projections from the lateral vestibular nucleus (*blue*) form the vestibulospinal tract. Fibers from the medial vestibular nucleus (*black*) enter the MLF and partially ascend and descend. Although ascending fibers in the MLF from this nucleus are shown as totally crossed, uncrossed fibers also are present. Descending fibers from the medial vestibular nucleus enter the MLF on both sides, but fibers in this bundle which project to spinal levels are mainly uncrossed.

Secondary vestibulocerebellar fibers (*black*) arise from caudal parts of the inferior and medial vestibular nuclei.

with the soma and dendritic stems of small cells (Mugnaini et al., '67). The large giant cells receive fewer synaptic endings from primary vestibular fibers. The dorsal half of the lateral vestibular nucleus is the largest regional area in this nuclear complex that is devoid of primary vestibular fibers (Lorente de Nö, '33a; Walberg et al., '58; Stein and Carpenter, '67). The medial vestibular nucleus receives primary vestibular fibers throughout large regions of its rostral part, but caudally terminations are mainly in lateral regions near the inferior vestibular nucleus (Fig. 12-13). Primary vestibular fibers are found throughout the rostrocaudal extent of the inferior vestibular nucleus, except in its ventrolateral part (Figs. 12-13 and 12-14). Of the so-called accessory vestibular nuclei, only the interstitial nucleus of the vestibular nerve receives primary vestibular fibers.

Studies of the central projections of cell groups of the vestibular ganglia that innervate distinctive parts of the labyrinth indicate a specific organization (Stein and Carpenter, '67). This organization in the monkey was determined by producing small lesions in specific parts of the vestibular ganglia and tracing degeneration: (1) distally to the receptor epithelium, and (2) centrally into the vestibular nuclei (Fig. 12-13). Cells of the superior vestibular ganglion, innervating the cristae of the anterior and lateral canals, give rise to central fibers which: (1) occupy rostral and lateral parts of the vestibular root, and (2) project mainly to the superior vestibular nucleus and oral portions of the medial vestibular nucleus (Fig. 12-13). Cells of the superior vestibular ganglion, innervating the macula of the utricle, mainly descend in the dorsomedial part of the inferior vestibular nucleus. Collaterals of these fibers pass to dorsolateral parts of the medial vestibular nucleus caudally. Cells of the inferior vestibular ganglion, innervating the crista of the posterior canal, pass in caudal parts of the vestibular root and terminate mainly in portions of the superior and medial vestibular nuclei. Central fibers from cells of the inferior vestibular ganglion, innervating the saccular macula, mainly descend in dorsolateral parts of the inferior vestibular nucleus. Cell groups within the vestibu-

lar ganglia, innervating selectively individual receptor components of the labyrinth, have major unique central projections within the ipsilateral vestibular nuclei and less extensive projections to all parts of the complex. The interstitial nucleus of the vestibular nerve appears distinctive in that this nucleus receive fibers from all cell groups of the vestibular ganglia (Fig. 12-14).

Primary vestibulocerebellar fibers traverse portions of the lateral and superior vestibular nuclei and enter the cerebellum via the juxtarestiform body. Most of these fibers are distributed to the cortex of the ipsilateral nodulus, uvula and flocculus (Brodal and Høivik, '64). Studies in the monkey, based upon discrete lesions in specific parts of the vestibular ganglia, indicate that cells in all parts of these ganglia project fibers to the ipsilateral nodulus and uvula (Carpenter et al., '72). These fibers appear to end as mossy fibers in the granular layer of cerebellar cortex. Cells of the vestibular ganglia innervating the cristae of the anterior and lateral canals and the maculae of the utricle and saccule have distinctive regions of termination in the folia of the ipsilateral flocculus. While many of these fibers appear to end as mossy fibers, others enter the molecular layer of the cerebellar cortex as climbing fibers. Although a few primary vestibular fibers end in the dentate nucleus, there is no conclusive evidence that such fibers terminate in the fastigial nucleus.

The vestibular system and its fiber projections constitute one of the most widely dispersed special sensory systems in the neuraxis. Fiber projections of this sensory system pass to all spinal and brain stem levels, and to specific parts of the cerebellum. The vestibular nuclei, which receive primary vestibular fibers, serve as a distributing center for secondary pathways. The vestibular nuclei do not receive descending fibers from the cerebral cortex, the corpus striatum, the superior colliculus or the nuclei of the posterior commissure (Pompeiano and Walberg, '57). Descending fibers from the interstitial nucleus of Cajal project via the medial longitudinal fasciculus to the medial vestibular nucleus. These fibers appear to be the only

descending vestibular afferent fibers arising from cells within the brain stem.

Secondary Vestibular Fibers. The vestibular nuclei give rise to secondary vestibular fibers which project to specific portions of the cerebellum, certain motor cranial nerve nuclei and to all spinal levels.
In addition to the primary vestibulocerebellar fibers described above, there are a
large number of secondary vestibulocerebellar fibers originating from specific portions of the inferior and medial vestibular
nuclei (Fig. 12-14). These fibers arise from
lateral and caudal parts of these nuclei,
traverse the juxtarestiform body and project to the nodulus, uvula, flocculus and
the fastigial nuclei. Within the cerebellum
these fibers are distributed bilaterally, but
with ipsilateral preponderance, except for
fibers passing to the flocculus. The latter
fibers are distributed ipsilaterally (Brodal
and Torvik, '57). The fastigial nuclei and
certain portions of the cerebellar cortex
give rise to fibers that project back to the
vestibular nuclei to be distributed in a selective manner (Thomas et al., '56; Carpenter, '59; Walberg et al., '62). These efferent
cerebellar fibers plus both primary and
secondary vestibulocerebellar fibers mainly
course medial to the inferior cerebellar peduncle in the *juxtarestiform body*. Thus the
vestibular nuclei serve as an important
relay station for the transmission of impulses to and from the cerebellum.

The cells of the lateral vestibular nucleus give rise to the uncrossed vestibulospinal tract, which descends throughout
the length of the spinal cord in the anterior
and lateral funiculi (Figs. 10-18, 10-19 and
12-14). These fibers arise from cells of all
sizes within the nucleus and are somatotopically organized (Pompeiano and Brodal,
'57b). In the brain stem, these fibers do not
have a direct course. Upon leaving the
lateral vestibular nucleus the fibers pass
ventromedially and caudally, successively
occupying positions dorsomedial to the motor nucleus of N. VII and the nucleus ambiguus; from a retro-olivary locus fibers
pass into the spinal cord. The vestibulospinal tract, derived exclusively from the
lateral vestibular nucleus, has a more important functional relationship with the
spinal cord than any other descending ves-

tibular fiber system. The lateral vestibular nucleus also receives a large number of
afferent fibers from the fastigial nucleus
and the cortex of the cerebellar vermis
(Fig. 14-20) which are somatotopically organized. Although crossed and uncrossed fastigiovestibular fibers are distributed differentially and asymmetrically within the lateral vestibular nucleus, they both supply
regions which project to all spinal levels
(Fig. 14-20). Most of these fibers establish
synaptic contact only with the smaller
cells of the lateral vestibular nucleus. Cerebellovestibular fibers from the vermis,
largely the anterior lobe, are distributed
ipsilaterally and terminate mainly in the
dorsal halves of the lateral and inferior
vestibular nuclei. These fibers terminate
upon cells of all sizes, but in the lateral
vestibular nucleus the majority make synaptic contact with large cells (Walberg and
Jansen, '61; Mugnaini and Walberg, '67).
Thus the lateral vestibular nucleus receives impulses from the vestibular nerve
and the cerebellum, and conveys impulses
to spinal levels that mediate responses in
axial and appendicular musculature (Brodal et al., '62). Impulses relayed to spinal
levels via the lateral vestibular nucleus
have important facilitating influences
upon extensor muscle tone and spinal reflex activity.

Medial Longitudinal Fasciculus (MLF).
Fibers from all of the vestibular nuclei pass
medially in the region of the abducens nucleus and enter the medial longitudinal
fasciculus. Vestibular fibers in the medial
longitudinal fasciculus are both crossed
and uncrossed and many bifurcate into ascending and descending branches (Figs.
10-18 and 12-14).

Descending vestibular fibers in the medial longitudinal fasciculus projecting to
spinal levels arise primarily, if not exclusively, in the medial vestibular nucleus.
These fibers, both crossed and uncrossed,
descend in the medial longitudinal fasciculus until they reach the pyramidal decussation, where they shift ventrolaterally to
enter the sulcomarginal region of the anterior funiculus. In their course they may
project fibers into the lower brain stem
reticular formation. Although these fibers
are present bilaterally in the medulla, at

spinal levels almost all fibers are ipsilateral. Some fibers may descend as far as upper thoracic segments, but most fibers end at cervical levels. Some vestibular fibers descending in the MLF synapse directly upon α motor neurons. Experimental evidence indicates that these fibers exert direct inhibitory influences upon cervical motor neurons (Wilson and Yoshida, '69). The superior, lateral and inferior vestibular nuclei do not contribute descending fibers to the medial longitudinal fasciculus that reach spinal levels (Pompeiano and Brodal, '57b; Carpenter, '60; Nyberg-Hansen, '64).

The medial longitudinal fasciculus also contains nonvestibular descending fibers. These include fibers from: (1) the interstitial nucleus of Cajal (interstitiospinal tract), (2) the superior colliculus (tectobulbar and tectospinal tracts, sometimes referred to as the predorsal bundle), (3) the pontine reticular formation (reticulospinal tract), and (4) more rostral brain stem nuclei projecting to particular portions of the inferior olivary complex. The largest group of descending fibers in the medial longitudinal fasciculus are the pontine reticulospinal fibers (Figs. 10-11 and 10-20).

Ascending fibers in the medial longitudinal fasciculus are mostly vestibular and arise from portions of all vestibular nuclei and the interstitial nucleus of the vestibular nerve (Brodal and Pompeiano, '57a). These ascending vestibular fibers project primarily to portions of the nuclei of the extraocular muscles (i.e., the abducens, trochlear and oculomotor) and bring the innervation of these muscles under the influence of vestibular, and possibly cerebellar, regulation. A small number of ascending fibers in the medial longitudinal fasciculus bypass the oculomotor nucleus to terminate in the interstitial nucleus of Cajal (lateral to the medial longitudinal fasciculus near the oculomotor nucleus) (Figs. 13-14, 13-15 and 13-16). Although it has been presumed that vestibular impulses projected rostrally to thalamic relay nuclei, identification of these nuclei has proved illusive. Physiological technics indicate that short latency vestibular responses are found in the monkey in the ventral posterior inferior (VPI) nucleus of the thalamus

(Deecke et al., '73, '74). VPI is a distinctive cytoarchitectonic subdivision of the ventral posterior nucleus of the thalamus, located ventral to VPL and VPM. These authors suggest that VPI is closely associated with somesthetic areas of the cortex.

Ascending fibers in the medial longitudinal fasciculus, arising from individual vestibular nuclei, have both differential and overlapping projections to the nuclei of the extraocular muscles (McMasters et al., '66; Carpenter, '71a). Fibers from the superior vestibular nucleus ascend exclusively (Fig. 12-14), enter the ipsilateral medial longitudinal fasciculus rostral to the abducens nucleus and project primarily to the trochlear nucleus and the dorsal nucleus of the oculomotor complex (i.e., inferior rectus muscle) (Fig. 13-11). Ascending fibers from the medial and lateral vestibular nuclei enter the medial longitudinal fasciculus at the level of the abducens nucleus, are both crossed and uncrossed, and project bilaterally, asymmetrically and differentially to the nuclei of the extraocular muscles. Projections of the medial vestibular nucleus are particularly prominent to: (1) the contralateral trochlear nucleus, (2) the contralateral intermediate cell column (i.e., inferior oblique muscle), and (3) the ipsilateral ventral nucleus (i.e., medial rectus muscle) of the oculomotor complex (Fig. 13-11). Ascending fibers from the lateral vestibular nucleus appear to arise only from ventral parts of the nucleus and have prominent projections to: (1) the contralateral abducens and trochlear nuclei, and (2) asymmetrical portions of the oculomotor nuclear complex. Ascending fibers from the inferior vestibular nucleus in the medial longitudinal fasciculus are relatively sparse. No ascending secondary vestibular fibers in the MLF appear to project to the caudal central nucleus (i.e., the levator palpebrae muscle; Fig. 13-11) or to the visceral nuclei of the oculomotor complex.

Besides the above listed fibers, it is presumed that there are other fibers in the medial longitudinal fasciculus concerned with the mediation of conjugate horizontal eye movements which interconnect the nuclei of the extraocular muscles (Crosby, '50, '53). It seems likely that these fibers arise from portions of the pontine reticular formation (Carpenter, '71).

The medial longitudinal fasciculus, together with the tectospinal and tectobulbar tracts, represents a complex system of fibers which becomes myelinated very early in development. This bundle extends from the rostral part of the midbrain to the caudal medulla, where fibers pass into the sulcomarginal part of the anterior funiculus of the spinal cord. Below the level of the abducens nuclei most fibers of the bundle are descending; above these nuclei ascending fibers predominate.

FUNCTIONAL CONSIDERATIONS

Physiological studies (Szentágothai, '50; Fluur, '59; Cohen et al., '64; Cohen, '71) indicate that secondary vestibular fibers contained in the medial longitudinal fasciculus are essential for most conjugate eye movements. The investigations cited have shown that selective stimulation of individual semicircular canals, or of the nerves from the canals, produces conjugate deviations of the eyes in specific directions. Primary responses obtained by this type of stimulation are abolished following section of the medial longitudinal fasciculi rostral to the abducens nuclei. The fact that nystagmus produced by labyrinthine stimulation is not abolished by section of the medial longitudinal fasciculi (Lorente de Nó, '28, '31; Spiegel, '29; Bender and Weinstein, '44) suggests that vestibular impulses involved in this phenomenon may pass via the reticular formation.

Clinically, lesions involving the medial longitudinal fasciculus rostral to the abducens nuclei produce a disturbance of conjugate horizontal eye movements known as *anterior internuclear ophthalmoplegia* (Spiller, '24; Spiegel and Sommer, 44; Cogan et al., '50; Christoff et al., '60). The salient features of this syndrome are: (1) a paresis or paralysis of ocular adduction on attempted lateral gaze to the opposite side, (2) horizontal nystagmus, either more pronounced or exclusively present in the abducting eye, and (3) preservation of ocular convergence. In most of the clinical cases examined pathologically, brain stem lesions have been so extensive as to preclude reliable anatomical correlations. Available data indicate that paresis of ipsilateral ocular adduction on attempted lateral gaze to the opposite side occurs with unilateral lesions of the medial longitudinal fasciculus. Bilateral lesions of the medial longitudinal fasciculus rostral to the abducens nuclei, in patients with demyelinating disease,.may result in dissociated horizontal eye movements on attempted lateral gaze to both the right and left sides. These findings have been confirmed experimentally in the monkey (Bender and Weinstein, '44, '50; Shanzer et al., '59). In the monkey the syndrome has been produced unilaterally and bilaterally by discrete lesions in the medial longitudinal fasciculus rostral to the abducens nucleus (Carpenter and McMasters, '63; Carpenter and Strominger, '65). Ascending degeneration resulting from unilateral lesions in the MLF rostral to the abducens nucleus is confined to the ipsilateral medial longitudinal fasciculus and is distributed differentially to the ventral nucleus of the oculomotor complex, a cell group that innervates the ipsilateral medial rectus muscle. Such lesions produce no degeneration in any of the contralateral nuclei of the extraocular muscles. An adequate explanation for the monocular horizontal nystagmus seen in this syndrome has eluded both clinicians and investigators. Large bilateral lesions of the medial longitudinal fasciculi between the abducens nuclei in the monkey may produce bilateral paresis of all horizontal eye movements (both abducting and adducting eye movements), without impairment of vertical eye movements or ocular convergence. It is of great interest that in the monkey unilateral lesions of individual vestibular nuclei do not produce dissociated (i.e., disconjugate) eye movements (McMasters et al., '66; Carpenter, '66; Uemura and Cohen, '73).

The mechanisms governing equilibrium (i.e., the maintenance of appropriate positions of the body in space) are largely of a reflex character and are activated by afferent impulses from several sources. Among the more important of these are the general proprioceptive impulses from the muscles, joints and tendons of the neck, trunk and lower limbs, and the special proprioceptive impulses from the vestibular end organ. Impulses from the retina which project to the visual cortex also make an important contribution to spatial orientation. In this equilibratory complex, the labyrinth constitutes a highly specialized proprioceptive mechanism that is stimulated by the *position* or *changes in position* of the head. When the head is moved, either by contraction of the neck muscles or by shifting the body as a whole, the cristae are stimulated and, through the central vestibular connections, effect the reflex compensatory adjustments of the eyes and limbs needed for the particular movement (kinetostatic reflexes). The new attitude, as long as the position of the head remains unchanged, is sustained by impulses originating in the macula of the utricle. The sustaining (static) reflexes are initiated by the gravitational pull of the otolithic membrane on the macular hair cells.

The vestibulospinal tracts and descending fibers from the pontine reticular formation exert a strong excitatory influence upon muscle tone, particularly extensor tone. Descending vestibular impulses in the MLF exert inhibitory influences upon cervical motor neurons (Wilson and Yoshida, '69). Normally muscle tone is maintained by a balance of inhibitory and facilitatory influences from higher centers, a large part of which are considered to be mediated by the brain stem reticular formation. If the influences of these higher centers are removed in an experimental animal, such as the cat, by transection of the brain stem at the intercollicular level (i.e., between the superior and inferior colliculi), a condition known as *decerebrate rigidity* develops. This condition is characterized by tremendously increased tone in the antigravity muscles. Increased muscle tone seen in this condition appears to be an expression of facilitation of γ motor neurons, which thereby increase the rate of firing of muscle spindles; this in turn influences the firing of α motor neurons to maintain the tonic state (Fig. 9-27). In this type of experimental preparation, the facilitatory pathways of the reticular formation and the vestibulospinal tract remain active, while inhibitory elements of the reticular formation no longer function. Inhibitory regions of the reticular formation are considered to be dependent upon descending impulses from higher levels, while the facilitating regions of the reticular formation receive impulses from ascending afferent systems. Thus this type of midbrain transection removes the input to the reticular inhibitory system, but has little effect upon the reticular facilitating system or the descending vestibular system. This form of rigidity can be abolished, or reduced, by a variety of different lesions, including destruction of the vestibular nuclei and section of the anterior part of the spinal cord.

Labyrinthine stimulation, irritation or disease cause, vertigo, and objective signs such as unsteadiness, staggering, postural deviation, deviations of the eyes and nystagmus. In some instances nausea, vomiting, vasomotor changes and prostration occur. The term *vertigo* refers to a subjective sense of rotation, either of the individual or his environment; this term should not be regarded as a synonym for dizziness or giddiness. *Nystagmus*, one of the most prominent objective signs, is a rhythmic involuntary oscillation of the eyes characterized by alternate slow and rapid ocular excursions. Clinically, nystagmus is named for the direction of the rapid phase, but the slow phase is the primary physiological movement. The nausea and vomiting which occur with motion sickness are mainly the result of stimulation of the utricle. Since the labyrinths are antagonistic to each other, the elimination of one causes the other to be overactive until accommodation takes place.

Tests for vestibular function, based upon stimulation of the semicircular canals or vestibular nerve endings, include: (1) the rotating chair test (Bárány chair), (2) the caloric test (i.e., thermal stimulation which changes the temperature of the endolymph), and (3) the galvanic test which stimulates nerve endings directly. In the first of these testing procedures, the slow phase of the nystagmus, deviation of the eyes, postural deviation and pastpointing are all in the direction of the previous rotation, and can be correlated with the direction of endolymphatic flow. The sensation of vertigo is in the opposite direction (DeJong, '58). It is not possible to test the otoliths directly.

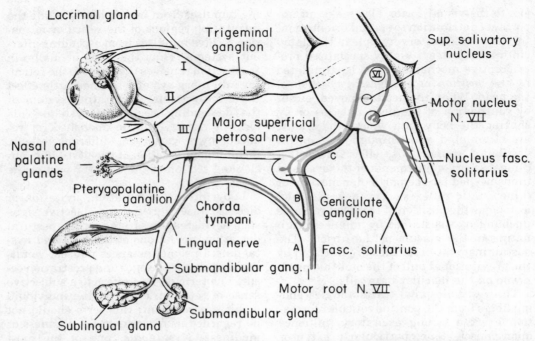

Fig. 12-15. Diagram showing the functional components, organization and peripheral distribution of the facial nerve. Special visceral efferent fibers (motor) are shown in *red*. General visceral efferent fibers (parasympathetic) are in *yellow*, and special visceral afferent fibers (taste) are in *blue*. *A*, *B* and *C* denote lesions of the facial nerve at the stylomastoid foramen, distal to the geniculate ganglion, and proximal to the geniculate ganglion. Disturbances resulting from lesions at these locations are described in the text (page 348).

THE FACIAL NERVE

The facial nerve and the intermediate nerve usually are discussed together although they subserve separate functions (Figs. 12-1 and 12-2). Functional components of these nerves include: (1) *special visceral efferent* (SVE, branchiomotor) *fibers,* (2) *general visceral efferent* (GVE, parasympathetic) *fibers,* (3) *special visceral afferent* (SVA, taste) *fibers,* and (4) a few *general somatic afferent* (GSA, sensory) *fibers.*

Special visceral efferent (SVE) *fibers* of the motor component innervate the muscles of facial expression, the platysma, the buccinator, the posterior belly of the digastric and the stapedius muscles. The motor nucleus of N. VII forms a column of multipolar neurons in the ventrolateral tegmentum dorsal to the superior olivary nucleus and ventromedial to the spinal trigeminal nucleus (Figs. 12-1, 12-2, 12-5 and 12-15).

The facial nucleus is composed of several distinct cell groups (Papez, '27; Vraa-Jensen, '42; Courville, '66b) which appear to innervate specific facial muscles. Most authors recognize at least four cell groups, designated as dorsomedial, ventromedial, intermediate and lateral. The dorsomedial cell group appears to give rise to the posterior auricular nerve which innervates auricular muscles and the occipital muscle. The ramus colli which innervates the platysma muscle arises from the ventromedial cell group. Cells in the medial group are considered to innervate the stapedius muscle (Borg, '73). The temporal and zygomatic branches of the facial nerve, related to the intermediate cell group, supply the frontalis, orbicularis oculi, the corrugator supercilli and the zygomaticus. The lateral cell group gives rise to the buccal branches which innervate the buccinator muscle and the buccolabial muscles. It is uncertain as to which cell groups innervate the stylohyoid and the posterior belly of the digastric muscle (Courville, '66b). Comparisons of the cell groups of the facial nucleus in animals and man (Vraa-Jensen, '42) reveal a close correspondence, except that in man the lateral cell group (buccolabial muscles) is especially prominent while the medial cell group is very small.

A few muscle spindles have been described in facial muscles (Bowden and Mahran, '56; Voss, '56). The presence of muscle spindles suggests the existence of γ efferent fibers, and leads to the assumption that γ neurons are mixed with α neurons in the facial nucleus.

Efferent fibers from the facial motor nucleus emerge from its dorsal surface and project dorsomedially into the floor of the fourth ventricle. These fibers pass medial to the abducens nucleus and ascend for a short distance longitudinally in the floor of the fourth ventricle dorsal to the medial longitudinal fasciculus (Fig. 12-7). Near the oral pole of the abducens nucleus, root fibers of the facial nerve make a sharp lateral bend around the rostral border of the abducens nucleus and pass ventrolaterally. In their course the fibers pass medial to the spinal trigeminal complex, lateral to the superior olivary nucleus and emerge from the brain stem near the caudal border of the pons, at the cerebellopontine angle (Figs. 11-25 and 12-1). Root fibers looping around the abducens nucleus form the *internal genu* of the facial nerve.

The facial motor nucleus receives afferent fibers from a number of sources. Among these are: (1) secondary trigeminal fibers from the spinal trigeminal nucleus (Cajal, '09; Carpenter and Hanna, '61) involved in corneal and other trigeminofacial reflexes, (2) direct corticobulbar fibers (Fig. 11-23) which project bilaterally, but with important regional differences (Kuypers, '58), (3) indirect corticobulbar fibers which convey impulses to the facial nucleus via relays in the reticular formation (Walberg, '57; Kuypers, '58, '58a), and (4) crossed rubrobulbar fibers (Courville, '66) which project only to cell groups (i.e., dorsomedial and intermediate) innervating the upper facial muscles. In addition it seems likely that descending fibers from the mesencephalic reticular formation project ipsilaterally to portions of the facial nucleus (Courville, '66). Secondary or tertiary auditory fibers, considered to reach

the facial nucleus, are thought to mediate certain acousticofacial reflexes. These reflexes include closing of the eyes in response to a sudden loud noise, and contraction of the stapedius muscle to dampen the movements of the ear ossicles. Recent studies of the neuronal organization of acoustic middle ear reflexes indicate that pathways involved in the stapedius reflex involve three or four neurons: (1) primary auditory neurons, (2) processes of cells of the ventral cochlear nucleus which form the trapezoid body, and (3) neurons in the ipsilateral and contralateral medial superior olivary nucleus which project to facial motor neurons that innervate the stapedius muscle (Borg, '73). On clinical grounds it has been suggested that impulses from the thalamus or globus pallidus may reach portions of the facial nucleus indirectly, since pathology involving these structures has been said to produce a *mimetic* or *emotional* type facial palsy (Monrad-Krohn, '24, '39). The pathways which may be involved in this type of facial palsy are unknown.

The *intermediate nerve,* which emerges between the facial motor root and the vestibular nerve (Fig. 12-2), contains afferent and general visceral efferent fibers. Afferent fibers (SVA and GSA) arise from cells of the geniculate ganglion, located at the external genu of the facial nerve (Fig. 12-15). *Special visceral afferent* (SVA) *fibers* convey gustatory sense (taste) from the anterior two-thirds of the tongue via the chorda tympani nerve. Centrally these fibers enter the solitary fasciculus and terminate upon cells in the rostral part of the solitary nucleus, sometimes referred to as the gustatory nucleus. General somatic afferent (GSA) fibers convey cutaneous sensory impulses from the external auditory meatus and the region back of the ear; centrally these fibers enter the dorsal part of the spinal trigeminal tract.

There are some observations which suggest that the facial nerve may carry impulses of deep pain and deep pressure from the face (Hunt, '15). In some cases in which the trigeminal nerve has been sectioned for the relief of facial neuralgia, deep pain sense due to pressure has persisted. The question is not settled, but most investigations suggest that both deep and superficial pain probably are mediated by the trigeminal nerve (Smyth, '39).

General visceral efferent (GVE) *fibers* in the intermediate nerve arise from the *superior salivatory nucleus,* which probably consists of scattered neurons in the dorsolateral reticular formation (Figs. 11-17, 11-18 and 12-15). This scattered visceral cell column is considered to extend caudally to levels near the nucleus ambiguus; the most caudal cells of this column constitute the inferior salivatory nucleus of the glossopharyngeal nerve. Preganglionic parasympathetic fibers from the superior salivatory nucleus pass peripherally as a component of the intermediate nerve, but near the external genu of the facial nerve they divide into two groups: (1) one group that passes to the pterygopalatine ganglion via the major superficial petrosal nerve, and (2) another group that projects via the chorda tympani nerve to the submandibular ganglion (Fig. 12-15). Synapses with postganglionic nerves occur in the pterygopalatine and submandibular ganglia. Postganglionic fibers from the pterygopalatine ganglion give rise to secretory and vasomotor fibers that innervate the lacrimal gland and the mucous membrane of the nose and mouth. Postganglionic parasympathetic fibers from the submandibular ganglion pass to the submandibular and sublingual salivary glands.

Lesions of the Facial Nerve (*Bell's palsy*). Lesions producing paralysis of facial movements, and sometimes disturbances of taste and secretory function, may involve fibers of the facial nerve within the brain stem or in their peripheral course. The particular deficits which result depend upon the location of the lesion and its extent. A complete lesion of the motor part of the facial nerve as it emerges from the stylomastoid foramen (*A*, Fig. 12-15) produces paralysis of all ipsilateral facial movements. The patient is unable to wrinkle the forehead, close the eye, show the teeth, purse the lips or whistle. On the side of the lesion the palpebral fissure is widened, the nasolabial fold is flattened and the corner of the mouth droops. Although corneal sensation is present, the corneal reflex is lost on the side of the

lesion because motor fibers participating in this reflex are destroyed. A lesion of this nerve distal to the geniculate ganglion (*B*, Fig. 12-15) produces all of the deficits found with a lesion at *A*, plus impairment of secretions from the sublingual and submandibular salivary glands, hyperacusis and sometimes impairment of taste over the anterior two-thirds of the tongue. Impairment of salivary secretion results from interruption of preganglionic parasympathetic fibers from the superior salivatory nucleus. *Hyperacusis* is caused by paralysis of the stapedius muscle, which normally functions to dampen the oscillations of the ear ossicles. Taste may not always be impaired by such lesions since some fibers may take an aberrant course with the major petrosal nerve. Lesions of the facial nerve proximal to the geniculate ganglion (*C*, Fig. 12-15) produce all of the deficits encountered with lesions at *A* and *B* and, in addition, invariably result in complete loss of taste over the anterior two-thirds of the tongue. Lacrimation also is impaired on the side of the lesion as a consequence of destruction of parasympathetic fibers to the pterygopalatine (sphenopalatine) ganglion. With complete lesions in this location no regeneration of sensory fibers takes place. Aberrant regeneration of preganglionic parasympathetic fibers may occur, since the cell bodies lie within the central nervous system. In this aberrant regeneration, fibers previously synapsing upon postganglionic neurons of the submandibular ganglion established new relationships with cells of the pterygopalatine ganglion. Thus a stimulus which previously produced a salivary response may provoke lacrimation on the side of the lesion (syndrome of "crocodile tears"). The true etiology of Bell's palsy is poorly understood. It is tacitly presumed that most facial palsies of this type are due to compression of the nerve secondary to an unexplained swelling in the bony facial canal.

Central lesions involving corticobulbar and corticoreticular fibers projecting upon reticular neurons, which in turn discharge upon cells of the facial nucleus, produce a marked weakness of muscles in the lower half of the face contralaterally, especially in the perioral region. Muscles of the upper facial region concerned with wrinkling the forehead, frowning and closing the eyes are not affected. The accepted explanation of this upper motor neuron facial paralysis is that corticobulbar fibers projecting to the upper part of the facial nucleus (supplying muscles of the upper face and forehead) are distributed bilaterally, while corticobulbar projections to the lower part of the facial nucleus (supplying muscles of the lower face) are predominantly crossed. Although a completely satisfactory explanation is still lacking as to why a capsular hemiplegia in man is accompanied by paresis only in the lower facial muscles, the anatomical observations of Kuypers ('58a) support the accepted thesis. This author found direct bilateral corticobulbar projections to the facial nucleus, but noted that ventral cell groups (regarded as innervating lower facial muscles) of the contralateral facial nucleus received more fibers than the same cell groups of the ipsilateral facial nucleus.

Even in the presence of a central type facial paralysis, as described above, mimetic or emotional innervation of the facial muscles may be preserved. In response to a genuine emotional stimulus, the muscles of the lower face will contract symmetrically while smiling or laughing. Actually, contractions of facial muscles on the paretic side may begin earlier and last longer than on the normal side (Monrad-Krohn, '39). Mimetic or emotional innervation of facial muscles is largely involuntary. Evidence suggests that impulses from higher levels of the neuraxis, other than those arising in the cerebral cortex, must reach the facial nuclei and bring about emotional facial expression. The neural mechanism for emotional facial innervation appears distinct and separate from that controlling voluntary facial movement. Thus two different types of central facial paresis are recognized, one concerned with voluntary facial movement, and another involving emotional facial expression. Each of these types of central facial paresis can occur alone, since the central pathways are different, but with certain lesions both voluntary and mimetic facial paralyses can occur together. The neuroanatomical pathways mediating emotional facial innervation are unknown.

THE ABDUCENS NERVE

The abducens is the motor nerve (GSE) innervating the lateral rectus muscle of the eye. The nucleus forms a column, about 3 mm in length, of typical somatic motor cells in the lateral part of the medial eminence (Figs. 12-3 and 12-7). Fibers of the facial nerve form a complicated loop about the nucleus. Root fibers of the abducens nerve emerge from the medial aspect of the nucleus and pass ventrally through the pontine tegmentum and lateral to the corticospinal tract (Figs. 12-1, 12-6 and 12-7). They emerge from the brain stem at the caudal border of the pons (Figs. 11-1, 11-17 and A-7). The nucleus receives, and is traversed by, crossed and uncrossed fibers from the vestibular nuclei entering the medial longitudinal fasciculi (Fig. 12-14). Impulses conveyed by these fibers are concerned with the vestibular control of eye movements. Corticobulbar fibers convey impulses to abducens nuclei bilaterally via intercalated neurons in the reticular formation (Fig. 11-23).

Lesions of the abducens nerve in the brain stem, or in its long intracranial course, cause ipsilateral paralysis of the lateral rectus muscle. Owing to the unopposed action of the medial rectus muscle, the affected eye is strongly adducted. The contralateral eye is unaffected and can move in all directions. The patient has diplopia (double vision) on attempting to gaze to the side of the lesion; two images are seen side by side. This is called horizontal diplopia. *Diplopia* results because light reflected by an object in the visual field does not fall upon corresponding points of the two retinae.

Discrete unilateral lesions of the abducens nucleus produce a weakness, or paralysis, of lateral gaze toward the side of the lesion. The syndrome of *"lateral gaze paralysis"* differs from a simple paralysis of the lateral rectus muscle in that both eyes are forcefully and conjugately directed to the side opposite the lesion, and movement of the eyes laterally toward the side of the lesion is severely limited, or impossible. The head may be tilted slightly to the opposite side. Ocular convergence usually is preserved. The abducens nucleus thus appears unique among the motor cranial nerve nuclei, since it is the only cranial nerve in which disturbances associated with lesions of root fibers and motor nucleus are not identical. This curious finding requires an explanation.

All ocular movements, whether horizontal, vertical or rotatory, require reciprocal activity in the extraocular muscles producing these movements. Conjugate lateral gaze requires simultaneous appropriate contractions of the lateral rectus on one side and the medial rectus of the opposite side. The central neural mechanism underlying conjugate lateral movements of the eyes is not fully understood, but it is generally accepted that fibers in the medial longitudinal fasciculus interconnecting the abducens nucleus and portions of the oculomotor nuclear complex are essential for these movements. It has been postulated that cells in the reticular formation adjacent to, or in, the abducens nucleus may give rise to these fibers. This cell group, referred to as the *parabducens nucleus,* often is called the pontine "center for lateral gaze." Although the theoretical existence of the parabducens nucleus has been acknowledged (Crosby, '53; Peele, '61), there is no definitive description or experimental evidence substantiating it as an entity. It also has been suggested that ascending vestibular fibers which are known to traverse and terminate in the abducens nuclei, and to project rostrally in the medial longitudinal fasciculus, might be implicated in the syndrome of "lateral gaze paralysis." Since oculomotor fibers supplying the medial rectus muscle are uncrossed (Fig. 13-11; Warwick, '53), it would be expected that ascending fibers from the pontine "center for lateral gaze" must cross in the vicinity of the abducens nucleus. In any case, axons destined for the contralateral medial longitudinal fasciculus are interrupted, and coordinating impulses do not reach appropriate cell groups in the oculomotor nucleus. It should be recalled that unilateral lesions of the medial longitudinal fasciculus rostral to the abducens nucleus produce a fragment of the syndrome of *lateral gaze paralysis,*

namely paralysis of ocular adduction on attempted lateral gaze to the opposite side. Thus lateral gaze paralysis due to lesions in the region of the abducens nucleus would appear to be a combination of two factors: (1) paralysis of the ipsilateral lateral rectus due to destruction of cells in the abducens nucleus, and (2) paralysis of adduction in the contralateral medial rectus muscle due to interruption of fibers which cross to the opposite side, and project via the medial longitudinal fasciculus to specific parts of the contralateral oculomotor nucleus.

Discrete lesions in the abducens nucleus in the monkey produce paralysis of ipsilateral lateral gaze that is enduring (Carpenter et al., '63). Such lesions produce degeneration in the root fibers of the abducens nerve and ascending degeneration in the medial longitudinal fasciculi, which is most profuse contralaterally. These ascending fibers are distributed differentially to the contralateral ventral nucleus of the oculomotor complex, a cell group innervating the medial rectus muscle on that side. Lesions of the medial longitudinal fasciculus rostral to the abducens nucleus (Carpenter and Strominger, '65) produce paresis of ipsilateral ocular adduction (i.e., anterior internuclear ophthalmoplegia) and similarly distributed degeneration in the ipsilateral oculomotor nucleus. Available evidence suggests that the paresis of ocular adduction, which forms a part of the "lateral gaze paralysis" syndrome, and anterior internuclear ophthalmoplegia probably have a common basis, namely, interruption of fibers of the medial longitudinal fasciculus at different locations and on different sides of the median raphe. However, lesions limited to individual vestibular nuclei do not produce paresis of ocular adduction (McMasters et al., '66). Thus it seems likely that the ascending fibers of the medial longitudinal fasciculus whose interruption produces these disturbances of conjugate horizontal eye movements probably do not arise from the vestibular nuclei.

Because of the proximity of emerging root fibers of the abducens nerve to the corticospinal tract, lesions in the caudal pons involving both of these structures produce the so-called *middle alternating hemiplegia* (Fig. 11-23). This syndrome is characterized by paralysis of the ipsilateral lateral rectus muscle and a contralateral hemiplegia. This condition resembles the *inferior alternating hemiplegia* seen with comparable medullary lesions which involve the hypoglossal nerve and the medullary pyramid.

ROSTRAL PONS

Transverse sections through the upper pons at the level of root fibers of the trigeminal nerve (Figs. 12-16, 12-17, 12-18 and A-8) reveal important changes when compared with sections at lower pontine levels (Figs. 12-2, 12-4 and 12-7). The fourth ventricle is narrower, although its roof is still formed by the cerebellum. Within the cerebellum portions of all the deep cerebellar nuclei can be seen (Fig. 12-16), and fibers of the inferior and middle cerebellar peduncles enter the cerebellum close to each other (Fig. 12-16). At slightly higher levels fibers of the superior cerebellar peduncle form the dorsolateral wall of the fourth ventricle (Fig. 12-18).

The ventral portion of the pons is larger than at lower levels but still contains transverse and longitudinal fibers, as well as large masses of pontine nuclei. Corticospinal and corticopontine tracts here consist of numerous fiber bundles less compactly arranged than in the caudal pons. Fibers within the raphe of the pons are probably reticulocerebellar fibers arising from cells in the pontine tegmentum (Fig. 12-17).

In the dorsal part of the pons the medial lemniscus is traversed by the transverse fibers of the trapezoid body. Lateral to the medial lemniscus and closely associated with fibers of the trapezoid body is the rostral pole of the superior olivary nucleus (Fig. 12-16). Ventrolaterally the lateral lemniscus is becoming a well-defined bundle (Figs. 12-17 and 12-18). The spinothalamic and anterior spinocerebellar tracts are located lateral to the medial lemniscus. The position of the medial longitudinal fasciculus is unchanged from lower levels. Longitudinally cut fibers of the facial genu appear lateral to the medial longitudinal fasciculus (Fig. 12-17). Fibers of the

central tegmental tract form a fairly discrete bundle in the reticular formation dorsal to the lateral part of the medial lemniscus (Fig. 12-17).

The Pontine Reticular Formation. This cell group, occupying the central core of the tegmentum, is somewhat reduced in size. Dorsal to the facial genu the nucleus of the medial eminence remains. The central reticular area contains the *nucleus reticularis pontis oralis*, the rostral continuation of the more caudal pontine reticular nucleus (Fig. 12-19). This cell group extends rostrally into the caudal mesencephalon, where its oral boundaries become indistinct. The more caudal part of this nuclear mass contains scattered giant cells, like those which characterize the medial two-thirds of the medullary reticular formation. Some of the larger cells at this level give rise to the uncrossed reticulospinal fibers; others give rise to ascending fibers which pass rostrally in the central tegmental tract. In many instances a single cell with a dichotomizing axon projects fibers both rostrally and caudally. Ascending fibers from parts of the nuclei reticularis pontis oralis and caudalis pass to parts of the intralaminar nuclei of the thalamus. These ascending fibers and those originating from more caudal brain stem regions participate in activation of broad regions of the cerebral cortex.

In the ventral part of the tegmentum immediately dorsal to the medial lemnisci is a moderately large group of multipolar cells known as the *nucleus reticularis tegmenti pontis*, or the reticulotegmental nucleus (Fig. 12-19). These cells have been considered as a medial tegmental extension of the pontine nuclei, which they resemble in certain respects. Portions of the reticulotegmental nucleus receive a bilateral and an ipsilateral projection from the frontal and parietal cortex (Brodal and Brodal, '71). In addition, this nucleus receives a large bundle of cerebellar efferent fibers via the descending division of the superior cerebellar peduncle (Carpenter and Nova, '60; Brodal and Szikla, '72). Since this nucleus projects virtually all its fibers to the cerebellum, it must play a role in integrating impulses from the cerebral cortex and from portions of the cerebellum, prior to

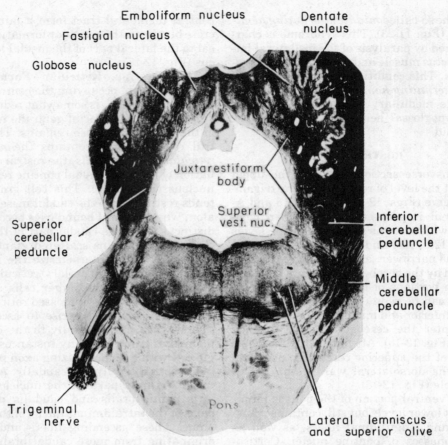

FIG. 12-16. Section of pons, pontine tegmentum and part of cerebellum through the root of the trigeminal nerve. One-month infant. Weigert's myelin stain. Photograph.

their projection to the cerebellum. Projections of this nucleus to the cerebellar vermis are both crossed and uncrossed, while those to the hemisphere are entirely crossed (Brodal and Jansen, '46). In the raphe region dorsal to the reticulotegmental nucleus is the *superior central nucleus,* a closely packed aggregation of relatively small cells. This nucleus is more prominent at isthmus levels (Figs. 12-19, 12-23 and 12-24).

Afferent root fibers of the trigeminal nerve traverse the lateral portion of the pons, reach the dorsolateral pontine tegmentum and terminate in specific nuclei of the trigeminal nerve. Lateral to the entering root fibers is a large gray cellular mass, the *nucleus sensorius principalis* of the trigeminal nerve (Fig. 12-19). Small groups of root fibers can be seen entering

this nucleus (Figs. 12-16 and 12-17). Medial to the trigeminal root fibers and the principal sensory nucleus is a smaller oval collection of large cells whose efferent fibers emerge medial to the afferent fibers. This is the *motor nucleus* of the trigeminal nerve. A small bundle of afferent fibers coursing dorsally between the motor and sensory nuclei toward the ventricular surface constitutes the *mesencephalic tract of the trigeminal nerve* (Fig. 12-17). Although these are afferent fibers, they arise from large unipolar cells situated in the central gray matter along the lateral border of the ventricle (Figs. 12-17 and 12-19).

THE TRIGEMINAL NERVE

The trigeminal, the largest cranial nerve, contains both sensory and motor fibers (Figs. 11-1 and 12-16). *General so-*

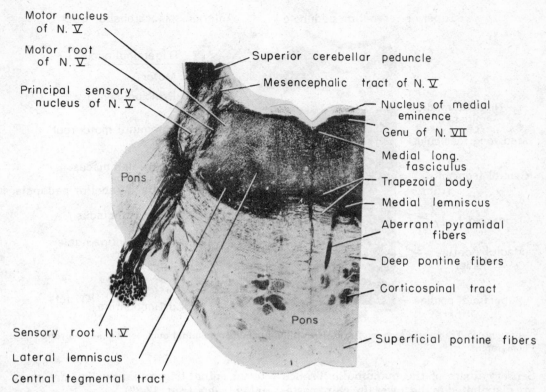

Motor nucleus of N. V
Motor root of N. V
Principal sensory nucleus of N. V
Pons
Sensory root N. V
Lateral lemniscus
Central tegmental tract

Superior cerebellar peduncle
Mesencephalic tract of N. V
Nucleus of medial eminence
Genu of N. VII
Medial long. fasciculus
Trapezoid body
Medial lemniscus
Aberrant pyramidal fibers
Deep pontine fibers
Corticospinal tract
Pons
Superficial pontine fibers

FIG. 12-17. Section of pons and pontine tegmentum of 1-month infant through entrance of trigeminal nerve. Weigert's myelin stain. Photograph.

matic afferent (GSA) *fibers* convey both exteroceptive and proprioceptive impulses. Exteroceptive impulses of touch, pain and thermal sense are transmitted from: (1) the skin of the face and forehead (Fig. 7-13), (2) the mucous membranes of the nose, the nasal sinuses and the oral cavity, (3) the teeth, and (4) extensive portions of the cranial dura. Proprioceptive impulses (deep pressure and kinesthesis) are conveyed from the teeth, peridontium, the hard palate and temporomandibular joint. In addition, afferent fibers convey impulses arising from stretch receptors in the muscles of mastication. *Special visceral efferent fibers* (SVE; branchiomotor) innervate the muscles of mastication, the tensor tympani and the tensor veli palatini. Afferent fibers constitute the sensory root (portio major), while efferent fibers form the smaller motor root (portio minor).

Trigeminal Ganglion. The afferent fibers, except those associated with proprioception and stretch receptors, have their cell bodies in the large, flattened, crescent-shaped *trigeminal ganglion* (Figs. 1-10 and 2-19). This semilunar-shaped ganglion, placed on the cerebral surface of the petrous bone in the middle cranial fossa, is composed of typical unipolar ganglion cells (Truex, '40; Figs. 12-21 and 12-22). The peripheral processes of these cells form the three main divisions of the trigeminal nerve: ophthalmic, maxillary and mandibular. The first two are wholly sensory, but incorporated in the mandibular branch is the entire motor root supplying the muscles of mastication. The ophthalmic branch innervates the forehead, upper eyelid, cornea, conjunctiva, dorsum of the nose, and mucous membranes of the nasal vestibule and the frontal sinus (Fig. 7-13). The maxillary division supplies the upper lip, lateral and posterior portions of the nose, upper cheek, anterior portion of the temple, and mucous membranes of the nose, upper jaw, upper teeth and roof of the mouth to the palatopharyngeal arch.

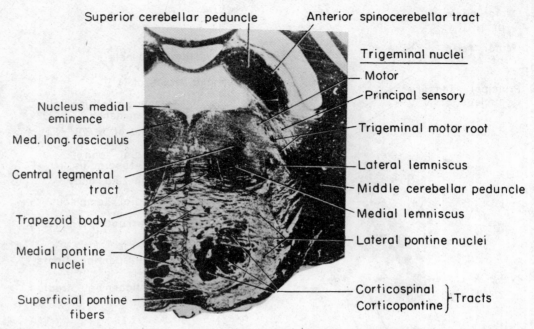

FIG. 12-18. Transverse section of adult pons through motor trigeminal nucleus. Weigert's myelin stain. Photograph.

Sensory fibers of the mandibular branch are distributed to the lower lip, chin, posterior portions of the cheek and the temple, external ear, and mucous membranes of the lower jaw, lower teeth, cheeks, anterior two-thirds of the tongue and floor of the mouth. All three divisions of the trigeminal nerve contribute sensory fibers to the dura. The dura of the posterior fossa also is innervated by fibers from the tenth cranial and the upper three spinal nerves (Penfield and McNaughton, '40; Kimmel, '61).

The central processes of cells in the trigeminal ganglion form the sensory root which passes through the lateral part of the pons and enters the tegmentum, where many fibers divide into short ascending and long descending arms (Figs. 11-18 and 12-20). Other fibers descend or ascend without bifurcation (Windle, '26). The short ascending fibers and their collaterals terminate in the principal sensory nucleus lying dorsolateral to the entering fibers. The long descending branches form the spinal trigeminal tract, whose longest fibers reach the uppermost cervical segments of the spinal cord; terminals and collaterals

to the spinal trigeminal nucleus are given off *en route* (Fig. 12-20).

Spinal Trigeminal Tract and Nucleus. Root fibers entering the spinal trigeminal tract have a definite topographical organization (Woodburne, '36; Kerr, '63; Kerr et al., '68). Fibers of the ophthalmic division are most ventral, fibers of the mandibular division are most dorsal and those of the maxillary division are intermediate (Fig. 12-21). This inverted laminar arrangement of fibers results from medial rotation of the trigeminal sensory root as it enters the brain stem and persists throughout the length of the tract. The tract extends from the level of the trigeminal root in the pons to the uppermost cervical spinal segments (Figs. 12-21 and 12-22). While it has been suggested that fibers in different divisions of the trigeminal nerve descend in the spinal trigeminal tract for different distances (Smyth, '39; McKinley and Magoun, '42), studies based upon better technics indicate that the laminar arrangement of fibers in the different divisions of the tract persists throughout its length with little intermingling of fibers (Darian-Smith and Mayday, '60; Kruger and

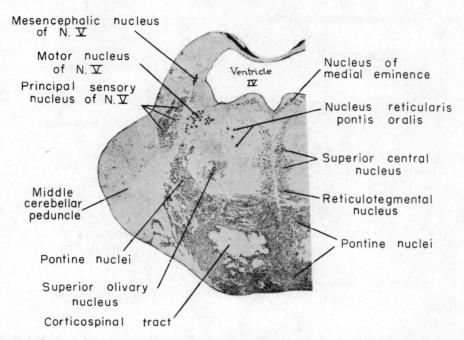

FIG. 12-19. Section through pons and pontine tegmentum of 1-month infant at about same level as Figure 12-17. Cresyl violet. Photograph, with cell groups schematically blocked in.

Michel, '62; Kerr, '63). Fibers of the spinal trigeminal tract terminate upon cells of the spinal trigeminal nucleus, which forms a long cell column medial to the tract. Rostrally the nucleus merges with the principal sensory nucleus, while caudally it blends into the substantia gelatinosa of the first two cervical spinal segments. Fibers of the spinal trigeminal tract project into that part of the spinal trigeminal nucleus immediately adjacent to it (Kerr, '63). Thus, there is a sharp segregation of terminal fibers within parts of the nucleus and virtually no overlap of fibers from the different divisions of the nerve. The mandibular division of the spinal trigeminal tract also contains small groups of GVA fibers from the facial, glossopharyngeal and vagus nerves which project dorsomedially into the nucleus solitarius (Torvik, '56; Kerr, '61; Rhoton et al., '66), a finding suggesting that some descending fibers in this tract may serve visceral functions.

In addition the spinal trigeminal tract contains some general somatic afferent (GSA) fibers from the facial, glossopha-

ryngeal and vagus nerves, most of which occupy dorsomedial locations.

Cytoarchitecturally the spinal trigeminal nucleus has been subdivided into three parts (Olszewski, '50): (1) a *pars oralis* extending caudally to the rostral third of the inferior olivary nucleus, (2) a *pars interpolaris* extending from the pars oralis to the decussation of the pyramids, and (3) a *pars caudalis* extending caudally as far as the second cervical spinal segment. Elaborate physiological studies (Wall and Taub, '62) in the cat reveal that a somatotopic map of the face exists at all levels within the spinal trigeminal nucleus. Throughout the nucleus the face is represented in upside down fashion with the jaw dorsal and the forehead ventral. Cells of the pars oralis receive impulses from the head, mouth, nose and eyes, have small receptive fields, and the dominant representation is of internal structures. The pars interpolaris has small receptive fields and is related mainly to cutaneous facial regions. The pars caudalis has large receptive fields and responds to light pressure over proximal parts of the face (i.e., forehead, cheeks and

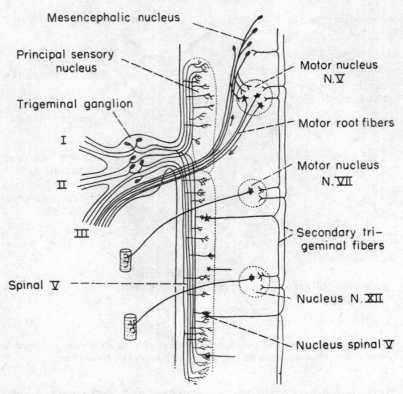

Fig. 12-20. Diagram of the trigeminal nuclei and some of the trigeminal reflex arcs. *I*, Ophthalmic division; *II*, maxillary division; *III*, mandibular division (modified from Cajal, '09).

region of the jaw angle). Although neuronal receptive field size generally is related to peripheral innervation density, an extensive study of the trigeminal nuclear complex in the monkey failed to demonstrate any consistent variation of receptive field size throughout its rostrocaudal extent (Kerr et al., '68).

In addition to fibers of the trigeminal nerve and general somatic afferent fibers from other branchiomeric cranial nerves, the spinal trigeminal nucleus receives corticobulbar fibers (Brodal et al., '56; Kuypers, '58; Kuypers and Tuerk, '64; Zimmerman et al., '64). These fibers arise mainly from the frontoparietal cortex and are predominantly crossed. Physiological studies (Darian-Smith and Yokota, '66) indicate that corticobulbar fibers projecting to the pars oralis and pars caudalis mediate both inhibitory and excitatory effects. Observations suggest that inhibitory effects are presynaptic in nature.

There is considerable clinical evidence that lesions of the spinal trigeminal tract result chiefly in loss, or diminution, of pain and thermal sense in the area innervated by the trigeminal nerve, but do not affect tactile sensibility. It is probable that the nonbifurcating descending fibers mediate exclusively pain and thermal sense, while the bifurcating ones convey tactile sensibility. Hence in lesions of the spinal trigeminal tract many tactile fibers may be destroyed, but the ascending branches of these fibers still reach the principal sensory nucleus and touch remains intact. Clinically there is no doubt that pain and thermal sense are handled entirely by the spinal trigeminal tract and nucleus, while touch and two-point discrimination are in large part related to the principal sensory nucleus (Figs. 12-20 and 12-22). However, physiological studies (Wall and Taub, '62; Kruger and Michel, '62a) indicate that it is extremely difficult to isolate and identify

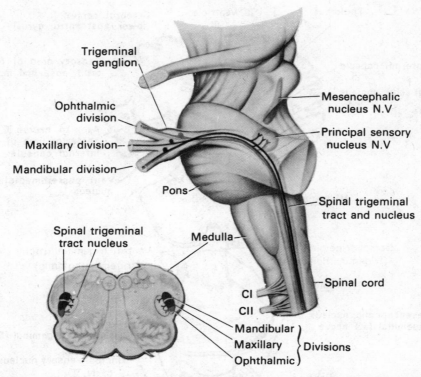

FIG. 12-21. Diagram of the topographical arrangement of the fibers in the spinal trigeminal tract. The laminar arrangement of fibers from the different divisions of the trigeminal nerve persists throughout its length, although fibers leave the tract at all levels to terminate upon cells of the spinal trigeminal nucleus. (From Carpenter, *Core Text of Neuroanatomy*, '72; courtesy of The Williams & Wilkins Company.)

neurons in the spinal trigeminal nucleus uniquely concerned with impulses related to pain. Neurons at nearly all levels of the nucleus respond to tactile stimuli (Kruger and Michel, '62).

The composition, location and relationships of the spinal trigeminal tract and nucleus are of considerable diagnostic and surgical importance. It should be noted that virtually no overlap exists between the cutaneous areas supplied by the three peripheral divisions of the trigeminal nerve, a finding in sharp contrast to the extensive overlap characteristic of spinal dermatomes (Fig. 7-13). Neurosurgical studies (Sjöqvist, '38) have demonstrated that trigeminal tractotomy can relieve various forms of facial pain including trigeminal neuralgia (tic douloureux). The importance of this procedure is that it selectively eliminates, or greatly reduces, pain and thermal sense without impairing tactile

sense. Meticulous examination of such patients (Walker, '39a; Weinberger and Grant, '42) frequently reveals that tactile sense is mildly impaired and that there is not a complete loss of any sensory modality. One notable advantage of this procedure is that corneal sensation is not abolished, and the corneal reflex is not lost (although it may not be as brisk). The fact that section of this tract caudal to the level of the obex has produced complete facial analgesia is cited as supporting the thesis that the caudal part of the nucleus is concerned chiefly with pain.

The Principal Sensory Nucleus. This nucleus lies lateral to the entering trigeminal root fibers in the upper pons (Figs. 12-17 and 12-20). Root fibers conveying impulses for tactile and pressure sense enter the principal sensory nucleus and are distributed in a manner similar to that described for the spinal trigeminal nucleus.

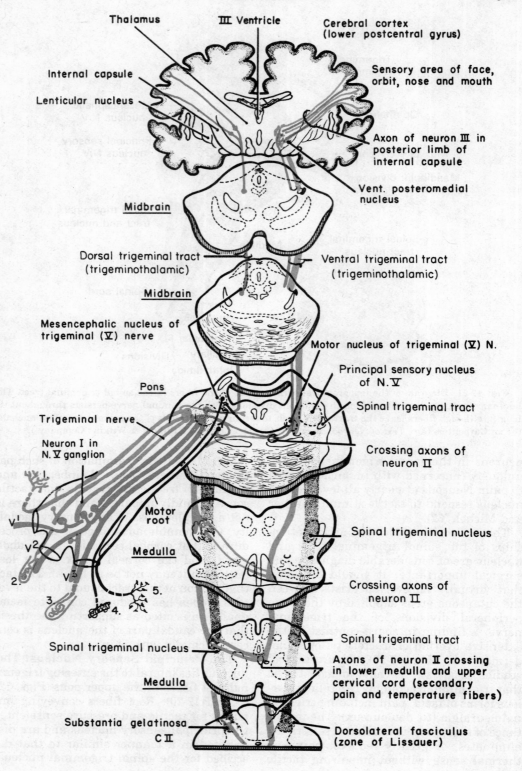

Thalamus

III Ventricle

Cerebral cortex
(lower postcentral gyrus)

Internal capsule

Sensory area of face,
orbit, nose and mouth

Lenticular nucleus

Axon of neuron III in
posterior limb of
internal capsule

Vent. posteromedial
nucleus

Midbrain

Dorsal trigeminal tract
(trigeminothalamic)

Ventral trigeminal tract
(trigeminothalamic)

Midbrain

Mesencephalic nucleus of
trigeminal (V) nerve

Motor nucleus of trigeminal (V) N.

Principal sensory nucleus
of N. V

Pons

Spinal trigeminal tract

Trigeminal nerve

Neuron I in
N. V ganglion

Crossing axons of
neuron II

V¹

Motor
root

Spinal trigeminal nucleus

V²

Medulla

2.

V³

3.

5.

4.

Crossing axons of
neuron II

Spinal trigeminal tract

Spinal trigeminal nucleus

Axons of neuron II crossing
in lower medulla and upper
cervical cord (secondary
pain and temperature fibers)

Medulla

Substantia gelatinosa
C II

Dorsolateral fasciculus
(zone of Lissauer)

Fibers of the ophthalmic division terminate ventrally, fibers of the maxillary division are intermediate and fibers of the mandibular division are most dorsal (Kerr, '63; Kerr et al., '68). Cells of the principal sensory nucleus have an ovoid configuration in transverse sections, and consist of small- to medium-sized neurons with relative large nuclei (Fig. 12-19). Caudally this nucleus merges with the pars oralis of the spinal trigeminal nucleus and the level of transition is indistinct (Fig. 12-20). Cells of the principal sensory nucleus have large receptive fields, show high spontaneous activity and respond to a wide range of pressure stimuli with little adaptation (Wall and Taub, '62).

The Mesencephalic Nucleus. This nucleus of the trigeminal nerve forms a slender cell column near the lateral margin of the central gray of the upper part of the fourth ventricle and cerebral aqueduct (Figs. 12-19, 12-20 and 12-21). The nucleus is composed of large unipolar neurons which extend from the level of the motor nucleus into the rostral midbrain. Studies of neurons in this nucleus have revealed many bipolar and multipolar cells as well, but most cells resemble those of the dorsal root ganglion (Pearson, '49, '49a). However, unlike dorsal root ganglion cells, these cells lie within the central nervous system, are not encapsulated and often have more than one process. The principal processes of these cells form a slender sickle-shaped bundle, the *mesencephalic tract of the trigeminal nerve* (Figs. 12-17, 12-20, 12-21, 12-22, 12-23 and A-8), which descends to the level of the trigeminal motor nucleus, provides collaterals to motor cells and appears to emerge as part of the motor root. Cells of this nucleus commonly

are regarded as afferent peripheral neurons which have been "retained" within the central nervous system, but proof that these cells arise from the neural crest in mammals is still lacking (Pearson, '49, '49a).

Afferent fibers of the mesencephalic nucleus of the trigeminal nerve convey proprioceptive impulses (pressure and kinesthesis) from the teeth, periodontium, hard palate, muscles of mastication and joint capsules (Allen, '19, '25; Pfaffmann, '39; Corbin, '40; Corbin and Harrison, '40). It appears likely that these fibers may be concerned with the mechanisms which control the force of the bite. The mesencephalic nucleus also receives afferent impulses from stretch receptors in the muscles of mastication. Action potentials can be recorded in the mesencephalic nucleus in response to stretching the masticatory muscles (Corbin and Harrison, '40; Cooper et al., '53a). Scattered ganglion cells found along the motor root appear related to the mesencephalic nucleus and are considered to convey impulses from stretch receptors in the mylohyoid and diagastric muscles. Although most afferent fibers of the mesencephalic nucleus course peripherally with fibers of the motor root, experimental evidence (Corbin, '40), indicates that some fibers from this nucleus pass peripherally in all three divisions of the trigeminal nerve. One author (Peele, '61) considers cells of the mesencephalic nucleus to be homologous to cells of the dorsal nucleus of Clarke, but some impulses relayed by this nucleus reach consciousness and must be relayed to thalamic levels.

Connections of the mesencephalic nucleus are more extensive than previously believed (Pearson, '49). Some fibers leave

---

FIG. 12-22. Diagram of the secondary trigeminal tracts. The ventral trigeminal tract (*red*) conveys pain, thermal and tactile sense. These fibers originate from the spinal trigeminal nucleus, cross in the lower brain stem at various locations and ascend in association with the contralateral medial lemniscus. Secondary trigeminothalamic fibers from the principal sensory nucleus, conveying touch and pressure (*blue*), ascend by two separate pathways. Fibers from the ventral part of the principal sensory nucleus of N. V cross and ascend in association with the contralateral medial lemniscus. Fibers from the dorsomedial part of the same nucleus ascend uncrossed as the dorsal trigeminal tract. Both the ventral and dorsal trigeminal tracts project to the ventral posteromedial nucleus of the thalamus. The brain stem location of the ascending lateral spinothalamic tract is indicated in *black* on the *right side*. The ophthalmic (V^1), maxillary (V^2) and mandibular (V^3) divisions of the trigeminal nerve are identified. *1,* Free nerve ending; *2,* thermal receptor; *3,* Meissner's corpuscle; *4,* neuromuscular spindle; *5,* motor end plate in muscle of mastication.

the mesencephalic tract and enter the white matter of the cerebellum, possibly connecting with the deep cerebellar nuclei. Other fibers have been traced to the roof of the cerebral aqueduct, the base of the cerebellum and to the region of the superior colliculi.

Some authorities have suggested that deep sensibility of the lingual, facial and extraocular muscles is mediated by fibers of the fifth nerve (Cooper et al., '53, '53a). Other studies indicate that a localized part of the trigeminal ganglion contains cells whose afferent fibers convey impulses from muscle spindles in the extraocular muscles (Manni et al., '66). Cells, in a part of the ganglion which forms the ophthalmic division, respond with a sustained increase in discharge rate when the extraocular muscles are stretched; the discharge ceases as soon as the stretched muscles are released. These short latency responses are abolished by section of the ophthalmic division of the trigeminal nerve. Deep sensibility from the face also is considered to be mediated by the trigeminal nerve, but the possibility remains that this may be supplemented by facial nerve afferents.

The Motor Nucleus. The motor nucleus of the trigeminal nerve forms an ovoid column of typical multipolar motor cells that lies medial to the motor root and the principal sensory nucleus (Fig. 12-19). Its coarse efferent fibers emerge internal to the entering sensory root and pass underneath the trigeminal ganglion to become incorporated in the mandibular branch (Figs. 12-20 and 12-22). Among the terminals ending in the nucleus are collaterals from the mesencephalic root and other afferent trigeminal fibers. These fibers furnish a two-neuron arc for reflex control of the jaw muscles. Additional secondary trigeminal fibers, both crossed and uncrossed, provide reflex control of the jaw muscles to superficial stimuli, especially from the lingual and oral mucous membranes. As in the case of other motor cranial nerve nuclei, many corticobulbar fibers do not terminate directly upon cells of the motor trigeminal nucleus but pass to reticular neurons, which in turn project to motor cells (Fig. 11-23).

Secondary Trigeminal Pathways. Secondary trigeminal pathways originate from cells in the principal sensory and spinal trigeminal nuclei and project to higher levels of the brain stem. Collaterals of these fibers provide numerous, largely uncrossed projections to motor nuclei of the brain stem involved in complex reflexes (Fig. 12-20).

Axons from cells within the spinal trigeminal nucleus pass ventromedially in the reticular formation, cross the median raphe and become associated with the contralateral medial lemniscus (Smyth, '39; Walker, '39, '42; Nauta and Kuypers, '58; Carpenter and Hanna, '61). These secondary trigeminal fibers retain their close association with the contralateral medial lemniscus as they ascend in the brain stem (Fig. 12-22). At thalamic levels these fibers leave the medial lemniscus and terminate in a selective manner about cells of the ventral posteromedial (VPM) nucleus of the thalamus. Crossed axons from cells of the spinal trigeminal nucleus which ascend in the brain stem with the medial lemniscus form the *ventral trigeminal tract* (ventral trigeminothalamic tract).

Some efferent fibers from the spinal trigeminal nucleus pass into the parvicellular part of the reticular formation, and others arborize about cells of the nucleus reticularis gigantocellularis; a moderate number of fibers project to the cerebellum via the inferior cerebellar peduncle.

The relationship of the spinal trigeminal tract and nucleus to the spinothalamic tracts in the brain stem should be noted in Figure 12-22. The location of the latter tract is represented in *solid black dots* on the right side at each level. Vascular lesions in the lower medulla involving structures in this dorsolateral area frequently interrupt these pathways and produce a syndrome characterized by: (1) loss of pain and thermal sense over the face ipsilaterally, and (2) loss of pain and thermal sense, and impairment of tactile sensation over the contralateral half of the body (Figs. 20-13 and 20-14). The involvement of other structures in this region produces additional neurological deficits.

Secondary trigeminal fibers originating from the principal sensory nucleus are both crossed and uncrossed. Cells in the dorsomedial part of the nucleus give rise to a small bundle of uncrossed fibers which ascends to ipsilateral thalamic nuclei (Torvik, '57; Carpenter, '57a). These uncrossed fibers, constituting the *dorsal trigeminal tract* (von Economo, '11; Winkler, '21; Papez and Rundles, '37; Walker, '39; Verhaart, '54), ascend in the dorsal pontine tegmentum; at mesencephalic levels they occupy a position near the periaqueductal gray (Fig. 12-22). At the level of the fasciculus retroflexus the fibers make a ventrolateral bend and enter the medial part of the ventral posteromedial (VPM) nucleus of the thalamus. Because afferent fibers terminating in the dorsal part of the principal sensory nucleus are associated primarily with the mandibular division (Kerr, '63), it has been suggested that fibers of the dorsal trigeminal tract may subserve a unique function.

Neurons in the ventral part of the principal sensory nucleus of N. V give rise to a larger crossed bundle of trigeminothalamic fibers which ascends in association with the contralateral medial lemniscus, in a manner similar to that described for the ventral trigeminal tract (Wallenberg, '05; Winkler, '21; Papez and Rundles, '37; Walker, '39; Russell, '54; Torvik, '57). These crossed secondary trigeminal fibers also terminate in the ventral posteromedial (VPM) nucleus of the thalamus.

As previously mentioned the mesencephalic nucleus of the trigeminal nerve is anomalous in that the primary sensory neurons are found in this brain stem nucleus rather than in the trigeminal ganglion. While there is convincing evidence that fibers from this nucleus convey impulses from pressure, joint and stretch receptors, the pathway by which these impulses are transmitted centrally remains obscure. It seems likely that processes of cells in the mesencephalic nucleus of the trigeminal nerve may project to the cerebellum (Woodburne, '36; Pearson, '49). Since a significant part of the input to this nucleus comes from stretch receptors, and impulses from most stretch receptors in other parts of the body are relayed to the cerebellum, this hypothesis seems reasonable.

Trigeminal Reflexes. The numerous secondary *reflex* fibers arising from the terminal nuclei of N. V ascend and descend in the dorsolateral part of the reticular formation, giving off terminals or collaterals to various motor nuclei (Fig. 12-20). These are largely uncrossed and provide connections for reflexes initiated by stimulation of the skin of the face, the oral and nasal mucous membranes, and muscles, tendons and bones of the jaw and face. Among the more important of these reflexes is the *corneal reflex*. Normally stimulation of the cornea with a wisp of cotton produces bilateral blinking and closing of the eyes. The blinking and closing of the eyes is effected by impulses reaching the facial nuclei on both sides. Evidence suggests that secondary trigeminal fibers project bilaterally to the facial nuclei. Following an injury to the ophthalmic division of the trigeminal nerve, corneal sensation and the corneal reflex are lost on that side because the afferent limb of the reflex arc has been destroyed. However, corneal sensation remains on the opposite side and stimulation of that cornea will produce bilateral blinking and eye closure, indicating that the efferent limb (facial nucleus and nerve) of the reflex arc is intact. In patients with peripheral facial palsies, corneal sensation will be present on both sides, but no corneal reflex can be elicited on the side of the lesion because the efferent limb of the reflex arc has been destroyed. However, stimulation of the cornea on the side of the lesion will cause blinking and closure of the opposite eye (consensual response).

Other reflexes involving secondary trigeminal fibers which project impulses to cranial nerve nuclei include: (1) the *lacrimal* or *tearing reflex*, in which impulses pass to the superior salivatory nucleus of the intermediate nerve; (2) *sneezing*, in which impulses probably pass to the nucleus ambiguus, respiratory centers in the reticular formation and into the spinal cord (i.e., phrenic nerve nuclei and anterior horn cells innervating the intercostal muscles); and (3) *vomiting*, in which impulses pass predominantly to vagal nuclei (i.e., dorsal motor, ambiguus and solitary).

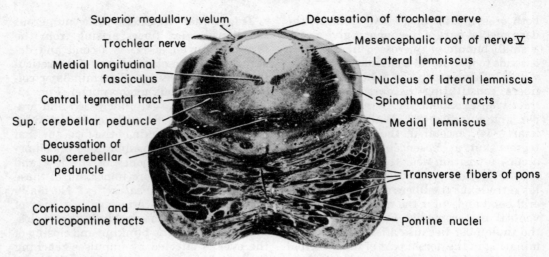

FIG. 12-23. Section of the isthmus of an adult brain at the level of the decussation and exit of the trochlear nerve. Weigert's myelin stain. Photograph.

The *jaw jerk,* or masseter reflex, is a monosynaptic myotatic reflex. This reflex is elicited by placing the examiner's index finger over the middle of the patient's chin (mouth slightly open) and tapping gently with a reflex hammer. The response is a bilateral contraction of the masseter and temporal muscles. This reflex involves the mesencephalic nucleus and collaterals given off by it to the motor nucleus.

ISTHMUS OF THE HINDBRAIN

The narrow portion of the hindbrain, situated rostral to the cerebellum, which merges with the midbrain is known as the *isthmus rhombencephali.* The most rostral levels of this region, near the junction with the midbrain, demonstrate characteristic features (Figs. 12-23, 12-24 and A-9). As in more caudal sections three regions are distinguishable, namely, a roof, the tegmentum and a ventral pontine portion. The roof consists of a thin membrane, the *superior medullary velum,* which covers the most superior portion of the fourth ventricle. The fourth ventricle is greatly reduced in size and resembles the *cerebral aqueduct* of the midbrain. The ventricle is bounded ventrally and laterally by the central gray matter. The root fibers of the *trochlear nerve* (N. IV) completely decussate in the superior medullary velum. They originate from nuclei which lie more rostrally in the ventral part of the central gray. The fibers arch dorsally and somewhat caudally around the fourth ventricle, decussate in the roof and emerge caudal to the inferior colliculus (Fig. 11-2). Only the decussation is seen at this level. The trochlear nerve innervates the superior oblique muscle of the eye.

The lateral lemniscus lies near the lateral surface of the tegmentum, forming the major part of the external structure known as the *trigonum lemnisci.* Groups of cells among its fibers constitute the *nucleus of the lateral lemniscus,* one of several intercalated nuclei in the auditory pathway (Figs. 12-10, 12-23 and 12-24). The medial lemniscus is a flattened band extending transversely in the ventrolateral tegmentum, and the spinothalamic tract is in its usual position between the two lemnisci. Included in the medial lemniscus are the secondary trigeminal fibers. The dorsal trigeminal tract ascends in the dorsal part of the reticular formation, lateral to the medial longitudinal fasciculus (Fig. 12-22). Thus at this level the principal ascending sensory pathways form a peripheral shell of fibers which enclose the pontine tegmentum. The ventral portion of the pons remains considerably larger than the tegmental portion (Figs. 12-23, A-26 and A-27). The pontine nuclei are extensive and lie in sheets between the numerous

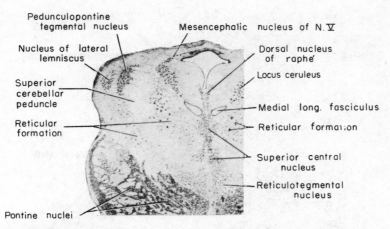

Pedunculopontine tegmental nucleus

Mesencephalic nucleus of N. Ⅴ

Nucleus of lateral lemniscus

Dorsal nucleus of raphé

Locus ceruleus

Superior cerebellar peduncle

Medial long. fasciculus

Reticular formation

Reticular formation

Superior central nucleus

Reticulotegmental nucleus

Pontine nuclei

FIG. 12-24. Section through isthmus of 3-month infant. Cresyl violet. Photograph, with cell groups schematically blocked in.

bundles of corticospinal and corticopontine fibers.

Superior Cerebellar Peduncle. This large bundle has passed from the hilus of the deep cerebellar nuclei into the dorsolateral part of the rostral pontine tegmentum. It forms a crescent-shaped bundle medial to the lateral lemniscus (Fig. 12-23). The superior cerebellar peduncle arises from the dentate, emboliform and globose nuclei and forms the most important efferent fiber system of the cerebellum. Emerging from the cerebellum, it first forms the dorsolateral wall of the fourth ventricle, then dips into the pontine tegmentum, and in the caudal midbrain undergoes a complete decussation (Figs. 12-23 and 14-16). Some of its fibers end in the red nucleus; others continue directly to the ventral lateral nucleus of the thalamus (Figs. 14-16 and 15-12). A relatively small number of fibers of the superior cerebellar peduncle descend lateral to the superior central nucleus to terminate in the reticulotegmental nucleus in the upper pons, and the paramedian reticular nuclei in the medulla (Carpenter and Nova, '60; Brodal and Szikla, '72). These cerebelloreticular fibers form part of a cerebelloreticular feedback pathway, since these reticular nuclei project fibers to parts of the cerebellum (Fig. 14-16).

Fibers of the anterior spinocerebellar tract which ascend in the lateral part of the reticular formation to levels of the up-

per pons become concentrated on the lateral surface of the superior cerebellar peduncle (Fig. 14-18). These fibers reverse their direction and enter the cerebellum by passing caudally along the dorsolateral border of the superior cerebellar peduncle. As these fibers descend in the superior medullary velum they terminate in the anterior lobe of the cerebellar vermis (Fig. 14-1). The majority of the fibers cross to the opposite side within the cerebellum. Part of the fibers of the rostral spinocerebellar tract also enter the cerebellum in association with the superior cerebellar peduncle.

In the upper pons the fibers of the superior cerebellar peduncle move ventromedially toward their decussation and divide the reticular formation into medial and lateral parts (Fig. 12-23). In the lateral part is a fairly dense collection of cells known as the *pedunculopontine tegmental nucleus* (i.e., the pedunculopontine nucleus). Cells of this nucleus are partially traversed by fibers of the superior cerebellar peduncle (Figs. 12-24 and 17-11). Compact and diffuse portions of this nucleus extend rostrally into the caudal midbrain (Olszewski and Baxter, '54). This nucleus receives cortical projections from the precentral gyrus (Kuypers and Lawrence, '67), and descending fibers from the globus pallidus (Nauta and Mehler, '66; Carpenter and Strominger, '67). The efferent projections of the pedunculopontine nucleus are unknown.

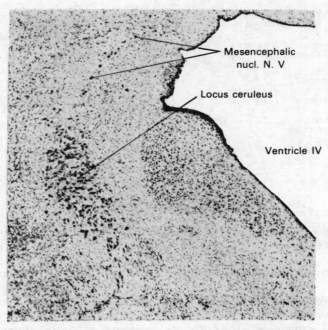

Mesencephalic
nucl. N. V

Locus ceruleus

Ventricle IV

FIG. 12-25. Photograph of the cell groups surrounding the periventricular gray at isthmus levels. Cells of the locus ceruleus contain melanin pigment granules and high concentrations of norepinephrine. Globular cells of the mesencephalic nucleus of N. V are present along the dorsal border of the locus ceruleus and extend dorsally and rostrally at the margin of the central gray.

Locus Ceruleus. Near the central gray of the upper part of the fourth ventricle is an irregular collection of medium-sized pigmented cells referred to as the *locus ceruleus* or *nucleus pigmentosus pontis* (Figs. 12-24 and 12-25). This nucleus, which first appears at levels slightly rostral to the principal sensory nucleus of N. V, lies ventromedial to the mesencephalic root and nucleus of the trigeminal nerve. The large globular neurons of the mesencephalic nucleus of N. V are partially intermingled with those of the locus ceruleus ventrally, but these cells extend further dorsally and rostrally in a linear fashion at the margin of the central gray (Fig. 12-25). Cells of the locus ceruleus are of at least two types: (1) medium-sized oval or round cells with eccentric nuclei and fairly large clumps of melanin pigment granules, and (2) small oval cells with scant cytoplasm which usually are free of pigment (Olszewski and Baxter, '54; Russell, '55). Ventrolateral to the locus ceruleus is a more diffuse collection of similar cells which forms the *nu-*

cleus subceruleus (Olszewski and Baxter, '54).

Although the locus ceruleus is a large structure which can be identified readily in gross sections of the brain stem, the significance of this pigmented nucleus long remained unknown. It had been postulated that it might be related to the trigeminal nuclei, that it might give rise to fibers descending in the reticular formation and that it might be associated with the pontine pneumotaxic center (Johnson and Russell, '52; Baxter and Olszewski, '55). By means of a sensitive fluorescence technic for demonstrating monoamine-containing neurons in the central nervous system, it was demonstrated that cells of the locus ceruleus contained catecholamines, practically all of which are norepinephrine (Dahlström and Fuxe, '64; Andén et al., '66; Olson and Fuxe, '71; Ungerstedt, '71). Using various anatomical and biochemical technics, norepinephrine pathways originating in the locus ceruleus have been mapped (Fig. 12-26). Norepinephrine path-

ways from the locus ceruleus ascend in
dorsal parts of the midbrain, and at diencephalic levels appear to join the medial forebrain bundle and pass rostrally into the
septal region (Figs. 18-4 and 18-5). Lesions
of the locus ceruleus and the dorsal bundle
ascending from it appear to distribute norepinephrine nerve terminals in wide regions of the cerebral and cerebellar cortex
and in the hippocampal formation (Ungerstedt, '71; Olson and Fuxe, '71; Maeda and
Shimizu, '72). Fibers originating from a
more disseminated group of pontine neurons which includes part of the locus ceruleus and the nucleus subceruleus ascend
as an intermediate norepinephrine pathway to the periventricular zone of the hypothalamus (Maeda and Shimizu, '72). The
precise manner in which these fine norepinephrine fibers are distributed so widely
in the forebrain is not entirely clear. Norepinephrine fibers projecting to the cerebellar cortex pass dorsally medial to the middle cerebellar peduncle. It has been stated
that collaterals from a single noradrenergic neuron in the dorsolateral part of
the locus ceruleus can monosynaptically
innervate both the cerebral and cerebellar
cortex (Olson and Fuxe, '71). Thus neurons
of the locus ceruleus appear organized to
simultaneously influence neural activity
in practically all cortical regions of the
brain. The extent to which the ascending
nonadrenergic pathways give collaterals
to subcortical structures remains to be determined.

Raphe Nuclei. In addition to the cell
groups of the pontine reticular formation
previously described, the pons contains
cell groups in the median raphe which
properly belong to the reticular formation,
but appear to serve distinctive functions
(Taber et al., '60; Brodal et al., '60).

The raphe nuclei of the human brain
have not been studied extensively, and the
variations in nomenclature used are confusing. Detailed cytological descriptions of
these nuclei in the cat (Taber et al., '60)
suggest similarities to the raphe nuclei in
man (Olszewski and Baxter, '54). The
raphe nuclei of the medulla (i.e., nucleus
raphe obscurus, nucleus raphe pallidus
and nucleus raphe magnus) are smaller

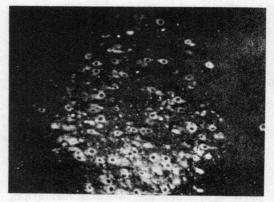

FIG. 12-26. Photomicrograph of catecholamine-
containing cell bodies in the locus ceruleus of the
squirrel monkey. Green fluorescence in the cytoplasm of these cells is considered to be due to norepinephrine. The nuclei of these cells are nonfluores-
cent. A few catecholamine-containing varicosities
are present in the background. ×200. (Courtesy of
Dr. David L. Felton, School of Medicine, Indiana
University.)

and more restricted than similar nuclei in
the pons. The *inferior central nucleus* appears in the median raphe at the junction
of pons and medulla (Fig. 11-24) and at
caudal pontine levels (Fig. 12-4). This nucleus may represent the rostral part of the
nucleus raphe magnus. The *nucleus raphe
pontis* consists of several small cell groups,
dorsal and rostral to the inferior central
nucleus. The rostral extension of the pontine raphe nuclei is the *superior central
nucleus* (Figs. 12-19 and 12-24), a large
aggregation of closely packed small- and
medium-sized cells. Decussating fibers of
the superior cerebellar peduncle pass
through the superior central nucleus (Fig.
12-23). On each side of the midline, dorsal
to the medial longitudinal fasciculus, is
the *dorsal nucleus of the raphe* (Fig. 12-
24). This nucleus extends rostrally in the
ventral central gray into the caudal midbrain and merges with the *dorsal tegmental nucleus* (Fig. 13-3). Anatomical studies
indicate that most of the raphe nuclei give
rise to long ascending projections (Brodal
et al., '60). The superior central nucleus
receives descending fibers from the medial
forebrain bundle and some fibers from the
fasciculus retroflexus (Fig. 18-5; Nauta,

'58). The dorsal tegmental nucleus receives fibers from the mammillotegmental tract and projects impulses back to the mammillary bodies.

Histofluorescence technics demonstrate that the nuclei of the raphe region have a yellow fluorescence distinctive for 5-hydroxytryptamine (5-HT, serotonin) which can be demonstrated best by the use of monoamine oxidase inhibitors (Dahlström and Fuxe, '64; Pin et al., '68). These cells present a sharp contrast with the norepinephrine-containing neurons in lateral parts of the pontine reticular formation, particularly the locus ceruleus, which have a green fluorescence. The 5-HT cell bodies in the raphe nuclei give rise to ascending axons which enter the ventral part of the medial forebrain bundle and pass to the septal region and limbic forebrain structures (Ungerstedt, '71).

Recent investigations indicate that both serotonin and norepinephrine-containing neurons in the reticular formation play roles in the active mechanisms that control sleep states (Jouvet, '69). Sleep is not a single phenomenon. Sleep states can be quantitatively measured and correlated with biochemical, pharmacological and structural alterations. Inhibition of serotonin synthesis, or total destruction of serotonin-containing neurons, in the raphe system leads to total insomnia. Serotonin appears to be involved in the mechanism of what is called *slow wave sleep,* a state characterized by the posture of sleep, myotic pupils and cortical electrical activity (electroencephalogram) which displays spindles and slow waves. In addition, serotonin-containing neurons appear to have a "priming" effect upon the cells of the locus ceruleus which serve as the "triggering" mechanism for what is called *paradoxical sleep* (Jouvet, '69; Chu and Bloom, '73). Paradoxical sleep occurs intermittently after variable periods of slow sleep and is characterized by: (1) abolition of antigravity muscle tone, (2) reductions in blood pressure, bradycardia and irregular respiration, (3) bursts of rapid eye movements (REM), and (4) an electroencephalogram (EEG) which resembles that of the waking state. Lesions in caudal portions of the raphe nuclei suppress paradoxical sleep relative to slow sleep, while bilateral lesions of the locus ceruleus cause a total selective suppression of paradoxical sleep.

At this point the student will find it instructive to review the blood supply of the medulla and pons (Chapter 20, page 616). Familiarity with the internal organization of the hindbrain and the connections of the cranial nerves should give the reader a better appreciation of the neurological syndromes which follow sudden occlusion of arteries of the vertebro-basilar system. Other lower brain stem lesions associated with syringobulbia, demyelinating diseases and tumors frequently begin in localized regions and produce specific neurological signs and symptoms.

CHAPTER 13

The Mesencephalon

The midbrain, or mesencephalon, is the smallest and least differentiated division of the brain stem. Like other parts of the brain stem it can be divided into three parts: (1) the *tectum* or quadrigeminal plate, dorsal to the cerebral aqueduct, (2) the massive *crura cerebri* on the ventrolateral surfaces, and (3) the *tegmentum*, centrally, representing the rostral continuation of the pontine tegmentum. The cerebral aqueduct, surrounded by the central gray substance (i.e., periaqueductal gray) separates the tectum from the tegmentum (Fig. 13-1). The term *cerebral peduncle*, according to the accepted nomenclature, denotes one half of the midbrain, excluding the tectum. The cerebral peduncle consists of two parts: (1) a dorsal part, the tegmentum, and (2) a ventral part, the crus cerebri. These two parts of the cerebral peduncle are separated from each other by a large pigmented nuclear mass, the *substantia nigra* (Figs. 13-1 and A-27).

The midbrain contains the nuclei of the trochlear and oculomotor nerves and neural structures concerned with ocular and visual reflexes. Relay nuclei constituting important parts of the auditory and visual systems are prominent, along with pathways inter-relating higher and lower portions of the neuraxis. The principal nuclear masses and fiber pathways can be observed and studied at two typical levels, namely, the levels of the inferior and superior colliculi. The latter level is shown diagrammatically in Figure 13-1.

INFERIOR COLLICULAR LEVEL

The transition from isthmus to midbrain is associated with changes mainly in the tectum and tegmentum (Figs. 12-23, 12-24, 13-2, 13-3, A-9 and A-10). Comparison of these levels reveals that: (1) the fourth ventricle has become the cerebral aqueduct, (2) the superior medullary velum is replaced by two rounded eminences, the inferior colliculi, and (3) fibers of the superior cerebellar peduncles have begun to decussate. The ventral part of the pons is reduced in size and, at slightly more rostral levels, undergoes a reorganization as the massive crura cerebri appear (Figs. 13-3 and 13-4). In some sections portions of the heavily pigmented substantia nigra are evident dorsal to the rostral pontine nuclei. Fibers of the lateral lemniscus, located near the lateral surface of the tegmentum, migrate dorsally and enter the inferior colliculus. These fibers envelop the inferior colliculus and form its capsule (Figs. 13-2 and 13-3).

The Inferior Colliculi. These distinctive large cellular masses can be divided into three main subdivisions: (1) an ovoid cell mass called the central nucleus, (2) a thin dorsal cellular layer referred to as the cortex, and (3) a pericollicular tegmentum which surrounds the central nucleus medially, laterally and ventrally, and contains most of the myelinated fibers passing to and from the inferior colliculus (Geniec and Morest, '71). The *central nucleus* con-

367

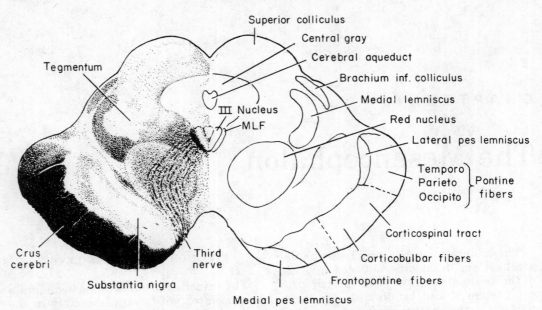

FIG. 13-1. Schematic transverse section through upper portion of midbrain.

sists of densely packed cell bodies of many sizes and shapes which appear intermingled (Figs. 13-3 and A-10). Golgi impregnations indicate a definite spatial orientation of dendrites. At least five types of neurons have been identified; three of these have stellate dendrites arranged in radial patterns, and two have disc-shaped dendritic fields. The cells with disc-shaped dendrites are layered obliquely, parallel to the incoming fibers of the lateral lemniscus. The cortex of the inferior colliculus extends its entire length, from the junction with the superior colliculus to the superior medullary velum. Like the cerebral cortex this collicular cortex is layered, consisting of four lamina. Dendrites of cortical neurons often extend more than one layer. Cortical neurons are mainly small, with the largest neurons in layer IV. Neurons of the pericollicular tegmentum may, in part, represent extensions of the lateral midbrain tegmentum.

The inferior colliculus receives fibers from the lateral lemniscus, the opposite inferior colliculus, the ipsilateral medial geniculate body and the auditory cortex (Fig. 12-10). The auditory cortex projects fibers bilaterally to the inferior colliculi; ipsilateral fibers pass to all three divisions of the inferior colliculus, while crossed fibers are fewer in number and restricted to the central nucleus and the dorsomedial cortex (Diamond et al., '69). Efferent fibers from the inferior colliculus project to the small-celled portion of the medial geniculate body via the brachium of the inferior colliculus (Figs. 12-10, 13-4, 13-17 and A-12). Other fibers pass to the opposite inferior colliculus, the superior colliculus and to lower relay nuclei in the auditory system (Rasmussen, '60). Few, if any, tectospinal fibers arise from the inferior colliculus (Woollard and Harpman, '40).

The inferior colliculi serve as relay nuclei in transmitting auditory impulses to thalamic levels and are involved in acoustic reflexes. Physiological studies (Rose et al., '63) in the cat indicate that a definite tonotopic localization is present in the inferior colliculus. Neurons in the central nucleus of the inferior colliculus are arranged in an orderly geometric manner with respect to frequencies. Advancement of an electrode from its point of penetration (dorsal, caudal and lateral) in a ventral, oral and medial direction consistently gives a sequence of frequencies from low to high in the central nucleus. In the lateral part of the inferior colliculus, near its capsule, frequencies follow a sequence from high to low, the reverse of that seen in the central nucleus. Other data (Rose et al., '66) have demonstrated that there are neurons in the inferior colliculus whose response is a sensitive function of interaural time relationships. Since it is well known that time and sound intensity cues are utilized for the localization of sound sources, these data suggest that the inferior colliculus may play a significant role in this function.

Ventrolateral to the inferior colliculus is a fairly well-defined zone known as the *parabigeminal area*, lying between the lateral lemniscus and the periphery (Fig. 13-2). It is composed mainly of obliquely, or transversely, running fibers, among which are scattered cells or groups of cells constituting the *parabigeminal nucleus*. Its connections are obscure, but apparently some fibers from the nucleus pass to the lateral nuclei of the pons. The more numerous fibers gathered at the lateral periphery of the area are regarded by some as corticopontine fibers from the occipital cortex.

The Trochlear Nerve. The nucleus of the trochlear nerve is a small compact cell group in the ventral part of the central gray that appears to indent the dorsal surface of the medial longitudinal fasciculus (Fig. 13-3). The nucleus consists of a column of typical somatic motor cells that in essence constitute a small caudal appendage to the oculomotor nuclear complex. Root fibers emerging from the nucleus curve dorsolaterally and caudally in the outer margin of the central gray, decussate completely in the superior medullary velum and exit from the dorsal surface of the brain stem caudal to the inferior colliculus (Figs. 2-18, 2-19, 11-2, 12-23, 13-2, 13-3 and A-9). Peripherally the slender nerve root curves around the lateral surface of the brain stem, passes between the superior cerebellar and posterior cerebral arteries and enters the cavernous sinus (Fig. 20-9). This cranial nerve innervates the superior oblique muscle that serves to: (1) intort the eye when abducted, and (2) depress the eye when adducted. Lesions involving the trochlear nerve alone are unusual and detection of resulting disturb-

ances of extraocular movement by inspection is difficult. Diplopia resulting from such a nerve lesion is vertical and maximal on attempted downward gaze to the opposite side. Patients with trochlear nerve lesions complain especially of difficulty in walking downstairs. Tilting of the head to the opposite side, seen in some patients with trochlear nerve lesions, is a posture which compensates for the weakness of ocular intortion on the lesion side (Cogan, '56).

Tegmental and Interpeduncular Nuclei. The narrow aqueduct, somewhat triangular in section, is surrounded by a broad layer of central gray substance that contains numerous diffuse cell groups. In the rapheal region several nuclei are present at this level (Fig. 13-3). The dorsal nucleus of the raphe has expanded into the *dorsal tegmental nucleus* (supratrochlear nucleus, Olszewski and Baxter, '54), composed of many small and some larger cells. It lies in the central gray dorsal to the trochlear nuclei. Immediately ventral to the medial longitudinal fasciculus, the cells near the raphe constitute the *ventral tegmental nucleus*, which appears to be a continuation of the superior central nucleus of the pons.

In the rapheal region of the ventral tegmentum is the *interpeduncular nucleus*, a collection of medium-sized, multipolar, slightly pigmented cells (Fig. 13-3). This nucleus, situated immediately dorsal to the interpeduncular fossa, is prominent in most mammals, but comparatively small in man. Fibers from the habenular nucleus project to the interpeduncular nucleus via the fasciculus retroflexus (Figs. 15-5 and 16-5); some fibers in this bundle bypass the interpeduncular nucleus and are distributed to the superior central nucleus, the dorsal tegmental nucleus and caudal regions of the central gray (Nauta, '58). The dorsal tegmental nucleus also receives fibers from the interpeduncular nucleus and from the mammillary bodies (via the mammillotegmental tract). The dorsal tegmental nucleus appears related to the *dorsal longitudinal fasciculus* (of Schütz), a small but complex pathway in the ventromedial part of the central gray

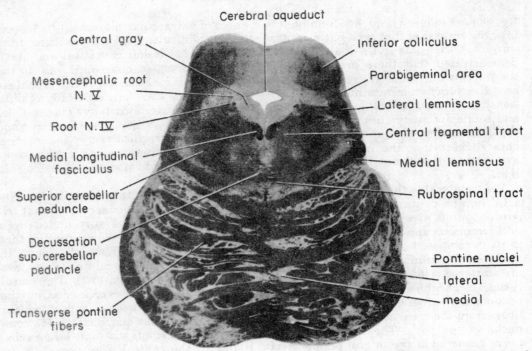

FIG. 13-2. Transverse section of the adult midbrain through the inferior colliculus. Large fascicles of corticospinal and corticopontine fibers (unlabeled), cut in cross section, are located among the bundles of transverse pontine fibers. Weigert's myelin stain. Photograph.

(Fig. 16-7). Although the prevailing direction of conduction appears to be ascending in this bundle, it contains some descending elements, but few of these reach pontine levels. The pathways described above constitute part of the complex system by which impulses related to the limbic system are projected to midbrain levels. Impulses conducted via these pathways are thought to be concerned primarily with visceral functions.

Corticofugal fibers (corticospinal, corticopontine and corticobulbar) on the ventral surface of the brain stem undergo a rearrangement and at higher levels begin to form the *crus cerebri* (Fig. 13-3). At slightly higher levels these fibers are separated from the tegmentum by a mass of gray matter, the *substantia nigra* (Figs. 13-4, A-10 and A-11).

SUPERIOR COLLICULAR LEVEL

Transverse sections of the rostral midbrain appear strikingly different from those through the inferior colliculus in

that: (1) the flattened superior colliculi form the tectum (Figs. 13-4, 13-5 and 13-6), (2) the oculomotor nuclei form a V-shaped complex ventral to the central gray and root fibers of the nerve emerge from the interpeduncular fossa (Figs. 13-1, 13-4 and 13-17), (3) the red nuclei, surrounded by fibers of the superior cerebellar peduncle, occupy the central tegmental region (Figs. 13-1, 13-4 and 13-10), and (4) the substantia nigrae achieve their maximum size ventral to the tegmentum and dorsal to the crura cerebri (Fig. 13-4). Fibers of the brachium of the inferior colliculus lie on the lateral surface of the tegmentum (Fig. 13-4). The medial lemniscus appears as a curved bundle dorsal to the substantia nigra and lateral to the red nucleus. The spinothalamic and spinotectal tracts lie together, medial to the most dorsal part of the medial lemniscus.

Superior Colliculi

The superior colliculi are two flattened eminences which form the rostral half of

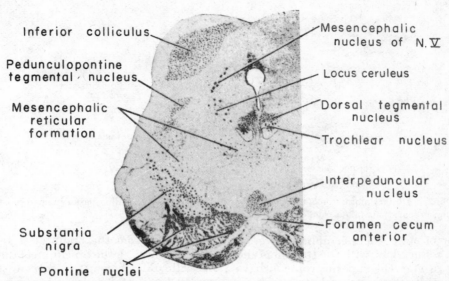

Inferior colliculus

Pedunculopontine
tegmental nucleus

Mesencephalic
reticular
formation

Substantia
nigra

Pontine nuclei

Mesencephalic
nucleus of N. V

Locus ceruleus

Dorsal tegmental
nucleus

Trochlear nucleus

Interpeduncular
nucleus

Foramen cecum
anterior

FIG. 13-3. Section through inferior colliculi of midbrain. Three-month infant. Cresyl violet. Photograph, with schematic representation of main cell groups.

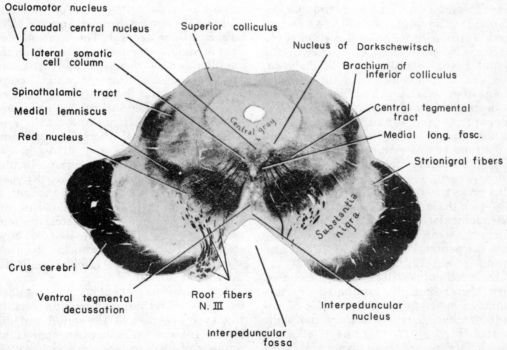

Oculomotor nucleus
  caudal central nucleus
  lateral somatic
  cell column

Spinothalamic tract
Medial lemniscus
Red nucleus

Crus cerebri

Ventral tegmental
decussation

Root fibers
N. III

Interpeduncular
fossa

Superior colliculus

Nucleus of Darkschewitsch

Brachium of
inferior colliculus

Central tegmental
tract

Medial long. fasc.

Strionigral fibers

Interpeduncular
nucleus

Central gray

Substantia nigra

FIG. 13-4. Transverse section of adult midbrain through exit of N. III. Weigert's myelin stain. Photograph.

the tectum (Figs. 2-18, 2-19, 13-4 and A-11). In submammalian vertebrates the optic tectum, a structure homologous with the mammalian superior colliculus, has a complex laminated structure resembling that of the cerebral cortex, and it is a primary way station in the optic tract. Beginning with reptiles, the importance of the superior colliculus in visual discrimination diminishes progressively as an increasing

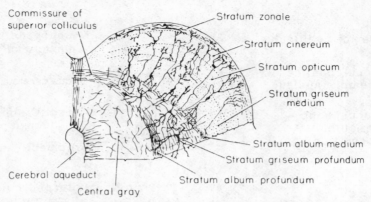

FIG. 13-5. Cellular lamination and organization of the superior colliculus based upon reconstruction from Golgi preparations taken from an 8-month human fetus.

number of optic fibers establish more extensive connections with the thalamus and cortex. In man the superior colliculi have become reduced in size and serve primarily as reflex centers, influencing the position of the head and eyes in response to visual, auditory and somatic stimuli (Gordon, '72). The superior colliculus is concerned primarily with the detection of the direction of movement of objects in the visual fields (Sterling and Wickelgren, '69), and in this way it facilitates visual orientation, searching and tracking. Cells in deeper layers of the superior colliculus appear to respond to auditory, somatic and visual stimuli, sometimes separately and sometimes in different combinations (Gordon, '72). Further efferent fibers arising in the superficial layers of the superior colliculus project to regions of the pulvinar and posterior thalamus that form parts of an extrageniculate visual pathway which parallels the geniculostriate system (Altman and Carpenter, '61; Graybiel, '72; Casagrande et al., '72; Harting et al., '73).

Each colliculus still shows in a rudimentary form the complex laminated structure found in lower forms and consists of several alternating layers of gray and white matter (Figs. 10-17, 13-5 and 13-6). From the surface inward these layers are: (1) the *stratum zonale* (mainly fibrous), (2) the *stratum cinereum* (outer gray layer), (3) the *stratum opticum* (superficial white layer), and (4) the *stratum lemnisci* consisting of middle and deep, gray and white layers (Figs. 13-5 and 13-6). The stratum zonale is composed of fine nerve fibers aris-

ing mainly from the occipital cortex and entering through the brachium of the superior colliculus. Among the fibers are small, mostly horizontal cells with tangentially or centrally directed axons. The stratum cinereum consists of radially arranged cells whose dendrites pass peripherally and whose axons project inward. The larger cells lie deepest. The stratum opticum is composed mainly of fibers from the ganglion cells of the retina, and corticostriate fibers arising from the visual cortex. These fibers enter the stratum opticum via the brachium of the superior colliculus and pass into the superficial and middle gray layers. Corticotectal fibers from the frontal lobe (Brodmann's area 8) reach deep and middle layers of the superior colliculus via a transtegmental approach (Kuypers and Lawrence, '67), and are thought to participate in mechanisms related to conjugate eye movements. The stratum lemnisci, composed of medium-sized and large stellate cells, receive spinotectal fibers and some fibers from the inferior colliculus (Mehler et al., '60).

The superior colliculus receives fibers from: (1) the retina, via the optic tract, (2) the cerebral cortex, (3) the spinal cord, and (4) the inferior colliculus. An appreciable number of *primary optic fibers* leave the optic tract rostral to its principal termination in the lateral geniculate body and project to the superior colliculus via its brachium. These fibers are predominantly crossed and terminate largely in the caudal two-thirds of the superior colliculus. Ganglion cells receiving impulses from the

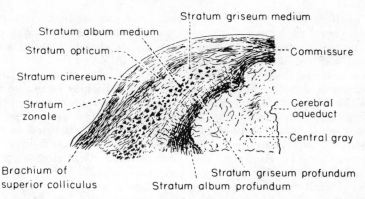

Stratum griseum medium

Stratum album medium

Stratum opticum

Commissure

Stratum cinereum

Stratum
zonale

Cerebral
aqueduct

Central gray

Brachium of
superior colliculus

Stratum griseum profundum

Stratum album profundum

FIG. 13-6. Drawing of the myelinated fiber structure of the adult superior colliculus based upon Weigert-stained sections.

macular region of the retina project no direct fibers to the superior colliculus (Brouwer and Zeeman, '26; Wilson and Toyne, '70). The visual field projects upon the superior colliculus in an orderly fashion so that homonymous halves of the visual field are represented in the contralateral superior colliculus (Fig. 15-21). The visual field is represented in a distorted fashion, with the central 30 degrees of the visual field occupying the rostral three-fourths of the superior colliculus and the remaining 60 degrees crowded into the caudal quarter.

Corticotectal fibers arise from portions of the frontal, temporal, parietal and occipital lobes. The most substantial and highly organized projection arises from the visual cortex (Kuypers and Lawrence, '67; Garey et al., '68). These fibers enter the stratum opticum and terminate in the superficial and middle gray layers of the superior colliculus, in the same manner as fibers from the retina. Corticotectal fibers from the visual cortex project ipsilaterally to rostral portions of the superior colliculus which do not receive retinal fibers (Wilson and Toyne, '70). Although retinal and visual cortical projections to the superior colliculus are similar, there are certain important differences: (1) retinal projections are bilateral and greatest contralateral, while (2) visual (striate) cortical projections are unilateral. Anatomical data suggest that portions of the visual cortex and superior colliculus related to particular regions of the retina are interconnected (Garey et al., '68; Wilson and Toyne, '70). Superior por-

tions of the retina (i.e., inferior half of the visual field) are represented superiorly in the visual cortex and laterally in the superior colliculus, while inferior portions of the retina (i.e., superior half of the visual field) are represented inferiorly in the visual cortex and medially in the superior colliculus. Thus many of the same cells of the superior colliculus receive distinct, but related, inputs from the ganglion cells of the retina and cells of the striate cortex. The macular representation in the superior colliculus, however, receives an input only from the striate cortex. Cells in the rostral part of the superior colliculus represent the macular area of the retina. At this brain stem level there is the possibility of a potent interaction and integration of peripheral visual impulses with the more complex output of the visual cortex. Corticotectal fibers from the auditory cortex project mainly to deeper layers in caudal parts of the superior colliculus (Diamond et al., '69). *Spinotectal* and other afferent fibers, including some from the inferior colliculus, end in the deeper layers.

Efferent fibers from the superior colliculus arise from large and medium-sized cells in deeper layers. Efferent projections include: tectothalamic, tectoreticular, tectopontine and tectospinal fibers. *Tectothalamic fibers* are considered to arise from the superficial layers of the superior colliculus and to project to subdivisions of the ipsilateral pulvinar, dorsal and ventral lateral geniculate nuclei and perhaps the pretectum (Altman and Carpenter, '61; Casagrande et al., '72; Graybiel, '72; Harting et al., '73). Part of these fibers form links in extrageniculate visual pathways. *Tectoreticular fibers* project profusely and bilaterally to dorsal regions of the midbrain reticular formation. Some of these fibers enter the accessory oculomotor nuclei (i.e., the nucleus of Darkschewitsch and the interstitial nucleus of Cajal), but none appear to enter the oculomotor complex (Papez and Freeman, '30; Rasmussen, '36; Marburg and Warner, '47; Szentágothai, '50; Altman and Carpenter, '61). *Tectopontine fibers* pass caudally beneath the inferior colliculus and terminate in the dorsolateral pontine nuclei on the same side.

Experimental studies (Jefferson, '58) have demonstrated that stimulation of the superior colliculus in the cat provokes a typical EEG arousal response (see page 390), suggesting that visual activation of the cerebral cortex may be mediated by tectoreticular fiber systems. Available data suggest that the tectopontine fibers may relay optic impulses to the cerebellum as described physiologically by Snider ('50).

Tectospinal and *tectobulbar fibers* cross in the dorsal tegmental decussation at midbrain levels and descend near the median raphe (Fig. 10-17); at medullary levels these fibers become incorporated within the medial longitudinal fasciculus. Tectospinal fibers continuing to cervical spinal segments descend in the medial part of the anterior funiculus (Fig. 10-21).

Functional Considerations. Each superior colliculus receives a visual input largely from the contralateral visual field. In addition it receives an ipsilateral projection from the visual cortex supplying information concerning only the contralateral visual field. These two systems are precisely and topographically organized at all levels. Unilateral lesions of the superior colliculus in a variety of animals produce: (1) relative neglect of visual stimuli in the contralateral visual field, (2) deficits in perception involving spatial discriminations and tracking of moving objects, (3) heightened responses to stimuli in the ipsilateral visual field, and (4) no impairment of eye movements (Sprague and Meikle, '65; Sprague, '72). These disturbances undergo considerable compensation in time,

but they suggest that the superior colliculus contributes to ability to use head and eye movements to localize and follow visual stimuli.

Physiological studies in the cat indicate that the collicular receptive fields are two to four times larger than receptive fields in the visual cortex. The receptive field in the visual system is defined as that region of the retina (or visual field) over which one can influence the firing of a particular ganglion cell (Kuffler, '53). The receptive field consists of a central circular region and a concentric surround. Most collicular cells respond only to moving stimuli and three-fourths of these cells show directional selectivity (Sterling and Wickelgren, '69). These cells respond well to movement in one direction, poorly, or not at all, to movement in the opposite direction, and are nonresponsive to stationary stimuli flashed on and off within the receptive field. In the superior colliculus the preferred directional selectivity is parallel to the horizontal meridian of the visual field and toward the periphery of the visual field. Thus most units in the right superior colliculus had receptive fields in the left visual field and responded best to stimuli moving from right to left. Cells in the superficial layers of the superior colliculus tend to be most responsive to small moving objects.

Thus the superior colliculus receives two major visual inputs, one from the retina and one from the visual cortex. In animals in which the visual cortex has been removed, cells of the superior colliculus lose their directional sensitivity to moving objects in the visual field (Wickelgren and Sterling, '69). While in the normal animal cells in the superior colliculus can be driven by stimuli to either eye, following ablations of the visual cortex, these cells respond only to stimuli in the contralateral eye. These studies suggest that the superior colliculus cannot perform its normal function as a detector of specific movements within the visual field when deprived of input from the visual cortex.

The Pretectal Region

This region lies immediately rostral to the superior colliculus at levels of the posterior commissure (Figs. 13-7 and 15-4). This

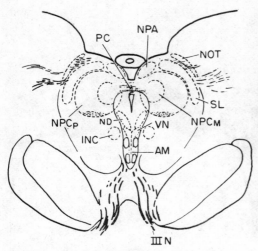

III N

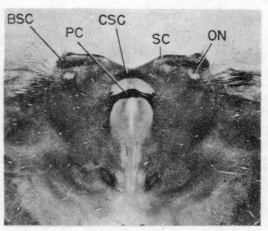

FIG. 13-7. Outline drawing of a brain stem section through the most compact portion of the posterior commissure (*PC*). At this level, the nucleus of the optic tract (*NOT*), the sublentiform nucleus (*SL*), the nucleus of the pretectal area (*NPA*) and the nuclei of the posterior commissure (*NPC*) are well developed. The anterior median nucleus (*AM*) is present, but the dorsal visceral nuclei (*VN*) of the oculomotor complex have not separated into medial and lateral cell columns. Additional abbreviations: *INC*, interstitial nucleus of Cajal; *ND*, nucleus of Darkschewitsch; *NPCm*, nucleus of posterior commissure, pars magnocellularis; *NPCp*, nucleus of posterior commissure, pars principalis; *III N*, oculomotor nerve. (Carpenter and Pierson, '73; courtesy of The Wistar Institute.)

FIG. 13-8. Photomicrograph of myelin-stained section at junction of pretectum and superior colliculus in the rhesus monkey. Abbreviations are as follows: *BSC*, brachium of the superior colliculus; *CSC*, commissure of the superior colliculus; *ON*, olivary nucleus; *PC*, posterior commissure; *SC*, superior colliculus. Weil stain. ×7. (Carpenter and Pierson, '73; courtesy of The Wistar Institute.)

area is composed of several distinct cell groups, most of which are related to the visual system. The nuclei of the pretectal region include: (1) the nucleus of the optic tract, (2) the sublentiform nucleus, (3) the nucleus of the pretectal area, (4) the olivary nucleus, and (5) the principal pretectal nucleus (Aronson and Papez, '34; Kuhlenbeck and Miller, '49). The nucleus of the optic tract consists of an irregular plate of large cells along the dorsolateral border of the pretectum at its junction with the pulvinar (Fig. 13-7). The sublentiform nucleus forms a crescent-shaped group of small- and medium-sized cells medial to the nucleus of the optic tract. The nucleus of the pretectal area occupies a dorsomedial part of the pretectum throughout its extent. The olivary nucleus (or olivary nucleus of the superior colliculus) forms a sharply delimited cell group at levels through cau-

dal parts of the posterior commissure and rostrolateral parts of the superior colliculus (Fig. 13-8). This nucleus and the nucleus of the optic tract are considered to be derived from a common ontogenetic matrix. The principal pretectal nucleus lies ventral to the sublentiform nucleus and its boundaries are difficult to distinguish. These nuclei receive fibers from the optic tract, the lateral geniculate body, certain areas of the cortex and probably from posterior thalamic nuclei (Garey et al., '68; Hendrickson et al., '70; Giolli and Tigges, '70; Giolli and Guthrie, '71; Scalia, '72; Pierson and Carpenter, '74). The pretectal region is considered as the principal midbrain center involved in the *pupillary light reflex* (Ranson and Magoun, '33; Magoun and Ranson, '35, '35a).

Studies in the monkey indicate that fibers from the olivary nucleus, which receives retinofugal fibers, cross in the posterior commissure and project to specific components of the visceral nuclei of the oculomotor complex (Carpenter and Pierson, '73). Fibers from the nuclei of the posterior commissure, projecting bilaterally to other visceral nuclei, partially decussate ventral to the cerebral aqueduct (Fig. 13-13). Because of the complex crossed and un-

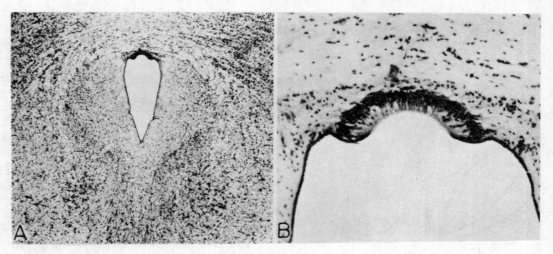

FIG. 13-9. Photomicrographs of the subcommissural organ in the rhesus monkey. *A*, shows the position of the structure in the roof of the aqueduct beneath the posterior commissure. *B*, contrasts the tall columnar cells of the subcommissural organ with the cells of the ependyma. Nissl stain. ×16; ×100.

crossed projection system to the visceral nuclei of N. III, only relatively large lesions involving multiple structures in the pretectum appear to impair the pupillary light reflex.

The Posterior Commissure

The region of transition from midbrain to diencephalon is marked dorsally by the *posterior commissure*. The posterior commissure lies immediately rostral to the superior colliculus at the place where the cerebral aqueduct becomes the third ventricle (Figs. 2-21, 13-7, 13-8, 13-9*A* and 13-12*B*). Fibers of the posterior commissure are surrounded rostrally, laterally and ventrally by cells known collectively as the nuclei of the posterior commissure (Fig. 13-7; Carpenter and Peter, '70/'71). Although the posterior commissure is a fairly good sized bundle and appears to contain several different fiber components, its entire composition is unknown. The posterior commissure is considered to contain: (1) fibers from the pretectal nuclei, (2) fibers from the nuclei of the posterior commissure (Fig. 13-7), and (3) fibers from the interstitial nucleus and the nucleus of Darkschewitsch (Fig. 13-7). Fibers from the olivary nucleus (Fig. 13-8) cross in the commissure to the same nucleus on the opposite side and give collaterals to the visceral nuclei of the oculomotor complex (Fig. 13-13). Lesions in the

posterior commissure are said to reduce, but not eliminate, the consensual pupillary light reflex in the cat (Magoun et al., '35). In the monkey interruption of fibers of the commissure in the midline produces no detectable change in the pupillary light reflex as measured in infrared pupillograms (Carpenter and Pierson, '73). Lesions in the nuclei of the posterior commissure, interrupting fibers from the interstitial nuclei of Cajal, produce bilateral eyelid retraction and impairment of vertical eye movements (Carpenter et al., '70).

The ependyma of the cerebral aqueduct immediately beneath the posterior commissure is modified to form a special plate of cells, the *subcommissural organ* (Wislocki and Leduc, '53). The subcommissural organ (Fig. 13-9) consists of tall, columnar ciliated cells which appear to have a secretory function. Evidence reviewed by Gilbert and Glaser ('61) suggests that the subcommissural organ may secrete aldosterone and serve as a volume receptor. The subcommissural organ is regarded as the only neurosecretory structure in the midbrain, and one of the few areas of the brain not included in the blood-brain barrier. This structure would seem capable of responding quickly to changes in effective circulating blood volume. Lesions of the subcommissural organ in rats result in an immediate and drastic reduction of water

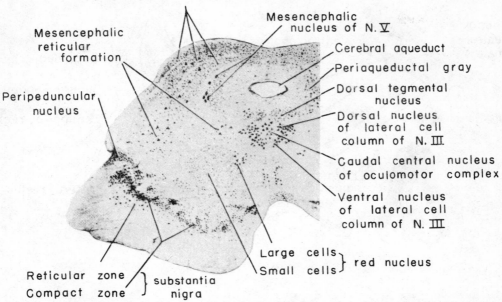

External, middle and deep
gray layers of superior colliculus

Mesencephalic
nucleus of N. Ⅴ

Mesencephalic
reticular
formation

Cerebral aqueduct

Periaqueductal gray

Peripeduncular
nucleus

Dorsal tegmental
nucleus

Dorsal nucleus
of lateral cell
column of N. Ⅲ

Caudal central nucleus
of oculomotor complex

Ventral nucleus
of lateral cell
column of N. Ⅲ

Large cells ⎫
Small cells ⎭ red nucleus

Reticular zone ⎫
Compact zone ⎭ substantia nigra

FIG. 13-10. Section through superior colliculi of midbrain. Three-month infant. Cresyl violet. Photograph, with main cell groups schematically blocked in.

consumption, and marked dehydration; because dehydration is more intense than could be accounted for on the basis of adipsia alone, an increase in the renal excretion of salt and water is postulated (Gilbert, '60).

The Oculomotor Nerve

The Oculomotor Nuclear Complex. This complex is a collection of cell columns and discrete nuclei which: (1) innervate all the extraocular muscles except the lateral rectus and the superior oblique, (2) supply the levator palpebrae muscle, and (3) provide preganglionic parasympathetic fibers to the ciliary ganglion. Functional components of the nerve are categorized as general somatic efferent (GSE) and general visceral efferent (GVE). This complex lies ventral to the central gray in the midline in a "V"-shaped trough formed by the diverging fibers of the MLF; it extends from the rostral pole of the trochlear nucleus to the upper limit of the midbrain (Figs. 13-4, 13-10 and 13-11). The complex consists of paired lateral somatic cell columns, midline and dorsal visceral nuclei and a discrete midline dorsal cell group, called the caudal central nucleus.

The *lateral somatic cell columns,* composed of large motor type neurons, innervate the extraocular muscles (Warwick, '53). The dorsal cell column (or nucleus) innervates the inferior rectus muscle, the intermediate cell column innervates the inferior oblique muscle and the ventral cell column supplies fibers to the medial rectus muscle (Fig. 13-11). Root fibers arising from these cell columns are uncrossed. A cell column medial to both the dorsal and intermediate cell columns, referred to as the medial cell column, provides crossed fibers that innervate the superior rectus muscle.

The *caudal central nucleus* is a midline somatic cell group found only in the caudal third of the complex (Warwick, '53a). This nucleus gives rise to crossed and uncrossed fibers that innervate the levator palpebrae muscle (Figs. 13-10 and 13-11).

Visceral nuclei of the oculomotor nuclear complex consist of two distinct nuclear groups which are in continuity rostrally, and often are collectively referred to as the *Edinger-Westphal nucleus* (Figs.

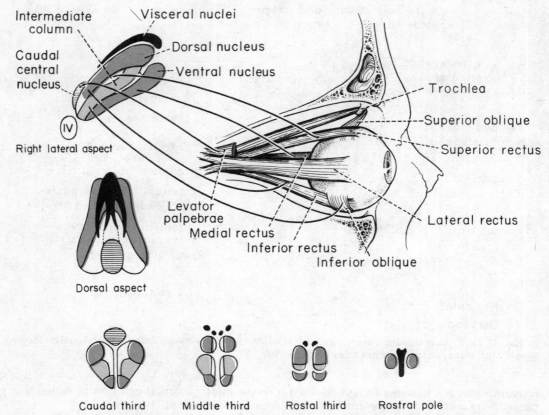

FIG. 13-11. Schematic representation of the localization of the extraocular muscles within the oculomotor nuclear complex, based upon studies in the rhesus monkey (Warwick, '53). Cell columns composing the complex are shown in lateral and dorsal views and in transverse sections through various levels. The visceral motor (parasympathetic) cell columns are shown in *black*. The ventral nucleus (*blue*) innervates the medial rectus muscle. The dorsal nucleus (*red*) innervates the inferior rectus muscle. The intermediate cell column (*yellow*) innervates the inferior oblique muscle. The cell column (*white*) medial to the dorsal and intermediate cell columns innervates the superior rectus muscle. The caudal central nucleus (*lined*) supplies fibers to the levator palpebrae superioris. Fibers innervating the medial rectus, inferior rectus and inferior oblique muscles are uncrossed; fibers supplying the levator palpebrae muscle are both crossed and uncrossed, while those to the superior rectus muscle are crossed. The *drawing in the upper right* shows the positions of all the extraocular muscles in relation to the globe and the bony orbit.

13-11 and 13-12A). The most rostral of these are the *anterior median nuclei*. The anterior median nuclei lie rostral to the somatic cell columns and consist of two slender, paired cell columns lying on each side of the median raphe (Fig. 13-7). Further caudally these nuclei elongate in a dorsoventral dimension and lie between rostral portions of the lateral somatic cell columns (principally the dorsal cell columns). Dorsally and rostrally cells of the anterior median nucleus merge with the dorsal visceral cell columns (Figs. 13-11 and 13-12A), which form the Edinger-West-

phal nucleus in the strict sense (Warwick, '54). The dorsal visceral cell columns lie dorsal to the rostral three-fifths of the somatic cell columns. Rostrally each nucleus is composed of two cell types: medium-sized round cells which occupy a medial region, and smaller lightly staining cells in a lateral region (Carpenter and Peter, '70/'71). Further caudally the cell group divides into a medial cell column of medium-sized cells and a distinct small-celled lateral cell column that lies slightly more dorsal. The anterior median nuclei and the lateral visceral cell column receive fibers from the contralateral olivary nuclei which cross in the posterior commissure (Fig. 13-13). The anterior median and medial visceral cell columns receive bilateral projections from the nuclei of the posterior commissure which partially decussate ventral to the aqueduct (Carpenter and Pierson, '73). Both the anterior median nucleus and the dorsal visceral cell columns give rise to uncrossed preganglionic parasympathetic fibers that emerge with somatic root fibers. These fibers pass to the ciliary ganglion and synapse upon postganglionic neurons which give rise to the short ciliary nerves. These postganglionic fibers innervate the ciliary body, concerned with the mechanism of accommodation, and the sphincter of the iris (pupillary light reflex). According to Warwick ('54), practically all of the cells of the ciliary ganglion (97%) innervate the intrinsic ocular musculature; only a small per cent of the cells supply axons to the sphincter pupillae.

The so-called central nucleus of Perlia has been regarded as a midline cell group particularly concerned with convergence. There has been great difficulty in identifying this nucleus in brains of man and monkey (Clark, '26; Warwick, '55). The existence and function of this nucleus remain in doubt.

Neuromuscular spindles identified in the extraocular muscles are thought to act as low threshold stretch receptors (Cooper and Daniel, '49; Cooper et al., '55). Recent evidence suggests that afferent impulses from eye muscle spindles are conveyed by cells in the trigeminal ganglion which form part of the ophthalmic division (Manni et al., '66).

The root fibers arising from the oculomotor nucleus pass ventrally in a number of bundles, some coursing medial to, and some traversing, the red nucleus. Ventrally the fibers converge and emerge in the interpeduncular fossa on the anterior aspect of the midbrain (Figs. 2-5, 2-19 and 11-1). This spreading of the root fibers through and around the red nucleus is an expression of the intraradicular expansion of the red nucleus during embryological development (Fig. 13-4).

The Accessory Oculomotor Nuclei. Grouped under this designation are three nuclei closely associated with the oculomo-

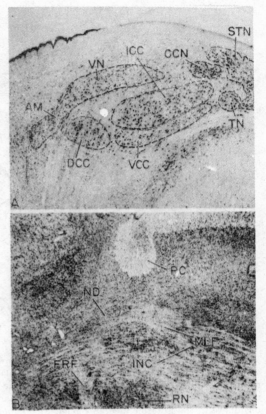

FIG. 13-12. *A*, Photomicrograph of a sagittal section through the oculomotor complex slightly removed from the midline in a rhesus monkey. The continuity of the anterior median (*AM*) and dorsal visceral cell columns (*VN*) is evident. Other nuclei identified are: *DCC*, dorsal (somatic) cell column; *VCC*, ventral (somatic) cell column; *ICC*, intermediate (somatic) cell column; *CCN*, caudal central nucleus; *TN*, trochlear nucleus; and *STN*, supratrochlear (dorsal tegmental) nucleus. Nissl stain. ×20. *B*, Parasagittal section through the posterior commissure (*PC*) and the medial longitudinal fasciculus (*MLF*) demonstrating the relationships between the nucleus of Darkschewitsch (*ND*), the interstitial nucleus of Cajal (*INC*) and the red nucleus (*RN*). *FRF*, indicates fasciculus retroflexus. Nissl stain. ×20. (Carpenter and Peter, '70/'71; courtesy of Akademie-Verlag, Berlin.)

tor complex. These nuclei are the interstitial nucleus of Cajal, the nucleus of Darkschewitsch and the nucleus of the posterior commissure. The *interstitial nucleus* is a small collection of multipolar neurons situated among, and lateral to, the fibers of the MLF in the rostral midbrain (Figs. 13-

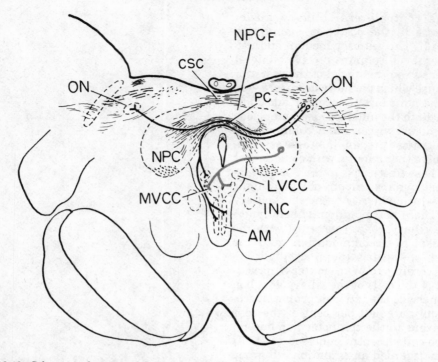

Fig. 13-13. Schematic drawing of the brain stem through the caudal part of the posterior commissure, showing the course of fibers projecting to the visceral nuclei of the oculomotor complex. Fibers (*red*) from the nuclei of the posterior commissure (*NPC*) enter the ipsilateral central gray and project primarily to the medial visceral cell columns (*MVCC*); these fibers partially cross ventral to the cerebral aqueduct and some terminate in the anterior median nuclei. Fibers (*black*) from the olivary nucleus (*ON*) pass through the posterior commissure (*PC*), enter the central gray and project to the contralateral lateral visceral cell column (*LVCC*) and bilaterally to the anterior median nuclei (*AM*). There is evidence of a commissural projection from *ON* to the corresponding nucleus contralaterally. Additional abbreviations: *CSC*, commissure of superior colliculus; *INC*, interstitial nucleus of Cajal; *NPCf*, nucleus of posterior commissure, pars infracommissuralis. (Carpenter and Pierson, '73; courtesy of The Wistar Institute.)

7, 13-9*A*, 13-12*B*, 13-15 and 13-16). This nucleus gives rise to fibers that cross in the ventral part of the posterior commissure and are distributed to all somatic cell columns of the oculomotor complex except the ventral (Carpenter et al., '70). In addition, it projects fibers bilaterally to the trochlear nuclei and ipsilaterally to the medial vestibular nucleus (Pompeiano and Walberg, '57) and spinal cord (Fig. 13-14).

The *nucleus of Darkschewitsch* is formed by small cells which lie inside the ventrolateral border of the central gray dorsal and lateral to the somatic cell columns of the oculomotor complex (Figs. 13-7, 13-9*A*, 13-12*B* and 13-16). The nucleus projects fibers into the posterior commissure, but does not send fibers into the oculomotor complex or to lower brain stem levels. The *nucleus of the posterior com-*

missure has been previously described (page 376).

Afferent Connections of the Oculomotor Complex. The oculomotor complex receives impulses from the cerebral cortex, the cerebellum, the vestibular nuclei, the superior colliculus, the reticular formation and certain accessory oculomotor nuclei. Although no direct corticobulbar fibers reach the oculomotor complex, impulses from the cerebral cortex are conveyed by corticoreticular fibers and reticular neurons which relay these impulses. A small number of fibers from ventral parts of the dentate nucleus cross in the midbrain and terminate in specific parts of the oculomotor complex (Carpenter and Strominger, '64). The vestibular nuclei give rise to a large number of fibers which ascend in the MLF and are distributed in a particular

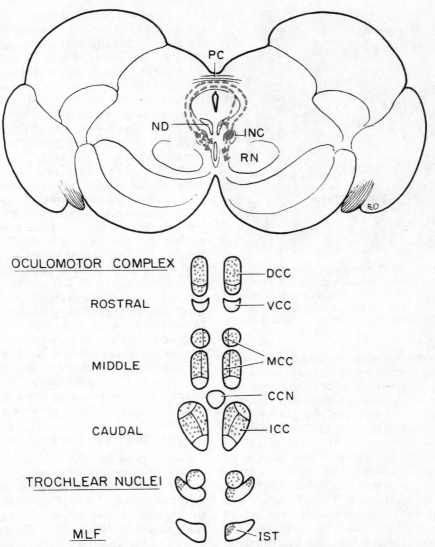

Fig. 13-14. Schematic diagram of degeneration resulting from a lesion (*red*) in the right interstitial nucleus (*INC*). The lesion destroyed: (1) cells which give rise to fibers that cross in the ventral part of the posterior commissure and fibers which descend in the ipsilateral *MLF*, and (2) fibers from the opposite interstitial nucleus which have crossed in the posterior commissure and traverse the lesion *en route* to the oculomotor complex. Fairly symmetrical differential degeneration (*red stippling*) in the oculomotor complex was greatest in the intermediate (*ICC*) and medial cell columns (*MCC*), somewhat less profuse in the dorsal cell columns (*DCC*) and absent in the ventral cell columns (*VCC*) and in the caudal central nucleus (*CCN*). Degeneration in the trochlear nuclei was bilateral but greatest ipsilaterally. Fibers of the interstitiospinal tract (*IST*) were concentrated in the dorsomedial part of the MLF (Carpenter et al., '70; courtesy of The Wistar Institute.)

manner to the lateral somatic cell columns of the oculomotor complex (Fig. 12-14; McMasters et al., '66). Ascending vestibular fibers also end in the interstitial nucleus of Cajal (Fig. 13-15). Vestibulo-oculomotor fibers reflexly correlate the position of the head and eyes, while internuclear fibers in the medial longitudinal fasciculus integrate activities of the abducens nucleus and subdivisions of the oculomotor complex (i.e., ventral cell column) in the performance of conjugate horizontal eye movements. The superior colliculus does not give rise to direct projections to the

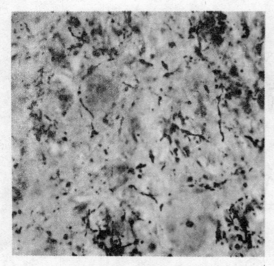

FIG. 13-15. Photomicrograph of terminal fiber degeneration passing around cells of the interstitial nucleus of Cajal. Ascending degeneration passing to this nucleus resulted from a lesion in the medial longitudinal fasciculus. Monkey. Nauta-Gygax stain. ×560.

oculomotor complex; it seems likely that impulses from this structure reach the oculomotor complex via either the interstitial nucleus of Cajal or the midbrain reticular formation (Altman and Carpenter, '61). The interstitial nucleus of Cajal gives rise to fibers that cross in the ventral part of the posterior commissure and pass to all somatic cell columns, except the ventral, on the opposite side (Fig. 13-14; Carpenter et al., '70; Carpenter, '71a). Although discrete lesions in the interstitial nucleus in monkeys do not produce detectable disturbances in oculomotor function, there is physiological evidence that this nucleus plays a role in vertical and rotatory eye movements (Markham et al., '66).

The fact that the conjugate eye movements (lateral, vertical and converging) cannot be dissociated voluntarily, or reflexly, suggests that the pyramidal, and many other fibers, act on internuncial cells. These in turn integrate the various motor neurons used in the eye movements. This certainly would seem to be the case with the conjugate lateral movements, which are controlled by two widely separated nuclei: N. VI for the lateral rectus, and N. III for the medial rectus.

Lesions of the Third Nerve. Lesions of this nerve produce an ipsilateral lower motor neuron paralysis of the muscles supplied by the nerve. There is an external strabismus (squint) due to the unopposed action of the lateral rectus muscle, inability to move the eye vertically or inward, drooping of the eyelid (ptosis), dilatation of the pupil (mydriasis), loss of the pupillary light reflex and convergence, and loss of accommodation of the lens. The nearness of the emerging root fibers of N. III to the corticospinal tract in the crus cerebri may lead to the inclusion of both structures in a single lesion, which causes an alternating hemiplegia similar to those already described for the sixth and twelfth nerves (Fig. 10-13). In this case, there is an ipsilateral lower motor neuron paralysis of muscles innervated by N. III, combined with a contralateral hemiplegia. Since at this level the corticobulbar and corticospinal fibers are close to each other, there also may be contralateral paresis (weakness) of the muscles innervated by the cranial nerves, especially those of the lower face and tongue. This constitutes the *superior* or *oculomotor alternating hemiplegia* clinically known as *Weber's syndrome*.

PUPILLARY REFLEXES

Light shone on the retina of one eye causes both pupils to constrict. The response in the eye stimulated is called the *direct pupillary light reflex,* while that in the opposite eye is known as the *consensual pupillary light reflex.* Pathways involved in the pupillary light reflex are not entirely known, but involve: (1) axons of retinal ganglion cells which pass via the optic nerve, optic tract and brachium of the superior colliculus to the pretectal area, (2) axons of pretectal neurons which partially cross in the posterior commissure and presumably terminate bilaterally in visceral nuclei of the oculomotor complex (Fig. 13-13), (3) preganglionic fibers from the visceral nuclei which course with fibers of the third nerve and synapse in the ciliary ganglion (Fig. 8-1), and (4) postganglionic fibers from the ciliary ganglion which project to the sphincter of the iris. Section of the posterior commissure re-

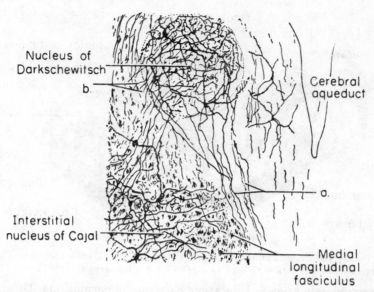

Nucleus of
Darkschewitsch

b.

Cerebral
aqueduct

a.

Interstitial
nucleus of Cajal

Medial
longitudinal
fasciculus

FIG. 13-16. Relationships of the nucleus of Darkschewitsch and the interstitial nucleus of Cajal to the central gray (surrounding the cerebral aqueduct) and the medial longitudinal fasciculus. Collateral fibers terminating in the nucleus of Darkschewitsch are indicated by *b*, while fibers indicated by *a* are leaving the nucleus. Drawing based upon Golgi preparations from a newborn kitten (after Cajal, '11).

duces, but does not abolish, the consensual pupillary light reflex.

The term *anisocoria* is used to denote pupillary inequality. In man and monkey the direct and consensual pupillary light reflexes are exactly equal (Lowenstein, '54). In the cat the direct pupillary light response is stronger than the indirect response, presumably because most retinofugal fibers are crossed. In man anisocoria results only from lesions involving the efferent pathways from the oculomotor complex or pretectal fiber systems passing to it.

The *accommodation-convergence reaction* occurs when gaze is shifted from a distant object to a near one. This reaction involves: (1) contractions of both medial recti muscles for convergence, (2) contraction of the ciliary muscles which relaxes the suspensory ligament of the lens and causes the lens to assume a more convex shape, and (3) pupillary constriction. In this reflex response retinal impulses must first reach the visual cortex and be relayed via corticofugal fibers to brain stem centers. It is presumed that the corticofugal fibers involved in this response reach the superior colliculus and pretectal region

and are relayed, directly or indirectly, to the oculomotor complex.

There is some physiological evidence suggesting that some preganglionic fibers in the motor pathway for accommodation may not synapse in the ciliary ganglion (Westheimer and Blair, '73). Although under normal circumstances accommodation always is accompanied by pupillary constriction, certain central nervous system lesions can impair or abolish the pupillary light reflex without affecting accommodation. Such lesions occur with central nervous system syphilis (tabes dorsalis) in which the pupils are small (miosis) and do not react to light, but the reaction to accommodation remains. This is the *Argyll-Robertson pupil*. The precise location of the responsible lesion is unknown.

In intense illumination, contraction of the pupil may be accompanied by closure of the eyelids, lowering of the brows and general contractions of the face, designed to shut out the maximal amount of light. In so far as they are not volitional, these reflex movements probably are mediated through the superior colliculi and the tectobulbar tracts.

The central pathways for pupillary dila-

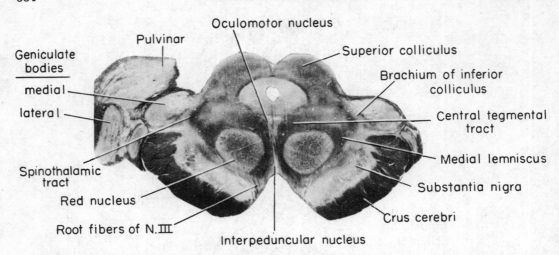

Fig. 13-17. Transverse section of the adult midbrain through the superior colliculus. Caudal portions of the thalamus are seen dorsolaterally. Weigert's myelin stain. Photograph.

tation are incompletely known. Dilatation occurs reflexly on shading the eye or scratching the side of the neck with a pin, and it is a constant feature in severe pain and extreme emotional states. Experimental evidence points to a path from the frontal cortex to the posterior region of the hypothalamus, one of the highest autonomic centers of the brain stem. Descending fibers from the hypothalamus passing in the reticular formation (and periventricular region) terminate upon reticular neurons in the brain stem, which in turn give rise to fibers that project to spinal levels. Impulses conveyed by these fibers, and probably relayed by spinal internuncial neurons, reach cells of the intermediolateral cell column in upper thoracic spinal (C8 to T1) segments. The latter send preganglionic fibers by way of the upper two or three rami communicantes and the sympathetic trunk to the superior cervical ganglion, from which postganglionic fibers go to the dilator muscle of the iris (Fig. 10-26). Interruption of these descending fibers, which probably course in the dorsolateral tegmentum, at any level of the brain stem caudal to the hypothalamus will produce a *Horner's syndrome*. In a Horner's syndrome due to a brain stem lesion, the pupil shows relatively little dilatation to adrenalin, but if the lesion producing this syndrome involves postganglionic sympathetic fibers, adrenalin causes mydriasis and lid retraction on the affected side but

not on the normal side. This hypersensitivity of the pupil to adrenalin seen with lesions involving the postganglionic fibers is an example of denervation sensitivity (Cogan, '56). See page 205 for a discussion of denervation sensitivity.

NUCLEI OF THE MESENCEPHALIC TEGMENTUM

The midbrain tegmentum, the region ventral to the cerebral aqueduct and dorsal to the substantia nigra, contains the trochlear and oculomotor nuclei, the mesencephalic reticular formation, the red nuclei and many scattered collections of cells. The functional significance of many smaller cell groups remains obscure. The most conspicuous structure in the midbrain tegmentum at the level of the superior colliculus is the red nucleus.

The Red Nucleus

The red nucleus, recognized as a part of the mesencephalic reticular formation, has been distinguished as an entity because of special anatomical characteristics. In fresh specimens it has a pinkishyellow color said to be due to its relatively high vascularity. The "capsule" of the nucleus, formed by fibers of the superior cerebellar peduncle, its central position within the mesencephalic reticular formation, and its color serve to sharply define the structure (Figs. 13-4, 13-10, 13-17, A-11, A-26 and A-27). The nucleus is a large ovoid column of cells extending from the caudal margin of the superior colliculus into the caudal diencephalon (Figs. 17-13 and A-12). In transverse sections the nucleus has a characteristic circular appearance.

Since the classic comparative studies of Hatschek ('07), it has been customary to recognize magnocellular (paleoruber) and parvocellular (neoruber) portions of the red nucleus. The magnocellular part tends to occupy more caudal parts of the structure; it is more extensive in lower mammals and has been considered by some as the only cellular group which gives rise to the rubrospinal tract. The small-celled, or parvocellular, portion forms the bulk of the nucleus (Fig. 13-10); its development has been considered to parallel the growth of the deep cerebellar nuclei, particularly the dentate nucleus. Between the cells of the nucleus are numerous small bundles of myelinated fibers which give a punctate appearance to the nucleus in transverse sections. These are primarily fibers from the superior cerebellar peduncle which traverse the nucleus, as well as terminate in parts of it. The red nucleus is traversed in several directions by different bundles of fibers. Fibers of the superior cerebellar peduncle traverse it in a caudorostral direction. Oculomotor root fibers pass through it *en route* to the interpeduncular fossa, and fibers of the fasciculus retroflexus traverse its rostral pole medially (Fig. 15-5).

Afferent fibers projecting to the red nucleus are derived from two principal sources, the deep cerebellar nuclei and the cerebral cortex. Fibers from both of these sources appear to terminate somatotopically within the red nucleus. Fibers of the superior cerebellar peduncle, arising from the dentate, emboliform and globose nuclei, undergo a complete decussation in the caudal midbrain and both enter and surround the contralateral red nucleus. According to Jansen and Jansen ('55), approximately half of the fibers arising from the dentate nucleus pass rostrally beyond the red nucleus, while little more than 10% of those arising from the interposed nuclei (i.e., emboliform and globose) project beyond the red nucleus. Fibers from the dentate nucleus terminate mainly in the rostral third of the red nucleus (Courville, '66a). On the basis of discrete lesions in the interposed nucleus (anterior part) in the cat, it is evident that fibers from this nucleus project to the caudal two-thirds of the red nucleus in a somatotopic fashion (Fig. 14-17; Courville, '66a). There is a complex mediolateral and caudorostral correspondence between portions of the interposed and the red nuclei. Since lesions destroying both the dentate and interposed nuclei produce degeneration in all parts of the contralateral red nucleus, it may be inferred that fibers from the dentate nucleus project particularly to rostral parts of the red nucleus (Fig. 14-16). The caudal portions of the red nucleus, which are linked somatotopically with the contralateral interposed nucleus (and paravermal cerebellar cortex), project somatotopically to spinal levels (Fig. 10-17). Thus indirect pathways are present by which impulses from the cerebellar cortex and interposed nucleus can be conveyed somatotopically to spinal levels via the red nucleus. This indirect pathway involves two midbrain decussations (i.e., the superior cerebellar peduncle and the rubrospinal tract).

Corticorubral fibers, mainly from the precentral gyrus (Rinvik and Walberg, '63; Kuypers and Lawrence, '67), project somatotopically upon cells in all parts of the red nucleus. These fibers are uncrossed. Fibers from the "motor" cortical forelimb area terminate in the dorsal part of the red nucleus, while fibers from the cortical hindlimb area end in the ventral part of the red nucleus. These regions of the red nucleus project fibers, respectively, to cervical and lumbosacral regions of the spinal cord (Pompeiano and Brodal, '57). Thus corticorubral and rubrospinal fiber systems together constitute a somatotopically linked nonpyramidal pathway from the motor cortex to spinal levels.

The efferent projections of the red nucleus are to the spinal cord, the brain stem and the cerebellum. Experimental data for the cat (Pompeiano and Brodal, '57) indicate that rubrospinal fibers arise chiefly, but not exclusively, from cells of all sizes in the caudal three-fourths of the red nucleus. In general, cells in dorsomedial parts of the nucleus project fibers to cervical spinal segments, while cells in ventral and ventrolateral locations project to lumbosacral spinal segments; fibers passing to thoracic regions of the spinal cord arise from intermediate parts of the red nucleus. Cervical spinal segments receive the largest number of rubrospinal fibers, probably as many as project to all other spinal regions. According to Kuypers and Lawrence ('67), the rubrospinal tract in the monkey arises almost exclusively from the caudal magnocellular part of the nucleus.

Rubrospinal fibers issue from the medial margin of the red nucleus, cross the median raphe in the *ventral tegmental decussation (of Forel)* and descend in the brain stem close to the branchiomeric motor cranial nerve nuclei (Fig. 10-17). In the upper pons some crossed descending rubral efferent fibers separate from the rubrospinal tract, traverse portions of the trigeminal nuclei and enter the cerebellum in association with the superior cerebellar peduncle. These *rubrocerebellar fibers,* originally described as projecting to the dentate nucleus (Brodal and Gogstad, '54; Hinman and Carpenter, '59), have been traced to the nucleus interpositus (anterior part) (Courville and Brodal, '66). This direct (and crossed) rubrocerebellar feedback is somatotopically organized. Other crossed descending rubral efferent fibers leave the rubrospinal tract in the lower brain stem and enter parts of the facial nucleus and the lateral reticular nucleus of the medulla. Rubral efferent fibers project only to the dorsomedial and intermediate cell groups of the facial nucleus (Courville, '66), cell groups which innervate upper facial muscles. In the medulla crossed rubral efferent fibers project to parts of the lateral reticular nucleus (Walberg, '58; Courville, '66), a cerebellar relay nucleus previously described (Fig. 10-17). Except for these fibers, which may be considered as *rubrobulbar,* no crossed descending rubral efferent fibers end upon portions of the brain stem reticular formation. Rubrospinal fibers in the retro-olivary area of the medulla pass caudally to enter the lateral funiculus of the spinal cord; the most dorsally situated fibers in the tract are intermingled with those of the lateral corticospinal tract.

Uncrossed descending rubral efferents, from the parvocellular part of the nucleus, enter the central tegmental tract and project to the dorsal lamella of the principal inferior olivary nucleus (Walberg, '56; Poirier and Bouvier, '66). These fibers, referred to as *rubro-olivary fibers,* constitute the largest contingent of the so-called rubrobulbar fibers. It is possible that some of these fibers may terminate in, or give off collaterals to, the brain stem reticular formation. From the above discussion it is apparent that descending rubral efferent fibers, other than those in the rubrospinal tract, are organized to project impulses to the cerebellum via: (1) direct rubrocerebellar fibers, or (2) rubrobulbar fibers which pass to cerebellar relay nuclei (i.e., the lateral reticular nucleus of the medulla and parts of the principal inferior olivary nucleus).

Information concerning ascending rubral efferent fibers is less specific because these fibers are intermingled with those of the superior cerebellar peduncle. Certain evidence (Carpenter, '56; Pompeiano and Brodal, '57; Kuypers and Lawrence, '67) has suggested that the majority of ascending fibers from the red nucleus arise from rostral portions of the nucleus. Because lesions in the red nucleus (Hinman and Carpenter, '59) produce degeneration in essentially the same thalamic nuclei as lesions of the superior cerebellar peduncle, it has been presumed that their projection was similar. Anatomical evidence that the red nucleus projects ascending fibers is based upon studies of retrograde cell changes in the nucleus produced by lesions at more rostral brain stem levels (Preisig, '04; von Monakow, '09; Pompeiano and Brodal, '57; Kuypers and Lawrence, '67). Electrophysiological evidence (Conde, '66) also suggests connections between the rostral part of the red nucleus and the thalamus. Morphological studies indicate that interruption of the central tegmental tract causes a complete cell loss in the parvocellular part of the ipsilateral red nucleus, and interruption of the rubrotegmentospinal tract produces complete loss of cells in the magnocellular part of the contralateral red nucleus. These observations suggest that virtually all of the projections of the red nucleus are descending (Poirier and Bouvier, '66). Evidence of scant, or absent, rubrothalamic projections is supported by data from autoradiographic tracing studies (Edwards, '72).

It is evident from the above that the red nucleus is a way station interposed in a variety of complex pathways. It would appear to relay cerebellar impulses to the spinal cord, as well as to participate in various neural mechanisms by which some cerebellar impulses can be fed back to the cerebellum. Impulses from the cerebral cortex also can be conveyed to the spinal cord and cerebellum via the red nucleus.

There is considerable evidence that in lower mammals the midbrain contains a center for the integration of complex postural reflexes which enable an animal to change from an abnormal to a normal position (righting reactions). This center may be located in the magnocellular portion of the red nucleus and in the adjacent reticular formation. The rubrospinal tract excites flexor motor neurons via polysynaptic pathways, and stimulation of the red nucleus during locomotion enhances flexor muscle activity during the swing phase (Orlovsky, '72a). Vestibulospinal influences have a similarly enhancing effect upon extensor muscles during the stance phase of the step (Orlovsky, '72). The cerebellum apparently modulates the activity of both rubrospinal and vestibulospinal neurons to provide appropriate locomotor rhythms.

Conflicting statements in the literature suggest that stimulation of the red nucleus in animals produces flexion of ipsilateral forelimb and extension of the contralateral forelimb. This reaction, generally known as "the tegmental response," frequently can be obtained from regions of the mesencephalic reticular formation dorsal and lateral to the red nucleus. The studies of Pompeiano ('56, '57) indicate that stimulation of the red nucleus *per se* elicits flexion in the contralateral extremities, which appears to be mediated by the rubrospinal tract (Pompeiano and Brodal, '57). It has been demonstrated that stimulation of the red nucleus in the decerebrate cat gives rise to: (1) excitatory postsynaptic potentials in the contralateral flexor α motor neurons, and (2) inhibitory postsynaptic potentials in contralateral extensor α motor neurons.

Because the red nucleus receives a large proportion of its afferents from the cerebellum by way of the superior cerebellar peduncle, it is possible to relate certain phenomena associated with cerebellar stimulation to the red nucleus. These observations concern mainly the nucleus interpositus, which projects the majority of its fibers to the caudal two-thirds of the contralateral red nucleus. Reciprocal somatotopic relationships exist between the nucleus interpositus and the contralateral red nucleus (Courville and Brodal, '66; Courville, '66a). Stimulation of specific parts of the nucleus interpositus (anterior part) in decerebrate preparations produces flexion in either the ipsilateral forelimb or hindlimb (Pompeiano, '59, 60a; Maffei and Pompeiano, '62). These flexor responses are mediated by the red nucleus and occur ipsilaterally because of the double crossing of the fiber systems involved (i.e., superior cerebellar peduncle and rubrospinal tract) (Fig. 14-17).

Lesions of the Red Nucleus. Clinically, unilateral lesions of the mesencephalic tegmentum involving the red nucleus are described as producing a syndrome characterized by contralateral motor disturbances that are variously designated as tremor, ataxia and choreiform activity, and an ipsilateral oculomotor palsy. The motor disturbances associated with this syndrome, known as the *syndrome of Benedikt* since the time of Charcot, have been attributed to destruction of the red nucleus. Experimentally produced lesions in the red nucleus in a variety of different animals (von Economo and Karplus, '09; Rademaker, '26; Mussen, '27; Ingram and Ranson, '32; Carpenter, '56) have not produced physiological disturbances equivalent to those reported in man. Isolated lesions of the red nucleus in the monkey (Carpenter, '56) produce transient tremor and ataxia, enduring hypokinesis and ipsilateral oculomotor disturbances. It is of interest that unilateral lesions in the red nucleus in monkeys, with virtually complete degeneration of the contralateral superior cerebellar peduncle, produce no additional neurological disturbances (Carpenter, '57). These findings suggest that motor disturbances resulting from lesions of the mesencephalic tegmentum, including the red nucleus, are primarily a consequence of interruption of cerebellar efferent fibers in the superior cerebellar peduncle. In the monkey, neither lesions of the red nucleus nor section of the rubrospinal tract in the spinal cord abolishes cerebellar disturbances produced by lesions of the deep cerebellar nuclei.

Mesencephalic Reticular Formation

The midbrain reticular formation is less extensive than the pontine reticular formation caudal to it. While the red nucleus is recognized as a distinctive part of the reticular formation, classically it is customary to reserve this term for structures lateral and dorsal to the red nucleus. According to detailed studies (Olszewski, '54; Olszewski and Baxter, '54), the principal reticular nuclei of the mesencephalon are: (1) the *nucleus tegmenti pedunculopontinus* (pedunculopontine nucleus), (2) the *nucleus cuneiformis*, and (3) the *nucleus subcuneiformis*. The pedunculopontine nucleus lies in the lateral part of the midbrain tegmentum ventral to the inferior colliculus (Fig. 13-3). The nucleus consists of two parts, a compact part located dorsolaterally and a small-celled diffuse part located ventrally. Fibers of the superior cerebellar peduncle traverse portions of the nucleus as they shift ventromedially to decussate. Although the connections of this nucleus are poorly understood, it would appear to be important in the integration of motor activities, since it receives descending pallidotegmental fibers (Fig. 17-11; Nauta and Mehler, '66; Carpenter and Strominger, '67) as well as corticofugal fibers from the precentral gyrus (Kuypers and Lawrence, '67). The nuclei cuneiformis and subcuneiformis lie between the tectum, dorsally, and the pedunculopontine nucleus. At more rostral levels only the cuneiform and subcuneiform nuclei are found. Medial to the latter nuclei are the fibers of the central tegmental tract. Also seen at this level is the interpeduncular nucleus, which occupies a small triangular space dorsal to the interpeduncular fossa (Figs. 13-3, 13-4 and 13-17). Cells of this nucleus are very

small, spindle-shaped, lightly staining and compactly arranged. The interpeduncular nucleus receives fibers from the habenular nuclei via the fasciculus retroflexus (Figs. 15-5 and 16-5).

The central gray substance (periaqueductal gray) surrounding the cerebral aqueduct is composed of small oval or spindle-shaped cells. The *nucleus of Darkschewitsch* is a rather indistinct cell group just inside the ventrolateral border of the central gray (Figs. 13-7, 13-12*B* and 13-16). The *dorsal tegmental nucleus* (supratrochlear nucleus) lies within the central gray, dorsal to the trochlear nucleus and the oculomotor complex (Figs. 13-3 and 13-12*A*). Fibers from this nucleus and from a collection of more caudally located cells known as the *ventral tegmental nucleus* ascend to the mammillary bodies, the lateral hypothalamic areas and the preoptic and septal areas (Guillery, '56; Nauta and Kuypers, '58). These fibers travel in the dorsal longitudinal fasciculus (of Schütz), the mammillary peduncle, and some continue rostrally in the medial forebrain bundle (Fig. 16-5).

FUNCTIONAL CONSIDERATIONS OF THE RETICULAR FORMATION

The anatomical organization of the medullary and pontine reticular formation has been described. It will be recalled that the medullary reticular formation consists essentially of three zones: (1) a median region containing the nuclei of the raphe and the paramedian reticular nuclei, (2) a medial region constituting roughly the medial two-thirds of the reticular formation and regarded as an "effector" area, and (3) a smaller lateral region referred to as the "sensory" or "receptive" part because of the large number of collateral fibers projected to it from secondary sensory pathways. The pontine reticular formation has essentially the same divisions, except that the "sensory" portion is smaller and clearly evident only in the caudal pons. Electrophysiological investigations in animals have yielded important information concerning the functions of the reticular formation. Magoun and Rhines ('46, '47) found that electrical stimulation of the ventromedial zone of the medullary reticular formation inhibited or reduced most forms of motor activity. Stimulation in this region produced inhibition of the patellar tendon reflex, the flexion reflex of the foreleg and the blink reflex. In addition, it caused inhibiton of extensor muscle tone in decerebrate animals and inhibited responses to stimulation of the motor cortex in intact animals. All inhibitory effects were bilateral, but ipsilateral inhibition sometimes could be obtained at a lower threshold. No inhibitory effects could be elicited from the most lateral part of the medullary reticular formation. Regions of the medullary reticular formation from which inhibitory responses are obtained correspond closely to the area occupied by the nucleus reticularis gigantocellularis (except for its most rostral part) and part of the nucleus reticularis ventralis. Since these nuclei give rise to medullary reticulospinal fibers, it would appear that these inhibitory influences are mediated directly by this fiber system (Torvik and Brodal, '57). This thesis is further supported by the fact that medullary inhibition can still be obtained by electrical stimulation following chronic midbrain and pontine hemisection (Niemer and Magoun, '47). Nevertheless, there is evidence that higher centers projecting to medullary reticular units may produce inhibition of motor activity and of extensor muscle tone. Such higher centers are thought to include the anterior lobe of the cerebellum, the corpus striatum and certain cortical regions (Magoun and Rhines, '47).

A far greater region of the reticular formation facilitates, or augments, reflexes at lower levels, and cortically induced movements in response to electrical stimulation. This facilitatory area extends rostrally uninterruptedly from the upper medulla through the pontine and mesencephalic tegmentum into the hypothalamic, subthalamic and intralaminar thalamic regions of the diencephalon. Bilateral facilitatory effects can be evoked at any level within this long stretch of the reticular formation. The facilitatory region of the reticular formation includes many areas from which no direct reticulospinal projections arise. Facilitatory effects produced by stimulation of the rostral and dorsal parts of the nucleus reticularis gigantocellularis, or of the nuclei reticularis pontis caudalis and oralis, presumably could reach spinal levels by direct reticulospinal fibers originating in these nuclei. Descending polysynaptic pathways would appear to mediate facilitatory effects obtained from regions of the midbrain and diencephalon, which have no direct reticulospinal projections.

The descending influences of the brain stem reticular formation are not limited to inhibition and facilitation of reflex activity or somatic motor function. As commented upon earlier, respiratory responses can be obtained by electrical stimulation of the reticular formation. Maximal inspiratory responses can be obtained from stimulating points within the nucleus reticularis gigantocellularis.(Torvik and Brodal, '57), while expiratory effects are evoked chiefly from the parvocellular reticular nucleus in the medulla. Vasomotor depressor effects generally are obtained from areas within the nucleus reticularis gigantocellularis and the most rostral part of the nucleus reticularis ventralis. Pressor effects usually are evoked by stimulations outside of the reticular regions which project fibers to spinal levels.

Although nearly all parts of the central nervous system are capable of exerting detectable influences upon the heart and blood vessels, the primary vasomotor control center is located in the reticular formation of the medulla. Transections of the brain stem as far caudal as the lower third of the pons have no significant effect upon arterial blood pressure or on the tonic discharge of the inferior cardiac nerve. Successively more caudal transections produce: (1) an increasing drop in blood pressure, and (2) a reduction in the discharge of cardiac accelerator impulses (Bard, '68). The bulbar pressor and depressor areas constitute a central cardiovascular mechanism which reflexly regulates blood pressure and the parameters of the heart rate. In the intact animal a normal arterial pressure is dependent upon the bulbar pressor area. There is no evidence that activity in the pressor area depends upon afferent influx. Vagal cardiac centers, assumed to lie in the dorsal motor nucleus of N. X, must be intimately integrated with neurons in pressor areas; activity of vagal units are subject to reflex excitation and inhibition.

While it is well known that α motor neurons can be influenced by stimulation of the reticular formation, the investigations of Granit ('55) indicate that these effects are not necessarily due to reticulospinal volleys impinging directly upon these neurons, since activity of γ motor neurons can influence α motor neurons through the γ loop (Fig. 9-27). Granit and Kaada ('52) demonstrated that repetitive electrical stimulation of the facilitating regions of the brain stem tegmentum increased the efferent discharge of γ motor neurons, and increased the rate of discharge from the muscle spindle. On the other hand, inhibition of the γ discharge was produced by stimulating the medullary inhibitory region. These data suggest that a large part of the excitation of α motor neurons results from firing of the γ efferents, which are actively controlled by the reticular formation. The inhibition of extensor muscle tone in a decerebrate animal by stimulation of the medullary reticular formation (Terzuolo and Terzian, '53) is a dramatic example of this potent influence.

The discovery that the activity of the muscle spindle could be modified by descending reticular influences suggested that the reticular formation might affect the initiation and transmission of other sensory impulses. Hagbarth and Kerr ('54) demonstrated that synaptic transmission of sensory impulses in the spinal cord could be depressed by stimulation of the reticular formation. Likewise, potentials evoked in the posterior column nuclei following stimulation of the posterior columns could be depressed or abolished by stimulation of the reticular formation. Although findings suggest that the inhibitory influence of the reticular formation acts upon the second order sensory neurons, it is possible that some of these effects may be a consequence of stimulation of corticofugal fibers projecting to sensory relay nuclei. Many of the latter fibers traverse portions of the reticular formation.

Moruzzi and Magoun ('49) have demon-

strated that the facilitatory region of the brain stem reticular formation also acts in an ascending direction to influence the electrical activity of the cerebral cortex. The pioneer investigations of Berger ('29, '30) showed that in man and lower mammals wakefulness, sleep, alertness and relaxation were characterized by strikingly different electroencephalographic patterns. Wakefulness and alertness are characterized by fast low voltage activity, while at least one form of sleep is associated with the appearance of slow high voltage waves.

Fundamental insight into the underlying brain mechanisms was provided by Bremer ('37) who compared the electroencephalograms (EEG) of animals following high spinal transections (*encéphale isolé*) and decerebration (i.e., transection of the midbrain at the intercollicular level, *cerveau isolé*). In the encéphale isolé preparation the EEG displayed the waking pattern, while the cerveau isolé preparation exhibited an EEG pattern characteristic of the sleeping state. These experiments pointed to a potent electrotonic influence which appeared to be generated in the lower brain stem. While it was well known that a variety of different stimuli could change the EEG from a synchronized pattern (i.e., sleep state) to a desynchronized one (i.e., alert state), the puzzling feature was how impulses channeled in the classic pathways could exert such broad and diffuse electrotonic changes in the cerebral cortex. The observations of Moruzzi and Magoun ('49) that stimulation of the brain stem reticular formation could activate and desynchronize the EEG and produce behavioral arousal without discharging the classic lemniscal pathways, suggested the concept of a second ascending system. This second ascending system which exerts powerful influences upon broad regions of the cerebral cortex has become known as the *ascending reticular activating system* (ARAS).

The ascending reticular activating system has been shown to respond to peripheral, splanchnic, trigeminal and vagal nerve stimulation, as well as to auditory, vestibular, visual and olfactory stimuli (Bremer, '36; Gerebtzoff, '40; McKinley and Magoun, '42; Moruzzi and Magoun, '49; Starzl et al., '51a; French et al., '52; Dell, '52; French et al., '53; Bernhaut et al., '53).

Furthermore, it has been shown that interruption of the long ascending sensory pathways in the brain stem does not prevent impulses from reaching the reticular activating system and provoking the characteristic EEG arousal response (Moruzzi and Magoun, '49; Starzl and Whitlock, '52; French et al., '53). Lesions in the rostromedial midbrain tegmentum abolish the EEG arousal elicited by sensory stimulation (French and Magoun, '52; Magoun, '52), even though the long ascending sensory pathways are intact. Thus, two functionally distinct, but inter-related, pathways must project to diencephalic levels. The long ascending sensory pathways, located laterally with respect to the reticular core, constitute the *lemniscal system*, which is concerned largely with the transmission of specific sensory impulses to particular thalamic relay nuclei. The lemniscal systems (i.e., the medial lemniscus, lateral lemniscus, spinothalamic tracts and secondary trigeminal projections) are regarded as oligosynaptic specific sensory pathways. Although electrical stimulation of the lemniscal systems produces arousal (Starzl et al., '51; French et al., '52; Magoun, '63), this is not considered a direct effect. The second pathway, the *ascending reticular activating system*, occupies more medial areas within the brain stem reticular formation and receives collateral fibers from surrounding specific sensory systems. Physiologically this system is regarded as a multineuronal, polysynaptic system within which collaterals from various sensory systems lose their specific indentities. The continuous subliminal facilitating effect of these nonspecific afferents upon the reticular activating system appears to be responsible for wakefulness, alerting and arousal.

Anatomical and physiological data are in agreement concerning the distribution of collaterals from secondary sensory fibers within the reticular formation. Collaterals are given off by secondary fibers in the auditory and vestibular systems, as well as from the nuclei of the solitary tract, the trigeminal nuclei, the vagal nuclei and the spinothalamic tracts. Visual impulses would appear to reach the reticular formation via tectoreticular fibers (Altman and Carpenter, '61). Anatomically it is significant that direct spinoreticular fibers are more numerous than collaterals from the spinothalamic tracts and have a wider distribution within the reticular formation. The medial lemniscus, unlike other long ascending systems, does not contribute collateral fibers to the reticular activating system. Experimental studies (Rossi and Zirondoli, '55; Roger et al., '56) indicate that the secondary trigeminal collaterals given off at pontine levels are a particularly potent source of tonic influence to the reticular activating system and exceed in importance the contribution by other cranial nerves.

Lastly, it has been shown that the cerebral cortex plays a role in altering the state of consciousness and alertness by influencing reticular neurons that mediate the arousal responses (Jasper et al., '52; Bremer and Terzuolo, '54; French et al., '55). Such a role has been suggested by the well known arousal effect of psychic stimuli. Areas of the cerebral cortex from which the arousal responses can be obtained by nonconvulsive electrical stimulation include loci on the orbitofrontal surface, the frontal convexity, the sensorimotor cortex, the posterior parieto-occipital cortex, the superior temporal gyrus and cingulate gyrus. Corticoreticular fibers, which originate from all parts of the cerebral cortex, convey excitatory impulses to the reticular neurons, whose ascending discharge may produce the arousal response. Anatomical evidence (Rossi and Brodal, '56) indicates that corticoreticular fibers are projected most abundantly to two regions of the brain stem reticular formation: (1) a pontine region corresponding to the nucleus reticularis pontis oralis, and (2) a medullary region corresponding to the nucleus reticularis gigantocellularis.

As noted earlier, the more lateral regions of the brain stem reticular formation are regarded as the "sensory" part, while the larger, more medial region, which projects numerous long ascending and descending fibers, is considered the "effector" portion. Although physiological studies support the view that ascending transmission in the reticular formation involves chains of neurons which fire successively, it has not been possible to demonstrate short-axoned, Golgi type II cells in the reticular formation (Scheibel and Scheibel, '58). Since approximately one-third of the cells in the "effector" reticular regions give rise to long ascending fibers in the reticular core, it appears likely that these fibers actually form the stuctural basis of the ascending reticular activating system (Brodal and Rossi, '55). Rapidly conducted impulses in the reticular core are transmitted by long ascending axons, while slowly conducted impulses are conveyed by fine caliber axons, or by circuitous pathways involving laterally dispersed collaterals. The main long ascending pathway of the brain stem reticular formation appears to be the *central tegmental fasciculus* (Figs. 12-4, 12-7 and 12-23), a large composite bundle that also contains descending fiber systems (Brodal, '57; Nauta and Kuypers, '58). This bundle occupies a large part of the bulbar tegmentum, but at mesencephalic levels it is displaced dorsally so that its fibers occupy a position adjacent to the central gray and dorsal to the red nucleus (Fig. 13-17). At diencephalic levels the central tegmental tract projects into the subthalamic region and to the intralaminar nuclei of the thalamus. Although the areas of origin of ascending fibers within this system have not been delineated precisely, most evidence indicates that ascending fibers originate throughout the longitudinal extent of the medulla and pons (Brodal and Rossi, '55); reticular pathways ascending beyond the midbrain appear to arise largely from levels rostral to the inferior olivary nuclei. The central tegmental tract also contains an abundance of short ascending fibers which appear to form a multineuronal system for intrareticular conduction (Nauta and Kuypers, '58).

Ascending reticular projections to the hypothalamus arise from medial regions of the caudal midbrain and are distinct from those contained in the central tegmental tract (Nauta and Kuypers, '58). These projections are represented largely by three bundles: (1) the dorsal longitudinal fasciculus (Schütz) situated near the central gray, (2) fibers of the mammillary peduncle (which originate in the medial tegmental region (Fig. 16-5) and terminate in the mammillary body and lateral hypothalamus (Nauta, '58), and (3) the medial forebrain bundle, which contains certain ascending components.

Anatomical and physiological data are in agreement concerning the diencephalic projections (hypothalamus, subthalamic region and intralaminar nuclei of the thalamus) of the ascending reticular activating system, but the manner in which these structures influence the activity of the cerebral cortex is not established (French et al., '52; Rossi and Zanchetti, '57; Bowsher, '66). While the EEG arousal response undoubtedly is mediated in part by the intralaminar nuclei (Moruzzi and Magoun, '49), the role of thalamic relay nuclei has been unclear. Recent evidence indicates that the intralaminar thalamic nuclei project profusely upon the neostriatum and give rise to an extensive system of collaterals that project diffusely upon the cerebral cortex (Jones and Leavitt, '74).

It is significant that bilateral interruption of lemniscal systems in the brain stem still leaves the animal with an electrocorticogram characteristic of the wakeful state. After lesions in the upper reticular core which spare the lemniscal system, the electroencephalogram changes to that of the sleeping state. After lesions in the rostral midbrain interrupting somatic and auditory pathways (without destroying the ascending reticular system), tactile and auditory stimuli produce and EEG arousal, although no tactile or auditory impulses reach the thalamus by the specific sensory pathways. The central reticular core might be regarded as a common system of neurons with multiple relays which are discharged equivalently by all sensory systems projecting collaterals to it. Such a common system would not be involved in the conscious perception of any one sensory modality, but would be involved with afferent functions common to all types of sensory experience, namely, alerting and attracting attention. The nonspecific sensory impulses ascending in the reticular activating system would appear to function by sharpening the attentive state of the cortex and creating optimal conditions for the conscious perception of sensory impulses mediated by the classical pathways.

A differential susceptibility of these two systems to the action of depressant drugs contributes to a considerable degree in the production of the anesthetic state (French et al., '53; Brazier, '54; Arduini and Arduini, '54; Killam and Killam, '58). The undiminished persistence of impulses in the lemniscal systems, and the blocking of impulses in the ascending reticular core, in anesthetic states (e.g., ether and certain barbiturates) suggest that many effects may be due to impairment or blockage of synaptic transmission in the multineuronal activating system.

Long term studies (Sprague et al., '63) of cats with extensive rostral midbrain lesions interrupting the specific lemniscal pathways bilaterally produce consistent alterations of behavior. Such animals exhibit: (1) a marked reduction of somatic and autonomic signs of affective behavior, (2) marked inattention to, and poor localization of visual, auditory, tactile and nociceptive stimuli, (3) stereotyped, hyperexploratory behavior, largely independent of stimuli in the external environment, and (4) changes in eating, grooming, excretory and sexual habits. In spite of these changes, these animals show essentially normal behavioral and EEG arousal.

In man lesions of the brain stem often produce disturbances of consciousness which range from fleeting unconsciousness to hypersomnia, and to deep and sustained coma (Cairns, '52). As Magoun ('54) has stated, "It is not easy for the physiologist to put his finger upon consciousness, though it is present abundantly and for long periods of time." One of the accepted working definitions of consciousness is, "an awareness of environment and of self" (Cobb, '48). In all forms of disturbed consciousness due to brain stem lesions, there is a loss of crude awareness. With lesions of the lower brain stem unconsciousness usually is accompanied by respiratory and cardiovascular disturbances, and often these are associated with increased muscle tone. The loss of consciousness frequently is sudden in onset and depression of vital functions leads to extreme states which may be rapidly fatal. Lesions of the upper brain stem most commonly produce hypersomnia characterized by muscular relaxation, slow respiration and an EEG pattern showing large amplitude slow waves. The level of unconsciousness usually is not deep and some patients can be aroused briefly. If the patient develops decerebrate rigidity, there is usually coma, but these phenomena are not always correlated. A variant of hypersomnia seen with upper brain stem lesions is referred to as *akinetic mutism* (coma vigil). In this variant the EEG pattern mainly resembles that associated with slow sleep, but eye movements remain normal. Many patients survive for months in this state. With lesions at all levels of the brain stem, liability to unconsciousness is related to the rapidity with which the lesions develop. Lesions associated with hemorrhage usually produce sudden unconsciousness and coma; slowly developing lesions, such as tumors, may not disturb consciousness for a considerable period of time. This subject has been reviewed extensively by Plum and Posner ('66). Although there is probably no center uniquely concerned with consciousness, there are indications that the functional integrity of the brain stem reticular formation is essential for its maintenance. This further suggests that a healthy cerebral cortex cannot by itself maintain the conscious state.

SUBSTANTIA NIGRA

The substantia nigra is the most voluminous nuclear mass of the human mesencephalon, extending throughout its length and into the caudal diencephalon (Figs. 13-1, 13-3, 13-4, 13-10 and 13-17). It is rudimentary in lower vertebrates, makes its definite appearance in mammals, and reaches its greatest development in man. In sections two zones are distinguishable: a dorsal compact or black zone, and a ventral reticular zone, which has a reddish brown color in the fresh condition similar to that of the globus pallidus (Fig. 13-10). The compact zone appears as an irregular band of closely packed, large polygonal or pyramidal cells containing granules of melanin

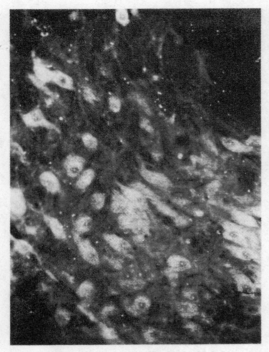

FIG. 13-18. Dopamine-containing cell bodies in the pars, compacta of the substantia nigra of the squirrel monkey. Fluorescence in the cell bodies extends into some of the large processes which contribute to the background fluorescence. Fluorescence photomicrograph. ×400. (Courtesy of Dr. David L. Felton, School of Medicine, Indiana University.)

pigment. Pigmented cells are found in the substantia nigra of a wide variety of mammals (Marsden, '61); the intensity of the pigmentation in primates is greater than in any other order and reaches maximum intensity in man. In man, pigmented cells in the substantia nigra do not appear until the 4th or 5th year. The compact zone extends to the most caudal part of the midbrain, where it is covered ventrally by the pontine nuclei (Fig. 13-3). The reticular zone, also known as the stratum intermedium, lies close to the crus cerebri and is composed of scattered cells of irregular shape that are rich in iron but contain no melanin pigment. Islands of such cells may be seen penetrating between the fibers of the crus cerebri. Within the stratum intermedium, especially in its lateral portion, are many bundles of descending myelinated fibers coming chiefly from the

corpus striatum (Fig. 13-4). This zone extends upward into the diencephalon, where it lies ventral to the subthalamic nucleus (Figs. 15-5 and 17-13).

Dorsal to the substantia nigra and ventrolateral to the red nucleus is a region containing scattered cells of various sizes and shapes, among which are large cells with melanin pigment. It is not certain whether some of these belong to the substantia nigra or to the tegmentum, but many authorities regard this region as a diffusely organized extension of the compact zone. Lateral to the substantia nigra a layer of small cells, the *peripenducluar nucleus*, caps the dorsal surface of the crus cerebri (Fig. 13-10).

The substantia nigra is implicated primarily in the metabolic disturbances considered to underlie parkinsonism and appears to be the principal source of striatal dopamine (Dahlström and Fuxe, '64; Anden et al., '64; Poirier and Sourkes, '65; Fuxe and Andén, '66; Hornykiewicz, '66; Hökfelt and Ungerstedt, '69; Bédard et al., '69; Moore et al., '71). Data based upon a histochemical fluorescence method (Falck, '62; Falck et al.,'62) indicated that dopamine, stored in varicosities in nerve terminals is mainly concentrated in three areas of the telencephalon: (1) the striatum (i.e., caudate nucleus and putamen), (2) the nucleus accumbens septi, and (3) the olfactory tubercle (Fuxe and Andén, '66). These terminal varicosities are fine, densely packed and exhibit a diffuse green fluorescence. Dopamine is believed to be synthesized in the large pigmented cells in the pars compacta. In contrast to the nerve terminals in the striatum, the concentrations of monoamines in large cells of the substantia nigra seem low, and monoamines occur mainly in the perinuclear cytoplasm (Fig. 13-18). Most of the dopamine-containing neurons are localized to the pars compacta of the substantia nigra (Ungerstedt, '71). There is convincing evidence that dopamine, synthesized in the substantia nigra, is continuously transported via axoplasmic flow to terminal varicosities in the striatum. At this time there is no direct evidence concerning the release of dopamine from these varicosities. Lesions in the substantia nigra cause

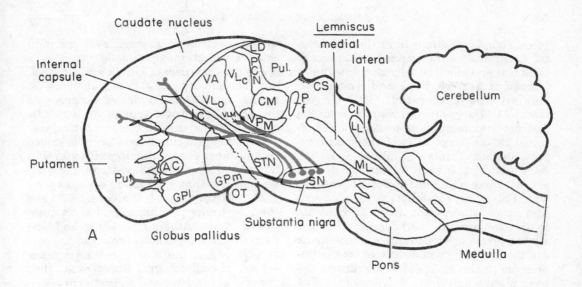

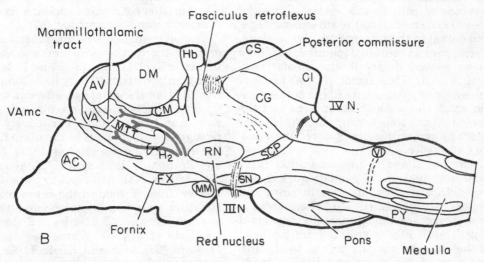

Fig. 13-19. Schematic drawings of the efferent projections (*red*) of the substantia nigra in sagittal sections. Ascending fibers from the substantia nigra (*SN*) pass rostrally into Forel's field H and divide into a small medial bundle (*B*) which projects to the thalamus and a larger lateral bundle (*A*) that courses through the internal capsule. Medially projecting nigral efferent fibers pass to the medial part of the ventral lateral (*VLm*) and the magnocellular part of the ventral anterior (*VAmc*) thalamic nuclei. These fibers parallel the course of the mammillothalamic tract. Nigrostriatal fibers pass laterally, mainly dorsal to the subthalamic nucleus (*STN*), cross through the internal capsule and enter the putamen and caudate nucleus via the globus pallidus and posterior limb of the internal capsule. Drawing *A*, lateral to *B*, shows the course of *nigrostriatal fibers*. Drawing *B*, relatively near the midline, shows *nigrothalamic fibers* (Carpenter and Strominger, '67; Carpenter and Peter, '72). Abbreviations indicate the following: *AC*, anterior commissure; *AV*, anterior ventral thalamic nucleus; *CG*, central gray; *CI*, inferior colliculus; *CM*, centromedian thalamic nucleus; *CS*, superior colliculus; *DM*, dorsomedial thalamic nucleus; *GPl* and *GPm*, lateral and medial segments of the globus pallidus; *H2*, lenticular fasciculus; *Hb*, habenular nucleus; *LD*, lateral dorsal thalamic nucleus; *MM*, mammillary body; *MTT*, mammillothalamic tract; *OT*, optic tract; *PCN*, paracentral thalamic nucleus; *Pf*, parafascicular nucleus; *Pul*, pulvinar; *Py*, medullary pyramid; *SCP*, superior cerebellar peduncle; *VA*, ventral anterior thalamic nucleus; *VLc* and *VLo*, ventral lateral thalamic nucleus (caudal and oral parts); *VPM*, ventral posteromedial thalamic nucleus; *ZI*, zona incerta. Compare with Figure 17-14.

conspicuous reductions in ipsilateral striatal dopamine as measured by fluorescent chemical and electron microscopic technics (Andén et al., '64; Fuxe and Andén, '66; Hökfelt and Ungerstedt, '69; Ungerstedt, '71). Large striatal lesions produce a distinct increase of monoamines (dopamine) in the large cells of the pars compacta which ultimately decreases as the cells undergo chromatolysis (Andén et al., '64; Fuxe and Andén, '66; Ungerstedt, '71). Following interruption of nigrostriatal axons, fluorescent material builds up in the axon proximal to the lesion. Ordinarily the levels of monoamines in the axons are too low to be demonstrated by the fluorescent technic. These observations appear highly significant in view of the fact that the brains of patients with parkinsonism show a virtual absence of dopamine in the striatum and substantia nigra.

Axons of cells in the *ventral tegmental area* (Tsai), medial to the substantia nigra and dorsal to the interpeduncular nucleus, also appear to contain dopamine, but these fibers ascend dorsal to the medial forebrain bundle (Ungerstedt, '71). At levels of the anterior commissure fibers of this bundle enter the nucleus accumbens and the nucleus of the stria terminalis, while other laterally projecting fibers enter the olfactory tubercle.

Afferent fibers to the substantia nigra arise mainly from the caudate nucleus and the putamen (Morgan, '27; Rundles and Papez, '37; Verhaart, '50). These *strionigral fibers* are topographically organized (Fig. 17-14). Fibers arising from the head of the caudate nucleus project to the rostral part of the nigra and have a mediolateral correspondence with portions of the caudate nucleus (Voneida, '60; Szabo, '62). The body of the caudate nucleus sends fibers to the most ventrolateral region of the nigra (Szabo, '70). The putamen projects fibers to portions of the substantia nigra posterior to the root fibers of the oculomotor nerve. Putaminonigral fibers are organized so that: (1) dorsal parts of the putamen project to lateral parts of the nigra, and (2) ventral parts of the putamen project to medial regions of the nigra (Szabo, '67). Most of the strionigral fibers end upon cells in the pars reticulata, al-

though electron microscopic evidence indicates terminations upon dendrites of cells of the pars compacta (Rinvik and Grofová, '70). The majority of strionigral fibers establish symmetrical types of synapses on the soma, dendritic trunks or dendritic spines of nigral cells in the pars reticulata.

Corticonigral fibers have been described by a number of investigators (Rinvik, '66); however, recent electron microscopic studies indicate that such fibers are absent in the cat (Rinvik and Walberg, '69), and their existence in other mammals is questioned. Most authors report that no fibers from the globus pallidus project to the substantia nigra, but this question is unresolved. If pallidonigral fibers exist, they are probably sparse and restricted in distribution (Nauta and Mehler, '66). Subthalamonigral fibers have been described (Woodburne et al., '46; Whittier and Mettler, '49), but this connection remains doubtful (Carpenter and Strominger, '67).

The efferent fibers of the substantia nigra project to the striatum and certain thalamic nuclei (Figs. 13-19 and 17-14). Although nigrostriatal fibers have long been regarded as the principal efferent bundle from this nucleus, evidence for their existence was based almost exclusively upon retrograde cell changes in the nigra following striatal lesions (Holmes, '01; Dresel and Rothman, '25; Ferraro, '25; Morrison, '29; Mettler, '43). Attempts to trace degeneration from lesions in the nigra into the striatum were usually unsuccessful (Ranson and Ranson, '42; Mettler, '42; Rosegay, '44; Cole et al., '64; Carpenter and McMasters, '64; Afifi and Kaelber, '65; Carpenter and Strominger, '67; Faull and Carman, '68). In view of the obvious discrepancies presented by these data and those based upon fluorescent histochemical technics, it was suggested that these axon terminals might be too fine to be resolved by the light microscope (Fuxe et al., '64) or refractory to silver staining technics (Faull and Carman, '68). These fibers were successfully demonstrated by one of the silver impregnation methods after relatively short survival times.

Nigrostriatal fibers project rostrally and dorsolaterally over the subthalamic nucleus, and cross through the internal capsule (Figs. 13-19 and 17-14). These fibers traverse parts of the globus pallidus *en route* to the caudate nucleus and putamen (Carpenter and Peter, '72). Available evidence indicates that nigrostriatal fibers are topographically organized in a manner reciprocal to that of strionigral fibers. Fibers in the caudal two-thirds of the nigra project to portions of the putamen, while rostral parts of the nigra appear related to the head of the caudate nucleus. Lateral parts of the caudal nigra project fibers to dorsal regions of the putamen, while medial regions are related to more ventral parts of the putamen. Nigrostriatal fibers appear to arise mainly from the large cells of the pars compacta. The large cells of the pars compacta apparently synthesize and transmit dopamine via axoplasmic flow to terminal varicosities in restricted and specific regions of the striatum. Electron microscopic evidence suggests that these fibers terminate predominantly upon dendritic spines (Kemp, '68). These findings suggest that strionigral and nigrostriatal fibers may form a closed feedback loop in which strionigral fibers form the afferent limb and nigrostriatal fibers constitute the efferent limb that conveys dopamine to terminal varicosities in the striatum (Fig. 17-14).

In patients with paralysis agitans, there is a virtual absence of dopamine in the striatum and the substantia nigra (Hornykiewicz, '66; Pinder, '73). An effective treatment for this metabolic disorder is large doses of L-dihydroxyphenylalanine (L-dopa), a precursor of dopamine, which passes the blood brain barrier. The effectiveness of this drug sometimes can be enhanced by the use of a peripheral decarboxylase inhibitor (Mars, '73) which prevents systemic decarboxylation of L-dopa to dopamine. Thus, adequate L-dopa will be left unmetabolized systemically to enter the brain where the desired decarboxylation to dopamine can occur.

It is unclear as to whether the substantia nigra projects fibers to the globus pallidus, although certain chemical studies suggest relationships between the nigra and pallidum (McGreer et al., '71). No nigral efferent fibers appear to terminate in the subthalamic nucleus.

Nigrothalamic fibers arise from the cells of the pars reticulata of the nigra and project rostrally to the large-celled part of the ventral anterior nucleus (VAmc) and to the medial part of the ventral lateral nucleus (VLm; Fig. 13-19). These thalamic projections in their course parallel closely the mammillothalamic tract (Carpenter and Peter, '72). Experimental lesions in the substantia nigra also interrupt large numbers of corticotegmental and corticothalamic fibers which descend in the internal capsule and crus cerebri and traverse portions of the nigra *en route* to specific terminations (Rinvik, '68). The significance of the nigrothalamic projection, which is easily demonstrated by silver impregnation technics, is unknown (Cole et al., '64; Afifi and Kaelber, '65; Carpenter and Strominger, '67; Faull and Carman, '68).

The substantia nigra is the brain stem nucleus most intimately related to the largest part of the basal ganglia, namely, the neostriatum. It is one of the structures that is affected with a high degree of consistency in paralysis agitans (Tretiakoff, '19; Foix, '21; Hassler, '39; Heath, '47). It is of interest that discrete lesions of the substantia nigra in the monkey, destroying up to 40% of the nucleus, do not produce alterations of muscle tone, impairment of associative movements, tremor or any detectable form of dyskinesia (Carpenter and McMasters, '64).

CRUS CEREBRI

The most ventral part of the midbrain contains a massive band of descending corticofugal fibers, the *crus cerebri*. According to Déjerine ('01), the medial three-fifths of the crus cerebri contain somatotopically arranged corticospinal and corticobulbar fibers. Other authors (Flechsig, '05; von Monakow, '05; Quensel, '10) indicate that smaller portions of the central part of the crus cerebri contain these fibers. Fibers in the most lateral part of the central region are concerned with the lower extremity; the larger middle region contains fibers concerned with the upper extremity; and the most medial fibers of the central region are associated with the musculature of the face, pharynx and larynx. The

extreme medial and lateral portions of the
crus cerebri contain *corticopontine fibers*.
Frontopontine fibers are medial, while corticopontine fibers from the temporal, parietal and occipital cortices are located laterally (Fig. 13-1).

Besides the above named tracts, there
often are two fiber bundles which descend
partly within the crus cerebri and partly in
the region of the medial lemniscus, known
as *pes lemnisci* (Fig. 13-1). The *medial* or
superficial pes lemniscus detaches itself
from the lateral portion of the crus cerebri,
winds ventrally around the crus and forms
a semilunar fiber bundle medial to the
frontal corticopontine tract (Fig. 13-1). At
lower levels the fibers leave the crus cerebri, pass dorsally through the substantia
nigra and descend in or near the ventromedial portion of the medial lemniscus. The
lateral or *deep pes lemniscus* detaches itself from the dorsal surface of the crus,
runs for some distance in the lateral portion of the substantia nigra, then turns
dorsally and descends in the region of the
medial lemniscus (Fig. 13-1). Certain authors (Déjerine, '01; Verhaart, '35) regarded these bundles as aberrant corticospinal fibers which during phylogenesis became separated from the main tract by the

increasing development of the dorsal pontine nuclei. According to Kuypers ('58a),
fibers of the pes lemnisci can be traced
caudally through the pons to the level of
the pyramidal decussation. A number of
these fibers are distributed to the tegmentum of the pons and medulla. These fibers,
which are undoubtedly corticobulbar, appear to project mainly into the reticular
formation; few, if any, of these fibers pass
directly to motor cranial nerve nuclei (Fig.
11-23).

At this juncture it is recommended that
the blood supply of the midbrain be reviewed (Chapter 20). A more complete
understanding of the structural organization of the midbrain should emphasize the
importance of the vessels that supply this
part of the brain stem. The principal vessels supplying parts of the midbrain include the posterior cerebral, the superior
cerebellar, the posterior communicating
and the anterior choroidal arteries (Figs.
20-14 and 20-15). The numerous veins
draining large portions of the diencephalon and basal regions enter the great cerebral vein in regions dorsal to the midbrain
(Fig. 20-19). These veins and their tributaries are of major importance.

CHAPTER 14

The Cerebellum

The cerebellum is concerned with the coordination of somatic motor activity, the regulation of muscle tone and mechanisms that influence and maintain equilibrium. It is derived embryologically from ectodermal thickenings about the cephalic borders of the fourth ventricle, known as the rhombic lip (Figs. 3-10 and 3-12). Although this portion of the brain is derived from tissue which lies dorsal to the sulcus limitans and receives sensory inputs from virtually all kinds of receptors, it is not concerned with sensory perception, and no information transmitted to it enters the conscious sphere. The sensory information transmitted to the cerebellum is utilized primarily in the regulation and control of motor functions. The cerebellum serves as an example of the important role sensory integrating mechanisms play in motor function. The cerebellum, a metencephalic derivative, functions in a suprasegmental manner in that its integrative influences can effect activities at all levels of the neuraxis. The cerebellum does not give rise to any known tract that projects directly to spinal levels. Thus cerebellar influences upon segmental parts of the nervous system are mediated indirectly by groups of neurons that relay impulses to these parts of the nervous system.

GROSS ANATOMY

The gross anatomy of the cerebellum has been described in Chapter 2. From this discussion, it will be recalled that the cerebellum consists of: (1) a superficial gray mantle, the *cerebellar cortex*; (2) an internal white mass, the *medullary substance*; and (3) four pairs of *intrinsic nuclei* (Figs. 12-6, 12-16 and 14-13). Grossly the cerebellum may be divided into a median portion, the *vermis*, and two expanded lateral lobes or *hemispheres*. The cerebellar cortex is composed of numerous narrow *laminae* or cerebellar *folia*, which in turn possess secondary and tertiary infoldings. Five deeper fissures divide the cerebellar vermis and hemispheres into lobes and lobules which can be identified in gross specimens as well as in midsagittal section (Figs. 2-23, 2-24, 2-25 and 2-26). These fissures are (1) the *primary*, (2) the *posterior superior*, (3) the *horizontal*, (4) the *prepyramidal*, and (5) the *posterolateral* (prenodular). They form the basis for all subdivisions of the cerebellum (Fig. 14-1). In spite of a wealth of histological detail concerning the structural organization of the cerebellum, precise anatomical localization within various lobules is difficult, except in gross specimens. Precise identification of cerebellar lobules, laminae and folia in microscopic sections is difficult even in serial sections. Detailed atlases of the human (Angevine et al., '61) and monkey (Madigan and Carpenter, '71) cerebella facilitate the microscopic study of cerebellar sections.

On developmental and functional bases, the cerebellum can be divided into three distinct parts. The *archicerebellum*, represented largely by the *nodulus*, the *two flocculi* and their peduncular connections

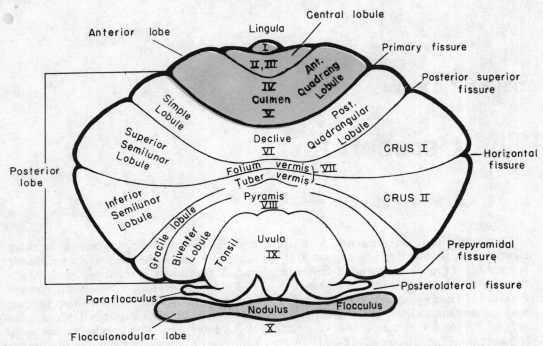

FIG. 14-1. Schematic diagram of the fissures and lobules of the cerebellum (Larsell, '51; Jansen and Brodal, '58; Angevine et al., '61). Portions of the cerebellum caudal to the posterolateral fissure (*blue*) represent the flocculonodular lobule (archicerebellum), while portions of the cerebellum rostral to the primary fissure (*red*) constitute the anterior lobe (paleocerebellum). The neocerebellum lies between the primary and posterolateral fissure. *Roman numerals* refer to portions of the cerebellar vermis only.

(i.e., *flocculonodular lobe*), is the oldest part of the cerebellum and is the subdivision most closely related to the vestibular nerve and nuclei (*blue* in Fig. 14-1). The flocculonodular lobe is separated from the corpus cerebelli by the posterolateral fissure, the first fissure to develop in the cerebellum. The *paleocerebellum*, consisting of all parts of the cerebellum rostral to the primary fissure, is referred to as the *anterior lobe* of the cerebellum (*red* in Fig. 14-1). In lower forms, the paleocerebellum forms the largest part of the cerebellum, while in man it constitutes a small subdivision which receives impulses primarily from stretch receptors. It is the part of the cerebellum considered to be most concerned with the regulation of muscle tone. Influences upon muscle tone mediated via the fastigial nuclei and cerebellovestibular projections reach spinal levels via the vestibulospinal and reticulospinal tracts. Impulses from the emboliform nucleus modify muscle tone by projecting upon cells of

the red nucleus which in turn project to spinal levels (Massion, '67). These fibers are shown in Figure 14-17.

The *neocerebellum* is phylogenetically the newest and the largest portion of the human cerebellum. It includes all parts of the cerebellum between the primary and posterolateral fissures in both the vermis and lateral lobes and comprises the posterior lobe (Fig. 14-1). Lateral parts of the cerebellum, between the primary and the posterior superior fissures, are known as the *simple lobule*. The portions of the lateral lobe between the posterior superior fissure and the gracile lobule constitute the *ansiform lobule*. The horizontal fissure divides the ansiform lobule into *crus I* (superior semilunar lobule) and *crus II* (inferior semilunar lobule). Between the prepyramidal and posterolateral fissures are the biventer lobule and the cerebellar tonsil in the hemisphere, and the pyramis and uvula in the vermis. The neocerebellum is the portion of the cerebellum considered to be related primarily to coordination of skilled movements initiated at cortical levels.

The cerebellum is attached to the medulla, the pons and the midbrain by three paired cerebellar peduncles (Figs. 2-18, 2-19 and 2-25). These compact fiber bundles interconnect the archicerebellum, paleocerebellum and neocerebellum with the spinal cord, brain stem and higher levels of the neuraxis. The extensive nature of these connections suggests that the cerebellum serves as a great integrative center for the coordination of muscular activity. Before examining the afferent and efferent fiber systems of the cerebellum, the structure of the cerebellar cortex will be considered.

CEREBELLAR CORTEX

The cerebellar cortex is uniformly structured in all parts and extends across the midline without evidence of a median raphe. The cortex is composed of three well-defined layers containing five different types of neurons. These layers from the surface are: (1) the molecular layer, (2) the Purkinje cell layer, and (3) the granular layer (Figs. 14-2, 14-3 and 14-4).

The Molecular Layer. This consists principally of dendritic arborizations, densely packed thin axons coursing parallel to the long axis of the folia and two types of neurons (Figs. 14-2, 14-4 and 14-5). The cell density of this layer is low. The two types of cell bodies in the molecular layer are the basket cell and the outer (superficial) stellate cell (Figs. 14-4 and 14-5). The dendritic ramifications of both of these neurons are confined to the molecular layer, as are the axons of the outer stellate cells. The axons of the basket cells lie mainly in the molecular and Purkinje cell layers, but penetrate short distances into the granular layer. The cell processes of both cells are oriented tranversely to the long axis of the folia. The *outer stellate cells,* located in the outer two-thirds of the molecular layer, have small cell bodies, short thin dendrites and fine unmyelinated axons (Figs. 14-4 and 14-5). The short thin dendrites ramify near the cell body, and fine unmyelinated axons extend trans-

versely to the folia to establish synaptic contacts with Purkinje cell dendrites. The *basket cells* (or deep stellate cells) are situated in the vicinity of the Purkinje cell bodies (Figs. 14-3, 14-4 and 14-5). These cells give rise to numerous branching dendrites that ascend in the molecular layer, and elaborate unmyelinated axons arising from one side of the cell body that course transversely to the folia. The axons of the basket cells, passing in the same plane as the dendritic arborizations of the Purkinje cells, give off one or more descending collaterals which form intricate terminal arborizations about the somata of about 10 Purkinje cells. A single descending axon collateral may furnish terminal arborizations for more than one Purkinje cell, and Purkinje cells may receive axonal collaterals from several different basket cells. Basket cell axons divide and form a dense plexus about the Purkinje cell axon hillock (Bell and Dow, '67). Thus a single basket cell may come in synaptic relationship with many Purkinje cells situated in a sagittal plane, its axon even extending to a neighboring folium (Fig. 14-4). It is evident from the above that besides the relatively few cells, the molecular layer is composed primarily of unmyelinated dendritic and axonal processes. These processes include the dendrites of the Purkinje cells, the transversely running axons of the granule cells, the axons of the outer stellate cells, the sagittally oriented axons of the basket cells, and the dendrites of basket and Golgi type II cells. Section of all these processes gives to the molecular layer its finely punctate appearance. Only in its deepest portion is there a narrow horizontal plexus of myelinated fibers composed of axonal collaterals of Purkinje cells (Fig. 14-4).

The Purkinje Cell Layer. This layer consists of a sheet of large flask-shaped cells relatively uniformly arranged along the upper margin of the granular layer (Figs. 14-2, 14-4, 14-5 and 14-6). Purkinje cells have a clear vesicular nucleus with a deeply staining nucleolus and irregular Nissl granules usually arranged concentrically (Fig. 14-3). Although the nucleus appears smooth and round in Nissl-stained sections, in electron micrographs the nu-

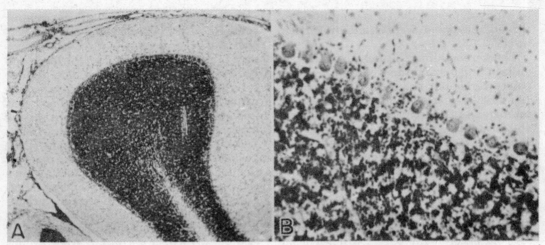

FIG. 14-2. Sections through a folium of monkey cerebellar cortex. In *A* the relative thickness of the three
cerebellar layers can be seen. Light spaces in the dark staining granular layer are the "cerebellar islands"
containing the glomeruli. A single row of Purkinje cells above the granular layer is shown in *B*. Nissl stain.
Photograph. ×20; ×50.

clear membrane is wrinkled or puckered
on the side facing the dendritic tree (Fig. 4-
9; Palay and Chan-Palay, '74). Each cell
gives rise to an elaborate dendritic tree
which arborizes in a flattened fanlike fashion in a plane at right angles to the long
axis of the folium (Figs. 14-4, 14-6 and 14-
7). The dendritic tree arises from the neck
of the cell as two or three large primary
dendrites which branch repeatedly. In the
depth of a furrow the dendritic branches
form a broad angle approximating 180 degrees, while near the crest of a folium
dendritic branches form more acute angles
(Eccles et al., '67). The full extent of the
dendritic arborization can be appreciated
only in sagittal sections of the cerebellum.
Primary and secondary dendritic branches
have a smooth surface, but tertiary
branches are characterized by short rather
thick spines, densely and regularly distributed over all surfaces. These thick dendritic spines are referred to as "spiny
branchlets" (Fox and Barnard, '57) or "gemmules" (Fig. 14-7). The axon arises from
the part of the Purkinje cell opposite to the
dendrites, acquires a myelin sheath and
passes through the granular layer to enter
the underlying white matter (Figs. 14-4
and 14-5); most, but not all, of these axons
pass to the deep cerebellar nuclei. Purkinje cell axons give rise to recurrent Pur-

kinje collaterals (Fig. 14-4) which establish
axo-somatic contacts with Golgi type II
cells in the granular layer (Hámori and
Szentágothai, '66). Some Purkinje cell collaterals may make synaptic contact with
basket cells but present evidence is not
conclusive. Occasionally somewhat
smaller, aberrantly placed Purkinje cells
may be found in the granular or molecular
layers. Since the axons of the Purkinje
cells are the only ones to enter the white
matter, it is evident that all impulses entering the cerebellar cortex must ultimately converge on these cells to reach the
efferent cerebellar paths.

The Granular Layer. In ordinary
stains the granular layer presents the appearance of closely packed chromatic nuclei, not unlike those of lymphocytes; irregular light spaces here and there constitute
the so-called "cerebellar islands" or "glomeruli" (Figs. 14-2, 14-3, 14-4 and 14-5).
The *granule cells* are so prodigious in number (3 million to 7 million granule cells/
mm³ of granular layer, Braitenberg and
Atwood, '58) that the residual space seems
insufficient to accommodate their processes, fibers of passage and other intrinsic
cells. Granule cell nuclei are round or
oval in shape, and range in diameter from
5 to 8 μ; chromatin granules are aggregated against their nuclear membrane as

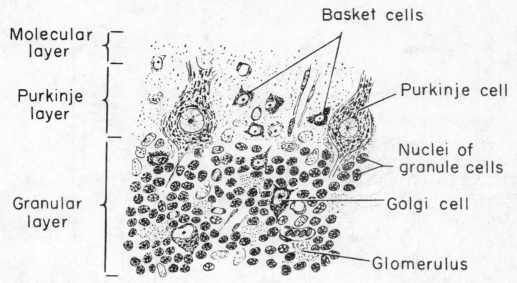

FIG. 14-3. Drawing of portions of the three layers of the human cerebellar cortex. Nissl stain (after Cajal, '11).

well as clustered centrally. The nakedness of granule cell nuclei is said to be due to: (1) the complete absence of discrete Nissl granules, and (2) the thinness of the rimming cytoplasm (Fox et al., '67). In silver preparations these cells give rise to four or five short dendrites, which arborize in clawlike endings within the "glomeruli" (Fig. 4-4*B*).

The scattered relatively clear areas in the granular layer, known as "cerebellar islands," contain glomeruli which are complex synaptic structures (Fig. 14-9). The unmyelinated axons of granule cells ascend vertically into the molecular layer, where each bifurcates into two branches which run parallel to the long axis of the folium. These parallel fibers practically fill the whole depth of the molecular layer and run transversely to the dendritic expansions of the Purkinje cells. In general parallel fibers are thicker in the lower third of the molecular layer. Granule cells in deep parts of the granular layer give rise to parallel fibers in deeper parts of the molecular layer, while cells in the more superficial parts of the granular layer provide parallel fibers in the upper part of the molecular layer (Palay and Chan-Palay, '74). Parallel fibers traverse layer after layer of Purkinje cell dendrites, like tele-

graph wires strung along the branches of a tree, and extend laterally in a folium (Fig. 14-4). Electron microscopic observations (Gray, '61; Fox et al., '64; Hámori and Szentágothai, '66) have shown that each dendritic spine of the Purkinje cell dendritic tree receives a synaptic connection from a parallel fiber in the so-called "crossing-over" synapse. In 1957 Fox and Barnard estimated that each Purkinje cell in the cerebellar cortex of the monkey had a total of 60,000 dendritic spines and that from 200,000 to 300,000 parallel fibers projected through the territory of its dendritic tree. More recent studies in cat, monkey and man (Fox et al., '67) indicate that the early estimate of 60,000 spines on a single Purkinje cell should be doubled. Each parallel fiber, extending about 1.5 mm from its bifurcation, has been estimated to traverse the dendritic trees of up to 500 Purkinje cells. The parallel fibers of the granule cells also make "crossing-over" synaptic contacts with the dendrites of outer stellate, basket and Golgi type II cells in the molecular layer (Fig. 14-5).

The *Golgi type* II cell usually is found in the upper part of the granular layer, but it is seen also in other parts of this layer. These cells have vesicular nuclei and definite chromophilic bodies (Fig. 14-3). The

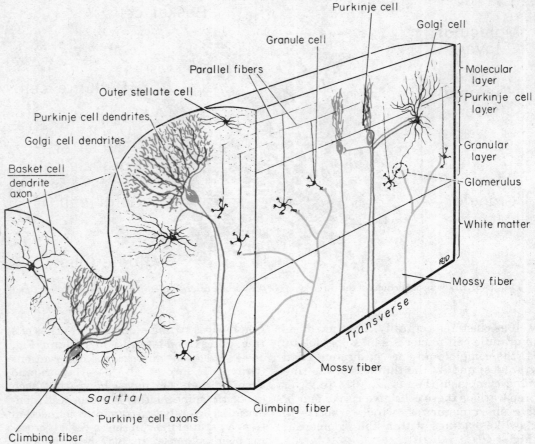

FIG. 14-4. Schematic diagram of the cerebellar cortex in sagittal and transverse planes showing cell and fiber arrangements. Purkinje cells and cell processes (i.e., axons and dendrites) are shown in *blue*. Mossy fibers are in *yellow*; climbing fibers are shown in *red*. Golgi cells, basket cells and outer stellate cells are in *black*. While the dendritic arborizations of Purkinje cells are oriented in a sagittal plane, dendrites of the Golgi cells show no similar arrangement. Layers of the cerebellar cortex are indicated.

dendritic branches of the Golgi cell extend throughout all layers of the cerebellar cortex, but are most extensive in the molecular layer. Unlike the dendrites of the Purkinje cell, arborizations are not restricted to a single plane (Figs. 14-4 and 14-5). In the molecular layer Golgi cell dendrites are contacted by parallel fibers; the cell body is in contact with collaterals of climbing fibers and recurrent collaterals of Purkinje cells (Scheibel and Scheibel, '54; Hámori and Szentágothai, '66). It has been estimated that there is one Golgi cell for every 10 Purkinje cells (Bell and Dow, '67). The axonal arborization of the Golgi cell is extremely dense; it extends throughout the width of the granular layer but is restricted laterally to a region immediately beneath the cell body. The axons of Golgi type II cells have complex relationships with the terminals of mossy fibers and the dendrites of granule cells.

In addition to the large Golgi cells described above, there is a small Golgi cell whose dendritic tree arises from several trunks which radiate outward from the cell body (Palay and Chan-Palay, '74). Groups of two or three small Golgi cells often are clustered together.

Cortical Afferent Input. Afferent fibers to the cerebellar cortex are supplied by tracts entering the cerebellum mainly

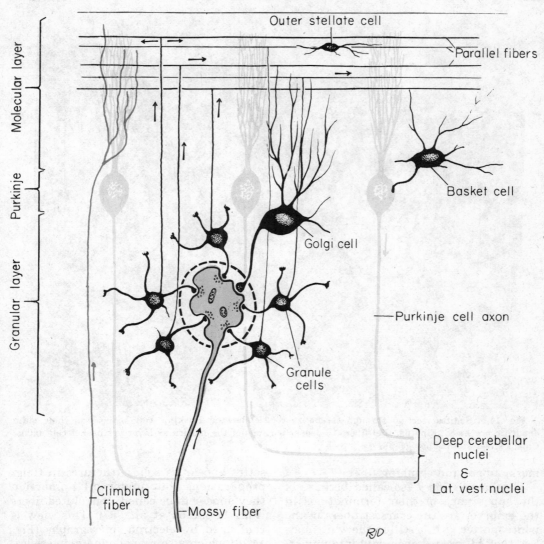

Molecular layer

Purkinje

Granular layer

Outer stellate cell

Parallel fibers

Basket cell

Golgi cell

Purkinje cell axon

Granule cells

Deep cerebellar nuclei & Lat. vest. nuclei

Climbing fiber

Mossy fiber

RJD

FIG. 14-5. Schematic diagram of the cellular and fiber elements of the cerebellar cortex in the longitudinal axis of a folium. Excitatory inputs to the cerebellar cortex are conveyed by the mossy fibers (*yellow*) and the climbing fibers (*red*). The *broken line* represents a glia lamella ensheathing a glomerulus, containing: (1) a mossy fiber rosette, (2) several granule cell dendrites, and (3) one Golgi cell axon. Axons of granule cells ascend to the molecular layer, bifurcate and form an extensive system of parallel fibers which synapse on the spiny processes of the Purkinje cells. Purkinje cells and their processes are shown in *blue*. Climbing fibers traverse the granular layer and ascend the dendrites of the Purkinje cells where they synapse on smooth branchlets. *Arrows* indicate the directions of impulse conduction. Outer stellate and basket cells are shown in the molecular layer, but the axons of the basket cells which ramify about Purkinje cell somata are not shown (based on Gray, '61; Eccles et al., '67).

via the inferior and middle cerebellar peduncles. These include the spinocerebellar, the cuneocerebellar, the olivocerebellar, the vestibulocerebellar and the pontocerebellar tracts as well as numerous smaller bundles. In addition there are cere-

bellar association fibers (Eager, '63a, '65) that pass from one folium to adjacent folia, and longer association fibers that connect different cortical regions on the same side. Structurally two types of afferent terminals are found in the cerebellar cortex,

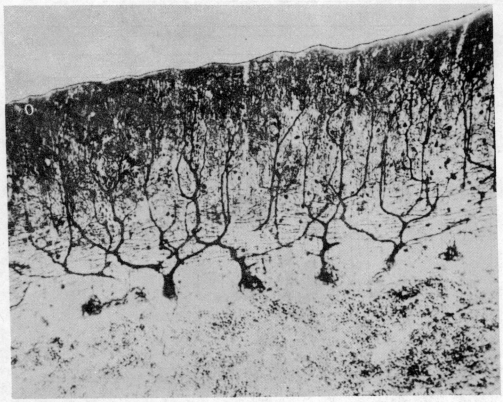

Fig. 14-6. Sagittal section through cerebellar cortex showing Purkinje cell bodies and their main dendritic processes. Fine parallel fibers in deeper portions of the molecular layer are basket cell axons. Cajal's silver stain. Photograph.

mossy fibers and climbing fibers.

The *mossy fibers,* so-called because of the appearance of their terminations in the embryo, are the coarsest fibers in the white matter. While still in the white matter, they bifurcate repeatedly into numerous branches, and enter the granular layer, where the branches of a single fiber often go to adjacent folia. They pass into the granular layer, lose their myelin sheath and give off many fine collaterals. According to electron microscopic evidence the mossy fiber retains its myelin sheath up to its point of continuity with a rosette (Gray, '61). Rosettes are the sites of synapses between mossy fibers and the claw-like terminals of granule cell dendrites. Mossy fiber rosettes are fine lobulated enlargements that occur along the course of branches and at terminals (Figs. 14-4, 14-5 and 14-8). Under low magnification ro-

settes appear as solid structures in Golgi preparations, but under oil immersion they appear to be coiled, convoluted fibers (Fig. 14-8; Fox et al., '67). This view is confirmed by electron micrographs (Fig. 14-10) which also reveal synaptic vesicles, a concentration of mitochondria and a conspicuous core of neurofilaments and neurotubules (Mugnaini, '72). A single mossy fiber rosette forms the center of each cerebellar glomerulus (Figs. 14-5 and 14-9). In the glomerulus it comes into synaptic relationship with granule cell dendrites and Golgi cell axon terminals.

A *glomerulus* is a complex synaptic structure contained within the "cerebellar islands" of the granular layer (Figs. 14-4, 14-5 and 14-9). A cerebellar glomerulus is a nodular structure formed by: (1) one mossy fiber rosette, (2) the dendritic terminals of numerous granule cells, (3) the terminals

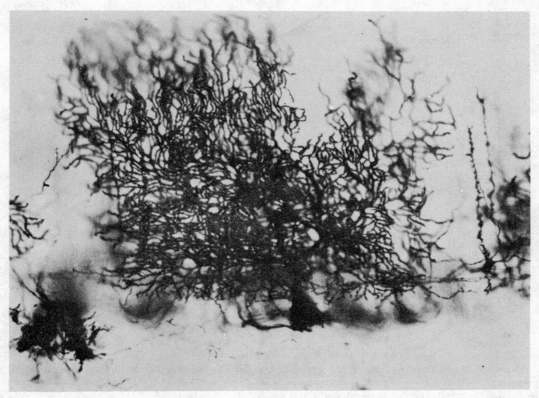

FIG. 14-7. Photograph of a single Purkinje cell and virtually all of its rich dendritic arborizations. ×300. (Courtesy of C. A. Fox, School of Medicine, Wayne State University.)

of Golgi cell axons, and (4) proximal parts of Golgi cell dendrites. The center of the glomerulus contains a single mossy fiber rosette with which the dendrites of about 20 different granule cells interdigitate (Figs. 14-8, 14-9 and 14-10). The axons of the Golgi cells form a plexus on the outer surface of the granule cell dendrites. The whole structure is encased by a single glial lamella (Eccles et al., '67; Bell and Dow, '67). Physiological evidence (Eccles et al., '66) indicates that in the glomerulus, the mossy fiber-granule cell synapse is excitatory, while the Golgi axon-granule cell junction is inhibitory. Thus a glomerulus is basically a cluster in which two types of presynaptic fibers enter into a complex relationship with one postsynaptic element. The granule cell and its dendrites constitute the postsynaptic element. The Golgi cell functions as a negative feedback to the mossy fiber-granule cell relay; the main

excitatory input to the Golgi cell is derived from the parallel fibers (Fig. 14-5).

Mossy fiber rosettes also establish a synapse *en marron* on Golgi type II cell bodies. In the region of contact the mossy fiber terminal appears pressed into the finger-like ridges of the Golgi II cell soma (Chan-Palay and Palay, '71). Dendritic claws of granule cells make contact with the surface of the mossy fiber rosette not in contact with the Golgi II cell soma.

Climbing fibers, according to classic descriptions (Cajal, '11), pass from the white matter through the granular layer and past the Purkinje cell bodies to reach the main dendrites of the latter. There they lose their myelin sheath and split into a number of small fibers which climb ivy-like along the dendritic arborization of the Purkinje cell, whose branchings they closely imitate (Figs. 14-4 and 14-5). Climbing fibers contact only the smooth branches of

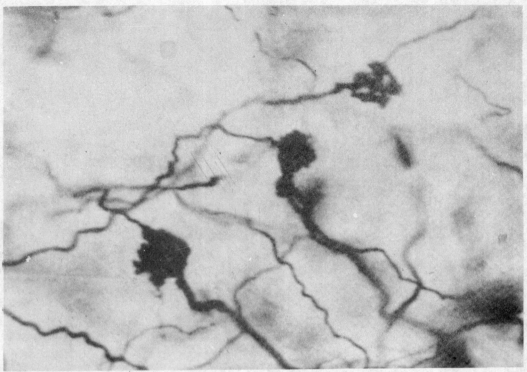

FIG. 14-8. Mossy fiber rosettes in the granular layer of the monkey cerebellum as seen in Golgi preparations. Although mossy fiber rosettes appear as solid structures under low magnifications, under oil immersion the rosettes appear as coiled, convoluted fibers. ×850. (Courtesy of C. A. Fox, School of Medicine, Wayne State University.)

the dendrites; they do not contact the spiny branchlets on which parallel fibers synapse (Fox et al., '67). Although Cajal considered each climbing fiber to be related to a single Purkinje cell, Scheibel and Scheibel ('54) have demonstrated that many fine collaterals leave the parent fiber and end on portions of the somata, or primary dendrites of adjacent Purkinje cells. Many climbing fibers have intracortical courses that change abruptly in the infraganglionic plexus (i.e., beneath the Purkinje cell layer). Some fibers may course transversely near the somata of five or six Purkinje cells before turning toward the surface to be deployed over the dendritic arbor of a single Purkinje cell (O'Leary et al., '70). Light and electron microscopic studies (Scheibel and Scheibel, '54; Hámori and Szentágothai, '66) indicate that climbing fiber collaterals also make contact with stellate, basket and Golgi cells. Recent electron microscopic

evidence indicates that although climbing fibers and basket cell axons partially overlap in their contact with portions of the Purkinje cell dendritic tree, there are no synaptic junctions between these fibers (Chan-Palay and Palay, '70). Climbing fibers articulate primarily with the smooth branchlets of the dendritic tree, while basket cell axons are restricted to dendritic shafts. Additional electron microscopic data establish that collaterals of climbing fibers given off in the granular layer synapse directly upon the shafts of granule cell dendrites and the somata of Golgi II cells (Chan-Palay and Palay, '71a).

Physiologically the climbing fiber system is remarkably specific. Each climbing fiber possesses an extensive all-or-none excitatory connection with the Purkinje cell dendrites. Whenever the climbing fiber discharges, the Purkinje cell also discharges (Eccles et al., '64, '66). Morphologi-

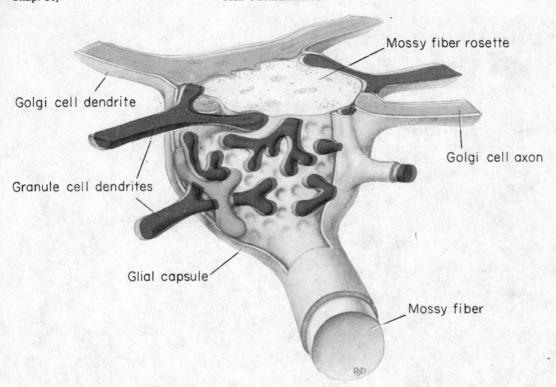

Fig. 14-9. Schematic reconstruction of a cerebellar glomerulus based upon electron microscopic studies. A cerebellar glomerulus is formed by one mossy fiber rosette, the dendritic terminals of numerous granule cells (*red*), and terminals of Golgi cell axons (*yellow*). Proximal parts of Golgi dendrites (*blue*) also enter the glomerulus and establish broad synaptic contacts with the mossy fiber rosette. The entire nodular structure is ensheathed in a glial capsule. In this reconstruction the glomerulus is shown in horizontal section, and in a schematic three-dimensional view (based on Eccles et al., '67).

cal information suggests that stimulation of a climbing fiber not only excites a single Purkinje cell, but also a number of granule cells whose axons (parallel fibers) in turn excite Purkinje cells in the long axis of the folium. Thus excitation carried by parallel fibers will influence Purkinje cells surrounding a particular Purkinje cell which is excited directly by a climbing fiber. The potential inhibitory influence that climbing fibers may exert via Golgi II cells is more difficult to understand, but it is possible that their output may inhibit granule cells not strongly excited by mossy or climbing fibers (Eccles et al., '67).

The respective sources of the mossy and climbing fibers have been difficult to determine. Experimental evidence indicates that the mossy fibers degenerate following interruption of spinocerebellar and ponto-

cerebellar tracts and lesions involving primary and secondary vestibulocerebellar fibers (Miscolczy, '31, '34; Snider, '36; Mettler and Lubin, '42; Brodal, '54; Brodal and Høivik, '64). Mossy fibers are considered to constitute the principal afferent system to the cerebellar cortex and are the mode of termination of most cerebellar afferent systems. The climbing fibers have been the center of great interest since their discovery by Cajal in 1888 because of their remarkable one-to-one relationship with dendritic branches of the Purkinje cell. These fibers have been thought to be recurrent axonal collaterals of Purkinje cells (Lorente de Nó, '24), or recurrent axons of the deep cerebellar nuclei (Carrea et al., '47). There is now general agreement that climbing fibers, like mossy fibers, have exogenous origins (i.e., from nuclei outside

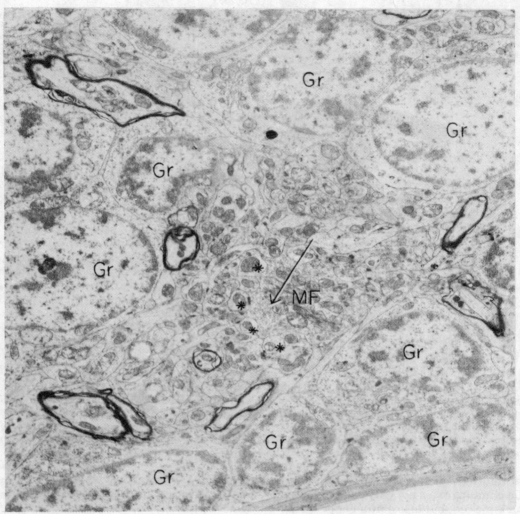

FIG. 14-10. Electron micrograph of cerebellar glomerulus in the monkey. A mossy fiber rosette (*MF*) with dispersed synaptic vesicles (*arrow*) is surrounded by granule cells (*Gr*). Granule cell dendrites are indicated by *asterisks*. ×5600. (Courtesy of R. C. Henrikson, College of Physicians and Surgeons, Columbia University.)

of the cerebellum). Silver impregnation technics originally suggested that most climbing fibers originated from the inferior olivary complex (Szentágothai and Rajkovits, '59). This view was strengthened by electrophysiological results which concluded that climbing fibers originated only from the inferior olivary complex (Eccles et al., '67; Carrea et al., '70; Thach, '70). More detailed light and electron microscopic investigations indicated that following unilateral lesions in the inferior oli-

vary complex, mossy fiber terminals bore the brunt of the degenerative changes, and that significant numbers of climbing fibers remained intact after long survivals (O'Leary et al., '70; Rivera-Dominguez et al., '74). New and more specific information concerning the origins of both mossy and climbing fibers has come from autoradiographic studies utilizing the principles of protein synthesis and axoplasmic flow (Murphy et al., '73). These studies indicate that radioactive labeling of: (1) the pontine nuclei permits the identification of both mossy and climbing fibers in the contralateral cerebellar cortex with a slight preponderance of mossy fibers, (2) the medial reticular formation identifies almost exclusively climbing fibers, and (3) the inferior olivary complex identifies both mossy and climbing fibers with a marked preponderance of climbing fibers. Findings with this new technic suggest that fibers projecting to the cerebellar cortex from the same nuclear mass may have more than one mode of termination.

Fluorescence microscopy has revealed a hitherto unrecognized fiber system in the cerebellar cortex which contains norepinephrine (Hökfelt and Fuxe, '69). These fibers, detectable by their green fluorescence, extend from the white matter into all layers of the cortex, are not restricted to any particular plane and are moderately concentrated in the Purkinje cell layer. This fiber system is considered to arise mainly from the locus ceruleus (Figs. 12-24, 12-25, 12-26 and 13-3) and probably establishes synaptic contacts with Purkinje cell dendrites (Olson and Fuxe, '71; Bloom et al., '71). The number of fibers in this system is small, and without their fluorescent marker they cannot be recognized by other technics (Palay and Chan-Palay, '74).

Structural Mechanisms. The intricate geometric relationships of the structural elements in the cerebellar cortex have furnished many hypotheses concerning intracortical impulse transmission and the possible functions of individual neurons. Studies of the microphysiology of cerebellar neurons have yielded spectacular findings. These observations indicate that the climbing fiber has an extremely powerful excitatory synaptic action on the primary and secondary dendrites of the Purkinje cell (Eccles et al., '64, '66). On the basis that different endings of the same neuron probably mediate similar effects, it seems likely that climbing fibers also excite basket cells, some granule cells and Golgi type II neurons. Stimulation of the superficial parallel fibers, representing axons of granule cells, produces excitation of Purkinje cells via crossing-over synapses with Purkinje

cell dendrites (Eccles et al., '66a). However, stimulation of deeper parallel fibers produces less marked excitatory effects on Purkinje cells because of the concomitant inhibitory influences of basket and outer stellate cells. Available evidence (Eccles et al., '66b) indicates that the outer stellate cells, basket cells and Golgi type II cells are inhibitory interneurons in the cerebellar cortex. Inhibitory influences of the outer stellate cells affect Purkinje cell dendrites in the molecular layer (Fig. 14-4). Basket cell inhibition appears to be effected by axosomatic synapses on Purkinje cell somata. Golgi type II cells appear to inhibit the afferent input to the cerebellar cortex at the mossy fiber-granule cell relay in the glomeruli (Eccles et al., '66a). Inhibitory influences of the outer stellate and basket cells would be mediated in a plane transverse to the folia; outer stellate cell inhibition would be relatively localized, but basket cell inhibition would involve 10 to 12 Purkinje cells (Fig. 14-4). Because Golgi cell axons reach glomeruli throughout the depth of the granular layer, they could inhibit input via mossy fibers to parallel fibers for a distance of about 3 mm longitudinally, and over a distance of 5 or 6 Purkinje cells transverse to the folium (Figs. 14-4, 14-5 and 14-9). Although Purkinje cell axons represent the principal discharge pathway from the cerebellar cortex, recurrent axonal collaterals exert important influences upon Golgi cells and basket cells (Fig. 14-4). Present evidence suggests that these axonal collaterals have a disinhibitory influence upon these cells (Hámori and Szentágothai, '66). The cerebellar cortex thus has an exceedingly elaborate structural and functional organization in which multiple interactions influence input, conduction, synaptic articulations and the output which ultimately must pass via Purkinje cell axons to the deep cerebellar nuclei. It has been estimated that the human cerebellar cortex contains 15 million Purkinje cells (Braitenberg and Atwood, '58). The combined surface area of the dendritic branchlets and spines of one Purkinje cell in the monkey is said to be about 200,000 μ^2 (Fox and Barnard, '57). A synaptic area of such magnitude on each of 15 million cells provides an index of the elaborate activity of the cerebellar cortex. The fact that all parts of the cerebellar cortex have a similar structure has been interpreted to mean that specific functions are not precisely localized.

Purkinje cell axons represent the efferent pathway from the cerebellar cortex. These axons project mainly to the deep cerebellar nuclei, although some fibers from certain cortical areas bypass the deep cerebellar nuclei and project to portions of the vestibular nuclear complex. Direct cerebellovestibular fibers arise from the flocculonodular lobe (Dow, '36, '38) and from portions of the vermis both anteriorly and posteriorly (Walberg and Jansen, '61; Eager, '63). Physiological studies indicate that the entire output of the cerebellar cortex is inhibitory (Ito and Yoshida, '64, '66; Ito et al., '64; Ito et al., '66; Eccles et al., '67). Thus the axons of the Purkinje cells inhibit the cells with which they synapse, namely those of the deep cerebellar nuclei and portions of the vestibular nuclei.

The majority of cerebellar cortical association fibers are short interconnections extending no more than two or three folia. Long association pathways have been traced only from the paravermal cortex, the lateral culmen and the lateral cortex of crus II (Eager, '63a). Anatomically the cortex of the vermis appears independent of that of the lateral hemispheres, in that association fibers in vermal cortex pass only to adjacent vermal folia, and the cortex of the lateral hemispheres does not project to the vermis (Clarke and Horsley, '05; Jansen, '33; Eager, 63a). Paravermal and lateral cortical areas of the anterior lobe give rise to long association fibers passing to the posterior folia of crus II on the same side. Long association fibers, crossing the midline, arise from lateral crus II, and terminate in folia of the contralateral crus II, the paramedian lobule and parts of the paraflocculus (Eager, '63). Long and short association fibers in the cerebellar cortex are regarded as myelinated axonal collaterals of Purkinje cells (Fox et al., '67).

Neuroglia. While most of the neuroglial elements in the cerebellar cortex are similar to those in other parts of the central nervous system, the architectonics of the neuroglia bear definite relationships to the three-layered neuronal structure (Fig. 14-11). Each cortical layer has a different population of neuroglial cell types, and one type, the Golgi epithelial cell, is unique to the cerebellar cortex. The cerebellar cortex contains both astrocytes and oligodendrocytes. Astrocytes are primarily protoplasmic and have been divided into three classes: (1) the Golgi epithelial cell, (2) the lamellar or velate astrocyte, and (3) the smooth astrocyte (Palay and Chan-Palay, '74). The Purkinje cell layer contains modified astrocytes known as the *Golgi epithelial cells* (Cajal, '11), or *Bergmann cells*. These neuroglial cells are true satellites of Purkinje cells in that they lie directly against the surface of Purkinje cells and form a nearly complete sheath around them. Purkinje cells also are surrounded by Fañanas cells (Fig. 14-11), which in thin sections do not appear different in the electron microscope (Sotelo, '67; Palay and Chan-Palay, '74). Each Bergmann cell gives rise to two or more processes which bifurcate and ascend in almost parallel lines to the pial surface. The upward prolongations of these processes course perpendicularly in the molecular layer and terminate at the surface of the cortex (i.e., limiting glial membrane) in conical expansions. These cells resemble miniature candelabra with their branches either clustered or spread out in parasagittal planes. The neuroglial processes of these cells were considered to be between the dendritic arborizations of consecutive Purkinje cells (Cajal, '11). Electron micrographs indicate that the ascending processes of neighboring Bergmann cells are interdigitated to form a dense forest, rather than alternating palisades. Processes of Bergmann cells have been considered to insulate the smooth branchlet of Purkinje cell dendrites from passing parallel fibers (Fox et al., '67). This insulation appears absent only where climbing fibers come into synaptic relationship with the smooth branchlets. These specialized glial processes also may serve to confine transmitter substances to a particular synaptic site and in

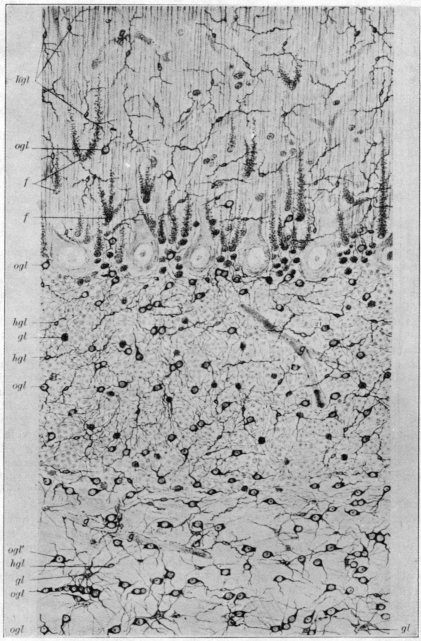

FIG. 14-11. Arrangement of neuroglia cells in human cerebellar cortex. *f*, Cells of Fañanas; *gl*, astroglia; *hgl*, microglia; *ogl* and *ogl'*, oligodendrocytes. (Jakob, '28, after Schröder.)

this way promote neuronal specificity (Peters et al., '70). The Golgi epithelial cell is characteristic of the Purkinje and molecular layers and is not found elsewhere. Electron microscopic studies indicate that Golgi epithelial cells, Fañanas cells and protoplasmic astrocytes of the cerebellar cortex probably are all variants of a single cell type (Palay and Chan-Palay, '74).

The lamellar astrocyte is found chiefly in the granular layer, while the smooth astrocyte may be found in any layer, but is most common in the granular layer. Lamellar astrocytes are about the same size as granule cells, have a bean-shaped nucleus and may contain one or two nucleoli. The distribution and form of the glial processes of these cells are unusual. Numerous lamellar neuroglial processes pass between adjacent granule cells, dendrites and axons, forming open and confluent compartments. The number and extent of these processes is greater than might be expected. The lamellar processes separate one glomerulus from another in the cerebellar islands, and interweave with the dendrites and Golgi cell axons on the periphery of the glomeruli (Palay and Chan-Palay, '74).

Smooth astrocytes with long radiating processes, found in the molecular and granular layers, resemble stellate neuroglial cells, but are much smaller. Processes of these cells are kinky, contorted and branch repeatedly. Oligodendrocytes are seen throughout the cerebellar cortex, but are most numerous in the granular layer and in the depths of the molecular layer where myelinated fibers are found.

THE DEEP CEREBELLAR NUCLEI

The corpus medullare is a compact mass of white matter, continuous from hemisphere to hemisphere, that is covered everywhere by the cerebellar cortex. It consists of afferent projection fibers to the cerebellar cortex, efferent projection fibers from the cerebellar cortex and, to a lesser extent, association fibers connecting the various portions of the cerebellum. Some of these fibers cross to the other side in two cerebellar commissures: (1) a posterior commissure in the region of the fastigial nuclei, and (2) an anterior commissure rostral to the dentate nuclei.

The corpus medullare is continuous with the three peduncles which connect the cerebellum with the brain stem: (1) the *inferior cerebellar peduncle*, which connects with the medulla; (2) the *middle cerebellar peduncle*, which connects with the pons; and (3) the *superior cerebellar peduncle*, which connects with the midbrain (Figs. 2-19 and 2-25). Medially and ventrally, near the roof of the ventricle, the corpus medullare splits into two white laminae, inferior

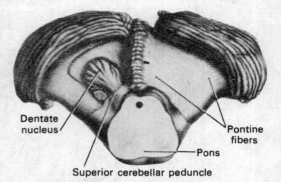

Dentate nucleus

Pontine fibers

Pons

Superior cerebellar peduncle

FIG. 14-12. Drawing of dissection of the superior surface of the cerebellum exposing the dentate nucleus (from Mettler's *Neuroanatomy*, '48; courtesy of The C. V. Mosby Company).

and superior, which separate at an acute angle to form a tentlike recess (i.e., fastigium) in the roof of the fourth ventricle (Figs. 2-20, 2-21 and 2-26). The inferior medullary lamina passes caudally over the nodulus and becomes continuous with the tela choroidea and the choroid plexus of the fourth ventricle (Fig. 2-20). Laterally the inferior medullary velum extends to the flocculi, forming a narrow bridge connecting these structures with the nodulus (Fig. 2-25). The largest part of the medullary substance is continued rostrally, forming the superior medullary velum (Figs. 2-21 and 2-25). The latter is a thin white plate joining the two superior cerebellar peduncles; together these structures form the roof and lateral walls of the upper part of the fourth ventricle.

Imbedded in the white matter of each half of the cerebellum are four nuclear masses (Figs. 12-6, 12-16 and 14-13). From medial to lateral these nuclei are the fastigial, the globose, the emboliform and the dentate.

The Dentate Nucleus. This nucleus, the largest of the deep cerebellar nuclei, lies in the white matter of the cerebellar hemisphere close to the vermis (Fig. 14-12). It is a convoluted band of gray having the shape of a folded bag with the opening or hilus directed medially and dorsally. In transverse section it has an appearance similar to that of the inferior olivary nucleus. It is found as a definite nucleus only in mammals, and it becomes greatly enlarged in man and the anthropoid apes. A

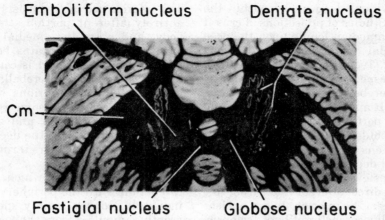

Emboliform nucleus   Dentate nucleus

Cm—

Fastigial nucleus   Globose nucleus

FIG. 14-13. Horizontal section through adult cerebellum showing portions of the deep cerebellar nuclei and the corpus medullare (*Cm*). Weigert's myelin stain. Photograph.

dorsomedial older portion may be distinguished from a newer and larger ventrolateral portion. The nucleus is composed mainly of large multipolar cells with branching dendrites. Axons of these cells acquire a myelin sheath while still in the nucleus and emerge from the cerebellum in the superior cerebellar peduncle. Between these large cells are small stellate cells whose axons apparently arborize within the nucleus. Afferent fibers from the Purkinje cells enter laterally and form a dense fiber plexus, the amiculum, around the nucleus.

The Emboliform Nucleus. This nucleus is a wedge-shaped gray mass close to the hilus of the dentate nucleus and often difficult to delimit from the latter. It is composed of clumps of cells resembling those of the dentate nucleus (Fig. 14-13).

The Globose Nucleus. This nucleus consists of one or more rounded gray masses lying between the fastigial and emboliform nuclei. It likewise contains large and small multipolar cells. In lower mammals the globose and emboliform nuclei form essentially a single structure referred to as the *nucleus interpositus*. Two parts of the nucleus interpositus have been distinguished in the cat and monkey: (1) an anterior nucleus interpositus located rostrally close to the dentate nucleus that appears homologous to the emboliform nucleus, and (2) a posterior nucleus interpositus located more medially that appears ho-

mologous to the globose nucleus.

The Fastigial Nucleus. This nucleus, the most medial of the deep cerebellar nuclei and the oldest, lies near the midline in the roof of the fourth ventricle (Figs. 12-16 and 14-13). This nucleus is characterized by a population of densely packed cells of varying sizes. Large, medium and small cells are intermingled in dorsal parts of the nucleus, while small cells predominate ventrally (Courville and Cooper, '70).

Quantitatively the largest number of afferent fibers to deep cerebellar nuclei arise from Purkinje cells in the cerebellar cortex. All parts of the cerebellar cortex project upon the intrinsic nuclei. The pattern of corticonuclear projection indicates that anterior and posterior vermal areas project fibers to the fastigial nuclei (Jansen and Brodal, '40, '42; Eager, '63). The paravermal cortex projects fibers mainly to the ipsilateral intermediate nuclei (i.e., the globose and emboliform), although fibers from some portions of this cortical region pass to parts of the dentate nucleus. Cortex of the lateral hemispheres gives rise to fibers projecting throughout the length of the dentate nucleus, and to caudal parts of the intermediate nuclei. Portions of the paraflocculus project fibers to the intermediate nuclei and to caudal parts of both fastigial nuclei. There have been suggestions that longitudinal zones of the cerebellar cortex (i.e., vermal, paravermal and lateral) project Purkinje cell axons to individual deep nuclei within the same zone. Studies of projections of crus II and the paramedian lobule upon the deep nuclei (Brodal and Courville, '73; Courville et al., '73) do not support this thesis, except in respect to the relationship between the cerebellar vermis and the fastigial nuclei. It appears that the lateral and paravermal portions of the 10 consecutive cerebellar lobules (Fig. 14-1) have distinctive projections to more than one of the more lateral deep cerebellar nuclei.

The intrinsic cerebellar nuclei, in addition, receive direct afferent fibers from specific portions of the inferior olivary nuclear complex. Olivocerebellar fibers, comprising one of the largest cerebellar afferent systems, pass to all parts of the cerebellar cortex and to the deep cerebellar nuclei. Other afferent fibers to the intrinsic cerebellar nuclei include: (1) secondary vestibular fibers to the fastigial nuclei, and (2) a small number of rubrocerebellar fibers to the interposed nuclei (Courville and Brodal, '66). If the Purkinje cells are inhibitory, as present evidence indicates, the deep cerebellar nuclei must be provided with some excitatory input. It is assumed that the deep cerebellar nuclei receive excitatory influences via collaterals of cortical afferents. It seems likely that the principal, but not the exclusive, source of this excitation may come from the inferior olivary complex (Eccles, '66; Fox et al., '67). Thus the deep cerebellar nuclei probably receive both excitatory and inhibitory impulses. The current assumption is that in these neurons tonic facilitation predominates over inhibition, and thus maintains a tonic discharge of impulses directed toward brain stem neurons (Eccles et al., '67).

CEREBELLAR CONNECTIONS

Afferent Fibers. Afferent cerebellar fibers are nearly three times more numerous than efferent ones (Snider, '50). They convey impulses from the periphery and from various levels of the neuraxis via relay nuclei in the brain stem. Most of the fibers enter the cerebellum through the inferior and middle cerebellar peduncles, although a small number enter in association with the superior cerebellar peduncle.

The inferior peduncle consists of a larger, entirely afferent portion, the restiform body, and a smaller, medial, juxtarestiform portion that contains both afferent and efferent fibers, and is concerned primarily with vestibulocerebellar and cerebellovestibular connections (Fig. 12-16). With the exception of some rubrocerebellar, vestibulocerebellar and olivocerebellar fibers, which go to the deep cerebellar nuclei, all afferent fibers terminate in the cerebellar cortex.

The afferent fibers which connect the cerebellum with the periphery, directly or indirectly, convey mainly special proprioceptive impulses from the vestibular end organ and impulses from stretch receptors in muscles and tendons (Lloyd and McIntyre, '50; Oscarsson, '65). However, electrophysiological experiments on several species, including the monkey, have shown that exteroceptive impulses, such as tactile, auditory and visual impulses, likewise reach the cerebellum, although the tracts conveying them are not fully known (Snider, '50). The projection of exteroceptive impulses to the cerebellar cortex is somatotopically organized in a definite way. Tactile stimulation evokes potential changes in the anterior lobe and simple lobule of the same side and in the paramedian lobules of both sides. The paramedian lobule corresponds to the gracile lobule (Fig. 14-1), but according to the accepted nomenclature is regarded as a part of the inferior semilunar lobule (Angevine et al., '61). The leg is represented in the central lobule, the arm in the culmen, and the head in the simple lobule. The orientation is reversed in the paramedian lobules, the leg area lying most caudally and the head area most rostrally (Fig. 14-14). Similarly, auditory and visual stimulation evokes potentials in limited areas of the cerebellar cortex, i.e., in the simple lobule, folium, and tuber and immediately adjacent portions of the hemispheres (Fig. 14-15).

Vestibulocerebellar fibers enter the cerebellum largely through the juxtarestiform body. Primary vestibulocerebellar fibers arise from the vestibular ganglion and project to the ipsilateral nodulus, uvula and flocculus (Brodal and Høivik, '64). In the monkey, fibers from all parts of the gan-

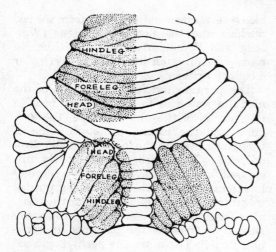

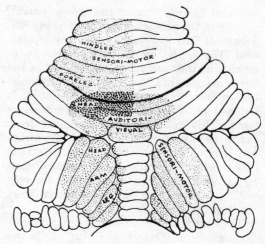

FIG. 14-14. Tactile areas of the cerebellum of the monkey as mapped out by discrete movement of hairs on the left side of the animal (Snider, '50).

FIG. 14-15. Corticocerebellar projections in the monkey (*Macaca mulatta*). Note the head, arm and leg areas receiving projections from the sensorimotor cortex. Note also the overlap of the head area with the area receiving projections from the audiovisual cortex (Snider, '50).

glion project to parts of the nodulus and uvula, while fibers from ganglion cells innervating the cristae of the semicircular canals and the maculae of the utricle and saccule project to different folia of the flocculus (Carpenter et al., '72). Some primary vestibulocerebellar fibers end as climbing fibers in the flocculus. Secondary vestibular fibers originate from the inferior vestibular nucleus and, to a lesser extent, from parts of the medial vestibular nucleus. Although primary and secondary vestibulocerebellar fibers have similar distributions, the number of secondary fibers is much greater. In addition secondary vestibular fibers pass bilaterally to the nodulus, uvula and the fastigial nuclei (Brodal and Torvik, '57; Carpenter et al., '59).

The *posterior spinocerebellar tract* enters the inferior cerebellar peduncle and projects upon the rostromedial part of the anterior lobe (lobules I to IV, Fig. 14-1) and the lateral part of the pyramis and the paramedian lobule (Grant, '62a; Oscarsson, '65; Larsell and Jansen, '72). Most of these fibers terminate ipsilaterally. The posterior spinocerebellar tract conveys impulses from stretch receptors via group Ia and Ib muscle afferents, exteroceptive impulses from touch and pressure receptors in the skin and slow adapting pressure receptors (Oscarsson, '65). Fibers of this tract do not convey impulses from low threshold joint receptors.

The *anterior spinocerebellar tract* ascends in the brain stem to rostral pontine levels and enters the cerebellum in association with the superior cerebellar peduncle (Figs. 10-10, 12-18 and 14-18). Fibers initially located dorsolateral to the superior cerebellar peduncle arch medially over this largely efferent bundle to enter the cerebellum. These fibers pass to essentially the same cortical areas as those of the posterior spinocerebellar tract. However, the main area of termination is in the anterior lobe; only a few fibers reach the pyramis and paramedian lobule (Grant, '62a). The majority of the fibers of this tract terminate in the cerebellum contralaterally with respect to the tract in the spinal cord (and ipsilateral to the cells of origin); about 15% of the fibers terminate bilaterally (Smith, '61; Grant, '62a; Oscarsson, '65; Larsell and Jansen, '72). The anterior spinocerebellar tract mainly conveys impulses from group Ib afferent fibers.

Cuneocerebellar fibers from the accessory cuneate nucleus in the lower medulla enter the inferior cerebellar peduncle and pass to the posterior part of the anterior lobe (lobule V, Fig. 14-1), the anterior folia of the simple lobule, the paramedian lobule and the depths of the prepyramidal fissure in the posterior vermis (Grant, '62). Fibers of this afferent system are ipsilateral. The accessory cuneate nucleus is regarded as the medullary equivalent of the dorsal nucleus of Clarke, and the cuneocerebellar tract is regarded as the forelimb equivalent of the posterior spinocerebellar tract. This tract conveys impulses from group Ia muscle afferents and exteroceptive impulses from cutaneous afferents (Fig. 10-10). Receptive fields for cutaneous impulses are smaller than those associated with the posterior spinocerebellar tract (Oscarsson, '65).

The *rostral spinocerebellar tract*, identified in the cat (Oscarsson, '64a, '65), is the forelimb functional equivalent of the anterior spinocerebellar tract, but is uncrossed. This tract arises from cells rostral to the dorsal nucleus of Clarke, ascends in the anterior part of the spinal cord and enters the cerebellum via both the inferior and superior cerebellar peduncles. Fibers of this tract are distributed almost exclusively to the anterior lobe of the cerebellum in lobules I to V (Fig. 14-1). Fiber terminations are predominantly ipsilateral (Oscarsson, '65, '67a). This tract is activated monosynaptically by group Ib muscle afferents and polysynaptically by flexor afferents.

Reticulocerebellar fibers arise from two distinctive reticular nuclei in the medulla. These fibers enter the cerebellum via the inferior cerebellar peduncle. The lateral reticular nucleus of the medulla projects uncrossed fibers to the anterior lobe and the paramedian lobule. The projection to the vermis is more abundant than to other parts of the cerebellum. Spinal fibers contained in the anterolateral funiculus terminate in a specific manner upon the small-celled part of this nucleus. Anatomical (Brodal, '49) and physiological (Combs, '56) evidence indicates that the lateral reticular nucleus is a relay in a spinocerebellar pathway transmitting somatotopically organized impulses to specific parts of the cerebellum. Fibers from this nucleus appear to mediate tactile impulses, and perhaps other types of impulses, to the cerebellum. The lateral reticular nucleus

also receives descending fibers from the red nucleus and the fastigial nucleus (Walberg and Pompeiano, '60), and thus, in part, may function in a cerebelloreticular feedback system.

The paramedian reticular nuclei of the medulla give rise to fibers which pass to the vermis of the anterior lobe, the pyramis and the uvula, although some of them terminate in the fastigial nuclei (Brodal, '53). These fibers are mostly uncrossed, and also may be part of a cerebelloreticular feedback. Another group of medullary nuclei not belonging to the reticular formation has cerebellar projections similar to those of the paramedian reticular nuclei. These are the perihypoglossal nuclei described in Chapter 11 (page 308).

Olivocerebellar fibers form the largest component of the inferior cerebellar peduncle. They arise from the contralateral inferior olivary nucleus and are distributed to all parts of the cerebellar cortex in an orderly pattern (Fig. 14-22A). In man, fibers from the medial portion of the principal olive and the accessory olives go to all portions of the vermis. A much larger component from the lateral portion of the principal olivary nucleus is distributed to the cerebellar hemisphere. The dorsal part of the olive projects to the superior surface of the cerebellum, while the ventral part projects to its inferior surface (Holmes and Stewart, '08). The olivocerebellar projection in young cats and rabbits has been worked out in detail by Brodal ('40). The intracerebellar nuclei, as well as all parts of the cortex, receive olivary fibers, and the distribution is localized exquisitely, each portion of the olive projecting to a specific cerebellar area.

The inferior olivary nucleus is a highly developed complex in man. It is the source of a large number of climbing fibers that have potent excitatory synapses on Purkinje cell dendrites (Szentágothai and Rajkovits, '59; Hámori and Szentágothai, '66; Eccles et al., '64, '66; Murphy et al., '73). The principal part of this nucleus receives descending fibers from the central tegmental tract, a composite bundle originating from multiple brain stem nuclei. Descending fibers in this tract passing to the principal part of the inferior olivary nucleus arise from the red nucleus, the central gray substance and the midbrain tegmentum. Fibers from the sensorimotor cortex pass to the ventral lamella of the principal olive via the crus cerebri and the pyramid (Walberg, '56). Spino-olivary fibers project to specific parts of the medial and dorsal accessory olivary nuclei. Spinal pathways belonging to the olivary system have been identified physiologically by their climbing fiber responses in the anterior lobe of the cerebellum (Miller and Oscarsson, '70). Several spino-olivocerebellar pathways have been described, all of which project to sagittal zones in the anterior lobe. These sagittal projection zones display a somatotopic pattern in lobules IV and V of the vermis. Spino-olivocerebellar pathways resemble the spinocerebellar tracts (Brodal et al., '50). Responses in these systems are evoked by stimuli activating groups II and III muscle afferents, cutaneous afferents and high threshold joint afferents with wide receptive fields. These impulses, referred to as *flexor reflex afferents*, also have actions upon segmental reflexes and are transmitted by several other ascending tracts. There is difficulty in interpreting the information transmitted by these pathways because it lacks modality specificity and permits only crude spatial discrimination. Certain evidence suggests that olivary neurons may convey specific information related to interneuronal activities at spinal and brain stem levels (Miller and Oscarsson, '70). The spino-olivary systems may be activated by either flexor reflex afferents or by the corticospinal tract through a common set of interneurons, which are assumed to influence motor neurons and to be part of the segmental reflex arc. Thus, the spino-olivocerebellar system may monitor the activity of interneurons at spinal levels and transmit such signals to the cerebellum.

Pontocerebellar fibers, contained in the massive middle cerebellar peduncle, convey impulses from the cerebral cortex to the cerebellum. The pontine nuclei receive cortical fibers from the frontal and temporal lobes and, to a lesser extent, from the parietal and occipital lobes. In the cat there

is evidence that corticopontine fibers arising from the sensorimotor complex project in a somatotopical manner onto two longitudinally oriented cell columns within the pontine nuclei (Brodal, '68). Each part of the cerebral cortex appears to project to several well-defined areas within the pontine nuclei (Brodal, '72, '72a). The fibers from the temporal cortex terminate in the caudal pons, those from the frontal cortex in the cranial portion of the pons. In man the pontocerebellar fibers are almost entirely crossed (Fig. 14-22B) and are distributed primarily to the ansoparamedian lobe and probably to the folium and tuber. According to Brodal and Jansen ('46), both uncrossed and crossed pontine fibers go to all parts of the vermis except the nodulus. Thus while the neocerebellum receives the bulk of the pontocerebellar projections, a considerable number of fibers go to the paleocerebellum as well.

Anatomically, the pontocerebellar projection does not show a definite pattern of localization. Electrical stimulation of the cerebral cortex in cats and monkeys evokes potentials in extensive cerebellar areas. These potentials are more definite and widespread from the motor and sensory cortex, but they may be elicited also from parietal, temporal and occipital regions (Dow, '42). Several investigators have obtained remarkably localized cerebellar projections, from certain cortical areas. The results have been summarized by Snider ('50). The motor area (area 4) and the somatic sensory areas (areas 3, 1 and 2) project to the anterior lobe and the simple lobule. Within the cerebellum the cortical leg area projects to the central lobule, the arm area to the culmen and the face area to the simple lobule (Fig. 14-15). These are the same cerebellar regions which receive tactile impulses from the leg, arm and face, respectively. Similarly the auditory and visual areas of the cortex project to the simple lobule, folium and tuber. Again these are the cerebellar regions receiving auditory and visual impulses from the periphery. The probable meaning of these projections will be discussed in the section on cerebellar function.

The reticulotegmental nucleus of the pons (Fig. 12-19) receives a bilateral, and an ipsilateral, projection from the frontal and parietal cortex (Brodal and Brodal, '71). This nucleus also receives part of the cerebellar output via the descending division of the superior cerebellar peduncle (Carpenter and Nova, '60; Brodal and Szikla, '72) and appears to constitute part of a reticular feedback system to the cerebellum (Fig. 14-16). Fibers from this reticular nucleus pass into the cerebellum via the middle cerebellar peduncle and are distributed to all parts of the vermis, except the nodulus, and to the ansoparamedian lobule. Evidence from different kinds of anatomical studies suggests that cerebellar projections from the reticulotegmental nucleus terminate largely as climbing fibers (Szentágothai and Rajkovits, '59; Murphy et al., '73).

Trigeminocerebellar fibers, both primary and secondary, from different subdivisions of the trigeminal nuclear complex have been described. Although primary trigeminocerebellar fibers have been observed in lower vertebrates (Larsell, '23, '47; Woodburne, '36; Herrick, '48), their areas of termination in the cerebellum have not been established. Secondary trigeminocerebellar fibers from the mesencephalic nucleus of N. V, studied in human fetal material (Pearson, '49, '49a), enter the cerebellum in association with the superior cerebellar peduncle and are distributed to the dentate and the emboliform nuclei. These fibers are believed to conduct impulses from stretch receptors in the muscles of mastication and possibly also from the facial muscles. Secondary trigeminocerebellar fibers from the principal sensory and spinal trigeminal nuclei (Woodburne, '36; Larsell, '47a; Carpenter and Hanna, '61) enter the cerebellum via the inferior cerebellar peduncle. Fibers from these nuclei terminate in the upper culmen and declive (Snider and Stowell, '44; Whitlock, '52; Carpenter and Hanna, '61; Larsell and Jansen, '72).

Tectocerebellar fibers, described as originating from the inferior and superior colliculi and entering the cerebellum in association with the superior cerebellar peduncle, do not appear to be accepted by all authors. The existence of such fibers has attracted attention because Snider and Stowell ('44) have shown that optic and auditory impulses give rise to action potentials in specific portions of the cerebellar cortex (Fig. 14-15). It seems likely that impulses from the superior colliculus pass via tectopontine fibers to pontine nuclei (Altman and Carpenter, '61), which in turn project to areas of the cerebellar cortex. The cerebellar projection area of the pontine nuclei receiving tectopontine fibers corresponds to loci from which optic and auditory responses have been evoked (Snider and Stowell, '44; Brodal and Jansen, '46).

Efferent Fibers. The principal efferent tracts of the cerebellum arise from the deep cerebellar nuclei. Cerebellar efferent fibers from the deep cerebellar nuclei are organized into two major systems contained in three separate bundles. The major efferent systems are the superior cerebellar peduncle and the fastigial efferent projection.

The *superior cerebellar peduncle* (Figs. 12-18, 12-23 and 14-16), the largest cerebellar efferent bundle, is formed by fibers from the dentate, emboliform and globose nuclei. This composite group of fibers emerges from the hilus of the dentate nucleus and passes rostrally into the upper pons where it forms a compact bundle along the dorsolateral wall of the fourth ventricle (Figs. 2-18 and 2-19). At isthmus levels fibers of the superior cerebellar peduncle sweep ventromedially into the tegmentum (Fig. 12-23). All fibers of the superior cerebellar peduncle decussate at levels through the inferior colliculus (Fig. 13-2). Most of these crossed fibers ascend to enter and surround the contralateral red nucleus. A relatively small part of the fibers from the dentate nucleus terminate in the rostral third of the red nucleus (Angaut and Bowsher, '65; Courville, '66a); the bulk of these fibers project to the thalamus and end in the ventral lateral (VLo) nucleus (Fig. 14-16) (Jansen and Brodal, '58; Carpenter, '67). A small number of fibers from the dentate nucleus project beyond VLo to the rostral intralaminar thalamic nuclei (Ranson and Ingram, '32; Mehler et al., '58).

The ventral lateral nucleus of the thalamus projects in a topical fashion upon the primary motor area of the cerebral cortex (Walker, '38, '49, '66). Thus impulses from the dentate nucleus are conveyed via contralateral thalamic nuclei to the motor cortex. In this manner, impulses from the dentate nucleus can influence activity of motor neurons in the cerebral cortex; impulses from the motor cortex are transmitted to spinal levels via the corticospinal tract. This system appears to be concerned primarily with the coordination of somatic motor function.

A relatively small number of cerebellar efferent fibers from the dentate nucleus decussate in the caudal mesencephalon, pass dorsally and are distributed differentially within the lateral somatic cell columns of the contralateral oculomotor nuclear complex (Carpenter and Strominger, '64). Most of these fibers terminate about cells which innervate the superior rectus muscle on the opposite side (Fig. 13-11). These cerebello-oculomotor fibers appear to constitute a unique example of cerebellar efferent fibers projecting directly to a lower motor neuron.

Another small group of fibers in the superior cerebellar peduncle decussate with the main bundle and descend in the ventromedial tegmentum of the brain stem near the median raphe. These fibers, constituting the descending division of the superior cerebellar peduncle, project largely to the reticulotegmental and the paramedian reticular nuclei (Carpenter and Nova, '60; Brodal and Szikla, '72). Because these nuclei are known to project to the cerebellum, this component of the superior cerebellar peduncle is a part of a cerebelloreticular feedback system (Fig. 14-16).

Fibers from the emboliform and globose nuclei enter the superior cerebellar peduncle, undergo a complete decussation and surround caudal portions of the contralateral red nucleus, where many of these fibers terminate. According to Courville ('66a) fibers from the anterior interposed nucleus in the cat (which corresponds to the emboliform nucleus in man; Flood and Jansen, '61) project somatotopically upon cells of the red nucleus. Two patterns of fiber organization have been recognized between these nuclei: (1) fibers distributed in a mediolateral sequence in the red nucleus have a caudorostral pattern of origin in the nucleus interpositus, and (2) fibers terminating in a rostrocaudal arrangement in the red nucleus have a corresponding lateromedial origin in the nucleus interpositus. However, only fibers from the interposed nucleus terminating in a mediolateral arrangement in the red nucleus are regarded as having a somatotopic distribution (Pompeiano and Brodal, '57; Courville, '66a; Massion, '67). Thus rostral parts of the interposed nucleus project to hindlimb regions of the red nucleus (ventral and ventrolateral areas), while caudal parts of the nucleus project to forelimb regions of the red nucleus (dorsal and dorsomedial areas; Fig. 14-17). Because of the topographical projections of cerebellar cortex upon the deep cerebellar nuclei (Jansen and Brodal, '58; Eager, '63) which are organized as three longitudinal zones, connections exist between: (1) the paravermal cortex and the red nucleus through the anterior interposed nucleus, and (2) cerebellar cortex of the hemisphere and the red nucleus through the dentate nucleus (Massion, '67).

The pathway from the paravermal cortex to the contralateral red nucleus via the anterior interposed nucleus forms part of a somatotopic linkage that extends to spinal levels. Somatotopically organized rubrospinal fibers cross in the midbrain and descend to spinal levels. This small system involves two decussations, that of the superior cerebellar peduncle and that of the rubrospinal tract (Fig. 14-17). Thus impulses conveyed from paravermal cortex to the spinal cord end on the same side. This system appears to be primarily concerned with mechanisms that can influence (i.e., facilitate) ipsilateral flexor muscle tone.

Physiological studies (Appelberg, '60; Eccles et al., '67) indicate that a number of axons from the interposed nucleus also project to the ventral lateral nucleus of the thalamus after giving off collaterals to the red nucleus.

Fastigial efferent projections emerge from the cerebellum via the *uncinate fasciculus (Russell)* and the *juxtarestiform body* (Figs. 14-18, 14-19 and 14-20). Fibers

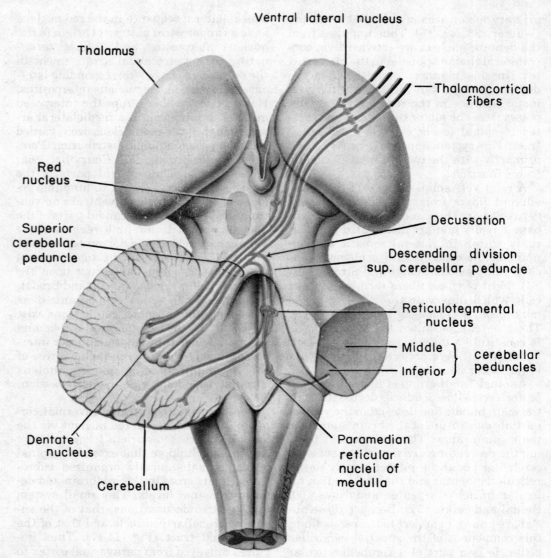

Fig. 14-16. Diagram of the efferent fibers of the dentate nucleus. These fibers, contained in the superior cerebellar peduncle, all decussate in the caudal mesencephalon. Ascending fibers project to the rostral part of the red nucleus and to the ventral lateral (*VLo*) nucleus of the thalamus. Fibers of the descending division of the superior cerebellar peduncle project to the reticulotegmental nucleus and the paramedian reticular nuclei of the medulla. Descending fibers of the superior cerebellar peduncle constitute part of a cerebelloreticular system that conveys impulses back to the cerebellum.

in the uncinate fasciculus, both crossed and uncrossed, arch around the superior cerebellar peduncle. Fibers of this bundle originating from the rostral part of the fastigial nucleus are uncrossed, while the more numerous fibers from the caudal part of the nucleus are mostly crossed (Carpen-

ter, '59; Walberg et al., '62). Fibers forming the descending component of the uncinate fasciculus sweep ventromedially to be distributed differentially in parts of all of the vestibular nuclei and in dorsomedial parts of the reticular formation of the pons and medulla (Figs. 14-19 and 14-20).

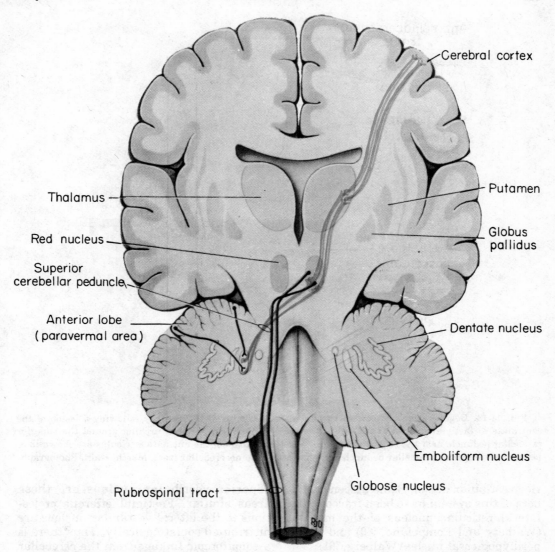

Fig. 14-17. Schematic diagram of connections between the emboliform nucleus (anterior interposed nucleus) and the red nucleus. Axons of Purkinje cells (*black*) in the paravermal cortex of the anterior lobe of the cerebellum project somatotopically upon the emboliform nucleus. The most rostral cortical regions, concerned with the lower extremity (Figs. 14-14 and 14-15), project to the rostral part of the emboliform nucleus, while caudal regions, concerned with the upper extremity, project to caudal parts of this nucleus. Fibers from the emboliform nucleus (*blue*) project via the superior cerebellar peduncle to caudal portions of the contralateral red nucleus, and to the ventral lateral nucleus of the thalamus. Projections from the emboliform nucleus to the red nucleus terminate somatotopically. Rubrospinal fibers (*red*) arising from dorsomedial regions of the red nucleus project to cervical spinal segments, while fibers from ventrolateral parts of this nucleus project to lumbosacral spinal segments. Thus the somatotopic linkage is maintained from cerebellar cortex to spinal levels (Courville, '66a; Massion, '67).

Within the vestibular nuclei crossed fibers of the uncinate fasciculus are distributed to the peripheral parts of the superior vestibular nucleus, the ventralmost part of the medial vestibular nucleus and the ventrolateral portions of the lateral and infe-

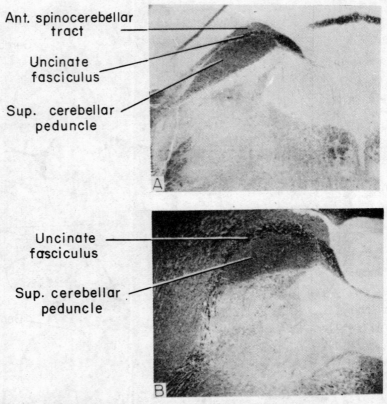

Ant. spinocerebellar tract

Uncinate fasciculus

Sup. cerebellar peduncle

Uncinate fasciculus

Sup. cerebellar peduncle

FIG. 14-18. Degeneration of fibers in the uncinate fasciculus of the monkey following a lesion of the contralateral fastigial nucleus. In *B*, all of the crossed fibers can be seen arching around the superior cerebellar peduncle near the site of emergence. Ascending fibers of the uncinate fasciculus are shown in *A* between the superior cerebellar peduncle and the anterior spinocerebellar tract. Marchi stain. Photograph.

rior vestibular nuclei. Some descending fibers of this system have been traced to the lateral reticular nucleus of the medulla (Walberg and Pompeiano, '60) and to the perihypoglossal nuclei (Walberg, '61).

Uncrossed fastigial efferent fibers contained in the uncinate fasciculus, and to a larger extent in the juxtarestiform body, arise from the rostral part of the fastigial nucleus and project largely to the vestibular nuclei, where they have a distribution distinctly different from that of the crossed fibers. In the inferior, medial and lateral vestibular nuclei these fibers terminate in more dorsal areas which do not receive crossed fastigial efferent fibers (Walberg et al., '62). There is relatively little overlap in the areas of terminal distribution of crossed and uncrossed fastigial efferent fibers in the vestibular nuclei. Only in the

superior vestibular nucleus are these areas similar. Fastigial efferent projections to the lateral vestibular nucleus are distributed somatotopically. Thus there is a somatotopic linkage from the cerebellar vermis to spinal levels, via vermal projections to the fastigial nuclei, fastigial efferents to the lateral vestibular nucleus and the vestibulospinal tract (Fig. 14-20). This system, in spite of certain crossings, exerts its principal influence (i.e., facilitation) upon ipsilateral extensor muscles.

Some fibers in the uncinate fasciculus bypass the vestibular nuclei and project to regions of the reticular formation known to serve inhibitory functions (Carpenter, '59; Walberg et al., '62). Fastigioreticular fibers do not appear to be somatotopically organized.

A small portion of the fibers in the uncinate fasciculus ascend in the dorsolateral part of the brain stem and project fibers to thalamic nuclei (Thomas et al., '56; Carpenter et al., '58). Ascending fibers in the uncinate fasciculus arise from cells in the caudal part of the fastigial nucleus, decussate within the cerebellum and ascend contralaterally (Angaut and Bowsher, '70). A number of these fibers are projected to the centromedian nucleus of the thalamus, but the largest bundle terminates in medial portions of the ventral lateral (VLo) nucleus (Kievit and Kuypers, '72). Thus at thalamic levels some fastigial efferent fibers terminate in the same nucleus (VLo) as fibers of the superior cerebellar peduncle (Fig. 14-19).

Although the flocculonodular lobe is classically regarded as the "vestibulocerebellum," primary vestibulocerebellar fibers have a more extensive distibution in that they also project to ventral parts of the uvula and to the ventral paraflocculus (Brodal and Høivik, '64). All of these parts of the "vestibulocerebellum," considered in its broadest sense, project fibers to the vestibular nuclear complex, except the paraflocculus (Angaut and Brodal, '67). The flocculus and nodulus project fibers to portions of the four main vestibular nuclei; the uvula gives rise to fibers passing to portions of the superior, lateral and inferior vestibular nuclei. These fibers have an ipsilateral distribution.

Direct *cerebellovestibular fibers* derived from the vermis of the anterior lobe appear to constitute the largest group of cortical efferents projecting to the vestibular nuclei (Walberg, '72). These fibers, representing Purkinje cell axons, end in parts of two nuclei, the lateral and inferior vestibular nuclei, and are considered to exert inhibitory influences.

CEREBELLAR ORGANIZATION

In spite of certain anatomical evidence indicating that cerebellar cortical projections to the deep cerebellar nuclei are not organized into strict longitudinal zones (Brodal and Courville, '73; Courville et al., '73), this concept provides an elementary view of the functional organization of the cerebellum. In this simplified scheme the cerebellar efferent systems are related to three longitudinal (sagittal) zones referred to as vermal, paravermal and lateral.

The *vermal zone* is the midline, unpaired portion of the cerebellum related to fastigial nuclei, and is concerned primarily with mechanisms that influence extensor muscle tone. To some extent this system is bilateral, and many efferent fibers cross within the cerebellum. This zone displays a somatotopic linkage from vermal cortex to fastigial nuclei and ultimately to the lateral vestibular nucleus. Excitatory impulses acting upon vestibular neurons are projected ipsilaterally to spinal levels (Fig. 14-20). A parallel direct projection from the anterior lobe to the lateral vestibular nucleus conveys inhibitory influences.

The *paravermal zone* relates the paravermal cortex with the emboliform nucleus, which has connections predominantly with the opposite red nucleus. This somatotopically organized system is concerned with mechanisms that can facilitate ipsilateral flexor muscle tone via the rubrospinal tract (Fig. 14-17).

The *lateral zone* relates the cortex of the cerebellar hemisphere with the dentate nucleus which has projections primarily to the ventral lateral nucleus of the thalamus on the opposite side (Fig. 14-16). This, the largest cerebellar efferent system, appears to be concerned with the coordination of ipsilateral somatic motor activity. Impulses conveyed to the ventral lateral nucleus of the thalamus are relayed to the motor cortex where they modify the activity of neurons projecting to spinal levels and to pontine nuclei.

Some relay nuclei at all brain stem levels, receiving part of the cerebellar output, project fibers back to the cerebellum. These pathways are referred to as feedback systems, and appear similar to those found in electronic systems which provide controlling and regulating effects. The motor cortex in turn gives rise to frontopontine fibers, which convey impulses back to the contralateral cerebellar hemisphere via the pontine nuclei and the middle cerebellar peduncle (Fig. 14-21). Other areas of the cerebral cortex also influence the activ-

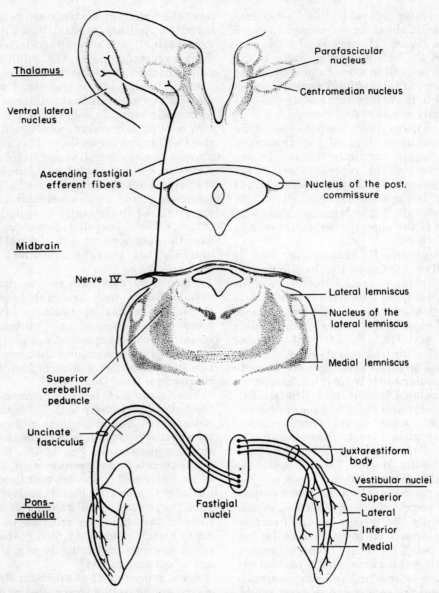

FIG. 14-19. Diagram of the fastigial efferent projections. Fastigiovestibular fibers are distributed differentially within the vestibular nuclei (Walberg et al., '62). Ascending fastigial efferents, predominately crossed, ascend to portions of the centromedian (*CM*) and ventral lateral (*VLo*) thalamic nuclei (Kievit and Kuypers, '72).

ity of the cerebellum via corticopontine and pontocerebellar pathways. The central tegmental tract conveys impulses from the red nucleus and the midbrain tegmentum which reach the contralateral cerebellar hemisphere by way of parts of the inferior

olivary nuclear complex. Certain fibers of the superior cerebellar peduncle that descend in the brain stem terminate upon reticular nuclei, which project fibers back to the cerebellum (Fig. 14-16). Efferent fibers from the red nucleus also project di-

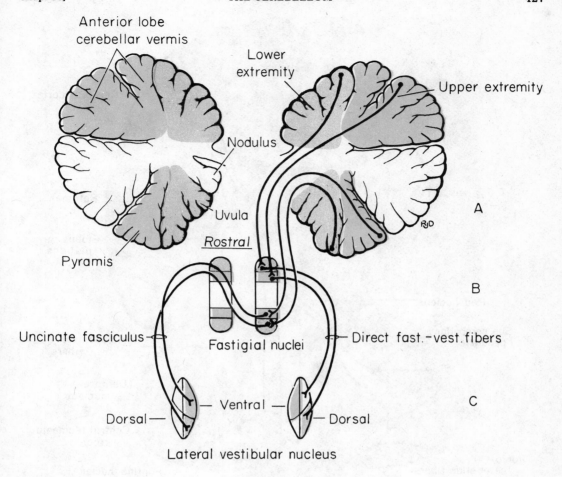

FIG. 14-20. Diagram of the somatotopic arrangements of the projections of the anterior and posterior cerebellar vermis upon the fastigial nuclei and the projections of the fastigial nuclei upon the lateral vestibular nuclei. The cerebellar vermis in *A* is shown in midsagittal section, with areas concerned with the lower extremity in *red* and those concerned with the upper extremity in *blue* (see Figs. 14-14 and 14-15). The fastigial nuclei in *B* are shown in horizontal section, while the lateral vestibular nuclei in *C* are shown in sagittal planes. The direct fastigiovestibular fibers which arise mainly from the rostral part of the fastigial nucleus are shown on the right: these fibers project mainly to dorsal parts of the lateral vestibular nucleus. Fibers of the uncinate fasciculus, arising mainly from caudal parts of the fastigial nucleus, are crossed and project to ventral parts of the lateral vestibular nucleus. These somatotopic relationships were determined in the cat by anatomical and physiological studies (Walberg et al., '62). *Blue* areas of the cerebellar vermis, fastigial nuclei and lateral vestibular nuclei are concerned with the upper extremity; *red* areas refer to the lower extremity.

rectly to the interposed nucleus (Courville and Brodal, '66). Parts of the inferior and medial vestibular nuclei which receive impulses from the fastigial nuclei give rise to secondary vestibular fibers that project back to the cerebellum (Fig. 12-14). Simi-

lar relationships exist between parts of the cerebellum and the brain stem reticular formation.

Some of the neocerebellar connections in man are especially evident in Figure 14-22, which shows sections through the me-

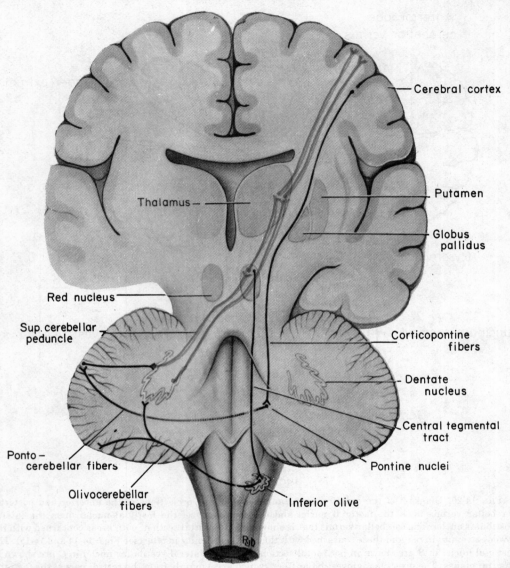

Fig. 14-21. Diagram of some of the principal afferent and efferent cerebellar connections. Cerebellar efferent fibers from the dentate nucleus are shown in *blue*. Corticopontine and pontocerebellar fibers (*black*) represent the most massive cerebellar afferent system. The principal inferior olivary nucleus receives uncrossed descending fibers from the red nucleus and periaqueductal gray via the central tegmental tract. Cortico-olivary fibers to the principal inferior olivary nucleus (not shown) pass via the medullary pyramids. Olivocerebellar fibers (*black*) cross, enter the inferior cerebellar peduncle and are distributed to: (1) the cerebellar cortex as climbing fibers, and (2) the deep cerebellar nuclei.

dulla, pons and isthmus from an individual in whom the left cerebellar hemisphere failed to develop (hemicerebellar agenesis). There was also a correlated agenesia of all the afferent and efferent pathways to and from the left cerebellar hemisphere. The left dentate nucleus was represented by a minute structure, the right inferior olive was greatly reduced and the right red nucleus (not shown) and pontine nuclei were practically absent. All of the cerebellar peduncles on the left were

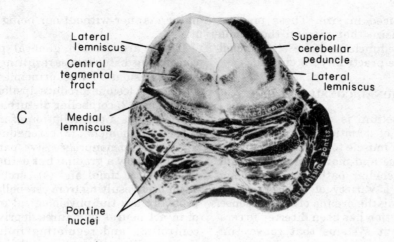

Lateral
lemniscus

Central
tegmental
tract

Medial
lemniscus

C

Superior
cerebellar
peduncle

Lateral
lemniscus

Pontine
nuclei

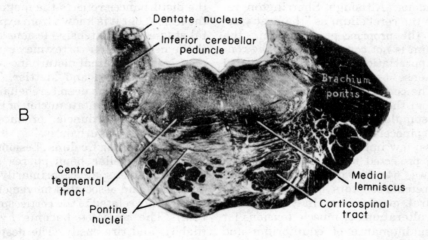

Dentate nucleus

Inferior cerebellar
peduncle

Brachium
pontis

B

Central
tegmental
tract

Pontine
nuclei

Medial
lemniscus

Corticospinal
tract

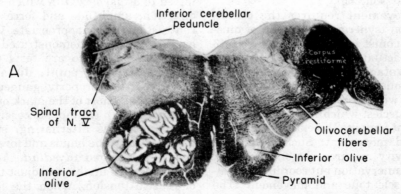

Inferior cerebellar
peduncle

Corpus
restiforme

A

Spinal tract
of N. V

Inferior
olive

Olivocerebellar
fibers

Inferior olive

Pyramid

FIG. 14-22. Transverse sections of the medulla (*A*), pons (*B*) and isthmus (*C*) from a case of left cerebellar agenesis (Strong, '15). These sections clearly demonstrate the crossed nature of olivocerebellar and pontocerebellar fibers. Weigert's myelin stain. Photograph.

greatly reduced in size. These preparations emphasize that in man the middle cerebellar peduncle and the olivocerebellar fibers are practically all crossed.

FUNCTIONAL CONSIDERATIONS

The cerebellum is concerned with the coordination of somatic motor activity, the regulation of muscle tone and mechanisms that influence and maintain equilibrium. Afferent cerebellar pathways convey impulses from a variety of different receptors, including the organs of special sense. Special attention has been directed to cerebellar afferent systems that convey impulses from stretch receptors in muscles and tendons. Although Sherrington referred to the cerebellum as "the head ganglion of the proprioceptive system," the cerebellum is not concerned with the conscious appreciation of muscle, joint and tendon sense, or any specific sensory modality. The cerebellum receives a massive input from the stretch receptors (i.e., the muscle spindle and Golgi tendon organ) via the spinocerebellar and cuneocerebellar tracts; few impulses from these receptors are projected to the cerebral cortex (Matthews, '64). The major afferent input from stretch receptors provides part of the neural mechanism that: (1) effects gradual alterations of muscle tensions for proper maintenance of equilibrium and posture, and (2) assures the smooth and orderly sequence of muscular contractions that characterize skilled voluntary movement (Oscarsson, '65).

Each movement requires the coordinated action (synergy) of a group of muscles. The agonist is the muscle which provides the actual movement of the part, while the antagonist is the opposing muscle which must relax to permit movement. Associated with these are other synergic or fixating muscles, which fix neighboring or even distant joints to the extent needed for the desired movement. Such synergistic motor activity requires not only complex reciprocal innervation but coordinated control of muscle tone and movement. The cerebellum provides this control for the somatic motor system in an efficient, automatic manner without our being aware of it.

There are certain general principles concerning disturbances resulting from cerebellar lesions. These principles are: (1) cerebellar lesions produce ipsilateral disturbances, (2) cerebellar disturbances usually occur as a constellation of intimately related phenomena, (3) cerebellar disturbances due to nonprogressive pathological changes show a gradual but definite attenuation with time, and (4) cerebellar disturbances resulting from cerebellar lesions probably are the physiological expression of intact neural structures deprived of the controlling and regulating influences of the cerebellum. To a degree the severity of the disturbances reflects the magnitude of the lesion, but it is known from experimental studies that extensive lesions confined to the neocerebellar cortex may cause only transient or minimal disturbances (Keller et al., '37; Carrea and Mettler, '47). Lesions involving the deep cerebellar nuclei, particularly the dentate nuclei, or the superior cerebellar peduncle, produce severe and enduring disturbances.

Neocerebellar Lesions. Lesions involving the cerebellar hemispheres and the dentate nucleus affect primarily skilled voluntary and associated movements (i.e., movements related to the corticospinal system). The muscles become *hypotonic* (flabby) and tire easily. The deep tendon reflexes tend to be sluggish and often have a pendular quality. There are severe disturbances of coordinated movement referred to as *asynergia* in which the range, direction, amplitude and force of muscle contractions are inappropriate. Cerebellar asynergia can be demonstrated by many tests. Among these are tests of precise movements to a point; distances frequently are improperly gauged (*dysmetria*) and fall short of the mark or exceed it (*pastpointing*). Rapid successive movements, such as alternating, supinating and pronating the hands and forearms, are poorly performed (*dysdiadochokinesis*). The patient is unable to adjust to changes of muscle tension. When the forearm is flexed at the elbow and held flexed against resistance, a sudden release of resistance causes the forearm to strike the chest. This is an example of the *rebound phenomenon*. These patients also demonstrate a *decomposition of movement* in which phases of complex movements are performed as a series of successive single simple movements.

The *tremor* seen in association with neocerebellar lesions occurs primarily during voluntary and associated movements (Holmes, '39). This tremor is referred to as "intention tremor" because it is not present at rest. It involves especially the proximal appendicular musculature, but is transmitted mechanically to distal parts of the extremities. Tremor is most evident in the upper extremities because weight-bearing masks the disturbance in the lower extremities. Cerebellar tremor frequently is contrasted with the tremor seen in paralysis agitans, which is referred to as a "rest tremor," meaning that the tremor is present in the absence of voluntary and associated movement. Each of these types of tremor has unmistakable features and occurs in different syndromes. Nevertheless, "rest tremor" may occur in association with certain cerebellar lesions (Holmes, '22). There are certain indications that the basic mechanisms involved in cerebellar tremor may underlie other kinds of tremor (Carpenter, '61).

Ataxia is an asynergic disturbance associated with neocerebellar lesions which results in a bizarre distortion of voluntary and associated movements. It involves particularly the axial muscles, and groups of muscles around the shoulder and pelvic girdles. This disturbance is evident during walking and is characterized by muscle contractions which are highly irregular in force, amplitude and direction, and which occur asynchronously in different parts of the body. There frequently is unsteadiness in standing, especially if the feet are close together. The gait is broad-based and the patient reels, lurches and stumbles.

Nystagmus commonly is seen in association with cerebellar disease; it is most pronounced when the patient directs the eyes laterally toward the side of the lesion. This disturbance consists of an oscillatory pattern in which the eyes slowly drift in one direction and then rapidly move in the opposite direction to correct the drift. Although nystagmus seen in association with cerebellar disease has been considered as an expression of asynergic phenomena in the extraocular muscles, many pathological processes which affect the cerebellum also involve the underlying brain stem and the vestibular nuclei located in the floor of the fourth ventricle.

Speech disturbances are common in association with cerebellar lesions of long standing. Speech often is slow and monotonous, and some syllables are unnaturally separated. There is a slurring of speech and some words are uttered in an explosive manner.

Archicerebellar Lesions. Lesions involving portions of the posterior cerebellar vermis (i.e., nodulus and uvula) and probably portions of the flocculus produce what has been called the *archicerebellar syndrome*. Such lesions affect the axial musculature and the bilateral movements used for locomotion and maintenance of equilibrium. The patient sways and is generally unsteady when standing; when walking he staggers and has a tendency to fall backwards or to either side. The gait resembles that of a drunken individual in that it is broad-based, jerky and highly incoordinate. If the muscles involved in speech are affected, articulation is jerky and words are slurred; the words are often shot out with unnecessary force. Nystagmus and abnormal attitudes, if present, are usually ascribed to injury of the vestibular structures. Muscle tone is little affected, there is usually no tremor and there is no incoordination of arm or leg movements when the patient is resting in bed. This particular syndrome most commonly occurs in children as a consequence of a midline cerebellar tumor (medulloblastoma) that probably arises from cell-rests in the inferior medullary velum at the base of the nodulus.

Experimental studies (Tyler and Bard, '49) indicate that ablations of the nodulus in dogs, demonstrated to be susceptible to motion sickness, render these animals immune to the emetic effects of motion. These findings suggest that the emetic responses of motion sickness involve neural mechanisms independent of the forebrain.

Anterior Lobe of the Cerebellum. Lesions of the anterior lobe of the cerebellum (paleocerebellum) in the dog and cat produce severe disturbances of posture and increased extensor muscle tone. These animals exhibit an extreme opisthotonus, tight closure of the jaw, hyperactive deep tendon reflexes, increased positive supporting mechanisms and periodic tonic seizures. Animals surviving these lesions regain the ability to walk without swaying of the head or trunk, and can perform voluntary movements without evident tremor (Fulton, '49). Conclusive information concerning ablations of the anterior lobe of the cerebellum in primates does not appear to be available. A clinical syndrome in man corresponding to that described in experimental animals has not been defined. The closest related phenomenon would appear to be the so-called "tonic seizure," which usually is related to compression of the brain stem. Other experimental studies (Bremer, '22) have shown that ablations of the anterior lobe of the cerebellum produce an exaggeration of decerebrate rigidity in the cat.

In what is now a classical experiment, Sherrington (1898) demonstrated that electrical stimulation of the anterior lobe of the cerebellum could inhibit the extensor muscle tone in a decerebrate animal. This experiment, confirming the early work of Loewenthal and Horsley (1897), indicated an important inhibitory action of the paleocerebellum upon muscle tone. Studies summarized by Moruzzi (Dow and Moruzzi, '58) indicate that facilitating effects also can be obtained by stimulation of the anterior lobe of the cerebellum, and that the rate of stimulation is critical in determining whether inhibition or facilitation occurs. With square wave stimulation, it was found that low repetitive rates (2 to 10 cycles/sec) caused a slow increase in ipsilateral extensor muscle tone, while rapid stimulation (30 to 300 cycles/sec) produced a relaxation of the muscles in the ipsilateral limbs. These apparently opposite effects originally were interpreted as indicating that inhibitory and facilitatory neu-

rons were intermingled in the cortex of the anterior lobe of the cerebellum. Further studies of these interesting phenomena (summarized by Brodal et al., '62) indicate that these inhibitory and facilitatory influences must involve different parts of the fastigial nuclei and their fiber projections, as well as cerebellovestibular fiber projections (Fig. 14-20). Following lesions near the rostrolateral part of the fastigial nucleus, stimulation of the ipsilateral vermis of the anterior lobe with high frequency square waves (300 cycles/sec) produced a clear-cut increase in extensor rigidity on the side stimulated. This finding suggested that most of the inhibitory pathways had been interrupted by the fastigial lesion, while the facilitatory pathways remained intact. Following lesions near the rostromedial part of the fastigial nucleus, stimulation of the vermis of the anterior lobe with low frequency square waves (2 to 10 cycles/sec) caused inhibitory effects upon ipsilateral decerebrate rigidity, indicating that facilitatory fiber systems were interrupted by the fastigial lesion. After a unilateral total lesion of the fastigial nucleus, stimulation of the surface of the ipsilateral vermis of the anterior lobe yielded no responses (Sprague and Chambers, '53, '54), and the same effect was seen when the lesion was limited to the rostral part of the ipsilateral fastigial nucleus (Moruzzi and Pompeiano, '56). Although a complete anatomical basis for these physiological observations cannot be provided, it seems likely that: (1) inhibitory influences obtained from stimulating the vermis of the anterior lobe of the cerebellum are mediated via the fastigial nucleus and act in part upon the ipsilateral reticular formation, and (2) facilitatory influences obtained from stimulation of the vermis of the anterior lobe are mediated by parts of the fastigial nucleus that act upon the lateral vestibular nucleus (Brodal et al., '62). Cerebellovestibular fibers which pass through regions near the rostrolateral part of the fastigial nucleus (Walberg and Jansen, '61) have been demonstrated to exert an inhibitory influence upon cells of the lateral vestibular nucleus (Ito and Yoshida, '66; Ito et al., '66; Eccles et al., '67).

This is an example of direct cerebellar cortical inhibition upon cells of the lateral vestibular nucleus. There is no direct fiber projection from the cerebellar cortex to the reticular formation.

The effects of discrete lesions in the fastigial nucleus upon decerebrate rigidity in the cat have demonstrated that fastigial efferent fibers exert potent influences upon muscle tone. Sprague and Chambers ('53) observed that isolated unilateral destruction of the fastigial nucleus caused an inhibition of ipsilateral extensor muscle tone in the decerebrate cat. This finding was confirmed by Moruzzi and Pompeiano ('56) who further demonstrated that: (1) unilateral destruction of the rostral pole of the fastigial nucleus caused an ipsilateral inhibition of extensor muscle tone, (2) unilateral destruction of the caudal pole of the fastigial nucleus caused an inhibition of contralateral extensor muscle tone, and (3) bilateral total, or symmetrical, destruction of the fastigial nuclei caused extensor rigidity to be reestablished symmetrically (if lesions were produced serially), or to be essentially unchanged (if simultaneously produced). These findings initially were explained on the basis of interruption of fastigial efferent fibers presumed to have a facilitatory influence upon portions of the reticular formation. Because the fastigial efferent fiber projections to the vestibular nuclei are more abundant than that to the reticular formation and have a definite somatotopic pattern of termination in the lateral vestibular nucleus (Walberg et al., '62), it seems likely that asymmetrical interruptions of fastigiovestibular fiber systems account for the observed modifications of muscle tone (Fig. 14-20). Bilateral symmetrical, or total, lesions of the fastigial nuclei interrupt fastigiovestibular fiber systems equally on both sides, and under these circumstances muscle tone is not modified. These observations indicate that fastigiovestibular fiber systems are not essential for the maintenance of extensor muscle tone in decerebrate rigidity, but that asymmetrical withdrawal of the facilitating influences mediated by this system causes detectable differences in muscle tone.

Other cerebellar mechanisms which can influence muscle tone involve the paravermal cortex, the nucleus interpositus and the contralateral red nucleus (Massion, '67); all of these structures are connected by somatotopically organized fibers. Stimulation of the rostral part of the interposed nucleus (anterior part) produces flexion in the ipsilateral hindlimb of the cat, while stimulation of the caudal part of this nucleus produces flexion in the ipsilateral forelimb (Pompeiano, '59; Maffei and Pompeiano, '62). These responses occur ipsilaterally because fibers of both the superior cerebellar peduncle and the rubrospinal tract are crossed (Fig. 14-17). Intracellular recordings in the red nucleus demonstrate that stimulation of the nucleus interpositus produces excitatory postsynaptic potentials with a monosynaptic latency (Tsukahara et al., '64; Massion, '67). The pathway between the interposed nucleus and the red nucleus is regarded as purely excitatory and impulses conveyed by this system have an important facilitatory influence upon flexor muscle tone; these impulses are conveyed to spinal levels by the rubrospinal tract. Although the Purkinje cell output from the cerebellar cortex is inhibitory, variations in the activity of these cells are responsible for the inhibition, or activation, of cells in the interposed nucleus which directly affects cells of the contralateral red nucleus.

Modification of Cerebellar Disturbances. Experimental studies in the monkey demonstrate that cerebellar dyskinesia, produced by lesions in the deep cerebellar nuclei, can be abolished by surgical section of the dorsal half of the lateral funiculus of the spinal cord at high cervical levels (Carpenter and Correll, '61). Selective section of the anterior half of the lateral funiculus and the anterior funiculus of the spinal cord in these animals has no appreciable effect on the dyskinesia. Bilateral selective destruction of the posterior funiculi tends to exaggerate ataxia and asynergic disturbances, including tremor. These data suggest that impulses essential to the neural mechanism of experimental cerebellar dyskinesia in the monkey probably are transmitted to segmental levels via the lateral corticospinal tract. Since no fibers of the corticospinal tract are infrapallial in origin, and most are crossed, this implies that the neocerebellum must exert its regulating and controlling influences upon the contralateral motor cortex through the mediation of certain thalamic relay nuclei. This hypothesis is in accord with the well established finding that neocerebellar disturbances occur ipsilateral to cerebellar lesions.

Clinical experiences indicate that lesions in the contralateral thalamic nuclei can significantly modify and ameliorate cerebellar dyskinesia in man (Cooper and Poloukhine, '59; Cooper, '60; Martin, '60). Experimental studies (Carpenter and Hanna, '62) in the monkey have demonstrated that lesions destroying significant parts of the ventral lateral nucleus of the thalamus can reduce the tremor associated with cerebellar lesions without destroying fibers of the corticospinal tract and without producing paresis. Thus this thalamic nucleus must be concerned with the mediation of certain cerebellar disturbances (Fig. 14-21). Physiological evidence also suggests that the cerebellothalamic cortical relay system may play an important role in the unconscious regulation of muscle tone. It seems likely that some impulses from stretch receptors may be conveyed to higher integrative levels of the neuraxis by these fibers. Furthermore, it seems likely that surgical interruption of the relay fibers of this system at thalamic levels may be responsible for the reduction in muscle tone seen in patients with paralysis agitans.

Computer Functions. Recent advances concerning the structural and functional components of the cerebellar cortex (Eccles et al., '67; Palay and Chan-Palay, '74) suggest that in some way the cerebellum functions as a type of computer particularly concerned with smooth and effective control of movement. Present evidence sug-

gests that the cerebellum integrates and organizes information flowing into it via numerous neural pathways, and that cerebellar output participates in the control of motor function by the transmission of impulses to: (1) brain stem nuclei (i.e., lateral vestibular and red nuclei) that project to spinal levels, and (2) thalamic nuclei which can modify the activity of cortical regions concerned with motor function.

Every part of the cerebellar cortex receives directly, or indirectly, two different inputs, that of the mossy fibers and that of the climbing fibers. Although these inputs differ in their structural and functional characteristics, they appear to convey very similar "sensory" information to particular areas of the cerebellar cortex. The only output of the cerebellar cortex, conveyed by Purkinje cell axons, is inhibitory. This inhibition is exerted upon the deep cerebellar nuclei and the lateral vestibular nucleus. The output of the deep cerebellar nuclei is excitatory, a fact which implies that excitatory, as well as inhibitory, impulses must reach these nuclei. Excitatory impulses passing to the deep cerebellar nuclei are difficult to define, but are thought to be conveyed to these nuclei via collaterals of both climbing and mossy fibers. The fact that the cerebellar cortex transforms all input into inhibition precludes the possibility of dynamic storage of information by impulses circulating in complex neuronal pathways, as in the cerebral cortex. The absence of reverberatory chains of neurons in the cerebellar cortex appears to enhance its performance as a special kind of computer, in that it can provide a quick and clear response to the input of any particular set of information. Thus the cerebellum processes its input information rapidly, conveys its output indirectly to other parts of the nervous system, and has virtually no short-term dynamic memory.

CHAPTER 15

The Diencephalon

The rostral end of the brain stem is the diencephalon, a nuclear complex composed of several major subdivisions. Although the diencephalon is relatively small, constituting less than 2% of the neuraxis (Jenkins and Truex, '63), it has long been regarded as the key to the understanding of the organization of the central nervous system. The diencephalon extends from the region of the posterior commissure rostrally to the region of the interventricular foramen. Laterally it is bounded by the posterior limb of the internal capsule, the tail of the caudate nucleus and the stria terminalis (Figs. 15-4, 15-6 and 15-7). The third ventricle separates the diencephalon into two symmetrical halves, except in the region of the interthalamic adhesion where the medial surfaces of the thalami may be in continuity. The diencephalon is divisible into four major parts: the epithalamus, the thalamus, the hypothalamus and the subthalamus or ventral thalamus. The medial and lateral geniculate bodies constitute distinctive subdivisions of the thalamus, referred to as the *metathalamus*. Adjacent to the diencephalon, but separated from it by the fibers of the internal capsule, are the basal ganglia.

The region can be approached best through a graded series of photomicrographs of transverse sections. The level and plane of each section are indicated in Figures 15-1 and 15-2.

MIDBRAIN-DIENCEPHALIC JUNCTION

Rostral transverse sections of the midbrain reveal the addition of several discrete nuclear masses of the caudal thalamus closely surrounding the posterior and lateral surfaces of the mesencephalon. These structures include the *medial* and *lateral geniculate bodies* and the *pulvinar*. External to all of these is the *retrolenticular* portion of the internal capsule (Figs. 15-3, 15-4 and A-12). The pineal body lies dorsally between the superior colliculi, while portions of the mammillary bodies can be seen in the interpeduncular fossa (Fig. 15-3). Fibers from thalamic nuclei pass laterally into the internal capsule, through which they are distributed to various parts of the cerebral cortex. The internal capsule also contains corticofugal fibers projecting to thalamic nuclei. Thus *thalamocortical* and *corticothalamic* fibers constitute a large part of the internal capsule referred to as the *thalamic radiations*.

The pulvinar is a large nuclear mass dorsal to the medial geniculate body. Its dorsal surface is covered by a thin plate of fibers, the *stratum zonale* (Fig. 15-6). Fibers passing laterally from this nucleus contribute to the retrolenticular portion of the internal capsule (Fig. 15-17) and are distributed to the posterior parietal and occipitotemporal cortex. The innermost portion of the internal capsule, wedged

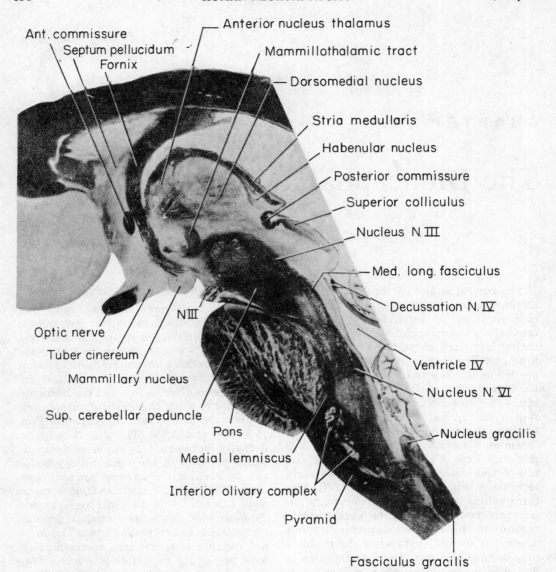

Ant. commissure
Septum pellucidum
Fornix
Anterior nucleus thalamus
Mammillothalamic tract
Dorsomedial nucleus
Stria medullaris
Habenular nucleus
Posterior commissure
Superior colliculus
Nucleus N. III
Med. long. fasciculus
Decussation N. IV
Ventricle IV
Nucleus N. VI
Optic nerve
Tuber cinereum
Mammillary nucleus
N III
Sup. cerebellar peduncle
Pons
Medial lemniscus
Inferior olivary complex
Pyramid
Nucleus gracilis
Fasciculus gracilis

FIG. 15-1. Sagittal section of brain stem through pillar of fornix and root of third nerve. Weigert's myelin stain. Photograph.

between the pulvinar and lateral geniculate body, forms a triangular area known as the *zone of Wernicke*. This zone, composed of a mixture of transverse and longitudinal fibers (Fig. 15-3), contains the optic radiations. Intermingled with these are fibers from the pulvinar and the medial geniculate body.

Sections through more rostral levels (Figs. 15-4 and A-12) reveal a great expansion of the diencephalic nuclei, as well as significant, although less marked, changes in the midbrain. The pulvinar is much larger, the medial geniculate body is smaller, and some fibers of the optic tract can be seen entering the lateral geniculate body. Lateral to the pulvinar is the body of the caudate nucleus, separated from the pulvinar by fibers of the *stria terminalis* (Figs. 15-3 and 15-4). The cerebral aqueduct expands into the deeper third ventricle; the posterior commissure marks the

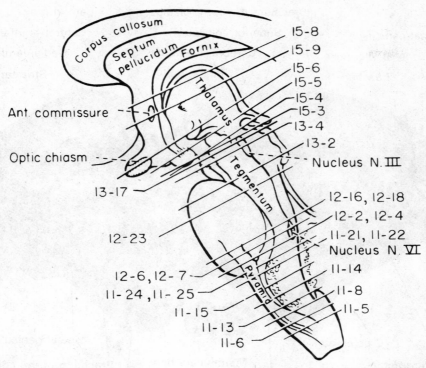

Fig. 15-2. Outline of paramedian sagittal section of the brain stem indicating level and plane of transverse sections. Figure numbers are opposite levels of section. Structures in this parasagittal outline are identified in Figure 15-1.

boundary between midbrain and diencephalon. Superior to the posterior commissure is the stalk of the pineal body, enclosing the pineal recess of the third ventricle. The superior colliculi are replaced by the pretectal areas, considered to be centers for the pupillary light reflex (Fig. 15-4). The connections of the pretectal area and posterior commissure have been discussed in Chapter 13.

The oculomotor nuclei and their root fibers have largely disappeared, although portions of the most rostral visceral nuclei of the oculomotor complex are present in the midline area below the ventricle. Lateral to the rostral part of the oculomotor complex is a collection of relatively large cells, the *interstitial nucleus of Cajal* (Figs. 13-12*B*, 13-14 and 15-4). The area lateral to the posterior commissure and ventral to the pretectum contains the *nuclei of the posterior commissure* (Fig. 13-12*B*).

The medial portion of the red nucleus is traversed by a vertical fiber bundle, the *fasciculus retroflexus or habenulopeduncular tract*. These fibers arise from the *habenular nucleus*, situated at a somewhat more rostral level (Figs. 15-5 and A-13). The capsular fibers of the red nucleus change from a longitudinal to a transverse direction and form a radiating bundle that extends from the dorsolateral surface of the red nucleus toward the ventral portion of the thalamus. This is the beginning of the *tegmental field H of Forel* or *prerubral field* (Fig. 15-5). Cells scattered among the fibers of Forel's field H and along its dorsal border constitute the *nucleus of the tegmental field of Forel* (nucleus of the prerubral field; Figs. 15-10 and 15-11).

CAUDAL DIENCEPHALON

Transverse sections through the habenular nuclei and the mammillary bodies (Fig. 15-5) reveal the structural organiza-

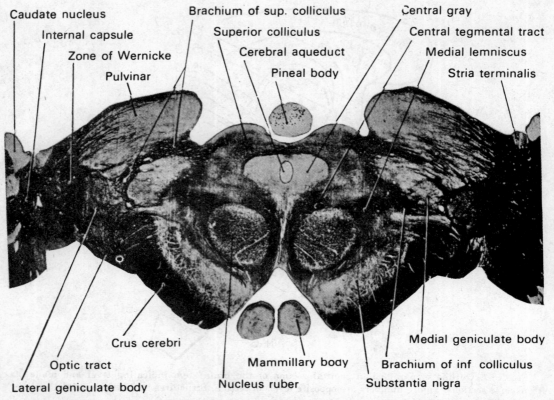

Fig. 15-3. Transverse section through rostral midbrain demonstrating relationship of midbrain and caudal portions of the thalamus. Weigert's myelin stain. Photograph.

tion of the caudal diencephalon. The *habenular nuclei* are two small gray masses forming triangular eminences on the dorsomedial surfaces of the thalami. These nuclei receive fibers mainly from the septal nuclei and the preoptic area via the striae medullares (Figs. 2-18, 2-22, 15-1 and 16-5). Some fibers crossing to the opposite side in the *habenular commissure* are not illustrated in Figure 15-5, but can be seen in Figures 2-18 and 2-22. Axons from the habenular nuclei form a well-defined bundle, the *fasciculus retroflexus,* which passes ventrally and caudally to terminate in the interpeduncular nuclei.

The third ventricle appears enlarged, and parts of it are seen in two locations (Figs. 15-5 and A-13). The main part of the third ventricle is present dorsally, where it is covered by a thin roof extending between the habenular nuclei and the striae medullares. The margins of this attachment (not shown in Fig. 15-5) on each side

constitute the *tenia thalami*. A small part of the third ventricle, referred to as the *infundibular recess,* is present ventral to the mammillary bodies and dorsal to the infundibulum. The mammillary bodies, tuber cinereum and infundibulum are parts of the hypothalamus.

A progressive increase in the size of the thalamus is evident (Figs. 15-5 and A-13). The pulvinar has reached its greatest extent, and part of the lateral thalamic nuclear group, with which the pulvinar is continuous rostrally, also may be present. Ventral to the pulvinar are the ventral tier thalamic nuclei and the *centromedian nucleus;* the latter nucleus is delimited by a thin fibrous capsule. The medial geniculate body has disappeared and the lateral geniculate is greatly reduced.

THE EPITHALAMUS

The epithalamus comprises the pineal body, the habenular trigones, the striae

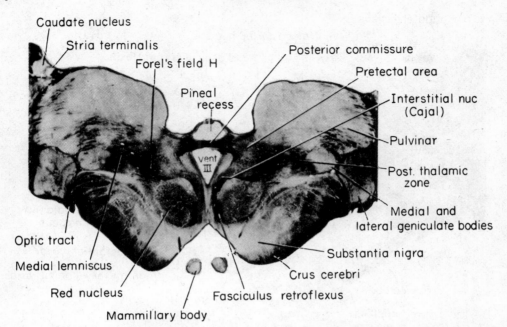

Caudate nucleus
Stria terminalis
Forel's field H
Pineal recess
Posterior commissure
Pretectal area
Interstitial nuc (Cajal)
Pulvinar
vent III
Post. thalamic zone
Medial and lateral geniculate bodies
Optic tract
Medial lemniscus
Red nucleus
Mammillary body
Fasciculus retroflexus
Crus cerebri
Substantia nigra

FIG. 15-4. Transverse section of the brain stem at the junction of mesencephalon and diencephalon. The posterior thalamic zone, which receives impulses from many sources concerned with painful and noxious stimuli, lies medial to the medial geniculate body. This cell group lies caudal to the ventral posterior thalamic nucleus (Fig. 15-5). Weigert's myelin stain. Photograph.

medullares and the epithelial roof of the third ventricle (Fig. 2-22). The habenular ganglion in man consists of a smaller medial and a larger lateral nucleus (Figs. 15-5 and 16-5). The medial nucleus consists of small, closely packed, deeply staining round cells; in the lateral nucleus, the cells are larger, paler and more loosely arranged. The ganglion receives the terminals of the stria medullaris (Figs. 15-1 and 15-7) and gives origin to the habenulopeduncular tract or fasciculus retroflexus, which terminates in the interpeduncular nucleus and certain midline reticular nuclei (Figs. 13-3, 15-5 and 16-5). The *stria medullaris* is a complex bundle composed of fibers arising from: (1) the septal nuclei, (2) lateral preoptic region (Nauta, '58), (3) the anterior thalamic nuclei, and (4) the globus pallidus (Nauta and Mehler, '66). The septal nuclei which receive fibers from both the hippocampal formation and the amygdaloid nuclear complex project profusely to the medial habenular nucleus. Fibers from the lateral preoptic nucleus and the globus pallidus pass to the lateral habenular nucleus (Fig. 16-5). Some of the

strial fibers cross to the opposite side in the habenular commissure. Thus the stria medullaris, habenula and fasciculus retroflexus form segments of visceral efferent pathways which convey impulses to rostral portions of the midbrain.

The pineal body, or *epiphysis,* is a small, cone-shaped body attached to the roof of the third ventricle in the region of the posterior commissure (Fig. 15-7). It appears to be a rudimentary gland whose function in the adult is not fully known. It consists of a network of richly vascular connective tissue trabeculae in the meshes of which are found glial cells and cells of a peculiar type, the *pineal* or *epiphysial cells*. These are cells of variable size with a pale nucleus, granular argentophilic cytoplasm and relatively few branching processes. They may represent modified nerve cells, since they have staining properties different than glial cells. True nerve cells do not appear to be present, although occasional cells with typical Nissl bodies have been observed by some investigators. The gland is said to receive fibers from the stria medullaris (Fig. 15-6), habenular gan-

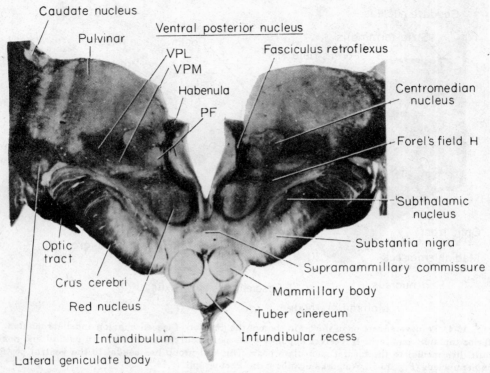

Fig. 15-5. Transverse section of the diencephalon through levels of the habenular ganglia, mammillary bodies and infundibulum. *VPL* and *VPM* indicate the ventral posterolateral and ventral posteromedial nuclei of the thalamus. *PF* indicates the parafascicular nucleus which surrounds the fasciculus retroflexus. Weigert's myelin stain. Photograph.

glion and posterior commissure; the fibers terminate in a plexus between the epiphysial cells.

Although the functions of the pineal body are not completely known, present information (Thiéblot, '65) indicates that it is an endocrine gland. Experimental and clinical evidence suggests that the pineal body directly or indirectly inhibits gonadal function. If this effect is indirect, it is probably mediated by way of the anterior hypophysis. The resultant effect seems to be inhibition of pituitary gonadotrophin. Pinealectomy in experimental animals or pineal tumors in young males cause precocious development of the gonads. After the age of 16 calcareous bodies frequently are present in the pineal body. These calcareous bodies, consisting of calcium and magnesium phosphates and carbonates, form large conglomerations which often are visible in skull roentgenographs. Identifica-

tion and measurements of the position of the pineal body in skull films can provide useful information, especially in the diagnosis of space occupying intracranial lesions.

THE THALAMUS

Transverse sections through the central part of the diencephalon demonstrate three major divisions of the diencephalon: (1) the thalamus, (2) the hypothalamus, and (3) the subthalamic region (Figs. 2-14, 2-22, 15-5 and 15-6).

The narrow third ventricle, extending from the region immediately ventral to the striae medullares to the optic chiasm, completely separates the thalami. A shallow groove on the ventricular surface, the hypothalamic sulcus (Fig. 15-6), separates the dorsal thalamus from the hypothalamus. The dorsal surface of the thalamus is covered by the stratum zonale. At the junc-

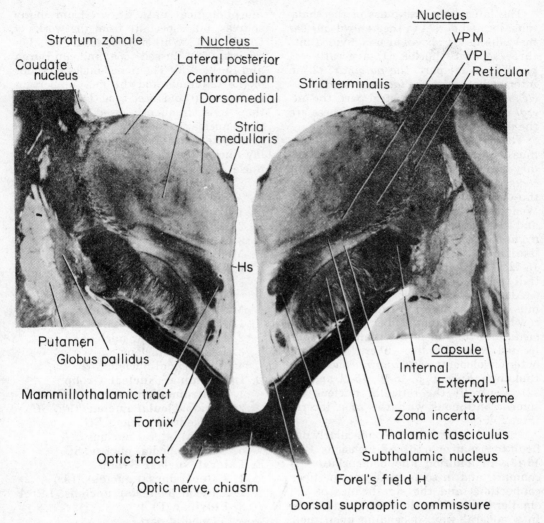

FIG. 15-6. Transverse section through the diencephalon and basal ganglia at the level of the optic chiasm. *HS* indicates the hypothalamic sulcus in the wall of the third ventricle. *VPM* and *VPL* refer to the ventral posteromedial and ventral posterolateral nuclei of the thalamus. Weigert's myelin stain. Photograph.

tion of the dorsal and medial thalamic surfaces, fibers of the striae medullares are cut transversely and appear as small bundles of myelinated fibers. The dorsal thalamus is divided into medial and lateral nuclear groups by a band of myelinated fibers, the internal medullary lamina of the thalamus (Fig. 2-22). In the lateral nuclear group, ventral and lateral (dorsal) nuclear masses can be distinguished (Figs. 15-6 and 15-12). The ventral nuclear mass, ex-

tending nearly the entire length of the thalamus, is divisible into three separate nuclei: (1) a caudal, *ventral posterior nucleus*, (2) an intermediate, *ventral lateral nucleus*, and (3) a rostral, *ventral anterior nucleus*. The ventral posterior nucleus is subdivided into a ventral posterolateral nucleus, located laterally, and a ventral posteromedial nucleus, located medially (Figs. 15-11 and 15-12). These are the ventral tier thalamic nuclei.

The lateral nuclear mass of the thalamus, located dorsal to the ventral nuclear mass discussed above, also is divided into three separate nuclei: (1) a greatly expanded caudal part, the *pulvinar*, (2) an intermediate part, the *lateral posterior nucleus*, and (3) a more rostral part, the *lateral dorsal nucleus* (Fig. 15-12). These are the dorsal tier thalamic nuclei.

The medial nuclear group of the thalamus, located medial to the internal medullary lamina, contains the *dorsomedial nucleus*, a nuclear mass intimately related to the cortex of the frontal lobe (Fig. 15-6). Wedged between the dorsomedial nucleus and the ventral nuclei caudally is the *centromedian nucleus*, the largest of the intralaminar nuclei (Figs. 15-5, 15-6, 15-11 and 15-12). The internal medullary lamina partially splits to surround this nucleus.

Along the lateral border of the thalamus, near the internal capsule, is a narrow band of myelinated fibers, the *external medullary lamina* of the thalamus. Cells located external to these fibers form a thin outer envelope, the *reticular nucleus* of the thalamus (Figs. 15-6, 15-10, 15-11 and 15-12). Ventrally the reticular nucleus becomes continuous with the zona incerta (Fig. 15-6).

The thalamic nuclei are particularly difficult to visualize in three dimensions (Fig. 15-12). In addition, the nomenclature is complex, and in some instances the fiber connections and the significance of the smaller thalamic nuclei remain unknown. In a general way, depending upon their fiber connections, most of the major thalamic nuclei can be classified either as specific relay nuclei (*R*), or as association nuclei (*A*). The specific relay nuclei project to, and receive fibers from, well defined cortical areas considered to be related to specific functions. The association nuclei of the thalamus do not receive direct fibers from ascending systems, but project to association areas of the cortex. Other thalamic nuclei have predominantly, or exclusively, subcortical (*SC*) connections. Physiological studies suggest that certain thalamic nuclei may have diffuse cortical connections, but these have not been established. The following classification of thalamic nuclei is based upon functional and morphological data drawn from many sources, but especially from the works of Clark ('32), Walker ('38, '38a, '66), Olszewski ('52), Russell ('55a) and van Buren and Borke ('72). The major nuclear groups of the thalamus and the most important nuclei are in bold faced type. The abbreviations most frequently used to designate these nuclear subdivisions are in parentheses. Letters in italics indicate specific relay nuclei (*R*), association nuclei (*A*) and nuclei with subcortical (*SC*) projections.

A. **Anterior Nuclear Group**
   1. **Anteroventral nucleus** (AV) *R*
   2. Anterodorsal nucleus (AD) *R*
   3. Anteromedial nucleus (AM)
B. **Medial Nuclear Group**
   1. **Dorsomedial nucleus** (DM)
      a. parvocellular part *A*
      b. magnocellular part *SC*
C. **Midline Nuclear Group**
   1. Paratenial nucleus
   2. Paraventricular nucleus
   3. Reuniens nucleus
   4. Rhomboidal nucleus
D. **Intralaminar Nuclear Group**
   1. **Centromedian nucleus (CM)** *SC*
   2. **Parafascicular nucleus** (PF) *SC*
   3. Paracentral nucleus *SC*
   4. Central lateral nucleus *SC*
   5. Central medial nucleus *SC*
E. **Lateral Nuclear Group**
   1. **Lateral dorsal nucleus** (LD) *A*
   2. **Lateral posterior nucleus** (LP) *A*
   3. **Pulvinar** (P) *A*
      a. medial part
      b. lateral part
      c. inferior part
F. **Ventral Nuclear Group**
   1. **Ventral anterior nucleus** (VA)
      a. parvocellular part (VApc) *R, SC*
      b. magnocellular part (VAmc) *R, SC*
   2. **Ventral lateral nucleus** (VL)
      a. **oral part** (VLo) *R*
      b. caudal part (VLc) *R*
      c. medial part (VLm) *R*
   3. **Ventral posterior nucleus** (VP) *R*
      a. **ventral posterolateral** (VPL) *R*
         aa. oral part (VPLo) *R*
         bb. caudal part (VPLc) *R*
      b. **ventral posteromedial** (VPM) *R*

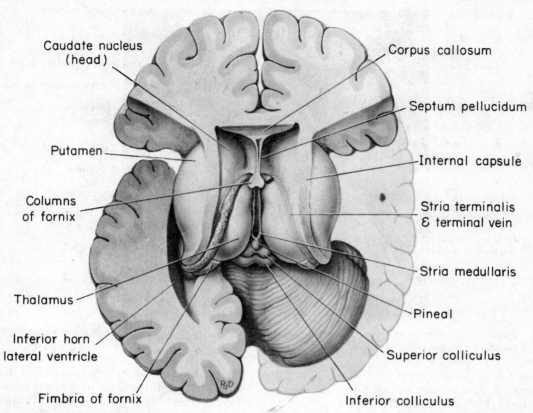

Caudate nucleus (head)

Corpus callosum

Septum pellucidum

Putamen

Internal capsule

Columns of fornix

Stria terminalis & terminal vein

Stria medullaris

Thalamus

Pineal

Inferior horn lateral ventricle

Superior colliculus

Fimbria of fornix

Inferior colliculus

FIG. 15-7. Drawing of a brain dissection showing gross relationships of the thalamus, internal capsule, basal ganglia and the ventricular system.

aa. parvocellular part (VPMpc) *R*

c. ventral posterior inferior (VPI) *R*

G. **Metathalamus**
  1. **Medial geniculate body** (MGB) *R*
    a. parvocellular part (MGpc) *R*
    b. magnocellular part (MGmc)
  2. **Lateral geniculate body** (LGB) *R*
    a. dorsal part *R*
    b. ventral part
H. **Unclassified Thalamic Nuclei**
  1. Submedial nucleus
  2. Suprageniculate nucleus
  3. Limitans nucleus
I. **Thalamic Reticular Nucleus** (RN) *SC*

The gross appearance of the dorsal surface of the diencephalon exposed by dissection is shown in Figure 15-7. This illustration demonstrates the relationships of the thalamus and epithalamus to surrounding structures. Figures 15-10 and 15-11 show

portions of many major thalamic nuclei at two important levels. The major subdivisions of the thalamus together with the established afferent and efferent thalamic projections are diagrammed in Figure 15-12. The cortical projection areas of the thalamic nuclei are diagrammatically represented in Figure 15-13. Examples of ascending thalamic afferent systems have been provided in diagrams for spinal pathways (Figs. 10-1, 10-7 and 10-8), for certain pathways originating in the brain stem (Figs. 12-10 and 12-22) and for the cerebellum (Figs. 14-16, 14-17 and 14-21). Review of these schematic diagrams will contribute to your understanding of thalamic organization. The illustrations in the atlas section provide additional material worthy of reference.

The Anterior Nuclear Group

The anterior nuclear group lies beneath the dorsal surface of the most rostral part

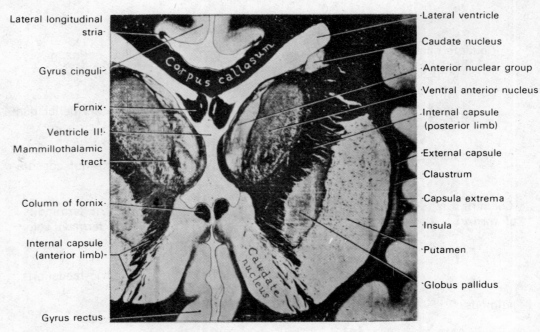

Lateral longitudinal stria

Gyrus cinguli

Fornix

Ventricle II

Mammillothalamic tract

Column of fornix

Internal capsule (anterior limb)

Gyrus rectus

Lateral ventricle

Caudate nucleus

Anterior nuclear group

Ventral anterior nucleus

Internal capsule (posterior limb)

External capsule

Claustrum

Capsula extrema

Insula

Putamen

Globus pallidus

Corpus callosum

Caudate nucleus

FIG. 15-8. Photograph of section transverse to the axis of the brain stem passing through rostral portions of the thalamus and portions of the basal ganglia. Weigert's myelin stain.

of the thalamus, where it forms a distinct swelling, the anterior tubercle (Figs. 15-8, 15-10, 15-12, A-16 and A-17). It consists of a large principal nucleus, the anteroventral (AV), and accessory nuclei, the anterodorsal (AD) and anteromedial (AM). The round or polygonal cells composing these nuclei are of medium or small size; they have little chromophilic substance and a moderate amount of yellow pigment. The anterior nuclei receive the mammillothalamic tract and may send some fibers to the mammillary body (Clark and Boggon, '33) by the same bundle (thalamomammillary; Fig. 15-12B). According to Fry et al. ('63), fibers from the medial mammillary nucleus project to the ipsilateral anteroventral and anteromedial nuclei, while the lateral mammillary nucleus projects bilaterally to the anterodorsal nucleus, but not to other subdivisions of the nuclear group. In addition, the anterior nuclei of the thalamus receive as many direct fibers from the fornix as from the mammillothalamic tract (Powell et al., '57). The cortical projections of the anterior nuclei are to the cingulate gyrus (areas 23, 24 and 32) via the

anterior limb of the internal capsule (Fig. 15-13). Although these cortical areas have been considered to project back to the anterior thalamic nuclei (Meyer et al., '47; Freeman and Watts, '48), the bulk of the projections are via the cingulum to the entorhinal cortex (Fig. 18-11) (Raisman et al., '65; Raisman, '66). Because the entorhinal cortex projects to the hippocampal formation, impulses following this course can affect hypothalamic activities. Fibers passing from the anterior nuclei to the habenular ganglion via the stria medullaris also have been described by some investigators.

The Dorsomedial Nucleus

The dorsomedial nucleus (DM) occupies most of the area between the internal medullary lamina and the periventricular gray (Figs. 15-9, 15-10, 15-11, 15-12A and A-16). Two cytologically distinct regions of the nucleus are recognized: (1) a magnocellular portion, located rostrally and dorsomedially, consisting of fairly large, polygonal, deeply staining cells; and (2) a larger dorsolateral and caudal parvocellular portion made up of small, pale-staining cells

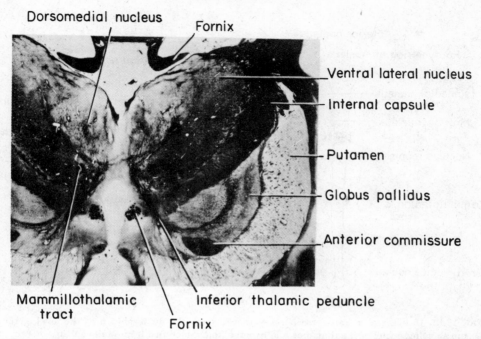

Dorsomedial nucleus   Fornix

Ventral lateral nucleus

Internal capsule

Putamen

Globus pallidus

Anterior commissure

Mammillothalamic   Inferior thalamic peduncle
       tract
                    Fornix

Fig. 15-9. Transverse section through the diencephalon and basal ganglia demonstrating fibers of the inferior thalamic peduncle. The inferior thalamic peduncle consists of fibers from the amygdaloid complex, temporal neocortex and possibly the substantia innominata, which project to the dorsomedial nucleus of the thalamus. The inferior thalamic peduncle, plus amygdaloid projections to the hypothalamus and preoptic regions, constitute the *ansa peduncularis*. Weigert's myelin stain. Photograph.

which tend to occur in clusters (Sheps, '45; Olszewski, '52; Dekaban, '53). The nucleus has connections with the centromedian and other intralaminar nuclei and with the lateral nuclear groups. The medial magnocellular division of the dorsomedial nucleus receives fibers from the amygdaloid complex, temporal neocortex and possibly the substantia innominata via the inferior thalamic peduncle (Fig. 15-9) (Whitlock and Nauta, '56; Nauta, '61; Powell et al., '63, '65). The caudal orbitofrontal cortex also has connections with the medial division of the dorsomedial nucleus (Nauta, '62). Most of these fibers constitute components of the so-called *ansa peduncularis*. The ansa peduncularis consists of fibers of the inferior thalamic peduncle, plus fibers interconnecting the amygdaloid complex and the preoptico-hypothalamic region (Nauta and Mehler, '66).

The much larger parvocellular portion of the dorsomedial nucleus is connected by a massive projection with practically the entire frontal cortex rostral to areas 6 and 32 (Figs. 15-12 and 15-13). After extensive prefrontal cortical lesions, or lesions interrupting fibers to this region, nearly all small cells of the dorsomedial nucleus degenerate (Walker, '36; Sheps, '45; Meyer et al., '47; Freeman and Watts, '48; McLardy, '50). Fibers projected by the parvocellular part of this nucleus are organized in such a way that cells in the rostral and caudal parts of the nucleus project to corresponding parts of the prefrontal cortex (Mettler, '47). The dorsomedial nucleus is thought to be concerned with integration of certain somatic and visceral impulses (Walker, '59). Some impulses relayed to the prefrontal cortex may enter consciousness and may thus influence or produce various feeling tones. Psychosurgical studies (i.e., prefrontal lobotomy) suggest that the dorsomedial nucleus may mediate impulses of an affective nature, and although these vary greatly among individuals,

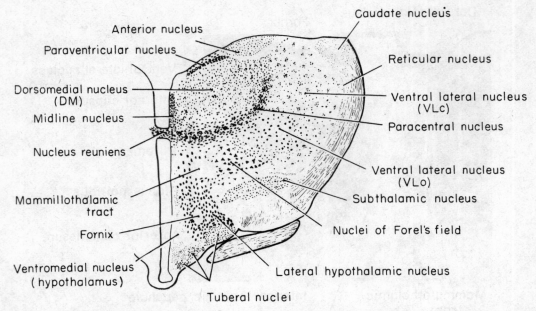

FIG. 15-10. Drawing of a transverse Nissl section through the diencephalon at the level of the tuber cinereum showing nuclei of the thalamus and hypothalamus (modified from Malone, '10).

they may constitute part of the emotional experience that contributes to the formation of personality. Prefrontal lobotomy and lesions in the dorsomedial nucleus of the thalamus modify the patient's reaction to chronic pain, but it is doubtful if they eliminate pain.

The Midline Nuclei

The midline nuclei are more or less distinct cell clusters which lie in the periventricular gray matter of the dorsal half of the ventricular wall and in the interthalamic adhesion (Figs. 15-10 and 15-11). They are small and difficult to delimit in man, but in the lower vertebrates they, together with some of the intralaminar nuclei, form the largest part of the thalamus (paleothalamus). They consist of small, fusiform, rather darkly staining cells resembling preganglionic autonomic neurons (Malone, '10), and are believed to be concerned with visceral activities. Their scanty connections are mainly with the hypothalamic region by fine myelinated and unmyelinated fibers which run in the periventricular gray substance. They also are related to the magnocellular por-

tion of the dorsomedial nucleus and to the intralaminar nuclei. The more distinct midline cell groups include the *paratenial nucleus,* near the stria medullaris, and the *paraventricular nucleus,* in the dorsal ventricular wall (Fig. 15-10). In an attempt to homologize these ill-defined nuclei with the more developed nuclei of lower mammals, some authorities recognize several cell groups in this periventricular gray: the *nucleus reuniens,* the *rhomboidal nucleus* and the *median central nucleus.* The reuniens, rhomboidal and median central nuclei all bear close relationships with the interthalamic adhesion (massa intermedia), when present. The latter structure is reported to be absent in about 30% of human brains (Morel, '47).

The Intralaminar Nuclei

The intralaminar nuclei (Figs. 15-5, 15-6, 15-10, 15-11 and 15-12) are cell groups of variable extent infiltrating the internal medullary lamina, which separates the medial from the lateral thalamic mass. Their cells, although varying in size in the different nuclei, are usually fusiform and darkly staining, and they resemble those of the

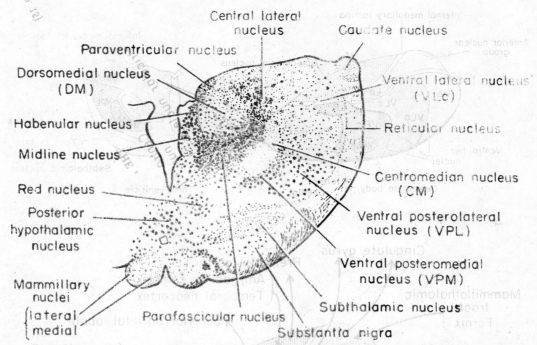

FIG. 15-11. Drawing of a transverse Nissl section through the diencephalon at the level of the habenular nuclei and the mammillary bodies showing the nuclei of the thalamus and hypothalamus (modified from Malone, '10).

midline nuclei. Their fiber connections are intricate and incompletely understood (Fig. 15-12*B*).

The Centromedian Nucleus (CM). This is the largest and most easily defined of the intralaminar thalamic nuclei (Figs. 15-5, 15-6 and 15-12); other intralaminar nuclei are smaller and some of their boundaries are indistinct. This prominent nucleus is located in the middle third of the thalamus between the dorsomedial nucleus above and the ventral posterior nucleus below (Figs. 15-5, 15-6 and 15-11). It is surrounded by fibers of the internal medullary lamina, except along its medial border, where it merges by interdigitations with the parafascicular nucleus (Figs. 15-5 and 15-11). It is composed of small, loosely arranged, ovoid or round cells containing a considerable amount of yellow pigment. Cells in the lateral portion of the nucleus are small, while those in more medial regions bordering the dorsomedial nucleus are larger and more densely arranged. There has been considerable controversy

concerning precise delimitation of the centromedian nucleus, particularly with respect to the border separating it from the parafascicular nucleus. According to Mehler ('66) only the ventrolateral small-celled region should be identified as the centromedian nucleus.

The Parafascicular Nucleus (PF). This nucleus lies medial to the centromedian nucleus and ventral to the caudal part of the dorsomedial nucleus (Figs. 15-5 and 15-11). Caudally the boundary between the parafascicular nucleus and the centromedian nucleus is indistinct and somewhat arbitrary. The most distinguishing feature of the parafascicular nucleus is that its larger, more deeply stained cells surround the dorsomedial part of the fasciculus retroflexus; portions of the nucleus medial and lateral to this tract show no cytological differences (Walker, '38a).

The paracentral, central lateral and central medial nuclei are all associated with the internal medullary lamina of the thalamus. The paracentral nucleus lies along

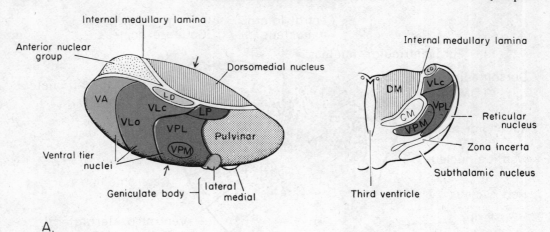

A.

B.

Fig. 15-12. Schematic diagrams of the major thalamic nuclei. An oblique dorsolateral view of the thalamus and its major subdivisions is shown on the *left* in *A*. A transverse section of the thalamus at level of *arrows* is shown on the *right* in *A* and indicates: (1) the relationships between *VPM* and *VPL*, and (2) the location of *CM* with respect to the internal medullary lamina of the thalamus. In *B*, the principal afferent and efferent projections of particular thalamic subdivisions are indicated. While most cortical areas project fibers back to the thalamic nuclei from which fibers are received, not all of these are shown.

the lateral border of the dorsomedial nucleus rostrally (Fig. 15-10); caudally, it is fused with the central lateral nucleus in its dorsal part and with the central medial nucleus in its medial part (Toncray and Krieg, '46).

Although it is widely recognized that the brain stem reticular formation probably is one of the principal sources of afferent impulses to the intralaminar nuclei of the thalamus, considerable controversy has developed concerning the manner in

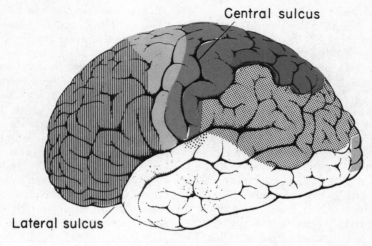

Central sulcus

Lateral sulcus

Lateral surface

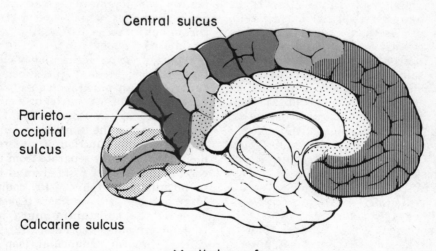

Central sulcus

Parieto-
occipital
sulcus

Calcarine sulcus

Medial surface

FIG. 15-13. Diagram of the left cerebral hemisphere showing the cortical projection areas of thalamic nuclei. The color code is the same as in Figure 15-12. The diffuse projection of the ventral anterior nucleus (*VApc*) to the frontal lobe appears to largely overlap the projection of the dorsomedial nucleus (*DM*). Information concerning the cortical projection areas of some thalamic nuclei is incomplete.

which these impulses are transmitted rostrally. This controversy centers around discrepancies between the results of anatomical and physiological investigations. According to physiological findings (Moruzzi and Magoun, '49; Starzl et al., '51), transmission of ascending impulses in the reticular formation takes place via a series of

reticular neurons with short axons. This type of impulse transmission involves a large number of neurons, is polysynaptic and is said to account for the long latency of responses. As mentioned previously (Chapter 13), Golgi studies of the intrinsic organization of the reticular core (Scheibel and Scheibel, '58) do not reveal neurons with short axons (Golgi type II cells) within the reticular formation, although such neurons might be expected on the basis of physiological evidence. Anatomical studies (Brodal and Rossi, '55; Papez, '56; 56a; Brodal, '57; Nauta and Kuypers, '58; Scheibel and Scheibel, '58) indicate that "effector" regions of the reticular formation give rise to long ascending fibers which enter the area of the central tegmental tract. Areas of the reticular formation from which the largest number of ascending fibers in this system originate correspond to parts of the nucleus reticularis gigantocellularis and nucleus reticularis ventralis (medulla) and to the nucleus reticularis pontis caudalis (pons) (Figs. 10-11, 11-9, 11-15 and 12-3). The most complete study of the diencephalic projection of this system is that of Nauta and Kuypers ('58) based upon silver staining methods. These authors traced fibers from the central tegmental fasciculus into: (1) the centromedian-parafascicular nuclear complex, as well as the paracentral and central lateral nuclei, and (2) the subthalamic region. These ascending reticular projections are said to be chiefly ipsilateral. The above findings have been confirmed in nearly every detail by Golgi studies (Scheibel and Scheibel, '58). Because action potentials in the brain stem reticular formation have been recorded with stimulation of almost every type of receptor, it has been presumed that activation of the ascending reticular system is due to "collateral" excitation derived from specific sensory pathways (Chapter 13).

As mentioned earlier (Chapter 10) with respect to the spinothalamic tract, anterolateral cordotomy (Mehler et al., '60; Bowsher, '61) produces ascending degeneration which passes not only to the ventral posterolateral nucleus and the posterior thalamic zone, but also to the intralaminar thalamic nuclei. Unilateral anterolateral cordotomy produces bilateral degeneration in these nuclei which is greatest ipsilaterally, except in the intralaminar nuclei where nearly equal bilateral degeneration is seen. Within the intralaminar nuclei these fibers are distributed to parts of the paracentral nuclei and

throughout the central lateral nuclei (Fig. 15-11). These spinal afferents to parts of the intralaminar nuclei follow pathways in the brain stem that are independent of the classic spinothalamic trajectory (Mehler et al., '60) and probably are related to a phylogenetically older system.

Other afferent fibers to the intralaminar nuclei appear to originate from the dentate (Hassler, '50; Cohen et al., '58) and the fastigial nuclei (Thomas et al., '56; Carpenter et al., '58; Kievit and Kuypers, '72). Although fibers of the superior cerebellar peduncle have been described as passing to the centromedian nuclei, most of these fibers merely pass through this nucleus to the more rostral intralaminar nuclei (Mehler et al., '58; Carpenter, '67). Many of these fibers appear to terminate in the central lateral nucleus.

The centromedian (CM) and parafascicular (PF) nuclei receive afferent fibers mainly from forebrain derivatives. Area 4 projects fibers which are distributed throughout the centromedian nucleus, while area 6 appears to project to the lateral part of the parafascicular nucleus (Petras, '64, '69; Mehler, '66). Fibers to the centromedian-parafascicular complex (CM-PF) reach these nuclei by a circuitous route described by Rinvik ('68). These fibers descend in the internal capsule as far caudally as the junction of midbrain and diencephalon; they separate from the crus cerebri and project rostrally and dorsally to terminate in the CM-PF complex. A large number of these fibers traverse portions of the substantia nigra in their course (Carpenter and Peter, '72). This so-called "cerebral peduncular loop" is the pathway taken by most corticofugal fibers to basal and inferior thalamic nuclei.

The centromedian nucleus (CM) also receives a large number of pallidal efferent fibers that separate from the thalamic fasciculus at nearly right angles (Nauta and Mehler, '66; Kuo and Carpenter, '73). A considerable part of these fibers may be collaterals of pallidofugal fibers passing to the ventral anterior and ventral lateral thalamic nuclei (Figs. 15-12 and 17-11).

While all of the efferent projections of the intralaminar nuclei are not known, the principal projection of the centromedian-parafascicular nuclear complex is to the putamen (Mettler, '47; Freeman and Watts, '47; McLardy, '48; Droogleever-Fortuyn and Stefens, '51; Nauta and Whitlock, '54; Powell and Cowan, '56). The smaller and most rostral intralaminar nuclei project fibers to the caudate nucleus. These thalamostriatal fibers follow a wide curved path through the ventral anterior and rostral reticular nuclei of the thalamus, but do not appear to establish terminal connections within the ventral anterior nucleus (Mehler, '66). Some of these fibers, however, may terminate in portions of the reticular nucleus. The majority of the afferent projections to the striatum course dorsal to the globus pallidus.

The intralaminar nuclei of the thalamus have long been regarded as having no cortical projections. This conclusion is based upon the absence of retrograde cell changes in these nuclei following virtually complete decortication (Walker, '38, '38a; Sheps, '45; Combs, '49; Powell, '52) and the absence of degeneration traceable from lesions in the centromedian nucleus to any part of the cortex (Clark and Boggon, '33, '33a; Nauta and Whitlock, '54). These observations have been difficult to reconcile with abundant physiological studies indicating that the intralaminar nuclei are of extreme importance in the control and regulation of electrocortical activity over broad regions of the cerebral cortex. Bowsher ('66) has described projections from the centromedian nucleus that passed beyond the thalamus into the subcortical white matter. Recent studies utilizing horseradish peroxidase provide evidence that thalamostriate fibers from the intralaminar nuclei give rise to collateral systems which project to the cortex (Jones and Leavitt, '74). These collateral fibers have overlapping cortical terminations with fibers of at least one cortical thalamic relay nucleus.

The striking development of the centromedian nucleus in primates, including man, in relation to that of the principal thalamic nuclei, suggests that the centromedian nucleus may constitute a complex intrathalamic regulating mechanism

(Clark, '32; Purpura and Cohen, '62; Cohen et al., '62).

The Lateral Nuclear Group

The lateral nuclear group begins as a narrow strip some distance from the anterior limit of the thalamus, enlarges posteriorly and merges caudally with the pulvinar. It consists of two small gray masses, the lateral dorsal and lateral posterior nuclei (Fig. 15-12A).

The Lateral Dorsal Nucleus (LD). This nucleus, which lies on the dorsal surface of the thalamus, extends along the upper margin of the internal medullary lamina (Fig. 15-12). Topographically this nucleus has been considered as a posterior extension of the anterior nuclear group (Locke et al., '61; Walker, '66). While many authors accept that this nucleus projects to the posterior parietal cortex (Fig. 15-13), recent data indicate that its fibers pass mainly to the cingulate gyrus, although some pass to the supralimbic cortex of the parietal lobe. Afferent fibers to this nucleus are poorly understood.

The Lateral Posterior Nucleus (LP). This nucleus lies caudal to the lateral dorsal nucleus and dorsal to the ventral posterior nucleus (Fig. 15-12). The small cells of this nucleus have a homogeneous appearance and project to the parietal cortex (Fig. 15-13). The input to this nucleus presumably is derived from internuncial neurons of adjacent primary relay nuclei, especially the ventral posterior nucleus (Walker, '66). Posteriorly the nucleus is difficult to delimit from the pulvinar.

These nuclei receive few ascending sensory fibers, but they possess reciprocal connections with a rather extensive area of the cortex. The lateral dorsal nucleus sends and receives fibers from the precuneal cortex, while the lateral posterior nucleus is intimately connected with the superior parietal lobule (areas 5 and 7).

The Pulvinar (P). This is a large nuclear mass forming the posterior portion of the thalamus. Caudally it overhangs the geniculate bodies and dorsolateral surface of the midbrain (Figs. 15-3, 15-4 and 15-5). The pulvinar is divided into a narrow lateral nucleus, a large medial nucleus and a more primitive inferior nucleus. The lateral nucleus of the pulvinar is traversed by fibers passing to and from the external medullary lamina. The medial nucleus occupies the dorsomedial two-thirds of the pulvinar, while the inferior nucleus is adjacent to the lateral geniculate body. The pulvinar does not receive long ascending sensory fibers; its input appears to be derived from internuclear relationships with other thalamic nuclei, especially the medial and lateral geniculate bodies and perhaps the ventral posterior nucleus. The cortical projections of the different parts of the pulvinar are specific (Simpson, '52; Walker, '66). The medial nucleus projects to the posterior parietal region, while the lateral nucleus sends fibers mainly to posterior parts of the temporal lobe. The inferior nucleus of the pulvinar sends fibers to the area surrounding the striate cortex (Fig. 15-13). There are suggestions that portions of the pulvinar which receive tectothalamic projections may transmit visual information to the extrastriate "visual" cortex (Harting et al., '73).

The Ventral Nuclear Mass

The ventral nuclear mass of the thalamus usually is divided into three separate nuclei: the *ventral anterior,* the *ventral lateral* and the *ventral posterior*. The ventral anterior nucleus is the most rostral and smallest of this group. The ventral posterior nucleus, the largest and most posterior of the group, is further subdivided into the *ventral posterolateral* and *ventral posteromedial* nuclei (Fig. 15-12). Although the *medial* and *lateral geniculate bodies* together constitute the *metathalamus,* these well defined nuclear masses may be considered as a caudal continuation of the ventral nuclear mass. The ventral nuclear group and the metathalamus constitute the largest division of the thalamus concerned with relaying impulses from other portions of the neuraxis to specific parts of the cerebral cortex. The most caudal parts of this complex are concerned with relaying impulses of specific sensory systems to cortical regions, while more rostral nuclei (ventral anterior and ventral lateral nuclei) relay impulses from the basal ganglia and cerebellum.

The Ventral Anterior Nucleus (VA).

This subdivision lies in the extreme rostral part of the ventral nuclear mass where it is bounded anteriorly and ventrolaterally by the thalamic reticular nucleus. Rostrally this nucleus occupies the entire thalamic region lateral to the anterior nuclear group (Fig. 15-8), but caudally it becomes restricted to a more medial region. The mammillothalamic tract passes through the ventral anterior nucleus but does not from its medial border. The nucleus is composed of large and medium-sized multipolar cells arranged in clusters. The clustering of cells is particularly evident in rostrolateral parts of the nucleus due to thick myelinated fiber bundles coursing longitudinally within the nucleus.

A distinctive part of the nucleus adjacent to the mammillothalamic tract and along the ventral border of the nucleus is composed of large, dark, densely arranged cells. This subdivision, called the magnocellular part (VAmc) (Olszewski, '52), extends further caudal than the principal part of the ventral anterior nucleus (VApc). Thus there are two distinctive cytological subdivisions of the ventral anterior nucleus. Each of these subdivisions receives fibers from different sources. Afferent fibers to the ventral anterior nucleus (VApc) arise from the medial segment of the globus pallidus and reach the nucleus via the lenticular fasciculus and ansa lenticularis (Ranson and Ranson, '42; Papez, '42; Nauta and Mehler, '66; Scheibel and Scheibel, '66a). These fibers enter the thalamic fasciculus, turn dorsolaterally and are distributed in a rostrolateral direction within the ventral anterior nucleus. Pallidothalamic fibers projecting to the rostral ventral tier thalamic nuclei (i.e., VApc and VLo) appear organized in a specific manner (Kuo and Carpenter, '73). Rostral parts of the medial pallidal segment project most profusely to VApc. More caudal parts of the medial pallidal segment project fibers to parts of the ventral lateral nucleus (VLo).

The magnocellular part of the ventral anterior nucleus (VAmc) receives a significant fiber projection from the substantia nigra (Cole et al., '64; Afifi and Kaelber,

'65; Carpenter and Strominger, '67; Faull and Carman, '68). Nigrothalamic fibers arise from the pars reticularis, pass medially and rostrally through Forel's field H and follow a course that parallels that of the mammillothalamic tract (Figs. 13-19, 15-1 and 15-8) (Carpenter and Peter, '72). Terminals of nigrothalamic fibers form a dense felt-work about groups of cells in VAmc.

Other afferent fibers to the ventral anterior nucleus appear to be collaterals of: (1) corticofugal fibers (Rinvik, '68), and (2) fibers arising from intralaminar and midline thalamic nuclei (Scheibel and Scheibel, '66a). The latter projections account for the characteristics of the nonspecific thalamic system exhibited by this nucleus.

Information concerning the efferent projections of the ventral anterior nucleus is conflicting and incomplete. Some experimental studies indicate that nearly all cells of the ventral anterior nucleus degenerate following hemidecortication (Bard and Rioch, '37; Papez, '38), while others indicate virtually no cell changes in this nucleus (Walker, '38a). Observations in man reveal that over 50% of the cells in this nucleus remain following hemispherectomy (Powell, '52). Data from Golgi studies tend to confirm this observation (Scheibel and Scheibel, '66a). It has been suggested that the ventral anterior nucleus projects to parts of the anterior insular cortex (Angevine et al., '62). A recent investigation indicates that no significant cell changes in VA follow ablations limited to single cortical areas, including area 6, frequently cited as receiving a projection from this nucleus (Freeman and Watts, '47; Carmel, '70). Cell loss and morphological alteration of remaining cells in VA were noted after large cortical ablations. This evidence suggested that the ventral anterior nucleus may have unusually widespread frontal cortical projections, perhaps on the basis of collateral systems. Although certain authors suggest that VAmc does not have a projection to the cerebral cortex (Yakovlev et al., '66), recent investigations reveal a projection from VAmc to the caudal and medial orbitofrontal cortex (Scheibel and Scheibel, '66a; Carmel, '70). Subcortical projections from VA have

been alluded to by many authors (Walker, '38a; Mettler, '47a), but their determination has been exceedingly difficult because this nucleus is traversed by fibers from many sources. In spite of these difficulties it appears established that: (1) VAmc projects fibers to VApc, although this connection is not reciprocal, and (2) portions of VApc project to the intralaminar nuclei and the dorsomedial nucleus (Carmel, '70). According to Scheibel and Scheibel ('66a), caudally projecting axons from VA give off a large number of collaterals to the intralaminar nuclei. Fibers from VA do not cross the midline to contralateral thalamic nuclei; none of the fibers from this nucleus project to the caudate nucleus, although this has been suggested by physiological evidence (Starzl and Magoun, '51).

Physiological data (Starzl and Magoun, '51; Jasper et al., '52; Jasper, '54) indicate that the ventral anterior nucleus may be functionally related to the intralaminar nuclei of the thalamus in that responses in widespread cortical areas can be evoked by repeated low frequency stimulation of the nucleus. Other authors have demonstrated that VA is essential for the recruiting response and that lesions in this nucleus block the responses elicited by stimulating the nonspecific thalamic nuclei (Skinner and Lindsley, '67). The *recruiting response* is a surface negative response evoked by repetitive stimulation of the midline and intralaminar nuclei that waxes and wanes and can be recorded over broad areas of the cerebral cortex. The ventral anterior nucleus appears to be the pre-eminent site among thalamic nuclei for production of the recruiting response. The system of efferent projections from VA seems to form an anatomical substrate well suited for diffuse synchronous discharge to large regions of the frontal cortex and thalamus. Anatomical and physiological data are in agreement concerning the special role projections of VAmc to the orbitofrontal cortex may play in "triggering" the recruiting response. This cortical response is abolished by ablations of the orbitofrontal cortex (Velasco and Lindsley, '65) and reversibly diminished by cryogenic blockade of this cortical region (Skinner and Lindsley, '67). The ventral anterior thalamic nucleus appears to exhibit characteristics of both the specific and nonspecific thalamic nuclei.

The Ventral Lateral Nucleus (VL). This nucleus, caudal to the ventral anterior nucleus, is composed of small and large neurons that show considerable differences in various parts of the nucleus (Figs. 15-9 and 15-10). This nucleus has been subdivided into three main parts (Olszewski, '52): (1) pars oralis (VLo), (2) pars caudalis (VLc), and (3) pars medialis (VLm). The largest subdivision (VLo) consists of numerous deep staining cells arranged in clusters. The pars caudalis (VLc) is less cellular but formed of scattered large cells. The pars medialis (VLm) begins ventral to VA and extends caudally to the subthalamic region. Cerebellar efferent fibers contained in the superior cerebellar peduncle decussate in the mesencephalon and project profusely to the contralateral ventral lateral nucleus, pars oralis (Olszewski, '52; Jansen and Brodal, '58). These fibers arise mainly from the dentate nucleus. The pars oralis also receives pallidofugal fibers via the thalamic fasciculus which are topographically organized (Kuo and Carpenter, '73). These fibers arise from the medial pallidal segment and appear to be most profuse from caudal regions of the pallidum.

The ventral lateral nucleus of the thalamus receives a considerable number of fibers from the precentral cortex (Clark, '32; Levin, '36, '49; Verhaart and Kennard, '40; Mettler, '47). These corticofugal fibers pass to both the pars oralis and the pars caudalis of VL (Olszewski, '52). Both areas 4 and 6 project profusely upon the ventral lateral nucleus, the thalamic reticular nucleus and the centromedian-parafascicular (CM-PF) complex (Auer, '56; Petras, '64, '66, '69; Rinvik, '68). Corticofugal fibers to VL and the reticular nucleus follow a different path than those passing to the CM-PF complex. The majority of fibers to VL leave the posterior limb of the internal capsule, enter the reticular nucleus and course medially and caudally. Cortical projections to the CM-PF complex follow the so-called "cerebral peduncle loop" in that they descend to levels of the mesence-

phalic-diencephalic junction, leave the crus cerebri and project rostrally and dorsally to their thalamic nuclei of termination (Rinvik, '68).

Connections of the ventral lateral nucleus with the precentral cortex are reciprocal and topically arranged. Medial parts of the nucleus send fibers to the face area, lateral parts send fibers to the leg area and fibers from intermediate portions of the nucleus pass to cortical regions representing the arm and trunk (Walker, '38, '49). Most of these fibers pass to area 4, but some may reach area 6 (Fig. 15-13). This topical arrangement of thalamocortical fibers passing to the precentral cortex is considered as the anatomical expression of the functional independence of different body parts in the primary motor area. The fact that impulses from the cerebellum and basal ganglia project in overlapping fashion upon VLo, which in turn projects to the motor cortex, suggests that the influence of these structures upon motor activity probably is effected primarily at a cortical level (Fig. 15-13). Different regions of the medial part of the ventral lateral nucleus (VLm) receive afferent fibers from the substantia nigra and a smaller number from the globus pallidus (Carpenter and Peter, '72; Kuo and Carpenter, '73).

The Ventral Posterior Nucleus (VP). This nucleus, whose cells are among the largest in the thalamus, is composed of two main portions, the *posteromedial* and the *posterolateral* (Figs. 15-6, 15-11 and 15-12). The ventral posterior nucleus is regarded universally as the largest primary somatic sensory relay nucleus of the thalamus.

The Ventral Posterolateral Nucleus (VPL). This has been subdivided into a pars oralis (VPLo), characterized by very large, relatively uniform cells sparsely distributed, and a pars caudalis (VPLc), containing large and small cells, and characterized by a wide range of cell size and a high cellular density. Both divisions of the nucleus contain medium-sized fiber bundles radiating in an oblique dorsal direction.

Two principal long ascending systems project to VPL, the medial lemniscus

(Clark, '36; Walker, '38a; Rasmussen and Peyton, '48; Matzke, '51; Bowsher, '58, '61) and the spinothalamic tracts (Clark, '36; Walker, '38a; Berry et al., '50; Bowsher, '57, '61; Mehler et al., '60). Fibers of the medial lemniscus course through the brain stem without supplying collateral or terminal fibers to the reticular formation, and terminate exclusively in the ventral posterolateral nucleus (Fig. 15-12). These fibers terminate profusely in all parts of the nucleus in a pattern presenting a sharp contrast with the parcellated distribution of the spinothalamic fibers. Fibers arising from the nucleus gracilis terminate lateral to those of the nucleus cuneatus (Clark, '36; Walker, '38a). Fibers of the medial lemniscus establish predominantly axodendritic contacts throughout the rostrocaudal extent of VPL.

Spinothalamic fibers in the monkey enter the caudal part of the nucleus and spread out laterally on the inner surface of the external medullary lamina; from this location bundles of fibers invade more medial regions of the nucleus (Mehler et al., '60). Other impressive contrasts between these ascending sensory pathways might be mentioned. The spinothalamic tracts contribute a large number of fibers and collaterals to the bulbar reticular formation, and project fibers to both a ventral relay nucleus (ventral posterolateral) and the nonspecific nuclei (intralaminar nuclei) of the thalamus. According to Bowsher ('57), spinothalamic fibers, interrupted by anterolateral cordotomy in man, project bilaterally to the ventral posterolateral nuclei.

Physiological studies (Mountcastle and Henneman, '49, '52; Rose and Mountcastle, '52, '59; Poggio and Mountcastle, '60) indicate the precise and orderly fashion in which the contralateral body surface is represented in the ventral posterolateral nucleus (external portion of the ventrobasal complex). There is a complete, although distorted, image of the body form; volume representation of a given part of the body is related to its effectiveness as a tactile organ (i.e., to its innervation density). Cervical segments are represented most medially and sacral segments most laterally.

The thoracic and lumbar regions are represented only dorsally, while the regions concerned with the distal parts of the limbs extend ventrally. Each neuron of this complex is related to a restricted, specific and unchanging receptive field on the contralateral side of the body. Each neuron of the ventrobasal complex can be activated by either tactile stimulation of the skin, or mechanical alteration of deep structures (especially joint rotation), but by only one of these. These neurons are regarded as place specific, modality specific, and concerned, almost exclusively, with the perception of tactile sense and position sense (kinesthesis). Few cells of the ventrobasal complex appear to be activated by noxious stimuli (Poggio and Mountcastle, '60). Although the terminology used by these authors differs from that used here, it is generally accepted that these superbly defined principles apply to man. The inner portion of the ventrobasal complex, known as the ventral posteromedial nucleus, contains the representation of the contralateral head, face and intraoral structures.

The Ventral Posteromedial Nucleus (VPM). This nucleus is located medial to the posterolateral nucleus, and the centromedian nucleus forms its medial boundary (Figs. 15-6, 15-11 and 15-12). The ventral posteromedial nucleus (VPM) contains one distinct subdivision in its medial apical region composed of small, light-staining, densely packed cells. This subdivision is known as the pars parvocellularis (VPMpc). The precise boundaries of VPM are best defined on the basis of its fiber connections. The ventral posteromedial nucleus receives afferent systems concerned with the head, face and intraoral structures. Ascending secondary trigeminal fibers include: (1) crossed fibers from the spinal and principal sensory trigeminal nuclei, which ascend in association with the medial lemniscus (Carpenter and Hanna, '61), and (2) uncrossed fibers of the dorsal trigeminal tract (Carpenter, '57a; Torvik, '57), originating from the dorsal part of the principal sensory nucleus of N. V. Some impulses from stretch receptors in the facial musculature also are believed to reach the ventral posteromedial nucleus, but the pathways are not known. Experimental evidence (Mountcastle and Henneman, '52; Berry et al., '56) indicates that tactile impulses from the face and intraoral structures are transmitted bilaterally to parts of the ventral posteromedial nucleus. Even though the central pathways conveying impulses mediating gustatory sense are not known, it seems likely that secondary fiber systems originating from the nucleus solitarius may reach the medial part of the ventral posteromedial nucleus (VPMpc), since electrical stimulation of the chorda tympani and glossopharyngeal nerves evokes localized responses (Blomquist et al., '62) in this nucleus. According to Rose and Mountcastle ('52) and Mountcastle and Henneman ('52), VPMpc was not found to respond to tactile stimuli of body surfaces. Benjamin and Akert ('59) have shown that ablations of the cortical taste area in the rat produce retrograde degeneration of thalamic neurons confined to VPMpc. Gustatory representation in thalamic neurons in the rat, cat and monkey (Blomquist et al., '62) is said to be bilateral, but apparently is predominantly ipsilateral in the cat and monkey. Emmers ('64) has found that the most medial portion of the thalamic taste projection does not relay any tactile afferent impulses and suggests that gustatory sense has an independent representation in the thalamus.

Lesions in the ventral posteromedial nucleus in experimental animals impair taste (Blum et al., '43; Patton et al., '44; Anderson and Jewell, '57). Some evidence supports this thesis in that degenerated fibers from lesions in the nucleus solitarius have been traced to the ventral posteromedial nucleus (Allen, '23). These fibers are described as ascending in association with the contralateral medial lemniscus. Clinical evidence (Adler, '33) suggests that gustatory sense in the thalamus may be represented only contralaterally.

The ventral posterior nucleus has a precise topical projection to the cortex (Clark and Boggon, '35; Walker, '38a; Clark and Powell, '53; Kruger and Porter, '58). Fibers project to the postcentral gyrus so that dorsal portions of the gyrus receive fibers from the lateral part of VPL; lower portions of the gyrus near the lateral sulcus are supplied by fibers from VPM. Intermediate parts of VP project to intermediate parts of the postcentral gyrus (Fig. 15-13). This thalamocortical projection correlates precisely with the termination of ascending somatosensory systems in the ventral posterior nuclear complex. Cortical areas 3, 1 and 2 receive the specific projections of VPL and VPM, with the majority of the cells projecting to area 3.

The Ventral Posterior Inferior Nucleus (VPI). This is a small subdivision of the ventral posterior nuclear mass that lies ventral to VPL and VPM near their junction. This nucleus, composed of scattered light-staining medium-sized cells, lies dorsal to fibers of the thalamic fasciculus (Olszewski, '52). Certain evidence suggests that these cells may serve to relay vestibular impulses to the cerebral cortex. Isolated stimulation of the vestibular nerve in the monkey evokes short latency responses in VPI which are abolished by vestibular nerve section, but are not affected by total cerebellectomy (Deecke et al., '73, '74). Antidromic stimulation of the parietal cortex suggests that neurons in VPI project to caudal portions of the postcentral gyrus, near the junction of Brodmann's areas 2 and 5 (Fig. 19-5). These authors (Deecke et al., '73, '74) regard this region of the parietal cortex as the primary vestibular area and suggest it may be associated with conscious vestibular perception.

The Posterior Thalamic Zone. Caudal to the ventral posterior nucleus there is a transitional diencephalic zone with a complex and varied cellular morphology. This posterior zone lies ventral to the lateral posterior nucleus and medial to the principal part of the medial geniculate body (Fig. 15-4). Part of this region contains the large cells of the magnocellular part of the medial geniculate body. This region is of interest because it receives spinothalamic fibers (Mehler et al., '60; Bowsher, '61) and appears to be concerned with the perception of painful and noxious stimuli (Poggio and Mountcastle, '60). Spinothalamic fibers project bilaterally about cells in this region (Mehler, '66b). Physiological evidence (Poggio and Mountcastle, '60; Emmers, '65) indicates that cells in this region are activated by somatic sensory stimuli, but that mechano-receptive cells are not place specific and there is only a vague representation of the body image within this region. Cells of this region are not modality specific in that many cells may respond to tactile, vibratory or auditory stimuli. None of the cells in this thalamic region has been observed to be activated by gentle rotation of joints. The majority of cells in this region respond to noxious stimuli. Neurons responding to nociceptive stimuli are related to large, and usually bilateral, receptive fields. Thalamic neurons of this region, which includes the magnocellular part of the medial geniculate body, are considered to project in a sustaining fashion upon the second somatic area of the cortex (Rose and Woolsey, '58). It seems likely that cells of this posterior thalamic zone have a diverse polysensory input and that it may be the locus of complex sensory interactions.

The Medial Geniculate Body

The medial geniculate body (MGB) usually is described as consisting of a small-celled dorsal nucleus (parvocellular part) and a large-celled ventral nucleus (magnocellular part) (Figs. 13-17, 15-3 and 15-4). More detailed cytoarchitectural studies of the medial geniculate body suggest that the pars principalis (parvocellular part) consists of two distinct divisions, designated as the dorsal and ventral parts (Morest, '64). Cells of the ventral division contain neurons with tufted dendrites considered to be typical of regions with a relatively homogeneous input. Cells of the dorsal division exhibit radiating dendrites similar to cells of the reticular formation which have a variety of dissimilar connections. Cells of the magnocellular division have radiating dendrites with branches occurring at irregular intervals; these cells appear to have the properties of an interstitial nucleus suited for relay of multiple fiber systems. In the ventral nucleus of the pars principalis dendrites of cells, and fibers of the brachium of the inferior colliculus, form laminae arranged as curved vertical sheets and spirals (Morest, '65). This lamination appears similar in some respects to that which is well known in the lateral geniculate body, but in the medial geniculate body this organization is evident only in Golgi preparations. Furthermore, this lamination in the MGB is seen only in the ventral division of pars principalis which is the major site of termination of axons from the central nucleus of the inferior colliculus.

The principal cortical projection of the medial geniculate body is to the superior temporal convolution (transverse gyrus of Heschl) via the geniculotemporal or auditory radiations (Figs. 12-10, 15-12 and 15-13). This cortical projection area (area 41) is presumed to have a tonotopic localization in which high tones are appreciated in medial regions and low tones in anterior and lateral regions. The tonotopic localization at the cortical level is neither simple nor easily defined (Whitfield, '67). While there is a well established tonotopic organization in the cochlear nuclei and in the inferior colliculus, little evidence has favored a similar organization in the medial geniculate body (Whitfield, '67). Studies in the cat suggest a clear tonotopic organization in the medial geniculate body in which low frequencies are represented laterally and high frequencies are located medially in the principal division (Aitkin and Webster, '71). The tonotopic sequence in the medial geniculate body conforms to the pattern of lamination described in Golgi material by Morest ('65). This lamination in part parallels the lateral convex surface of the medial geniculate body and is traversed in sequence by an electrode passing medially from the lateral surface.

Some fibers from the medial geniculate nucleus also pass to the ventral and lateral thalamic nuclei, as well as to parts of the pulvinar. In addition parts of the medial geniculate body project fibers or collaterals to the inferior colliculus, the nucleus of the lateral lemniscus, the trapezoid body and the superior olivary nucleus (Ades, '41). One of the characteristic features of the auditory pathways (Rasmussen, '60) is that ascending fibers connecting the nuclei at various levels are to a degree paralleled by similar, although less extensive, descending pathways, which may serve as a regulatory feedback mechanism.

The magnocellular part of the medial

geniculate body is reported to be unresponsive to supramaximal click stimuli (Rose and Galambos, '52), but as previously mentioned, part of this subdivision is related to the posterior thalamic zone which receives a polysensory input. Regions ventral to the medial geniculate body give rise to fibers of the ventral supraoptic decussation (Gudden) which cross to the opposite side and terminate in the medial geniculate body and its capsule (Fig. 16-10).

The Lateral Geniculate Body

The lateral geniculate body (LGB), which is intimately associated with the optic tract, consists in most mammals of a dorsal and a ventral nucleus. The former is connected with the ventral thalamic nucleus, pulvinar and striate area of the cortex. The ventral nucleus apparently represents a subthalamic structure related to the zona incerta. In man the ventral nucleus is represented by the pregeniculate nucleus located rostral to the principal nucleus (Polyak, '57). The principal nucleus is a laminated mass with the shape of a horseshoe, whose hilus is directed ventromedially (Figs. 15-3, 15-4 and 15-14). It is composed of six concentrically arranged cell layers that are separated by intervening fiber bands. The four outer layers consist of small and medium-sized cells; in the two narrower, inner layers the cells are large and more loosely arranged (magnocellular nucleus of Malone, '10). According to the scheme of numbering shown in Figure 15-14, crossed fibers of the optic tract terminate on laminae 1, 4 and 6, while uncrossed fibers end in laminae 2, 3 and 5. Phylogenetically, the nucleus first differentiates into three cell layers. It becomes six-layered in forms where the optic tracts show a partial decussation, the uncrossed and crossed portions each terminating upon three different laminae (Minkowski, '13; Clark, '32).

Retinal projections to the lateral geniculate body are highly organized and have a sharply defined topographical representation (Noback and Laemle, '70). Minute lesions in the retina produce transneuronal degeneration in small, well delimited clusters of cells in three layers of the LGB on

Dorsolateral

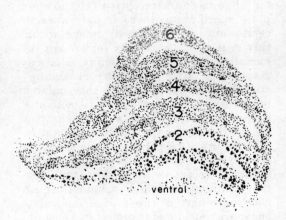

Ventromedial

FIG. 15-14. Drawing of the cellular lamination of the lateral geniculate body. Laminae *1* and *2* constitute the magnocellular layers; the *ventral nucleus* is shown *below*. Crossed fibers of the optic tract terminate in laminae *1, 4* and *6;* uncrossed fibers terminate in laminae *2, 3* and *5.*

each side; the layers in which these cell changes occur differ in accordance with the disposition of crossed and uncrossed retinal fibers (Polyak, '57; Matthews et al., '60). Each neuron of the lateral geniculate body receives a direct input from the retina and projects directly to the visual cortex (striate cortex, area 17). Cells within this nucleus exhibit both convergence and divergence. A retinofugal fiber may synapse with several neurons in the LGB (divergence), and each neuron of the LGB may receive inputs from several retinofugal fibers (convergence). Retinofugal fibers from ganglion cells of the retina establish different types of synaptic articulations with LGB neurons (Colonnier and Guillery, '64; Campos-Ortega et al., '68). These fibers terminate axosomatically and axodendritically upon primary and secondary dendrites, in boutons *en passage* and in complex glomerular endings. Glomeruli in the LGB constitute a synaptic complex of interlocking nerve processes of various origins which are arranged in a specific manner and separated from the environment by a capsule of glial processes (Fig. 15-15) (Szentágothai, '70). The axon termi-

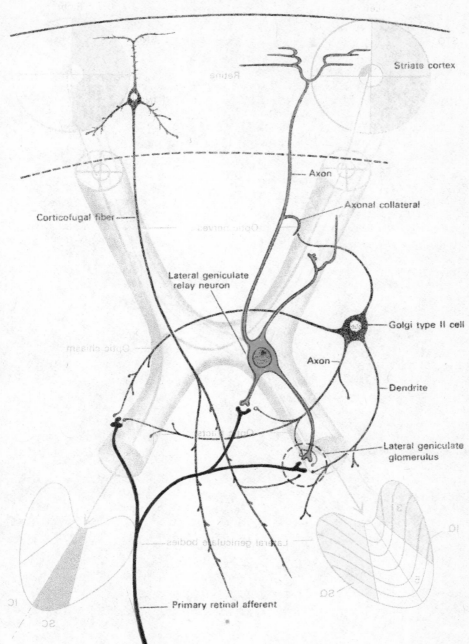

Fig. 15-15.　Schematic diagram of the neuronal arrangements in a glomerulus of the lateral geniculate body. A primary retinal afferent is indicated in *red*, while the *LGB* relay neuron is in *blue*. A corticofugal fiber and a Golgi type II cell are shown in *black*. The glomerulus contains a terminal of a primary retinal afferent, several club-shaped terminals of a *LGB* relay neuron and contributions from both Golgi type II neurons and corticofugal fibers. This synaptic complex is enclosed in a capsule of glial processes, indicated by the *dashed line* (modified from Szentágothai, '70).

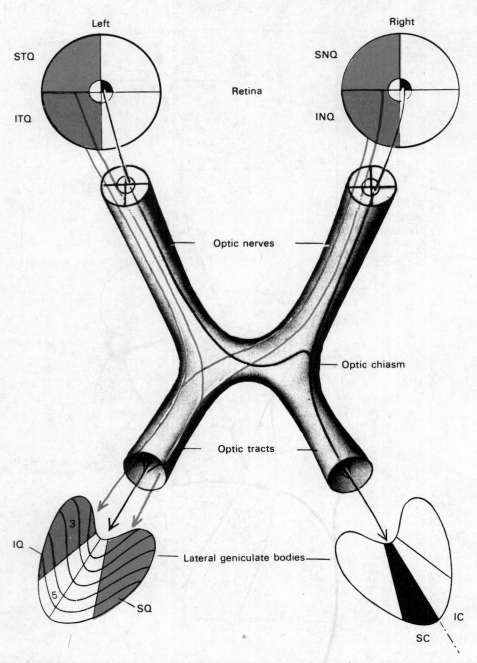

Left

Right

STQ

SNQ

Retina

ITQ

INQ

Optic nerves

Optic chiasm

Optic tracts

IQ

3

5

SQ

Lateral geniculate bodies

IC

SC

FIG. 15-16. Schematic diagram of retinal ganglion cell projections through the optic nerves, optic chiasm and optic tracts to terminations within the lateral geniculate bodies. Superior peripheral quadrants of the retina on both sides (*SNQ*, superior nasal quadrant; *STQ*, superior temporal quadrant) shown in *red* project to the medial part (*SQ*) of the left lateral geniculate body (*red*). Inferior peripheral quadrants of the retina (*INQ*, inferior nasal quadrant; *ITQ*, inferior temporal quadrant) shown in *blue* project to the lateral part (*IQ*) of the left lateral geniculate body (*blue*). Superior central regions of the retina on nasal and temporal sides (*black*) on the opposite side project to the region of the right lateral geniculate body indicated by *SC*. Inferior central regions of the retina project in the same fashion to the region of the right lateral geniculate body indicated by *IC*. *Numbers* in the left lateral geniculate body indicate two of the six laminae. (Based on Hoyt and Luis, '62; Noback and Laemle, '70.)

nals of retinal afferents occupy the central position in these glomeruli. Unlike the cerebellar glomeruli which contain only one mossy fiber rosette, several club-shaped retinal afferents may occur in a LGB glomerulus. Other contributions to the glomeruli arise from Golgi type II cells and corticofugal fibers. Glomeruli often are located at the bifurcation of stem dendrites of a LGB neuron. Axons of Golgi type II cells enter the glomeruli and establish synapses with relay cell (LGB neuron) dendrites; these cells are considered to be inhibitory in nature. The LGB glomerular complex contains: (1) axodendritic synapses on stem, secondary and peripheral dendrites, and (2) axoaxonic synapses in which the presynaptic portion is contributed by terminals of the retinofugal fibers. The most remarkable feature of these glomeruli is the frequent occurrence of axoaxonic synapses. It is assumed that the synaptic arrangements within the glomeruli are effective in the versatile processing of information. The interpretation of the structural arrangement within the LGB glomeruli suggests that optic afferents by depolarizing Golgi cell terminals would presynaptically inhibit the inhibitory influence exerted by these cells upon geniculate body neurons (Szentágothai, '70). This concept of presynaptic disinhibition by retinal afferents appears attractive because LGB neurons exhibit less activity if the visual field is uniformly illuminated than if there is a sharp contrast of light and dark projected upon the retina.

Information concerning the retinotopic organization of retinofugal fibers in the optic nerve, chiasm, tract and lateral geniculate body in man and monkey is based upon extensive research (Brouwer and Zeeman, '26; Polyak, '57; Hoyt and Luis, '62, '63). Nonmacular fibers from the retina maintain their retinal topography throughout the optic nerve. At the chiasm retinal projections shift their positions so that in the optic tract: (1) uncrossed fibers from the superior temporal quadrant of the retina occupy a dorsomedial location and fibers from the lower temporal quadrant occupy an inferior lateral location, and (2) crossed fibers from the superior nasal quadrant of the retina occupy a medial location, while fibers from the inferior nasal quadrant assume a ventrolateral position (Fig. 15-16). Macular fibers pass through central and peripheral regions of the optic nerve, and after decussating in the chiasm, both crossed and uncrossed fibers occupy superior parts of the optic tract. The macular projection is extensively mixed with that from peripheral retinal areas in all but the most distal part of the optic nerve (Hoyt and Luis, '62). Macular axons are mainly fine caliber fibers while those from nonmacular regions are large caliber fibers.

In the lateral geniculate body fibers from the superior nonmacular quadrants of the retina project to medial regions, while inferior nonmacular quadrants of the retina project to lateral regions (Fig. 15-16). The macular region of the retina projects to a wedge-shaped sector in the posterior two-thirds of the LGB.

The lateral geniculate nucleus is the main end station of the optic tract. It projects to the calcarine cortex (area 17) by the geniculocalcarine tract or visual radiations. It has been generally accepted that corticogeniculate fibers arising from the primary visual cortex project back to the LGB (Garey et al., '68; Giolli and Guthrie, '71). This view has been challenged by Holländer ('72), who found that area 18 rather than 17 projected to the LGB. Intranuclear connections of the LGB are with the pulvinar, and the ventral and lateral thalamic nuclei.

The Thalamic Reticular Nucleus

The thalamic reticular nucleus (RN) is a thin neuronal shell which surrounds the lateral, antero-superior and antero-inferior aspects of the dorsal thalamus (Figs. 15-6, 15-10, 15-11 and 15-12). This thalamic nuclear envelope develops embryologically from the mantle layer of the subthalamus and migrates dorsally between the external medullary lamina of the thalamus and the internal capsule (Kuhlenbeck, '48; Dekaban, '54). Thus this nucleus actually is a derivative of the ventral thalamus, although it surrounds the lateral aspect of the dorsal thalamus. Cells of this nucleus are said to resemble those of adjacent thalamic nuclei (Walker, '38). According to

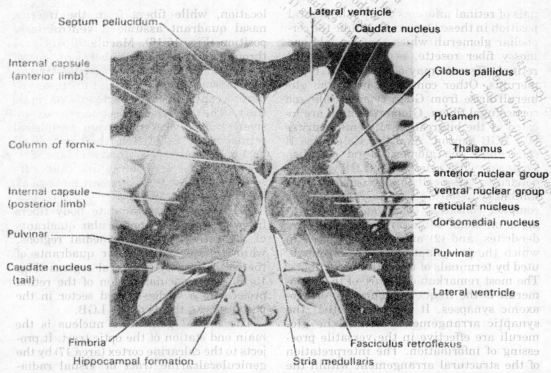

Septum pellucidum

Internal capsule
(anterior limb)

Column of fornix

Internal capsule
(posterior limb)

Pulvinar

Caudate nucleus
(tail)

Fimbria

Hippocampal formation

Lateral ventricle

Caudate nucleus

Globus pallidus

Putamen

Thalamus

anterior nuclear group

ventral nuclear group

reticular nucleus

dorsomedial nucleus

Pulvinar

Lateral ventricle

Fasciculus retroflexus

Stria medullaris

FIG. 15-17. Horizontal section through thalamus, internal capsule and basal ganglia. Weigert's myelin stain. Photograph.

Scheibel and Scheibel ('66), Golgi studies of the reticular nucleus show that its neurons are similar to those of the brain stem reticular formation in that they are multipolar, vary in size from medium to large and lie immersed in a complex neuropil. Dendrites of cells are long, relatively unramified and without specific orientation. The main axons of the majority of cells turn caudally and penetrate deeply into the thalamus, although some axons appear to run exclusively within the reticular nucleus. About one-fifth of the axons from cells in the reticular nucleus, directed caudally, are said to enter the mesencephalic tegmentum and end among clusters of reticular neurons. Golgi preparations (Scheibel and Scheibel, '66) provide no evidence that fibers of this nucleus have cortical terminations. Although cells in the reticular nucleus are said to undergo degeneration following cortical ablations (Rose and Woolsey, '43; Rose, '52), degeneration occurs late and is less severe than in cortically dependent thalamic nuclei. It

has been suggested that cell changes and cell loss in the reticular nuclei under these conditions may be transneuronal. The reticular nucleus of the thalamus receives cortical afferent fibers which are organized topographically (Carman et al., '64). Thus the reticular nucleus of the thalamus does not appear to be part of a nonspecific thalamic pathway to the cortex. Since its major projections are to specific and nonspecific thalamic nuclei, it may serve to integrate intrathalamic activities.

THE THALAMIC RADIATIONS AND INTERNAL CAPSULE

Fibers which reciprocally connect the thalamus and the cortex constitute the thalamic radiations. These thalamocortical and corticothalamic fibers form a continuous fan that emerges along the whole lateral extent of the caudate nucleus. Fiber bundles, radiating forward, backward, upward and downward, form large portions of various parts of the internal capsule (Figs. 2-8, 2-9, 2-10, 15-17 and 15-18). Al-

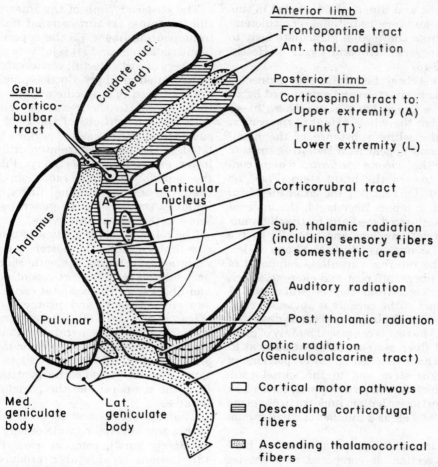

FIG. 15-18. Schematic diagram of the right internal capsule as seen in a horizontal section similar to that shown in Figure 15-17. The blood supply of the thalamus, internal capsule and basal ganglia is shown in Figures 20-11 and 20-12.

though the radiations connect with practically all parts of the cortex, the richness of connections varies considerably for specific cortical areas. Most abundant are the projections to the frontal granular cortex, the precentral and postcentral gyri, the calcarine area and the gyrus of Heschl. The posterior parietal region and adjacent portions of the temporal lobe also have rich thalamic connections, but relatively scanty radiations go to other cortical areas (Walker, '38) (Fig. 15-13).

The thalamic radiations are grouped into four subradiations designated as the thalamic *peduncles* (Fig. 15-18). The *anterior* or *frontal peduncle* connects the frontal lobe with the medial and anterior tha-

lamic nuclei. The *superior* or *centroparietal peduncle* connects the Rolandic area and adjacent portions of the frontal and parietal lobes with the ventral tier thalamic nuclei. The fibers, carrying general sensory impulses from the body and head, form part of this radiation and terminate in the postcentral gyrus (Figs. 15-12, 15-13 and 15-18). The *posterior* or *occipital peduncle* connects the occipital and posterior parietal convolutions with the caudal portions of the thalamus. It includes the optic radiations (geniculocalcarine) from the lateral geniculate body to the calcarine cortex (striate area). The *inferior* or *temporal peduncle* is small and includes the scanty connections of the thalamus with the temporal lobe and the insula. Included in this are the auditory radiations (geniculotemporal) from the medial geniculate body to the transverse temporal gyrus of Heschl (Fig. 15-18).

The cerebral hemisphere is connected with the brain stem and spinal cord by an extensive projection system. These fibers arise from the whole extent of the cortex, enter the white substance of the hemisphere and appear as a radiating mass of fibers, the *corona radiata,* which converges toward the brain stem (Figs. 2-8 and 2-10). On reaching the latter they form a broad, compact fiber band, the *internal capsule,* flanked medially by the thalamus and caudate nucleus and laterally by the lenticular nucleus (Figs. 15-17 and 15-18). Thus the internal capsule is composed of all the fibers, afferent and efferent, which go to, or come from, the cerebral cortex. A large part of the capsule is obviously composed of the thalamic radiations described above. The rest is composed mainly of corticofugal fiber systems (efferent cortical fibers) which descend to lower portions of the brain stem and to the spinal cord. These include the corticospinal, corticobulbar, corticoreticular and corticopontine tracts, as well as a number of smaller bundles.

The internal capsule, as seen in a horizontal section, is composed of a shorter *anterior* and a longer *posterior limb,* which meet at an obtuse angle, forming a junctional zone known as the *genu* (Figs. 2-9, 2-10, 15-17 and 15-18). The anterior limb lies between the lenticular and caudate nuclei. The posterior limb of the internal capsule *(lenticulothalamic portion)* lies between the lenticular nucleus and the thalamus. A *retrolenticular* part of the internal capsule extends caudally for a short distance behind the lenticular nucleus. In this caudal region a number of fibers passing beneath the lenticular nucleus to reach the temporal lobe collectively form the *sublenticular* portion of the internal capsule.

The *anterior limb* of the internal capsule contains the anterior thalamic radiation or peduncle, and the prefrontal corticopontine tract. The *genu* contains corticobulbar and corticoreticular fibers.

The *posterior limb* of the internal capsule contains: (1) corticospinal fibers, (2) frontopontine fibers, (3) the superior thalamic radiation, and (4) relatively smaller numbers of corticotectal, corticorubral and corticoreticular fibers. Corticospinal fibers are organized in a specific manner so that those closest to the genu are concerned with cervical portions of the body, while succeeding, more caudal regions are related to the upper extremity, trunk and lower extremity, respectively. Fibers of the superior thalamic radiation, located caudal to the corticospinal fibers, project impulses concerned with general somatic sense to the postcentral gyrus.

The *retrolenticular portion* of the posterior limb contains the posterior thalamic radiations, including the optic radiations, parietal and occipital corticopontine fibers and fibers from the occipital cortex to the superior colliculi and pretectal region (Figs. 15-3 and 15-18). The *sublenticular portion,* difficult to separate from the retrolenticular, contains the *inferior thalamic peduncle* (Fig. 15-9), the auditory radiations (Fig. 15-18) and corticopontine fibers from the temporal and the parieto-occipital areas.

Thalamocortical and corticofugal fibers within the internal capsule occupy a comparatively small, compact area (Fig. 15-18). Lesions in this area produce more widespread disability than lesions in any other region of the nervous system. Thrombosis or hemorrhage of the anterior choroidal, striate or capsular branches of the middle cerebral arteries (Fig. 20-12) are responsible for most injuries to the internal capsule. Vascular lesions in the posterior limb of the internal capsule may result in contralateral hemianesthesia of the head, trunk and limbs due to injury of thalamocortical fibers *en route* to the sensory cortex. There is also a contralateral hemiplegia due to injury of the corticospinal tracts. If the genu of the internal capsule is involved in the injury, corticobulbar fibers also are destroyed. Lesions in the posterior third of the posterior limb may include the optic and auditory radiations. In such instances there may be a contralateral triad consisting of hemianesthesia, hemianopsia and hemihypacusis. More extensive vascular lesions may include the thalamus or corpus striatum, so that affective changes and symptoms due to injury of the basal ganglia may be added to those characteristic of injury to the internal capsule.

THE VISUAL PATHWAYS

The Retina. The retina arises as an evaginated portion of the brain, the optic pouch, which secondarily is invaginated to form the two-layered optic cup. The outer layer gives rise to pigmented epithelium. The inner layer forms the neural portion of the retina, from which are differentiated the bipolar rod and cone cells, the bipolar and horizontal neurons (confined within the retina itself) and the multipolar ganglionic neurons whose axons form the optic nerve (Fig. 15-19). The inner layer thus constitutes a fiber tract connecting two parts of the brain. Its fibers possess no Schwann sheaths, and its connective tissue investments represent continuations of the meningeal sheaths of the brain (i.e., pia, arachnoid and dura).

The rod and cone cells are visual receptors which react specifically to physical light. The cones, numbering some 7 million in the human eye, have a higher threshold of excitability and are stimulated by light of relatively high intensity. They are responsible for sharp visual definition and for color discrimination in adequate illumination. The rods, whose number has been estimated at more than 100 million, react to low intensities of illumination and subserve twilight and night vision. Close to the posterior pole of the eye, the retina shows a small, circular, yellowish area, the *macula lutea,* in direct line with the visual axis. The macula represents the retinal area for central vision, and the eyes are fixed in such a manner that the retinal image of any object is always focused on the macula. The rest of the retina is concerned with paracentral and peripheral vision. In the macular region the inner layers of the retina are pushed apart, forming a small central pit, the *fovea centralis,* which constitutes the point of sharpest vision and most acute color discrimination. Here the retina is composed entirely of closely packed slender cones.

The rods and cones are composed of an outer segment, a narrow neck, an inner segment, a cell body and a synaptic base (Fig. 15-20). Photopigments are present in the outer segments, where the photochemical reactions to light take place that give rise to the generator potential. The outer segment is composed of a series of laminated discs derived from the infolding of the plasma membrane. The photopigments, bound to the membranes of the discs, are constantly renewed. Rhodopsin is the photopigment of the rods in primates, and three pigments with maximum absorptions for blue, green and red are present in the cones (Wald, '68). The synaptic base of the cone is called a pedicle, while that of the rod is referred to as a spherule. Each cone pedicle has several invaginations which contain terminals of horizontal, midget bipolar and flat bipolar cells in a specific arrangement. Rod spherules have a single invagination containing multiple processes of horizontal and rod bipolar cells (Fig. 15-20) (Noback and Laemle, '70). Each midget ganglion cell makes several synaptic contacts with a single midget bipolar cell. Diffuse ganglion cells establish synaptic contacts with all types of bipolar cells (Dowling and Boycott, '66). Horizontal cells and amacrine cells constitute retinal interneurons. It is difficult to determine whether processes of horizontal cells are axons or dendrites, and it is possible that each process may be capable of both receiving and transmitting signals. Amacrine cells in the inner plexiform layer have no axon, but make synaptic contacts with all types of bipolar cells, other amacrine cells and the dendrites and somata of ganglion cells. The axons of ganglion cells, at first unmyelinated, are arranged in fine radiating bundles which run parallel to the retinal surface and converge at the optic disc to form the optic nerve. On emerging from the eyeball the fibers immediately acquire a myelin sheath, and there is a consequent increase in the size of the optic nerve.

The Optic Nerves. These nerves enter the cranial cavity through the optic foramina and unite to form the optic chiasm,

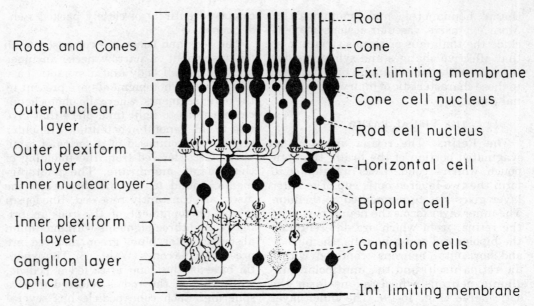

Fig. 15-19. Neural elements of the human retina as schematically drawn from Golgi preparations. *A* represents an amacrine cell (modified from Walls, '63).

beyond which they are continued as the optic tracts. Within the chiasm a partial decussation occurs, the fibers from the nasal halves of the retina crossing to the opposite side, and those from the temporal halves of the retina remaining uncrossed (Fig. 15-21). In binocular vision each visual field, right and left, is projected upon portions of both retinae. Thus the images of objects in the right field of vision (*red* in Fig. 15-21) are projected on the right nasal and the left temporal half of the retina. In the chiasm the fibers from these two retinal portions are combined to form the left optic tract, which represents the complete right field of vision. By this arrangement the whole right field of vision is projected upon the left hemisphere, and the left visual field upon the right hemisphere.

The Optic Tract. On each side the optic tract sweeps outward and backward, encircling the hypothalamus and the rostral portions of the crus cerebri. Most of its fibers terminate in the lateral geniculate body, although small portions continue as the brachium of the superior colliculus to the superior colliculi and pretectal area (Fig. 15-21). Although the existence of retinohypothalamic fibers has been suggested by many authors, only recently have these assumptions been confirmed. Using autoradiographic technics it has been possible to establish that retinal fibers terminate bilaterally in the suprachiasmatic nucleus of the hypothalamus in a variety of mammals, including the monkey (Moore and Lenn, '72; Moore, '73; Pierson and Carpenter, '74). This direct projection from the retina has functional relevance to mechanisms of neuroendocrine regulation.

The lateral geniculate body gives rise to the geniculocalcarine tract which forms the last relay to the visual cortex. The superior colliculus is concerned with detection of movement with the visual fields and with the coordination of eye and head movements. The pretectal region is concerned with the pupillary light reflex.

The Geniculocalcarine Tract. This tract arises from the lateral geniculate body, passes through the retrolenticular portion of the internal capsule and forms the optic radiations, which end in the striate cortex (area 17), located on the medial surface of the occipital lobe. These fibers terminate on both banks of the calcarine sulcus (Figs. 2-4, 15-13 and 15-21). All fibers of this radiation do not reach the cortex by the shortest route (Figs. 15-21 and 15-22). The most dorsal fibers pass almost

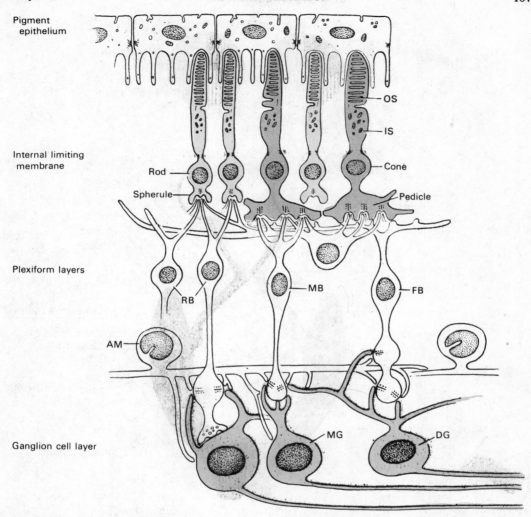

Pigment epithelium

OS

IS

Internal limiting membrane

Rod

Cone

Spherule

Pedicle

Plexiform layers

MB

FB

RB

AM

Ganglion cell layer

MG

DG

Fig. 15-20. Schematic diagram of the ultrastructural organization of the retina. Rods (*blue*) and cones (*red*) are composed of an outer segment (*OS*), an inner segment (*IS*), a cell body and a synaptic base. Photopigments are present in the outer segments (*OS*) which are composed of laminated discs. The synaptic base of the rod is called the spherule, while the synaptic base of the cone is called the pedicle. In the plexiform layers *RB* indicates rod bipolar cells, *MB* a midget bipolar cell and *FB* a flat bipolar cell. *AM* indicates an amacrine cell. Ganglion cells (*MG*, midget ganglion cell; *DG*, diffuse ganglion cell) and retinal afferents are in *yellow* (modified from Dowling and Boycott, '66; Noback and Laemle, '70).

directly backward to the striate area. Those placed more ventrally first turn forward and downward into the temporal lobe, and spread out over the rostral part of the inferior horn of the lateral ventricle; these fibers then loop backward and run close to the outer wall of the lateral ventricle (external sagittal stratum) to reach the occipital cortex (Fig. 2-16). The most ventral fibers make the longest loop; some

of these extend into the uncal region of the temporal lobe before turning backwards (Figs. 15-21 and 15-22).

The retinal areas have a precise point-to-point relationship with the lateral geniculate body, each portion of the retina projecting on a specific and topographically limited portion of the geniculate body (Fig. 15-16). The fibers from the upper retinal quadrants (representing the lower visual

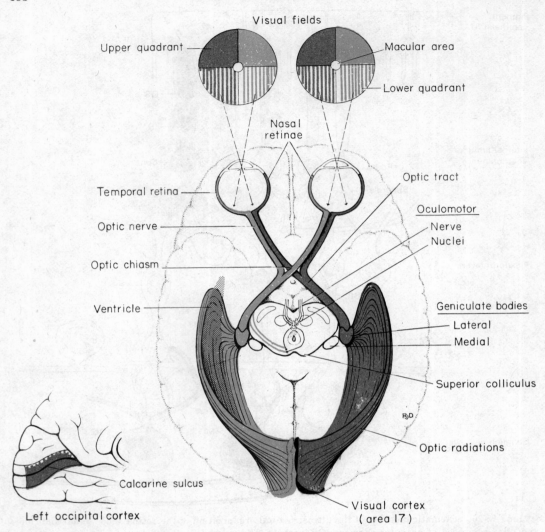

Visual fields

Upper quadrant

Macular area

Lower quadrant

Nasal
retinae

Temporal retina

Optic tract

Optic nerve

Oculomotor
Nerve
Nuclei

Optic chiasm

Ventricle

Geniculate bodies
Lateral
Medial

Superior colliculus

Optic radiations

Calcarine sulcus

Left occipital cortex

Visual cortex
(area 17)

FIG. 15-21. Diagram of the visual pathways viewed from the ventral surface of the brain. Light from the upper half of the visual field falls on the inferior half of the retina. Light from the temporal half of the visual field falls on the nasal half of the retina, while light from the nasal half of the visual field falls on the temporal half of the retina. The visual pathways from the retina to the striate cortex are shown. The plane of the visual fields has been rotated 90 degrees toward the reader. The insert shows the projection of the quadrants of the visual field upon the left calcarine (striate) cortex. The macular area of the retina is represented nearest the occipital pole. Fibers mediating the pupillary light reflex leave the optic tract and project to the pretectal region; other fibers relay impulses to the visceral nuclei of the oculomotor complex.

field) terminate in the medial half, those from the lower quadrants in the lateral half of the geniculate body. The macular fibers occupy the central portion, flanked medially and laterally by fibers from the paracentral and peripheral retinal areas. A similar point-to-point relation exists between the geniculate body and the striate

cortex. The medial half of the lateral geniculate body, representing the upper retinal quadrants (lower visual fields), projects to the superior lip of the calcarine sulcus, and these fibers form the superior portion of the optic radiations (Fig. 15-21). The lateral half of the lateral geniculate body, representing the lower retinal quad-

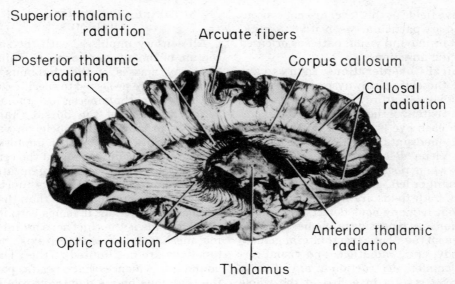

Superior thalamic radiation

Arcuate fibers

Posterior thalamic radiation

Corpus callosum

Callosal radiation

Optic radiation

Anterior thalamic radiation

Thalamus

FIG. 15-22. Dissection of brain from medial surface, showing internal capsule (thalamic radiations) and portions of callosal radiation. Photograph.

rants (upper visual field), projects to the inferior lip of the calcarine sulcus. These fibers occupy the inferior portion of the optic radiations. The macular fibers, which constitute the intermediate part of the optic radiations, terminate in the caudal third of the calcarine cortex. Those from the paracentral and peripheral retinal areas end in respectively more rostral portions.

Experimental studies (Kuffler, '53) with stationary spots of light indicate that the receptive fields of ganglion cells in the retina are organized in concentric zones with either an "on" or "off" type of discharge in the center and the reverse in the periphery or surround (Fig. 19-15). The concept of receptive fields in the visual system has been critically reviewed by Jacobs ('69). In the retina the receptive field consists of those receptors, rods and cones, and retinal neurons, which influence the excitability of a single ganglion cell. The retina is a composite of as many receptive fields as there are ganglion cells. Each receptive field is organized into two zones: (1) a small circular central zone, and (2) a surrounding concentric zone referred to as the periphery or surround. These two zones are functionally antagonistic. Two general types of receptive fields have been de-

scribed: (1) those with an "on" center and an "off" surround, and (2) those with an "off" center and an "on" surround. If a light stimulus illuminates (or is withdrawn from) an "on" center, or an "on" surround, the ganglion cell will fire vigorously. If the light stimulus illuminates both "on" and "off" zones, which exhibit mutual inhibition, the stimuli cancel each other. According to Dowling and Boycott ('66), retinal connections account for the concentric circular receptive fields at the ganglion cell level. Impulses from the central zone are said to be mediated by direct connections between receptor cells, bipolar cells and ganglion cells, while the antagonistic surround zone has interposed connections with amacrine cells (i.e., between bipolar and ganglion cells).

The receptive fields of neurons in the lateral geniculate body appear similar with stationary spots of light (Hubel and Wiesel, '61). The major difference between the receptive fields for ganglion cells and lateral geniculate cells is that cells of the LGB show a greater suppression of the receptive field periphery (Jacobs, '69). This suggests that LGB neurons receive multiple inputs from the optic tract. However, studies (Hubel and Wiesel, '62, '63) of single units in the striate cortex reveal that receptive fields at this level are not concentric and are particularly sensitive to "slits" of light or moving visual patterns oriented in specific directions.

Clinical Considerations. Injury to any part of the optic pathway produces visual defects whose nature depends on the location and extent of the injury. During examination each eye is covered in turn as the retinal quadrants of the opposite eye are tested. Visual defects are said to be *homonymous* when restricted to a single visual field, right or left, and *heteronymous* when parts of both fields are involved. It is evident that homonymous defects are caused by lesions on one side anywhere behind the chiasm (i.e., optic tract, lateral geniculate body, optic radiations and visual cortex). Complete destruction of any of these structures results in a loss of the whole opposite field of vision (*homonymous hemianopsia*) (Fig. 15-23C); partial injury may produce *quadrantic homonymous* defects. Lesions of the temporal lobe, by compressing or destroying the looping fibers in the lower portion of the optic radiations, are likely to produce such quadrantic defects in the upper visual field. Injury to the parietal lobe may involve the more superiorly placed fibers of the radiations and cause similar defects in the lower field of vision.

Lesions of the chiasm may cause several kinds of heteronymous defects. Most commonly the crossing fibers from the nasal portions of the retina are involved, with consequent loss of the two temporal fields of vision (*bitemporal hemianopsia*) (Fig. 15-23D). Rarely, both lateral angles of the chiasm may be compressed; in such cases the nondecussating fibers from the temporal retinae are affected, and the result is loss of the nasal visual fields (*binasal hemianopsia*). Injury of one optic nerve naturally produces blindness in the corresponding eye with loss of the pupillary light reflex (Fig. 15-23A). The pupil will, however, contract consensually to light entering the other eye, since the pretectal reflex center is related bilaterally to visceral nuclei of the oculomotor complex. The pupillary reflex will not be affected by lesions of the visual pathway above the brachium of the superior colliculus (Fig. 15-21).

FUNCTIONAL CONSIDERATIONS OF THE THALAMUS

All sensory impulses, with the sole exception of the olfactory ones, terminate in the gray masses of the thalamus, from which they are projected to specific cortical areas by the thalamocortical radiations. While portions of the dorsal thalamus serve as primary relay nuclei in various sensory pathways in which impulses are projected to specific regions of the cerebral cortex, the structure and organization of the thalamus indicate that its function is more complex and elaborate than that of a simple relay station. It seems certain that the thalamus is the chief sensory integrating mechanism of the neuraxis, but its functions are not limited to this. There is abundant evidence that specific parts of the thalamus play a dominant role in the maintenance and regulation of the state of consciousness, alertness and attention, through widespread functional influences upon the activity of the cerebral cortex. The thalamus is concerned not only with general and specific types of awareness, but with certain emotional connotations that accompany, or are associated with, most sensory experiences. Other data suggest that some thalamic nuclei serve as integrative centers for motor functions, since they receive the principal efferent projections from the cerebellum and the basal ganglia.

In terms of physiological functions the thalamus and related neuronal subsystems are concerned with high fidelity transmission of sensory information, with input selection, output tuning, synchronization and desynchronization of cortical activity, parallel processing of information and signal storing and modification (Purpura, '70).

The Specific Sensory Relay Nuclei. Specific sensory relay nuclei of the thalamus are in the ventral tier of the lateral nuclear group. These include the medial and lateral geniculate bodies and the two divisions of the ventral posterior nucleus. The medial geniculate body receives fibers from the inferior colliculus. The parvocellular part of the nucleus, concerned with audition, projects fibers via the geniculotemporal radiations to the transverse tem-

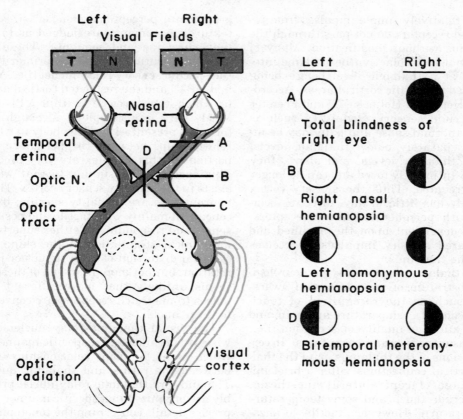

FIG. 15-23. Diagram of common lesions within the visual pathway. On the *left, A* through *D* indicate lesions. Corresponding visual field defects are shown on the *right* (modified from Haymaker, '56).

poral gyrus of Heschl, the *primary auditory area* (Figs. 12-10 and 15-13). The lateral geniculate body, receiving both crossed and uncrossed fibers of the optic tract, gives rise to the geniculocalcarine fibers, which project in a specific way to the cortex surrounding the calcarine sulcus; this represents the *primary visual area* (Fig. 15-21). As mentioned earlier, the two divisions of the ventral posterior nucleus project to the cortex of the postcentral gyrus. In the postcentral gyrus all parts of the body are represented in a definite sequence (Penfield and Rasmussen, '50); this cortical region is referred to as the *primary somesthetic area* (somatic sensory area I). The sensory representation of the body in somatic sensory area I is duplicated in reverse sequence at the base of the postcentral gyrus along the border of the lateral sulcus (Penfield and Boldrey, '37; Woolsey, '58). This second topographi-

cal body representation, known as *somatic sensory area II* (somatic area II), receives fibers from the posterior part of the ventral posterior nucleus and the posterior thalamic zone caudal to it (Fig. 15-4) (Knighton, '50; Rose and Woolsey, '58; Poggio and Mountcastle, '60; Mehler, '66a). Some intercalated thalamic neurons also may project impulses to this area (Rose and Mountcastle, '59). While ablation experiments indicate that somatic area II is not essential for somatic discrimination, the observations of Poggio and Mountcastle ('60) indicate that somatic area II is concerned in a special way with pain sensibility. This finding does not mean that pain sensations project exclusively to this area, for it is well known that electrical stimulation of the postcentral gyrus in man may evoke painful sensations, and ablations of the postcentral gyrus may eliminate certain types of pain.

The relatively simple impulses from peripheral receptors do not pass through the thalamus without modification. Many of the impulses become synthesized and integrated at a thalamic level before being projected to specific cortical areas. According to Head and Holmes ('11) and Foerster ('27), crude sensory modalities such as touch, thermal sense and pain may be injured separately below thalamic levels, but at thalamic levels, and above, they become intimately fused and can no longer be segregated. Thus the sensory cortex probably has little, if any, direct association with peripheral sensory receptors, and is dependent upon the modified and integrated sensory impulses it receives from the thalamus.

The thalamus represents the neurological substratum of a crude sort of awareness, such as the recognition of touch (mere contact), temperature and pain, and of the affective quality of sensation (i.e., its pleasantness or unpleasantness). In certain lesions of the thalamus, or of the thalamocortical connections, after a brief initial stage of contralateral anesthesia, pain, crude touch and some temperature sense return. However, tactile localization, two-point discrimination and the sense of position and movement are lost or severely impaired. The sensations recovered are poorly localized and are accompanied by a great increase in "feeling tone," most commonly of an unpleasant character. Although the threshold of excitability is raised on the affected side, tactile and thermal stimuli previously not unpleasant now evoke disagreeable sensations (dysesthesias), not easily characterized by the patient. Often the patient cannot endure innocuous cutaneous stimulation, yet he cannot tell the nature of the exciting stimulus. Occasionally the reverse occurs: a previously indifferent stimulus evokes a most pleasant feeling. These feeling states may even be induced by other sensations, for instance auditory ones (Head, '20).

There are two aspects to sensation: the discriminative and the affective. In the former, stimuli are compared with respect to intensity, locality and relative position in space and time. These impulses are integrated into perceptions of form, size and texture; movements are judged as to extent, direction and sequence. These aspects of sensation are related primarily to the specific sensory relay nuclei (i.e., VPL and VPM) and the restricted cortical areas to which they project. Within VPL and VPM there is a complete, although distorted, representation of the body in which relationships between the periphery and portions of this complex are very precise. This specificity is similar to that which exists in the primary sensory cortex. These neurons also are modality specific, being concerned mainly with tactile and position sense, and responding to either superficial mechanical stimulation of the skin, mechanical distortion of deep tissues or joint rotation, but not more than one of these. It seems unlikely that many afferent impulses from stretch receptors are conveyed to these nuclei.

The visual thalamic relay nuclei likewise are organized in a specific manner in which point for point relationships exist between the retina and thalamic nuclei. The auditory thalamic relay nuclei probably are organized in a specific manner, but precise details concerning the tonotopic arrangement in the medial geniculate body in man are lacking. Data from studies in the cat suggest that an orderly arrangement of frequency representation conforms to the laminar pattern of the medial geniculate body evident in Golgi preparations (Morest, '65; Aitkin and Webster, '71).

"Affective" sensation is concerned with pain, agreeableness and disagreeableness. Pain is a subjective sensation that often is difficult to describe and almost impossible to measure. The localization of different types of pain is often inexact and clinical judgment of its intensity must take into account the personality of the patient. Temperature and many tactile sensations likewise have a marked affective tone. This is especially true for visceral sensations, in which the discriminative element is practically absent. This affective quality, which forms the basis of general bodily well-being or *malaise*, and of the more intense emotional states, is believed to be "appreciated" by the thalamus rather than the cortex, although it may be profoundly modified and controlled by the latter. The appreciation of pain, crude touch and some temperature sense is retained even after complete destruction of the sensory cortical areas of both sides.

The Cortical Relay Nuclei. Cortical relay nuclei of the thalamus receive impulses from specific subcortical structures and project to well defined cortical regions. These nuclei include: (1) the anterior nuclei, (2) the ventral lateral nucleus, and (3) the ventral anterior nucleus (in part). The anterior nuclei of the thalamus receive the largest efferent fiber bundle from the hypothalamus, the mammillothalamic tract and direct projections from the hippocampal formation via the fornix (Figs. 15-1, 15-8, and 16-5). These nuclei in turn project to the cingulate gyrus, a cortical area demonstrated to produce a variety of visceral responses upon stimulation (Kremer, '47; Ward, '48). Impulses from the cingulate gyrus are relayed to the hippocampal formation via the entorhinal area (Raisman et al., '65). The hippocampal formation projects to the hypothalamus and to the anterior thalamic nuclei.

The ventral lateral nucleus of the thalamus, which receives cerebellar and pallidal efferent fibers, relays impulses from these sources to the precentral gyrus. Fibers from the dentate nucleus and the globus pallidus projecting to VLo represent the major outputs of the cerebellum and the basal ganglia. Anatomical data suggest that these systems overlap within this nucleus, but the physiological nature of their interaction is unknown. Since the ventral lateral nucleus is the principal subcortical structure projecting to the motor cortex, it is apparent that signals conveyed to it have profound effects upon cortical neurons that give rise to impulses that underlie the most important aspects of motor function. It seems likely that neocerebellar disturbances resulting from cerebellar lesions may be the physiological expression of release of the ventral lateral thalamic nucleus from the controlling and regulating influences normally provided by the cerebellum. With respect to the basal ganglia the situation is different in that dyskinesia (disturbances of movement) due to disease processes seems to be dependent upon the integrity of pallidothalamic fibers systems. However, lesions in the ventral lateral nucleus can ameliorate aspects of both cerebellar and basal gangliar dyskinesia, presumably by reducing the output of VL to the motor cortex.

Although the distinctive parts of the ventral anterior nucleus receive substantial and nonoverlapping projections from the globus pallidus (VApc) and the pars reticularis of the substantia nigra (VAmc), only part of the cells of this nucleus relay impulses to the cerebral cortex. VAmc has, in part, a specific projection to the caudal and medial orbitofrontal cortex (Carmel, '70), which appears to be involved in the "triggering" mechanism of the recruiting response (Velasco and Lindsley, '65). Cells of VApc which receive some input from VAmc appear to have a widespread frontal cortical projection (Fig. 15-13). In addition this rostral ventral tier thalamic nucleus has connections with the intralaminar and dorsomedial thalamic nuclei. Thus the ventral anterior nucleus exhibits characteristics of both the specific and the nonspecific thalamic nuclei.

As a group the cortical relay nuclei of the thalamus possess common features, although the ventral anterior nucleus presents certain exceptions: (1) all receive substantial projections from specific parts of the neuraxis, (2) all, except for parts of VA, project to well defined cortical areas, and (3) all, except VA, undergo extensive cell change following ablation of their cortical projection areas. These nuclei, with the exception of certain parts of VA, constitute the *specific thalamic relay nuclei*. Low frequency electrical stimulation of individual specific sensory relay nuclei, and certain cortical relay nuclei (i.e., the ventral lateral nucleus), evokes a primary surface potential followed by an augmenting sequence which is limited to the cortical projection area. This response is called the augmenting response. Characteristically, *augmenting responses*: (1) have a short latency, (2) are diphasic and increase in magnitude during the initial four or five stimuli of a repetitive train, and (3) are localized to the primary cortical projection area of the specific thalamic nucleus stimulated (Dempsey and Morison, '42).

The Association Nuclei. The association nuclei of the thalamus receive no direct fibers from the ascending systems, but have abundant connections with other diencephalic nuclei. They project largely to association areas of the cerebral cortex in the frontal and parietal lobes and, to a lesser extent, in the occipital and temporal lobes. The principal association nuclei include the dorsomedial nucleus (DM), the lateral dorsal nucleus (LD), the lateral posterior nucleus (LP) and the pulvinar (P) (Fig. 15-13). The dorsomedial nucleus, the most prominent gray mass of the medial thalamus, is highly developed in primates, especially man (Fig. 15-12). It is connected with the lateral thalamic nuclei, the amygdaloid nuclear complex and temporal lobe neocortex; moreover, it has a strong reciprocal connection with the frontal granular cortex (Fig. 15-13). It has been suggested that in this nucleus somatic impulses forming the basis for discriminative cortical sensibility are blended with the feeling tone engendered by visceral activities. These somatovisceral impulses are projected to the prefrontal cortex, which constitutes a large, phylogenetically new cortical area highly developed in man. While the significance of the prefrontal cortex is not fully understood, it has been regarded as the place where the discriminative cortical activities may attain their highest elaboration.

Large injuries to the frontal lobes of both hemispheres are likely to cause defects in complex associations, as well as certain changes in behavior, expressed by loss of acquired inhibitions and more direct and excessive emotional responses. Similar alterations in emotional behavior may be produced when the pathways between the dorsomedial nucleus and the frontal cortex are severed (e.g., in frontal lobotomy).

The lateral dorsal and lateral posterior nuclei receive afferent fibers principally from the ventral nuclei and apparently are concerned with complex somesthetic association mechanisms related to various parts of the body. These nuclei project largely to parietal association areas (Fig. 15-13). The pulvinar, considered as an outgrowth of the lateral posterior nucleus, appears relatively late in phylogenetic development. Development of this huge nuclear mass seems to be correlated with increasing complexity in the integration of somatic and special senses, especially vision and audition. The cortical projections of this thalamic nuclear mass are to portions of the posterior parietal and occipitotemporal cortex. The pulvinar and the lateral posterior nucleus also are involved in extrageniculate visual pathways which parallel the geniculocalcarine projection (Schneider, '69; Casagrande et al., '72; Harting et al., '73). Defects in this system result in impairments of certain patterned visual discriminations.

The Intralaminar and Midline Nuclei. The intralaminar and midline nuclei of the mammalian dorsal thalamus have long constituted an unexplored and poorly understood region. Phylogenetically these nuclei are older than the specific relay nuclei, composing such a large and conspicuous part of the human thalamus. In man and primates many of these nuclei are small and indistinct. Most of these nuclei have been regarded anatomically as having no cortical projections, although they appear to have connections with other thalamic nuclei (Nauta and Whitlock, '54), the hypothalamus (Bodian, '40), the globus pallidus (Nauta and Mehler, '66; Kuo and Carpenter, '73) and the striatum (Powell and Cowan, '56). As previously described, many of the afferent fibers to the intralaminar nuclei ascend from the brain stem in the central tegmental fasciculus, a composite bundle containing predominantly long axons originating from neurons in the reticular formation. Stimulation of the ascending reticular activating system and various kinds of sensory stimuli result in a generalized desynchronization and activation of the electroencephalogram, and behavioral arousal. These phenomena are comparable to those associated with arousal from natural sleep. It is presumed that the electroencephalographic (EEG) arousal response, which produces dramatic effects upon cortical activity, is mediated, in part, by the intralaminar nuclei. Physiological studies suggest that impulses producing these changes in cortical activity reach the cortex via a diffuse thalamic projection system (Moruzzi and Magoun, '49; Jasper, '49; Starzl and Magoun, '51; Jasper et al., '52), the exact nature of which has been in doubt. Studies utilizing retrograde axonal transport of horseradish peroxidase indicate that the nonspecific cortical projections arise as collaterals of fibers from the intralaminar thalamic nuclei; the principal projection from these nuclei is to the neostriatum (Jones and Leavitt, '74). Ascending reticular fibers also pass to the hypothalamus and the subthalamic region (Nauta and Kuypers, '58; Scheibel and Scheibel, '58), suggesting that the so-called diffuse thalamic projection system should not be regarded as the only relay by which impulses from the reticular formation can influence electrocortical activity. It has been suggested that some impulses to the cerebral cortex may follow alternate extrathalamic pathways involving basal diencephalic nuclei that project fibers into the internal capsule (Starzl et al., '51). Golgi studies also indicate that the principal axons from the centromedian and parafascicular nuclei project only to the putamen, but that collaterals of these fibers probably project to the overlying cortex (Scheibel and Scheibel, '67). Axons from the rostral intralaminar nuclei pass through medial parts of the ventral anterior nucleus and through ventral parts of the thalamic reticular nucleus. Some of these fibers can be followed into the white matter of the orbitofrontal cortex.

The classical studies of Dempsey and Morison ('42, '43) and of Morison and Dempsey ('42) showed that stimulation of the so-called nonspecific thalamic nuclei, and the basal diencephalic region, produced widespread and pronounced effects upon electrocortical activity. The *nonspecific*, or *diffuse*, thalamic nuclei include the intralaminar and midline nuclei and, in part, the ventral anterior nucleus of the ventral tier. Repetitive stimulation of these thalamic nuclei alters spontaneous electrocortical activity over large areas and, under certain conditions, resets the frequency of brain waves by eliciting responses that are time-locked to the thalamic stimulus. The most characteristic effect of stimulating the nonspecific thalamic nuclei is the *recruiting response*. When the frequency of stimulation is in the range of 6 to 12 cycles/sec, predominantly surface negative cortical responses rapidly increase to a maximum (by the fourth to sixth stimulus of the train) and then decrease over a broad area; continued stimulation causes the evoked responses to wax and wane. Stimulation of one of the nonspecific thalamic nuclei causes all others to be activated in a mass excitation (Starzl and Magoun, '51). Bilateral cortical responses do not appear to be dependent upon transmission by fibers of the corpus callosum or anterior commissure, nor does spread from one cortical area to another depend upon intracortical propagation (Morison and Dempsey, '42; Jasper, '49). Available evidence suggests that cortical spread involves intrathalamic activities, including conduction across midline gray masses of the thalamus. Although stimulating the nonspecific thalamic nuclei produces changes in electrocortical activity over broad areas, these effects are not indiscriminate or equal in all cortical areas. Responsive cortical zones appear to be relatively specific in the frontal, cingulate, orbital, parietal and occipital association areas. The so-called diffuse thalamic projection system appears capable of exerting a massive influence mainly upon areas of the associational cortex, but with a great preponderance of its effects upon the frontal association cortex (Starzl and Whitlock, '52). No recruiting responses or other evoked potentials are recorded in rhinencephalic structures (i.e., olfactory tubercle, pyriform lobe, amygdaloid complex or hippocampal formation) upon stimulation of the intralaminar nuclei. Interruption of this nonspecific thalamocortical system has been produced by lesions, or reversible cryogenic blockade, at three sites: (1) the ventral anterior nucleus, (2) the inferior thalamic peduncle, and (3) the orbitofrontal cortex (Skinner and Lindsley, '67).

Stimulation of the nonspecific thalamic nuclei demonstrates that these nuclei also exert a potent influence upon subcortical structures, particularly the thalamic association nuclei, such as the dorsomedial nucleus, the lateral dorsal nucleus, the lateral posterior nucleus and the pulvinar (Starzl and Whitlock, '52). Effects may be observed also in the anterior nuclei. Stimulation of midline thalamic nuclei is capable of eliciting recruiting activities in mesencephalic reticular regions, which apparently do not depend on cortical connections (Schlag and Faidlerbe, '61). Recruiting responses are said to be observed in the head of the caudate nucleus upon thalamic stimulation of this system (Starzl and Magoun, '51; Starzl and Whitlock, '52; Verzeano et al., '53), but they are rarely found in the putamen and do not occur in the globus pallidus. It is possible that stimulation of the head of the caudate nucleus may produce this response as a result of current spread to fibers in the anterior thalamic radiation. Attempts to analyze the functional relationships between subcortical structures and the nonspecific thalamic nuclei have shown that recruiting responses are not dependent upon: (1) the thalamic association nuclei, (2) the specific relay nuclei of the thalamus, or (3) the striatum, if these structures are destroyed individually (Hanberry and Jasper, '53; Hanberry et al., '54; Koella and Gellhorn, '54; Kerr and O'Leary, '57). The above statement does not imply that recruiting responses remain after all of these structures have been destroyed collectively.

The observation of Moruzzi and Magoun ('49) that cortical recruiting responses induced by low frequency stimulation of the nonspecific thalamic nuclei could be reduced, or blocked, by stimulation of the bulbar reticular formation provides experimental evidence that the nonspecific nuclei of the thalamus are within the sphere of influence of the ascending reticular formation. This finding together with anatomical evidence (Nauta and Kuypers, '58; Scheibel and Scheibel, '58) supports the thesis that EEG arousal reactions elicited by ascending reticular volleys are mediated, at least in part, via the nonspecific thalamic nuclei.

Some idea of the complex physiological relationship between the brain stem reticular formation and nonspecific thalamic nuclei is provided by the antagonistic effects of reticular activation on the recruiting responses and other varieties of electrocortical synchronization elicited by stimulation of the nonspecific thalamus, as noted above. However, it must be pointed out that electrocortical synchronization also may be obtained by stimulation of caudal as well as rostral regions of the brain stem reticular formation and that, conversely, electrocortical desynchronization may be obtained with high frequency stimulation of nonspecific thalamic nuclei. The overt electroencephalographic effects appear to depend in part on both the frequency and the intensity of stimulation at different sites within the mesencephalic and diencephalic reticular system (Moruzzi, '63).

Physiological evidence (Cohen et al., '62; Frigyesi and Purpura, '64; Purpura et al., '66) indicates that transmission of cerebellofugal impulses projecting to the motor cortex via the ventral lateral nucleus of the thalamus may be markedly altered by synaptic activities at multiple sites. Of the pathways studied, those arising in the nonspecific thalamic nuclei appear especially potent. Low frequency stimulation (8 cycles/sec) of the nonspecific thalamic nuclei produces short latency facilitation and prolonged inhibition of specific evoked responses in VLo, the motor cortex and the corticospinal tract. Present findings suggest that the modulation of cerebellar influences on the motor cortex may be the consequence of facilitatory and inhibitory effects of the nonspecific thalamic nuclei upon synaptic activities in the ventral lateral nucleus.

The thalamus is played upon by two great streams of afferent fibers: the peripheral and the cortical. The former brings sensory impulses from all parts of the body concerning changes in the external and internal environment. The cortical connections link the thalamus with the associative memory mechanism of the pallium and bring it under cortical control. The thalamus has subcortical efferent connections with the hypothalamus and striatum (i.e., caudate nucleus and putamen) through which the thalamus can influence visceral and somatic effectors. The functional nature of these subcortical efferent thalamic pathways is unknown, but they are considered to serve primarily affective reactions. These pathways, like the thalamus itself, are under the control of the cerebral cortex. Corticothalamic projections usually are considered to exert inhibitory influences upon thalamic activity. It has been suggested that corticothalamic fibers may constitute part of a complex neural mechanism for the selective regulation of the integrative actions of the thalamus, permitting certain subdivisions to function while inhibiting the activity of others.

CHAPTER 16

The Hypothalamus

The hypothalamus is the part of the diencephalon concerned with the central control of visceral, autonomic and endocrine functions, and with affective behavior. This structure lies in the walls of the third ventricle below the hypothalamic sulci and is continuous across the floor of this ventricle (Figs. 2-22 and 16-1). On the ventral surface of the brain the *infundibulum*, to which the hypophysis is attached, emerges posterior to the optic chiasm (Figs. 2-5, 2-6 and 16-1). A slightly bulging region posterior to the infundibulum is the *tuber cinereum* (Fig. 16-6). The *mammillary bodies* are found posteriorly near the interpeduncular fossa (Figs. 2-5, 2-6, 2-21 and 16-1). The hypothalamus can be described as extending from the region of the optic chiasm to the caudal border of the mammillary bodies. Anteriorly it passes without sharp demarcation into the basal olfactory area (diagonal gyrus of the anterior perforated substance) (Fig. 18-2). The region immediately in front of the optic chiasm, extending rostrally to the lamina terminalis and dorsally to the anterior commissure, is known as the preoptic area (Fig. 16-1). The preoptic area, classically regarded as a forebrain derivative (Clark et al., '38), is considered by Kuhlenbeck ('69) to arise from a rostral hypothalamic anlage and to be structurally and functionally a part of the hypothalamus. Caudally the hypothalamus merges imperceptibly into the central gray and tegmentum of the midbrain. The thalamus lies dorsal to the hypothalamus; the subthalamic region is lateral and caudal (Figs. 2-22 and 15-6).

THE HYPOTHALAMIC NUCLEI

Pervading the whole hypothalamic area is a diffuse matrix of cells constituting the central gray substance, in which are found a number of more or less distinct nuclear masses. A sagittal plane passing through the anterior column of the fornix roughly separates the medial and lateral hypothalamic areas (Fig. 16-2).

The Lateral Hypothalamic Area. This area is bounded medially by the mammillothalamic tract and the anterior column of the fornix; the medial edge of the internal capsule and the subthalamic region form its lateral boundary (Figs. 16-2 and 16-3). Rostrally this area is continuous with the lateral preoptic nucleus, while caudally it merges with the ventral tegmental area of the midbrain. Rostral and caudal portions of this area are narrow, but the tuberal region is expanded. The lateral hypothalamic area contains several groups of cells, the largest of which is the *tuberomammillary nucleus* which caudally extends lateral and ventral to the mammillary body (Nauta and Haymaker, '69). The *lateral tuberal nuclei* (nuclei tuberis lateral or tuberales) consists of two or three sharply delimited cell groups which often produce small visible eminences on the basal surface of the hypothalamus (Fig. 15-10). They consist of small, pale, multipolar

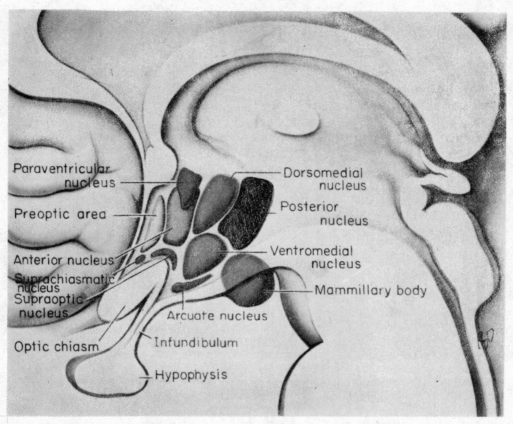

Paraventricular
nucleus
Preoptic area
Anterior nucleus
Suprachiasmatic
nucleus
Supraoptic
nucleus
Optic chiasm
Arcuate nucleus
Infundibulum
Hypophysis
Dorsomedial
nucleus
Posterior
nucleus
Ventromedial
nucleus
Mammillary body

FIG. 16-1. Schematic diagram of the medial hypothalamic nuclei. Nuclei in the supraoptic region are in *blue*. The paraventricular and supraoptic nuclei are *dark blue*; the suprachiasmatic and anterior nuclei of the hypothalamus are *light blue*. Nuclei of the middle or tuberal region of the hypothalamus are *yellow*. Nuclei of the caudal or mammillary region are in shades of *red*. The preoptic area lies rostral to the anterior hypothalamic region and classically is regarded as a forebrain derivative functionally related to the hypothalamus.

cells surrounded by a delicate fiber capsule about which are found the large cells of the lateral hypothalamic nucleus (Figs. 16-2 and 16-3).

The Preoptic Area. This area constitutes the periventricular gray of the most rostral part of the third ventricle (Figs. 16-1, 16-2 and 16-3). The *preoptic periventricular nucleus* surrounds the walls of the third ventricle in the region of the preoptic recess. The diffusely arranged small cells are poorly differentiated from the ependymal lining. The *medial preoptic nucleus*, composed of predominantly small cells, lies lateral to the preoptic periventricular nucleus and extends ventrally to the optic chiasm (Fig. 16-3). The *lateral preoptic nu-*

cleus, rostral to the lateral hypothalamic area, is composed of diffusely dispersed medium-sized cells (Figs. 16-2 and 16-3) and is regarded as the interstitial nucleus of the median forebrain bundle (Kuhlenbeck, '69).

Caudal to the preoptic area three hypothalamic regions are recognized. In rostrocaudal sequence these are: (1) an anterior or *supraoptic region*, lying above the optic chiasm and continuous rostrally with the preoptic area, (2) a middle or *tuberal region*, and (3) a posterior or *mammillary region*, which is continuous caudally with the central gray of the midbrain (Fig. 16-1).

The Supraoptic Region. This region

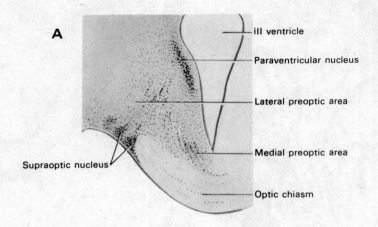

A
- III ventricle
- Paraventricular nucleus
- Lateral preoptic area
- Medial preoptic area
- Optic chiasm
- Supraoptic nucleus

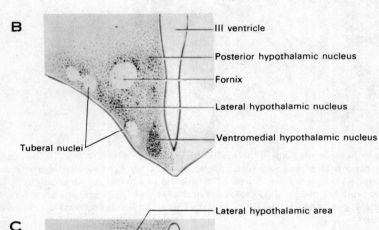

B
- III ventricle
- Posterior hypothalamic nucleus
- Fornix
- Lateral hypothalamic nucleus
- Ventromedial hypothalamic nucleus
- Tuberal nuclei

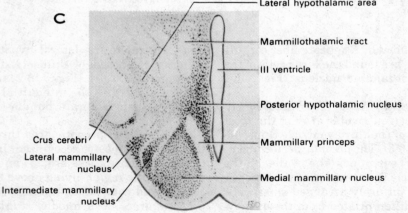

C
- Lateral hypothalamic area
- Mammillothalamic tract
- III ventricle
- Posterior hypothalamic nucleus
- Mammillary princeps
- Medial mammillary nucleus
- Crus cerebri
- Lateral mammillary nucleus
- Intermediate mammillary nucleus

FIG. 16-2. Drawings of transverse sections through portions of the human hypothalamus. *A*, Supraoptic region; *B*, infundibular region; *C*, mammillary region (after Clark et al., '38).

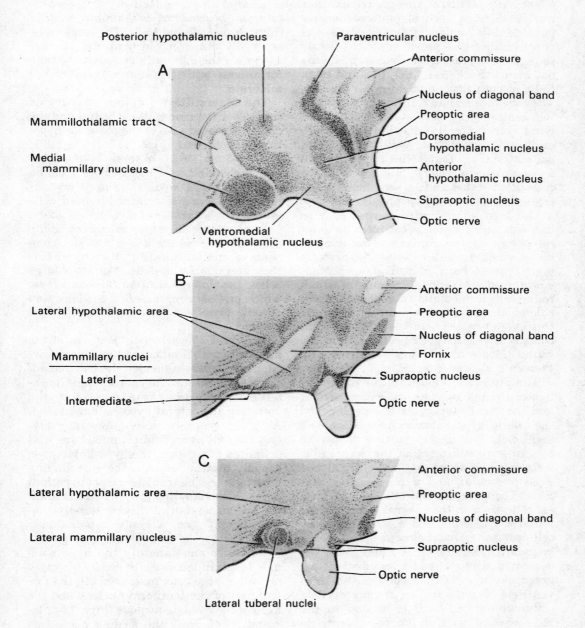

FIG. 16-3. Sagittal drawings of the human hypothalamus. *A*, Near ventricular surface. *B*, Through the anterior column of the fornix. *C*, Near lateral border of hypothalamus (after Clark et al., '38).

contains two of the most striking and sharply defined hypothalamic nuclei, the *paraventricular nucleus* and the *supraoptic nucleus*. Cells of the paraventricular nucleus form a vertical plate of densely packed cells immediately beneath the ependyma of the third ventricle, while cells of the supraoptic nucleus straddle the optic tract (Figs. 16-1, 16-2, 16-3 and 16-4). Cells in both these nuclei appear similar. They are larger than cells in the surrounding central gray and stain deeply. The Nissl substance is distributed peripherally, and cytoplasmic inclusions of colloidal material are found which are regarded as the neurosecretory product of these cells. Both of these nuclei send fibers to the posterior lobe of the hypophysis.

The less differentiated central gray in the supraoptic region constitutes an *anterior hypothalamic* nucleus. This nucleus merges imperceptibly with the preoptic area (Figs. 16-1 and 16-3). The *suprachiasmatic nucleus* forms a group of small round cells immediately dorsal to the optic chiasm and close to the ventral part of the third ventricle (Fig. 16-1). This small nucleus receives direct projections from the retina (Moore and Lenn, '72; Moore, '73; Pierson and Carpenter, '74).

The Tuberal Region. In this region the hypothalamus reaches its widest extent and the fornix separates the medial and the lateral hypothalamic areas (Figs. 16-2 and 16-6). The medial portion forms the central gray substance of the ventricular wall, in which there may be distinguished a *ventromedial* and a *dorsomedial nucleus*. The ventromedial nucleus, the largest cell group in the tuberal region, has a round or oval shape and is surrounded by a cell-poor zone that helps to delineate its boundaries (Figs. 16-1, 16-2 and 16-3). The dorsomedial nucleus is a less distinct aggregation of cells that borders the third ventricle (Fig. 16-3). The *arcuate nucleus* (infundibular nucleus) is located in the most ventral part of the third ventricle near the entrance to the infundibular recess, and extends into the median eminence (Fig. 16-1). The small cells of this nucleus are in close contact with the ependyma lining the ventricle. In coronal sections the nucleus has an arcuate shape

(Nauta and Haymaker, '69). In the caudal part of the tuberal region many large oval or rounded cells are scattered in a matrix of smaller ones; collectively they constitute the *posterior hypothalamic nucleus* (Figs. 16-1, 16-2 and 16-3). The large cells, especially numerous in man, extend caudally over the mammillary body to become continuous with the central gray of the midbrain.

The Mammillary Region. This region consists of the mammillary bodies and the dorsally located cells of the posterior hypothalamic nucleus (Figs. 15-5, 15-11, 16-1, 16-2, 16-3 and 16-6). In man the mammillary body consists almost entirely of the large, spherical *medial mammillary nucleus*, composed of relatively small cells invested by a capsule of myelinated fibers. Lateral to this is the small *intermediate (intercalated) mammillary nucleus* composed of smaller cells (Fig. 16-2). Even further lateral is a well-defined group of large cells, the *lateral mammillary nucleus*, which probably represents a condensation of cells from the posterior hypothalamic nucleus.

The most characteristic features of the human hypothalamus are the sharply circumscribed tuberal nuclei, the large size of the medial mammillary nuclei and the extensive distribution of the large cells in the posterior and lateral hypothalamic areas. Although synthetic descriptions may suggest that all hypothalamic nuclei are well delimited structures, the hypothalamus is broadly continuous with the surrounding gray matter. The transition from hypothalamus to surrounding gray matter is gradual and tissue continuities contain the major afferent and efferent hypothalamic pathways.

Rostrally and laterally the hypothalamus is continuous with the *basal olfactory region*, a large gray mass beneath the rostral part of the lentiform nucleus and the head of the caudate nucleus (Figs. 16-3, 18-2 and A-24). Near the median plane this region extends dorsally, rostral to the anterior commissure, where it becomes the *septal region* (Figs. 18-4 and A-23). Beneath the lentiform nucleus the gray mass extends toward the amygdaloid complex; this region contains cell islands and

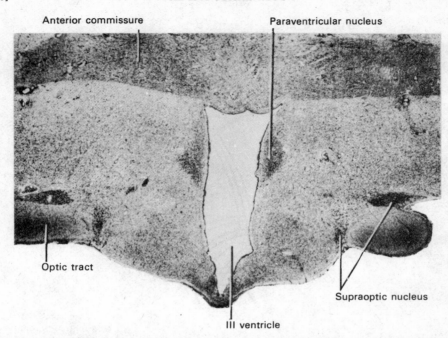

Anterior commissure · Paraventricular nucleus · Optic tract · Supraoptic nucleus · III ventricle

FIG. 16-4. Photograph of human hypothalamus at the level of the anterior commissure demonstrating the periventricular and supraoptic nuclei. Nissl stain.

groups referred to as the *substantia innominata* (Fig. A-22). The rostral part of the substantia innominata lies under the cortex of the anterior perforated substance (Figs. 2-6 and 18-2). The base of the septal region (i.e., the part ventral to the anterior commissure) is continuous with the substantia innominata laterally and with the preoptic region caudally. The dorsal part of the septum forms the septum pellucidum (Figs. 2-4, A-23 and A-24). The septal region contains the *medial septal nucleus,* composed of fairly large neurons, and the *lateral septal nucleus*, which consists of smaller neurons. One of the largest nuclei in this region is the *nucleus accumbens septi* (Fig. A-24), which leans against the base of the septum and is situated medially at the junction of caudate nucleus and putamen.

CONNECTIONS OF THE HYPOTHALAMUS

The hypothalamus, in spite of its small size, has extensive and complex fiber connections. Some fibers are organized into definite and conspicuous bundles, while others are diffuse and difficult to trace.

The Afferent Connections of the Hypothalamus

The afferent connections of the hypothalamus which have been established are: (1) the *medial forebrain bundle*, a complex group of fibers arising from the basal olfactory regions, the periamygdaloid region and the septal nuclei, that pass to, and through, the lateral preoptic and hypothalamic regions (Fig. 16-5). The bundle is formed, at levels rostral to the anterior commissure, mainly of fibers from the septal region, and in its parasagittal course receives contributions from the substantia innominata and amygdalo-pyriform cortex. The bundle is a loose-textured fiber system, in part composed of relatively short fibers, although some longer axons continue caudally into the midbrain tegmentum. The medial forebrain bundle conducts both rostrally and caudally. (2) *Hippocampohypothalamic fibers*, originating from the hippocampal formation, form the fornix (Figs. 16-5, 16-6 and 18-4). In the septal region fibers of the fornix form two distinct bundles: (a) a compact fornix col-

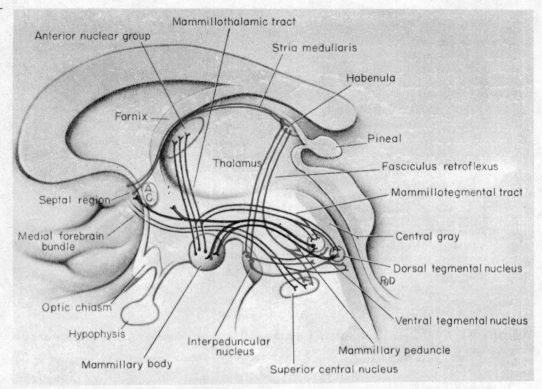

FIG. 16-5. Semischematic diagram of limbic pathways inter-relating the telencephalon and diencephalon with medial midbrain structures. The medial forebrain bundle and efferent fibers of the mammillary body are shown in *black*. The *medial forebrain bundle* originates from the septal and lateral preoptic regions, traverses the lateral hypothalamic area and projects into the midbrain tegmentum. The mammillary princeps divides into two bundles, the *mammillothalamic tract* and the *mammillotegmental tract*. Ascending fibers of the *mammillary peduncle*, arising from the dorsal and ventral tegmental nuclei, are shown in *red*; most of these fibers pass to the mammillary body, but some continue rostral to the lateral hypothalamus, the preoptic region and the medial septal nucleus. Fibers arising from the septal nuclei project caudally in the medial part of the stria medullaris (*blue*) to terminate in the medial habenular nucleus. Impulses conveyed to the habenular nucleus are distributed to midbrain tegmental nuclei via the *fasciculus retroflexus* (based on Nauta, '58).

umn or *postcommissural fornix,* which arches caudal to the anterior commissure, and (b) a more diffuse *precommissural fornix* (Daitz and Powell, '54; Powell et al., '57). Precommissural fibers are distributed to the septal nuclei, the lateral preoptic region, the nucleus of the diagonal band and the dorsal hypothalamic area (Nauta, '56). Postcommissural fibers of the fornix project to the medial mammillary nucleus, except for those which leave the bundle and terminate in thalamic nuclei. (3) *Amygdalo-hypothalamic fibers,* arising from different parts of the amygdaloid nuclear complex (Fig. 2-6) and following distinctive pathways to the hypothalamus,

are: (a) the *stria terminalis* (Figs. 15-6 and 15-7), and (b) the *ventral amygdalofugal pathway* (Gloor, '55). The stria terminalis arises principally from the corticomedial group of the amygdaloid nuclei (Fig. 18-12) and distributes terminals in the medial preoptic area, medial parts of the anterior hypothalamic area and in the ventromedial and arcuate nuclei (Nauta, '56, '61; Hall, '63; Heimer and Nauta, '67; Dreifuss et al., '68; Nauta and Haymaker, '69). The ventral amygdalofugal pathway arises from the pyriform cortex and the basolateral amygdaloid nuclei and supplies the whole extent of the medial forebrain bundle region, as well as having terminations

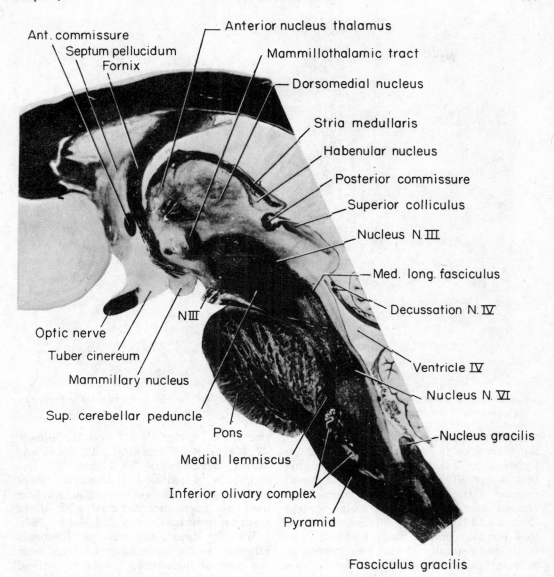

FIG. 16-6. Sagittal section of brain stem through the pillar of fornix, the mammillothalamic tract and the stria medullaris. Weigert's myelin stain. Photograph.

in the lateral hypothalamic nucleus (Fig. 16-8) (Hall, '63; Cowan et al., '65; Valverde, '65; Raisman, '66). (4) *Thalamo-hypothalamic fibers* that arise chiefly from the midline thalamic nuclei. Fibers from periventricular thalamic nuclei are considered to descend into the dorsal hypothalamic area, but relatively little is known about this system (Fig. 16-7). (5) *Brain stem reticular afferent fibers* ascend to the hypothalamus via: (a) the *mammilliary*

peduncle, and (b) the *dorsal longitudinal fasciculus*. The mammillary peduncle arises from the dorsal and ventral tegmental nuclei of the midbrain and projects mainly to the lateral mammillary nucleus (Fig. 16-5). In this course the mammillary peduncle passes rostrally through the rootlets of the third nerve and lies lateral to the interpeduncular nucleus. A few of these fibers ascend in the medial forebrain bundle beyond the hypothalamus. The as-

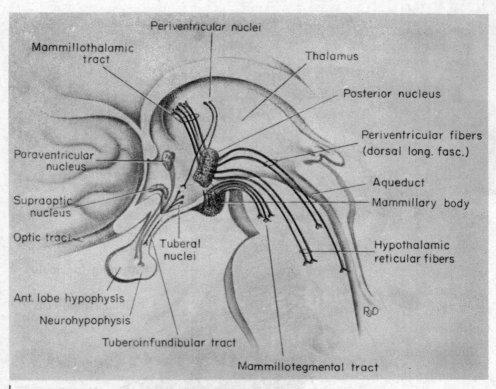

Fig. 16-7. Diagram of some of the efferent hypothalamic pathways. Color code is the same as in Figure 16-1. Terminations of the mammillotegmental tract are shown in Figure 16-5.

cending component of the dorsal longitudinal fasciculus is formed from cells in the central gray of the midbrain. Fibers in this bundle spread out over caudal and dorsal regions of the hypothalamus where they become part of a periventricular system (Nauta and Haymaker, '69). Since fibers of this bundle conduct impulses both rostrally and caudally, it may be regarded as a reciprocally organized association system between the hypothalamus and the midbrain central gray (Fig. 16-7). (6) *Retinohypothalamic fibers,* arising from the ganglion cells of the retina, project to the suprachiasmatic nucleus and are thought to convey impulses relating ambient light to hormonal control of the reproductive cycle in animals (Sawyer, '69; Moore, '73).

Opinion is varied concerning *corticohypothalamic fibers,* usually described as arising from portions of the frontal lobe and passing directly to the hypothalamus. The region from which these fibers seem to be described most consistently is the poste-

rior orbital cortex (Ward and McCulloch, '47; Meyer, '49; Sachs et al., '49; Clark and Meyer, '50; Showers, '58; Nauta, '62). Descriptions of pallido-hypothalamic fibers projecting to the ventromedial nucleus have not been substantiated with silver staining technics (Nauta and Mehler, '66).

Broadly stated, the principal forebrain afferents to the hypothalamus arise from the two phylogenetically oldest cortical areas, the pyriform cortex and the hippocampal formation (Fig. 16-8; Raisman, '66). In each instance the cortical projection is reinforced by a corresponding subcortical projection, the amygdala in the case of the pyriform cortex, and the septum in the case of the hippocampal formation. Each of these subcortical nuclei is reciprocally connected with the overlying cortical area. Of the phylogenetically newer cortical areas the cingulate gyrus appears particularly favored to influence the hypothalamus indirectly through the entorhinal cortex and the hippocampal formation. The cingulate

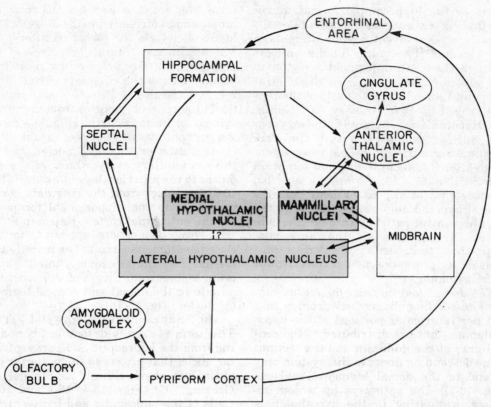

FIG. 16-8. A schematic diagram of the principal fiber connections of the hypothalamus. The principal afferents to the hypothalamus from the forebrain arise from two phylogenetically older cortical areas, the pyriform cortex and the hippocampal formation. Each of these projections is reinforced by a second projection from a related subcortical nuclear mass; this secondary projection arises from the amygdaloid complex in the case of the pyriform cortex, and from the septal nuclei in the case of the hippocampal formation. Reciprocal connections exist between the hypothalamus and these subcortical nuclei. The cingulate gyrus and the pyriform cortex can exert influences upon the hypothalamus via the entorhinal area and the hippocampal formation. The mammillary nuclei and the hippocampal formation project to the anterior thalamic nuclei which in turn influence activities in the cingulate gyrus (modified from Raisman, ' 66).

cortex can in turn be influenced by hypothalamic projections to the anterior nuclear group of the thalamus.

The Efferent Connections of the Hypothalamus

The efferent connections of the hypothalamus appear, in part, to be reciprocal to the afferent systems. There are reciprocal connections in the medial forebrain bundle which provide indirect connections between the lateral hypothalamus and the hippocampal formation (Raisman, '66a). In addition, there are hypothalamic projections to the amygdaloid nuclear complex

via both the stria terminalis (Fig. 18-4) and the ventral pathway. Reciprocal connections with the midbrain tegmentum and central gray are conducted by the dorsal longitudinal fasciculus and via pathways projecting to and from the mammillary bodies. In addition, there are several efferent hypothalamic pathways which have no counterpart among afferent systems.

The medial forebrain bundle conveys impulses from the lateral hypothalamus rostrally to the nuclei of the diagonal band and to the medial septal nuclei (Guillery, '57; Raisman, '66a), which in turn send fibers to the hippocampal formation via the fimbria of the fornix (Daitz and Powell, '54). Descending hypothalamic efferents in the medial forebrain bundle project through the ventral tegmental region to the superior central nucleus, the ventral tegmental nucleus and to parts of the central gray (Fig. 16-5; Guillery, '57; Nauta, '58). Hypothalamic efferents to the amygdaloid nuclear complex via both the stria terminalis and the ventral pathway degenerate after lesions in the medial forebrain bundle (Nauta, '58; Cowan et al., '65; Szentágothai et al., '68). Fibers from the lateral hypothalamic region appear to follow the ventral pathway through the substantia innominata to the amygdala, while those that pass via the stria terminalis arise from more medial cells (Nauta and Haymaker, '69).

The dorsal longitudinal fasciculus contains descending fibers mostly from medial and periventricular portions of the hypothalamus, that are distributed to the central gray of the midbrain and the tectum. Some descending fibers in this system may extend to the dorsal tegmental nucleus (Fig. 16-7). The pathways by which impulses originating in the hypothalamus are relayed to nuclei in the medulla and spinal cord are poorly understood. It is presumed that impulses are projected to cells in the reticular formation which relay the impulses to the medulla and to spinal levels (Fig. 16-7). Evidence concerning pupillodilator pathways in the brain stem supports this thesis (Loewy et al., '73).

Mammillary efferent fibers, arising from the medial mammillary nucleus, and to a lesser extent from the lateral and intermediate mammillary nuclei, form a well-defined bundle, the *fasciculus mammillaris princeps* (Figs. 16-5 and 16-6). This bundle passes dorsally for a short distance and divides into two components: the *mammillothalamic tract* and the *mammillotegmental tract* (Figs. 16-5, 16-6 and A-20). The mammillothalamic tract contains fibers from the medial mammillary nucleus which project to the ipsilateral anteroventral and anteromedial nuclei, and fibers from the lateral mammillary nucleus that pass bilaterally to the anterodorsal nucleus (Fry et al., '63). Superimposed

upon this are direct projections from the hippocampal formation to the anterior thalamic nuclei via the fornix (Guillery, '56; Valenstein and Nauta, '59). Each of the anterior thalamic nuclei in turn projects to subdivisions of the cingulate cortex (Figs. 2-4, 18-4 and 18-13). Thus the main neocortical projection of impulses from the hippocampal formation is to the cingulate cortex via postcommissural fibers of the fornix to: (1) the anterior thalamic nuclei, and (2) the mammillary body which relays impulses to the anterior thalamic nuclei (Fig. 16-8). Impulses from the cingulate cortex pass back to the hippocampal formation via the entorhinal cortex (Raisman et al., '65). These connections appear to form a closed anatomical circuit. The mamillotegmental tract curves caudally into the midbrain tegmentum. Fibers of this tract terminate in the dorsal and ventral tegmental nuclei (Fig. 16-5).

The Supraopticohypophysial Tract. This term is used to designate fibers arising from the supraoptic and paraventricular nuclei that project to the posterior lobe of the hypophysis (Pines, '25; Stengel, '26; Greving, '35) (Figs. 16-4, 16-7 and 16-9). Cells of the supraoptic and paraventricular nuclei are *neurosecretory* and transmit colloid droplets which are liberated at their endings in the neurohypophysis. Following transection of the hypophysial stalk, stainable colloid substance accumulates above the cut, and disappears distally. Electron microscopic studies reveal that the neurosecretory material consists of aggregates of granules, 500 to 2000 Å in diameter (Palay, '57; Bodian, '63, '66). The neurosecretory substance, assumed to be the posterior lobe hormones, or their precursors, is liberated near capillaries of the neurohypophysis. There is evidence which suggests that the supraoptic nucleus is related to vasopressin (antidiuretic hormone) and the paraventricular nucleus to oxytocin (Olivecrona, '57; Heller, '66; Pickford, '69).

The Tuberohypophysial (Tuberoinfundibular) Tract. This tract arises from the tuberal region, mainly from the arcuate nucleus (Fig. 16-1), and can be traced only to the median eminence and the infundibular stem (Szentágothai et al., '68;

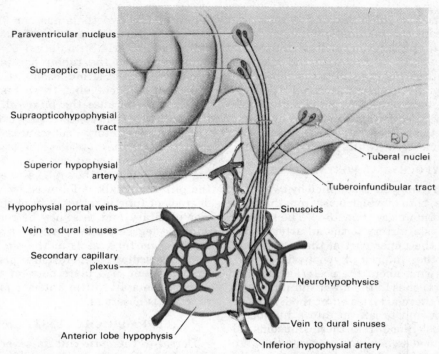

Paraventricular nucleus

Supraoptic nucleus

Supraopticohypophysial
tract

Superior hypophysial
artery

Hypophysial portal veins

Vein to dural sinuses

Secondary capillary
plexus

Anterior lobe hypophysis

Tuberal nuclei

Tuberoinfundibular tract

Sinusoids

Neurohypophysics

Vein to dural sinuses

Inferior hypophysial artery

FIG. 16-9. Diagram of the hypophysial portal system, the tuberoinfundibular tract and the supraopticohypophysial tract. The hypophysis is supplied by the superior and inferior hypophysial arteries. Branches of these arteries form sinusoidal capillaries about the infundibulum. Blood from the sinusoids passes to the anterior lobe of the hypophysis via the portal vessels which give rise to a second capillary plexus in the anterior lobe. The tuberoinfundibular tract ends in the sinusoids of the infundibular stem and transports neurosecretory substances, called *releasing factors*, which enter the sinusoids. The supraopticohypophysial tract contains fibers from the supraoptic and paraventricular nuclei which pass to the neurohypophysis. Neurosecretory products of cells in these hypothalamic nuclei are conveyed directly to the neurohypophysis. The supraoptic nucleus is concerned with the antidiuretic hormone, while the paraventricular nucleus gives rise to oxytocin.

Haymaker, '69). According to Szentágothai et al. ('68), these fibers properly should be referred to as the tuberoinfundibular tract (Figs. 16-7 and 16-9). Although these fibers accompany those of the supraoptic-hypophysial tract in part of their course, they end upon capillary loops near the sinusoids of the hypophysial portal system (Fig. 16-9). These are fine fibers, but secretory granules can be demonstrated in their axons (provided tissues are not fixed in formalin). Fibers of the tuberoinfundibular tract are assumed to convey "releasing" hormones rather than hormones in their active form (Haymaker, '69). Functionally, the tuberoinfundibular tract and the hypophysial portal system establish the neurohumoral link between the hypothalamus and the anterior pituitary. Under stressful conditions neurosecretory gran-

ules disappear from nerve fibers, and adrenocorticotrophic hormone (ACTH) releasing factor is present in the plasma obtained from portal vessels (Porter and Jones, '56). The infundibulum also contains high concentrations of acetylcholine (Haymaker, '69), and the cell bodies and fibers of the tuberoinfundibular system contain dopamine (Fuxe and Hökfelt, '70). Although a direct action of dopamine on the anterior pituitary seems to have been excluded, increases in dopamine in the arcuate nucleus occur in pregnancy, pseudopregnancy and during lactation.

Hypothalamic efferent projections fall into three main categories: (1) those that emerge via the medial forebrain bundle, (2) those concerned with neurosecretion which convey hormones to the neurohypophysis, and hormonal releasing factors to the median eminence, and (3) those that arise from the mammillary nuclei which project to the anterior nuclear group of the thalamus and to nuclei in the midbrain tegmentum. Relatively little is known concerning the inter-relationships between medial and lateral hypothalamic nuclei and how hypothalamic impulses are transmitted to lower levels of the brain stem and spinal cord (Nauta, '72).

HYPOPHYSIAL PORTAL SYSTEM

The hypophysis is supplied by two sets of arteries, both of which arise from the internal carotid artery (Fig. 16-9). The superior hypophysial artery forms an arterial ring around the upper part of the hypophysial stalk; the inferior hypophysial artery forms a ring about the posterior lobe and gives branches to the lower infundibulum. Both of these arteries enter the hypophysial stalk and break up into a number of sinusoids. Blood from these sinusoids collects into vessels which pass into the anterior lobe of the hypophysis. The anterior lobe of the pituitary receives almost all of its blood supply via these vessels. These vessels are referred to as the hypophysial portal vessels (Popa and Fielding, '30). The flow of blood from the hypophysial stalk and median eminence to the anterior lobe of the hypophysis has been demonstrated in living animals (Green and Harris, '49). By exerting vasomotor control over the portal vessels the hypothalamus may regulate the blood supply of the anterior lobe and in turn regulate its activity.

There is considerable evidence that hypothalamic influences upon the anterior lobe of the hypophysis are conveyed by humoral substances, transported along the tuberoinfundibular tract to the sinusoids, that reach the anterior lobe via the portal system (Harris, '55; Harris and George, '69). This generally accepted concept implies that hypothalamic control of the anterior lobe of the hypophysis also is neurosecretory.

The hypothalamus appears intimately concerned with mechanisms that influence the hormonal activity of the anterior lobe and cause the secretion of gonadotrophic, adrenocorticotrophic (ACTH) and thyrotrophic (TSH) hormones. Electrical stimu-

lation of the hypothalamus can increase the discharges of gonadotrophic hormone, TSH and ACTH. Stimulation of the tuberal region in the rabbit has produced ovulation. Direct stimulation of the anterior lobe does not elict these responses, presumably because the humoral part of this pathway is not electrically excitable. The neurosecretory substances acting upon cells of the anterior lobe are called *releasing factors,* and are named according to the hormone they release. Section of the pituitary stalk is followed by varying degrees of functional activity of the anterior pituitary and this may be correlated with the degree of preservation, or regeneration, of portal vessels at the site of section. If vascular regeneration is prevented by placement of a plate between the cut ends of the stalk, little anterior pituitary function is observed.

SUPRAOPTIC DECUSSATIONS

Dorsal to the optic chiasm several bundles of fine fibers cross the midline. These fiber bundles constitute the supraoptic decussations. Three decussations or commissures are recognized, although little is known concerning their origin, course, termination or function.

The most rostral of these decussations is the anterior hypothalamic commissure (Ganser; Figs. 16-10, 17-9 and 17-10). Fibers of this commissure are most readily identified as they project ventromedially from Forel's field H and arch over the fibers of the fornix. These fibers pass ventrally in the hypothalamus, cross the midline ventral to the third ventricle and contralaterally fan out into the lateral preopticohypothalamic area (Nauta and Haymaker, '69). Fibers of the anterior hypothalamic commissure are considered to arise from the reticular formation of the rostral pons and to ascend in association with fibers of the medial longitudinal fasciculus (Bucher and Bürgi, '53).

Two decussations lie along the dorsal aspect of the optic chiasm, the *dorsal supraoptic decussation* (Meynert) and the *ventral supraoptic decussation* (Gudden; Figs. 15-6, 16-10, 17-9 and 17-10). The precise origin of both of these bundles is obscure. Lesions in the subthalamic nucleus

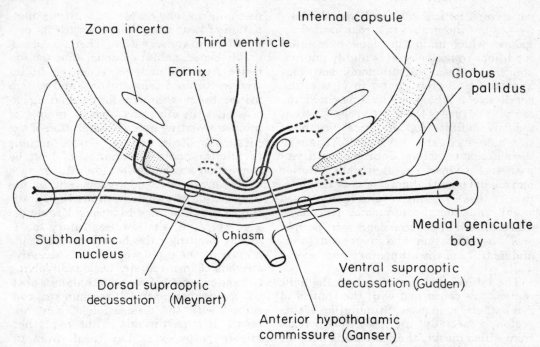

Fig. 16-10. Schematic diagram of the anterior hypothalamic commissure and the supraoptic decussations. Fibers of the *anterior hypothalamic commissure* (Ganser), presumed to arise from the reticular formation of the upper pons and isthmus (*dashed lines*, ascending fibers), become readily detectable as the fibers arch ventromedially over the fornix. These fibers cross ventral to the third ventricle and are distributed contralaterally to the lateral preopticohypothalamic region. Part of the dorsal supraoptic commissure (Meynert) consists of fibers that appear to arise from the subthalamic nucleus, pass through the internal capsule and course along the dorsal border of the optic chiasm and tract; part of these fibers may enter the contralateral globus pallidus. The ventral supraoptic decussation contains fibers from the tectum (*dashed lines*) and medial geniculate body which pass to the region of the contralateral medial geniculate body.

produce degeneration in the dorsal supraoptic decussation which passes into the contralateral globus pallidus (Carpenter and Strominger, '67), but it has been suggested that fibers in this bundle may arise from the hindbrain (Bucher and Bürgi, '53; Nauta and Haymaker, '69). The ventral supraoptic decussation is closely applied to the dorsal surface of the optic chiasm and tract. Fibers of this commissure appear related to both the tectum and the medial geniculate body. According to Papez ('37), ascending fibers from the inferior colliculus are joined by fibers from the ventral part of the medial geniculate body, cross the midline dorsal to the optic chiasm and project to the capsule of the contralateral medial geniculate body. Other observations suggest that fibers in this decussation arise, in part, from the superior colliculus, cross dorsal to the optic chiasm and project toward the opposite medial geniculate body (Bucher and Bürgi, '53; Altman and Carpenter, '61).

FUNCTIONAL CONSIDERATIONS

Experimental evidence and clinical observations have demonstrated that the hypothalamus and immediately adjoining regions are related to all kinds of visceral activities. The most diverse disturbances of autonomic functions involving water balance, internal secretion, sugar and fat metabolism and temperature regulation, all can be produced by stimulation or destruction of hypothalamic areas. Even the mechanism for normal sleep may be altered by such lesions. It is established that the hypothalamus is the chief subcortical center for the regulation of both sympathetic and parasympathetic activities. These dual activities are integrated into coordinated responses which maintain adequate internal conditions in the body. It is highly improbable that each of the autonomic activities has its own discrete center in view of the small size of the hypothalamus and the complex nature of these activities. There is a fairly definite topographical organization as regards the two main divisions of the autonomic system. Control of parasympathetic activities is related to the anterior and medial hypothalamic regions. Stimulation of these regions results in increased vagal and sacral autonomic responses, characterized by reduced heart rate, peripheral vasodilatation and increased tonus and motility of the alimentary and vesical walls.

The lateral and posterior hypothalamic regions are concerned with the control of sympathetic responses. Stimulation of this region, especially the posterior portion from which most of the descending efferent fibers arise, activiates the thoracolumbar outflow. This results in increased metabolic and somatic activities characteristic of emotional stress, combat or flight. These responses are expressed by dilatation of the pupil, piloerection, acceleration of the heart rate, elevation of blood pressure, increases in the rate and amplitude of respiration, somatic struggling movements and inhibition of the gut and bladder. All these physiological correlates of emotional excitement can be elicited when the hypothalamus is released from cortical control. Removal of the cortex, or interruption of the cortical connections with the hypothalamus, induces many of the above visceral symptoms which are collectively designated as "sham rage" (Fulton and Ingraham, '29; Bard, '39). On the other hand, destruction of the posterior hypothalamus produces emotional lethargy, abnormal sleepiness and a fall in temperature due to a general reduction of visceral and somatic activities.

The coordination of sympathetic and parasympathetic responses is strikingly shown in the regulation of body temperature. This complex function, involving widespread physical and chemical processes, is mediated by two hypothalamic mechanisms, one concerned with the dissipation of heat and the other with its production and conservation. There is considerable experimental evidence that the anterior hypothalamus is sensitive to increases in blood temperature, and sets in motion the mechanisms for dissipating excess heat. In man this consists mainly of profuse sweating and vasodilatation of the cutaneous blood vessels. These actions permit the rapid elimination of heat by convection and radiation from the surface of the engorged blood vessels, and by the evaporation of sweat. In animals with fur this is supplemented to a considerable degree by rapid, shallow respiratory movements (panting); the heat loss is effected mainly by the rapid warming of successive streams of inspired air. Lesions involving the anterior part of the hypothalamus abolish the neural control of mechanisms concerned with the dissipation of heat and result in hyperthermia. Thus hyperthermia (hyperpyrexia) may result from tumors in, or near, the anterior hypothalamus.

The posterior hypothalamus, on the other hand, is sensitive to conditions of decreasing body temperature, and controls mechanisms for the conservation and increased production of heat. The cutaneous blood vessels are constricted and sweat secretion ceases, so that heat loss is reduced. Simultaneously there is augmentation of visceral activities, and the somatic muscles exhibit shivering. All these activities tremendously increase the processes of oxidation, with a consequent production and conservation of heat. Bilateral lesions in posterior regions of the hypothalamus usually produce a condition in which body temperature varies with the environment (poikilothermia), since such lesions effectively destroy all descending pathways concerned with both the conservation and dissipation of heat.

These two intrinsically antagonistic mechanisms do not function independently but are continually inter-related and balanced against each other to meet the changing needs of the body; the coordinated responses always are directed to the maintenance of a constant and optimum temperature.

The supraoptic nuclei are specifically concerned with the maintenance of body water balance (Figs. 16-2, 16-3, 16-4, 16-7 and 16-9). Destruction of these nuclei, or their hypophysial connections, invariably is followed by the condition known as *diabetes insipidus*, in which there is an increased consumption of fluids and an increased secretion of urine (polyuria), without an increase in the sugar content. The antidiuretic hormone (vasopressin) is secreted directly by the cells of the supraoptic nuclei. The secretion is conducted to the posterior lobe along the unmyelinated axons of the supraopticohypophysial tract (Bargmann et al., '50). Experimental evidence indicates that the antidiuretic hormone is stored in the posterior lobe of the pituitary. The production of antidiuretic hormone varies in accordance with changes in the osmotic pressure of the blood. An increase in the osmotic pressure of the blood which supplies the supraoptic nuclei increases the activity of these neurons and the release of antidiuretic hormone. In states of experimental dehydration there is a depletion of the hormone in the posterior lobe and increased secretory activity in the supraoptic nuclei. After reestablishment of water balance, there is a reaccumulation of the hormone in the posterior lobe (Hild, '56).

Evidence suggests that the antidiuretic hormone acts specifically on the kidneys rather than on tissues in general (Pickford, '69). Although the exact mechanism by which the antidiuretic hormone brings about reabsorption of renal water is still under discussion, it appears likely that the active reabsorption of sodium, chloride and bicarbonate ions is followed by passive reabsorption of water. The antidiuretic hormone also appears to alter the permeability to water of the distal and collecting tubules of the kidney.

There is evidence that a region of the hypothalamus is responsible for the regulation of water intake. Electrical stimulation of anterior regions of the hypothalamus in goats creates fantastic "thirst" and results in consumption of large volumes of water (Andersson, '57). This is probably part of a more extensive system which regulates the consumption of both food and water. An increase in the osmotic pressure of body fluids may be an effective stimulus for water intake. According to Verney ('47), osmoreceptors probably are situated close to the cells of the supraoptic nucleus which have an abundant blood supply. Localized lesions in the lateral hypothalamus at the level of the ventromedial nucleus in rats cause a reduction in water intake without affecting food intake (Stevenson, '69), but larger lesions in the lateral hypothalamus may cause adipsia as well as aphagia. According to Emmers ('73), the lateral hypothalamic area can excite cells of the supraoptic nucleus which in turn inhibit the lateral hypothalamic area in a negative feedback circuit.

The paraventricular nuclei apparently produce oxytocin, which chemically is related closely to the antidiuretic hormone, but causes contractions of uterine muscle and myoepithelial cells surrounding the alveoli of the mammary gland (Olivecrona, '57; Heller, '66).

The important role of the hypothalamus in maintaining and regulating the activity of the anterior lobe of the hypophysis has been described in relation to the hypophysial portal system (Fig. 16-9). It should be emphasized that this is a humoral control mechanism in which releasing factors are transmitted via the portal system (Harris and George, '69). There are no hypothalamic efferent fibers that reach the anterior lobe of the pituitary. The anterior pituitary stands in marked contrast to other endocrine organs, such as the ovary, testis, thyroid and adrenal cortex, which may be transplanted to distant sites and still retain their endocrine functions. The anterior lobe of the pituitary cannot be transplanted to distant locations and retain its function, because it is dependent upon its close relationships with the hypothalamus. The essential hypothalamic structures are the tuberoinfundibular tract and the hypophysial portal system (Fig. 16-9). Thus the hypothalamus is considered the site of elaboration of releasing factors related to gonadotrophic, adrenocorticotrophic (ACTH), thyrotrophic (TSH) and growth hormones (Harris and George, '69; Sawyer, '69). Attempts to determine the loci within the hypothalamus concerned with particular releasing factors suggest that the neural area related to TSH appears to lie on either side of the midline between the paraventricular nucleus and the median eminence (Greer and Erwin, ' 56). Electrical stimulation of the anterior median eminence also results in increased thyroid activity, probably mediated by releasing factors (Harris and Woods, '58). Similarly, electrical stimulation of the hypothalamus in the rabbit can cause the discharge of gonadotrophic hormone (Markee et al., '46; Harris, '48) and of ACTH (De Groot and Harris, '50). While bilateral lesions in almost any region near the base of the hypothalamus will reduce ACTH release, the median eminence-tuberal region was found to have the most important controlling influence (Brodish, '64). It was concluded that control of ACTH secretion lies in a diffuse hypothalamic region rather than in a discrete localized center.

The brain plays an important role in the initiation and coordination of reproductive functions, and these functions are different in the two sexes. The tuberal region of the hypothalamus appears essential for the maintenance of basal levels of gonadotrophic hormone, but the integrity of the preoptic area is necessary for the cyclic surge of gonadotrophin which precedes ovulation (Sawyer, '59; Everett, '64; Raisman and Field, '73). Electrical stimulation of the preoptic area, or the corticomedial nuclear group of the amygdaloid complex, produces ovulation in rabbits and cats. The effects of preoptic stimulation are abolished by lesions separating this area from the tuberal hypothalamus, and the effects of amygdaloid stimulation are blocked by section of the stria terminalis. These observations suggest a functional linkage between the amygdala and medial preoptic area via the stria terminalis, and fiber systems from the medial preoptic area to the tuberal region of the hypothalamus. However, the amygdaloid input to the preoptic area is not essential for ovulation, for bilateral destruction of the stria terminalis does not prevent ovulation (Brown-Grant and Raisman, '72).

Tumor and other pathological processes involving the hypothalamus frequently modify sexual development. Such lesions may be associated with precocious puberty or hypogonadism associated with underdevelopment of secondary sex characteristics. Although hypergonadism has been attributed to tumors of the pineal, most tumors of the brain associated with precocious puberty actually involve, or impinge upon, the hypothalamus. These lesions frequently destroy the posterior hypothalamus and leave the anterior hypothalamus intact; the intact hypothalamic regions functioning in the absence of inhibitory influences from posterior regions leads to increased pituitary function (Weinberger and Grant, '41).

It has been known for a long time that certain lesions near the base of the brain are associated with obesity. Localized bilateral lesions in the hypothalamus involving primarily, or exclusively, the ventromedial nucleus in the tuberal region produce *hyperphagia* (Hetherington and Ranson, '40; Stevenson, '49, '69; Ingram, '52). Such animals eat voraciously, consuming two or three times the usual amount of food. In addition, most animals with such lesions exhibit savage and vicious behavior. Obesity appears to be the direct result of increased food intake. Lesions destroying portions of the lateral hypothalamic nucleus bilaterally impair, or abolish, the desire to feed in hyperphagic and normal animals (Anand and Brobeck, '51, '51a; Stevenson, '69). Because lesions in the lateral hypothalamic area concomitantly destroy the medial forebrain bundle, its importance in aphagia was investigated. It was concluded that only lesions in this bundle in the vicinity of the ventromedial nucleus produced aphagia. These data suggest that the ventromedial nucleus of the hypothalamus is concerned with *satiety*, while the lateral hypothalamic nucleus may be regarded as a *feeding center*.

The hypothalamus is regarded as one of the principal centers concerned with emotional expression. Since it is acknowledged that the physiological expression of emotion is dependent, in part, upon both sympathetic and parasympathetic components of the autonomic nervous system, it is evident that the hypothalamus, intimately relating both of these, probably is involved directly or indirectly in most emotional reactions. As mentioned above, lesions in the ventromedial nucleus of the hypothalamus produce savage behavior and extreme rage reactions (Wheatley, '44; Glusman, ' 74). Stimulation of the hypothalamus in unanesthetized cats with implanted electrodes (Masserman, '43; Hess, '54; Glusman, '74) provokes responses resembling rage and fear which can be increased by graded stimuli of different intensities. These reactions, referred to by some as "pseudo-affective," are "stimulus-bound" in that they are present only during the period of stimulation. Different types of responses are elicited from different parts of the hypothalamus; flight responses are most readily evoked from lateral regions of the anterior hypothalamus, while aggressive responses characterized by hissing, snarling, baring of teeth and biting are seen most commonly with stimulation of the region of the ventromedial nucleus (Nakao, '58; Glusman, '74). Because the emotional reactions provoked by electrical stimulation of the hypothalamus are directed, it seems likely that the thalamus, cerebral cortex and many forebrain structures play important roles in these responses. In these reactions the hypothalamus cannot be regarded as a simple efferent mechanism influencing only lower levels of the neuraxis.

Observations that selective stimulation and lesions of the ventromedial hypothalamic nucleus both produce aggressive and savage behavior raises basic questions concerning the mechanisms involved. Studies in the cat suggest that the savage behavior after bilateral lesions of the ventromedial nucleus cannot be assumed to result from a release of inhibitory influences (Glusman, '74). Because animals with bilateral lesions in the ventromedial hypothalamic nuclei never show spontaneous outbursts of aggressive behavior, unless disturbed, and this hyperirritable state develops gradually, it has been postulated that destruction of these nuclei may lead to a state of supersensitivity similar to that described by Cannon and Rosenblueth ('49). Furthermore, it was demonstrated that secondary midbrain lesions involving many structures, including the central gray, the reticular formation and the lemniscal systems, had "taming" effects upon this savage behavior.

Other studies, based upon electrical stimulation of unrestrained animals, indicate that the perifornical region and the central gray of the midbrain play important roles in expression of anger (Hunsperger, '56). The fact that hypothalamically induced rage reactions may be blocked by midbrain lesions suggests that certain midbrain structures are essential for the elaboration of aggressive behavior (Chi and Flynn, '71). Finally, electrical stimulation of the amygdaloid nuclear complex also produces behavioral changes in which fear and rage are prominent. It appears generally accepted that the morphophysiological substrates of abnormal and aggressive behavior involve, in some differential and selective fashion, predominantly brain structures rostral to the rhombencephalon. This part of the central nervous system contains the neural structures concerned with goal-directed behavior, and the motivational and emotional concomitants that make such behavior possible. Impulses generated in sensory systems, the cerebral cortex and still undetermined neural structures may trigger mechanisms that excite visceral and somatic systems whose activities in concert provide the physiological expression of aggressive behavior.

Although hypothalamic lesions produce somnolence resembling normal sleep (Ranson, '39; Cairns, '52), the fact that sleep and sleeplike states can be produced by electrical and chemical stimulation in a variety of structures within the brain stem makes it unlikely that there is a single "sleep center." The intralaminar thalamic nuclei seem to be the pre-eminent structures concerned with inducing sleep. Sleep induced by thalamic stimulation lasts for long periods of time and is comparable to that occurring naturally. The pontine reticular formation and the raphe nuclei constitute a lower center concerned with the triggering of paradoxical sleep (see page 366).

CHAPTER 17

The Basal Ganglia

In close relationship to parts of the diencephalon, but separated from it by the internal capsule, are the large nuclear masses that constitute the basal ganglia (Figs. 17-1 and 17-2). The basal ganglia represent massive subcortical nuclei derived from the telencephalon. Structures composing the basal ganglia are the *caudate nucleus*, the *putamen*, the *globus pallidus* and the *amygdaloid nuclear complex*. Because the terms designating components of the basal ganglia are used in various ways, it is appropriate to clarify them at the outset.

The *amygdaloid nuclear complex*, phylogenetically the oldest part of the basal ganglia, is known as the *archistriatum*. This structure is located internal to the uncus in the temporal lobe (Figs. 2-6 and 17-2). The amygdaloid nuclear complex has primarily an olfactory input via: (1) the lateral olfactory tract, and (2) relays in the prepyriform cortex (Powell et al., '65). Its efferent projections are largely to the hypothalamus (Nauta, '61; Raisman, '66; Heimer and Nauta, '67). Because the amygdaloid complex is primarily concerned with visceral, endocrine and behavioral functions, it is considered in detail in Chapter 18.

The *globus pallidus*, consisting of medial and lateral segments oriented along the lateral surface of the internal capsule, is designated the *paleostriatum*, but commonly is referred to simply as the pallidum (Figs. 2-9, 15-17, 17-1 and 17-2). The term *neostriatum* refers to the caudate nucleus and putamen, which together form the largest and newest component of the basal ganglia (Figs. 2-9, 15-7, 15-17, 17-1 and 17-2). The neostriatum commonly is called the striatum. Collectively the neostriatum (striatum) and the paleostriatum (pallidum) form the *corpus striatum*. The globus pallidus plus the putamen are referred to as the lenticular (lentiform) nucleus, mainly for descriptive purposes; the use of this term for other purposes is confusing for it groups together, in an incomplete way, two structures that are anatomically and physiologically distinct.

THE CORPUS STRIATUM

The part of the basal ganglia considered to be concerned with somatic motor function, or disturbances of somatic motor function, is the corpus striatum. Arising as a single gray mass during early development, the corpus striatum becomes secondarily divided by the fibers of the internal capsule into two cellular masses, the *lenticular nucleus* and the *caudate nucleus*. This separation is incomplete. The head of the caudate nucleus is continuous rostroventrally with parts of the putamen. In more posterior regions portions of the caudate nucleus and dorsal parts of the putamen are connected by a number of slender gray (striatal) bridges between fibers of the internal capsule (Figs. 17-1, 17-2, 17-3 and 17-4).

The Caudate Nucleus

The caudate nucleus is an elongated, arched gray cellular mass related throughout its extent to the ventricular surface of the lateral ventricle (Figs. 2-9, 15-7, 17-1, 17-2 and 17-3). Its enlarged anterior portion, or *head*, lies rostral to the thalamus and bulges into the anterior horn of the lateral ventricle. The *body* of the caudate nucleus extends along the dorsolateral border of the thalamus, from which it is separated by the stria terminalis and the terminal vein (Fig. 15-7). This part of the caudate nucleus is regarded as suprathalamic (Szabo, '70). The *tail* of the caudate nucleus is the long, attenuated caudal portion which sweeps into the temporal lobe in the roof of the inferior horn of the lateral ventricle and comes into relationship with the central nucleus of the amygdaloid complex (Figs. 2-9, 15-17, 17-2, 17-4, 18-9 and 18-12).

The Lenticular Nucleus

The lenticular nucleus has the size and form of a Brazil nut. In frontal sections this nucleus appears as a wedge with its broad convex base directed laterally and its blade medially. It has no ventricular surface but lies deeply buried in the white matter of the hemisphere, closely applied to the lateral surface of the internal capsule, which separates it from the caudate nucleus (rostrally) and the thalamus (caudally) (Figs. 2-9, 15-17, 17-1 and 17-2). A vertical plate of white matter, the lateral medullary lamina, divides the lenticular nucleus into an outer larger portion, the *putamen*, and an inner portion, the *globus pallidus*.

The Putamen. The putamen, the largest and most lateral part of the basal ganglia, lies between the external capsule and the lateral medullary lamina of the globus pallidus. In transverse sections it appears lightly stained and is traversed by fascicles of myelinated fibers directed ventromedially toward the globus pallidus. The caudate nucleus and putamen, which are continuous rostrally, have essentially the same cytological structure.

Two types of cells usually are described in the neostriatum: small round or spindle-shaped cells, and large multipolar cells. The smaller cells have been said to outnumber the large cells by a ratio of about 20 to 1 (Foix and Nicolesco, '25), but more recent data suggest that this ratio should be doubled or tripled (Namba, '57). In Nissl-stained sections the caudate nucleus and putamen have a fairly homogeneous appearance and no lamination or special grouping of cells is seen. Golgi and electron microscopic observations in the monkey indicate that striatal neurons fall into two groups: (1) those with spiny dendrites, and (2) those with smooth, or aspiny dendrites (Fox et al., '71; Fox et al., '71/'72). The *neurons with spiny dendrites* occur in enormous numbers, are readily impregnated with silver chromate and correspond to so-called small striatal neurons. Dendrites of spiny neurons radiate in all directions and encompass a spheroid space 300 to 400 μ in diameter (Fig. 17-5A). There is considerable overlap of the spheroid province of each neuron by that of adjacent neurons. Cell bodies of spiny neurons are round, ovoid or fusiform and give rise to a delicate axon having several collaterals that terminate a short distance from the cell body. Because axons of spiny neurons have never been followed for distances much greater than 150 μ, these neurons have been classified as Golgi type II neurons (Fox et al., '71). Almost all synapses on spiny neurons are upon dendritic spines and upon dendrites. It has been postulated that the dendritic spines provide a postsynaptic region effectively isolated from other synapses. The *aspiny striatal neurons* (i.e., neurons without dendritic spines) are of two types. Large aspiny neurons with elongated, bulbous cell bodies contain large masses of Nissl substance and correspond to the so-called large striatal cells (Fig. 17-5B and C). These cells have robust axons which acquire a myelin sheath and give rise to several collaterals. The other type of aspiny striatal neuron is smaller, has a round cell body and gives rise to numerous spindly dendrites; cells of this type have been referred to as "spidery" neurons (Fig. 17-5D). In Golgi preparations axons of "spi-

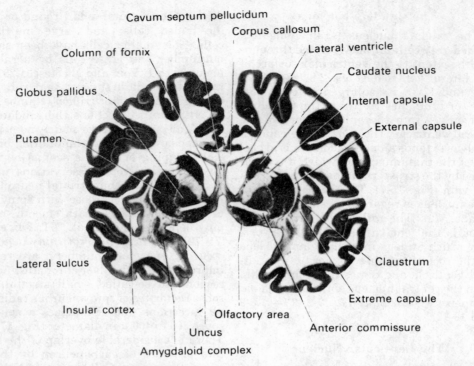

Cavum septum pellucidum

Corpus callosum

Column of fornix

Lateral ventricle

Caudate nucleus

Globus pallidus

Internal capsule

External capsule

Putamen

Lateral sulcus

Claustrum

Insular cortex

Extreme capsule

Olfactory area

Uncus

Anterior commissure

Amygdaloid complex

FIG. 17-1. Photograph of a frontal section of the brain passing through the columns of the fornix and the anterior commissure.

dery" neurons seem never to be impregnated. A conspicuous feature of the striatal neuropil is the very high proportion of nonmyelinated fibers (Kemp, '68a). However, striatal efferent fibers are myelinated and project radially like the spokes of a wheel (Papez, '42) into both segments of the globus pallidus and to parts of the substantia nigra (Nauta and Mehler, '66; Szabo, '62, '67, '70). The only striatal neurons with myelinated axons are the large aspiny neurons.

The striatum contains high concentrations of catecholamines, principally dopamine (Dahlström, '71). Dopamine and other monoamines in the striatum are contained in small granular vesicles in terminal boutons (Hökfelt and Ungerstedt, '69). These boutons are considered to be terminals of nigrostriatal fibers (Andén et al., '64; Poirier and Sourkes, '65; Hornykiewicz, '66; Ungerstedt, '71).

The Globus Pallidus. This nucleus forms the smaller and most medial part of the lentiform nucleus. This structure lies medial to the putamen throughout most of its extent; the dorsomedial margin of the pallidum borders the posterior limb of the internal capsule. A thin *lateral medullary lamina* is found on the external surface of the pallidum at its junction with the putamen. A *medial medullary lamina* divides the globus pallidus into medial and lateral segments (Figs. 17-2, 17-3, 17-7 and 17-8). A less distinct *accessory medullary lamina* (Kuo and Carpenter, '73) divides the medial pallidal segment into outer and inner portions which appear to give rise to efferent fibers that have distinctive courses (Fig. 17-7). The globus pallidus, phylogenetically older than the striatum, is well developed in lower vertebrates. Many bundles of myelinated fibers traverse the globus pallidus, which in fresh preparations give it a paler appearance than the putamen or caudate nucleus. Cells of the globus pallidus are large fusiform neurons with long, relatively smooth dendrites which are contacted by plexuses of afferent fibers that establish longitudinal axoden-

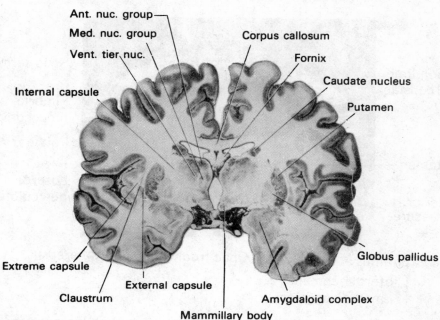

Thalamus

Ant. nuc. group

Med. nuc. group

Vent. tier nuc.

Internal capsule

Corpus callosum

Fornix

Caudate nucleus

Putamen

Extreme capsule

External capsule

Claustrum

Amygdaloid complex

Mammillary body

Globus pallidus

FIG. 17-2. Photograph of a frontal section of the brain at the level of the mammillary bodies. In this section the main nuclear groups of the thalamus are identified and portions of all components of the basal ganglia are present. The amygdaloid nuclear complex lies in the temporal lobe internal to the uncus and ventral to the lentiform nucleus.

dritic connections (Fox et al., '66, '74). Axons of these cells form the principal efferent system of the corpus striatum.

The Claustrum. This is a thin plate of gray matter lying in the medullary substance of the hemisphere between the lenticular nucleus and the insular cortex which is separated from these structures by two white laminae, the external capsule medially and the extreme capsule laterally (Figs. 2-9, 15-17, 17-1 and 17-2). Although some consider the claustrum as a part of the striatum, it seems likely that it arises from the deeper layers of the insular cortex. Its function and connections remain obscure.

STRIATAL CONNECTIONS

Striatal Afferent Fibers

These fibers arise primarily from the cerebral cortex, the intralaminar thalamic nuclei and the substantia nigra (Fig. 17-6).

Corticostriate Fibers. The question as to whether or not the striatum receives fibers from the cerebral cortex remained unanswered for many years because of a lack of a suitable histological technic for demonstrating degenerated axons. The observation that, at least, the intrastriatal portion of the corticostriate fibers is unmyelinated probably accounts for many discrepancies and the failure of the Marchi method to demonstrate these fibers. Silver staining methods indicate that nearly all regions of the cortex contribute fibers to the striatum (Webster, '61, '65; Carman et al., '63, '65; Kemp and Powell, '70). Corticostriate fibers are organized in both dorsoventral and mediolateral dimensions. The anterior half of the hemisphere, including the sensorimotor cortex, is related to a larger part of the striatum than is the posterior half of the hemisphere. The greater part of the cortex is connected to both the caudate nucleus and the putamen, but cortex along the dorsomedial margin of the hemisphere projects exclusively to dorsal parts of the caudate nucleus (Fig. 17-6). It further has been found

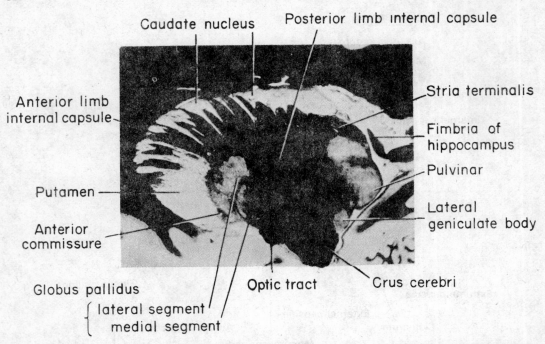

Caudate nucleus

Posterior limb internal capsule

Stria terminalis

Fimbria of hippocampus

Anterior limb internal capsule

Pulvinar

Putamen

Lateral geniculate body

Anterior commissure

Globus pallidus
{ lateral segment
  medial segment

Optic tract

Crus cerebri

FIG. 17-3. Sagittal section through the basal ganglia, internal capsule and thalamus. Note the relationships of the caudate nucleus to the fibers of the anterior limb of the internal capsule. Weigert's myelin stain. Photograph.

that in the rat, cat and rabbit the sensorimotor cortex projects bilaterally to the caudate nucleus and putamen (Carman et al., '65). Fibers projecting contralaterally cross the midline in the corpus callosum and enter the caudate nucleus via the subcallosal fasciculus, and the putamen via the external capsule. Most of these fibers pass to caudal parts of the head of the caudate nucleus and corresponding parts of the putamen. Less numerous bilateral corticostriate fibers in the monkey arise from the supplementary motor area and from area 5 (Jones and Powell, '69; Kemp and Powell, '70); none of the corticostriate fibers projecting contralaterally in the monkey arise from area 4 or the somatic sensory cortex. Corticostriate fibers from other regions have only an ipsilateral projection. Electron microscopic observations indicate that corticostriate fibers end predominantly upon the dendritic spines of spiny neurons (Kemp, '68; Fox et al., '71/'72).

Thalamostriate Fibers. These constitute one of the largest and most important groups of afferent fibers passing to the cau-

date nucleus and putamen (Figs. 17-6 and 17-8). The largest number of these fibers originate from the centromedian-parafascicular nuclear complex, traverse the internal capsule and enter the putamen (Mettler, '47; Nauta and Whitlock, '54; Powell and Cowan, '56). The most conclusive study of this subject (Powell and Cowan, '67) shows that the centromedian nucleus projects exclusively to the putamen and that cells in particular parts of the nucleus pass to selective parts of the putamen. None of these fibers appear to project to the globus pallidus or the claustrum. The parafascicular nucleus also has a topographical projection to the putamen and shows a similar organization. Afferent fibers to the caudate nucleus originate from the smaller intralaminar thalamic nuclei (medial central, paracentral and lateral central) found in more rostral and dorsal locations. Available evidence suggests that terminals of thalamostriate fibers have small synaptic vesicles and end exclusively upon the dendritic spines of spiny neurons (Fox et al., '71/'72). Studies utiliz-

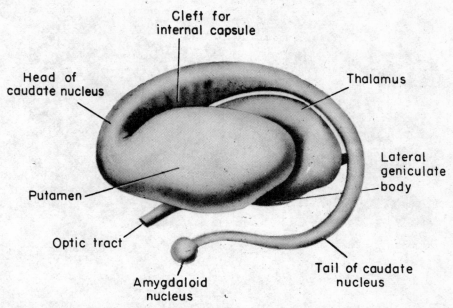

Fig. 17-4. Semischematic drawing of the isolated striatum, thalamus and amygdaloid nucleus showing: (1) the continuity of the putamen and head of the caudate nucleus rostrally, and (2) the relationships between the tail of the caudate nucleus and the amygdaloid nucleus. The cleft occupied by fibers of the internal capsule is indicated. The anterior limb of the internal capsule is situated between the caudate nucleus and the putamen (Figs. 15-17, 15-18 and 17-3), while the posterior limb of the internal capsule lies between the lentiform nucleus and the thalamus.

ing the principle of retrograde axonal transport indicate that collaterals of thalamostriate fibers project diffusely upon broad regions of the cerebral cortex (Jones and Leavitt, '74).

Nigrostriate Fibers. Until recently evidence concerning nigrostriatal fibers has been based almost entirely upon retrograde cell changes produced in the substantia nigra following large striatal lesions (von Monakow, 1895; Holmes, '01; Dresel and Rothman, '25; Ferraro, '25, '28; Morrison, '29; Mettler, '43). Attempts to trace fiber degeneration from lesions in the substantia nigra to the striatum in Marchi preparations and silver impregnated material (Cole et al., '64; Afifi and Kaelber, '65; Carpenter and Strominger, '67; Faull and Carman, '68) either failed to demonstrate these fibers, or indicated that they were extremely sparse. However, use of the fluorescence technic for the demonstration of monoamines (Falck, '62; Carlsson et al., '62) indicates that cells in the pars compacta of the substantia nigra (Fig. 13-18) send axons to the striatum (Hökfelt and

Ungerstedt, '69; Ungerstedt, '71). After lesions in the substantia nigra or internal capsule, the histochemical fluorescence and dopamine content of the striatum are markedly reduced (Andén et al., '64; Poirier and Sourkes, '65). Some electron microscopic evidence suggests that terminals of nigrostriatal fibers have medium-sized synaptic vesicles and end upon the cell bodies of spiny neurons and the dendrites of spidery neurons (Fox et al., '71/'72). If this observation is confirmed, it would indicate that dopaminergic terminals from the nigra end upon striatal interneurons.

Recent studies in the monkey based upon a modified silver staining method (Wiitanen, '69) indicate that nigrostriatal fibers arise almost exclusively from cells of the pars compacta and are topically arranged (Figs. 13-10, 13-19 and 17-6; Carpenter and Peter, '72). Nigrostriatal fibers appear organized in a manner reciprocal to that of strionigral fibers (Szabo, '62, '67, '70). Available data indicate that caudal parts of the nigra project primarily to the putamen and that there is a correspond-

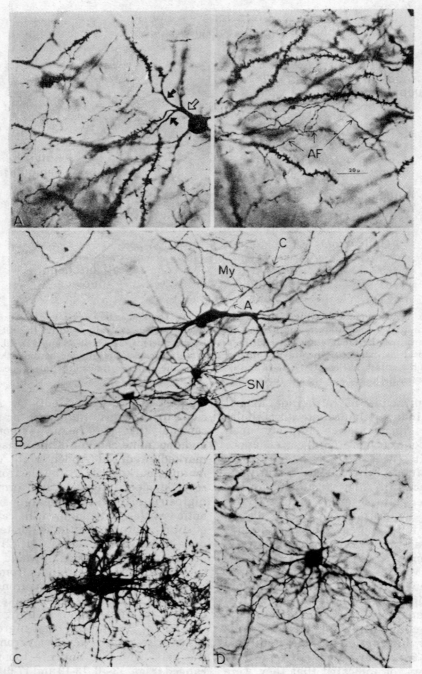

Fig. 17-5. *A*, Montage of a spiny striatal neuron in a Golgi preparation of the rhesus monkey. "Boutons en passage" of afferent fibers (*AF*) cross over its dendrites. The *open arrow* and the *closed arrows* indicate the spine-free dendritic trunk, and the initial, spine-free dendritic branches. Golgi stain. ×700. *B*, A large aspiny striatal neuron. *A*, axon; *MY*, initial segment of myelin sheath; *C*, axon collateral. *SN*, indicates spiny striatal neurons. Golgi stain. ×300. *C*, A large aspiny neuron in the putamen. Golgi stain. ×300. *D*, A spidery aspiny neuron in the putamen. Golgi stain. ×300. (Courtesy of Dr. C. A. Fox, Wayne State University, and Akademie-Verlag, Berlin.)

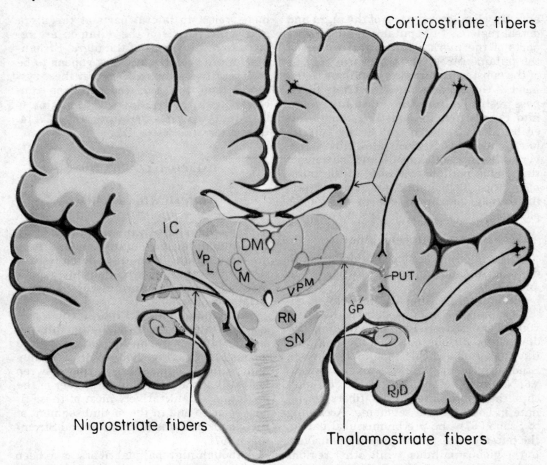

Corticostriate fibers

Nigrostriate fibers

Thalamostriate fibers

FIG. 17-6. Semischematic diagram of striatal afferent fibers. *Corticostriate fibers (black)* arising from broad cortical regions on the convexity of the hemisphere project to the putamen. Cortex on the medial surface projects largely to the caudate nucleus. *Nigrostriatal fibers (red)* arise from cells of the pars compacta. *Thalamostriate fibers (blue)* arise from the centromedian-parafascicular complex. All of these striatal afferent systems are topographically organized.

ence between lateral parts of the nigra and dorsal regions of the putamen, and medial parts of the nigra and ventral regions of the putamen (Fig. 17-14). Rostral regions of the substantia nigra project fibers to the head of the caudate nucleus. These fibers pass rostrally from the substantia nigra into Forel's field H and then course laterally, dorsal and rostral to the subthalamic nucleus. Nigrostriatal fibers traverse the internal capsule and portions of the globus pallidus *en route* to the putamen (Figs. 13-19 and 17-14). Some of these fibers may end upon cells in the globus pallidus.

Striatal Efferent Fibers

These fibers project to the globus pallidus and the substantia nigra (Figs. 17-14 and 17-15).

Striopallidal Fibers. These fibers are topographically organized in both dorsoventral and rostrocaudal sequences and radiate into various parts of the pallidum like spokes of a wheel (Figs. 15-9 and 17-3). Studies in the monkey (Cowan and Powell, '66; Nauta and Mehler, '66; Szabo, '67) indicate that putaminopallidal fibers terminate in both pallidal segments. According to Szabo ('67), the precommissural part of the putamen appears to project exclusively to the globus pallidus, while other regions of the striatum project to both globus pallidus and substantia nigra. Striopallidal fibers from the caudate nucleus pass ventrally through the internal capsule, while fibers from the putamen project medially to the globus pallidus. The bundles of myelinated fibers which are most numerous in medial parts of the putamen are collections of striopallidal fibers (Fig. 17-13). These bundles of striopallidal fibers are referred to as Wilson's pencils (Wilson, '14).

Strionigral Fibers. Experimental studies have convincingly demonstrated that strionigral fibers are topographically organized and end predominantly upon cells of the pars reticulata (Nauta and Mehler, '66; Szabo, '62, '67, '70). Fibers from the head of the caudate nucleus project to rostral parts of the nigra. Putaminonigral fibers pass to more caudal parts of the nigra and are arranged so that dorsal parts of the puta-

men project to lateral parts of the nigra and ventral parts of the putamen are related to medial parts of the nigra. Strionigral and nigrostriatal fibers appear to be reciprocally organized. Together these systems form a closed feedback loop concerned with the transport of dopamine to terminals in the striatum (Fig. 17-14; Carpenter and Peter, '72).

PALLIDAL CONNECTIONS

Pallidal Afferent Fibers

These fibers arise primarily from cells in the caudate nucleus and putamen. These are *striopallidal fibers* distributed to both segments of the globus pallidus in an organized manner. They are discussed under striatal connections.

Subthalamopallidal Fibers. These project ventrolaterally through the internal capsule to enter the medial segment of the globus pallidus (Fig. 17-8). Within the medial pallidal segment these fibers sweep ventrally toward the inferior border of the pallidum. Quantitatively most of these fibers seem to end in the medial segment of the globus pallidus (Carpenter and Strominger, '67).

Although nigropallidal fibers have been described in the literature (Ranson and Ranson, '42; Kimmel, '42; Mettler, '43, '70; Fox and Schmitz, '44), details concerning these fibers are meager. Definitive information concerning such fibers would seem to require evidence obtainable at the electron microscopic level. Certain chemical studies suggest a relationship (i.e., pallidonigral fibers) between the nigra and the globus pallidus in that lesions in the pallidum cause a significant reduction in glutamic acid decarboxylase (GAD) activity in the nigra, while no reduction in GAD activity occurs with striatal lesions (McGeer et al., '71). Whether corticofugal fibers terminate in the globus pallidus or not is unresolved. In most studies of corticostriate fibers little mention is made of corticopallidal projections. A few authors (Webster, '61; Petras, '65, '69) report no evidence of such fibers, but admit the problem requires further investigation.

Pallidofugal Fiber Systems

These systems represent the principal efferent system of the corpus striatum. Impulses from nuclei projecting upon the globus pallidus are ultimately transmitted from the pallidum by an intricate pallidofugal fiber system. Pallidal efferent fibers can be divided into four bundles: (1) the *ansa lenticularis*, (2) the *lenticular fasciculus*, (3) the *pallidotegmental fibers*, and (4) the *pallidosubthalamic fibers* (Figs. 17-7, 17-8, 17-9, 17-10 and 17-11). The first three of these arise exclusively from the medial pallidal segment (Figs. 17-7, 17-8, 17-9, 17-10 and 17-11; Ranson and Ranson, '42; Nauta and Mehler, '66; Carpenter and Strominger, '67). Pallidosubthalamic fibers arise predominantly, but not exclusively, from the lateral pallidal segment (Fig. 17-8; Carpenter et al., '68). Pallidofugal fibers are arranged in a rostrocaudal sequence with the ansa lenticularis most rostral, the lenticular fasciculus in an intermediate position and pallidosubthalamic fibers most caudal.

The Ansa Lenticularis. These fibers arise from lateral portions of the medial segment of the globus pallidus and form a well defined bundle on the ventral surface of the pallidum (Figs. 17-7, 17-8 and 17-9). Fibers sweep ventromedially and rostrally around the posterior limb of the internal capsule, and then course posteriorly to enter Forel's field H.

The Lenticular Fasciculus. These fibers arise from the inner part of the medial pallidal segment, issue from the dorsomedial margin of the pallidum slightly caudal to the ansa lenticularis and traverse ventral parts of the internal capsule in a number of small fascicles (Figs. 17-7, 17-8 and 17-10). These fibers cross through the internal capsule immediately rostral to the subthalamic nucleus and form a relatively discrete bundle ventral to the zona incerta. (Fig. 17-10). Although most of the lenticular fasciculus lies rostral to the subthalamic nucleus, some fibers of this bundle can be seen coursing along the dorsal capsule of this nucleus at more caudal levels. Fibers of the lenticular fasciculus are referred to as Forel's field H_2. While fibers of the lenticular fasciculus pursue a distinc-

tive course through the internal capsule, they pass medially and caudally to join fibers of the ansa lenticularis in Forel's field H (prerubral field). The majority of the fibers of the lenticular fasciculus (H_2) and the ansa lenticularis merge in Forel's field H and ultimately enter the thalamic fasciculus (Forel's field H_1) located dorsal to the zona incerta.

Investigations of the origin of pallidothalamic fibers in the monkey indicate that fibers emerging via the ansa lenticularis and the lenticular fasciculus arise from specific portions of the medial pallidal segment (Kuo and Carpenter, '73). These data indicate that fibers of the ansa lenticularis arise predominantly, and perhaps exclusively, from the outer part of the medial pallidal segment (i.e., from that part of the medial pallidal segment lateral to the accessory medullary lamina). These fibers course rostrally, ventrally and medially, and traverse portions of the inner pallidal segment (Fig. 17-7). Fibers of the lenticular fasciculus appear to arise exclusively from the inner pallidal segment (i.e., from the portion medial to the accessory medullary lamina). These fibers course dorsally, rostrally and medially, and traverse the peduncular part of the internal capsule (Fig. 17-7).

The Thalamic Fasciculus. Pallidofugal fibers from Forel's field H pass rostrally and laterally along the dorsal surface of the zona incerta where they form part of the thalamic fasciculus (Figs. 17-8 and 17-10). Most of the pallidothalamic fibers in the lenticular fasciculus merely make a "C"-shaped loop around the medial part of the zona incerta and enter the thalamic fasciculus (Figs. 17-8, 17-11 and 17-15). The thalamic fasciculus is a complex bundle containing pallidothalamic fibers, as well as dentatothalamic fibers which ascend through the prerubral region. Fibers of this composite bundle pass dorsolaterally over the zona incerta to enter parts of the rostral ventral tier thalamic nuclei. In the region dorsal to the zona incerta, where fibers of this bundle are distinct and separate from those of the lenticular fasciculus (Figs. 17-8 and 17-10), the thalamic fasciculus is designated as bundle H_1 of Forel. Pallidofugal fibers in the thalamic fascicu-

HORIZONTAL

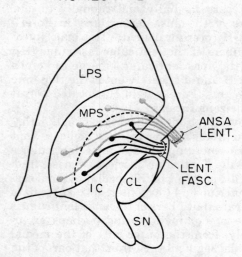

TRANSVERSE

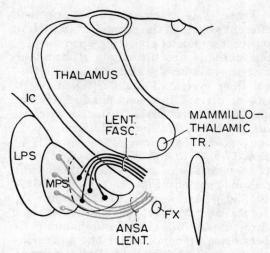

Fig. 17-7. Diagrammatic representation of origin and course of pallidothalamic fibers forming the *ansa lenticularis* and *lenticular fasciculus*. Fibers of the ansa lenticularis (*red*) arise from the outer portion of the medial pallidal segment (lateral to the accessory medullary lamina, *dashed line*) and course rostrally, ventrally and medially. Fibers of the lenticular fasciculus (*black*) arise from the inner portion of the medial pallidal segment (medial to the accessory medullary lamina, *dashed line*) and course dorsally and medially through the fibers of the internal capsule (Kuo and Carpenter, '73; courtesy of the Wistar Institute).

lus project rostrally and dorsally into the ventral anterior (VApc) and ventral lateral (VLo and VLm) thalamic nuclei (Figs. 15-12 and 17-11). Some of the pallidofugal fibers separate from the thalamic fasciculus and course dorsally, caudally and medially to enter the centromedian (CM) nucleus of the thalamus. In their course, these latter fibers pass through portions of the ventral posteromedial (VPM) nucleus of the thalamus. Fibers projecting to the centromedian nucleus may be collaterals of fibers passing to the rostral ventral tier thalamic nuclei (Nauta and Mehler, '66). Dentatothalamic fibers coursing with the thalamic fasciculus pass largely to the ventral lateral (VLo) nucleus of the thalamus, but some of these cerebellar efferent fibers project to the more rostral intralaminar nuclei.

Studies of pallidothalamic fibers in the monkey indicate that this projection to the rostral ventral tier thalamic nuclei (i.e., VApc, VLo and VLm) is topographically organized in three cardinal dimensions (Kuo and Carpenter, '73). Rostral parts of the medial pallidal segment project predominantly to parts of VApc, while caudal parts of this pallidal segment project primarily to VLo. There also is a dorsoventral and mediolateral correspondence in the pallidal projection to VApc and VLo which exhibits some overlap. Pallidothalamic projections to the centromedian nucleus (CM) terminate predominantly in rostral and medial regions, and a definite correspondence between the medial pallidal segment and parts of CM is seen only in the dorsoventral dimension.

Thus the thalamic fasciculus contains two main afferent systems projecting to the ventral tier thalamic nuclei: (1) fibers from the contralateral dentate nucleus (Fig. 14-16), and (2) fibers from the ipsilateral medial pallidal segment (Figs. 17-8, 17-11 and 17-15). These projections appear to be overlapping in the ventral lateral (VLo) nucleus and distinctive with respect to the intralaminar thalamic nuclei. Fibers from the deep cerebellar nuclei project mainly to the rostral intralaminar thalamic nuclei, while the globus pallidus projects exclusively to the centromedian nucleus. It has been suggested that some degree of integration of cerebellar and pallidal impulses probably occurs in the ven-

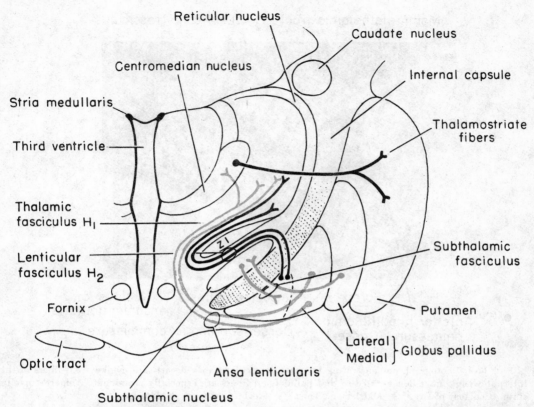

Fig. 17-8. Schematic diagram of pallidofugal fiber systems in a transverse plane. Fibers of the ansa lenticularis (*red*) arise from the outer portion of the medial pallidal segment, pass ventrally, medially and rostrally around the internal capsule and enter the prerubral field. Fibers of the lenticular fasciculus (H_2, *black*) issue from the dorsal surface of the inner part of the medial pallidal segment, traverse the posterior limb of the internal capsule and pass medially dorsal to the subthalamic nucleus to enter the prerubral field. The ansa lenticularis and the lenticular fasciculus merge in the prerubral field (field H of Forel, not labeled here) and project dorsolaterally as components of the thalamic fasciculus (H_1). Fibers of the thalamic fasciculus (H_1) pass dorsal to the zona incerta (*ZI*). The subthalamic fasciculus (*blue*) consists of pallidosubthalamic fibers arising from the lateral pallidal segment, and subthalamopallidal fibers that terminate largely in the medial pallidal segment. Both components of the subthalamic fasciculus traverse the internal capsule. Thalamostriate fibers from the centromedian nucleus (*black*) project to the putamen, as part of a feedback system. Compare with Figures 17-6, 17-7 and 17-11.

tral lateral (VLo) nucleus of the thalamus. It is highly significant that the ventral lateral nucleus of the thalamus projects upon the motor cortex (area 4).

Pallidotegmental Fibers. This small group of descending pallidofugal fibers (Fig. 17-11), derived from the medial segment of the globus pallidus (Nauta and Mehler, '66), becomes identifiable as a separate bundle dorsomedial to the subthalamic nucleus. This bundle descends along the ventrolateral border of the red nucleus. In the caudal midbrain tegmentum

these fibers sweep dorsolaterally to terminate upon large cells of the pedunculopontine nucleus (Figs. 12-24 and 13-3). No pallidofugal fibers descend to more caudal regions of the brain stem.

A small number of pallidal efferent fibers, emerging from the point of union of the lenticular fasciculus and the ansa lenticularis, pass ventromedially over the columns of the fornix and project toward the hypothalamus. Fibers, regarded as *pallidohypothalamic*, have been described as projecting to the ventromedial nucleus in the

Mammillothalamic tract   Lenticular fasciculus

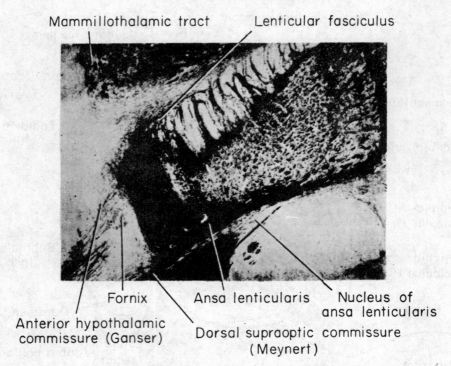

Fornix   Ansa lenticularis   Nucleus of
                                  ansa lenticularis

Anterior hypothalamic
commissure (Ganser)   Dorsal supraoptic commissure
                              (Meynert)

Fig. 17-9. Photograph demonstrating the ansa lenticularis in a decorticate monkey. All fibers of the internal capsule have degenerated so that pallidofugal fibers are especially prominent. Weigert's myelin stain. (Courtesy of Dr. F. A. Mettler and The C. V. Mosby Company, St. Louis.)

tuberal region of the hypothalamus (Ranson and Ranson, '42). These fibers are partially intermingled with those of the anterior hypothalamic decussation (Fig. 16-10; Ganser's commissure) but have not been traced across the midline (Fig. 17-10). According to Nauta and Mehler ('66) fibers, previously regarded as pallidohypothalamic, take off in the direction of the hypothalamus but loop back to join the principal bundle of pallidofugal fibers in their projection to thalamic nuclei. A small number of pallidofugal fibers caudal to the level of formation of the thalamic fasciculus are distributed to cells in Forel's field H (nucleus campi Foreli or prerubral field (Fig. 17-11); Papez, '42; Woodburne et al., '46; Johnson and Clementi, '59). No pallidofugal fibers pass to the red nucleus or the zona incerta.

The Subthalamic Fasciculus. This bundle consists of pallidofugal fibers that pass through the internal capsule to enter the subthalamic nucleus, and of fibers from the subthalamic nucleus that project back

to the globus pallidus. *Pallidosubthalamic fibers* arising from the lateral segment of the globus pallidus project exclusively upon cells of the subthalamic nucleus (Ranson and Ranson, '42; Nauta and Mehler, '66; Carpenter and Strominger, '67). These fibers are topographically organized, predominantly in mediolateral and dorsoventral sequences (Carpenter et al., '68), so that: (1) rostral and central regions project fibers to the rostral two-thirds of the subthalamic nucleus, (2) rostral regions project fibers primarily to the medial half of the nucleus, (3) central regions project fibers primarily to the lateral half of the nucleus, and (4) caudal regions of the lateral pallidal segment project fibers to caudal and dorsal parts of the nucleus. A small number of pallidal efferent fibers originating in the medial segment may terminate in the caudomedial part of the subthalamic nucleus. Pallidosubthalamic fibers traverse ventromedial and caudal parts of the internal capsule, caudal to both the ansa lenticularis and the lenticu-

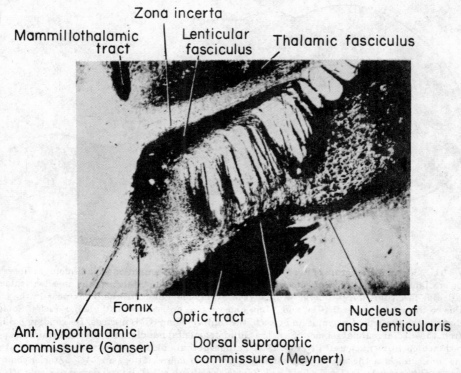

Fig. 17-10. Photograph demonstrating the lenticular fasciculus in a decorticate monkey. Fibers of this bundle can be seen passing through the degenerated internal capsule. At this level, immediately rostral to the subthalamic nucleus, the lenticular fasciculus lies on the inner aspect of the internal capsule ventral to the zona incerta. Weigert's myelin stain. (Courtesy of Dr. F. A. Mettler and The C. V. Mosby Company, St. Louis.)

lar fasciculus (Figs. 17-8 and 17-11). *Subthalamopallidal fibers* traverse the same part of the internal capsule in the opposite direction, and are distributed primarily to parts of the medial pallidal segment (Carpenter and Strominger, '67).

THE SUBTHALAMIC REGION

The subthalamic region lies ventral to the thalamus, medial to the internal capsule and lateral and caudal to the hypothalamus (Figs. 2-22, 15-5, 15-6 and 17-8). Nuclei found within the subthalamic region include the subthalamic nucleus, the zona incerta and the nuclei of the tegmental fields of Forel (nucleus campi Foreli, Forel's field H). Prominent fiber bundles passing through this region include the ansa lenticularis, the lenticular fasciculus (Forel's field H_2), the thalamic fasciculus (Forel's field H_1) and the subthalamic fasciculus.

The Subthalamic Nucleus (*corpus Luysi*). This nucleus, located on the inner surface of the peduncular portion of the internal capsule, has the shape of a thick biconvex lens (Figs. 2-22, 15-5, 15-6, 15-10, 15-11, 17-8, 17-11, 17-12, 17-13 and A-20). Caudally the medial part of the nucleus overlies the most rostral portions of the substantia nigra. Cells of the subthalamic nucleus are spindle-shaped, pyramidal or round with branching processes. Cells vary in size, shape and concentration in different parts of the nucleus, and all contribute to a rich neuropil. In medial parts of the nucleus cells tend to be round, smaller and more concentrated than in lateral regions. The nucleus has a café-au-lait color in fresh sections, and a rich blood supply derived from branches of the posterior communicating, posterior cerebral and anterior choroidal arteries (Foix and Hillemand, '25).

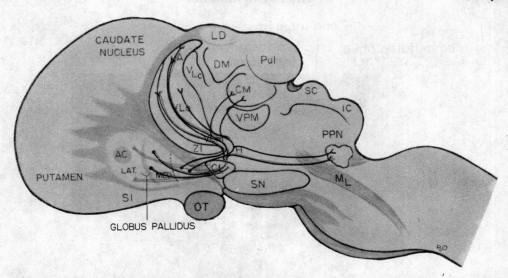

Fig. 17-11. Schematic diagram of the efferent projections and terminations of pallidofugal fibers arising from the medial and lateral pallidal segments shown in a sagittal plane. Fibers of the ansa lenticularis (*red*) and lenticular fasciculus (*black*) merge in field H of Forel. The bulk of these fibers pass in the thalamic fasciculus to the ventral lateral (VLo and VLm) and ventral anterior (VA) thalamic nuclei. Some fibers separate from the thalamic fasciculus and pass to the centromedian (CM) nucleus. Descending pallidofugal fibers from the medial pallidal segment form the pallidotegmental bundle; these fibers terminate upon cells of the pedunculopontine nucleus (PPN; Fig. 13-3). Pallidosubthalamic fibers arising from the lateral pallidal segment (*blue*) project to the subthalamic nucleus (*CL*). Other abbreviations are: *AC*, anterior commissure; *DM*, dorsomedial nucleus; *H*, Forel's field H; *IC*, inferior colliculus; *LD*, lateral dorsal nucleus; *ML*, medial lemniscus; *OT*, optic tract; *Pul*, pulvinar; *SC*, superior colliculus; *SI*, substantia innominata; *SN*, substantia nigra; *VLc*, ventral lateral nucleus, pars caudalis; *VPM*, ventral posteromedial nucleus; *ZI*, zona incerta.

Although there is no structure with which the subthalamic nucleus can be homogenized in reptiles and birds (Huber and Crosby, '29), the nucleus has a consistent distribution in mammals. This nucleus is rudimentary in carnivores, but well developed in primates. While the nucleus is small in the monkey, its relative size is essentially the same as in man (Whittier and Mettler, '49a; von Bonin and Shariff, '51).

The principal afferent fibers of the subthalamic nucleus come from the lateral segment of the globus pallidus via the subthalamic fasciculus. These fibers have a specific topographical distribution within the nucleus (Carpenter et al., '68). Data obtained from studies of human frontal lobotomy (Meyer et al., '47; Meyer, '49) suggest that corticofugal fibers project to the subthalamic nucleus. According to Petras ('65), ablations of area 4 produce abundant degeneration in Forel's fields H_1 and

H_2 and the zona incerta, but only scant degeneration in the subthalamic nucleus. Ablations of cortical areas 3, 1 and 2 produce only sparse degeneration in Forel's fields and the zona incerta and no degeneration in the subthalamic nucleus. Experimental studies (Verhaart and Kennard, '40; Mettler, '47b; Levin, '49) utilizing the Marchi method have failed to demonstrate corticofugal fibers passing into the subthalamic nucleus. Thus available evidence suggests that few, if any, corticofugal fibers project to the subthalamic nucleus.

Efferent fibers from the subthalamic nucleus traverse the internal capsule and project mainly to caudal parts of the medial segment of the globus pallidus (Fig. 17-8). A few of these fibers enter the medial and lateral medullary laminae of the pallidum. A small number of efferent fibers traverse the apex of the globus pallidus, enter the dorsal supraoptic decussation and pass toward the contralateral glo-

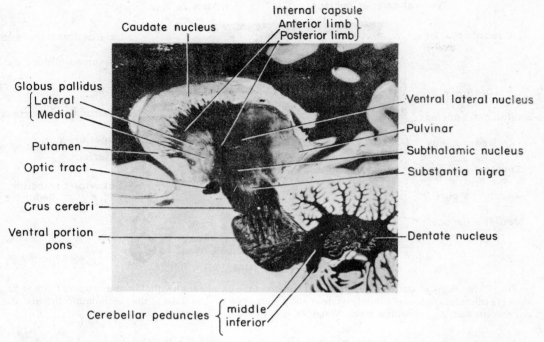

Caudate nucleus

Internal capsule
Anterior limb }
Posterior limb }

Globus pallidus
{ Lateral
{ Medial

Putamen

Optic tract

Crus cerebri

Ventral portion
pons

Ventral lateral nucleus

Pulvinar

Subthalamic nucleus

Substantia nigra

Dentate nucleus

Cerebellar peduncles { middle
{ inferior

FIG. 17-12. Sagittal section through the basal ganglia, thalamus, upper brain stem and cerebellum. Relationships between the basal ganglia, the subthalamic nucleus and the substantia nigra are evident. Weigert's myelin stain. Photograph.

bus pallidus (Fig. 16-10; Carpenter and Strominger, '67). Some authors believe that the subthalamic nucleus sends fibers to the substantia nigra (Glees and Wall, '46; Whittier and Mettler, '49a), but this connection remains in doubt. No fibers from the substantia nigra project to the subthalamic nucleus (Cole et al., '64; Carpenter and McMasters, '64). So-called subthalamotegmental fibers (Papez, '42; Woodburne et al., '46) appear to actually be pallidotegmental fibers. No fibers from the subthalamic nucleus project to the thalamus.

In man relatively discrete lesions in the subthalamic nucleus, usually hemorrhagic, give rise to violent, forceful and persistent choroid movements, referred to as *hemiballism*. These unusually violent involuntary movements occur contralateral to the lesion and involve primarily the proximal musculature of the upper and lower extremities, although they may involve the facial and cervical musculature as well (Jakob, '23; Martin, '27; von San-

tha, '28; Martin and Alcock, '34; Whittier, '47).

The Zona Incerta. This structure is a strip of gray matter situated between the thalamic and lenticular fasciculi (Figs. 15-6, 17-8, 17-10 and 17-11). It is a diffuse cell group which laterally is continuous with the thalamic reticular nucleus. This zone receives corticofugal fibers from the precentral cortex; its efferent projections are unknown.

The lenticular fasciculus, ansa lenticularis and thalamic fasciculus constitute the largest and best defined fiber bundles of passage in the subthalamic region. Scattered along and between the fibers of the ansa lenticularis are strands of cells which collectively constitute the so-called *nucleus of the ansa lenticularis* (Riley, '43).

Forel's Field H (*prerubral field*). This field contains pallidofugal fibers and scattered cells which constitute the nucleus of the prerubral field (nucleus campi Foreli). The nuclei of the prerubral field (Figs. 15-6, 15-10 and 17-11), together with similar

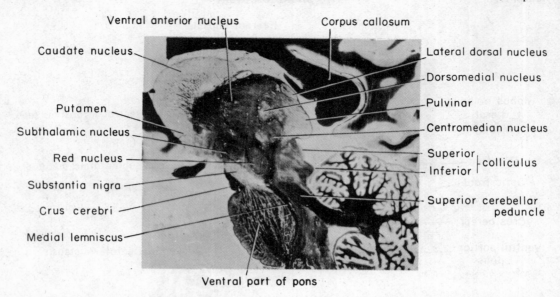

Ventral anterior nucleus
Corpus callosum
Caudate nucleus
Lateral dorsal nucleus
Dorsomedial nucleus
Putamen
Pulvinar
Subthalamic nucleus
Centromedian nucleus
Red nucleus
Superior | colliculus
Inferior |
Substantia nigra
Crus cerebri
Superior cerebellar peduncle
Medial lemniscus
Ventral part of pons

FIG. 17-13. Sagittal section through medial regions of the basal ganglia, thalamus and upper brain stem, showing the relationships of caudate nucleus and putamen as well as those of the subthalamic nucleus, the red nucleus and the substantia nigra. Weigert's myelin stain. Photograph.

cells scattered along pallidofugal pathways, have been referred to collectively as the *subthalamic reticular nucleus*.

FUNCTIONAL CONSIDERATIONS

Since the term basal ganglia refers to the subcortical telencephalic nuclei, neurologists have found it convenient to use the term "extrapyramidal" motor system to group together the corpus striatum and certain related brain stem nuclei, considered to subserve somatic motor functions. Even though there are many objections to the use of this term, which was coined but not defined by Wilson ('12), it has been used widely for over half a century. It serves mainly to emphasize important functional relationships between the corpus striatum and specific brain stem nuclei. Because the term "extrapyramidal" literally includes the entire central nervous system, except the corticospinal system, a more practical and precise designation is needed. According to many authors nuclei of the brain stem forming a part of this so-called system, in addition to the corpus striatum, include: (1) the subthalamic nucleus, (2) the substantia nigra, (3)

the red nucleus, and (4) the brain stem reticular formation. However, definite anatomical relationships with the corpus striatum have been established only for the subthalamic nucleus and the substantia nigra. The subthalamic nucleus has reciprocal connections with different portions of the globus pallidus. Afferent fibers to the subthalamic nucleus arise almost exclusively from the lateral pallidal segment, while subthalamic efferent fibers project mainly to the medial pallidal segment. Connections between the striatum and the nigra appear truly reciprocal, and topographically inter-relate specific regions of both nuclei. These anatomical relationships appear essential to the function of the corpus striatum. Similar relationships between the red nucleus, the brain stem reticular formation and the corpus striatum are less clear. Both the red nucleus and the reticular formation receive corticofugal fibers from the motor cortex, and portions of both project fibers to spinal levels. In this way these nuclei form part of a nonpyramidal motor pathway, but neither is related to the corpus striatum.

The so-called extrapyramidal system is phylogenetically older than the corticospinal system. It is interesting that the older motor system is defined with respect to the corticospinal system, even though the latter is present only in mammals. In reptiles and birds the neopallium is rudimentary, and descending fibers from the cortex are few in number. The corpus striatum, on the other hand, is an older part of the forebrain found in all vertebrates. The paleostriatum, comparable to the globus pallidus, is already well developed in fish. It receives mainly olfactory impulses and gives rise to the "basal forebrain bundle," which discharges into the thalamus, hypothalamus and midbrain (i.e., a lateral forebrain bundle). This bundle probably is homologous with the ansa lenticularis and lenticular fasciculus of mammals. In reptiles and birds a neostriatum (the caudate and putamen of higher vertebrates) develops and receives impulses mainly from the thalamus. In birds the striatal complex becomes highly differentiated and enlarged to form the most massive portion of the cerebrum. In animals without a cortex, or with a poorly developed one, the corpus striatum is the most important forebrain center. Largely instinctive activities, such as locomotion, defense, feeding and courting, depend upon the integrity of the striatum. Motor activities in these submammalian forms are highly stereotyped and resemble well patterned reflex movements. In birds these activities are practically unaffected after ablation of the primitive cortex, but they are severely impaired by lesions of the corpus striatum (Rogers, '22). Thus in submammalian forms the diencephalon and corpus striatum together constitute the highest sensorimotor integrating mechanism of the forebrain. The thalamus of such animals represents the receptive center; the corpus striatum and hypothalamus are related to motor and visceral control.

With the evolution of the neopallium in mammals the functions of the corpus striatum become subordinated to those of the cerebral cortex. However, the old motor system continues to be utilized for the more or less automatic movements concerned with postural adjustments, defensive reactions and feeding. Many mammals are able to perform their normal activities after destruction of both pyramidal tracts. Even chimpanzees recover sufficiently to feed themselves and to execute movements of walking and climbing. Whether the human striatum has similar functions is still disputed. Destruction of the corticospinal tract in man causes a far more complete and lasting paralysis, but the grosser movements are affected less severely and recover to a considerable extent. According to Wilson ('28), the corpus striatum maintains a postural background for voluntary activities, reinforcing and steadying movements, and postures of cortical origin, but is incapable of initiating such movements.

Physiological studies of the activity of pallidal neurons in unanesthetized monkeys revealed distinctly different discharge patterns in the medial and lateral pallidal segments at rest (De Long, '71). It was also found that neurons in both pallidal segments discharged phasically in relation to limb movement, particularly of the contralateral limbs. Pallidal units most closely related to contralateral limb movements were located in lateral portions of both pallidal segments, and units in extreme rostral and caudal portions of the pallidum failed to show relationships to movement.

Although the corpus striatum and related nuclei are considered to play an important role in motor function, none of these nuclei projects fibers to spinal levels. The corpus striatum consists of two parts, the striatum which receives the principal input, and the globus pallidus which gives rise to efferent systems. Striatal afferent systems arising from the cerebral cortex, the intralaminar thalamic nuclei and the substantia nigra are all topographically organized. Striatal output is conveyed to two structures, the globus pallidus and the substantia nigra, and each of these systems is topographically organized. Strionigral and nigrostriatal fibers are reciprocally organized and appear to constitute a closed feedback loop concerned with the transport of dopamine to localized regions of the striatum (Fig. 17-14). Striopallidal fibers projecting to both segments of the

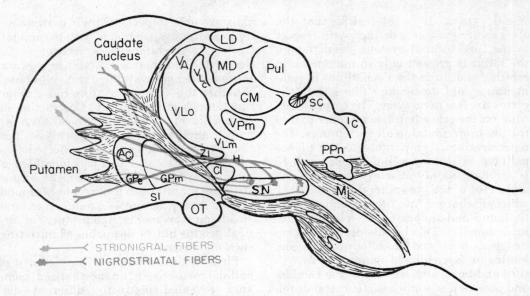

Fig. 17-14. Schematic diagram of the strionigral feedback system in a sagittal plane. Strionigral fibers (*blue*) project topographically upon cells of the pars reticulata of the nigra. Cells of the pars compacta of the nigra give rise to reciprocally arranged nigrostriatal fibers (*red*) considered to convey dopamine to specific loci with the striatum (Carpenter and Peter, '72). Abbreviations used: *AC*, anterior commissure; *Cl*, subthalamic nucleus; *CM*, centromedian nucleus; *GPe*, lateral segment globus pallidus; *GPm*, medial segment globus pallidus; *IC*, inferior colliculus; *LD*, lateral dorsal nucleus; *MD*, dorsomedial nucleus; *ML*, medial lemniscus; *OT*, optic tract; *PPn*, pedunculopontine nucleus; *Pul*, pulvinar; *SC*, superior colliculus; *SI*, substantia innominata; *SN*, substantia nigra; *VA*, ventral anterior nucleus; *VLo* and *VLm*, ventral lateral nucleus, pars oralis and pars medialis; *VPM*, ventral posterior medial nucleus; *ZI*, zona incerta.

pallidum thus represent the major striatal efferent system. The medial segment of the globus pallidus gives rise to the ansa lenticularis and the lenticular fasciculus which project to rostral ventral tier thalamic nuclei, and together constitute the major efferent system of the corpus striatum (Fig. 17-15). Pallidal impulses conveyed to the ventral lateral (VLo) nucleus of the thalamus are relayed to the motor cortex. Thus the contributions of the corpus striatum to motor function must be mediated by cortical motor neurons that project to spinal levels via the corticospinal tract. Because the efferent systems of the corpus striatum convey impulses which are relayed to the motor cortex on the same side, and most fibers of the corticospinal system cross at medullary levels, disturbances of motor function, due to pathological involvement of the corpus striatum, are manifest contralateral to the lesion.

Clinically two basic types of disturbances are associated with diseases of the corpus striatum. These disturbances are: (1) various types of abnormal involuntary movements, collectively referred to as *dyskinesia,* and (2) disturbances of muscle tone. Types of dyskinesia occurring in association with these diseases include *tremor, athetosis, chorea* and *ballism*.

Tremor. This is a rhythmical, alternating, abnormal involuntary activity having a relatively regular frequency and amplitude. A major clinical criterion used to describe and classify different tremors is whether the tremor occurs "at rest" or during voluntary movement. The type of tremor commonly seen in paralysis agitans (parkinsonism), involving primarily the digits and the lips, occurs during the absence of voluntary movement. During the course of voluntary movements the tremor ceases. Tremor classically associated with cerebellar lesions becomes evi-

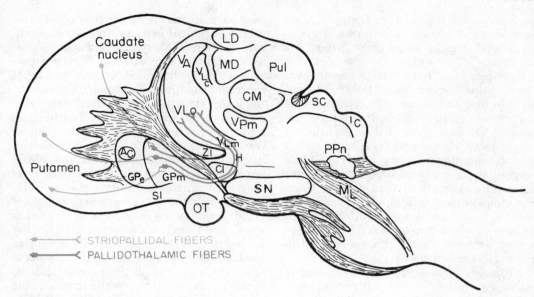

FIG. 17-15. Schematic diagram of striopallidal (*blue*) and pallidothalamic (*red*) fibers which together constitute the principal efferent system of the corpus striatum. The ventral lateral (*VLo*) nucleus of the thalamus projects upon the motor cortex. Abbreviations are the same as in Figure 17-14.

dent during voluntary and associated movements and ceases when the patient is "at rest." Although this criterion is of great importance in clinical neurology, it is acknowledged that tremor "at rest" and tremor during voluntary movement sometimes occur together in various degrees in association with diseases involving primarily either the corpus striatum, or the cerebellum.

Athetosis. Athetosis (Hammond, 1871) is the term used to designate slow, writhing, vermicular involuntary movements involving particularly the extremities, but in many instances also the muscles of the face and neck. The movements blend with each other to give the appearance of a continuous mobile spasm. Athetoid movements involving primarily the axial musculature produce severe torsion of the neck, shoulder girdle and pelvic girdle. This disturbance, referred to as *torsion spasm* or *torsion dystonia,* is considered by some (Jacob, '25; Alexander, '42) as a form of athetosis; differences between torsion dystonia and athetosis are considered to be due largely to inherent mechanical differences between axial and appendicular musculature.

Chorea. Chorea is a brisk, graceful series of successive involuntary movements of considerable complexity which resemble fragments of purposeful voluntary movements. These movements involve primarily the distal portions of the extremities, the muscles of facial expression, the tongue and the deglutitional musculature. Sydenham's chorea occurs in childhood in association with rheumatic heart disease, and most patients recover from the chorea in a relatively short time. Huntington's chorea is a hereditary disorder characterized by choreiform movements and progressive dementia. Although sporadic cases occur, the disorder is inherited as a Mendelian dominant.

Ballism. Ballism, a violent, forceful flinging movement, involves primarily the proximal appendicular musculature and muscles about the shoulder and pelvic girdles. It represents the most violent form of dyskinesia known. Ballism is almost invariably associated with discrete lesions in the subthalamic nucleus or its connections. The dyskinesia occurs contralateral to the lesion and is associated with marked hypotonus.

Although athetosis, chorea and ballism

each present distinguishing features, basic resemblances among these forms of dyskinesia are greater than their differences (Charcot, 1879; Wilson, '25; Mettler, '55; Carpenter, '58). Characteristics common to these dyskinesias include: (1) variable amplitude and frequency, (2) occurrence of movements in immediate and delayed sequence, (3) variations in the duration of single movements, and (4) a highly integrated, complex activity pattern. While each of these types of involuntary motor activity is specialized to a degree, there are indications that athetosis, chorea and ballism may form a spectrum of choreoid activity in which athetosis and ballism represent extreme forms possessing distinguishing characteristics.

Although it is customary to associate increased muscle tonus with most syndromes of the corpus striatum, this is not always found. The initial symptom of paralysis agitans is frequently a rigidity of the muscles, which gradually increases over a period of years. The augmentation of muscle tone is not selective, as in hemiplegia, but is present to a nearly equal degree in antagonistic muscle groups (i.e., in both flexor and extensor muscles). The rigidity in the early stages can be demonstrated by passively flexing or extending the muscles of the extremities, or by attempting to rotate the hand in a circular fashion at the wrist. These movements are interrupted by a series of jerks, referred to as *cog-wheel phenomenon*. In later stages of the disease rigidity may be so severe as to completely incapacitate the patient. Athetosis usually is associated with variable degrees of paresis and spasticity. It is suggested that the slow, writhing character of this dyskinesia may be due in part to the spasticity. Although muscle tone is increased greatly during athetoid movements and persists after the completion of the movement, muscle tone may thereafter gradually diminish (Herz, '31). Chorea and ballism usually are associated with variable degrees of hypotonus (Martin, '27).

The various types of dyskinesia and excesses of muscle tone associated with diseases of the basal ganglia are regarded as positive disturbances since they involve an excess of neural activity and the expenditure of energy (Martin, '59). Such disturbances cannot arise directly from destruction of specific neural structures, but must represent the functional capacity of surviving intact structures. According to this thesis, which is supported by experimental and clinical data, positive disturbances (i.e., tremor, athetosis, chorea and ballism) are believed to be the result of *release phenomena*. A lesion in one structure removes the controlling and regulating influences which that structure previously exerted upon an associated neural mechanism, and thus leads to overactivity of the second neural structure. The theory forms the basis of most neurosurgical attempts to alleviate and abolish dyskinesia and excesses of muscle tone without producing paresis. However, not all of the disturbances associated with diseases of the basal ganglia can be regarded as positive phenomena, particularly in paralysis agitans. Patients with paralysis agitans also exhibit a masklike face, infrequent blinking of the eyes, a slow dysarthric speech, a stooped posture, a slow shuffling gait, loss of associated movements (e.g., swing of the arms while walking) and general poverty of movement. Some patients may have excessive secretion of saliva, unusual oiliness of the skin, difficulty in holding the head erect and disturbances of equilibrium. According to certain authors (Martin and Hurwitz, '62; Martin et al., '62; Martin, '67), the negative symptoms of parkinsonism largely concern disorders of postural fixation, equilibrium, locomotion, phonation and articulation. Negative symptoms are considered to be deficits due to loss of function of destroyed neural structures.

Clinicopathological studies of most forms of dyskinesia categorized as extrapyramidal indicate widespread neuropathological changes. In these disorders the corpora striata suffer severe pathological alterations, but specific brain stem nuclei and parts of the cerebral cortex may be affected also. In paralysis agitans, pathological changes most consistently affect the substantia nigra, but significant altera-

tions may be found also in the globus pallidus, the cerebral cortex and the brain stem
reticular formation (Benda and Cobb, '42;
Heath, '47; Denny-Brown, '62). In the parkinsonian syndrome there is a virtual absence of dopamine in the neostriatum and
substantia nigra (Hornykiewicz, '66; Pinder, '73). In this syndrome there is a decreased ability of the affected brain tissues
to form dopamine. Dopamine, formed in
the large cells of the pars compacta of the
nigra, is conveyed to the neostriatum via
nigrostriatal fibers and stored in terminals. The manner in which dopamine is
liberated in the striatum is unknown, but
Fox et al. ('71/'72) suggest that terminals of
dopaminergic fibers establish connections
with striatal interneurons. Neurophysiological evidence suggests that dopamine
has an inhibitory effect upon single neurons (Hornykiewicz, '66), which suggests
that in parkinsonism there may be an impairment of neostriatal inhibition which
normally acts upon pallidal neurons. In
this sense the dyskinesia and increased
muscle tone seen in parkinsonism may be
regarded as release phenomena (i.e., a removal of inhibitory influences). The above
rationale forms the basis for giving L-dopa
in the treatment of parkinsonism. This
compound passes the blood-brain barrier
and is a precursor of dopamine. L-Dopa can
be given in smaller dosages when used
with a peripheral decarboxylase inhibitor
which prevents systemic decarboxylation
of L-dopa to dopamine (Mars, '73).

Athetosis most frequently is associated
with pathological processes involving the
striatum and cerebral cortex, although lesions are sometimes found in the globus
pallidus and thalamus (Carpenter, '50).
Hemiathetosis may develop after a hemiparesis, or in association with it, as a consequence of a necrotizing cerebrovascular lesion destroying portions of the internal capsule and striatum Athetoid activity occurs
contralateral to the lesion.

With respect to chorea, there is relatively little information available, except
that concerning chronic progressive chorea, or Huntington's chorea. This hereditary disease is characterized by an insidi-
ous onset in adult life. Pathological

changes are widespread but have a special
predilection for the cerebral cortex and
striatum. A study of postmortem brain tissue in a large series of patients dying with
Huntington's chorea (Bird and Iversen,
'74) demonstrated that striatal neurons
have reduced concentrations of glutamic
acid decarboxylase (GAD), γ-aminobutyric
acid (GABA) and choline acetyltransferase
(ChAc). Glutamic acid decarboxylase
(GAD) is the enzyme responsible for the
biosynthesis of GABA and is localized
mainly in inhibitory neurons which release GABA as their transmitter (Iversen,
'72). In these same patients concentrations
of tyrosine hydroxylase (T-OH) and dopamine were normal in the corpus striatum.
The most consistent lesion in Huntington's
chorea appears to be a loss of GABA-con-
taining neurons in the corpus striatum,
along with a loss of cholinergic neurons in
some cases. It is well known that L-dopa
given in large doses to patients with Parkinson's disease may cause choreiform
movements to appear. L-Dopa also tends to
exacerbate choreiform activity in patients
with Huntington's chorea. The most effective drugs for ameliorating choreiform dyskinesia are those which deplete catecholamines, such as reserpine, and dopamine
receptor antagonists. It thus seems that
the presence of normal dopaminergic systems in association with reduced availabil-
ity of GABA (and often acetylcholine) may
be the key neuropharmacological feature
of Huntington's chorea (Bird and Iversen,
'74).

Ballism appears to be the only form of
dyskinesia resulting from a discrete lesion. The lesion, usually hemorrhagic, is
confined to the subthalamic nucleus or its
immediate connections (Whittier, '47).

Attempts to produce dyskinesia in experimental animals by creating lesions in the
corpus striatum have been notoriously unsuccessful (Wilson, '14; Liddell and Phillips, '40; Mettler, '42). Experimental attempts to provoke dyskinesia in animals
by striatal or pallidal lesions have been
criticized on the basis of Meltzer's ('06–'07)
principle of physiological safety. This principle states that in biological organisms
more tissue is found in individual organs

and structures than is required for the maintenance of their essential functions. If this principle is applied to the neuraxis, it would seem to mean that a lesion cannot be expected to produce the symptoms and signs characteristic of a specific tissue deficit unless the amount of destruction includes some of the irreducible minimum necessary for normal function. Failure to produce athetoid or choreoid activity in animals by striatal lesions has been said to be due to the rather limited volumes of tissue destroyed. This explanation does not appear valid in all cases. Wilson ('14) succeeded in destroying selectively virtually the entire putamen in the monkey without producing dyskinesia. The experiments of Mettler ('42) indicate that large bilateral striatal lesions produce forced progression and cursive hyperkinesia, but no dyskinesia. This form of hyperactivity implies that the striatum normally may inhibit other neural mechanisms subserving motor function.

Unilateral lesions of the globus pallidus in monkeys produce minimal disturbances of motor function. Bilateral lesions of the globus pallidus, inflicted simultaneously, produce profound hypokinesis, loss of associated movements and disturbances of posture. Bizarre and enforced postures are maintained for long periods of time, with only feeble or ineffective attempts to establish a normal attitude. These animals bear certain striking resemblances to patients with paralysis agitans, but there is no tremor or rigidity. Evidence suggests that the globus pallidus makes a positive contribution to motor function, and may in some way be involved in all forms of dyskinesia because: (1) it is the source of the principal output of the corpus striatum, and (2) it is the only part of the corpus striatum that projects to thalamic nuclei which in turn project to the motor cortex (Kuo and Carpenter, '73). The validity of this thesis is demonstrated by the gratifying amelioration of various forms of dyskinesia, in selected patients, following stereotaxic lesions produced in either the globus pallidus or the ventral lateral (VLo) nucleus of the thalamus (Wycis and Spiegel, '52; Spiegel and Wycis, '54, '58; Cooper, '56, '60;

Narabayashi et al., '56). Destruction of portions of the globus pallidus appears most effective in relieving contralateral rigidity in paralysis agitans, while thalamic lesions are often most successful in alleviating contralateral tremor. Similar clinical evidence indicates that lesions in these locations can ameliorate symptoms in dystonia (Cooper, '57, '59; Cooper and Bravo, '58), chorea (Spiegel and Wycis, '50) and ballism (Talairach et al., '50; Roeder and Orthner, '56; Cooper, '57; Martin and McCaul, '59; Andy and Brown, '60).

The only form of dyskinesia, other than cerebellar tremor, produced in experimental animals which resembles that occurring in man is that resulting from discrete lesions in the subthalamic nucleus. In the monkey violent choreoid and ballistic activity occurs contralateral to localized lesions in the subthalamic nucleus which: (1) destroy approximately 20% of the nucleus, and (2) preserve the integrity of surrounding pallidofugal fiber systems (Whittier and Mettler, '49a; Carpenter et al., '50). This form of experimental abnormal involuntary activity has been referred to as *subthalamic dyskinesia*. Both clinical and experimental studies suggest somatotopic relationships between portions of the subthalamic nucleus destroyed and the portions of the body exhibiting dyskinesia (von Sántha, '28, '32; Carpenter and Carpenter, '51). In the monkey subthalamic dyskinesia involves the contralateral lower extremity most frequently and most severely, and involvement of the facial, glossal, deglutitional and cervical musculature was never observed. Dyskinesia in the lower extremity was associated with destruction of the rostral part of the subthalamic nucleus, while dyskinesia, predominantly in the upper extremity, was related to lesions in caudal parts of the nucleus. Studies of subthalamic dyskinesia in the monkey indicate that it can be abolished contralaterally without producing paresis by lesions destroying: (1) portions of the medial segment of the globus pallidus, (2) the lenticular fasciculus, or (3) the ventral lateral nucleus of the thalamus (Carpenter et al., '50). This form of dyskinesia can be abolished, but with concomitant paresis, by ablations of the contralateral motor cortex (area 4), or by surgical section of the ipsilateral corticospinal tract at high cervical spinal levels (Carpenter and Mettler, '51; Carpenter et al., '60; Carpenter, '61). No significant modification of this form of dyskinesia in the monkey results from: (1) ablation of area 6, (2) destruction of the centromedian nucleus, or (3) large lesions in the red nucleus (Carpenter and Mettler, '51; Carpenter and Brittin, '58; Carpenter et al., '65). Selective partial cordotomies in animals with this form of dyskinesia indicate that surgical interruption of the rubrospinal, vestibulospinal and reticulospinal tracts has little or no effect upon ipsilateral dyskinesia (Carpenter et al., '60). Multiple dorsal root sections (i.e., dorsal rhizotomy), virtually abolishing afferent input from an entire extremity, cause an increase in amplitude of the dyskinesia (Stein and Carpenter, '65). This increase in amplitude appears to be due to loss of conscious proprioceptive sense and increased loss of muscle tone.

These experimental results have been interpreted to mean that the subthalamic nucleus normally exerts inhibitory and regulating influences upon the globus pallidus. A lesion in the subthalamic nucleus releases the globus pallidus from this controlling influence; removal of this controlling influence is expressed physiologically by bursts of irregular, forceful, large amplitude ballistic movements on the opposite side of the body. Impulses from the globus pallidus reach the ipsilateral motor cortex via the ventral lateral (VLo) nucleus of the thalamus. Dyskinesia occurs contralaterally because impulses responsible for this dyskinesia are conveyed to segmental levels of the spinal cord via the corticospinal tract (Carpenter et al., '60), and most fibers of this system decussate at medullary levels. These experimental results, relative to the effects of pallidal and thalamic lesions, have been confirmed upon human ballism (Talairach et al., '50; Roeder and Orthner, '56; Martin and McCaul, '59).

Attempts to abolish various forms of dyskinesia and excesses of muscle tone by surgery are based on the thesis that these disturbances are the physiological expression of release phenomena. This implies that disease or pathological alterations of certain neural structures has removed inhibitory influences normally acting upon other intact neural structures, and that this overactivity, or excessive function of intact structures, is responsible for the dyskinesia.

Although subthalamic dyskinesia in the monkey represents a special form of dyskinesia, it may share an underlying common feature with the dyskinesia seen in parkinsonism. Since dopamine is considered to inhibit neuronal activity (Hornykiewicz, '66), and most physiological evidence suggests that the striatum subserves an inhibitory function (Mettler, '42), the tremor seen as part of the parkinsonian syndrome may be the physiological expression of diminished striatal inhibition upon the globus pallidus. Thus in these strikingly different forms of dyskinesia the basic mechanism may be the same, namely the removal of inhibitory influences which normally act upon the medial segment of the globus pallidus.

The fact that the medial and lateral segments of the globus pallidus have unique connections suggests that they may have distinctive functions. The medial pallidal segment may be involved in all forms of dyskinesia due to pathological involvement of the corpus striatum, since it gives rise to the major efferent system which connects with thalamic relay nuclei. For this reason lesions in the medial pallidal segment ameliorate most forms of the basal ganglia dyskinesia. Evidence from pathological studies suggests that extensive bilateral destruction of the lateral pallidal segment may provoke choreoid dyskinesia (Carpenter and Strominger, '65). It has been postulated that the dyskinesia associated with such lesions is due to the interruption of pallidal efferent fibers, all of which project to the subthalamic nucleus (Papez et al., '42).

There is abundant evidence that the cerebral cortex must play an important role in neural mechanisms of dyskinesia. It is well known that almost all forms of abnormal involuntary movement cease during sleep and are abolished by general anesthesia. Most forms of dyskinesia are exaggerated in situations where the patient becomes self-conscious, overly anxious or excited. The fact that ablations of motor cortex and interruption of the corticospinal tract at various locations abolish dyskinesia suggests that impulses from centers considered to be responsible for dyskinesia must be transmitted to segmental levels via the corticospinal tract (Bucy, '57, '58, '59; Carpenter et al., '60). These observations imply that the so-called extrapyramidal system is not a complete and independent motor unit.

CHAPTER 18

Olfactory Pathways, Hippocampal Formation and Amygdala

RHINENCEPHALON

The term *rhinencephalon* refers to the olfactory brain. Although some authors use this term broadly to include those regions of the brain concerned with both the reception and integration of olfactory impulses, it is apparent that not all regions of the brain from which potentials can be recorded in response to olfactory stimulation are concerned exclusively with olfactory sense. Higher order pathways of the olfactory system are complex and subject to modifying influences from many sources. Some of these pathways, involving multiple synapses, are subject to other influences and have lost their original olfactory specificity. For this reason use of the term "rhinencephalon" should be restricted to those structures of the central nervous system that receive fibers from the olfactory bulb (Brodal, '63). In this strict sense the rhinencephalon includes the olfactory bulb, tract, tubercle and striae, the anterior olfactory nucleus, parts of the amygdaloid complex and parts of the prepyriform cortex. The term rhinencephalon, in this restricted sense, is equivalent to the *paleopallium* or primitive olfactory lobe (Valverde, '65).

Although the rhinencephalon is large and conspicuous in the lower vertebrates, including many macrosmatic mammals, in man it is overshadowed and comparatively reduced by the tremendous development of the *neopallium*. *The archipallium,* the oldest cortical derivative, is represented by the hippocampal formation, the dentate gyrus, the fasciolar gyrus and the indusium griseum (supracallosal gyrus). The hippocampal formation reaches its greatest development in microsmatic man and is well formed in certain anosmatic aquatic mammals (e.g., porpoise, whale).

OLFACTORY PATHWAYS

Olfactory Receptors. The olfactory membrane is a yellowish brown patch of specialized epithelium in the upper posterior part of the nasal cavity. Olfactory receptors are located in this membrane (Fig. 18-1). Slender sensory cells scattered among supporting cells in the olfactory epithelium have two processes, a coarse peripheral one, passing to the surface, and a fine central one, projecting through the basement membrane. From the coarse peripheral processes ("olfactory rods") a variable number of fine olfactory hairs arise. The delicate central processes, which constitute the unmyelinated *olfactoria fila*, converge to form small fascicles and pass from the nasal cavity via foramina in the cribriform plate of the ethmoid bone.

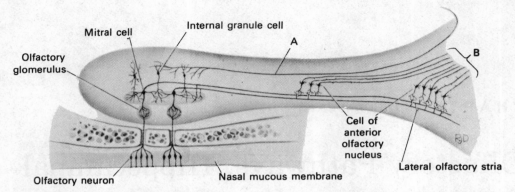

Fig. 18-1. Diagram of the olfactory bulb and tract showing relationships of the olfactory receptors and neurons in the nasal mucosa with cells in the olfactory bulb. Cells of the anterior olfactory nucleus form scattered groups caudal to the olfactory bulb. Centrally projecting fibers from the anterior olfactory nucleus are labeled B, while a fiber from the contralateral anterior olfactory nucleus is labeled A (after Cajal, '11).

These exceedingly small fibers, said to have the slowest conduction rate of any nerves, enter the ventral surface of the olfactory bulb (Figs. 18-1 and 18-2). The olfactory fila, representing the central processes of bipolar cells in the olfactory epithelium, collectively constitute the olfactory nerve (N. I).

Morphologically the olfactory epithelium represents a primitive type of sensory cell and supports the thesis that olfaction is phylogenetically the oldest and most primitive of all senses (Brodal, '69). The extent of the olfactory area in the nasal cavity varies greatly in different animals. Although there is some degree of histological differentiation of olfactory receptor cells, attempts to distinguish morphologically distinct types have been unsuccessful (Clark, '56; de Lorenzo, '63)

Olfactory Bulb. This flattened ovoid body resting on the cribriform plate of the ethmoid bone is the terminal "nucleus" of the olfactory nerve (Figs. 18-1 and 18-2). The paired olfactory bulbs are parts of the central nervous system evaginated from the telencephalon. Most of the fibers of the olfactory nerve enter the anterior tip of the olfactory bulb. Structurally the olfactory bulb has a laminar organization, but in man this is difficult to demonstrate. Within the gray matter of the olfactory bulb are several types of nerve cells, the most striking of which are the large, triangular *mitral cells,* so named because of their resemblance to a bishop's mitre (Figs. 18-1 and 18-3). Primary olfactory fi-

bers synapse with the brushlike terminals of vertically descending dendrites of the mitral cells to form the *olfactory glomeruli.* Smaller cells of the olfactory bulb, known as *tufted cells,* have a number of dendrites, one of which participates in the formation of the glomerulus. The number of glomeruli and mitral cells is rather modest with respect to the large number of receptor cells, suggesting an extensive convergence of impulses (Allison and Warwick, '49). Granule cells of various sizes, found throughout the olfactory bulb, appear to serve associative function. Although the arrangement of afferent fibers in the olfactory bulb does not appear to be localized in any patterned way (Clark and Warwick, '46), a regional organization of olfactory nerve projections to the olfactory bulb has been demonstrated in mammals (Adrian, '42; Clark, '51, '57). Localized lesions in different regions of the olfactory epithelium produce degeneration in specific regions of the glomerular layer (Land, '73). Groupings of glomeruli show marked variations in the intensity of degeneration and some normal glomeruli are present in regions containing degeneration. It has been suggested that a selective projection from receptors in small regions of the olfactory epithelium to specific glomeruli, or groups of glomeruli, could provide the anatomical basis for selective responses to odors. Axons of mitral and tufted cells enter the olfactory tract as *secondary olfactory fibers* (Fig. 18-1).

Caudal to the olfactory bulb are scat-

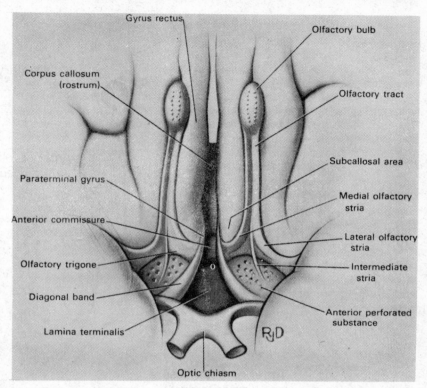

FIG. 18-2. Diagram of olfactory structures on the inferior surface of the brain. The optic nerves and chiasm have been retracted caudally to expose the olfactory area.

tered groups of neurons, intermediate in size between mitral and granule cells, that form the *anterior olfactory nucleus* (Figs. 18-1 and 18-3). Some cells of this loosely organized nucleus are found along the olfactory tracts near the base of the hemisphere. Dendrites of these cells pass among the fibers of the olfactory tract, from which they receive impulses. Axons of the cells of the anterior olfactory nucleus pass centrally, cross in the anterior part of the anterior commissure and enter the contralateral anterior olfactory nucleus and olfactory bulb (Lohman, '63; Powell et al., '65; Valverde, '65; Fig. 18-3). These neurons are thought to serve as part of a reinforcing mechanism for olfactory impulses.

Olfactory Tract. This tract passes toward the anterior perforated substance and divides into well defined *lateral* and *medial olfactory striae*. A thin covering of gray substance over the olfactory striae composes the *lateral* and *medial olfactory gyri* (Figs. 18-2 and 18-3). The lateral olfac-

tory stria and gyrus pass along the lateral margin of the anterior perforated substance to reach the prepyriform region (Fig. 18-4). Fibers of the lateral olfactory stria arising in the olfactory bulb give collaterals to the anterior olfactory nucleus and the anterior perforated substance (which corresponds to the olfactory tubercle in animals). These fibers terminate in the prepyriform cortex and in the corticomedial part of the amygdaloid nuclear complex (Clark and Meyer, '47; Allison, '53; Powell et al., '65). Terminations of these fibers are axodendritic in relation to pyramidal cells of the plexiform layer of the prepyriform cortex and axosomatic in the corticomedial part of the amygdaloid nuclear complex (Allison, '53; Powell et al., '65). Terminations also are present in the nucleus of the lateral olfactory tract and in parts of the anterior amygdaloid nucleus. The prepyriform cortex and the periamygdaloid area, which receive fibers from the lateral olfactory stria, constitute the *primary olfactory cortex*. Olfaction appears

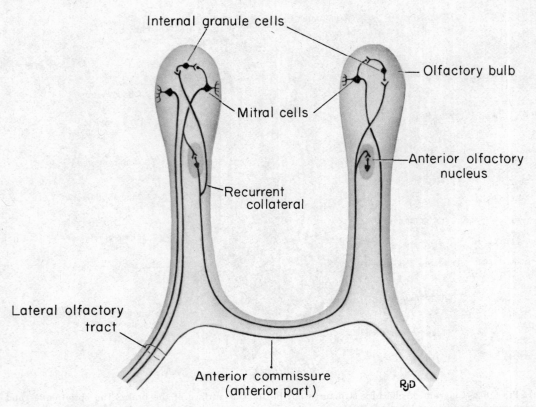

FIG. 18-3. Schematic diagram of interconnections of the olfactory bulbs and anterior olfactory nuclei. Collaterals of mitral cell axons synapse upon apical dendrites of pyramidal-shaped cells of the anterior olfactory nucleus. These cells give rise to fibers that cross in the anterior part of the anterior commissure (Fig. 18-7) and synapse upon cells in the contralateral anterior olfactory nucleus and internal granule cells in the olfactory bulb. Recurrent collaterals of axons of the anterior olfactory nuclei project back to the ipsilateral olfactory bulb to terminate upon internal granule cells, which can in turn activate mitral cells. The principal axons of mitral cells enter the lateral olfactory tract (based on Valverde, '65).

unique among the sensory systems in that impulses in this system reach the cortex without being relayed by thalamic nuclei.

Olfactory Lobe. This lobe makes its appearance in the 2nd month as a narrow longitudinal bulge on the basal surface of the developing cerebral hemisphere, ventral and medial to the basal ganglia (Fig. 3-9A). It is demarcated from the lateral surface of the pallium by the *rhinal sulcus* (Fig. 2-6), and soon differentiates into anterior and posterior portions. The anterior portion, at first containing an extension of the lateral ventricle, elongates into a tubular stalk which becomes solid by the end of the 3rd month, and forms the rudiment of the olfactory tract and bulb. The posterior portion differentiates into the olfactory

area (anterior perforated substance) and certain other olfactory structures closely related to the anteromedial portion of the temporal lobe, collectively known as the *pyriform lobe.*

At the point of division of the olfactory tract into lateral and medial olfactory striae, there is a rhomboid-shaped region, bounded by the olfactory trigone and the optic tract, known as the *anterior perforated substance* (Figs. 2-6, 18-2 and 18-6). This region is studded with numerous perforations made by entering blood vessels (Fig. 20-9). The posterior border of this region, near the optic tract, has a smooth appearance and forms an oblique band, the *diagonal band of Broca* (Fig. 18-2). In macrosmatic animals, especially those with well developed snouts or muzzles, the rostral portion of the area is marked by a prominent elevation, *the olfactory tubercle* (Fig. 18-4). Only rudiments of this structure are present in man. The region of the olfactory tubercle receives fibers from the olfactory bulb, the anterior olfactory nucleus and the amygdaloid nuclear complex. It projects fibers into the stria medullaris and the medial forebrain bundle.

The medial olfactory stria extends toward the medial hemispheric surface and becomes continuous with a small cortical field known as the *subcallosal area* (parolfactory area), located beneath the rostrum of the corpus callosum (Figs. 18-2 and 18-4). This area is limited in front by the anterior parolfactory sulcus, while behind it is separated by the posterior parolfactory sulcus from another strip of cortex, the *paraterminal gyrus* (subcallosal gyrus), which is closely applied to the rostral lamina of the corpus callosum.

The subcallosal area and the paraterminal gyrus together constitute the *septal area* (paraterminal body). The term septal area refers to the cortical part of this region. The subcortical part of the septal region consists of the *medial* and *lateral septal nuclei*, which are found rostral to the anterior commissure (Fig. 18-4). The medial septal nucleus becomes continuous with the nucleus and tract of the diagonal band (Fig. 18-2) and thus establishes connections with the amygdaloid nuclear complex (Fig. 18-4). The lateral septal nucleus appears continuous over the anterior commissure with scattered neurons of the septum pellucidum. The septal nuclei receive a large number of afferent fibers from the hippocampal formation via the fornix (Nauta, '56, '58; Raisman, '66) and some fibers from the amygdaloid complex. The medial septal nucleus also receives fibers from the medial midbrain reticular formation; these fibers ascend in the mammillary peduncle (Fig. 18-5) and continue rostrally in the medial forebrain bundle (Guillery, '56, '57; Nauta and Kuypers, '58). It is uncertain whether the septal nuclei receive olfactory impulses. Evidence suggests that fibers from the olfactory tubercle passing to the septal region are largely nonolfactory. Efferent fibers from the sep-

tal nuclei enter the medial part of the stria medullaris and pass to the habenular nucleus (Figs. 18-4 and 18-5). In addition, axons from these nuclei enter the medial forebrain bundle to be distributed caudally to the entire lateral extent of the hypothalamic region (Fig. 16-7); some fibers of this group extend into the midbrain tegmentum (Nauta, '56, '58). The medial septal nucleus projects fibers back to the hippocampal formation via the fornix (Daitz and Powell, '54; Raisman, '66). The studies of Nauta ('56, '58) indicate that the septal region constitutes a nodal area in the limbic projection system through which primary hippocampal and amygdaloid projections appear to overlap. Two distinct and separate pathways originating from this region conduct impulses to the midbrain tegmentum. These tracts are: (1) the stria medullaris which synapses upon the habenular nuclei (which in turn give rise to the fasciculus retroflexus), and (2) the medial forebrain bundle (Fig. 18-5).

The *pyriform lobe* consists of the lateral olfactory stria, the uncus and the anterior part of the parahippocampal gyrus. The rostral part of the parahippocampal gyrus is rolled inward and upward as a consequence of the tremendous development of the neopallium. The rostromedial protrusion of this gyrus is the *uncus* (Figs. 2-6 and 18-6). The shallow rhinal sulcus, a rostral continuation of the collateral sulcus, separates the anterior part of the parahippocampal gyrus from the more lateral neocortex (Figs. 2-4, 2-6 and 18-8). In man the caudal limits of this area are indistinct, and it is uncertain how much of the parahippocampal area should be included.

The pyriform lobe, so named because of its pear shape in certain species, is divided into several regions. These include the *prepyriform*, the *periamygdaloid* and the *entorhinal areas*. The prepyriform area, often referred to as the lateral olfactory gyrus, extends along the lateral olfactory stria to the rostral amygdaloid region (Fig. 18-4). Since its afferent fibers are derived from the lateral olfactory stria, it is regarded as an olfactory relay center. The periamygdaloid area is a small region dorsal and rostral to the amygdaloid nuclear complex; it is intimately related to the prepyriform

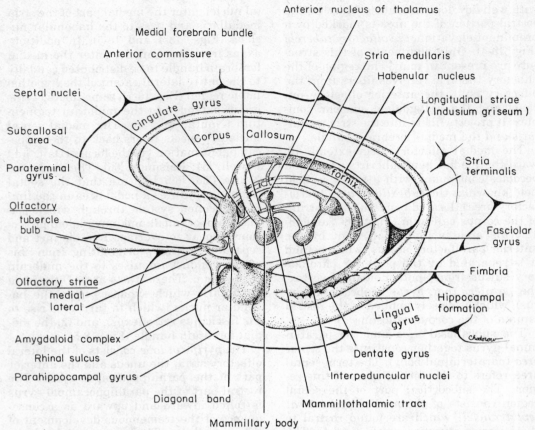

FIG. 18-4. Semischematic drawing of rhinencephalic structural relationships as seen in medial view of the right hemisphere. Both deep and superficial structures are indicated. Modified from a drawing by Krieg ('53).

area. The entorhinal area, the most posterior part of the pyriform lobe, corresponds to area 28 of Brodmann and constitutes a major portion of the anterior parahippocampal gyrus in man (Fig. 19-5). This area, relatively large in primates and in man, is composed of a six-layered cortex of a transitional type. The entorhinal cortex does not receive direct fibers from the olfactory bulb or tract (Cajal, '11; Humphrey, '36; Fox, '40; Clark and Meyer, '47; Powell et al., '65).

The prepyriform cortex projects fibers to the entorhinal cortex (area 28), the basal and lateral amygdaloid nuclei, the lateral preoptic area, the nucleus of the diagonal band, the medial forebrain bundle and to parts of the dorsomedial nucleus of the thalamus (Powell et al., '65). The entorhi-

nal cortex is regarded as a *secondary olfactory cortical area* (Figs. 18-11 and 19-5), although no fibers of the lateral olfactory tract project directly to this area. Efferent fibers from the entorhinal cortex are projected to the hippocampal formation, and to the anterior insular and frontal cortex via the uncinate fasciculus. No fibers from the prepyriform cortex pass to the hippocampal formation.

Different parts of the amygdaloid nuclear complex receive olfactory inputs. Direct projections from the olfactory bulb pass to the corticomedial amygdaloid nuclei, while indirect, but substantial, olfactory impulses pass to the basal and lateral amygdaloid nuclei, via relays in the prepyriform cortex. It is of interest that direct and indirect olfactory pathways to the

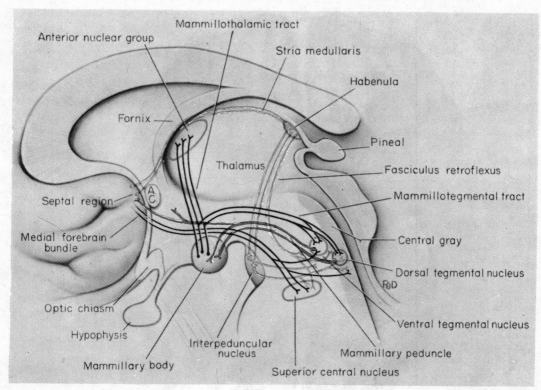

FIG. 18-5. Semischematic diagram of limbic pathways inter-relating the telencephalon and diencephalon with medial midbrain structures. The medial forebrain bundle and efferent fibers of the mammillary body are shown in *black*. The *medial forebrain bundle* originates from the septal and lateral preoptic regions, traverses the lateral hypothalamic area and projects into the midbrain tegmentum. The mammillary princeps divides into two bundles, the *mammillothalamic tract* and the *mammillotegmental tract*. Ascending fibers of the *mammillary peduncle*, arising from the dorsal and ventral tegmental nuclei, are shown in *red*; most of these fibers pass to the mammillary body, but some continue rostrally to the lateral hypothalamus, the preoptic regions and the medial septal nucleus. Fibers arising from the septal nuclei project caudally in the medial part of the *stria medullaris (blue)* to terminate in the medial habenular nucleus. Impulses conveyed by this bundle are distributed to midbrain tegmental nuclei via the fasciculus retroflexus (based on Nauta, '58).

amygdaloid complex terminate in different components, and that these two pathways probably influence the entire amygdaloid complex, except the central nucleus. The central nucleus of the amygdaloid complex contains high concentrations of dopamine (Ungerstedt, '71) and appears to be related to the tail of the caudate nucleus.

Clinical Considerations. The ability of the human nose, in concert with the brain, to discriminate thousands of different odor qualities is well known, but the physiological and psychological bases for such discriminations are unknown. Olfactory discrimination does not appear to be based

upon morphologically distinct types of receptors, but there is some evidence that certain odors may be distinguished by their relative effectiveness in stimulating particular regions of the olfactory epithelium (Mozell, '64; Land, '73). Current theories suggest that spatial and temporal factors probably play important roles in the neural coding of olfactory responses (Moulton and Beidler, '67). Other evidence indicates that the sense of smell is based upon the geometry of molecules (Amoore et al., '64). Two optical isomers, molecules identical in every respect except that one is the mirror image of the other, may have differ-

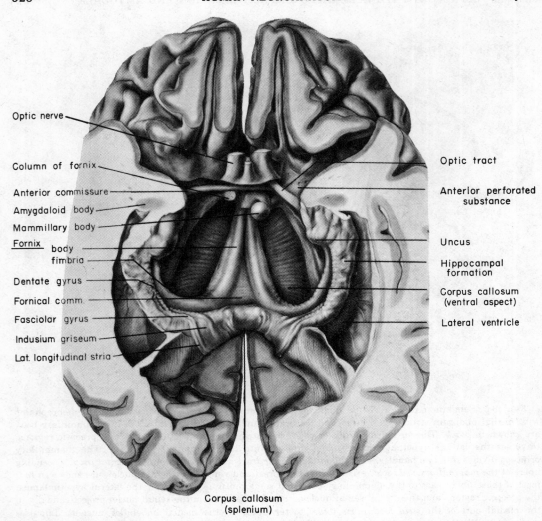

Optic nerve

Column of fornix

Anterior commissure

Amygdaloid body

Mammillary body

Fornix body

fimbria

Dentate gyrus

Fornical comm.

Fasciolar gyrus

Indusium griseum

Lat. longitudinal stria

Optic tract

Anterior perforated substance

Uncus

Hippocampal formation

Corpus callosum (ventral aspect)

Lateral ventricle

Corpus callosum (splenium)

FIG. 18-6. Dissection of the inferior surface of the brain showing the configuration of the fornix, the hippocampal formation, the dentate gyrus and related structures. (Mettler, *Neuroanatomy*, 2nd ed., '48. Courtesy of Dr. F. A. Mettler and The C. V. Mosby Company, St. Louis.)

ent odors. Seven primary odors have been distinguished (i.e., camphoraceous, musky, floral, pepperminty, ethereal (ether-like), pungent and putrid) and are considered to be equivalent to the three primary colors because every known odor can be produced by appropriate mixtures of primary odors. Molecules with the same primary odor appear to have particular configurations, and these configurations are thought to fit appropriately shaped receptors in olfactory nerve endings. Some molecules may fit more than one receptor in different fash-

ions and these are considered to signal a complex odor.

From a clinical viewpoint the importance of the olfactory system is slight in man, since this special sense plays a less essential role than in lower vertebrates. In certain instances valuable clinical information can be obtained by testing olfactory sense by appropriate methods. Olfaction is tested in each nostril separately by having the patient inhale or sniff nonirritating volatile oils or liquids with characteristic odors. Substances which stimulate gusta-

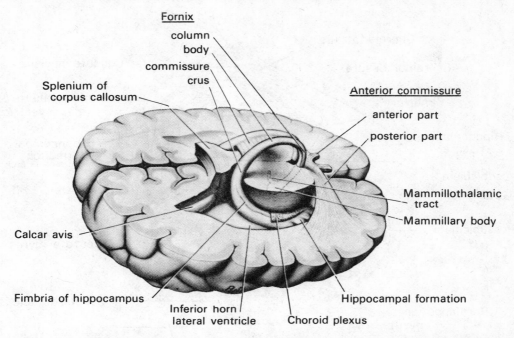

Fornix
column
body
commissure
crus

Splenium of
corpus callosum

Anterior commissure

anterior part

posterior part

Mammillothalamic
tract

Mammillary body

Calcar avis

Fimbria of hippocampus

Inferior horn
lateral ventricle

Choroid plexus

Hippocampal formation

FIG. 18-7. Drawing of a brain dissection showing the hippocampal formation, the fornix system and the anterior and posterior parts of the anterior commissure. In this drawing only postcommissural fibers of the fornix are shown projecting to the mammillary body.

tory end organs, or peripheral endings of the trigeminal nerve in the nasal mucosa, are not appropriate for testing olfaction. Comparisons between the two sides are of great importance. While the olfactory nerves are rarely the seat of disease, they frequently are involved by disease or injury of adjacent structures. Fractures of the cribriform plate of the ethmoid bone or hemorrhage at the base of the frontal lobes may cause tearing of the olfactory filaments. The olfactory nerves may be involved as a consequence of meningitis or abscess of the frontal lobe. Unilateral anosmia may be of important diagnostic significance in localizing intracranial neoplasms, especially meningiomas of the sphenoidal ridge or olfactory groove. Hypophysial tumors affect the olfactory bulb and tract only when they extend above the sella turcica. Olfactory "hallucinations" frequently are a consequence of lesions involving or irritating the parahippocampal gyrus, the uncus or adjoining areas around the amygdaloid nuclear complex. The olfactory sensations which these patients experience

usually are described as disagreeable in character and may precede a generalized convulsion. Such seizures are referred to as "uncinate fits."

THE ANTERIOR COMMISSURE

The anterior commissure crosses the median plane as a compact fiber bundle immediately in front of the anterior columns of the fornix (Figs. 2-10, 2-13, 15-1, 18-4, 18-5, 18-6 and A-25). Proceeding laterally it splits into two portions. The small anterior, or olfactory portion, greatly reduced in man, loops rostrally and connects the gray substance of the olfactory tract on one side with the olfactory bulb of the opposite side (Fig. 18-7). Fibers in this part of the anterior commissure arise from the anterior olfactory nucleus, cross to the opposite side and project to the contralateral anterior olfactory nucleus and to granule cells in the olfactory bulb (Fig. 18-3). It has been suggested (Powell and Cowan, '63) that these centrifugal fibers may subserve reflex control of activity in the olfactory

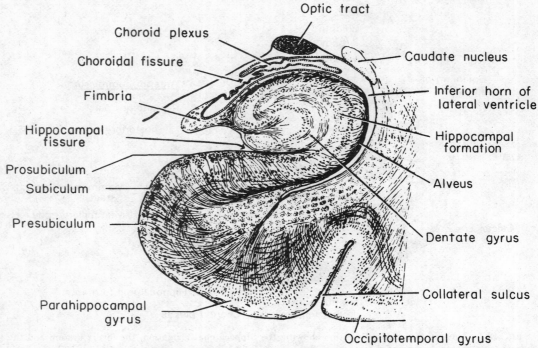

Fig. 18-8. Transverse section through human hippocampal formation and parahippocampal gyrus.

bulb, and in principle may be comparable to the efferent system at spinal levels.

The larger posterior portion forms the bulk of the anterior commissure. From its central region fibers of the anterior commissure pass laterally and backward through the most inferior parts of the lateral segment of the globus pallidus and putamen, a relationship most obvious in sagittal sections of the brain (Figs. A-31 and A-32). Further laterally the fibers of the anterior commissure enter the external capsule and come into apposition with the inferior part of the claustrum. On entering the external capsule the fibers of the commissure twist so that posterior fibers pass ventrally. Fibers of the posterior portion of the anterior commissure mainly interconnect the middle temporal gyri, although some pass into the inferior temporal gyrus (Fox et al., '48). Similar findings have been reported in physiological studies in the monkey (McCulloch and Garol, '41) and in the chimpanzee (Bailey et al., '41). The findings of Whitlock and Nauta ('56), who used silver impregnation

methods, appear similar to those of Fox and his associates.

THE HIPPOCAMPAL FORMATION

The hippocampal formation is laid down in the embryo on the medial wall of the hemisphere along the hippocampal fissure, immediately above and parallel to the choroidal fissure, which marks the invagination of the choroid plexus into the ventricle (Fig. 3-13). With the formation of the temporal lobe, both these fissures are carried downward and forward, each forming an arch extending from the region of the interventricular foramen to the tip of the inferior horn of the lateral ventricle (Fig. 3-15). The various parts of the hippocampal arch do not develop to the same extent. The upper or anterior portion of the hippocampal fissure is invaded by the crossing fibers of the corpus callosum and ultimately becomes the callosal fissure, which separates this massive commissure from the overlying pallium. The corresponding part of the hippocampal formation, which lies above the corpus callosum,

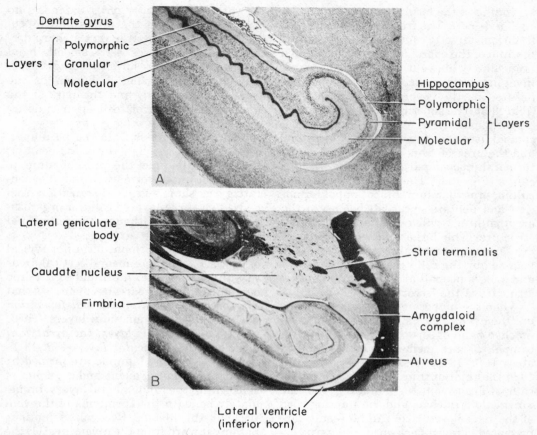

FIG. 18-9. Sagittal sections through the hippocampal formation and dentate gyrus in the rhesus monkey showing the relationships of these structures to the inferior horn of the lateral ventricle, the neostriatum and the amygdaloid nuclear complex. In *A*, the cellular layers of the hippocampal formation and dentate gyrus are identified. In *B*, the alveus, fimbria, tail of the caudate nucleus, stria terminalis, amygdaloid complex and part of the lateral geniculate body are identified. *A*, Nissl stain, ×8; *B*, Weil stain, ×9.

undergoes little differentiation; in the adult, it forms a thin vestigial convolution, the *indusium griseum* (Figs. 18-6 and 18-7). The lower temporal portion of the arch, which is not affected by the corpus callosum, differentiates into the main structures of the hippocampal formation. The hippocampal fissure deepens, and the invaginated portion, which bulges deeply into the inferior horn, becomes the *hippocampus*, while the lips of the fissure give rise to the *dentate* and the *parahippocampal gyri*. The relationships of these structures are best illustrated in a frontal section through this area, or in special dissections (Figs. 18-6 and 18-8). Proceeding from the collateral sulcus, the *parahippocam-*

pal gyrus extends to the hippocampal fissure, where it dips into the ventricle to form the *hippocampal formation*. The latter curves dorsally and medially and, on reaching the medial surface, curves inward again to form a semilunar convolution, the *dentate gyrus* or *fascia dentata* (Fig. 18-9). The whole ventricular surface of the hippocampal formation is covered by a white layer, the *alveus*, which is composed of axons from cells of the hippocampus (Figs. 18-8, 18-9 and 18-10). These fibers converge on the medial surface of the hippocampus to form a flattened band, the *fimbria*, lying medial to the hippocampus and the dentate gyrus. Fibers from the alveus entering the fimbria constitute the beginning of the fornix system (Figs. 18-4, 18-6 and 18-7). The free thin border of the fimbria is directly continuous with the epithelium of the choroidal fissure, which lies immediately above it. The choroid plexus, invaginated into the ventricle along this fissure, partly covers the hippocampus (Fig. 18-8). The superior portion of the parahippocampal gyrus adjoining the hippocampal fissure is known as the *subiculum*, and the area of transition between it and the parahippocampal gyrus, as the *presubiculum* (Fig. 18-8). The presubiculum, subiculum, prosubiculum, hippocampal formation and dentate gyrus all belong to the archipallium, which has an allocortical structure. The larger inferior portion of the parahippocampal gyrus, which is bounded by the collateral sulcus (Figs. 2-4 and 2-6), is neopallial and has the general structure of the isocortex.

When the hippocampal fissure is opened up, the *dentate gyrus* is seen as a narrow, notched band of cortex between the hippocampal fissure below and the fimbria above (Fig. 18-6). In sagittal sections (Fig. 18-9) the relationships between the hippocampal formation, the dentate gyrus, the amygdaloid nucleus and the inferior horn of the lateral ventricle can be readily appreciated. Traced backward, the gyrus accompanies the fimbria almost to the splenium of the corpus callosum. There it separates from the fimbria, loses its notched appearance, and as the delicate *fasciolar gyrus*, passes on to the superior surface of the corpus callosum (Fig. 18-6). It spreads out into a thin gray sheet representing a vestigial convolution, the *indusium griseum* or *supracallosal gyrus* (Figs. 18-4 and 18-6). Imbedded in the indusium griseum are two slender bands of myelinated fibers which appear as narrow longitudinal ridges on the superior surface of the corpus callosum. These are the *medial* and *lateral longitudinal striae (Lancisii)*, which constitute the white matter of these vestigial convolutions (Figs. 2-7 and 18-6). The indusium griseum and the longitudinal striae extend the whole length of the corpus callosum, pass over the genu and become continuous with the paraterminal gyrus, which is in turn prolonged into the diagonal band of Broca (Fig. 18-2). Traced

forward, the dentate gyrus extends into the notch between the uncus and hippocampal gyrus. Here it makes a sharp dorsal bend and passes as a smooth band across the inferior surface of the uncus. This terminal portion is known as the *band of Giacomini*, and the part of the uncus lying posterior to it often is designated as the *intralimbic gyrus*.

The cortical zones from the parahippocampal gyrus through the presubiculum, the subiculum and the prosubiculum to the hippocampal formation and the dentate gyrus show a gradual transition from a six- to a three-layered cellular organization (Fig. 18-8). Although the entorhinal region (area 28) is six-layered cortex, it represents a transitional form not typical of neocortex. In more medial cortical areas certain layers of the entorhinal cortex drop out and undergo rearrangement, so that the cortex of the *hippocampal formation* has only three fundamental layers. These are the *polymorphic layer*, the *pyramidal layer* and the *molecular layer* (Fig. 18-9). Several secondary laminae are formed by the arrangement of axons and dendrites of cells within the fundamental layers. Immediately beneath the ependyma of the ventricle is the alveus. Recognized laminae passing inward from the alveus are: (1) the stratum oriens, (2) the stratum pyramidale, (3) the stratum radiatum, (4) the stratum lacunosum, and (5) the stratum moleculare (Fig. 18-10). The last three laminae are considered to correspond to the molecular layer of the neocortex (Lorente de Nó, '33, '34). The most characteristic layer of the hippocampal formation is the pyramidal layer consisting of large and small pyramidal and Golgi type II cells (Fig. 18-11). *Large* and *small pyramidal cells* exhibit many morphological differences, especially in dendritic development. Some of the cells are described as double pyramids because of the rich dendritic plexuses arising from both poles (Fig. 4-4*J*). Basal and apical dendrites of the pyramidal cells enter adjacent layers, while axons of these cells pass through the stratum oriens to enter the alveus (Fig. 18-11). *Hippocampal basket cells*, similar to the pyramidal cells, are found mainly near the border between the stratum pyramidale and the stratum oriens (Raisman et al., '65). Their axons do not enter the alveus, but loop back through the stratum radiatum to form a dense basket plexus about pyramidal cell bodies. The stratum oriens, containing fibers and polymorphic cells, has been divided into outer and inner zones. Cells of the outer zone distribute axons to the molecular layer. Cells of the inner zone send some axons into the alveus, while others ramify within this layer or pass into the pyramidal layer. The stratum radiatum is made up largely of interlacing and branching processes which appear to radiate from the bordering pyramidal layer. The stratum lacunosum and stratum moleculare, sometimes considered as a single lamina, contain a rich plexus of fibers from other layers.

Although the architectonics of the hippocampal formation is uniform throughout its extent, there are variations in cell morphology, differences in the relative development of various cortical regions and differences in the pathways followed by various fiber systems. On the basis of these differences Lorente de Nó ('34) subdivided the hippocampal formation into sectors designated as CA1, CA2, CA3 and CA4. The position of these various sectors is shown in Figure 18-10.

The *dentate gyrus*, like the hippocampus, consists of three layers: a *molecular layer*, a *granular layer* and a *polymorphic layer* (Figs. 18-9 and 18-10). Layers of the dentate gyrus are arranged in a "U"- or "V"-shaped configuration in which the open portion is directed toward the fimbria in transverse sections (Figs. 18-8 and 18-11). Thus layers are present on both sides of sector CA3 of the hippocampus which extends into the hilus of the dentate gyrus. The molecular layer of the dentate gyrus is continuous with that of the hippocampus in the depths of the hippocampal fissure. The granular layer, made up of closely arranged spherical or oval neurons, gives rise to axons which pass through the polymorphic layer to terminate upon dendrites of pyramidal cells in the hippocampus. Dendrites of granule cells enter mainly the molecular layer. Cells of the polymorphic layer are of several types, including modified pyramidal cells and so-called basket cells. The dentate gyrus does not give rise to fibers passing beyond the hippocampal formation (Raisman et al., '66).

The *area dentata* (Blackstad, '56) is bounded by imaginary lines extending from the tip of the pyramidal cell layer of the hippocampus to the extremities of the granular layer of the dentate gyrus (Fig. 18-10). Within this line is the hilus of the fascia dentata containing polymorphic neurons; this region has been designated as sector CA4 by Lorente de Nó. The term *fascia dentata* applies only to the molecular and granular layers of the area dentata.

Studies of the hippocampal region utilizing autoradiographic technics (Angevine, '65) have provided new information concerning the development and migration of neurons in this cortical region. This technic is based upon the injection of tritiated thymidine into pregnant animals, which becomes incorporated into the DNA of premitotic cells. ^{3}H-Thymidine remains in the nuclei of daughter cells as a permanent label, providing a radioactive marking of neuroblasts. This makes it possible to study the proliferation and migration of neuroblasts destined for various parts of the brain. Studies of neurogenesis show that active displacement and migration of neurons is the rule. Neurons in all components of the hippocampal formation but one arise in a general, but not rigid, "inside-out" sequence. The outstanding exception in this cortical region is the granular layer of the dentate gyrus. Granule cells originating prenatally, or perinatally, migrate to the granular layer in an "outside-in" pattern, and postnatally granule cells arise by proliferation of deeply situated neuroblasts in the granular layer itself.

This "inside-out" sequence of neuron origin applies to the majority of cells in most cortical areas. Thus neurons arising late in gestation, and destined for superficial locations in a given cortical area, must traverse an extensive population of neurons which originated at earlier times. This same sequence of cell differentiation has been demonstrated in the hippocampal formation in human embryos (Humphrey, '66).

Even though the hippocampal formation

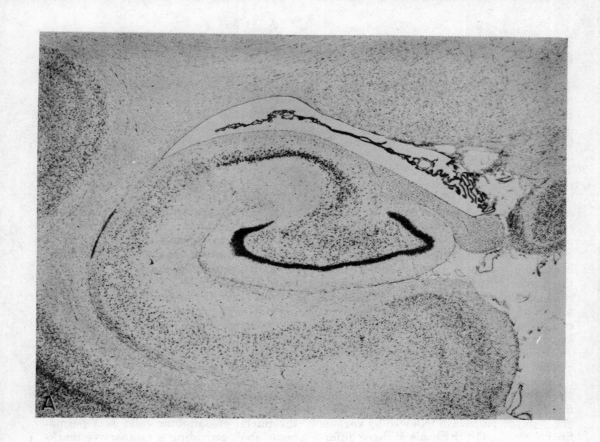

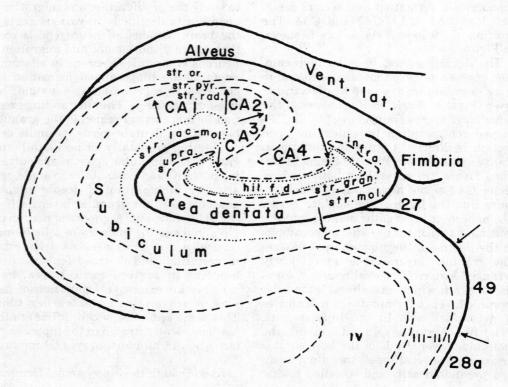

Alveus

Vent. lat.

str. or.
str. pyr.
str. rad.

CA1

CA2

CA3

str. lac-mol.

supra

CA4

infra

Fimbria

hil. f. d

str. gran.

Area dentata

str. mol.

27

S
u
b
i
c
u
l
u
m

49

IV

III-II-I

B

28a

has in the past been considered as an important olfactory center, there is no decisive evidence to support this concept (Brodal, '47). The anatomical connections of this structure indicate that it does not receive fibers from the olfactory bulb or the anterior olfactory nucleus (Rose and Woolsey, '43a; Fox et al., '44; Clark and Meyer, '47) and suggest that it is largely an effector structure.

Afferent fibers to the hippocampal formation arise mainly from the entorhinal area (Cajal, '11; Lorente de Nó, '33, '34), a portion of the pyriform lobe which does not receive direct olfactory fibers. Fibers from the entorhinal area (area 28) are distributed to the dentate gyrus and hippocampus in their entire posterior portion (Lorente de Nó, '34). Fibers arising from the medial part of the entorhinal area follow the so-called "alvear path" to enter the hippocampus from its ventricular surface (Fig. 18-11). These fibers are distributed to the deep layer of the subiculum and to sector CA1 of the hippocampus. Fibers from the lateral parts of the entorhinal cortex pursue the so-called "perforant path" and traverse the subiculum (Fig. 18-11). These fibers are distributed to all sectors of the hippocampus except the region transitional to the dentate gyrus (CA4). Afferent fibers following these pathways establish synaptic contacts with dendrites of pyramidal cells in the hippocampus, but do not come into direct contact with the granule cells in the dentate gyrus (Raisman et al., '65).

Other afferent fibers to the hippocampal formation have been described. The medial septal nucleus projects fibers via the fimbria (Daitz and Powell, '54) to sectors CA3 and CA4 of the hippocampus and to the dentate gyrus. The cingulum (Figs. 2-7 and 2-12), a massive fiber bundle derived from cells of the cingulate cortex, projects to the presubiculum and the entorhinal area (Raisman et al., '65), but not to the hippocampal formation. Since the entorhinal area projects to the hippocampus proper, these findings imply that impulses from the cingulate cortex are relayed to the hippocampus via the entorhinal area. Although it has been postulated that the indusium griseum contributes fibers to the hippocampus, these fibers are not numerous. In addition, some fibers crossing in the hippocampal commissure may interconnect the two hippocampi. None of these afferent pathways to the hippocampal formations appears to transmit olfactory impulses. The pyriform cortex gives rise to deep and superficial pathways that project to the lateral entorhinal cortex, but no fibers that pass directly to the hippocampal formation (Powell et al., '65).

Fornix. This band of white fibers constitutes the main efferent fiber system of the hippocampal formation, including both projection and commissural fibers (Figs. 18-6 and 18-7). It is composed of axons from the large pyramidal cells of the hippocampus, which spread over the ventricular surface as the *alveus* and then converge to form the *fimbria*. Proceeding backward, the fimbriae of the two sides increase in thickness. On reaching the posterior end of the hippocampus, they arch under the splenium of the corpus callosum as the *crura* of the fornix, at the same time converging toward each other. In this region a number of fibers pass to the opposite side, forming a thin sheet of crossing fibers, the *fornical commissure* (hippocampal commissure, or psalterium), a structure rather poorly developed in man (Fig. 18-6). The two crura then join to form the *body of the*

FIG. 18-10. Hippocampal region in the rhesus monkey in horizontal section showing the respective layers of the hippocampal formation and dentate gyrus. *A*, Nissl stain. Photograph, ×20. In *B*, the layers are drawn and the sectors of the hippocampal formation according to Lorente de Nó ('33, '34) are indicated. Abbreviations used are: *28a*, entorhinal area; *hilf. d.*, hilus fasciae dentatae; *49*, parasubiculum; *27*, presubiculum; *str. gran.*, stratum granulosum; *str. lac-mol.*, stratum lacunosum-moleculare; *str. mol.*, stratum moleculare; *st. or.*, stratum oriens; *str. pyr.*, stratum pyramidale; *str. rad.*, stratum radiatum; *supra* and *infra*, suprapyramidal and infrapyramidal limbs of the stratum granulosum. *Roman numerals* refer to layers of cortical areas 27, 49 and 28a. (The assistance of Dr. J. B. Angevine of the University of Arizona, College of Medicine, is acknowledged for delimiting the cell layers and sector boundaries.)

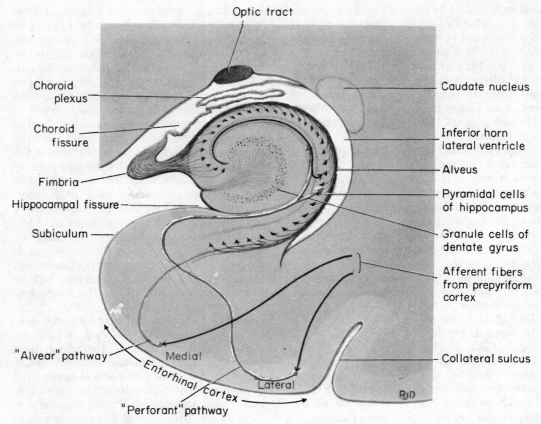

FIG. 18-11. Semischematic diagram of the hippocampal formation, dentate gyrus and entorhinal area. In the dentate gyrus only the granular layer is indicated. In the hippocampal formation only pyramidal cells and their axons projecting into the alveus are shown. Afferent fibers from prepyriform cortex projecting to the entorhinal cortex are shown in *black*. Projections of the entorhinal cortex to the hippocampal formation follow two pathways: (1) the lateral region gives rise to fibers which follow the so-called "perforant" pathway (*red*), and (2) the medial region gives rise to fibers which follow the so-called "alvear" pathway (*blue*). Axons of pyramidal cells in the hippocampal formation entering the alveus pass to the fimbria of the hippocampus. The dentate gyrus gives rise to fibers that project only to the hippocampal formation. (Based on Lorente de No, '34, and a schematic diagram by Peele, '61.)

fornix, which runs forward under the corpus callosum to the rostral margin of the thalamus (Fig. 15-1). Here the bundles separate again, and as the *anterior columns of the fornix*, arch ventrally in front of the interventricular foramina and caudal to the anterior commissure. The fimbriae, thin bands of fibers situated laterally, accompany the fornices throughout most of their extent (Figs. 18-6 and 18-7), but rostrally they become incorporated within the main bundles as the latter form the anterior columns of the fornix. Approximately half of the fibers descend caudal to the

anterior commissure as the *postcommissural fornix* (Daitz and Powell, '54; Powell et al., '57). Remaining fibers of the fornix pass rostral to the anterior commissure as the *precommissural fornix*.

Postcommissural fornix fibers traverse the hypothalamus *en route* to the mammillary body, but in their course give off fibers to the thalamus (Fig. 15-1). Fornix fibers passing directly to the mammillary body terminate mainly in the medial nucleus. Fibers leaving the postcommissural fornix rostral to the hypothalamus are distributed mainly to the anterior and the rostral intralaminar thalamic nuclei (Guillery, '56; Nauta, '56; Valenstein and Nauta, '59). According to Powell et al. ('57), the anterior nuclei of the thalamus receive as many direct fibers from the fornix as from the mammillothalamic tract. Some postcommissural fornix fibers descend caudally beyond the mammillary bodies to enter the midbrain tegmentum (Guillery, '56; Nauta, '56, '58).

Precommissural fornix fibers, constituting a less compact bundle than the postcommissural fibers, are distributed to the septal nuclei, the lateral preoptic area, the anterior part of the hypothalamus and the nucleus of the diagonal band (Nauta, '56). Part of these direct fibers, continuing beyond these nuclei, are distributed to rostral parts of the midbrain central gray. The latter fibers represent a direct hippocampo-mesencephalic projection (Nauta, '58). Caudally continuing fibers of the precommissural fornix are joined by numerous fibers from the septal nuclei to form a large part of one of the most massive roots of the medial forebrain bundle (Zuckerkandl's "olfactory bundle of Ammon's horn").

Detailed studies (Raisman et al., '66) provide data concerning the differential origin and distribution of hippocampal efferent fibers contained in the fornix and fimbria. *Postcommissural fornix fibers* arise from hippocampal sectors CA1 (anterior part) and CA2. Those from the anterior part of CA1 project via the fornix to terminate in the anterior thalamic nuclei and the medial and lateral mammillary nuclei. Sector CA2 distributes fibers via the fimbria to essentially the same nuclei. *Precommissural fornix fibers* arise from the posterior part of CA1 and from sectors CA3 and CA4. Fibers from sectors CA3 and CA4 are distributed via the fimbria, while those from sector CA1 (posterior part) pass via both the fornix and fimbria. These precommissural fibers terminate ipsilaterally in the medial septal nuclei, and bilaterally in the lateral septal nuclei and the diagonal band nuclei. The dentate gyrus does not have an extrahippocampal projection.

The above anatomical connections indicate the complex pathways by which impulses from the hippocampal formation can be projected to different parts of the neuraxis. Thus both direct and indirect pathways connect the hippocampal formation with certain thalamic nuclei (i.e., the anterior and the intralaminar), the hypothalamus and the midbrain reticular formation (Fig. 18-5). The anterior nucleus of the thalamus in turn projects to the cingulate gyrus, from which impulses can reach the hippocampus via the cingulum and the entorhinal cortex. One of many circuitous pathways involving the hippocampus is thus completed.

Functional Considerations. Although the hippocampal formation is a large structure and considerable information is available concerning its anatomical connections, relatively little is known about its function. Abundant anatomical and physiological evidence indicates that the hippocampus has no olfactory function (Brodal, '47). Comparative anatomists have long known that development of the hippocampus in mammals does not proceed parallel to the development of olfaction. The hippocampus and dentate gyrus are well developed in anosmatic cetaceans that lack olfactory bulbs and nerves (Addison, '15; Ries and Langworthy, '37). Animal experiments have shown that olfactory discrimination is not affected by ablations of the hippocampus (Swann, '34, '35), and that olfactory-conditioned reflexes persist after removal of the hippocampus (Allen, '40, '41).

Localized lesions in the hippocampus and local stimulation of this structure in conscious cats tend to produce similar phenomena (Green, '60). Behavioral changes observed in these animals resemble those occurring in psychomotor epilepsy, and it seems likely that the abnormal fears, hyperesthesia and pupillary dilatation seen may represent fragments of a seizure. The behavioral changes noted initially after lesions tend to disappear within several weeks, but recur at a later time. The hippocampus is recognized as having an exceedingly low threshold for seizure activity, and afterdischarge is prolonged (Green and Shimamoto, '53; MacLean, '55, '57a; Green, '60). Seizure discharges spread from the hippocampus to other parts of the limbic lobe and ultimately to the neocortex.

Considerable evidence indicates that the hippocampus may be concerned with recent memory (Green, '64). Relatively large bilateral lesions of the hippocampus (Bechterew, '00; Glees and Griffth, '52; Victor et al., '61; Drachman and Arbit, '66) are associated with profound impairment of memory for recent events and with relatively mild behavioral changes, such as persistent inactivity, indifference and loss of initiative. Memory for remote events usually is unaffected. Although general intellectual functions may remain at a fairly high level, these patients demonstrate an inability to learn new facts and skills. These findings are in accord with those found after bilateral resection of the medial parts of the temporal lobe. According to Scoville and Milner ('57), lesions of the most anterior portion of the temporal lobe do not impair memory; impairment of memory occurs only when the lesions extend far enough posteriorly to involve the hippocampal formation, the dentate gyrus and parts of the parahippocampal gyrus. It is generally felt that loss of memory occurs only if lesions of the hippocampal formation and parahippocampal gyrus are bilateral (Penfield and Milner, '58), but some patients may show mild verbal disorders or disturbances of memory following resections of parts of the temporal lobe of the dominant hemisphere. In these cases unsuspected lesions of the opposite hippocampus have been thought to be present. Some evidence suggests that in certain cases of senile dementia, characterized mainly by loss of memory, the most prominent lesions are found in the hippocampus. Experimental studies (Stepien et al., '60; Orbach et al., '60) in the monkey indicate that bilateral removals of the amygdaloid complex and portions of the hippocampus impair memory and learning that depend upon visual and auditory discriminations. Experiments in the rat (Kaada et al., '61) showed that bilateral lesions of the hippocampus, the fornix and mammillary bodies result in severe disturbances of recent memory, as demonstrated by interference with maze learning and retention.

Even though the fornix contains most of the efferent fibers from the hippocampal formation, evidence that interruption of these fibers produces memory loss is meager. No discernible deficits of memory have been reported after section of both fornices in the monkey (Garcia-Bengochea et al., '51) or in man (Dott, '38; Akelaitis et al., '42; Akelaitis, '43). One human case reported by Sweet et al. ('59) showed severe and lasting memory loss, apathy and lack of spontaneity following section of both columns of the fornix to facilitate removal of a third ventricular tumor. The mammillary bodies, like the fornix, would seem to be implicated in memory function, but it must be remembered that the entire projection of the fornix does not reach the mammillary bodies. According to Thompson and Hawkins ('61), bilateral lesions in the mammillary nuclei do not affect memory in the rat; but lesions in the lateral hypothalamic area or the caudal portion of the fasciculus retroflexus significantly impair memory.

Korsakoff's syndrome (amnestic confabulatory syndrome), appearing as a sequel to Wernicke's encephalopathy and probably caused by a thiamine deficiency associated with alcoholism, is characterized by severe impairment of memory, without clouding of consciousness, confusion and confabulatory tendencies. Lesions in this syndrome almost always involve the mammillary bodies and adjacent areas (Symonds, '66). However, it has been suggested that the amnesia of Korsakoff's syndrome is present only if there is additional involvement of the thalamus (Victor, '64).

Although it is not possible to further define the functions of the hippocampus, there are suggestions that it also may be concerned with: (1) emotional reactions or control of emotions, (2) certain visceral activities, and (3) regulation of reticular activating influences upon the cerebral cortex (Green, '64). Particularly prominent among concepts relating the hippocampal formation to emotion is the theory proposed by Papez ('37), which attempts to provide an anatomical basis for emotion. Realizing that the term "emotion" denotes both subjective feelings and the expression of these feelings by appropriate autonomic and somatic responses, Papez concluded, as have others, that the cortex is essential for subjective emotional experience and that emotional expression must be dependent upon the integrative actions of the hypothalamus. He expressed the belief that the hippocampal formation and its principal projection system, the fornix, provide one of the main pathways by which impulses from the cortex reach the hypothalamus (Figs. 15-1, 16-7 and 16-8). Impulses reaching the hypothalamus could be projected caudally through the brain stem to effector structures, as well as rostrally to thalamic, and ultimately cortical levels. The "central emotive process of cortical origin" was considered to be built up in the hippocampal formation, and transmitted to the mammillary bodies, the anterior nuclei of the thalamus and the cingulate gyrus. He regarded the cingulate cortex as the receptive region for impulses concerned with emotion and suggested that radiation of impulses from the cingulate gyrus to other cortical regions added emotional coloring to the psychic process. This circuitous inter-relation between cortex and diencephalon was thought to explain how emotional responses could result from either psychic or hypothalamic activity. Although this hypothesis has been criticized from several different viewpoints, it has served as a potent stimulus for further research and has drawn attention to the so-called limbic system.

AMYGDALOID NUCLEAR COMPLEX

The amygdaloid nuclear complex is a gray mass situated in the dorsomedial portion of the temporal lobe, in front of, and partly above the tip of the inferior horn of the lateral ventricle (Figs. 2-6, 2-14, 18-4, 18-6, 18-9 and 18-12). It is covered by a rudimentary cortex and caudally is continuous with the uncus of the parahippocampal gyrus (Figs. 2-4, 2-6, 2-12 and 18-12).

The amygdaloid complex usually is divided into two main nuclear masses, a corticomedial nuclear group and a basolateral nuclear group (Crosby and Humphrey, '41; Gloor, '60; Crosby et al., '62; Valverde, '65). A rather poorly defined central nucleus is regarded as a separate subdivision, but sometimes is included as part of the corticomedial nuclear group. In man the *corticomedial nuclear group* constitutes a dorsal or dorsomedial part of the complex due to a medial rotation of the temporal lobe. Nuclear subdivisions of the corticomedial group include: (1) the anterior amygdaloid area, (2) the nucleus of the lateral olfactory tract, (3) the medial amygdaloid nucleus, and (4) the cortical amygdaloid nucleus. The nucleus of the lateral olfactory tract is the least well developed of the amygdaloid nuclei in man. The anterior amygdaloid area, representing the most rostral part of the amygdaloid complex, is rather poorly differentiated (Fox, '40). The corticomedial amygdaloid nuclear group lies closest to the putamen and tail of the caudate nucleus.

The largest and best differentiated part of the amygdaloid complex in man is the *basolateral nuclear group*. Subdivisions of this nuclear group are: (1) the lateral amygdaloid nucleus, (2) the basal amygdaloid nucleus, and (3) an accessory basal amygdaloid nucleus. The amygdaloid complex is related medially to the area olfactoria and laterally to the claustrum, while dorsally it is hidden partially by the lentiform nucleus. Caudally the amygdaloid complex is in contact with the tail of the caudate nucleus, which sweeps rostrally in the roof of the inferior horn of the lateral ventricle (Figs. 2-9, 17-4 and 18-9). The amygdaloid complex is found in all mammals and has been homologized with the olfactory striatum (archistriatum) of submammalian forms.

The central amygdaloid nucleus contains nerve terminals with high concentrations of dopamine (Ungerstedt, '71) and appears closely related to the neostriatum.

Among the afferent connections of the amygdaloid complex, olfactory fibers are the best established. Fibers originating in the olfactory bulb project via the lateral olfactory tract to terminate in the corticomedial nuclear group (Clark and Meyer, '47; Adey and Meyer, '52; Allison, '54; Gloor, '60; Powell et al., '65). No fibers from the lateral olfactory tract appear to enter the basolateral nuclear group. The basolateral amygdaloid nuclei receive an indirect olfactory input via relays in the prepyriform cortex (Powell et al., '65; Valverde, '65). Thus nearly all parts of the amygdaloid nuclear complex receive either

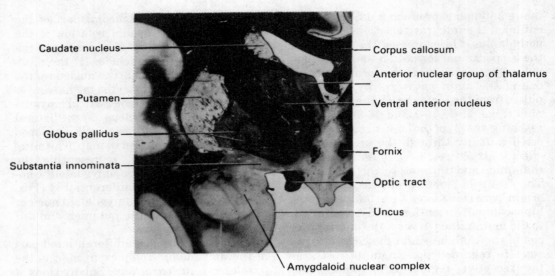

Caudate nucleus

Putamen

Globus pallidus

Substantia innominata

Corpus callosum

Anterior nuclear group of thalamus

Ventral anterior nucleus

Fornix

Optic tract

Uncus

Amygdaloid nuclear complex

Fig. 18-12. Photograph of transverse section through the thalamus, basal ganglia and amygdaloid nuclear complex. Weil stain.

direct or indirect olfactory pathways. The central nuclear group appears to be the exception.

Experimental evidence indicated important diencephalic projections to the amygdala that follow pathways which parallel efferent systems. Fibers arising in the rostral half of the hypothalamus pass via the stria terminalis and pathways ventral to the basal ganglia (ventral amygdalopetal) to all amygdaloid nuclei, except the central nucleus (Cowan et al., '65; Szentágothai et al., '68). This diencephalic input to the amygdaloid nuclear complex passes to all nuclei which receive direct or indirect olfactory afferents.

Although opinions differ, there are suggestions that the amygdala receives fibers from neocortical areas (Lammers, '72). Neocortical projections from the inferior temporal gyrus to the basolateral and central nuclei of the amygdala have been described in both the cat and monkey (Whitlock and Nauta, '56; Lammers and Lohman, '57). In the monkey there appear to be reciprocal relationships between the amygdala and this neocortical area (Nauta, '61). The orbitofrontal cortex also has been described as a source of afferent fibers to the amygdala (Valverde, '56), and van Alphen ('69) has found a limited number of afferent fibers from parietal, occipi-

tal and temporal areas that pass to the lateral amygdaloid nucleus via the posterior limb of the anterior commissure. The fact that neocortical amygdaloid afferents were not found in the rat (Powell et al., '65) has suggested possible species differences.

Anatomical evidence concerning nonolfactory sensory afferents to the amygdaloid complex is meager, although electrophysiological studies suggest such connections. Evoked potentials can be elicited in the amygdaloid complex in response to stimulation of nearly all sensory receptors (Gerard et al., '36; Machne and Segundo, '56). These responses are recorded mainly in the basolateral nuclear group. Impulses originating from distant parts of the body surface, as well as impulses concerned with different sensory modalities, were found to converge upon the same cells (Gloor, '60). Additional subcortical structures projecting afferent fibers to the amygdaloid complex include the brain stem reticular formation (Machne and Segundo, '56), and the pyriform cortex (Fox, '40).

The Stria Terminalis (stria semicircularis). This is the most prominent efferent pathway from the amygdaloid nuclear complex (Figs. 2-18, 2-22, 15-4, 15-6, 15-7, 17-3 and 18-4). Most, but not all, of the fibers in this bundle originate from the corticomedial part of the amygdaloid complex (Fox,

'40; Hall, '63; Cowan et al., '65; Valverde, '65; Raisman, '66; Lammers, '72; De Olmos, '72). Fibers of the stria terminalis arch along the entire medial border of the caudate nucleus near its junction with the thalamus (Fig. 15-7). Rostrally these fibers pass into and terminate in the nuclei of the stria terminalis located lateral to the columns of the fornix and dorsal to the anterior commissure (Heimer and Nauta, '69; De Olmos, '72). This is the most massive termination of the stria terminalis. Part of these fibers, which belong to the postcommissural part of the stria terminalis, also end in the anterior hypothalamic nucleus, and some of the fibers may join the medial forebrain bundle. Fibers of the precommissural part of the stria terminalis terminate in the medial preoptic area and continue caudally to end in a cell-poor zone surrounding the ventromedial hypothalamic nucleus (Hall, '63; Dreifuss et al., '68; Heimer and Nauta, '67, '69; De Olmos, '72).

The Ventral Amygdalofugal Projection. This projection, considered to arise from both the basolateral amygdaloid nuclei and the pyriform cortex, emerges from the dorsomedial part of the amygdala and spreads medially and rostrally beneath the lentiform nucleus (Gloor, '55; Nauta, '61; Cowan et al., '65). These fibers pass through the substantia innominata (Figs. 18-12 and A-22) and enter the lateral preoptic and hypothalamic areas, the septal region and the nucleus of the diagonal band (Broca). Evidence in the rat suggests that fibers in this projection arise mainly form the periamygdaloid cortex (Valverde, '65; Leonard and Scott, '71); some evidence suggests that ventral amygdaloid fibers are unique to higher mammals.

Amygdalofugal fibers, bypassing the preoptic region and hypothalamus, enter the inferior thalamic peduncle (Fig. 15-9) and project to the magnocellular part of the dorsomedial nucleus of the thalamus (Fox, '43; Nauta, '61). It has been suggested that these fibers arise from the basolateral amygdaloid nuclei, but Valverde ('65) reports they arise chiefly from the anterior amygdaloid area. Fibers with this course are joined by projections arising from temporal neocortex (Fig. 15-12). According to Nauta ('61), there are reciprocal connections between the dorsomedial nucleus of the thalamus and the amygdala.

Functional Considerations. Electrical stimulation of the olfactory bulb evokes potentials over the entire extent of the amygdaloid complex (Berry et al., '52), but this complex is only part of a larger cortical and subcortical field activated by such stimuli. Even though the amygdaloid complex receives an olfactory input, the importance of this complex for olfactory sense is uncertain. Most evidence suggests that the amygdaloid complex cannot be closely related to olfactory sense since it is well developed in anosmatic aquatic mammals, and bilateral destruction of it does not impair olfactory discrimination (Swann, '34; Allen, '41).

Electrical stimulation and ablation of the amygdaloid nuclear complex in animals have produced a wide variety of behavioral, visceral, somatic and endocrine changes (MacLean and Delgado, '53; Shealy and Peele, '57; Gloor, '60; Kaada, '51, '72). The most pronounced behavioral changes are elicited by stimulation in unanesthetized animals. The most common response to amygdaloid stimulation under such conditions is an "arrest" reaction in which all spontaneous ongoing activities cease as the animal assumes an attitude of aroused attention. This response is indistinguishable from the arousal reaction obtained from brain stem reticular activation and is associated with cortical desynchronization (Feindel and Gloor, '54; Ursin and Kaada, '60). The "arrest" reaction appears as the initial phase of flight and defense reactions obtained by amygdaloid stimulation. Flight (fear) and defensive (rage and aggression) reactions, termed agonistic behavior, have been elicited from different regions of the amygdaloid complex (Ursin and Kaada, '60). In the amygdaloid complex the intensity of the electrical current determines the intensity of the response, but unlike similar hypothalamic stimulation, the response builds up gradually and always outlasts the period of stimulation (Zbrożyna, '72). The reactions of fear and rage can be intense and are associated with pupillary dilatation, piloerection, growling, hissing and unmistakable signs of emotional involvement and participation of the autonomic nervous system. Electrical stimulation of the stria terminalis, or of the ventral amygdalofugal fibers, produces components of the defense reaction, but lesions of the stria terminalis do not alter the responses obtained by stimulating the amygdala (Hilton and Zbrożyna, '63). After lesions completely interrupting the ventral amygdalofugal projections, defense reactions can no longer be obtained by stimulating the amygdaloid complex (Zbrożyna, '72). These findings suggest that the basolateral part of the amygdaloid complex may play an important role in defense reactions. In man stimulation of the amygdaloid region produces feelings of fear, confusional states, disturbances of awareness and anmesia for events taking place during the stimulation (Feindel and Penfield, '54; Mullan and Penfield, '59; Gloor, '72). Although rage is the most common behavioral response to amygdaloid stimulation in animals, it rarely is associated with temporal lobe seizures or deep stimulation of the temporal lobe in man (Gloor, '72). On a few occasions rage has been elicited by amygdaloid stimulation in man (Heath et al., '55; Mark et al., '72).

Visceral and autonomic responses resulting from amygdaloid stimulation include alterations of respiratory rate, rhythm and amplitude, as well as inhibition of respiration. The most common response of amygdaloid stimulation in unanesthetized animals is an acceleration of the respiratory rate associated with a reduction in amplitude (Kaada, '72). Inhibition of respiration in animals and man has been elicited particularly from ventral parts of the amygdala (Kaada, '51; Shealy and Peele, '57). Cardiovascular responses involve both increases and decreases in arterial blood pressure and alterations of heart rate. Pressor responses appear to predominate following amygdaloid stimulation in the unanesthetized animals (Reis and Oliphant, '64). Gastrointestinal motility and secretion may be inhibited or activated, and both defecation and micturition may be induced. Piloerection, salivation, pupillary changes and alterations of body temperature can occur. These responses are both sympathetic and parasympathetic in nature.

Somatic responses obtained by stimulation of the amygdaloid complex include turning of the head and eyes to the opposite side, and complex rhythmic movements related to chewing, licking and swallowing. It is of interest that the varied somatic and autonomic effects of electric stimulation of the amygdaloid complex constitute an insignificant part of the syndrome produced by lesions in this complex.

Endocrine responses to stimulation of the amygdaloid nuclear complex include the release of ACTH and gonadotrophic hormone, and lactogenic responses. As might be expected stimulation of amygdaloid areas that produce arousal and emotional responses also produce increased adrenocortical output (Kaada, '72; Zolovick, '72). Bilateral lesions in the medial amygdaloid nuclei produce an elevation of serum levels of ACTH (Eleftheriou et al., '66) presumably due to release of an inhibitory influence upon the secretion of ACTH (Bovard and Gloor, '61; Eleftheriou et al., '66). More extensive damage to the amygdala or its hypothalamic projection system may attenuate, but not abolish corticosteroid responses (Zolovick, '72). Stimulation of the corticomedial division of the amygdala may induce ovulation; this response is abolished by transection of the stria terminalis (Shealy and Peele, '57; Everett, '59; Velasco and Taleisnik, '69). The amygdala also is concerned with the luteinizing (LH) and follicle-stimulating (FSH) hormones, but evidence is somewhat conflicting (Kaada, '72). However, evidence is quite clear that the amygdala participates with the hypothalamus in the control and regulation of hypophysial secretions.

Bilateral lesions, fairly well confined to the amygdaloid complex, in monkeys and cats consistently produce disturbances of emotional behavior (Thomson and Walker, '51; Anand and Brobeck, '52; Poirier, '52; Pribram and Bagshaw, '53; Green et al., '57; Green, '58; Gloor, '60; Kaada, '72). The animals become placid and display no reactions of fear, rage or aggression. Previously dominant and abusive animals become tame and do not retaliate to the threats or molestations of other animals. Hypersexuality has been noted as a prominent feature in some experimental studies (Schreiner and Kling, '54; Green et al., '57), but not in all. There are some indications that hypersexual behavior may occur only when the lesions concomitantly involve the pyriform cortex, since amygdaloid lesions sparing this region do not alter sexual behavior. In most instances hypersexual behavior following bilateral lesions develops after a latent period of several weeks. Castration will prevent hypersexuality, or cause it to disappear, following bilateral amygdalectomy (Schreiner and Kling, '54), but this should not necessarily be interpreted as indicating that an increased production of sex hormone is the basic cause of hypersexuality in these animals (Gloor, '60).

In a number of studies, all in cats, removal of the amygdala has led to increased aggressiveness (Bard and Rioch, '37; Bard and Mountcastle, '48; Green et al., '57). Cats displaying postoperative rage frequently developed seizures which were considered to play a role in the savage behavior. Theoretically, the aggressive savage behavior is caused by removals of structures exerting inhibitory influences, but their identification has been elusive.

Observations in man concerning the effects of bilateral lesions in the amygdaloid complex indicate that these lesions cause a decrease of aggressive and assaultive behavior (Green et al., '51; Pool, '54; Scoville, '54). Reports concerning stereotaxic lesions in the amygdaloid complex in man (Narabayashi et al., '63; Narabayashi, '72) suggest that such lesions produce a marked reduction in emotional excitability and tend to normalize social behavior and adaptation of individuals with severe behavior disturbances. Unilateral lesions in some cases proved sufficient to bring about definite improvement. Bilateral lesions did not produce signs and symptoms suggestive of the Klüver-Bucy syndrome. The *Klüver-Bucy syndrome* is characterized by conversion of wild intractable animals (monkeys) to docile beasts which show no evidence of fear, rage or aggression (Klüver and Bucy, '39). In addition, these animals display apparent "psychic blindness," a compulsion to examine objects visually, tactually and orally, bizarre sexual behavior and certain changes in dietary habits. These animals appear unable to distinguish between food and potentially dangerous objects. Almost all objects are examined, smelled and mouthed; if the object is not edible, it is discarded. Hypersexuality is characterized by the indiscriminate partnerships sought with both male and female animals. Tendencies to explore objects orally and docile behavior persist for years in these animals (Klüver, '52). The Klüver-Bucy syndrome has been described in man following large bilateral removals of portions of the temporal lobe (Terzian and Ore, '55; Terzian, '58).

The amygdaloid complex also plays an important role in food and water intake. Bilateral ablations of the amygdala may result in striking hyperphagia, or in hypophagia. Lesions of the basolateral nucleus of the amygdala result in hyperphagia (Fonberg, '68), while stimulation of this part of the amygdala produces an arrest of feeding behavior (Fonberg and Delgado, '61). It has been postulated that this part of the amygdaloid complex inhibits the lateral hypothalamic area, which is regarded as the feeding center of the hypothalamus (Oomura et al., '70; Kaada, '72).

The corticomedial part of the amygdaloid complex is a facilitatory area concerned with food intake. Stimulation of this region produces increases in food intake, as does stimulation of the stria terminalis (Robinson and Mishkin, '62, '68). The amygdala appears to exert its influence upon feeding by modulating the activity of hypothalamic mechanisms. As might be expected, the effects of amygdaloid lesions are less severe than those involving the hypothalamus. Hypophagia is produced by bilateral lesions of the corticomedial amygdaloid nucleus and is more severe in the rat than in the cat; it is not found in the monkey (Kling and Schwartz, '61).

LIMBIC SYSTEM

On the medial surface of the cerebral hemisphere, a large arcuate convolution formed primarily by the cingulate and para-

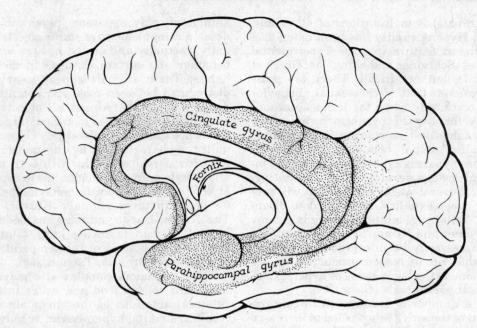

Fig. 18-13. Drawing of the medial surface of the hemisphere. *Shading* indicates the limbic lobe which encircles the upper brain stem. Although the cortical areas designated as the limbic lobe have some common structural characteristics, the extent to which they form a functional unit is not clear.

hippocampal gyri surrounds the rostral brain stem and interhemispheric commissures. These gyri, which encircle the upper brain stem, constitute what Broca (1878) referred to as the *grand lobe limbique*.

Limbic Lobe. The limbic lobe includes the subcallosal, cingulate and parahippocampal gyri, as well as the underlying hippocampal formation and dentate gyrus (Fig. 18-13). From a phylogenetic and cytoarchitectural point of view, the limbic lobe consists of *archicortex* (hippocampal formation and dentate gyrus), *paleocortex* (pyriform cortex of the anterior parahippocampal gyrus), and *juxtallocortex* or *mesocortex* (cingulate gyrus). The latter represents a type of cortex that is transitional between allocortex and neocortex. Some authors (Kaada, '60) in addition have included the cortex of the posterior orbital surface of the frontal lobe, the anterior insular region and the temporal polar region, because of cytoarchitectural and functional similarities. One of the striking features of the limbic lobe is the constancy of its gross and microscopic structure throughout phylogeny, compared with

that of the expanding neopallium which surrounds it (MacLean, '54). Although the cortical areas designated as the limbic lobe have some common structural characteristics, the extent to which they form a functional unit is not understood.

An even more extensive and inclusive designation is the *limbic system*. This term is used to include all components of the limbic lobe (Fig. 18-13) as well as associated subcortical nuclei (Fig. 18-4), such as the amygdaloid complex, septal nuclei, hypothalamus, epithalamus, anterior thalamic nuclei and parts of the basal ganglia (MacLean, '52, '54). Nauta ('58) regards the medial tegmental region of the midbrain as part of the limbic system, since anatomical connections, both ascending and descending, relate this region to the hippocampal formation and the amygdaloid complex. Despite the heterogeneity and diffuse nature of the so-called limbic system, there are compelling observations that structures comprising this system are involved in a neural circuitry that gives rise to a subcortical continuum that begins in the septal area and extends in a paramedian zone through the preoptic region and hypothalamus into the rostral mesencephalon. In this view the hypothalamus is regarded as the central part of this system which suggests the term "septo-hypothalamo-mesencephalic continuum" (Nauta, '72). The principal pathways inter-relating the thalamic nuclei and the brain stem reticular formation with the hippocampus and an amygdaloid complex appear to come together in this region (Figs. 18-4 and 18-5).

The role of the cerebral cortex in the subjective aspects of emotion has been emphasized repeatedly, yet the neocortex appears to have relatively few hypothalamic connections and comparatively little autonomic representation. The intimate relationship of the limbic lobe with the hypothalamus, and the inclusion of these neural structures within the limbic system, have caused many authors to refer to the limbic system as the "visceral brain." Papez's proposed mechanism of emotion, which implicated structures of the limbic system, received experimental support from the studies of Klüver and Bucy ('39) on monkeys deprived of parts of both temporal lobes.

Various visceral, somatic and behavioral responses also are obtained by electrical stimulation of the anterior cingulate cortex and the orbital-insular-temporal cortex. Elevation, as well as depression, of arterial blood pressure results from electrical stimulation of these regions in experimental animals (Kaada et al., '49; Anand and Dua, '56; Kaada, '60). Points from which pressor and depressor effects can be obtained frequently are only a few millimeters apart; most authors report that declines in blood pressure are more frequent and of greater magnitude. Effects upon arterial pressure do not appear to be secondary to associated respiratory changes. Other autonomic responses obtained in experimental animals include inhibition of peristalsis in the pyloric antrum, pupillary dilatation, salivation and bladder contraction. Perhaps the most striking effect of stimulating these regions is profound inhibition of respiratory movements (Smith, '45), which involves mainly the inspiratory

phase of the respiratory cycle, occurs almost instantaneously and cannot be held in abeyance for longer than 35 sec. Acceleration of respiratory movements, produced most readily in the dog, can be elicited by stimulating portions of the cingulate gyrus posterior to the zone yielding maximum inhibitory effects (Kaada, '60).

Somatic effects obtained by stimulating the anterior cingulate and orbital-insular-temporal cortex include: (1) inhibition of spontaneous movements, (2) inhibition and facilitation of cortically induced and reflex movements, and (3) chewing, licking and swallowing movements. Inhibition of spontaneous movements is associated with muscular relaxation and inhibition of respiration. Cortically induced movements appear to be more readily facilitated than spinal reflexes. According to some authors (Showers and Crosby, '58; Showers, '59), a pattern of somatotopic movements obtained by stimulating the anterior cingulate region in the monkey can be elicited in reverse order in the posterior cingulate region; a double somatic representation is thus indicated in this area. These movements are obtained only under light anesthesia and can be induced after ablations of the motor areas.

The behavioral changes observed in unanesthetized animals with stimulation of the cingulate gyrus, which are referred to as an "arrest reaction," consist of an immediate cessation of other activities, an expression of attention or surprise and movements of the head and eyes to the opposite side (Kaada, '51, '60). Animals remain alert during stimulations and respond to external stimuli. Stimulation of posterior cingulate areas may induce sexual reactions, enhanced grooming and seemingly pleasurable reactions (MacLean, '54, '58). Neither unilateral nor bilateral ablations of the cingulate cortex, or of the cortex of the orbitial-insular-temporal polar region, appear to disturb basic somatomotor or autonomic functions to any marked degree. These ablations do not alter: (1) voluntary or reflex motor performance, (2) muscle tone, or (3) respiratory, cardiovascular or gastrointestinal functions (Kaada, '60). Some observers have noted alterations of body temperature, pilo-erection and increased sudomotor activity following lesions of the anterior and posterior cingulate cortex in the monkey (Showers and Crosby, '58).

Experiments have shown that electrical stimulation of certain parts of the limbic system via implanted electrodes in unanesthetized rats, cats and monkeys produce apparent pleasurable effects (Olds and Milner, '54; Brady, '60). In these studies the experimental arrangement is such that the animals can deliver an electrical stimulus to localized areas of their own brains by pressing a pedal or bar. Self-stimulations of the septal region, the anterior preoptic area and the posterior hypothalamus by bar pressing may be at rates as high as 5000/hr in the rat (Olds, '60). The compulsive behavior seen in these situations, where the only reward is an electric shock to a localized region of the brain, suggests that the stimulus may provide a primary reinforcement for drives related to food or sex. Repeated self-stimulation may occur in the monkey from electrodes implanted in a variety of subcortical sites, such as the head of the caudate nucleus, the amygdaloid complex, the medial forebrain bundle and the midbrain reticular formation (Brady, '60). Self-stimulation of certain regions of the thalamus and hypothalamus may produce unpleasant or avoidance reactions, but these regions appear relatively small in number compared to those from which some gratification appears to result.

There is general agreement that the limbic lobe and system occupy central positions in the neural mechanisms that govern behavior and emotion. The components of the limbic system appear to have their main afferent and efferent relationships with two great functional realms, the neocortex and the viscero-endocrine periphery. Among the most prominent neocortical connections are the fibers of the cingulum which arise from the cingulate cortex (Figs. 2-7 and 2-12) and project to the entorhinal cortex along with fibers from other neocortical areas. The entorhinal cortex is a major site of convergence of cortical inputs to the hippocampal formation. Stated broadly and simply, impulses generated in sensory systems, the cerebral cortex and still undetermined neural structures appear to activate triggering mechanisms that in turn excite visceral and somatic systems whose activities in concert provide the physiological expression of behavior and emotion.

The functions of the so-called limbic system are complex and multiple, and the functions of the separate parts may be expressed through distinctive neural structures. Visceral functions appear to predominate in the amygdaloid complex, the anterior cingulate gyrus and the cortex of the orbital-insular-temporal region. Amygdaloid efferent fibers contained in the stria terminalis and the ventral amygdalofugal pathways projecting to the septal region, the preoptic region and portions of the hypothalamus mediate most of the responses produced by stimulation of the amygdaloid complex. However, it must be recalled that amygdalofugal fibers also project to the dorsomedial nucleus of the thalamus via the inferior thalamic peduncle and to specific cortical regions (Nauta, '61). Although the limbic system has been referred to as the "visceral brain," there are some parts of the system in which no visceral function has been demonstrated. In addition certain somatic functions appear to be intermingled inseparably with visceral functions.

CHAPTER 19

The Cerebral Cortex

STRUCTURE OF THE CORTEX

The cerebral cortex develops from the telencephalon which in early stages of histogenesis resembles other parts of the neural tube. The suprastriatal portion of the early telencephalic vesicle is composed of three concentric zones in its smooth-surfaced (lissencephalic) stage: (1) a *germinal zone* surrounding the lateral ventricle, (2) the *intermediate zone* which becomes the white matter of the cerebral hemispheres, and (3) a *marginal zone* which becomes the cortical zone or plate. The original columnar epithelial cells extend through all zones (Sidman, '70). At the end of the 2nd month cells migrate from the intermediate zone into the marginal zone, where they form a superficial gray layer, the *cerebral cortex*. As the cerebral cortex gradually thickens by the addition and differentiation of the migrating cells, it assumes a laminated appearance. The cells become organized into horizontal layers, and between the 6th and 8th months, six such layers may be distinguished (Brodmann, '09). The deeper pyramidal layer, rich in cells, forms layer II to VI, while the outermost layer, composed mostly of fibers, becomes the molecular layer (I). Cells formed at the same time tend to remain in the same layer, and newly formed cells migrate through these layers to more superficial locations (Angevine and Sidman, '61). This "inside-out" sequence of neuronal migration applies to the majority of cortical cells. This six-layered cellular arrangement is characteristic of the entire neopallial cortex, which is referred to as *neocortex, isocortex* (Vogt and Vogt, '19) or *homogenetic cortex* (Brodmann, '09). The *paleopallium* (olfactory cortex) and the *archipallium* (hippocampal formation and dentate gyrus) do not show six layers in either the developing or adult stage. The paleopallium and archipallium together constitute the *allocortex* or *heterogenetic cortex*.

The cerebral cortex has an area of approximately 2200 cm² (2.5 sq ft), but only one-third of this is found on the free surface; the remaining cerebral cortex is hidden in the depths of the sulci. The thickness of the cortex varies from about 4.5 mm in the precentral gyrus to about 1.5 mm in the depths of the calcarine sulcus. The cortex is always thickest over the crest of a convolution and thinnest in the depth of a sulcus. It has been estimated that besides nerve fibers, neuroglia and blood vessels, the cerebral cortex contains nearly 14 billion neurons (von Economo, '29).

The cerebral cortex contains: (1) *afferent fibers* and *terminals* from other parts of the nervous system (e.g., thalamocortical fibers), (2) *association* and *commissural neurons* whose axons inter-relate cortical regions of the same or opposite hemisphere, and (3) *projection neurons* whose axons conduct impulses to other parts of the neuraxis (e.g., corticospinal, corticoreticular or corticopontine fibers). Most projection fibers arise from the deeper layers of the cortex, while the association fibers

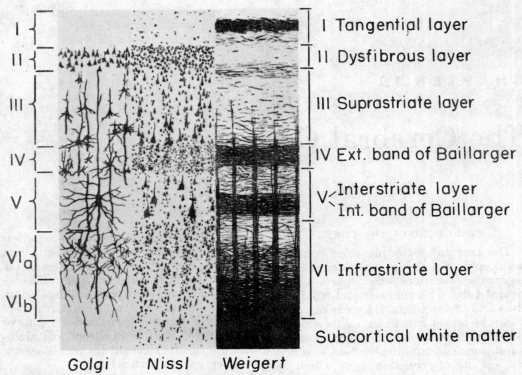

I		I Tangential layer
II		II Dysfibrous layer
III		III Suprastriate layer
IV		IV Ext. band of Baillarger
V		V Interstriate layer / Int. band of Baillarger
VIa		VI Infrastriate layer
VIb		
		Subcortical white matter

Golgi   Nissl   Weigert

FIG. 19-1. The cell layers and fiber arrangement of the human cerebral cortex. Semischematic (after Brodmann, '09).

come mainly, although not exclusively, from the more superficial ones. A striking feature of pallial structure is the relatively small number of projection fibers compared with the enormous number of cortical neurons.

Cortical Cells and Fibers. Although the cerebral cortex contains an enormous number of cells, the number of cell types is small (Colonnier, '67). The principal types of cells found in the cortex are pyramidal, stellate and fusiform neurons (Figs. 4-5, 19-1 and 19-2). The *pyramidal cells,* which are most characteristic of the cortex, have the form of an isosceles triangle whose upper pointed end is continued toward the surface of the brain as the *apical dendrite.* Besides the apical dendrite, a number of more or less horizontally running *basal dendrites* spring from the cell body and arborize in the vicinity of the cell. The axon emerges from the base of the cell and descends toward the medullary substance, either terminating in the deeper layers of

the cortex, or entering the white matter as a projection, or association fiber. The pyramidal cells have large vesicular nuclei, prominent Nissl granules and usually are classified as small, medium and large. The height of the cell body varies from 10 to 12 μ for the smaller neurons to 45 or 50 μ for the larger ones. The giant pyramidal cells of Betz, found in the precentral gyrus, may be more than 100 μ in height.

The *stellate* or *granule cells* are small, polygonal or triangular in shape and have dark-staining nuclei and scanty cytoplasm. These cells, ranging from 4 to 8 μ, have a number of dentrites passing in all directions and a short axon which ramifies close to the cell body (Golgi type II). Other larger stellate cells have longer axons which may enter the medullary substance. Some resemble pyramidal cells in that they have an apical dendrite which extends to the surface. These cells are known as *stellate or star pyramidal cells* (Lorente de Nó, '49). Stellate cells are found

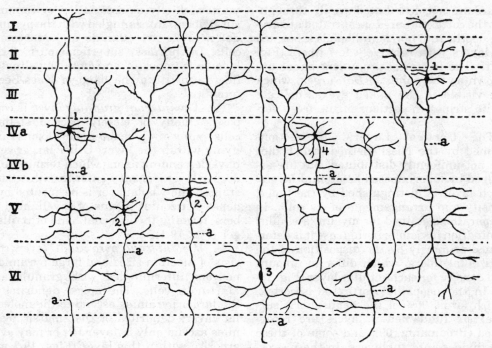

Fɪɢ. 19-2. The dendritic and axonal branchings of several types of cortical neurons with descending axons. Semischematic. *1*, Pyramidal cells of superficial layers; *2*, pyramidal cells from ganglionic layer; *3*, spindle cells; *4*, stellate cells; *a*, axon. Based on data by Cajal ('11) and Lorente de Nó ('49).

throughout all layers of the cortex but are especially numerous in layer IV.

The *fusiform cells* are found mainly in the deepest cortical layer, with their long axis vertical to the surface. The two poles of the cell are continued into dendrites; the lower dendrite arborizes within the layer, while the upper one ascends toward the surface. The axon arises from the middle or lower part of the cell body, and enters the white matter as a projection or association fiber. The large fusiform cells have been classified as "modified pyramidal" cells (Sholl, '56).

Other cell types found in the cortex are the *horizontal cells of Cajal*, and the *cells with ascending axons*, known as the *cells of Martinotti* (*M* in Fig. 19-3). The former are small fusiform cells found in the most superficial cortical layer; their long axons run horizontally for considerable distances and arborize within that layer. Martinotti cells, present in practically all cortical layers, are small triangular cells whose axons are directed toward the surface. Some fi-

bers arborize in the same layer; others send collaterals to a number of layers.

Fibers in the cerebral cortex are disposed both radially and tangentially. The former are arranged in delicate radiating bundles running vertically from the medullary substance toward the cortical surface (Fig. 19-1). They include the axons of pyramidal, fusiform and stellate cells, which leave the cortex as projection or association fibers, and the entering afferent and association fibers, which terminate within the cortex. Ascending axons of the Martinotti cells likewise have a vertical course.

The tangential fibers, running horizontal to the surface, are composed principally of the terminal branches of the afferent and association fibers, the axons of the horizontal and granule cells and the terminal branches of collaterals from the pyramidal and fusiform cells. The horizontal fibers represent, in large part, the terminal portions of the radial fibers, which bend horizontally to come into synaptic relation with cortical cells. The tangential

fibers are not distributed evenly throughout the cortex but are concentrated at varying depths into horizontal bands separated
by layers with relatively few fibers (Fig.
19-1). The two most prominent bands are
known as the *bands of Baillarger,* which
are visible to the naked eye as delicate
white stripes in sections of the fresh cortex.

The Cortical Layers. In sections
stained by the Nissl method, cell bodies
are not uniformly distributed, but are arranged in superimposed horizontal layers.
Each layer is distinguished by the types,
density and arrangements of its cells. In
preparations stained for myelin, a similar
lamination is visible; in this case it is determined primarily by the disposition of the
horizontal fibers, which differ in amount
and density for each cellular layer (Fig. 19-
1). In the neopallial cortex or isocortex,
which forms 90% of the hemispheric surface, six fundamental layers are recognized (Brodmann, '09), and some of these
are divided into sublayers. In the neocortex the following layers are distinguished
in passing from the pial surface to the
underlying white matter: I, molecular; II,
external granular; III, external pyramidal; IV, internal granular; V, internal pyramidal; and VI, multiform.

I. The *molecular* or *plexiform layer* contains cells with horizontal axons and Golgi
type II cells. Within it are found the terminal dendritic ramifications of the pyramidal and fusiform cells from the deeper layers, and the axonal endings of Martinotti
cells. These dendritic and axonal branches
form a fairly dense tangential fiber plexus;
hence the name plexiform layer.

II. The *external granular layer* consists
of numerous closely packed small granule
cells whose apical dendrites terminate in
the molecular layer and whose axons descend to the deeper cortical layers. This
layer is poor in myelinated fibers.

III. The *external pyramidal layer* is composed mainly of well formed pyramidal
neurons. Two sublayers are recognized: a
superficial layer of medium-sized pyramids, and a deeper layer of larger ones.
Their apical dendrites go to the first layer,
while most of their axons enter the white

matter, chiefly as association or commissural fibers. Intermingled with the pyramidal neurons are granule and Martinotti
cells. In the most superficial part of the
layer a number of horizontal myelinated
fibers constitute the band of Kaes-Bechterew.

IV. The *internal granular layer* is composed chiefly of closely packed stellate
cells, many of which have short axons ram-
ifying within the layer. Other larger cells
have descending axons which terminate in
deeper layers, or may enter the white substance. The whole layer is permeated by a
dense horizontal plexus of myelinated fibers, forming the external band of Baillarger (Fig. 19-1).

V. The *internal pyramidal layer* consists of medium-sized and large pyramidal
neurons intermingled with granule and
Martinotti cells. The apical dendrites of
the larger pyramids ascend to the molecular layer; dendrites of the smaller pyramids ascend only to layer IV, or may even
arborize within this layer (Figs. 19-2 and
19-3). Axons of these cells enter the white
matter chiefly as projection fibers, although a considerable number of callosal
fibers are furnished by the smaller pyramidal cells. The horizontal fiber plexus in the
deeper portion of this layer constitutes the
internal band of Baillarger.

VI. The *multiform* or *fusiform layer* contains predominantly spindle-shaped cells
whose long axes are perpendicular to the
cortical surface. Like the pyramidal neurons of layer V, the spindle cells vary in
size; the larger ones send a dendrite into
the molecular layer, while the dendrites of
the smaller ones ascend only to layer IV,
or arborize within the fusiform layer. Thus
the dendrites of many pyramidal and spindle cells from layers V and VI come into
direct relation with the endings of sensory
thalamocortical fibers, which ramify
chiefly in the internal granular layer. Axons of the spindle cells enter the white
substances, as both projection and association fibers. Many of the short arcuate association fibers connecting adjacent convolutions are furnished by the deep stellate
cells of layer VI (Lorente de Nó, '49). The
multiform layer may be divided into an

upper sublayer of densely packed larger cells, and a lower one of loosely arranged small cells. The whole layer is pervaded by fiber bundles which enter or leave the medullary substance (Fig. 19-3).

Besides the horizontal cellular lamination, the cortex also exhibits a vertical radial arrangement of the cells, which gives the appearance of slender vertical cell columns extending the thickness of the cortex (Fig. 19-9). This vertical lamination, quite distinct in the parietal, occipital and temporal lobes, is practically absent in the frontal lobe. The arrangement into vertical cell columns is produced by the radial fibers of the cortex, just as the horizontal lamination is largely determined by the distribution of the tangential fibers.

The internal granular layer, which receives the main specific afferent projections and is best developed in the primary sensory areas, has been used to distinguish supragranular and infragranular layers. *The supragranular layers* (II and III) are the last to arise, the most highly differentiated and the most extensive in man (Kaes, '07). These layers are considered to be concerned mainly with associative cortical functions since they receive and project association fibers. *The infragranular layers* (V and VI) are well developed in all mammals, are connected with subcortical structures by projection fibers and appear to be concerned with efferent mechanisms, particularly motor function. The supragranular layers are not present in the archipallium or paleopallium.

The Interrelation of Cortical Neurons. The structure of the cerebral cortex as seen in Nissl or myelin sheath stained sections is incomplete, for these stains reveal only the type and arrangement of cell bodies, or the course and distribution of myelinated fibers. These methods give no information regarding terminal dendritic and axonal arborizations, which constitute the synaptic junctions through which nerve impulses are transmitted. An understanding of the neuronal relationships, and of intracortical circuits, can be obtained only by impregnation methods which give a total picture of the cell body

and all its processes. With the Golgi technic the distribution of dendritic and axonal terminals has been worked out by a number of investigators, notably Cajal. Lorente de Nó ('49) has given a detailed account for the elementary pattern of cortical organization that is applicable to the parietal, temporal and occipital isocortex. According to this investigator, the arrangement of the axonal and dendritic branchings forms the most constant feature of cortical structure.

The afferent fibers to the cortex include projection fibers from the thalamus, association fibers from other cortical areas of the same side and commissural fibers from the opposite side. The thalamocortical fibers, especially the specific afferent ones from the ventral tier thalamic nuclei and the geniculate bodies, pass unbranched to layer IV (Figs. 10-1, 10-7, 10-8 and 12-22). Here the axons form a dense terminal plexus (Colonnier, '67); some of the fibers extend to layer III where they arborize (Fig. 19-3B). Specific afferent fibers in layer IV establish both axodendritic and axosomatic synapses upon stellate neurons which are fantastically profuse on some cells (Fig. 19-4; Colonnier, '68).

Fibers of the so-called nonspecific thalamocortical system, related to the intralaminar thalamic nuclei and indirectly to the ascending reticular activating system, also reach the cerebral cortex. Histological data concerning the origin, course and termination of these afferent fibers have been meager (Hanberry and Jasper, '53; Nauta and Whitlock, '54; Bowsher, '66). Recently it has been shown that the intralaminar thalamic nuclei, which project mainly to the striatum, project collateral fibers diffusely to broad regions of the cerebral cortex (Jones and Leavitt, '74). It is thought that the potent effects of the stimulation of the intralaminar thalamic and the brain stem reticular formation upon electrocortical activity probably are mediated by these diffuse collateral projections. These collateral projections to the cerebral cortex appear the same as the nonspecific cortical afferent fibers with diffuse connections described previously by Lorente de Nó ('49). According to Jasper ('60), the synaptic ter-

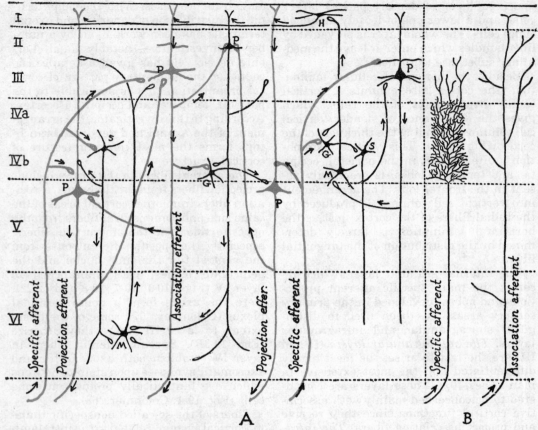

I

II

III

IVa

IVb

V

VI

Specific afferent

Projection efferent

Association efferent

Projection effer.

Specific afferent

Specific afferent

Association afferent

A

B

FIG. 19-3. *A*, Diagram showing some of the intracortical circuits. Synaptic junctions are indicated by *loops*. *Red*, Afferent thalamocortical fibers; *blue*, efferent cortical neurons; *black*, intracortical neurons; *G*, granule cell; *H*, horizontal cell; *M*, Martinotti cell; *P*, pyramidal cell; *S*, stellate cell; *B*, mode of termination of afferent cortical fibers. Based on data by Lorente de Nó ('49).

mination of fibers of this nonspecific system in the cortex is chiefly axodendritic and widely distributed in all layers, but the principal physiological effects appear to be within the superficial layers. Evidence favors the concept that recruiting waves recorded from the cerebral cortex may be a reflection of dendritic electrical activity, which implies that they are graded responses not dependent on the all-or-none firing of cortical cells (Clare and Bishop, '56; Purpura and Grundfest, '56). The association and callosal fibers, on the other hand, give off some collaterals to layers V and VI, and ramify mainly in layers II and III, and to a lesser extent in layer IV. The further course of the entering impulses naturally depends on the ax-

onal branching of the cells which have synaptic relations with the afferent fibers.

The cortical neurons may be grouped into cells with descending, ascending, horizontal and short axons. The last three types serve wholly for intracortical connections (Fig. 19-3). The cells with descending axons (pyramidal, fusiform and larger stellate cells) furnish all the efferent projection and association fibers, and their axonal collaterals form extensive intracortical connections. Some descending axons which do not reach the medullary substance have only intracortical branches.

The pyramidal cells of layers II, III and IV have a similar pattern of dendritic and axonal branchings (Fig. 19-2). They have a number of basilar dendrites which arbor-

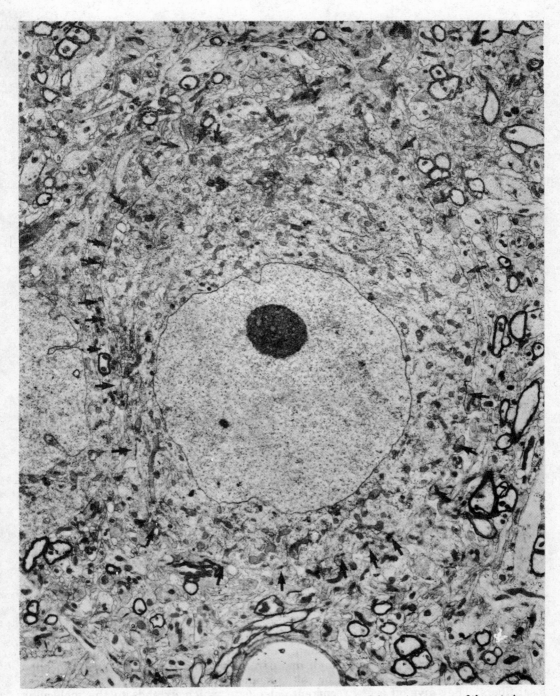

FIG. 19-4. Electron micrograph of a stellate cell in the fourth layer of the striate cortex of the cat. Arrows indicate the large number of synaptic contacts. ×5000. (Courtesy of Dr. Marc Colonnier, School of Medicine, University of Ottawa, and Elsevier Publishing Company, Amsterdam).

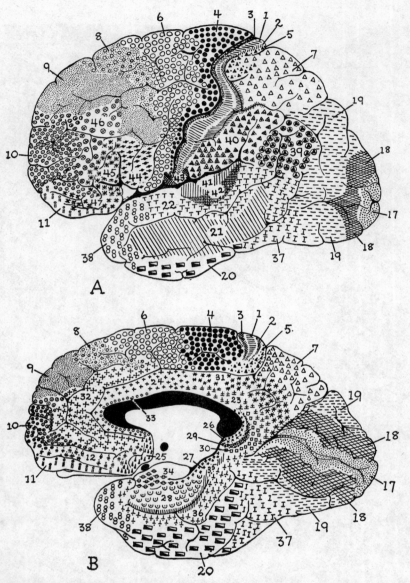

Fig. 19-5. Cytoarchitectural map of human cortex. *A*, Convex surface; *B*, medial surface (after Brodmann, '09).

ize in the same layer, and an apical dendrite which ends in the molecular layer. Their descending axons in part terminate in the deeper layers of the cortex and, in part, are continued as association or callosal fibers. They give off a few recurrent collaterals to their own layers, chiefly II and III, and numerous horizontal collaterals to layers V and VI, where they contribute to the horizontal plexuses.

The pyramidal and fusiform cells of layers V and VI have a characteristic pattern of dendritic and axonal branchings. All the pyramidal cells of layer V give off basilar dendrites to their own layer and an apical dendrite which extends to the molecular layer. There are, however, medium-sized pyramidal neurons, whose apical dendrites terminate in layer IV, and short pyramidal cells, whose dendrites all ra-

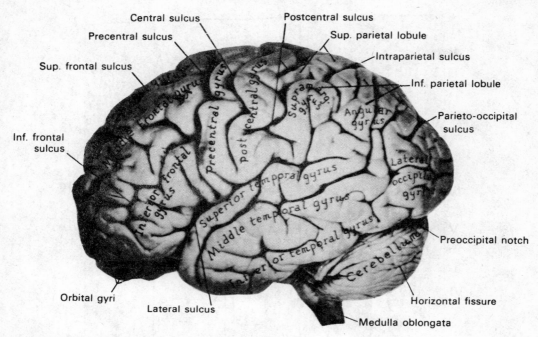

Central sulcus
Precentral sulcus
Sup. frontal sulcus
Postcentral sulcus
Sup. parietal lobule
Intraparietal sulcus
Inf. parietal lobule
Parieto-occipital sulcus
Inf. frontal sulcus
Inferior frontal gyrus
Middle frontal gyrus
Precentral gyrus
Postcentral gyrus
Supramarginal gyrus
Angular gyrus
Lateral occipital gyrus
Superior temporal gyrus
Middle temporal gyrus
Inferior temporal gyrus
Cerebellum
Preoccipital notch
Orbital gyri
Lateral sulcus
Horizontal fissure
Medulla oblongata

FIG. 19-6. Lateral view of human brain. Photograph.

mify in layer V (Fig. 19-2). The spindle cells of layer VI have similar branches. Axons of pyramidal and spindle neurons, and some of deep stellate cells, are continued as projection, association or callosal fibers. All these axons send horizontal collaterals to layers V and VI, where they contribute to the horizontal plexuses, especially those of layer V (internal band of Baillarger). In addition, one or more recurrent collateral ascends unbranched to arborize in layers II and III, and some even extend to the molecular layer (Fig. 19-2).

Although the most striking feature of Nissl-stained sections of the cerebral cortex is its horizontal lamination, physiological studies of the somatic sensory and visual cortex indicate that a vertical column of cells, extending across all cellular layers, constitutes the elementary functional cortical units (Mountcastle, '57; Powell and Mountcastle, '59a; Hubel and Wiesel, '62, '63). This conclusion is supported by the following evidence: (1) neurons of a particular vertical column are all related to the same, or nearly the same, peripheral receptive field, (2) neurons of the same vertical column are activated by the same peripheral stimulus, and (3) all cells of a vertical column discharge at more or less the same latency following a brief peripheral stimulus. The topographical pattern present on the cortical surface extends throughout its depth. Studies of the visual (striate) cortex demonstrate similar discrete functional columns extending from the pial surface to the white matter that are responsive to a specific kind of retinal stimulation in the form of long narrow rectangles of light ("slits"), dark bars against a light background, or straight-line borders, all of which must have a particular axis of orientation (Hubel and Wiesel, '62, '63). Microelectrode recordings indicate that functional columns of cells are arranged radially and perpendicular to the cortical layers. Columns display variations in size and cross-sectional area, and the receptive field axis of orientation varies in a continuous manner as the surface of the cortex is traversed. Anatomically an elementary functional unit of the cortex, represented by a column of cells, must contain the afferent, efferent and internuncial fiber

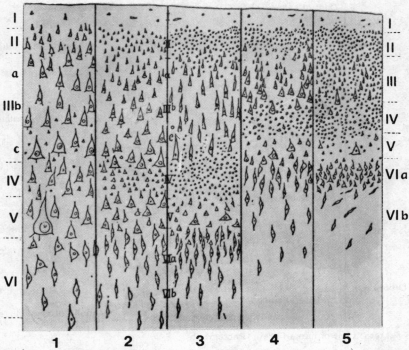

FIG. 19-7. The five fundamental types of cortical structure. *1*, Agranular; *2*, frontal; *3*, parietal; *4*, polar; *5*, granulous (koniocortex) (von Economo, '29).

systems necessary for the formation of a complete cortical circuit. In the basic columnar units the internal circuitry must vary with differences in cytoarchitecture. The convergence of specific afferents upon specific cells in the columnar unit appears to imprint a specific modality which is relayed by intracortical connections to other cells in the column. The complex axonal branching suggests that intracortical circuits involve cells in all parts of the column. These vertical circuits are interconnected by short neuronal links, represented primarily by the short axon granule cells whose processes arborize within a single layer. Through these short links, cortical excitation may spread horizontally and involve a progressively larger number of vertical units (Fig. 19-3). Thus a specific afferent fiber may not only fire vertical columns of cells in its immediate vicinity, but may reach other units through Golgi type II cell relays. These vertical units are fundamentally similar in all mammals. However, the columns of cells with short relays increase in complexity in the higher

forms, especially man. According to Cajal the unique morphological feature of the human cortex is the enormous number of Golgi type II cells, considered to interrelate vertical cell columns.

CORTICAL AREAS

The cerebral cortex does not have a uniform structure. It has been mapped and divided into a number of distinctive areas that differ from each other in total thickness, in the thickness and density of individual layers and in the arrangement and number of cells and fibers. In certain areas the structural variations are so extreme that the basic six-layered pattern is practically obscured. Such areas are termed *heterotypical*, as opposed to *homotypical*, which describes cortex in which the six layers are easily distinguished (Brodmann, '09). Histological surveys, based on differences in the arrangement and types of the cells, and in the pattern of the myelinated fibers, have furnished several fundamentally similar cortical maps, in which the number of distinctive areas has

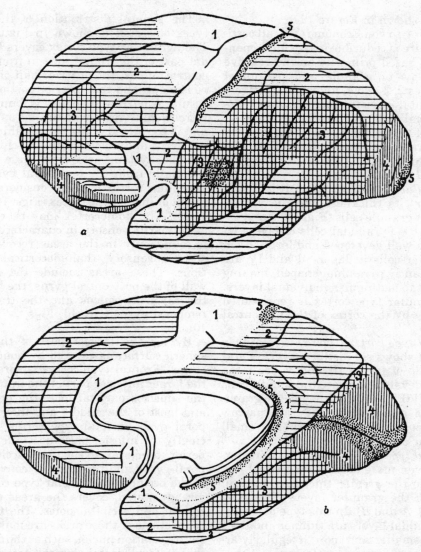

FIG. 19-8. Distribution of the five fundamental types of cortex (Fig. 19-7) over the convex (a) and the medial (b) surfaces of the hemisphere. 1, Agranular; 2, frontal; 3, parietal; 4, polar; 5, granulous (koniocortex) (von Economo, '29).

been estimated variously. Campbell ('05) described some 20 cortical fields; Brodmann ('09) increased the number to 47, and von Economo ('29) to 109; the Vogts ('19) parcelled the human cerebral cortex into more than 200 areas. Even the last number is apparently insufficient, since other investigators have found a number of distinctive cytoarchitectural fields in regions previously considered homogeneous (Beck, '29; Rose, '35). The brain map of Bailey and

von Bonin ('51) utilizes various colors to distinguish distinctive cytoarchitectural features. These authors felt that the concept of absolutely sharp areal boundaries has been carried to absurd lengths and that most brain maps failed to properly represent transitional areas. Brodmann's chart, which is the most widely used for reference, is shown in Figure 19-5. This cytoarchitectural map of the human cortex can be compared with the lateral view of the brain shown in Figure 19-6.

According to von Economo ('29), all cortical structure is reducible to five fundamental types, based primarily on the relative development of granule and pyramidal cells. Types 2, 3 and 4, known respectively as the frontal, parietal and polar types, are homotypical and constitute by far the largest part of the cortex. Types 1 (agranular) and 5 (granulous) are heterotypical and limited to smaller specialized regions (Figs. 19-7 and 19-8).

Agranular type cortex (type 1) is distinguished by its thickness and the virtual absence of granule cells (Figs. 19-7 and 19-9, *A* and *B*). Pyramidal cells of layers III and V are well developed and large. Even the smaller cells in layers II and IV are predominantly pyramidal-shaped, making it difficult to distinguish individual layers. The agranular type cortex is represented classically by the cortex of the precentral gyrus.

Frontal type cortex (type 2) is relatively thick and shows six distinct layers. Pyramidal cells of layers III and V are large and well developed, as are the spindle cells of layer VI (Fig. 19-7). Although the granular layers are distinct, they are narrow and composed of loosely arranged small triangular cells.

Parietal type cortex (type 3) is characterized by even more distinctive cortical layers due to the greater thickness and cell density of the granular layers (Figs. 19-7 and 19-10, *A* and *B*). In this type of cortex, the pyramidal layers are thinner and their cells are smaller and more irregularly arranged.

Polar type cortex (type 4), found near the frontal and occipital poles, is characterized by its thinness, its well developed granular layers and its comparative wealth of cells.

Granulous type cortex or *koniocortex* (type 5) is extremely thin and is composed mainly of densely packed granule cells (Figs. 19-7 and 19-10C). These are found not only in layers II and IV, but the other layers, especially layer III, show large numbers of such small cells and a consequent reduction of the pyramidal cells. The most striking example of this type is the calcarine cortex (Fig. 19-10C).

The general distribution of these five types of cortex is shown in Figure 19-8. The agranular type cortex covers the caudal part of the frontal lobe in front of the central sulcus, the anterior half of the gyrus cinguli and the anterior portion of the insula. A narrow strip also is found in the retrosplenial region of the gyrus cinguli and is continued along the parahippocampal gyrus and uncus. Since the chief efferent fiber systems arise from these regions, especially from the precentral gyrus, the agranular cortex may be considered as efferent or motor type cortex (Figs. 10-13 and 11-23). The koniocortex may be regarded as primarily sensory in character, since it is found only in the areas receiving the specific sensory thalamocortical projections. These areas include the anterior wall of the postcentral gyrus, the banks of the calcarine sulcus and the transverse temporal gyrus (Heschl; Figs. 2-7 and 12-10).

By far the largest part of the hemispheric surface is covered by homotypical cortex. Frontal type cortex is spread over the larger anterior part of the frontal lobe, the superior parietal lobe, the precuneus and most of the middle and inferior temporal gyri. Parietal type cortex includes chiefly the inferior parietal lobule, the superior temporal gyrus, the occipitotemporal gyrus and the anterior convex parts of the occipital lobe. Polar type cortex, as already stated, covers the areas near the frontal and occipital poles. The thalamic connections of these areas are mainly with the association nuclei, such as the dorsomedial, lateral dorsal, lateral posterior and the pulvinar.

Practically every part of the cerebral cortex is connected with subcortical centers by afferent and efferent projections. Strictly speaking there are no circumscribed cortical areas which are purely associative or projective in character. However, there are regions from which the more important descending tracts arise, which directly or through intercalated centers reach the lower motor neurons for the initiation and control of both somatic and visceral activities (Penfield and Jasper, '54). These primarily efferent or motor areas, from which muscular movements can be elicitated by electrical stimulation, are concentrated chiefly in the precentral part of the frontal lobe, but they also are found to a lesser extent in the cortex of other lobes. Similarly those cortical regions which receive direct thalamocortical sensory fibers from the ventral tier thalamic nuclei and from the geniculate bodies represent the primary receptive or sensory areas. The remaining cortical areas which constitute the largest part of the cerebral cortex in man are referred to as "association areas." Although the primary sensory and motor areas are predominant in lower mammals in that they constitute unusually large parts of the neocortex, there is considerable intermingling of functions. In higher mammals, the primary sensory and motor areas become more specific, and there is an absolute increase in the association cortex (Woolsey, '58). Afferent fibers to the association areas are derived from association nuclei of the thalamus and from primary sensory areas of the cortex.

SENSORY AREAS OF THE CEREBRAL CORTEX

Primary Sensory Areas. The localized regions to which impulses concerned with specific sensory modalities are projected are the primary sensory areas of the cerebral cortex. Although certain aspects of sensation probably enter consciousness at thalamic levels, the primary sensory areas are concerned especially with the integration of sensory experience and with the discriminative qualities of sensation. With the exception of olfaction, impulses involved in all forms of sensation reach localized areas of the cerebral cortex via thalamocortical projection systems. The organization of the thalamus is such that all of the specific sensory relay nuclei are located caudally in the ventral tier (Figs. 15-12 and 15-13). The cortical projections of the specific sensory relay nuclei are to localized areas of the parietal, occipital and temporal lobes. Although there is probably a primary cortical receptive area for each sensory modality, each modality is not represented separately, and the primary sensory areas for some forms of sensation are poorly defined. Established primary sensory areas in the cerebral cortex are: (1) the *somesthetic area,* consisting of the postcentral gyrus and its medial extension in the paracentral lobule (areas 3, 1 and 2), (2) the *visual* or *striate area,* located along the lips of the calcarine sulcus (area 17), and (3) the *auditory area,* located on the two transverse gyri (Heschl; areas 41 and 42; see Figs. 2-3, 2-7, 12-10 and 19-5). The *gustatory area* appears to be localized to the most ventral part (opercular) of the postcentral gyrus (area 43). The primary *olfactory area* consists of the allocortex of the prepyriform and periamygdaloid regions and is not assigned numbers under the Brodmann parcellation. A vestibular projection to the human cerebral cortex has not been established.

Secondary Sensory Areas. The primary sensory areas of the cerebral cortex undoubtedly receive the principal projections of the specific sensory relay nuclei of the thalamus, and are the focal regions in the cerebral cortex where specific sensory modalities are most extensively and critically represented. Evidence suggests that near each primary receptive area there are cortical zones which may receive sensory inputs directly, or indirectly, from the thalamus. These cortical zones, adjacent to primary sensory areas, but outside of the principal projection area of the specific sensory relay nuclei of the thalamus, are referred to as the *secondary sensory areas.* These areas have been defined and mapped in experimental animals by recording evoked potentials in response to peripheral stimulation (Adrian, '40, '41; Woolsey and Walzl, '42; Woolsey and Fairman, '46; Thompson et al., '50). Studies of these secondary sensory areas indicate that sequential representation of parts of the body, or of the tonotopic pattern in the case of the auditory areas, is not the same as in the primary areas (Woolsey, '58; Rose and Woolsey, '58). The secondary sensory areas are smaller than the primary sensory areas, and the order of representation is the reverse, or different from that found in the primary areas. Removals of the primary somesthetic area do not abolish potentials evoked in the secondary somatic sensory area (Woolsey and Wang, '45; Buser and Borenstein, '56). Evidence sug-

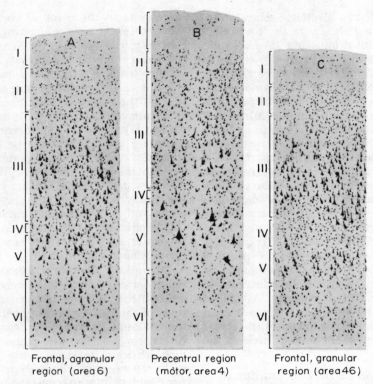

Frontal, agranular   Precentral region   Frontal, granular
region (area 6)   (mótor, area 4)   region (area 46)

FIG. 19-9. Cytoarchitectural picture of several representative cortical areas (after Campbell, '05).

gests that ablations of secondary sensory areas produce relatively minor sensory disturbances compared with those resulting from ablations of primary sensory areas. In the monkey ablations of the secondary somatic area do not appear to interfere with the performance tests based upon somesthetic discrimination (Orbach and Chow, '59).

Secondary sensory areas, which have been defined primarily in experimental animals, include: (1) a *secondary somatic sensory area* (somatic sensory area II; SS II), located ventral to the primary sensory and motor areas along the superior lip of the lateral sulcus (Fig. 19-13), (2) a *secondary auditory area* (auditory area II; A II), located ventral to the primary auditory area (auditory area I) in the cat (Rose and Woolsey, '58; Ades, '59), and (3) a *secondary visual area* (visual area II; V II), described in the rabbit, cat and monkey (Talbot and Marshall, '41; Woolsey, '47; Thompson et al., '50; Hubel and Wiesel, '65) as anterolateral to visual area I, and identical to the area defined anatomically as area 18 (Fig. 19-13). A secondary somatic sensory area has been demonstrated in man (Penfield and Rasmussen, '50), stimulation of which produces various sensations in the upper and lower extremities. Representation of the extremities is chiefly contralateral, although ipsilateral representation also is present. In man no cortical representation for the face, tongue, mouth or throat has been found in SS II. Because of the intimate functional relationships between the primary and secondary sensory areas, these will be discussed together.

The Primary Somesthetic Area. The cortical area subserving general somatic sensibility, superficial as well as deep, is located in the postcentral gyrus and in the posterior part of the paracentral lobule. Histologically the gyrus is composed of three narrow strips of cortex (areas 3, 1, 2) which differ in their architectural structure (Fig. 19-5). In the postcentral region there is a definite anteroposterior gradient of morphological change, but the gradient

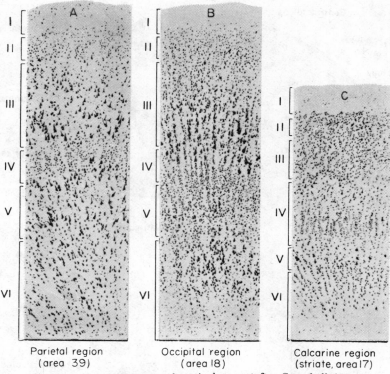

Parietal region	Occipital region	Calcarine region
(area 39)	(area 18)	(striate, area 17)

FIG. 19-10. Cytoarchitectural picture of several cortical areas (after Campbell, '05).

is not uniformly gradual. The anterior part, area 3, is clearly distinguishable from the posterior part; areas 1 and 2 show more gradual morphological changes. Area 3, for the most part, lies along the posterior wall of the central sulcus; its transition with area 4 anteriorly is not sharp and it lies in the posterior part of the depth of the central sulcus (Fig. 19-11). The cortex of area 3 is characterized by its thinness and by the fact that layers II, III and IV tend to fuse with each other (Powell and Mountcastle, '59) and are composed of densely packed granule cells (von Economo, '29). Areas 1 and 2, forming respectively, the crown and posterior wall of the postcentral gyrus, have a six-layered structure characteristic of homogenetic cortex (Fig. 19-11). The most marked differences between area 3 and area 1 are found in layer III; cells in layer III all become pyramidal in shape and there is a reduction in cell density. The transition from area 1 to area 2 is not defined sharply, but is characterized by an increase in the thickness of

the cortex and an increase in the number of large pyramidal cells in layers III and V. The transition from area 2 to areas 5 and 7 is gradual; in the latter areas layers II and IV are sharply demarcated and a pronounced columnar arrangement of cells is seen.

The postcentral gyrus receives the thalamic projections from the ventral posterior nuclei, which relay impulses from the medial lemniscus, the spinothalamic tracts and the secondary trigeminal tracts. Experimental studies (Clark and Powell, '53) in the monkey indicate that areas 3, 1 and 2 receive the specific cortical projection from the ventral posterolateral (VPL) and ventral posteromedial (VPM) nuclei. The majority of the cells of the ventral posterior nuclei project to area 3. Area 1, however, receives the exclusive projections of about 30% of the cells in these nuclei, but it also receives collaterals of fibers passing to area 3. Most of the fibers projecting to area 2 appear to be collaterals of fibers passing primarily to areas 3 and 1.

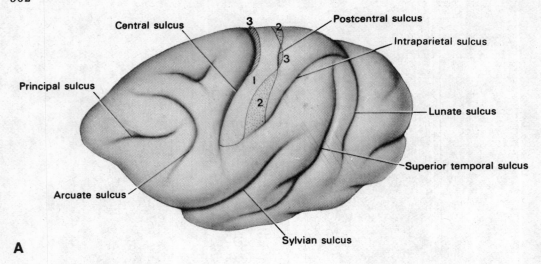

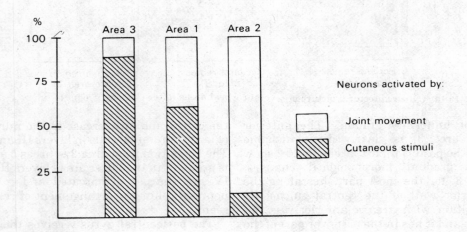

FIG. 19-11. *A*, Diagram of the lateral surface of the monkey cerebral hemisphere showing the extent of the three areas which compose the primary somesthetic cortex. *Area 3*, which forms the posterior wall of the central sulcus, is hidden, except for a small dorsomedial region indicated in the diagram. *Areas 1* and *2* form the crown and posterior wall of the postcentral gyrus. *B*, Bar graph indicating the relative prevalence in each cytoarchitectural area of the postcentral gyrus of neurons activated by cutaneous stimuli and joint movement. (Based upon Powell and Mountcastle, '59; and Mountcastle and Powell, '59.)

Although most of the information concerning thalamocortical projections is based upon retrograde cellular degeneration (Clark and Boggon, '35; Walker, '38a), studies of discrete lesions in the ventral posterior thalamic nuclei reveal additional details in that cells of VPL and VPM have an organized projection to both the pri-mary somesthetic area and somatic sensory area II (Jones and Powell, '70). The projection to area 3 is composed of thick coarse fibers, while fine fibers project to areas 1 and 2 and somatic sensory area II.

The various regions of the body are represented in specific portions of the postcentral gyrus, the pattern corresponding to

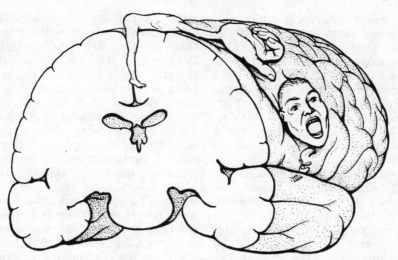

FIG. 19-12. Somatotopic localization of parts of the body in the motor cortex. Parts of the body are drawn in proportion to the extent of their cortical representation. The resulting disproportionate figure is called the motor "homunculus." A similar pattern of localization with respect to somesthetic sense is found in the postcentral gyrus (after Penfield and Rasmussen, '50).

that of the motor area (Fig. 19-12). Thus the face area lies in the most ventral part, while above it are the sensory areas for the hand, arm, trunk, leg and foot in the order named; the lower extremity extends into the paracentral lobule. The cortical areas representing the hand, face and mouth regions are disproportionally large. The digits of the hand, particularly the thumb and index finger, are well represented. The cortical area related to sensations from the face occupies almost the entire lower half of the postcentral gyrus; the upper part of the face is represented above, while the lips and mouth are represented below. The tongue and pharyngeal region are localized in more ventral areas. The distorted representation of the body surface in the primary sensory area reflects the peripheral innervation density. Those regions of the body with higher densities of receptor elements have extensive cortical representation, while those regions with relative few receptors have a minimal representation. According to Penfield, sensations from intra-abdominal structures are represented near the opercular surface of the postcentral gyrus. Most of our information concerning the pattern of representation in the somesthetic cortex has been obtained from stimulating this region in pa-

tients operated upon under local anesthesia (Penfield and Boldrey, '37; Penfield and Rasmussen, '50; Penfield and Jasper, '54). In attempts to present a readily apparent visual pattern of the sequence of sensory representation in the cerebral cortex, Penfield has drawn the "sensory homunculus" relating different parts of the body to appropriate areas of the cortex. The "sensory homunculus" corresponds to the "motor homunculus" (Fig. 19-12).

Using the evoked potential technic, Adrian ('41) found that touch, pressure and movements were the only stimuli which evoked well marked responses in the contralateral postcentral gyrus in the cat. No responses were observed to pain or thermal stimuli. Pressure applied to a foot produced a sustained discharge which increased in frequency as the pressure was increased and gradually declined with a constant stimulus. Tactile stimuli produced brief discharges that were not sustained. The fact that one cortical locus frequently could be activated by touching hairs within a relatively large skin area indicates a considerable degree of convergence at a cortical level. This convergence of pathways in the sensory cortex was observed also by Marshall et al. ('41). These authors found that one cortical point could be activated maximally, and also submaximally, from a considerable area of skin. It would appear that a restricted stimulus can activate a number of afferent units projecting to the cortex, and that slight differences in latency may be due to spread of excitation among thalamic neurons. Cortical responses were evoked contralaterally from all stimuli, except in the face area, where some ipsilateral responses were recorded.

Physiological studies (Powell and Mountcastle, '59a; Mountcastle and Powell, '59) in the monkey indicate that the majority of neurons in the postcentral gyrus are activated by mechanical stimulation, and are selectively excited by stimulation of receptors within either skin or deep tissues, but not by stimulation of both (Fig. 19-11). Over 90% of the neurons in area 2 are related to receptors in deep tissues of the body, while the majority of neurons in area 3 are activated only by cutaneous stimuli; different neurons in area 1 are related to either cutaneous or deep receptors. This differential representation of sensory modalities appears closely correlated with the gradient of morphological change that characterizes these three cytoarchitectural areas. Further evidence (Mountcastle and Powell, '59a) indicates that afferent impulses from receptors in joint capsules and pericapsular tissues, stimulated by joint movement, are conveyed by the posterior columns, the medial lemniscus and thalamic relay neurons to particular cell columns in the postcentral gyrus (Fig. 10-1). Impulses conveyed by this system subserve position sense and kinesthesis. Stretch receptors in muscle and tendons probably do not provide information useful in the perception of joint position; furthermore, most of the afferent impulses from stretch receptors are projected to the cerebellum (Oscarsson, '65). However, the rostral margin of the primary somesthetic area, designated as area 3a, receives a projection from deep tissues via the ventrobasal complex of the thalamus (Jones and Powell, '69). Evidence in the cat suggests that some group I muscle afferents from the forelimb pass to area 3a (Oscarsson and Rosén, '66).

Studies of cell columns of the postcentral

gyrus responsive to cutaneous stimuli (Mountcastle and Powell, '59a) indicate that receptive fields on the body surface are constant. The size and position of the receptive fields are not changed by variations in the depth of anesthesia. Furthermore, there is no evidence that the position of the stimulus within the receptive field is coded in terms of the temporal characteristics of the response. The majority of cortical neurons driven by cutaneous stimuli adapt quickly to steady stimuli. The above observations pertain only to the somatic afferent system composed of primary dorsal root afferents in the posterior columns, lemniscal fibers arising from the posterior column nuclei and thalamocortical fibers arising from the ventral posterolateral nucleus. This is a system of great synaptic security, poised for action at high frequency levels, and possessing the neural attributes required for discriminatory functions.

Although fibers of the spinothalamic tract project to the ventral posterolateral nucleus of the thalamus, fibers of this system also project bilaterally upon posterior portions of the thalamus near the magnocellular part of the medial geniculate body known as the posterior thalamic zone (Mehler et al., '60; Bowsher, '61; Whitlock and Perl, '61). Cells of this posterior thalamic zone differ from those of the ventral posterior nuclear complex in that they are only crudely place or modality specific. These cells have large receptive fields, frequently bilateral, and the majority of cells respond to noxious stimuli (Poggio and Mountcastle, '60). Experimental evidence (Knighton, '50; Mehler, '66a) indicates that cells in this posterior thalamic zone project to the secondary somatic sensory area (somatic area II). However, cortical cells with properties similar to those of the posterior thalamic zone probably are not confined to somatic area II. Mountcastle and Powell ('59a) observed a small percentage of cells in the postcentral gyrus of the monkey which responded only to noxious stimuli and were related to wide receptive fields.

Recent findings in the monkey disclose that the primary somesthetic area and somatic sensory area II (SS II) are reciprocally and topographically connected with each other and with the motor cortex (area 4) within the same hemisphere (Jones and Powell, '69). Each of these sensory areas also sends an organized projection to the supplementary motor area. Only the primary somesthetic area projects to parietal cortex and this projection is restricted to area 5. The most remarkable feature of these somatic sensory areas is the interlocking of topographical subdivisions. Parts of the primary somesthetic area, the somatic sensory area II and the motor cortex, related to the same portion of the periphery, are interconnected. Commissural connections also exist for the somatic sensory cortex. The primary somesthetic area has connections with its counterpart, and with somatic sensory area II on the opposite side; somatic sensory area II projects to its counterpart on the opposite side but only to regions of the primary somesthetic cortex which represent perioral regions (Jones and Powell, '69a).

Stimulation of the postcentral gyrus in man produces sensations described by the patient as numbness, tingling or a feeling of electricity. Occasionally the patient may report a sensation of movement in a particular part of the body, although no actual movement is observed. A sensation of pain is rarely produced by these stimulations. Sensations described are referred to contralateral parts of the body, except in response to stimulations of the face area. Evidence suggests that the face and tongue are represented bilaterally. It is of interest that essentially the same sensations can be elicited by stimulating the precentral gyrus. According to Penfield and Rasmussen ('50), 25% of the locations giving sensory responses are in the precentral gyrus, but the ratio of sensory responses obtained from the postcentral gyrus to those from the precentral gyrus varies in different parts of the sensory sequence. Sensation referable to the eyes is obtained, almost exclusively, by stimulating the precentral gyrus, while sensation in the lips is associated almost invariably with stimulations of the postcentral gyrus. Sensory responses are reported only rarely with stimulations at points greater than 1 cm from the central sulcus. That stimula-

tion of the precentral gyrus still produces sensory responses after removal of the postcentral gyrus indicates that these responses are not dependent upon the postcentral gyrus or collateral fibers to it. Even though sensation can be produced by stimulating the precentral gyrus, ablation of it produces no clinically detectable sensory deficits.

There are other observations which suggest that the somesthetic cortical area is not limited to the postcentral gyrus, but may include portions of the superior and inferior parietal lobules. The clinical observations of Foerster ('36) indicate that destructive processes in the superior parietal lobule are followed by sensory disturbances similar to those associated with lesions of the postcentral gyrus. Other authors (Penfield and Rasmussen, '50) report no detectable somatic sensory deficits following cortical removals of large parts of the superior and inferior lobules in the nondominant hemisphere, although their patient tended to ignore the contralateral hand and had difficulty performing complex maneuvers with it.

Available evidence indicates that position sense and kinesthesis are represented only contralaterally. Whether the discriminative aspects of tactile sensibility are represented bilaterally in the human cortex is not known definitely. Clinically the sensory deficits caused by lesions in the postcentral gyrus are detectable only on the opposite side.

The sensory cortex is not concerned primarily with the recognition of crude sensory modalities, such as pain, thermal sense and mere contact. These apparently enter consciousness at the level of the thalamus, and their appreciation is retained even after complete destruction of the sensory area. "The sensory activity of the cortex . . . endows sensation with three discriminative faculties. These are: (1) recognition of spatial relations, (2) a graduated response to stimuli of different intensity, (3) appreciation of similarity and difference in external objects brought into contact with the surface of the body" (Head, ' 20). Hence in lesions of the primary somesthetic area there is loss of appreciation of passive movement, of two-point discrimination and of ability to differentiate various intensities of stimuli. In severe lesions the patient, although aware of the stimulus and its sensory modality, is unable to locate accurately the point touched, to gauge the direction and extent of passive movement and to distinguish between different weights, textures or degrees of temperature; as a result, he is unable to identify objects by merely feeling them (astereognosis). The more complicated the test, the more evident the sensory defect becomes. With all this there is a variability of response so that a definite threshold for a given sensation cannot be established.

Somatic Sensory Area II (*SS II*). As described in experimental animals, somatic sensory area II lies along the superior bank of the lateral sulcus and extends posteriorly into the parietal lobe (Woolsey, '58). In the monkey the greater part of SS II lies buried in the lateral sulcus (Jones and Powell, '69, '69a, '70). Representation of the various parts of the body is in reverse sequence to that found in the primary somesthetic area, and the regions of the two face areas are adjacent (Fig. 19-13). Parts of the body are represented bilaterally in the secondary somatic sensory area, although contralateral representation predominates. In man the face, tongue, mouth and throat regions have not been verified as yet in somatic sensory area II, presumably because of proximity to the primary face area (Penfield and Rasmussen, '50). Stimulation of somatic sensory area II in the unanesthetized patient produces sensations in the extremities similar to those obtained by stimulating the primary somesthetic cortex. The secondary somatic sensory area in animals appears to concide with the so-called secondary motor area (Welker et al., '57). The studies of Penfield indicate that the concept of a precise secondary motor area in man is not yet justified.

Somatic sensory area II appears to have functional characteristics of both the lemniscal and spinothalamic systems. Representation of the body form in somatic sensory area II is nearly as detailed as that in the postcentral gyrus (Woolsey, '58), and single unit analysis (Carreras and Levitt, '59) has revealed many cells in this area to be both mode and place specific. Other functional characteristics of this area resemble those of the posterior thalamic zone in that they are neither place specific, nor modality specific, and they respond to more than one form of somatic stimulation. Certain cells in this cortical area respond only to noxious peripheral stimuli. Although our understanding of the functional significance of somatic sensory area II is incomplete, present evidence suggests it is related primarily to the spinothalamic system (or ascending sensory pathways which conduct impulses in the anterolateral portion of the spinal cord), and may be concerned in some special way with pain sensibility (Poggio and Mountcastle, '60). This statement should not be interpreted as implying that impulses concerned with pain do not reach the postcentral gyrus. In a broad sense it suggests that while the lemniscal system (ventral posterolateral thalamic nucleus and the postcentral gyrus) and the spinothalamic system (posterior thalamic zone and somatic area II) each have predominant characteristics, each also possesses to a certain extent the properties of the other system. It is also evident that the somatic sensory area II is not wholly independent because of reciprocal connections with the primary somesthetic area (Jones and Powell, '69).

The Primary Visual Area. Area 17, located in the walls of the calcarine sulcus and adjacent portion of the cuneus and lingual gyrus, represents the primary visual area. It occasionally extends around the occipital pole on to the lateral surface of the hemisphere (Figs. 15-13 and 19-5). The exceedingly thin cortex of this area (1.5 to 2.5 mm) is the most striking example of the heterotypical granulous cortex (type 5). Layers II and III are narrow and contain numerous small pyramidal cells that are hardly larger than typical granule cells (Fig. 19-10C). Layer IV, which is very thick, is subdivided by a light band into three sublayers. The upper and lower sublayers are packed with small granule cells. In the middle, lighter layer, fewer small cells are scattered between the large stellate cells (giant stellate cells of Meynert).

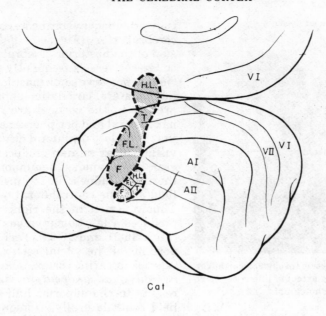

Cat

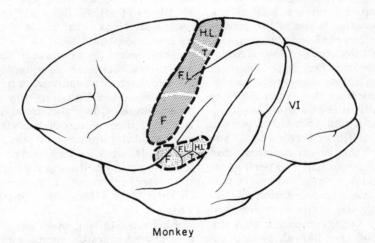

Monkey

Primary sensory area   Secondary sensory area

FIG. 19-13. Diagrams of the primary and secondary sensory areas in the cortex of the cat and monkey. Somatotopic representation of different parts of the body are indicated in the primary and secondary somatic sensory areas: *F*, face area; *T*, trunk; *FL*, forelimb; *HL*, hindlimb. Primary and secondary auditory (*A I* and *A II*) and visual (*V I* and *V II*) areas in the cat brain are shown. The medial aspect of the cat brain is represented *above* (after Woolsey, '58).

This light layer is occupied by the greatly thickened outer band of Baillarger, known here as the band of Gennari. This band, visible to the naked eye in sections of the fresh cortex, has given this region the name *area striata* (Fig. 19-14). Layer V is relatively narrow and poor in small cells, but scattered among these cells are isolated large pyramidal cells which may reach a height of 60 μ (Fig. 19-10C).

The visual cortex receives the geniculocalcarine tract, whose course and exact projection have been discussed in an earlier chapter (Fig. 15-21). Geniculocalcarine

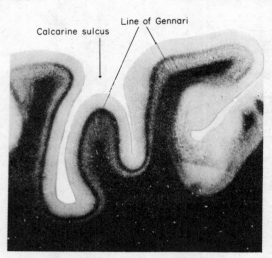

Fig. 19-14. Frontal section through calcarine cortex (area striata) showing extent of line of Gennari. Weigert's myelin stain. Photograph.

fibers pass in the *external sagittal stratum* which is separated from the wall of the inferior and posterior horns of the lateral ventricle by the *internal sagittal stratum*, and by fibers of the corpus callosum designated as the *tapetum* (Fig. 2-16). Fibers of the internal sagittal stratum are corticofugal fibers passing from the occipital lobe to the superior colliculus and the lateral geniculate body (Altman, '62; Garey et al., '68). The macular fibers terminate in the caudal third of the calcarine area, and those from the paracentral and peripheral retinal areas end in respectively more rostral portions. The representation of the macular area in the occipital cortex appears relatively large compared with the macular area of the lateral geniculate body (Fig. 15-16).

Because some unilateral lesions of the visual cortex result in a sparing of macular vision, certain authors have suggested that the macula is represented bilaterally. Anatomical evidence supports the thesis that parts of each macular area are represented only in the visual cortex of one hemisphere, since unilateral lesions of the visual cortex result in retrograde cell changes, or cell loss, only in the ipsilateral lateral geniculate body. Clinically, sparing of macular vision associated with vascular lesions involving the occipital cortex usually is attributed to collateral circula-

tion provided by branches of the middle cerebral artery (Fig. 20-6). Following occlusion of the posterior cerebral artery, these collateral vessels frequently may be sufficient to preserve some macular vision. Similar collateral circulation apparently is not present in the cortical area representing paracentral and peripheral parts of the retina. Complete unilateral destruction of the visual cortex in man produces a contralateral homonymous hemianopia in which there is blindness in the ipsilateral nasal field and the contralateral temporal field. Thus a lesion in the right visual cortex produces a left homonymous hemianopsia (Figs. 15-21 and 15-23). Lesions involving portions of the visual cortex, such as the inferior calcarine cortex, produce an *homonymous quadranopsia,* in which blindness results in the superior half of the visual field contralaterally. Homonymous hemianopsia can result from lesions involving all fibers of either the optic tract or the optic radiations (Fig. 15-23C), but lesions in these locations tend to be incomplete and the visual field defects in the two eyes are rarely identical. Frequently patients are unaware of homonymous hemianopsia and complain of bumping into people and objects on the side of the visual field defect. Bilateral destruction of the striate areas causes total blindness in man, but other mammals, such as dogs and monkeys, retain the ability to distinguish light intensities after ablations of the visual cortex (Klüver, '42; Glees, '61; Snyder et al., '66).

An image falling upon the retina initiates a tremendously complex process that results in vision. The transformation of a retinal image into a perceptual image occurs partly in the retina but mostly in the brain. The complexity of this process makes the achievement of a camera seem modest. Recent elegant experimental studies by Hubel and Wiesel in the cat have provided the first real insight into the functional organization of the visual cortex. The receptive field of a cell in the visual system is defined as the region of the retina (or visual field) over which one can influence the firing of that cell. In the retina the receptive field comprises those receptor sets (i.e., rods and cones) and other retinal neurons which influence the firing of one retinal ganglion cell. Receptive fields of retinal ganglion cells are circular, vary somewhat in size and are of two types: (1) those with an "on" (excitatory) center and an "off" (inhibitory) surround, and (2) those with an "off" (inhibitory) center and an "on" (excitatory) surround (Kuffler, '53). It is well known that retinal ganglion cells fire at a fairly steady rate even in the absence of stimulation. An "on" response is characterized by an increased firing rate of the cell to a light stimulus; in an "off" response the cell's firing rate diminishes when the light stimulus decreases. The physiological basis for the "on" and "off" retinal responses are the concentric receptive fields with either an "on" or "off" center and the reverse type of surround (Fig. 19-15). Lighting up the entire retina diffusely does not affect retinal ganglion cells as strongly as a small circular spot that covers the excitatory region of the receptive field center.

Cells of the lateral geniculate body are of two types and have physiological characteristics similar to retinal ganglion cells, in that: (1) each cell is driven from a circumscribed retinal region (receptive field), and (2) each receptive field has either an "on" or "off" center with an opposing surround (Hubel and Wiesel, '61). Lateral geniculate neurons are more specialized than retinal ganglion cells in that they are more sensitive to the differences in retinal illumination than to the illumination itself. Cells in different laminae of the lateral geniculate body are driven from receptive fields in one eye, either ipsilaterally or contralaterally, depending upon the uncrossed or crossed connections. In the lateral geniculate body only a minority of the cells are influenced binocularly (Hubel and Wiesel, '62). Visual processing by the brain begins in the lateral geniculate body.

The striate cortex, anatomically far more complex than the retina or lateral geniculate body, does not have cells with concentric receptive fields. Cells of the striate cortex show marked specificity in their responses to restricted retinal stimulation (Hubel and Wiesel, '59, '62, '63). The most effective stimulus shapes are long narrow rectangles of light ("slits"), dark bars against a light background ("dark bars") and straight line borders separating areas of different brightness ("edges"). A given cell responds vigorously when an appropriate stimulus is shone on its receptive field, or moves across it, provided the stimulus is presented in a specific orientation. This orientation is referred to as the *"receptive field axis of orientation,"* and it is critical and constant for any particular cell, but it may differ for different cells.

The visual cortex is subdivided into discrete columns extending from the surface to the white matter; all cells within each column have the same receptive field axis of orientation. The many varieties of cells in the striate cortex have been grouped into two main functional types, but it is apparent that other subtypes or varieties also exist. The main functional cell types are referred to as *"simple"* and *"complex."*

"Simple" type cells respond to slits of light having the proper receptive field axis of orientation. A slit of light oriented vertically in the visual field may activate a given "simple" cell, whereas the same cell will not respond, although other cells will, if the orientation of the slit of light is moved out of the vertical position. The retinal region over which a "simple" type cell can be influenced is, like the receptive fields of retinal and geniculate cells, divided into "on" and "off" areas (Fig. 19-15). In "simple" cells these "on" areas are not circular but are narrow rectangles, adjoined on each side by larger "off" regions. The magnitude of the "on" response depends upon how much of the region is coverd by the stimulating light. A narrow slit of light that just fills the elongated "on" region produces a powerful "on" response; stimulation with a slit of light having a different orientation produces a weaker response, because it includes part of the antagonistic "off" regions. A slit of light at right angles to the optimum orientation for a particular cell usually produces no response (Fig. 19-16). Thus a large spot of light covering the whole retina evokes no response in "simple" cortical cells, because "on" and "off" effects apparently balance. A particular cortical cell's optimum receptive field axis of orientation appears to be a

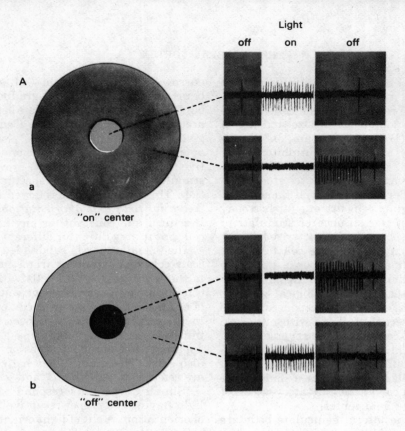

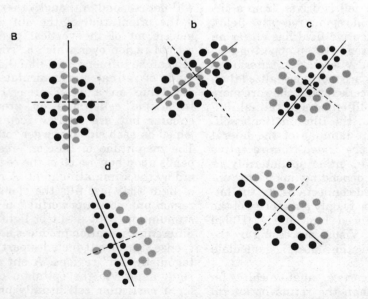

FIG. 19-15. *A*, *Receptive fields* of retinal ganglion cells and lateral geniculate neurons are concentric with either an "on" (excitatory) center and an "off" (inhibitory) surround, or the reverse. In *a*, a spot of light (*red*) filling the "on" center causes the cell to fire vigorously. If the spot of light strikes the surrounding "off" zone, firing of the neuron is suppressed until the light is turned off. In *b*, the responses of a cell with an "off" center and an "on" surround are the reverse. *B*, *Simple cells* of striate cortex receive their input from sets of lateral geniculate neurons whose "on" or "off" centers are arranged in straight lines. The receptive field **axis of** orientation varies for simple cells, as in *a*, *b* and *c*, with excitatory areas represented by *red dots* and inhibitory areas by *black dots*. Although simple cells always have excitatory and inhibitory areas **parallel** and in a straight line, these areas may be asymmetrical as in *d* and *e* (based on Hubel and Wiesel, '62).

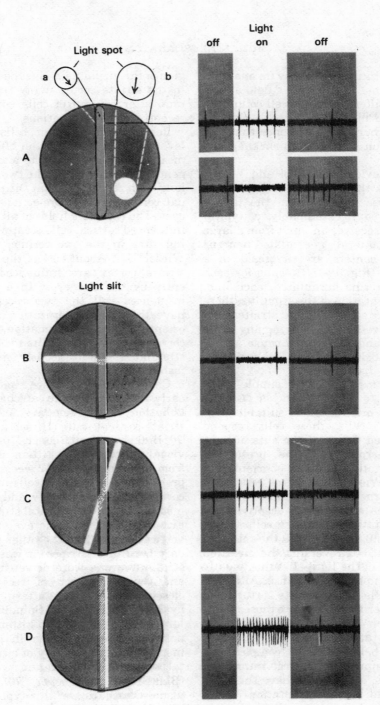

FIG. 19-16. Schematic diagram of the functional characteristics of "simple" cells in the striate cortex. In *A*, a small circular spot of light (*a*) shone on the excitatory part of the receptive field (*red*) of a simple cortical cell produces a weak response. A larger spot of light (*b*) shone on the inhibitory surround produces no response. Small spots of light (*a*) produce vigorous responses in retinal ganglion cells and lateral geniculate neurons. The receptive field of the simple cell shown above is similar to *a* in Figure 19-15*B*.

A narrow slit of light shone perpendicular to the receptive field axis of orientation (*red*) in *B* produces virtually no response. Tilting the slit of light, as in *C*, produces a weak response, while a vertical slit of light, as in *D*, which corresponds to receptive field axis of the simple striate cell, produces a vigorous response (after Hubel, '63).

property built into the cells by its anatomical connections. The receptive field axis of orientation differs from one cell column to the next, and may be vertical, horizontal or oblique. There is no evidence that any one orientation is more common than any other.

Available evidence (Hubel and Wiesel, '62) suggests that "simple" cells receive their impulses directly from the lateral geniculate body. Presumably a typical "simple" cell receives an input from a large number of lateral geniculate neurons whose "on" centers are arranged in a straight line (Fig. 19-15B). Thus for each area of the retina stimulated, each line, and each orientation of the stimulus, there is a particular set of "simple" striate cortical cells that respond. Changing any of the stimulus arrangements will cause an entirely new and different population of "simple" striate cells to respond.

"Complex" type cells, like "simple" cells, respond best to "slits," "bars" or "edges," provided the orientation is suitable. Unlike "simple" cells, these cells respond with sustained firing as the slits of light are moved across the retina, preserving the same receptive field axis of orientation (Hubel and Wiesel, '62). These cells have peculiar characteristics in that a slit of light with the appropriate receptive field axis of orientation can cause cells to fire vigorously as it moves across the retina in one direction, but reversing the direction of movement of the light stimulus usually produces a diminished response. Although "complex" cells in the striate cortex have some characteristics similar to those of simple cells, their receptive fields cannot be mapped into antagonistic "on" and "off" regions. It is believed that a "complex" cell receives its input from a large number of "simple" cells, all of which have the same receptive field axis of orientation. These findings imply that a vast network of intracortical connections relate "simple" and "complex" cells in the striate cortex in a very specific fashion, and that similar arrangements must exist for all receptive field axes of orientations. Since columns of cells constitute the fundamental functional units of the cortex, each small region of the visual field must be represented in the striate cortex many times, in column after column of cells with different receptive field orientations.

Recording from single cells at various levels of the visual system offers a direct means of determining the site of convergence of impulses from the two eyes. It has long been recognized that the primary visual cortex receives projections from both eyes. The receptive fields of all binocularly influenced cortical cells occupy corresponding sites in the two retinas (Hubel and Wiesel, '62). About 80% of the cells in the striate cortex are influenced independently by the two eyes. In a binocularly influenced cell the two receptive fields have the same organization and axis of orientation, and a summation occurs when corresponding parts of the two retinas are stimulated simultaneously in the same fashion.

Considerable evidence indicates that early visual experience can change the distribution of the selective orientation of striate cortical units (Hirsch and Spinelli, '70; Blakemore and Cooper, '70). If the total visual experience of kittens is controlled from birth until 10 or 12 weeks of age, the preferred orientation of cells in the striate cortex can be selectively and predictably modified by environmental stimulation. In kittens reared with one eye viewing only vertical stripes and the other eye viewing only horizontal stripes, it was found that striate neurons were driven monocularly and the orientation of receptive fields closely matched the pattern experienced by that eye (Hirsch and Spinelli, '70). Similar results were found in kittens permitted normal binocular vision in an environment consisting entirely of either horizontal or vertical black and white stripes (Blakemore and Cooper, '70). Controlled visual deprivation of this type causes certain physiological deficits. Such animals follow moving objects with clumsy, jerky head movements, exhibit poor judgment of distances and appear virtually blind for contours perpendicular to their controlled visual orientation experience. These animals show a striking lack of striate cells which can be activated by stimuli to both eyes and whose preferences for stimulus orientation cover the full range around the clock (Pettigrew et al., '73). An important question concerns the fate of cells which appear to be missing in the striate cortex in animals with a restricted and selective visual experience. It seems unlikely that controlled visual deprivation of this type causes cellular degeneration because no "silent areas" are encountered by recording electrodes traversing long distances in the cell columns of the striate cortex (Hubel and Wiesel, '63a; Blakemore and Cooper, '70). Cells of the striate cortex in kittens with controlled visual deprivation appear to adapt functionally to the restricted visual orientations to which they have exposed during the early critical period (Pettigrew et al., '73). Cell columns in the striate cortex show a persistence of ocular dominance, which usually is related to the contralateral eye. It is generally agreed that binocular connections are the result of years of normal visual experience. Studies of controlled visually deprived kittens, permitted normal binocular viewing after the critical period, show a dramatic increase in the number of striate cells which are binocularly activated (Spinelli et al., '72). These impressive studies suggest that visual experience is not only crucial during the critical period of development (i.e., the first 3 months of life), but that it has a continuing and lasting effect upon the functional connectivity of cells in the striate cortex.

The secondary visual area (visual area II) has been mapped in the rabbit, cat and monkey by recording the potentials evoked by flashing photic stimulation of the retina (Talbot and Marshall, '41; Woolsey, '47; Thompson et al., '50). Visual area II is a smaller mirror image representation of the primary visual area, located anterolaterally, which appears to be anatomically identical to area 18 in the cat (Fig. 19-13). Lateral to visual areas I and II is a third systematic projection of the contralateral visual field (visual area III), which in the cat appears to be identical with area 19 (Hubel and Wiesel, '65). Cells in visual area I (area 17) project to both visual area II (area 18), and visual area III (area 19)

bilaterally, indicating that visual impulses to the latter areas are transmitted from visual area I, the only area receiving direct fibers from the lateral geniculate body (Garey et al., '68). Fibers crossing to the opposite side pass in the splenium of the corpus callosum. Visual area II (area 18) sends fibers back to cortical areas 17 and 19.

Cells in visual areas II and III, like those in visual area I, respond best to slits, dark bars and edges which have a specific orientation. The majority (over 90%) of cells in visual area II are "complex" and over half of the cells in visual area III are "complex"; other cells in these areas, referred to as "hypercomplex", demonstrate more elaborate response properties. Both visual areas II and III are organized in columns, extending from the surface to the white matter, containing both "complex" and "hypercomplex" cells, all of which have the same receptive field orientation. These cells, however, differ in the precise position and arrangement of receptive fields. Hypercomplex cells have been divided into two types: (1) lower order hypercomplex cells which behave as though their input was derived from two sets of complex cells, one excitatory and one inhibitory, and (2) higher order hypercomplex cells which behave as though they receive their input from a large number of lower order hypercomplex cells. In visual area II, 5 to 10% of the cells were lower order hypercomplex cells, while in visual area III they comprised about half of the cells.

In visual area III there are columns in which some cells have one receptive field orientation, others with an orientation at 90 degrees to the first, and still others, which respond to both of these orientations. The majority of cells in visual areas II and III are driven from both eyes. Thus there appears to be as much binocular representation in visual areas II and III as in visual area I.

Area 18 is six-layered granular cortex which lacks the band of Gennari and rostrally merges with area 19 without distinct demarcation (Figs. 19-5 and 19-10B). This area interrelates areas 17 and 19 of the same and opposite hemispheres by association and commissural fibers. Projection fibers from area 18 enter the superior longitudinal and inferior occipitofrontal fasciculi (Fig. 2-11).

The Primary Auditory Area. This area (areas 41 and 42) is located on the two transverse gyri (Heschl) which lie on the dorsal surface of the superior temporal convolution. The primary auditory area is buried in the floor of the lateral sulcus (Figs. 2-3, 2-7, 12-10 and 19-5). The middle part of the anterior transverse gyrus and a portion of the posterior gyrus constitute the principal auditory receptive areas (area 41). Remaining parts of the posterior transverse gyrus and adjacent portions of the superior temporal gyrus compose area 42, which is largely an auditory association area. In order to visualize these gyri in an intact brain, it is necessary to separate widely the banks of the lateral sulcus (Fig. 2-3). These two cortical areas are cytoarchitecturally distinct. Although area 41 is typical koniocortex, resembling that of areas 3 and 17, it is relatively thick (3 mm) and distinguished by the thickness of the granular layers. Granular cells are arranged in perpendicular columns. Area 42 is six-layered cortex of the parietal type (type 3, Fig. 19-7). A distinguishing feature is the presence of a number of large pyramidal cells in layer III.

The auditory area receives geniculotemporal fibers (auditory radiation) from the medial geniculate body. The auditory radiation reaches its cortical projection site by passing through the sublenticular portion of the internal capsule (Fig. 15-18). The greater part of the auditory radiation projects to area 41, although fibers also project to area 42. One of the characteristic features of the auditory system is its tonotopic localization. The tonotopic localization present in the cochlea appears to be preserved through all of the relay nuclei of the auditory system to levels of the inferior colliculus (Neff, '61; Rose et al., '63; Whitfield, '67). Although a tonotopic organization in the medial geniculate nucleus exists, evidence of such organization is particularly impressive for the cochlear nuclei and the inferior colliculi. The number of neurons exhibiting frequency specificity

varies at different levels of the auditory system. While a large proportion of the fibers of the auditory nerve show a sharply restricted frequency specificity at threshold intensity, the number of neurons retaining this characteristic progressively diminishes at higher levels of the auditory pathway. At higher levels of the auditory system there is an increasing proportion of neural elements not directly concerned with the parameter of stimulus frequency, even though they respond to complex sounds (i.e., noise click) covering broad bands of the audible spectrum (Ades, '59).

In the cerebral cortex two areas showing tonotopic localization have been defined in the cat by determining the loci of potentials evoked in response to stimulation of nerve fibers in the cochlea, or different sound frequencies (Woolsey and Walzl, '42; Ades, '43, '59). The pattern of tonotopic localization in these two areas has been studied in detail. In the more dorsal area, referred to as auditory area I (A I), the basal coils of the cochlea (high frequencies) are represented rostrally, and the apical region of the cochlea (low frequencies) caudally. In the more ventral auditory area (A II) the tonotopic localization is reversed (Fig. 19-17). A third cortical zone designated EP (i.e., posterior ectosylvian area) lies posterior to auditory areas I and II and appears to be related functionally to auditory area I. Anatomical studies of ablations of these auditory areas have provided information concerning the origin of afferent fibers from the medial geniculate body (Rose and Woolsey, '49, '58). Auditory area I receives an essential projection from the anterior portion of the principal division of the medial geniculate body, while auditory areas II and EP receive only sustaining projections from the pars principalis of the medial geniculate body. This conclusion is based on the fact that removals of auditory area I cause severe degeneration in the anterior part of the principal division of the medial geniculate body, while ablations of auditory area II and EP do not cause marked cellular changes. However, simultaneous ablations of auditory areas I, II and EP result in more profound cellular degeneration in the medial geniculate

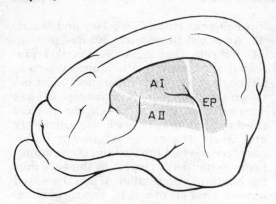

FIG. 19-17. Diagram of the auditory areas in the cat. In the primary auditory area (*A I*) the basal coils of the cochlea are represented rostrally, and the apical part of the cochlea caudally. A reverse tonotopic pattern is found in the secondary auditory area (*A II*). Area *EP* (posterior ectosylvian area) represents a third auditory area (after Ades, '59).

body than ablations of auditory area I alone. Auditory areas I and II have also been identified in the monkey (Ades and Felder, '42; Pribram et al., '54), although studies of the primate brain are less numerous. In the chimpanzee tones of low frequency are represented anterolaterally, while tones of high frequency are represented posteromedially (Bailey et al., '43). It seems likely that a similar tonotopic localization exists in man.

Some studies of the auditory cortex of the cat based upon a single unit analysis have raised doubts concerning its tonotopic organization (Erulkar et al., '56; Evans and Whitfield, '64; Evans et al., '65; Whitfield, '67). These investigators found many units did not respond at all to tones, even though they responded to complex sounds. A number of cortical units responded over such a wide frequency range that it was impossible to assign any particular characteristic frequency to them, although other units could be assigned a characteristic frequency. While high frequencies were located anterior in A I, low frequencies seemed to be distributed evenly throughout the auditory cortex.

Since studies of the somesthetic and visual cortex indicate that a vertical column of cells constitutes the elementary functional unit, it might be expected that a similar arrangement would exist in the auditory cortex. A study based upon the functional architecture of the auditory cortex in unanesthetized cats has indicated that: (1) units responsive to noise bursts are randomly distributed, (2) different regions respond to a high or low proportion of click stimuli which do not follow the direction of vertical columns, and (3) narrowly tuned units aligned with vertical columns tend to occur in clusters (Abeles and Goldstein, '70). Recent microelectrode studies of the auditory cortex in the cat and monkey have revealed a rather precise tonotopic organization (Merzenich and Brugge, '73; Merzenich et al., '73). In these studies the best frequencies at different cortical depths were averaged because of the small variations within individual penetrations. In the cat a highly ordered tonotopic organization was found in A I in which higher frequencies were represented rostrally and lower frequencies caudally (Fig. 19-17). The primary auditory area in the monkey lies caudally on the superior surface of the superior temporal gyrus and can be exposed by resection of the overlying parietal cortex (Fig. 19-18). Best frequencies in the full auditory range for the monkey were represented in an orderly fashion in the primary auditory area in a cytoarchitectonic field coextensive with the koniocortex. Lowest frequencies were represented rostrally and laterally, whereas highest frequencies were found caudally and medially (Fig. 19-18). In the monkey the primary auditory cortex is surrounded by a belt of auditory cortex which cytoarchitectonically is not uniform and can be parcelled into several divisions. This cortical belt, which appears to represent the secondary auditory area, has been divided topographically into three main areas designated as the rostrolateral, lateral and caudomedial fields (Fig. 19-18). The progression of best frequencies in the lateral field parallels that in the primary auditory area.

Electrical stimulation of the cortical areas in the temporal lobe near the primary auditory area (i.e., areas 42 and 22) in man produces sounds described as the noise of a cricket, a bell or a whistle. These

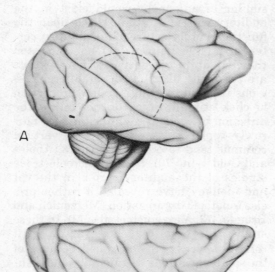

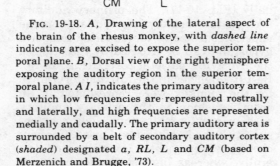

FIG. 19-18. *A,* Drawing of the lateral aspect of the brain of the rhesus monkey, with *dashed line* indicating area excised to expose the superior temporal plane. *B,* Dorsal view of the right hemisphere exposing the auditory region in the superior temporal plane. *A I,* indicates the primary auditory area in which low frequencies are represented rostrally and laterally, and high frequencies are represented medially and caudally. The primary auditory area is surrounded by a belt of secondary auditory cortex (*shaded*) designated *a, RL, L* and *CM* (based on Merzenich and Brugge, '73).

sounds are elementary tones which may be high or low pitched, continuous or interrupted, but always are devoid of complicated or changing qualities (Penfield and Rasmussen, '50). Most of these auditory responses are referred to the contralateral ear.

One of the distinctive features of the auditory system, in contrast to other sensory systems, is the large number of actual and potential sites at which impulses from one side can be transmitted to contralateral relay nuclei. The largest and most important fiber crossing is in the trapezoid body at the level of the cochlear nuclei, but others also are present (Fig. 12-10), including fibers from auditory cortical areas that cross in the corpus callosum (Mettler, '32).

Physiological studies (Woolsey and Walzl, '42; Ades and Brookhart, '50; Rosenzweig, '54) indicate that each cochlea is represented bilaterally in the auditory cortex, although some slight differences exist between the two sides. Rosenzweig ('54) has demonstrated that although the cortical effects of stimulating each ear separately are nearly the same, significant differences occur when the position of the stimulus is varied with respect to the ears during bilateral stimulation. When the sound is presented on one side, the cortical response is greatest in the contralateral hemisphere. If the sound is presented in a median plane, the cortical activity in the two hemispheres is equal. These studies suggest a correlation between auditory localization and differential responses in the auditory cortex.

Because audition is represented bilaterally at a cortical level, unilateral lesions of the auditory cortex cause only a partial deafness. The deficits, however, are bilateral, and the greatest loss is contralateral. According to Penfield and Evans ('34), removal of one temporal lobe impairs sound localization on the opposite side, especially judgment of the distance of sounds. Clinically, unilateral lesions of the auditory cortex are difficult to recognize. Experimental studies indicate that bilateral ablations of auditory areas I, II and EP in the cat do not abolish auditory localization of sound in space, although discriminations of this kind are impaired (Neff et al., '56; Neff and Diamond, '58). Sound localization in space is most critically impaired by bilateral ablations of A I (Strominger, '69). Bilateral ablations of the auditory cortical areas mentioned above reportedly have little or no effect on the ability of cats to discriminate changes in frequency (Meyer and Woolsey, '52; Butler et al., '57; Neff and Diamond, '58). Meyer and Woolsey ('52) reported that following bilateral ablations of auditory areas I, II and EP, and somatic area II, cats could not relearn to discriminate changes in frequency, but could discriminate changes in sound intensity. Studies by Goldberg and Neff ('61) suggest that cats can relearn an auditory frequency discrimination after more extensive cortical ablations that include all the areas mentioned above and portions of insular-temporal cortex as well. Although ability to localize sound in space depends to a degree upon the auditory cortex, it is not affected by section of the corpus callosum and is affected very little by section of the commissure of the inferior colliculus, but it is severely affected by section of the trapezoid body (Neff and Diamond, '58; Jerger, '60).

Brodmann's area 22, bordering the primary auditory area (Fig. 19-5) and representing typical six-layered isocortex, receives fibers from areas 41 and 42 and has connections with areas of the parietal, occipital and insular cortex (Bailey et al., '43; Sugar et al., '48, '50). Lesions of area 22 in the dominant hemisphere, or bilateral lesions, produce word deafness or sensory aphasia (see page 596). Although patients with these lesions can hear, they cannot interpret the meaning of sounds, especially speech. This form of sensory aphasia usually is associated with lesions in the posterior part of area 22.

The Gustatory Area. This area has not been established conclusively, although numerous cortical locations for taste sensibility have been suggested. Clinical and experimental evidence indicates that taste sensibility probably is represented in the parietal operculum (area 43) and in the adjacent parainsular cortex (Börnstein, '40, 40a; Patton and Ruch, '46; Penfield and Rasmussen, '50; Bagshaw and Pribram, '53). Ablations of the precentral and postcentral opercula in the monkey and chimpanzee reportedly cause a loss of taste. Similar lesions involving the anterior insular cortex, the postcentral operculum and the anterior supratemporal cortex in the monkey impair taste sensibility (Bagshaw and Pribram, '53). Stimulations of the parietal operculum (Penfield and Boldrey, '37) and adjacent insular cortex (Penfield and Rasmussen, '50) in conscious patients produce gustatory sensations. A particularly interesting report of an epileptic patient who experienced a gustatory aura characterized by a sour or bitter taste is cited as providing information concerning localization of taste in the cerebral cortex (Shenkin and Lewey, '44). Although this patient could recognize bitter and salty substances

bilaterally, he was unable to perceive sweet substances on one side of his tongue. A vascular anomaly was found in the parietal opercular region contralateral to the taste deficit.

Electrophysiological studies (Landgren, '61; Emmers et al., '62; Blomquist et al., '62; Emmers, '64) in the rat, cat and squirrel monkey indicate that afferent taste impulses conveyed by the chorda tympani and glossopharyngeal nerves are projected to the most medial and caudal part of the ventral posteromedial (VPM) nucleus of the thalamus. In the rat this projection was bilateral and symmetrical; in the cat and squirrel monkey this projection was predominantly ipsilateral. Direct lesions, destroying this thalamic region, produce gustatory deficits in the monkey (Blum et al., '43; Patton et al., '44) and goat (Andersson and Jewell, '57). Available evidence suggests that thalamic cell groups subserving taste probably are separated spatially from those related to other sensory modalities (Emmers, '66). Anatomical studies (Benjamin and Akert, '59) in the rat indicate that unilateral ablations of the cortical area in which potentials could be evoked by stimulating the chorda tympani and glossopharyngeal nerves (i.e., the parietal operculum) did not impair normal taste discrimination. Bilateral ablations of this area produced a partial loss of taste. Ablations of this cortical taste area produced retrograde degeneration of thalamic neurons confined to the most medial, parvocellular subdivision of the ventral posteromedial (VPMpc) nucleus. In an extensive study of thalamic projections to the insular and opercular cortex in the monkey, it was established that VPMpc projects to the parietal operculum and the insular cortex (Roberts and Akert, '63). The gustatory representation in the cerebral cortex is adjacent to the somesthetic area for the tongue (Cohen et al., '57), suggesting that taste may not have an exclusive primary receiving area. Although some cortical neurons in the taste area respond only to tactile, thermal or taste stimuli, others respond to more than one form of stimulation (Landgren, '57, '61). Different observations in the squirrel monkey (Benjamin, '63) suggest cortical areas concerned with taste may be separated from somesthetic areas; however, ablations of these areas have failed to produce detectable impairment of gustatory sense in this animal.

Vestibular Representation. In the cerebral cortex vestibular sense is poorly defined in comparison with other sensory modalities. In man, electrical stimulation of portions of the superior temporal gyrus, particularly regions rostral to the auditory area, provoke sensations of turning movements of the whole body, referred to as *vertigo* (Penfield and Rasmussen, '50). These sensations are comparatively mild in contrast with the violent vertigo produced by direct stimulation of the labyrinth. Nausea is comparatively infrequent during these vertiginous sensations, and when present may be the result of spread of the stimulus to portions of the underlying insular cortex. Less distinct illusions of body movement have been reported following stimulation of parietal cortex (Penfield, '57). Sensations of dizziness may be elicited from stimulating a variety of cortical sites, although these sensations most commonly are associated with subcortical stimulation.

Experimental studies of the vestibular system indicate that vestibular impulses are projected to cortical areas in the cat, dog and monkey. Either electrical stimulation of the vestibular nerve, or rotation of the animal, evokes potentials at cortical levels (Kempinsky, '51; Mickle and Ades, '52; Andersson and Gernandt, '54). In the cat responses are evoked in the anterior ectosylvian gyrus and the posterior bank of the anterior suprasylvian gyrus, regions which correspond to portions of the temporal lobe in primates. Cortical responses following stimulation of the vestibular nerve are principally contralateral.

Physiological studies indicate that short latency responses to isolated vestibular nerve stimulation are recorded chiefly in the contralateral ventral posterior inferior (VPI) thalamic nucleus (Deecke et al., '73, '74). Projections of VPI to portions of the postcentral gyrus were demonstrated by antidromic stimulation (Fredrickson et al., '66; Deecke et al., '73, '74). Apparently most of the impulses project to the face subdivision of Brodmann's area 2, a region concerned chiefly with the perception of sensation from deep tissues and joints. These results suggest a functional relationship between the vestibular and somatosensory systems at both thalamic and cortical levels.

CORTICAL AREAS CONCERNED WITH MOTOR FUNCTION

Corticofugal fibers arise from all regions of the cerebral cortex. These projections convey impulses concerned with motor function, modifications of muscle tone and reflex activity, modulation of sensory input and alterations of awareness and the state of consciousness. Corticofugal fibers, originating largely from the deeper layers of the cerebral cortex, are projected to the spinal cord, the brain stem nuclei at all levels, and to parts of the corpus striatum. The principal corticofugal fibers can be grouped under the following designations: (1) corticospinal, (2) corticoreticular, (3) corticopontine, (4) corticothalamic, and (5) corticonuclear (a composite grouping of different fibers passing to parts of the corpus striatum, the red nucleus and various sensory relay nuclei). Cortical efferent fibers projecting to other cortical areas of the same hemisphere are designated as associational, while those projecting to cortical areas of the opposite hemisphere are commissural.

The Primary Motor Area. Area 4 of Brodmann, commonly designated as the motor area, is located on the anterior wall of the central sulcus and adjacent portions of the precentral gyrus (Fig. 19-5). Broad at the superior border of the hemisphere, where it spreads over a considerable part of the precentral gyrus, it narrows inferiorly and, at the level of the inferior frontal gyrus, is practically limited to the anterior wall of the central sulcus. On the medial surface of the hemisphere it comprises the anterior portion of the paracentral lobule. The unusually thick cortex of the motor area (3.5 to 4.5 mm) is agranular in structure, and its ganglionic layer contains the giant pyramidal cells of Betz, whose cell bodies may reach a height of 60 to 120 μ (Figs. 4-5 and 19-9*B*). These cells are largest in the paracentral lobule, and smallest in the inferior opercular region.

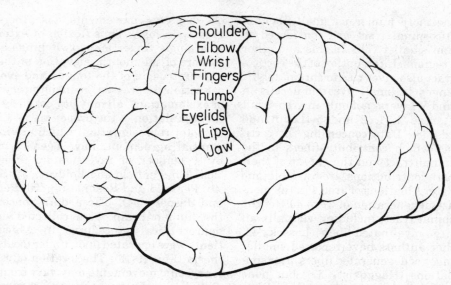

FIG. 19-19. Representation of parts of the body in the motor area on the lateral surface of the hemisphere. According to Scarff ('40), the leg usually is represented only in the anterior part of the paracentral lobule.

The density of Betz cells also varies in different parts of area 4 (Lassek, '40). Approximate percentages of Betz cells in different topographical subdivisions of area 4 are: 75% in the leg area, 18% in the arm area and 7% in the face area. According to Lassek ('40, '47), 34,000 giant pyramidal cells with cross-sectional areas between 900 and 4100 μ^2 have been counted in area 4 in the human brain. Cytoarchitecturally area 4 represents a modification of the typical six-layered isocortex in which the pyramidal cells in layers III and V are increased in number and the internal granular layer is obscured. For this reason the cortex is called agranular.

The rostral border of area 4 has been distinguished physiologically as a distinct subdivision, referred to as area 4S (Hines, '36, '37). Ablation of this narrow strip of cortex along the rostral border of area 4 in the monkey was said to produce a transient spastic paralysis, and stimulation of this area was reported to inhibit extensor muscle tone. Subsequent studies indicated that area 4S was one of a number of cortical areas from which suppressor effects could be obtained in response to stimulation (Dusser de Barenne and McCulloch, '39). Although some investigators suggested that this subdivision could be distinguished from other parts of area 4, anatomically it is not regarded as a separate entity. Physiological aspects of this region are discussed in more detail on pages 583 and 585.

The corticospinal tract, which is considered to transmit impulses for highly skilled volitional movements to lower motor neurons, arises in large part from area 4. The larger corticospinal fibers are probably the axons of giant pyramidal cells, for these cells undergo chromatolysis following section of the pyramid (Holmes and May, '09; Levin and Bradford, '38). Since the number of fibers in the human corticospinal tract at the level of the pyramid is approximately 1,000,000, axons of the giant cells of Betz could account for only a little over 3% of these fibers, assuming that each cell gives rise to a single corticospinal fiber (Lassek, '40). Studies of the fiber spectrum of the human corticospinal tract, indicating about 30,000 fibers with diameters between 9 and 22 μ (Lassek and Rasmussen, '39, '40; Lassek, '54), strongly support the view that these fibers are the parent axons of the giant pyramidal cells. Approximately 90% of the fibers of the corticospinal tract range from 1 to 4 μ in diameter. Of the total number of fibers in the tract, about 40% are poorly myelinated. The more numerous small fibers of the corticospinal tract are considered to arise from smaller cells in this and other cortical regions. Interruption of the corticospinal tract also gives rise to chromatolytic cell changes in small pyramidal cells in the III and V layers, not only in area 4, but also in areas 3, 1, 2 and 5 (Levin and Bradford, '38). Data concerning the cortical areas which contribute fibers to the corticospinal tract and the extent of their individual contributions are variable and incomplete. Ablations of area 4 in the monkey cause degeneration of 27 to 40% of the corticospinal tract, including virtually all of the large myelinated fibers (Lassek, '42, '54). Other authors have reported smaller percentages of degenerated fibers after similar ablations (Häggqvist, '37), but none report complete degeneration of the corticospinal tract (Mettler, '44a; Welch and Kennard, '44). Ablations of parietal cortex (areas 3, 1, 2, 5 and 7) also produce degeneration of myelinated fibers in the corticospinal tract (Minkowski, '23, '24; Peele, '42). Combined ablations of the precentral and postcentral gyri cause degeneration of 50 to 60% of the fibers in the corticospinal tract (Lassek, '42, '42a; Russell and DeMyer, '61). A quantitative study of the origin of corticospinal fibers in the monkey based on silver staining methods (Russell and DeMyer, '61) indicates that virtually all fibers of the corticospinal tract arise from area 4, area 6 and parts of the parietal lobe. Approximate percentages of corticospinal fibers arising from these areas are as follows: (1) area 4, 31%; (2) area 6, 29%; and (3) parietal lobe, 40%. Complete decortication, or hemispherectomy, causes all fibers of the corticospinal tract to degenerate in man (Lassek and Evans, '45) and in the monkey (Mettler, '44a; Russell and DeMyer, '61).

Electrical stimulation of the motor area evokes discrete isolated movements on the opposite side of the body. Usually the contractions involve the functional muscle groups concerned with a specific movement, but individual muscles, even a single interosseus, may be contracted separately. While the pattern of excitable foci is nearly the same for all mammals, the number of such foci, and hence the number of discrete movements, is increased greatly in man. Thus flexion or extension at a single finger joint, twitchings at the corners of the mouth, elevation of the palate, protrusion of the tongue and even vocalization, expressed in involuntary cries or exclamations, all may be evoked by careful stimulation of the proper areas. Charts of motor representation, which are in substantial agreement, have been furnished by a number of investigators (Foerster, '36a, 36b; Penfield and Boldrey, '37; Scarff; '40; Penfield and Rasmussen, '50; Penfield and Jasper, '54). These data concerning the human brain were collected during neurosurgical procedures in which patients were operated upon under local anesthesia (Fig. 19-19). The location of centers for specific movements may vary from individual to individual, but the sequence of motor representation appears constant (e.g., the point which on stimulation produces a movement of the pharynx always lies nearer to the lateral sulcus than that producing a movement of the lips, and so on). Ipsilateral movements have not been observed in man, but bilateral responses occur in the muscles of the eyes, face, tongue, jaw, larynx and pharynx. According to Penfield and Boldrey ('37), the center for the pharynx (swallowing) lies in the most inferior opercular portion of the precentral gyrus; it is followed, from below upward, by centers for the tongue, jaw, lips, larynx, eyelid and brow, in the order named (Fig. 19-12). Next come the extensive areas for finger movements, the thumb being lowest and the little finger highest; these are followed by areas for the hand, wrist, elbow and shoulder. Finally, in the most superior part, are the centers for the hip, knee ankle and toes. The last named are situated at the medial border of the hemisphere and extend into the paracentral lobule, which also contains the centers for the anal and vesicle sphincters (Fig. 19-12).

There has been considerable controversy regarding the location of representation of the lower extremity, due mainly to difficulties in stimulating the medial surface. According to Foerster ('36a), the paracentral lobule (Fig. 2-4) contains foci related to the foot, the toes, the bladder and the rectum. Penfield and Boldrey ('37) reported leg movements in 23 cases produced by stimulation of superior portions of the precentral gyrus, but Scarff ('40) was unable to elicit any leg movements by stimulating the lateral surface of the hemisphere. According to Scarff ('40) the leg, as a rule, is represented only on the medial surface of the hemisphere (i.e., in the paracentral lobule). This upward shift of the motor area, which appears unique to man, is considered to be due to the great expansion of cortical areas on the lateral surface of the hemisphere representing the tongue, mouth, lips, face and upper extremity (Fig. 19-19).

The movements elicited by electrical stimulation of the motor cortex probably are not equivalent to voluntary movements, although they are interpreted as "volitional" by the patient. These movements are never skilled movements, comparable to those of complex acquired movements, but consist largely of either simple flexions or extensions at one or more joints. The threshold in different topographical parts of area 4 varies. The region representing the thumb appears to have the lowest threshold, while the face area has the highest threshold. Excessive stimulation of area 4 produces either a focal seizure, or one resembling a Jacksonian convulsion.

Ablations of the motor cortex in mammals produce increasingly greater neurological deficits at progressively higher levels of the phylogenetic scale (Walker and Fulton, '38). In the cat removals of the motor cortex, or even hemidecortication, do not impair the animal's ability to walk upon recovery from anesthesia. Ablations of area 4 in the monkey produce a contralateral flaccid paralysis, marked hypotonia and areflexia. Within a relatively short time myotatic reflexes reappear, along with withdrawal responses to nociceptive stimuli (Fulton and Keller, '32). Recovery of movement begins in the proximal musculature and progresses distally, but the digits tend to remain permanently paralyzed. Studies by Travis ('55) in the monkey confirm these findings, except that recovery of motor function in the distal parts of the extremity was as rapid as

that in proximal parts. Although considerable improvement of motor function occurred, skilled movements were performed slowly and with some deliberation. Atrophy present in the paretic limbs during the period of greatest disuse disappeared after maximal functional recovery. No significant spasticity developed in these animals. Other results (Denny-Brown and Botterell, '48; Denny-Brown, '60) differ from the above in that some degree of spasticity accompanied the paretic manifestations after all lesions of the precentral gyrus in the monkey. Relatively mild spasticity developed first in proximal muscle groups and was described as most enduring following total ablations.

Because the precentral gyrus gives rise to a large number of nonpyramidal fibers, and is the source of only a part of the corticospinal tract, it is instructive to compare the motor deficits described above with those which follow surgical section of the pyramids. Selective pyramidotomy in the monkey and chimpanzee, accomplished by an anterior approach, produces a contralateral paresis which is somewhat more severe in the chimpanzee than in the monkey (Tower, '40, '49). In neither animal is the paresis so severe that the affected limbs are useless. The relatively stereotyped movements of progression are impaired, and there is a severe poverty of movement. The usage which survives is stripped of all the finer qualities which contribute to the skill, precision and versatility of motor performance. Although remaining stereotyped movements are useful, execution of purposeful movements appears to require deliberation and critical attention. Pyramidotomy is associated with hypotonia and loss of superficial abdominal and cremasteric reflexes. The myotatic reflexes are increased in threshold and somewhat pendular. Tonic neck reflexes are absent, and clonus does not occur. A forced grasp reflex is prominent and may be so severe as to interfere with climbing. In the chimpanzee, a persistent and enduring Babinski sign can be elicited. Observations on monkeys with bilateral pyramidal lesions by Lawrence and Kuypers ('68) also indicate that considerable recovery of independent limb movements occurs, but recovery of individual finger movements never returns. All movements are slower and the muscles fatigue more rapidly than in normal animals. These findings indicate that corticospinal pathways conduct impulses concerned with speed and agility of movement, and fractionation of movements, as exemplified by individual finger movements. Motor function remaining after bilateral pyramidotomy must be mediated by brain stem pathways projecting to spinal levels.

Lesions of the motor cortex in man produce neurological deficits similar to those described in the primate, although anatomical details are not so precise. Since conclusions based upon pathological lesions of various types are difficult to interpret, reliable data are limited to instances in which all, or parts, of the precentral gyrus have been removed surgically (Foerster, '36a; Bucy, '49, '59; Penfield and Rasmussen, '50). Ablations limited to the "arm" or "leg" area of the precentral gyrus result in a paralysis of a single limb (i.e., monoplegia). The ultimate loss of movement is always greatest in the distal muscle groups, but motor recovery in the affected limb usually is more complete than that associated with nearly total lesions of the motor area (Bucy, '49). Immediately after complete or partial lesions of the precentral gyrus, there is a flaccid paralysis of the contralateral limbs or limb, marked hypotonia and loss of superficial and myotatic reflexes. Within a relatively short time the Babinski sign can be elicited. The myotatic reflexes generally return early in an exaggerated form. There are differences of opinion concerning whether removals of area 4 in man result in a permanent spastic paralysis (Foerster, '36a; Bucy, '49, '59; Penfield and Rasmussen, '50). According to Bucy ('49), the spasticity is not severe and is less intense than that commonly associated with hemiplegias resulting from large capsular lesions. Although there is considerable restitution of function in proximal muscle groups, relatively little recovery of skilled motor function occurs in the smaller distal muscles of the extremities. The neural mechanisms underlying this partial recovery of function are not known.

The Premotor Area. This area (area 6) lies immediately in front of the motor area, runs dorsoventrally along the lateral aspect of the frontal lobe and is continued on the medial surface to the sulcus cinguli (Fig. 19-5). Near the superior border it is quite broad and includes the caudal portion of the superior frontal gyrus. Inferiorly the premotor area narrows, and near the operculum it is limited to the precentral gyrus. Its histological structure resembles that of the motor area; it is composed principally of large well formed pyramidal cells, but there are no giant cells of Betz (Fig. 19-9A). The presence of pyramidal cells in layers III and V and the narrowness of layer IV make it difficult to distinguish an internal granular layer. For this reason area 6, like area 4, is referred to as agranular frontal cortex. Area 6 has been subdivided into various portions, as shown in Figure 19-20 (Foerster, '36b). According to this parcellation, area 6aα lies immediately rostral to area 4 along the convexity of the hemisphere, while area 6aβ occupies the region of the superior frontal gyrus on both the lateral and medial surfaces of the hemisphere. A small area designated 6b lies in front of the face area.

Electrical stimulation of area 6aα in man produces responses similar to those obtained from area 4, although stronger currents are required (Foerster, '31, '36a). It is probably that area 6aα discharges via the corticospinal tract. Stimulation of area 6aβ elicits more general movement patterns characterized by rotation of the head, eyes and trunk to the opposite side, and synergic patterns of flexion or extension in the contralateral extremities. These general movement patterns appear independent of area 4, since they can be obtained after its removal. Portions of area 6aβ on the medial aspect of the hemisphere are considered to constitute part of the *supplementary motor area.* Stimulation of area 6b is reported to produce rhythmic coordinated movements of a complex type involving facial, masticatory, laryngeal and pharyngeal musculature.

Unilateral ablations of area 6, including portions on the medial aspect of the hemisphere, produce transient grasp reflexes in the monkey (Richter and Hines, '32). Bilat-

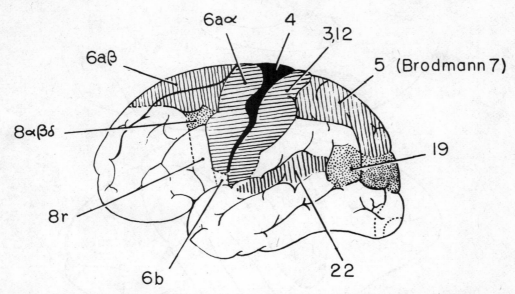

FIG. 19-20. The areas of electrically excitable cortex on the lateral surface of the human brain. The motor area is shown in *black*, and the so-called "extrapyramidal areas" are *hatched* except for the eye fields, which are *stippled* (after Foerster, '36b).

eral removals of area 6 produce more enduring grasp reflexes (Kennard and Fulton, '33; Welch and Kennard, '44). Unilateral destruction of area 6aβ in man produces little or no motor deficit (Foerster, '36a). Evidence in man and monkey emphasizes that only lesions involving the supplementary motor areas produce grasping phenomena (Erickson and Woolsey, '51; Travis, '55a). Ablations of area 6, not involving the precentral or supplementary motor areas, do not produce paresis, grasp reflexes or hypertonia.

Experimental studies in the monkey have suggested that combined ablations of areas 4 and 6 produce a contralateral spastic paralysis (Kennard and Fulton, '33; Fulton and Kennard, '34; Kennard, '49). Similar findings were reported in man following ablations of area 6, which undoubtedly included parts of area 4, as well as so-called area 4S (Kennard et al., '34). Attempts to clarify these results by Hines ('37) indicated the removal of area 4S in the monkey produced only a temporary paresis, but a permanent increase in tone in the contralateral antigravity muscles. Ablations of the posterior part of area 4 result in a contralateral flaccid paresis. These studies suggested that ablation of

area 4S probably was responsible for the release phenomena expressed as spasticity. Subsequent investigations (Travis, '55a) explain the spasticity resulting from combined lesions of areas 4 and 6 on the basis of simultaneous destruction of precentral and supplementary motor areas, which are known to produce a contralateral spastic paralysis. This same investigator has shown that bilateral removals of area 4S in the monkey do not produce spasticity until the lesions in the strip area (4S) encroach upon the supplementary motor area. These results appear to resolve a long-standing controversy, and eliminate apparent discrepancies concerning the effects of ablations of motor cortex and pyramidotomy.

Supplementary Motor Area. Observations by early investigators indicated that motor responses in different parts of the body could be elicited by electrical stimulation of the medial surface of the frontal lobe rostral to the primary motor area. This motor area, identified in the human brain, has been designated as the supplementary motor area (Penfield and Rasmussen, '50). The supplementary motor area in man and monkey occupies the medial surface of the superior frontal gyrus rostral to

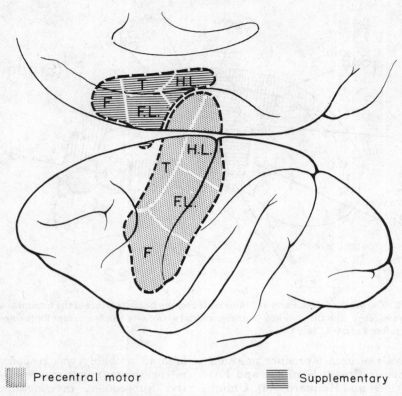

Fig. 19-21. Diagram of the precentral and supplementary motor areas in the monkey. The somatotopical representation of different parts of the body are shown: *F*, face area; *T*, trunk; *FL*, forelimb; *HL*, hindlimb. The precentral motor area on the lateral convexity extends over onto the medial aspect of the hemisphere; the *outlined area* shown posterior to the central sulcus represents cortex hidden in the depths of the central sulcus. The supplementary motor area, largely on the medial aspect of the hemisphere, is shown *above* (after Travis, '55a).

area 4. Detailed descriptions of somatotopic respresentation within the supplementary motor area of the monkey have been provided by Woolsey et al. ('51). The sequential representation of body parts in this area is shown in Figure 19-21. The threshold for stimulation of the supplementary motor area in man and monkeys is slightly higher than for the precentral region, but the motor effects are not due to spread of excitation across the cortex. Stimulation of the supplementary motor area in man produces raising of the opposite arm, turning of the head and eyes and bilateral synergic contractions of the muscles of the trunk and legs. Movements provoked by stimulation of the supplementary motor area have been divided into three types: (1) assumption of postures, (2) maneuvers consisting of a series of com-

plex patterned movements, and (3) infrequent rapid incoordinate movements. The whole pattern of movement seems to be bilateral and synergistic, but most movements are described as tonic contractions of the postural type. Other responses obtained included pupillary dilatation, cardiac acceleration, vocalization and occasional sensory phenomena. Although the visceral responses resemble those commonly obtained from the cingulate gyrus, these are not due to spread of the stimulus. Unilateral ablations of the supplementary motor area in man produce no permanent deficit in the maintenance of posture or the capacity for movement (Penfield and Rasmussen, '50; Penfield and Welch, '51).

Systematic studies in the monkey of removals of the supplementary motor area alone, and in combination with the precentral motor area, have contributed information concerning its function (Travis, '55, '55a). Unilateral ablations of the supplementary motor area in the monkey produce weak transient grasp reflexes in the contralateral limbs, and moderate bilateral hypertonia of the shoulder muscles, but no paresis. Bilateral simultaneous ablations of this area result in disturbances of posture and tonus, but produce no paresis. Gradually increasing hypertonia, resulting in muscle contracture, develops in a period of 2 to 4 weeks. The hypertonia is mainly in flexor muscles. Myotatic reflexes are hyperactive, and clonus can be demonstrated. The developed spasticity demonstrates a topographical localization according to the portions of the supplementary motor area removed. Ablations of the supplementary motor area and the precentral motor area on the same side result in an immediate contralateral hypotonic paresis with impaired myotatic reflexes. Within a period of 2 weeks, the hypotonus changes to hypertonus and the myotatic reflexes become exaggerated. These studies suggest that spasticity can be dissociated from paresis and paralysis, and that these phenomena need not always occur together.

As mentioned previously, physiological findings concerning the supplementary motor area appear to explain the controversy regarding ablations of areas 4 and 6, and the relationships of so-called area 4S to muscle tonus. All evidence indicates that the supplementary motor area is a bilaterally functioning entity concerned primarily with mechanisms of posture and movement. Other observations (Coxe and Landau, '65) following bilateral simultaneous ablations of the supplementary motor area in the monkey indicate that such lesions produce a milder increase in muscle tone, inconsistent reflex changes and no evidence of joint contracture. The explanation for these discrepancies in not obvious, but differences in the location and extent of the cortical lesions seem likely.

The neural pathways underlying responses from the supplementary motor area are poorly understood. Ablations of the supplementary motor area do not produce degeneration passing to the spinal cord, but electrical stimulation of the supplementary motor area in the monkey evokes potentials bilaterally in the region of the corticospinal tracts at spinal cord levels (Bertrand, '56). The bilateral features of this system are striking and appear to explain why unilateral lesions of the supplementary motor area cause only minor deficits. Penfield and Jasper ('54) report that motor responses from the supplementary motor area can be elicited after removal of the precentral gyrus.

According to Bates ('53), stimulation of this motor area in man, following hemispherectomy, induces ipsilateral movements similar to those which can be produced voluntarily.

Cortical Eye Fields. In front of the premotor area is a cortical region particularly concerned with voluntary eye movements. The *frontal eye field* in man occupies principally the caudal part of the middle frontal gyrus (corresponding to parts of area 8, shown in Fig. 19-20) and extends into contiguous portions of the inferior frontal gyrus. The entire frontal eye field does not lie within a single cytoarchitectonic area. Cytoarchitecturally, area 8 is typical six-layered isocortex of the frontal type in which the granualr layers are distinct (Fig. 19-7). Electrical stimulation of the frontal eye field in man causes conjugate deviation of the eyes, usually to the opposite side (Foerster, '31; Penfield and Rasmussen, '50). This cortical field is believed to be a center for voluntary eye movements not dependent upon visual stimuli. The conjugate eye movements commonly are called "movements of command," since they can be elicited by instructing the patient to look to the right or left (Cogan, '58). Some studies in man and primates suggest a double representation of specific eye movements in each frontal eye field (Crosby, '53; Crosby et al., '62; Lemmen et al., '59).

The concept of an *occipital eye center* for conjugate eye movements is based upon the fact that stimulation of occipital cortex produces conjugate eye movements to the opposite side, and lesions in this area are associated with transient deviation of the eyes to the side of the lesion. Unlike the frontal eye field, the occipital eye center is not localized to a small area. Eye responses can be obtained from a wide region of the occipital lobe in the monkey, but the lowest threshold is found in area 17 (Walker and Weaver, '40). The occipital eye centers are presumed to subserve movements of the eyes induced by visual stimuli, such as following moving objects. These pursuit movements of the eyes are largely involuntary, although they are not present in young infants. The occipital eye centers, unlike the frontal eye fields, are interconnected by fibers passing in the splenium of the corpus callosum. The threshold for excitation is higher in the occipital lobe than in the frontal eye fields; the latency of responses is longer, and eye movements tend to be smoother and less brisk.

The pathways by which responses from the frontal and occipital eye fields are mediated are not known, but it seems likely that the superior colliculus is involved. The frontal eye field projects fibers to deeper layers of the superior colliculus via a transtegmental projection (Kuypers and Lawrence, '67). The most substantial and highly organized projection to the superior colliculus arises from the visual cortex (Garey et al., '68). These fibers mainly enter the stratum opticum via the brachium of the superior colliculus. Although the superior colliculus does not project direct fibers to the nuclei of the extraocular muscles, it has projections to both the reticular formation and the accessory oculomotor nuclei (Carpenter, '71).

NONPYRAMIDAL CORTICOFUGAL FIBERS

These cortical projections consist largely of corticoreticular, corticopontine, corticothalamic and corticonuclear fibers.

Corticoreticular Fibers. These originate from all parts of the cerebral cortex, but the largest number arise from the motor and premotor areas (Rossi and Brodal, '56). Inferior cortical areas (basal) and parts of the cortex on the medial surface of the hemisphere also contribute to the corticoreticular projection, but few fibers arise from the auditory and visual areas. Corticoreticular fibers descend in association with fibers of the corticospinal tract, but they leave this bundle to enter specific areas of the brain stem reticular forma-

tion. The number of corticoreticular fibers is not large and the major part of these fibers terminate in two fairly well circumscribed areas in the medulla and in the pons. The terminal area in the medulla corresponds to the nucleus reticularis gigantocellularis, while the pontine area coincides with the nucleus reticularis pontis oralis (Fig. 10-20). Unilateral cerebral lesions produce an approximately equal distribution of degenerated corticoreticular fibers on both sides of the reticular formation. Some corticoreticular fibers also reach reticular cerebellar relay nuclei, such as the reticulotegmental nucleus, the lateral reticular nucleus and the paramedian reticular nuclei of the medulla.

Corticopontine Fibers. These fibers arise from extensive regions of the frontal, temporal, parietal and occipital regions of the cortex (Beck, '50; Nyby and Jansen, '51; Brodal, '68, '72, '72a). The massive *frontopontine tract* (bundle of Arnold) arises mainly from the lateral and superior convexity of the whole prefrontal cortex (areas 10, 9, 8, 45 and 46), with the exception of the orbital region and the extreme frontal pole. A smaller contingent comes from the precentral region (areas 4 and 6). The prefrontal fibers pass through the anterior limb of the internal capsule, while the precentral fibers pass in the posterior limb. On reaching the midbrain, the frontopontine tract forms the medial fifth of the crus cerebri, and is distributed to the medial pontine nuclei (Fig. 13-1 and 14-21). Corticopontine fibers from the "motor" and "sensory" areas in the cat project in a somatotopical manner onto two longitudinally oriented columns in the pontine nuclei (Brodal, '68). One column is located medial and one is lateral. Within the medial column, the hindlimb is represented ventrally and the face dorsally, while in the lateral column, the hindlimb is represented caudally and the forelimb rostrally.

Other corticopontine tracts arise from the superior, middle and inferior temporal gyri (*temporopontine*), and from the superior and inferior parietal lobules (*parietopontine*). An *occipitopontine* bundle comes chiefly from area 18 of the occipital lobe (Nyby and Jansen, '51). Recent studies in the cat indicate that corticopontine fibers arise from areas 17, 18 and 19 (Brodal, '72, '72a). The projection from area 17 comes mainly from regions representing peripheral parts of the visual field, and projects to several sharply delimited bands in the rostral half of the pontine nuclei. Fibers from area 18 terminate in the same region within the pontine nuclei. The temporal, parietal and occipital fibers, collectively known as the *bundle of Türck*, descend through the retrolenticular and sublenticular portions of the internal capsule. These fibers occupy the lateral fifth of the crus cerebri and are distributed mainly to the lateral and dorsolateral cell groups of the pons. Through these tracts the cerebral cortex is brought into intimate association with the synergic regulating mechanism of the cerebellum. The transient ataxia and hypotonia sometimes observed in frontal and temporal lesions may be due to injury of these corticocerebellar connections.

Corticothalamic Fibers. These constitute a large and impressive group of corticofugal fibers which arise from specific regions of the cortex and project upon particular thalamic nuclei. In general, cortical areas receiving projections from particular thalamic nuclei give rise to reciprocal fibers which pass back to the same nuclei. Areas of granular frontal cortex project primarily to the dorsomedial nucleus of the thalamus, although some fibers pass to the submedial nucleus (Clark, '48; Meyer, '49). Particularly prominent among these fibers are those arising from frontal areas 9 and 10. According to Mettler ('47), corticofugal fibers to the dorsomedial nucleus come from areas 11, 9, 8 and 6 in the monkey. Most of these fibers reach the thalamus via the anterior limb of the internal capsule.

Fibers from the cingulate gyrus are described as passing to the anterior nucleus of the thalamus (Pribram and Fulton, '54; Showers, '59). Most of these fibers come from the supracallosal part of the cingulate gyrus at the transition of areas 24 and 23 and pass through the anterior thalamic radiation. A larger number of fibers from the cingulate gyrus enter the cingulum (Fig. 2-12) and pass to the entorhinal cortex (Raisman et al., '65).

Corticothalamic fibers from the precentral area project to the ventral lateral nucleus of the thalamus (Clark, '32; Levin, '36, '49; Verhaart and Kennard, '40; Mettler, '47b; Hines, '49; Rinvik, '68; Rispal-Padel et al., '73). Olszewski ('52) makes an important point that cortical efferent fibers from the precentral gyrus pass to both the pars oralis and the pars caudalis of the ventral lateral nucleus. Thus corticofugal fibers pass to regions of this nucleus that receive fibers from the cerebellum and globus pallidus (VLo), as well as to regions (VLc) which do not. According to physiological studies inhibitory effects upon VL neurons resulting from stimulation of the motor cortex can be graded by varying the intensity of the stimulation (Rispal-Padel et al., '73). Furthermore, stimulation of various cortical sites can induce inhibitory effects in single neurons, suggesting considerable convergence.

Several investigators report that the motor cortex and portions of the premotor cortex also project upon portions of the intralaminar thalamic nuclei, principally the centromedian-parafascicular nuclear complex (Auer, '56; Niimi et al., '60; Petras, '64, '66, '69). The most extensive study of these corticothalamic fibers in the cat indicates that fibers from the pericruciate and coronal gyri (which collectively represent the primary sensorimotor area) follow different routes to individual thalamic nuclei (Rinvik, '68). The majority of corticofugal fibers to VL and the ventrobasal complex (VB) leave the posterior limb of the internal capsule, enter the reticular nucleus of the thalamus and course caudally and medially to be distributed to restricted areas of VL and the VB complex. Certain fibers arising from the sensorimotor cortex follow a more circuitous course which has been referred to as the "cerebral peduncle loop." Fibers following this pathway descend in the internal capsule and the crus cerebri to levels of the midbrain-diencephalic junction; at this level fibers leave the crus cerebri, pass through parts of the substantia nigra and project rostrally and dorsally to basal and inferior thalamic regions (Carpenter and Peter, '72). Corticothalamic fibers projecting to the centromedian-parafascicular complex, parts of VPM and caudal parts of DM follow this circuitous route (Rinvik, '68).

Efferent fibers from the parietal cortex in the monkey pass by way of the sensory radiations to the thalamic nuclei, from which they receive fibers. Corticothalamic fibers from the primary somesthetic cortex project to the ventral posterolateral (VPL) and posteromedial (VPM) nuclei, and have been described as ending in a somatotopic fashion within these nuclei (Peele, '42; Krieg, '54; Jones and Powell, '68). Both the primary somesthetic area and somatic sensory area II in the cat project in a topographically organized manner upon VPL and VPM, and in addition each cortical area projects upon the same part of the posterior thalamic zone (Jones and Powell, '68). The ventral posterior thalamic nucleus gives rise to a thalamocortical projection to the somatic sensory cortex and appears to receive a reciprocal corticothalamic projection. It is considered likely that reciprocating corticothalamic fibers may have an influence upon transmission of impulses to the cortex that is similar to that exerted by corticofugal fibers upon the posterior column nuclei and neurons of the trigeminal nuclear complex. Area 5 of the parietal cortex does not receive fibers from VPM, nor does it project to that thalamic nucleus (Jones and Powell, '68); this cortical area sends fibers to the lateral posterior and the suprageniculate nuclei.

Fibers from parts of the auditory cortex project back to the medial geniculate body through sublenticular parts of the internal capsule (Papez, '36; Riley, '43; Krieg, '47; Walther and Rasmussen, '60). In the cat fibers from auditory cortex pass to the medial geniculate body (MGB), the posterior thalamic zone, the inferior colliculi (bilaterally) and the pontine nuclei (Diamond et al., '69). While all fields of the auditory cortex contribute to this projection there are different patterns in the subdivisions of the medial geniculate body and the posterior thalamic zone; auditory area I sends the greatest number of fibers to the ventral nucleus of MGB, while the fewest come from EP.

The striate cortex, area 17, sends axons to the lateral geniculate body (LGB) and to the lateral posterior thalamic nucleus (Nauta and Bucher, '54; Altman, '62). Lesions in either area 17 or 18 produce degeneration in the dorsal and ventral nuclei of the lateral geniculate body (Garey et al., '68; Giolli and Guthrie, '71). Because geniculocortical and corticogeniculate fibers are reciprocally organized, the question arises as to whether some of the degeneration seen in the LGB after striate lesions might be retrograde fiber degeneration. Electron microscopic evidence and degeneration after short survival periods suggests that corticogeniculate fibers exist. Projections from the visual cortex also pass to parts of the pulvinar. According to Holländer ('72) area 18 in the cat projects to the LGB, but area 17 does not. Although species differences may exist, no projection to LGB from area 17 was found in the squirrel monkey, if the lesion spared the underlying white matter (Spatz et al., '70).

While reciprocal relationships exist between the principal thalamic nuclei and their cortical projection sites, a different relationship pertains to the reticular and intralaminar thalamic nuclei. The thalamic reticular nucleus, which forms an envelope about the lateral surface of the thalamus, receives afferents from almost all areas of the cerebral cortex (Carman et al., '64). These corticothalamic fibers are organized so that rostral cortical regions project to rostral parts of the reticular nucleus and posterior cortical regions project to posterior portions of the nucleus. There is no evidence that the reticular nucleus of the thalamus projects to the cerebral cortex (Scheibel and Scheibel, '66). The intralaminar thalamic nuclei, like the reticular thalamic nucleus, receive corticofugal fibers. According to Powell and Cowan ('67), most of the prefrontal cortex projects fibers to the rostral intralaminar thalamic nuclei. The premotor and motor cortex project fibers to centromedian and parafascicular nuclei; parietal and occipital cortex do not project fibers to the intralaminar thalamic nuclei. These nuclei have long been regarded as projecting exclusively to the neostriatum (Powell and Cowan, '56), but recent studies based upon retrograde axonal transport suggest they give rise to collateral fibers that project diffusely upon the cerebral cortex (Jones and Leavitt, '74).

Other nonpyramidal corticofugal fibers, collectively grouped together as corticonuclear fibers, pass to the neostriatum and certain brain stem nuclei. Cortical projections to the neostriatum and related brain stem nuclei are discussed in Chapter 18.

Corticofugal fibers, arising largely from the precentral and postcentral gyri, that leave the corticospinal tract in the lower brain stem and terminate upon certain secondary sensory relay nuclei, convey cortical impulses that modify the central propagation of afferent impulses (Hagbarth and Kerr, '54; Hernández-Péon and Hagbarth, '55). These fibers pass to the nuclei gracilis and cuneatus, the sensory trigeminal nuclei and the nucleus of the solitary fasciculus (Brodal et al., '56; Torvik, '56; Walberg, '57; Kuypers, '58, '58a, '58b, '60; Kuypers et al., '61). These corticobulbar fibers are discussed in Chapter 11.

PHENOMENON OF CORTICAL SUPPRESSION

Certain specific areas of the cerebral cortex, whose electrical stimulation is said to suppress the spontaneous electrical activity of area 4 and to inhibit responses from the motor cortex, have been described as suppressor areas. The first suppressor area in the monkey was defined as a narrow strip of cortex (so-called area 4S) lying between areas 4 and 6 (Hines, '36, '37). Area 4S generally is not recognized as a separate entity in cytoarchitectonic studies of the cortex. Subsequent studies based upon strychnine neuronography and electrical stimulation revealed several other areas (8S, 2S, 19S and 24) from which suppressor effects could be elicited in the monkey and chimpanzee (Dusser de Barenne et al., '42; McCulloch, '49). Although the predominant effect of stimulating these areas is suppression of motor responses, data also indicate that the suppressor areas influence afferent impulses to the cortex, and lead to a reduction in the amplitude of the EEG (Baker and Gellhorn, '47).

The phenomenon of cortical suppression appears to be somewhat inconstant and variable, depends to a degree on the depth of anesthesia, begins several minutes after the application of the stimulus and persists for a relatively long time (i.e., up to 30 min). It has been postulated that suppressor activity of these cortical areas involves corticocaudate fibers. Direct corticocaudate projections from all suppressor areas have been demonstrated physiologically in the monkey and chimpanzee (Dusser de Barenne et al., '42). The concept of specific localized suppressor areas in the cortex has been challenged with the implication that the suppression observed in stimulating these areas probably is identical with that of the spreading depression of Leão (Sloan and Jasper, '50; Druckman, '52). The latter phenomenon is not restricted to specific cortical areas, but is related to unfavorable experimental conditions. Leão ('44) described a depression of cortical rhythms in the rabbit which spreads slowly outward from the site of a weak mechanical, electrical or chemical stimulus to the cortex. Neither evoked potentials nor motor responses to cortical stimulation could be observed when the depression reached the sensorimotor cortex. Species differences in susceptibility of the cortex to spreading depression have been noted in that depression is more easily produced in the rabbit than the cat, and is seen only occasionally in the monkey. Substantial evidence indicates that cortical depression results from exposure of the brain to less than optimal physiological conditions, such as dehydration, cooling or prolonged experimentation (Marshall, '50; Marshall and Essig, '51; Marshall et al., '51; Marshall, '59). The existence of specific suppressor areas in the cerebral cortex of either animals or man appears doubtful.

CONSIDERATION OF CORTICAL FUNCTIONS

Cerebral Dominance

Although the two cerebral hemispheres appear as mirror images, or duplicates of each other, there are many functions which are not represented equally at a cortical level. This appears true even though impulses from receptors on each side of the body seem to project nearly equally, although largely contralaterally, to symmetrical cortical areas, and certain information received in the cortex of one hemisphere can be transferred to the other via interhemispheric commissures (Meyers, '56). In certain higher functions, believed to be cortical in nature, one hemisphere appears to be the "leading" one and, in this sense, is referred to as the *dominant hemisphere*. The most remarkable feature of cerebral dominance in man is the fact that in the adult the capacity for speech is overwhelmingly controlled by the left hemisphere. There is no known example in any other mammal of a class of learning so predominantly controlled by one half of the brain (Geschwind, '70). With respect to most of the higher functions, cerebral dominance appears to be one of degree (Zangwill, '60). According to Henschen ('26), cerebral dominance is most complete in relation to the complex and highly evolved aspects of language. Handedness also is related to cerebral dominance, although its relationship is less clear cut than has been assumed in the past. It seems likely that handedness is a graded characteristic. Left-handedness, in particular, is less definite than right-handedness, and less regularly associated with dominance in either hemisphere. There also appears to be a group of disturbances related to language that are said to be commonly associated with imperfectly developed cerebral dominance. These include the improper development of reading, writing and drawing abilities, poor spatial judgment and imperfect directional control (Zangwill, '60). In true right-handed individuals, it is nearly always the left hemisphere which is dominant and governs language and related processes, but the converse of this is not necessarily true. The degree of cerebral dominance appears to vary widely, not only among individuals, but with respect to different functions. Although a degree of "cerebral ambilaterality" would appear to be a distinct advantage with respect to recovery of speech following a unilateral cerebral injury, it appears to carry the risk or possibility of difficulty in learning to read, spell and draw. The relationship between handedness and speech is perhaps a more natural one than is commonly realized, since some gesturing often accompanies speech and in

certain situations may substitute for it. Although most clinicians relate handedness and speech to the dominant hemisphere, Penfield and Roberts ('59) report that there is no difference in the incidence of aphasia after operation on the left hemisphere between left- and right-handed patients, provided patients with cerebral injury occurring early in life are excluded. With this same exclusion there is said to be no significant difference in the frequency of aphasia after operations on the right hemisphere between right- and left-handed patients. Nevertheless, these authors regard the left hemisphere as dominant for speech regardless of handedness. Cerebral dominance is considered to have a genetic basis, but its hereditary determination probably is not absolute. Pathological and psychological factors also influence handedness, and many determining factors remain unknown.

It has been suggested that the normal neonate in a sense has a split-brain because the corpus callosum is incompletely developed and not fully functional (Gazzaniga, '70). Thus interhemispheric communication at birth probably is slight, but it increases with development of the corpus callosum which becomes reasonably complete about the 2nd or 3rd year of life. Until this level of development is reached, each hemisphere may process and record some linguistic information. Hand use probably reinforces hemisphere use, and the development of a special competence in one hemisphere results in a mutual reinforcement that establishes a life pattern. The major differences between the right and left hemispheres concern the analysis of language and the ability to speak. The fact that large left hemisphere lesions in young children do not cause total disruption of speech indicates that the right hemisphere has developed some linguistic competence. Surgical section of the interhemispheric commissure sheds light on certain problems of cerebral dominance, and indicates that in the adult the left hemisphere speaks for both hemispheres.

Many cortical functions are concerned only with contralateral regions of the body, and unilateral lesions affecting these functions produce a disturbance contralaterally, regardless of cerebral dominance. This appears particularly true of the primary motor and sensory areas. It also is the case with lesions of the parietal cortex which result in *astereognosis,* or inability to recognize the form, size, texture and identity of an object by touch alone. In certain parietal lobe lesions there is evidence that particular deficits occur more commonly in the nondominant hemisphere. One such syndrome is characterized by a disorder of the body image in which the patient: (1) fails to recognize part of his own body, (2) fails to appreciate the existence of hemiparesis, and (3) neglects to wash, shave or cover the part of his body which he denies (Critchley, '53).

Interhemispheric Transfer

Although the corpus callosum is the largest of the interhemispheric commissures, relatively little has been known of its functions until recently. The first convincing evidence regarding its function was the demonstration of its importance in interhemispheric transfer of visual discrimination learning in cats with longitudinal section of the optic chiasm (Meyers, '56). Following section of the optic chiasm and corpus callosum, cats trained with one eye masked were unable to remember simple visual discriminations learned with the first eye. The untrained eye could be trained to make a reverse type of discrimination without interfering with the patterned discrimination learned on the opposite side. This functional independence of the surgically separated cerebral hemispheres with respect to learning, memory and other gnostic activity has been the stimulus for considerable investigation (Mountcastle, '62). The results originally suggested that section of the corpus callosum prevented the spread of learning and memory from one hemisphere to the other. It was as if each hemisphere existed independently and had a complete amnesia for the experience of the other (Sperry, '62). Extension of these transfer studies in the monkey from visual to somesthetic and motor learning (Sperry, '61, '62; Gazzaniga, '70) have indicated that the independence of the surgically separated hemispheres may be less clear cut than originally supposed. In man and monkey, a subcallosal route may be active in transmitting high-order tactile information. Furthermore, both hemispheres may learn to discriminate simultaneously, one via a contralateral sensory system and the other by an ipsilateral sensory system (Gazzaniga, '70).

Observations of the functional effects of surgical separation of the hemispheres in man (Gazzaniga et al., '65; Gazzaniga and Sperry, '67) by complete transection of the corpus callosum, anterior and hippocampal commissures, and separation of the thalamic adhesion (massa intermedia) have been reported. These patients show a striking functional independence of the gnostic activities of the two hemispheres. Perceptual, cognitive, mnemonic, learned and volitional activities persist in each hemisphere, but each can proceed outside the realm of awareness of the other hemisphere. Subjective experiences of each hemisphere are known to the other only indirectly through lower level and peripheral effects. Disconnection of the hemispheres produces little disturbance of ordinary, daily behavior, temperament or intellect. Functional deficits tend to be compensated for by development of bilateral motor control from each hemisphere, as well as by the bilaterality of some sensory pathways. Information perceived exclusively, or generated exclusively, in the minor (right) hemisphere could not be communicated in speech or in writing; it was expressed entirely by nonverbal responses. There was no detectable impairment of speech or writing with reference to information processed in the major (left) hemisphere. These authors found linguistic expression to be organized almost exclusively in the dominant hemisphere.

In contrast to the above, comprehension of language, both spoken and written, was found to be represented in both hemispheres, with the minor hemisphere a little less proficient. In an analysis of the visual fields, with fixation assured, subjects verbally described only those small spots of light presented in the right half of the visual field (Gazzaniga, '70). A similar light stimulus present in the left half of the visual field produced no verbal responses. With double field stimulation, only spots of light falling in the right visual field were reported. In these subjects, the visual fields stopped exactly in the midline and no macular sparing was evident. Thus it would appear that no visual information can be transferred from one hemisphere to the other after section of the corpus callosum.

Certain lesions involving portions of the corpus callosum, or association areas of the cortex which give rise to commissural fibers, produce disturbances of higher brain functions collectively recognized as *disconnection syndromes* (Geschwind, '65, '65a, '70). Word blindness without agraphia presumably results from lesions which interrupt fibers from the visual association areas which cross in the splenium of the corpus callosum and project to the left angular gyrus. Pure word deafness may result from subcortical lesions in the left temporal lobe which interrupt the left auditory radiation, as well as callosal fibers from the contralateral auditory region. Similar syndromes manifested by various forms of agnosia or apraxia may result from lesions involving portions of the corpus callosum and association fiber systems.

Nonspecific Thalamocortical Relationships

Even though anatomical details concerning the manner in which impulses from the nonspecific thalamic nuclei reach the cortex are poorly understood, there is abundant physiological evidence that these nuclei play an important role in the regulation of the electrical activity of the cerebral cortex. The fact that repetitive stimulation of the nonspecific thalamic nuclei gives rise to widespread, diffuse cortical responses of a recruiting nature (Dempsey and Morison, '42, '43; Morison and Dempsey, '42, '42a) has served to distinguish this system from the short latency, local cortical responses which characterize the specific thalamic nuclei. The ascending reticular activating system, related physiologically to alerting, attention and general excitement, appears to exert its activating influences upon broad areas of the cerebral cortex, in part through the mediation of

the nonspecific thalamic nuclei. This conclusion is based on the fact that cortical recruiting responses can be blocked by stimulation of portions of the ascending reticular activating system (Moruzzi and Magoun, '49; Machne et al., '55). There is considerable evidence that the ventral anterior thalamic nucleus may play an important role in the recruiting response. Efferent fibers from the ventral anterior nucleus appear to have a widespread, diffuse projection to the frontal cortex (Fig. 15-13), and VAmc has a specific projection to the caudal and medial orbitofrontal cortex (Scheibel and Scheibel, '66a; Carmel, '70). Furthermore, the orbitofrontal cortex has been demonstrated to play a role in "triggering" the recruiting response (Velasco and Lindsley, '65; Skinner and Lindsley, '67).

Lorente de Nó ('49) described two types of cortical afferent fibers. Specific afferent fibers, forming the main projection system from the sensory relay nuclei of the thalamus, were described as terminating principally in layer IV of the cortex. What he referred to as "unspecific" fibers originated from: (1) undetermined regions of the thalamus independent of the specific thalamic nuclei, and (2) cortical cells giving rise to transcortical and commissural fibers. The nonspecific fibers ("unspecific") tended to terminate in all layers of the cortex. Most of these nonspecific fibers were regarded as terminating axodendritically in the cortex. Although the view is widely held that the nonspecific cortical afferents described by Lorente de Nó have their origin in the intralaminar thalamic nuclei, only recently has direct evidence for this thesis been presented (Murray, '66; Jones and Leavitt, '74). Utilizing the retrograde axonal transport of the enzyme horseradish peroxidase from injection sites in the cerebral cortex and striatum, it has been shown that: (1) injections in the medial, frontal and parietal cortex result in light labeling of cells in the intralaminar nuclei, and (2) injections in the striatum produce intense labeling of cells in the same thalamic nuclei. These results are consistent with the thesis that the intralaminar thalamic nuclei project profusely to the striatum, and sparsely and diffusely upon the cerebral cortex. It has been suggested that the cortical projections from the intralaminar thalamic nuclei may be small collaterals given off by thalamostriate fibers. It is of interest that in labeling neurons with horseradish peroxidase, at least one main cortical thalamic relay nucleus was always labeled in addition to portions of the intralaminar nuclei, indicating that two thalamocortical projection systems must overlap in their cortical terminations.

Electrophysiological evidence suggests that a large proportion of the nonspecific thalamocortical fibers probably terminate in the more superficial layers of the cerebral cortex (Jasper, '60), although activation of cortical neurons at all depths has been observed during recruiting responses. According to current concepts, the recruiting waves recorded in the cortex following repetitive stimulation of the nonspecific thalamic nuclei (i.e., the intralaminar thalamic nuclei) probably represent dendritic responses or activity (Clare and Bishop, '56; Purpura and Grundfest, '56). These responses do not depend upon all-or-none firing of cortical cells; they are graded, and they have no refractory period. The absence of a refractory period implies that these waves may be summated over wide ranges, with amplitude and duration being functions of the stimulus. Recruiting responses are attributed to axodendritic depolarizing and hyperpolarizing postsynaptic potentials, mainly in the superficial layers of the cortex (Purpura, '59). Microelectrode studies indicate that recruiting responses can be obtained in the absence of unit discharges in the depths of the cortex.

Repetitive stimulation of the nonspecific thalamic nuclei produces changes in electrocortical activity over broad areas. These nonspecific thalamic nuclei are capable of exerting a massive excitation, mainly upon areas of associational cortex with a great preponderance of effects upon frontal associational cortex (Starzl and Whitlock, '52). These cortical responses are not dependent upon transmission by fibers of the corpus callosum or upon intracortical propagation. It seems generally accepted that the nonspecific thalamocortical projection

system regulates the local and general excitability of the cortex and therefore the state of consciousness and awareness. As Magoun ('54) has stated, "It is not easy for the physiologist to put his finger upon consciousness, though it is present abundantly and for long periods." The most pronounced alterations of consciousness accompany the transition from sleep to wakefulness. Recordings of the electrical activity of the cerebral cortex provide objective evidence of this marked change of the conscious state. Although the whole brain must participate in what is called consciousness, the reticular formation and the nonspecific thalamocortical system appear to be the principal integrators, since it is through these systems that the cortical electrical activity is regulated (Gastaut, '54; Jasper, '58).

Sleep

Until recently, sleep has been considered a unique passive state, interpreted physiologically as the expression of functional deafferentation of the ascending reticular activating system. The awake state was explained in terms of increased activity of this ascending activating system, while sleep was correlated with passive dampening of this system. Recent advances indicate that sleep is an active, complex neural phenomenon initiated by sleep-inducing structures and mediated, in part, by biochemical transmitters. Sleep is not a single phenomenon, but a series of successive functionally related states, which depend upon different active mechanisms, some of which can be quantified, selectively modified or suppressed (Lindsley, '60; Kleitman, '63; Jouvet, '67, '69). In mammals two recurring, distinctive and related sleep states can be readily recognized. These are referred to as slow sleep and paradoxical sleep.

Slow sleep is characterized in the EEG by synchronized cortical activity consisting of spindles (11 to 16 cycles/sec) and high voltage slow waves. There are no specific behavioral criteria for slow sleep because the relationship between synchronized, or slow cortical activity, and sleep behavior is not absolute. During slow sleep, tone remains in the neck muscles, spinal reflex activity is present and changes in autonomic activity are minimal. After a time, this state is succeeded by a totally different sleep state, known as paradoxical sleep.

Paradoxical sleep is characterized by an EEG pattern with low voltage fast activity which resembles that of the alert, waking state. This sleep state occurs intermittently after variable periods of slow sleep and has precise behavioral criteria: (1) abolition of antigravity muscle tone (especially in cervical muscles), (2) depression of spinal reflex activity, (3) characteristic autonomic changes (i.e., reduction in blood pressure, bradycardia and irregular respiration), and (4) bursts of rapid eye movements (REM). The fact that paradoxical sleep is "deeper" than slow sleep, but associated with an EEG pattern similar to that of the waking state, gave rise to the term paradoxical sleep. Rapid eye movements (REM) of 50 to 60/min occur in a stereotyped pattern different from that seen in the waking state. These rapid eye movements are associated with subcortical and cortical activity, which have been termed *pontogeniculo-occipital* (PGO) *activity*. These phasic activities of high voltage can be recorded from the pontine reticular formation, the lateral geniculate body and the occipital cortex. This activity occurs transiently during slow sleep, and always precedes paradoxical sleep. During paradoxical sleep, PGO waves are fairly constant (about 60 waves/min), and it has been suggested that electrical events are triggering both these activities and the rapid eye movements (Jouvet, '69). Bursts of ascending impulses from the medial and inferior vestibular nuclei have been implicated in the REM occurring during paradoxical sleep (Pompeiano and Morrison, '65; Pompeiano, '67). Median rates of spontaneous discharge of units in these nuclei were two to four times higher during desynchronized sleep than during quiet waking. Lesions in the medial and inferior vestibular nuclei abolish the bursts of REM, but desynchronized sleep is still characterized by low voltage, fast activity in the EEG. The conclusion drawn is that the medial and inferior vestibular nuclei represent the causal link leading to activation of the extraocular motor nuclei which are responsible for the bursts of REM. So-called REM sleep (paradoxical sleep) occurs periodically during a night of sleep, with longer periods during the latter part of the night. If the subject is awakened during or immediately after a period of rapid eye movements, 80% of the subjects will report that they have been dreaming, and can relate the content of the dream (Lindsley, '60).

Recent advances in neuroanatomy, neurophysiology and neuropharmacology concerning the biogenic amines have provided a more complete understanding of their role in sleep states (Jouvet, '67, '69). In the cat reserpine, which depletes both serotonin and noradrenalin, produces a tranquil state and suppresses both slow and paradoxical sleep for different periods of time. Most monoamine oxidase (MAO) inhibitors have a suppressive effect upon paradoxical sleep and increase slow sleep. Histofluorescence techniques have demonstrated that most serotonin-containing neurons are located in the raphe system (Ungerstedt, '71; Felten et al, '74), and norepinephrine-containing neurons are located principally in the locus ceruleus (Ungerstedt, '71; Dahlström and Fuxe, '64). Inhibition of serotonin synthesis at the level of tryptophan hydroxylase leads to total insomnia which is reversible; injections of the immediate precursor of serotonin (5-hydroxy-tryptophan) causes a return to normal sleep. Nearly total destruction of serotonin-containing neurons in a raphe system also produces insomnia. Pharmacological studies suggest that serotonin may be most intimately associated with slow sleep, but many intricate facets of the sleep process are still poorly defined.

The relationship between slow sleep and paradoxical sleep is not simple, but recent studies suggest that serotonergic neurons involved in slow sleep may act as part of the priming mechanism for triggering paradoxical sleep (Jouvet, '69). Serotonergic neurons triggering paradoxical sleep are located in caudal regions of the pontine raphe, since lesions at this level severely depress paradoxical sleep relative to slow sleep. The structures responsible for paradoxical sleep, however, lie outside of the raphe system, and specifically include the locus ceruleus. Cells of the locus ceruleus contain norepinephrine and monoamine oxidase. Monamine oxidase inhibitors and bilateral lesions of the locus ceruleus selectively suppress paradoxical sleep without altering slow sleep. The fact that numerous drugs which act upon the synthesis of norepinephrine suppress paradoxical sleep suggests that noradrenergic neurons located in the locus ceruleus may trigger paradoxical sleep. Certain cholinergic mechanisms also have been implicated in the mechanism of paradoxical sleep, in that atropine suppresses this form of sleep, while direct injections of acetylcholine in the locus ceruleus produce paradoxical sleep. Thus the complex neuropharmacological events which underlie paradoxical sleep involve sequentially serotonergic, cholinergic and noradrenergic mechanisms.

Higher Cortical Functions

The most striking features of the human brain are its elaborate neural mechanisms for complex correlations, the discrimination of sensory impulses and the utilization of former reactions. The principal function of these mechanisms may be termed *associative memory* and the *reactions* they use, *mnemonic* (memory) *reactions*. In man, the acquired changes which occur in the cortex after birth permit the neurons to alter subsequent stimuli reaching the cortex. This ability to retain, modify and reuse neuronal chains probably provides the basis of conscious and unconscious memory, of personal experience and of individually acquired neural mechanisms. Other animals also utilize individual experience to "learn." However, it is doubtful if any animal other than man summates experience by transmitting it to other individuals and new generations. The symbolization necessary for this summation probably requires the pallial mechanism for associative memory. It has been estimated that the cerebral cortex contains nearly 14 billion nerve cells, and the largest number of these may be utilized for the above activities.

In a general way, the central sulcus divides the brain into a posterior receptive portion and an anterior portion related closely to efferent or motor functions. The posterior part contains all the primary receptive areas, which receive specific sensory impulses from the lower centers of the brain and hence indirectly from the peripheral sensory receptors. Impulses entering these primary areas produce sensations of a sharply defined character, such as distinct vision and hearing, sharply localized touch and accurate sensations of position and movement. However, these sensations probably have not attained the perceptual level necessary for the recognition of an object. This requires the integration of primary stimuli into more complicated sensory patterns. The regions in immediate contact with the receptive centers, known as *parasensory areas*, serve for the combination and elaboration of the primary impulses into more complex unisensory perceptions which can be recalled under appropriate conditions. In the more distant association areas the various sensory fields overlap (e.g., the inferior parietal lobule and adjacent portions of the occipital and temporal lobes). In these areas the combinations are more complicated and are expressed as multisensory perceptions of a higher order. Thus tactile and kinesthetic impulses are built up into perceptions of form, size and texture (stereognosis). Visual impulses similarly are compounded into perceptions of visual object recognition. Hence any object comes to be represented ultimately by a constellation of memories compounded from several sensory channels which are dependent upon previous experience. When sensory impulses initiated by feeling, or seeing, an object excite these memory constellations, the object is "recognized" (i.e., remembered as having been seen or felt before). This arousal of the associative mnemonic complexes of afferent cortical impulses may be termed "gnosis," and it forms the basis of understanding and knowledge. Disorders of this mechanism caused by lesions in the association areas usually are known as gnostic disturbances or *agnosias*. The tactile, visual or auditory stimuli evoked by an object no longer arouse the appropriate memories; hence the object and its uses appear unfamiliar and strange. When such gnostic disturbances involve the far more complicated associative mechanisms underlying the comprehension of language, they form part of a complex known as the *aphasias*. Closely related to both agnosia and aphasia is another group of disorders characterized by difficulty in performing learned complex or skilled movements even though no paralysis, sensory loss or ataxia is present. These disorders, which affect the motor side of higher sensory-motor integration, are referred to as the *apraxias*. One must realize that there are only two ways in which a patient can show that he recognizes an object: (1) by naming the object or describing its use, and (2) by demonstrating its use. These simple methods demonstrate that agnosia in part underlies both aphasia and apraxia. If the patient can demonstrate the use of an object, but is unable to name or describe it, he has an aphasia. If he can name or describe an object, but does not know how to use it, he has an apraxia.

Agnosia. The term agnosia means a failure to recognize. Various types of agnosias have been defined according to the particular sensory modality affected. Of the many types of agnosia classified on this basis with respect to both objects and space, three may properly be considered here, namely, *tactile agnosia, visual agnosia* and *auditory agnosia*.

Tactile agnosia is a failure to recognize objects by means of tactile and proprioceptive sensibilities when both are normal in the part of the body being tested. Astereognosis is the inability to recognize objects owing to sensory impairment at a cortical level. According to Brain ('61), tactile agnosia is associated especially with lesions of the supramarginal gyrus in the left cerebral hemisphere, which probably is the dominant hemisphere for tactile recognition.

Visual agnosia is a failure to recognize objects that cannot be attributed to a defect of visual acuity or to intellectual impairment. Although a patient with visual agnosia is unable to recognize an object by sight, he may recognize it by other sensibilities, and he can still recognize people. The disability usually is limited to small objects and varies somewhat from day to day.

In some instances the visual agnosia may extend to surroundings; it then results in spatial disorientation. Lesions associated with visual agnosia involve the lateral visual association areas in the dominant hemisphere. The term *alexia* denotes a special form of visual agnosia in which the patient is unable to read because he fails to recognize written or printed words. Lesions in this syndrome interrupt pathways conveying impulses from the visual cortex of both sides to the angular gyrus of the left hemisphere.

Auditory agnosia is the term used to describe the condition in which a patient with unimpaired hearing fails to recognize or distinguish what he hears. This type of agnosia may involve speech, musical sounds or familiar noises, such as the telephone bell or running water. One form of auditory agnosia, known as word deafness, constitutes a type of receptive aphasia. Lesions associated with auditory agnosia involve parts of the superior temporal convolution posteriorly (area 22) in the dominant hemisphere, although these disturbances are more severe when the injury is bilateral.

Aphasia. This disorder is characterized by receptive and expressive disturbances in the faculty of using symbols and signs to communicate. It results from organic neural lesions involving cerebral memory mechanisms for language without impairment of cortical or subcortical structures essential for the relay of impulses, or the innervation of speech organs (i.e., the muscles of the larynx, tongue, and lips). The aphasias usually are divided into two basic types: receptive (sensory) and expressive (motor). In receptive aphasia the disturbance involves an impairment in the appreciation of the meanings of both spoken and written words. Expressive aphasia is characterized by impairment or lack of ability to express thoughts in a meaningful way in speech or writing. Less severe forms of expressive aphasia may involve primarily the incorrect choice of words or grammatical confusion. The division of the aphasias into two types suggests a more clear cut distinction than our understanding permits, since common disturbances of memory and language must be involved in both types. While relatively pure receptive or expressive forms of aphasia do occur, mixed varieties are the most common. Certain patients with severe expressive forms of aphasia may be capable of making meaningful gestures which suggest some degree of thought comprehension.

It is extremely difficult to locate precisely the site, or sites, of lesions which result in different forms of aphasia. Most evidence suggests that the disorder is associated with lesions involving the posterior temporoparietal region, and the so-called Broca's area (portions of the pars opercularis and triangularis of the inferior frontal gyrus) in the dominant hemisphere (Penfield and Roberts, '59; Brain, '61). Penfield and Roberts ('59) report that any large lesion in the posterior temporoparietal region involving the cortex and underlying projection areas of the thalamus causes a severe aphasia. Although Broca's speech area has long been considered the cortical site of lesions in expressive aphasia, several observers have questioned its significance (Marie, '06; Mettler, '49; Jefferson, '50). According to these authors, this area can be sacrificed in the adult without eventual loss of normal speech. Penfield and Roberts ('59) also suggest that it is less important than the posterior temporoparietal region.

Apraxia. The inability to perform certain learned complex movements, in the absence of paralysis, sensory loss or disturbance of coordination, is known as apraxia. Since complex voluntary movements require the utilization of cerebral processes in formulating the nature of the act to be performed, movements of this nature are considered separate from those which are more or less automatic. Formulation of these movement complexes is largely unconscious and appears to depend upon memory constellations of similar acts previously performed. Complex learned movement patterns are organized in space and time, and follow sequences requiring close attention. Multiple sensory systems contribute to the skill of these movement patterns. Apraxia has been regarded as a disorganization of the underlying complex movement patterns. Many varieties of apraxia have been proposed as distinct en-

tities, although some tend to have common features.

Kinetic apraxia is characterized by an inability to execute fine acquired motor movements; there is no paresis, and automatic and associated movements can be carried out: This disturbance may be confined to one limb. It has been interpreted as an expressive defect, most frequently associated with lesions of the precentral cortex. The defect usually occurs contralateral to the lesion (De Jong, '58).

Ideomotor apraxia is caused by an interruption of pathways between the center for formulation of a motor act and the motor areas necessary for its execution. Although the patient may know what he wants to do, he is unable to do it. He can perform many complex acts automatically, but he may fail to perform the same acts on command. Spontaneous gestures may be normal. Ideomotor apraxia is often bilateral and affects the extremities equally. It is said to be associated with lesions of the parietal lobe, particularly the supramarginal gyrus, in the dominant hemisphere.

Ideational apraxia is the term used to describe loss of ability to formulate the ideational plan for the execution of the components of a complex act. While simple isolated movements may be performed normally, the component movements of a complex act are not synthesized into a purposeful plan and individual movements may be performed in a faulty sequence. Since kinesthetic memory and appreciation of the act to be performed are defective, ideational apraxia may be a variety of agnosia. This form of apraxia has been considered to result from lesions in the dominant parietal lobe, or in the corpus callosum (Geschwind and Kaplan, '62), but frequently it is associated with rather diffuse pathological processes.

Constructional apraxia is a disorder characterized by loss of visual guidance, impairment of the visual image and disturbances of revisualization. A patient suffering from this form of apraxia is unable to reproduce simple geometric figures by drawing or by the arrangement of blocks. Although this form of apraxia is included with expressive disorders of motor function, it is rarely a pure motor disorder. As a rule the patient is unaware of his inability to perceive spatial relationships. This variety of apraxia appears to be related to interruption of pathways between the occipital and parietal cortex (Critchley, '53).

Certain curious combinations of agnosia and apraxia occur as a consequence of lesions involving primarily the inferior parietal lobe, usually in the dominant hemisphere (Gerstmann, '40; Critchley, '53). This syndrome is characterized by: (1) finger agnosia, (2) right-left disorientation, (3) agraphia or dysgraphia, and (4) acalculia or dyscalculia. Patients suffering from this syndrome have difficulty in differentiating their fingers, in naming the individual fingers and in pointing to particular fingers. Right-left disorientation, unlike finger agnosia, may affect all parts of the body, as well as inanimate objects and other individuals. The disturbance in writing does not extend to copying, which can be accomplished without difficulty. Inability to solve arithmetical problems is most evident with written figures, but it involves mental calculations as well.

Prefrontal Cortex

The frontal lobe rostral to areas 6 and 8 represents a relatively late phylogenetic acquisition which is well developed only in primates, especially in man. These areas of cortex, including that on the orbital surface, are referred to as the prefrontal cortex. Areas of cortex on the lateral convexity of the brain (particularly areas 9 and 10) receive a large number of fibers from the dorsomedial nucleus of the thalamus, which may bring impulses from certain autonomic centers. These areas are connected by the cingulum and the uncinate fasciculus with anterior portions of the temporal lobe and, directly or indirectly, with parietal and adjacent occipitotemporal association areas. It is the opinion of some that complex memory patterns formed in areas caudal to the central sulcus may be transmitted to the prefrontal areas and synthesized into mnemonic constellations, which perhaps form the basis of abstract thinking and of certain higher intellectual activities. In the prefrontal region, these highly discriminative cortical activities are blended with the activities of medial nuclear groups of the thalamus, which appear associated with more primitive affective components of consciousness, and probably play an important role in emotional responses. Russell ('48) believes that the prefrontal areas are not primarily concerned with memory or general intelligence, but rather with the establishment and conditioning of emotional reactions. They are of great importance during childhood and the growing years, when behavioral patterns are being formed. Emotional reactions become less prominent after maturity, when behavior patterns have become established.

A procedure known as prefrontal *lobotomy* or *leucotomy* was used widely some years ago in attempts to modify the behavior of severely psychotic patients. The basic operation involved bilateral sectioning of the fiber connections to and from the prefrontal area. Lobotomy, introduced by Moniz ('36), was performed in the United States and elsewhere in the 1940's (Freeman and Watts, '49). This neurosurgical procedure permitted many institutionalized patients to return home and even to resume their former activities. Moreover, a considerable number of lobotomies were performed for the relief of chronic intractable pain of organic origin when other measures, such as massive doses of narcotics and even cordotomy, had proved of no avail (Falconer, '48; Freeman and Watts, '49; Scarff, '49). After the operation, the patient no longer complained spontaneously of pain and no longer appeared to be in distress, although when asked he acknowledged that pain was still present. Relief apparently was due to removal of the anxiety and fear usually associated with pain. Since prefrontal lobotomy, and numerous technical variations of it (Mettler, '49; Green et al., '52), was performed on a large number of patients, it afforded an opportunity to study the associated intellectual and behavioral effects of these lesions.

The results of numerous lobotomies have been critically discussed in a number of publications (Freeman and Watts, '49; Partridge, '50; Denny-Brown, '51). These studies are difficult to evaluate because of lack of agreement concerning the extent of the changes in behavior and intellect. Most striking are the alterations in emotional behavior, which were characterized by Freeman and Watts as a lessening of "consciousness of the self," and a narrowing of the patient's mental horizon to the immediate present and to his own person. The patient was easily amused, careless in personal habits, unconcerned in social relations and little affected by criticism. His emotional reactions were abrupt, transient and superficial, and they often were accompanied by outspoken tactlessness. Pain and hardship were not associated with anxiety, nor was there much concern about financial or domestic difficulties. There was inability to gauge or appreciate the gravity of a situation and to maintain a responsible attitude toward it. These were the most enduring changes which can be attributed to the operation, and they probably were responsible for the successful abolition of morbid anxiety and obsessional states (Freeman and Watts, '49).

Intellectual damage is especially difficult to evaluate. General memory returns rapidly, and standard psychometric tests are accurately performed. Nearly all agree that the capacity for abstract thought is reduced and that the patient develops a more concrete attitude. Easy distractibility is common, judgment is poor and initiative is reduced. Mental concentration and the capacity for sustained intellectual effort are impaired, especially with respect to solving complex problems. The most reliable data concerning the effects of lobotomy upon intelligence are those obtained from nonpsychotic patients in whom this procedure was done for relief of pain. On the basis of thorough studies of patients before and after operation, Rylander ('48) concluded that intellectual and emotional deterioration may be severe. The results of the operation necessarily depend upon the intelligence of the patient and the extent of the operative procedure. This conclusion appears to be supported by others (Koskoff et al., '48). Other forms of prefrontal lobe surgery, such as topectomy and orbitofrontal lobotomy, were not reported to produce such severe impairment of intellectual function (Landis et al., '50; Green et al.,

'52). The fact that the extent of intellectual deterioration following prefrontal lobotomy cannot be measured in specific terms reflects the exceedingly complex nature of what is called intellect and suggests that the criteria used to evaluate it may not be adequate. The unpredictable effects of the procedure upon intellect and severe personality changes associated with the irreversible nature of surgery have caused this procedure to be rarely used.

In spite of the difficulties in evaluating the behavior changes and the intellectual alterations of prefrontal lobotomy, some patients were considered to have benefitted from the operation. Perhaps the greatest problem, and one of the reasons why this form of psychosurgery is done only rarely now, was the difficulty in determining preoperatively which patients might be expected to be improved by it. Another important factor in the decline of psychosurgery was the introduction of the so-called tranquilizing drugs which have facilitated the treatment of severe behavioral disorders.

The human nervous system has evolved slowly, and although many of the details of its anatomical structure appear firmly established, concepts concerning the functional significance and interrelation of its various subdivisions change as a result of continuing research. Many so-called "electronic brains" have been constructed which can perform certain functions faster and more efficiently than the human brain. The more complex the performed function, the more elaborate the programming of the computer must be. "Electronic brains" are impressive in appearance and function; yet they do not approach in versatility or scope the fantastic potentialities of the human brain. The human brain is unique in that it provides its own programming; in fact, it is programmed throughout life by daily experiences. It seems likely that "electronic brains" will in the future perform many more of the functions now performed by human brains, but this change must be regarded as a redistribution of labor. This "electronic brain" is after all only one of the many expressions of the ingenuity of the human brain.

CHAPTER 20

Blood Supply of the Central Nervous System

The central nervous system is metabolically one of the most active systems of the body. Its metabolism depends almost entirely upon the aerobic combustion of glucose. Since there is little storage of glucose or oxygen in the brain, even brief interference with cerebral circulation can cause permanent neurological or mental disturbances. Neural tissue deprived of an adequate blood supply undergoes necrosis. Impairment of local or regional blood supply constitutes the most common cause of central nervous system lesions. The duration of consciousness after complete cessation of brain circulation is less than 10 sec.

Estimates of cerebral blood flow based on the nitrous oxide method of Kety and Schmidt ('48) indicate a normal blood flow of about 50 ml/100 g of brain tissue per min. Thus a brain of average weight has a normal blood flow of about 750 ml/min. The mean oxygen consumption in the normal conscious individual is about 3.3 ml/100 g of brain tissue, or about 46 ml/min for the entire brain. Thus the brain, constituting about 2% of the body weight, requires about 17% of the normal cardiac output and consumes about 20% of the oxygen utilized by the entire body. Since the brain is not a homogeneous organ, the metabolic activity and nutritive requirements of various regions differ greatly.

If adequate circulation is not maintained to local regions of the brain or spinal cord, the neural tissue deprived of its blood supply undergoes softening, necrosis and degeneration. Vascular lesions most commonly result from disease of the cerebral vessels (arteriosclerosis) which leads to thrombosis of particular vessels. Occlusions of cerebral vessels due to embolism may result from fragments of blood clots, fat, tumor or in some instances, from air bubbles. Hemorrhage into the brain or meninges may result from pathological changes in cerebral vessels. One of the most common causes of spontaneous hemorrhage into the brain and the subarachnoid space is rupture of abnormal sacculations (aneurysms), most of which are of congenital origin. Localized neural lesions resulting from interruptions of blood supply often can be correlated with specific sensory and motor changes which are characteristic for different cerebral vessels.

BLOOD SUPPLY OF THE SPINAL CORD

The spinal cord is supplied by: (1) branches of the *vertebral arteries* that descend, and (2) multiple *radicular arteries* derived from segmental vessels (Fig. 20-1). As the vertebral arteries ascend along the anterolateral surfaces of the medulla, each gives rise to two descending vessels: (1) posterior spinal artery, and (2) the ante-

600

rior spinal artery. The paired *posterior spinal arteries* descend on the posterior surface of the spinal cord, receive variable contributions from the posterior radicular arteries and form two longitudinal plexiform channels near the dorsal root entry zone. The *anterior spinal arteries* unite to form a single descending midline vessel that supplies midline rami to the lower medulla and sulcal branches that enter the anterior median fissure of the spinal cord. The continuity of the anterior spinal artery is dependent upon anastomotic branches which it receives from the anterior radicular arteries (Suh and Alexander, '39). The anterior and posterior spinal arteries are anastomotic channels extending the length of the spinal cord which receive branches from the radicular arteries. Branches of the vertebral arteries provide the principal blood supply of virtually the entire cervical spinal cord.

Radicular arteries derived from segmental vessels (i.e., ascending cervical, deep cervical, intercostal, lumbar and sacral arteries) pass through the intervertebral foramina, divide into *anterior* and *posterior radicular arteries* and provide the principal blood supply of thoracic, lumbar, sacral and coccygeal spinal segments (Fig. 20-2). The larger anterior radicular arteries course along the ventral roots and anterior surface of the spinal cord; in the anterior median fissure their branches enter the anterior spinal artery. The smaller posterior radicular arteries course along the anterior surface for the dorsal roots and give rise to branches which unite with those from adjoining segments to form the paired plexiform posterior spinal arteries. A plexus of smaller arteries within the pia mater, interconnecting the surface vessels, forms an *arterial vasocorona* (Fig. 20-2).

The blood supply of the spinal cord may be jeopardized in certain transitional regions where its arterial supply is derived from more than one source. For example, the cervical segments are supplied primarily by branches of the vertebral artery and to a lesser extent by small branches of the ascending cervical artery. The upper segments of the thoracic spinal cord, on the other hand, are dependent upon the radicular branches of the intercostal arteries. If one or more of the parent intercostal vessels are compromised by injury or ligature, segments of the spinal cord Tl to 4 could not be adequately maintained by the small sulcal branches of the anterior spinal artery (Fig. 20-1*A*). For this reason, thoracic segments T1 to 4, particularly T4, are considered vulnerable areas in the distribution of the anterior spinal artery (Zülch, '54). Spinal cord segment L1 is another vulnerable region. The posterior surface of the cord most susceptible to vascular insult is also in segments T1 to 4 (Fig. 20-1*B*). Such vascular injuries may result in necrosis of an entire segment and produce neurological symptoms comparable to complete cord transection.

The *anterior spinal artery* gives off a number of *sulcal* branches which enter the anterior median fissure of the cord and pass alternately to the right and left (Gillilan, '58). Only in the lumbar and sacral segments does an occasional single sulcal artery in the fissure divide into left and right branches. The anterior sulcal arteries are most numerous in the lumbar region and least numerous in the thoracic region, where the segmental blood supply is poorest. In the thoracic region only one sulcal artery may enter an entire segment (Herren and Alexander, '39).

The anterior spinal artery, through its sulcal branches, supplies the anterior and lateral horns, the central gray and the base of the posterior horn (Fig. 20-2). It also supplies the anterior and lateral funiculi, including the lateral corticospinal tract. To a lesser degree, the lateral funiculus also is supplied by branches from the arterial vasocorona. The posterior spinal arteries nourish the posterior gray horn and posterior funiculus (Fig. 20-2).

Spinal veins have a general distribution similar to that of spinal arteries. Anterior longitudinal venous trunks consist of anteromedian and anterolateral veins (Fig. 20-2). Sulcal veins entering the anteromedian vein drain anteromedial portions of the spinal cord; each sulcal vein drains regions on both sides of the spinal cord. Anterolateral regions of the spinal cord

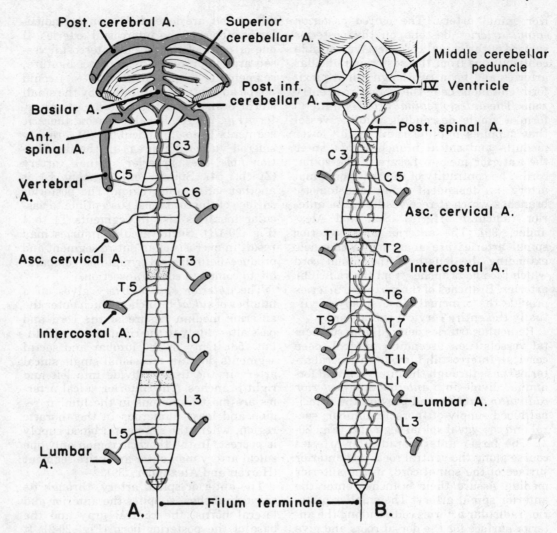

Fig. 20-1. Diagram of vessels that contribute arterial blood to the spinal cord. *A*, Anterior surface and arteries; *B*, posterior surface and arteries. Vulnerable segments of the spinal cord are *stippled*. *Letters* and *numbers* indicate most important radicular arteries (based on the work of Bolton, '39; Suh and Alexander, '39; and Zülch; '54).

drain into anterolateral veins and into the *venous vasocorona*. The *anteromedian* and *anterolateral spinal veins* are drained by 6 to 11 anterior radicular veins which empty into the epidural venous plexus. One large radicular vein in the lumbar region is referred to as the *vena radicularis magna* (Suh and Alexander, '39); other smaller radicular veins are distributed along the spinal cord.

Posterior longitudinal venous trunks, consisting of a *posteromedian vein* and

paired *posterolateral veins*, drain the posterior funiculus, the posterior horns (including their basal regions) and the white matter in the lateral funiculi adjacent to the posterior horn (Fig. 20-2). The posterior longitudinal veins are drained by 5 to 10 posterior radicular veins that enter the epidural venous plexus. The longitudinal veins are connected with each other by coronal veins (venous vasocorona) which encircle the spinal cord.

The *internal vertebral venous plexus* (epi-

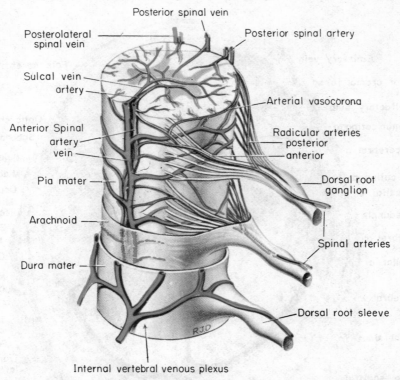

FIG. 20-2. Blood supply and venous drainage of the spinal cord shown with respect to the meninges and internal structure.

dural venous plexus), located between the dura mater and the vertebral periosteum, consists of two or more anterior and posterior longitudinal venous channels which are interconnected at many levels. At each intervertebral space there are connections with thoracic, abdominal and intercostal veins, as well as with the external vertebral venous plexus. Since there are no valves in this spinal venous network, blood flowing these channels may pass directly into the systemic venous system.

BLOOD SUPPLY OF THE BRAIN

The entire brain is supplied by two pairs of arterial trunks, the internal carotid arteries and the vertebral arteries. On the left the common carotid artery arises directly from the aortic arch; the right common carotid is one of the two branches which arises from the bifurcation of the brachiocephalic artery. The common carotid artery bifurcates at the upper level of

the thyroid cartilage forming the internal and external carotid arteries.

The Internal Carotid Artery

The internal carotid artery can be divided into four segments: cervical, intrapetrosal, intracavernous and supraclinoid. The *cervical segment,* which has no branches, extends from the bifurcation of the common carotid to the point where the vessel enters the carotid canal in the petrous bone. The *intrapetrosal segment* of this vessel is surrounded by dense bone. The *intracavernous segment* of the internal carotid artery lies close to the medial wall of the cavernous sinus, courses nearly horizontally, and bears important relationships to cranial nerves III, IV, V and VI which are within this sinus (Fig. 20-17). The *supraclinoid segment* of the internal carotid begins as the artery emerges from the cavernous sinus and passes medial to the anterior clinoid process. This portion of

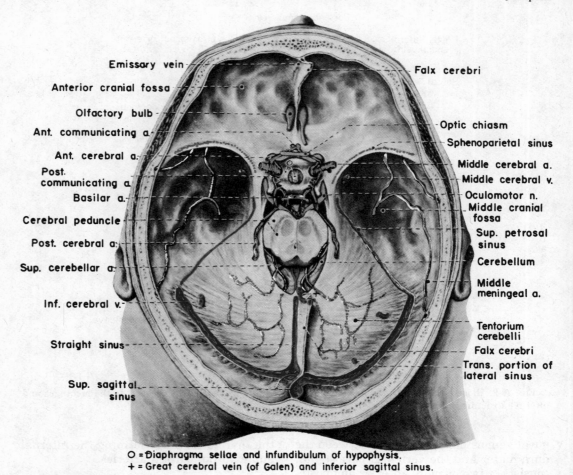

O = Diaphragma sellae and infundibulum of hypophysis.
+ = Great cerebral vein (of Galen) and inferior sagittal sinus.

Fig. 20-3. Cranial cavity after brain was removed to demonstrate relationship of the cerebral arterial circle, adjacent neural structures and reflections of the dura mater. (Truex and Kellner, *Detailed Atlas of the Head and Neck*, '48; courtesy of Oxford University Press.)

the artery usually extends upward and backward toward its bifurcation, but variations are common. The intracavernous and supraclinoid portions of the internal carotid artery are referred to as the "carotid siphon" by neuroradiologists (demonstrated but unlabeled in Fig. 20-7; Taveras and Wood, '64). Although all major branches of the internal carotid artery arise from the supraclinoid portion of this vessel, numerous small branches are given off from the intrapetrosal and intracavernous portions. These include branches to the tympanic cavity (caroticotympanic), the cavernous and inferior petrosal sinuses, the trigeminal ganglion and the meninges of the middle fossa.

Major branches of the internal carotid artery, originating from the supraclinoid portion, are the ophthalmic, posterior communicating and anterior choroidal arteries (Figs. 20-3 and 20-4). The *ophthalmic artery* enters the orbit through the optic foramen, ventral and lateral to the optic nerve. The *posterior communicating artery* arises from the dorsal aspect of the carotid siphon and passes posteriorly and medially to join the posterior cerebral artery. The *anterior choroidal artery* usually arises from the internal carotid artery distal to the posterior communicating artery and passes backward across the optic tract and then laterally to enter the choroidal fissure in the temporal lobe (Carpenter et

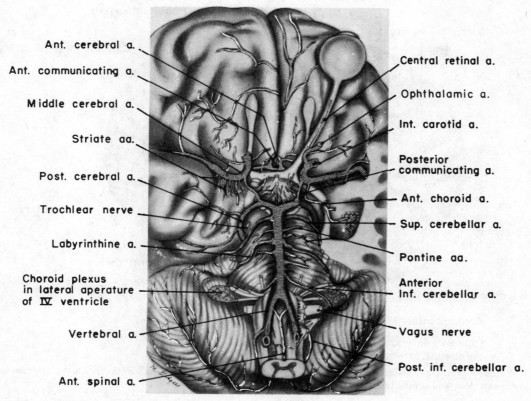

Ant. cerebral a.

Ant. communicating a.

Middle cerebral a.

Striate aa.

Post. cerebral a.

Trochlear nerve

Labyrinthine a.

Choroid plexus
in lateral aperature
of IV ventricle

Vertebral a.

Ant. spinal a.

Central retinal a.

Ophthalamic a.

Int. carotid a.

Posterior
communicating a.

Ant. choroid a.

Sup. cerebellar a.

Pontine aa.

Anterior
Inf. cerebellar a.

Vagus nerve

Post. inf. cerebellar a.

FIG. 20-4. Formation and branches of the arterial circle on the inferior surface of the brain. The relationships of the arterial circle to structures on the base of the skull are shown in Figure 20-3.

al., '54). Lateral to the optic chiasm the internal carotid artery divides into its two terminal branches: the smaller *anterior cerebral artery* and the larger *middle cerebral artery*, which is regarded as the direct continuation of the internal carotid artery.

Most of the arterial blood within the internal carotid artery is distributed by the more mobile branches of the anterior and middle cerebral arteries. The rostral parts of the brain normally supplied by these two arteries are the anterior half of the thalamus, the corpus striatum, the corpus callosum, most of the internal capsule, the medial and lateral surfaces of the frontal and parietal lobes and the lateral surface of the temporal lobe (Figs. 20-4, 20-5 and 20-6).

The Vertebral Artery

The vertebral artery originates as the first branch of the subclavian artery on each side, enters the foramen transversar-

ium of the sixth cervical vertebra and ascends in the foramina transversaria in all higher cervical vertebrae. This artery curves posteriorly around the superior articular process of the atlas, passes forward and medially to pierce the atlanto-occipital membrane and dura and enters the posterior fossa through the foramen magnum. The cervical part of the vertebral artery gives rise to spinal and muscular branches. Thin radicular branches of the vertebral artery pass through the intervertebral foramina to supply the meninges and portions of the cervical spinal cord (Fig 20-1). The relationships of the two vertebral arteries to the anterior and posterior surfaces of the caudal brain stem are shown in Figures 1-4, 1-10, 20-1 and 20-4. The two vertebral arteries unite at the caudal border of the pons to form the basilar artery. Branches of these three arteries normally provide the sole arterial blood supply to the caudal structures of the

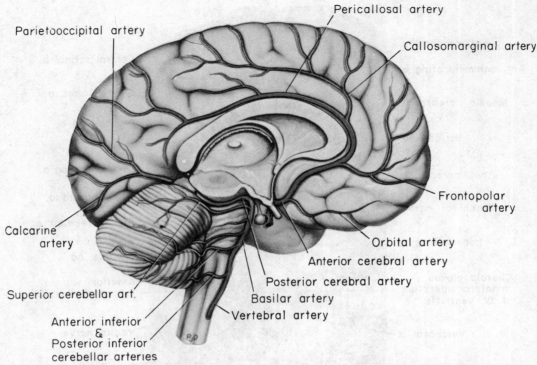

Parietooccipital artery

Pericallosal artery

Callosomarginal artery

Frontopolar artery

Calcarine artery

Orbital artery

Anterior cerebral artery

Posterior cerebral artery

Superior cerebellar art.

Basilar artery

Vertebral artery

Anterior inferior & Posterior inferior cerebellar arteries

Fig. 20-5. Principal arteries on the medial surface of the cerebrum shown together with the arteries of the brain stem and cerebellum.

brain, including the cervical spinal cord, medulla, pons, midbrain, cerebellum, posterior portions of the thalamus, occipital lobe and medioinferior surfaces of the temporal lobe (Fig. 20-4). The slender labyrinthine branch of the basilar artery follows the course of the vestibulocochlear nerve and nourishes internal ear structures through its vestibular and cochlear rami.

The Cerebral Arterial Circle

The cerebral arterial circle (Willis) is an arterial wreath encircling the optic chiasm, the tuber cinereum and the interpeduncular region formed by anastomotic branches of the internal carotid artery and the most rostral branches of the basilar artery (Figs. 20-3, 20-4 and 20-9). This arterial circle is formed by anterior and posterior communicating arteries and proximal portions of the anterior, middle and posterior cerebral arteries. The *anterior cerebral arteries* run medially and rostrally toward the interhemispheric fissure; in the region in front of the optic chiasm

these two arteries are joined by a short connecting vessel, the *anterior communicating artery*. At the rostral border of the pons the basilar artery bifurcates forming the two *posterior cerebral arteries*. The *posterior communicating arteries* arise from the internal carotid arteries and anastomose with proximal portions of the posterior cerebral arteries. The posterior cerebral arteries give rise to numerous small branches that enter the interpeduncular fossa and hypothalamus, while the main vessels pass laterally, rostral to the root fibers of the oculomotor nerve, and encircle part of the mesencephalon before passing above the tentorium cerebelli (Figs. 20-3 and 20-4). The cerebral arterial circle formed by the anastomoses of these vessels is said to equalize blood flow to various parts of the brain, but normally there is little exchange of blood between the right and left halves of the arterial circle because of the equality of blood pressure. Alterations of blood flow in the arterial circle undoubtedly occur following occlusion of one or more of the arteries contrib-

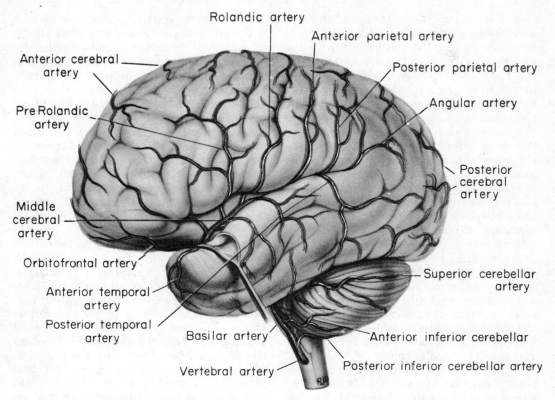

Rolandic artery

Anterior parietal artery

Anterior cerebral artery

Posterior parietal artery

Pre Rolandic artery

Angular artery

Posterior cerebral artery

Middle cerebral artery

Orbitofrontal artery

Superior cerebellar artery

Anterior temporal artery

Posterior temporal artery

Basilar artery

Anterior inferior cerebellar

Vertebral artery

Posterior inferior cerebellar artery

FIG. 20-6. Principal arteries on the lateral surface of the cerebrum and cerebellum.

uting to the circle. However, the communicating arteries of the arterial circle often form functionally inadequate anastomoses which account for the high incidence of serious disturbances in blood flow following unilateral occlusion or compression of the internal carotid artery, especially in elderly individuals.

Relationships of the arterial circle and its branches to the inferior surface of the brain and the origins of the respective cranial nerves are shown in Figure 20-4. The *in situ* surgical relationships of the arterial circle to the base of the skull following removal of the brain can be appreciated by comparing Figure 20-3 with the relationships illustrated in Figure 20-4.

From the arterial circle and the main cerebral arteries (anterior, middle and posterior) two types of branches arise: the *central* or *ganglionic,* and the *cortical* or *circumferential.* The central and cortical arteries form two distinct systems. The *central* arteries arise from the circle of

Willis and the proximal portions of the three cerebral arteries, dip perpendicularly into the brain substance and supply the diencephalon, corpus striatum and internal capsule (Fig. 20-9). For a long time these penetrating vessels have been referred to as terminal or end arteries. Studies by Scharrer ('44) indicate that the vast majority of arteries in the brains in lower animals are end arteries but in the human brain there are no end arteries. Precapillary anastomoses have been observed in man and animals, but these anastomoses usually are not sufficient to maintain adequate circulation if a major vessel is occluded suddenly. Thus occlusion of one of these arteries produces a softening in the area deprived of an adequate blood supply. The anterior and posterior choroidal arteries, respectively, branches of the internal carotid and posterior cerebral arteries, may be included in this group.

The larger *cortical* branches of each cerebral artery enter the pia mater, where they form a superficial plexus of more or less freely anastomosing vessels, which in some places may be continuous with the plexuses derived from the other main arteries. From these plexuses arise the smaller terminal arteries which enter the brain substance at right angles and run for variable distances. The shorter ones arborize in the cortex, while the longer ones supply the more deeply placed medullary substance of the hemisphere. Owing to the anastomoses of the larger cortical branches, the occlusion of one of these vessels is compensated to a variable extent by the blood supply from neighboring branches, although such collateral circulation is rarely sufficient to prevent brain damage. The great majority of vascular occlusions occur in the cerebral vessels before they enter the substance of the brain. Areas of the cerebral cortex, internal capsule, or basal ganglia which lie between the territorial distributions of two primary arteries are the sites most severely involved after vascular injury (Mettler et al., '54). The degree of brain damage is variable and depends upon several factors (e.g., site of injury, amount of vascular overlap and confluence and the rapidity with which an occlusion develops).

The Cortical Branches

The cortical branches of the cerebral hemisphere are derived from the anterior, middle and posterior cerebral arteries.

The Anterior Cerebral Artery. This artery originates at the bifurcation of the internal carotid artery, passes rostromedially, dorsal to the optic nerve, and approaches the corresponding artery of the opposite side with which it connects via the anterior communicating artery (Figs. 20-4, 20-5 and 20-9). The artery enters the interhemispheric fissure, passes upward on the medial surface of the hemisphere, curves around the genu of the corpus callosum and continues posteriorly on the superior surface of the corpus callosum. The anterior cerebral artery gives rise to: (1) the medial striate artery, (2) orbital branches, (3) the frontopolar artery, (4) the callosomarginal artery, and (5) the pericallosal artery. The pericallosal artery may be considered as the terminal part of the

anterior cerebral artery. The first portion of the anterior cerebral artery gives rise to many small branches which supply the rostrum of the corpus callosum, the septum pellucidum and the head of the caudate nucleus.

The *medial striate artery* (recurrent artery of Heubner) arises proximal to the anterior communicating artery, courses caudally and laterally and enters the anterior perforated space. This vessel supplies the anteromedial part of the head of the caudate nucleus, adjacent parts of the internal capsule and putamen and parts of the septal nuclei (Figs. 20-9, 20-11 and 20-12). The medial striate artery is said to anastomose with the lenticulostriate arteries and surface branches of the anterior and middle cerebral arteries (Kaplan, '58).

Orbital branches of the anterior cerebral artery arise from the ascending portion of this vessel just below the corpus callosum. These branches extend forward to supply the orbital and medial surfaces of the frontal lobe (Figs. 20-4 and 20-5). A *frontopolar branch* of the anterior cerebral artery is given off as the anterior cerebral artery curves around the genu of the corpus callosum. Two or three branches of the frontopolar artery supply medial parts of the frontal lobe and extend laterally on reaching the convexity of the hemisphere. A major branch of the anterior cerebral artery, the *callosomarginal artery*, arises distal to the frontopolar artery and passes backward and upward in the callosomarginal sulcus, dorsal to the cingulate gyrus (Fig. 20-5). Branches of this artery supply the paracentral lobule and parts of the cingulate gyrus. The *pericallosal artery*, as the terminal branch of the anterior cerebral artery, continues caudally along the dorsal surface of the corpus callosum; its terminal branches supply the precuneus (Salmon and Lazorthes, '71). Anomalies of the anterior cerebral artery occur in about 25% of brains; these include unpaired arteries and instances where branches are given off to the contralateral hemisphere (Baptista, '63). Occlusion of the trunk of one anterior cerebral artery produces a contralateral hemiplegia which is greatest in the lower limb. Obstruction of both anterior cerebral arteries is associated with bilateral paralysis, especially in the lower limbs, and impaired sensation that mimics spinal cord disease.

The Middle Cerebral Artery. The middle cerebral artery, the continuation of the internal carotid artery, passes laterally over the anterior perforated substance to the lateral cerebral fossa between the temporal lobe and the insula (Fig. 20-6). This artery divides into a number of large branches in the insular region which course upward and backward; as these arteries reach the uppermost portions of the insula, they reverse their course abruptly and pass downward to the lower margin of the lateral sulcus. The course of the branches of the middle cerebral artery in the insular region is of great importance in the interpretation of cerebral angiograms (Traveras and Wood, '64). In the insular region 5 to 8 branches of the middle cerebral artery lie within what is called the Sylvian triangle. The Sylvian point (or apex) is established angiographically by the most posterior branch of the middle cerebral artery to emerge from the lateral sulcus. The inferior margin of the Sylvian triangle is formed by the lower branches of the middle cerebral artery, while the superior margin is formed by looping branches of this artery that are reversing their course (Fig. 20-7). Displacement of branches of the middle cerebral artery in the Sylvian triangle by mass lesions can be detected readily in cerebral angiograms and the direction of displacement provides important information concerning localization of these lesions.

Branches of the middle cerebral artery emerge from the lateral sulcus and are distributed in a "fanlike" fashion over the lateral convexity of the hemisphere. These cortical branches supply lateral portions of the orbital gyri, the inferior and middle frontal gyri, large parts of the precentral and postcentral gyri, the superior and inferior parietal lobules and the superior and middle temporal gyri, including the temporal pole. In many instances the territory of the middle cerebral artery is extended caudally to supply most of the lateral gyri of the occipital lobe. Branches of the middle cerebral artery include: (1) the lenticulostriate arteries, (2) the anterior temporal artery, (3) the orbitofrontal artery, (4) pre-Rolandic and Rolandic branches, (5) anterior and posterior parietal branches, and (6) a posterior temporal branch which extends caudally to supply lateral portions of the occipital lobe.

The first branches to arise from the middle cerebral artery are the *lenticulostriate arteries* which enter the anterior perforated substance (Fig. 20-9). These vessels will be considered with the central or ganglionic branches. The next branches to arise from the middle cerebral artery are the anterior temporal artery and the orbitofrontal artery (Fig. 20-6). The *anterior temporal artery* frequently anastomoses with temporal branches of the posterior cerebral artery, while the *orbitofrontal artery* may anastomose with the frontopolar branch of the anterior cerebral artery. Ascending branches of the middle cerebral artery, given off more distally, include *pre-Rolandic branches,* a *Rolandic branch*, an *anterior parietal* (or post-Rolandic) *branch* and a *posterior parietal branch*. A *posterior temporal branch* extends backwards to supply lateral portions of the occipital lobe. The angular branches supplying the angular gyrus constitute the terminal part of the middle cerebral artery.

Thus the extensive and important territory nourished by the middle cerebral artery includes the motor and premotor areas, the somesthetic and auditory projection areas and the higher receptive association areas. Occlusion of the middle cerebral artery near the origin of its cortical branches, when not fatal, produces a contralateral hemiplegia most marked in the upper extremity and face, and a contralateral sensory loss of the cortical type, in which there may be astereognosis and inability to distinguish between different intensities of stimuli. When the left or dominant hemisphere is involved, there also are severe aphasic disturbances both in the (motor) formulation of speech (verbal aphasia) and the comprehension of spoken or written words (page 596).

The Posterior Cerebral Arteries. These arteries, formed by the bifurcation of the basilar artery, pass laterally over the crus cerebri (Figs. 20-3, 20-4 and 20-5).

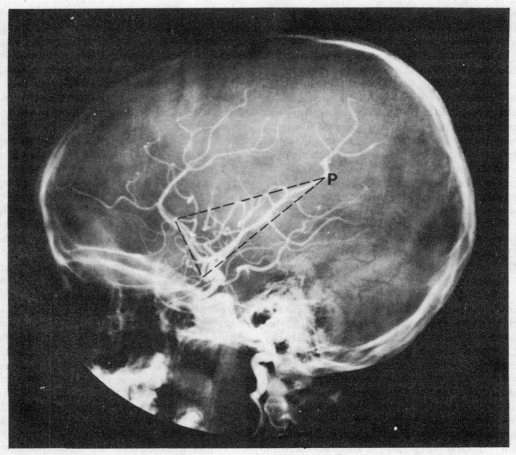

FIG. 20-7. Cerebral angiogram demonstrating the Sylvian triangle. There are 5 to 8 branches of the middle cerebral artery on the surface of the insula. As they course upward, they reach the deepest portion of the sulcus formed by the junction of the insula and the frontoparietal operculum. Upon reaching this point, the middle cerebral branches change direction and proceed downward a short distance to emerge from the lateral sulcus (Sylvian fissure). The points of reversal can be identified in the angiogram and a line is drawn from the most anterior to the most posterior point (P) forming the upper margin of the Sylvian triangle. The inferior margin of the triangle is a line from the most posterior point (the angiographic Sylvian point, P) to the anterior extremity of the middle cerebral artery. The anterior aspect is drawn from the rostral extremity of the middle cerebral artery up to the turn of the first opercular branch. The triangle contains the middle cerebral vessels as they are disposed on the insula (Courtesy of Dr. Ernest H. Wood, Columbia University, College of Physicians and Surgeons; Taveras and Wood, '64).

After receiving anastomoses from the posterior communicating arteries, these arteries continue along the lateral aspect of the midbrain, and then pass dorsal to the tentorium to course on the medial and inferior surfaces of temporal and occipital lobes. Branches of the posterior cerebral artery extend onto the lateral surfaces of the hemisphere to supply part of the inferior temporal gyrus, variable portions of the occipi-

tal lobe and portions of the superior parietal lobule (Fig. 20-6).

The posterior cerebral artery divides into two main branches, the posterior temporal (temporo-occipital) and the internal occipital arteries. The *posterior temporal artery* gives off an anterior temporal branch which supplies anterior portions of the inferior surface of the temporal lobe and frequently anastomoses with branches of the anterior temporal artery derived from the middle cerebral artery (Figs. 20-5 and 20-8B). More posterior branches of this vessel supply the occipito-temporal and lingual gyri. The *internal occipital artery* divides into the *parieto-occipital artery* and the *calcarine artery*, both of which supply different regions on the medial aspect of the occipital lobe. Thus the cortical branches of the posterior cerebral artery supply the medial and inferior surfaces of the occipital lobe and the inferior surface of the temporal lobe, except for the temporal pole (Figs. 20-5 and 20-8B). Branches of these arteries extend onto the lateral surface of the brain and supply the inferior temporal gyrus and variable portions of the lateral occipital region; some of the branches from the medial surface supply a considerable part of the superior parietal lobule. In these regions branches of the posterior cerebral artery anastomose with marginal branches of the anterior and middle cerebral arteries. The calcarine branch of the posterior cerebral artery is of major importance because it supplies the primary visual cortex. The extensive anastomoses mentioned above appear to explain why occlusion of the posterior cerebral artery rarely produces softening (encephalomalacia) in the total distribution of this vessel. Occlusion of the posterior cerebral artery produces a contralateral homonymous hemianopsia (Fig. 15-23), frequently with sparing of macular vision. Anastomoses between branches of the middle and posterior cerebral arteries in the region of the occipital pole probably account for the preservation of macular vision.

The introduction of cerebral angiography as a diagnostic technic in clinical neurology (Moniz, '31, '34) has emphasized the great importance of the anatomical distribution, course and variations of individual cerebral vessels. This technic is based upon the injection of radiopaque solutions into the internal carotid or vertebral arteries, and the taking of rapid serial roentgenograms showing various phases of the passage of the radiopaque solution through cerebral vessels. Cerebral angiography is particularly useful in localizing aneurysms and vascular malformations, and

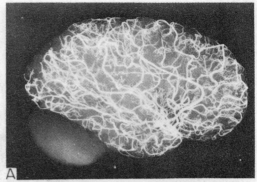
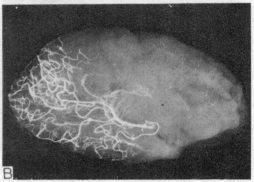

FIG. 20-8. Roentgenograms of fresh cadaver brains in which cerebral vessels have been injected with radiopaque material. *A*, Injections of the anterior, middle and posterior cerebral arteries. *B*, Injection of the posterior cerebral artery. Note the filling of the thalamoperforating branches. (Courtesy of Dr. Harry A. Kaplan.)

often it provides specific information concerning occlusive vascular disease and space-occupying intracranial masses. Cerebral aneurysms are mostly of congenital origin and appear to arise frequently from vessels on the inferior surface of the brain. Although it has been stated that aneurysms arise only at the point of bifurcation of an artery, Dandy ('47) found that many were not associated with arterial branching. Vascular malformations are of many types; arteriovenous malformations are characterized by an abnormal nest of blood vessels in which there are direct anastomoses of arteries and veins. Cerebral angiography is of importance in diagnosing occlusive vascular disease in the internal carotid (both cervical and intracranial portions) and in the vertebral and basilar ar-

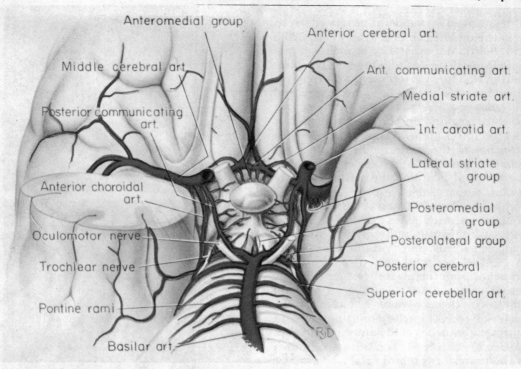

FIG. 20-9. The cerebral arterial circle (Willis) at the base of the brain showing the distribution of the ganglionic branches. These vessels form *anteromedial, posteromedial, posterolateral* and *lateral striate groups*. The *medial striate* and *anterior choroidal arteries* also are shown.

teries, as well as in the trunk of the middle cerebral artery. It is more difficult to ascertain the presence of vascular occlusions in the distal branches of the anterior, middle and posterior cerebral arteries (Taveras, '61) because of direct end-to-end anastomoses between branches of these vessels on the surface of the brain. While intracerebral hemorrhage cannot be distinguished angiographically from cerebral edema or other avascular space-occupying lesions, intracranial hemorrhage sometimes can be localized on the basis of occlusion of certain vessels and displacement of cerebral vessels. Certain highly vascular brain tumors may produce what is called a "tumor stain" in the cerebral angiogram.

While cerebral angiography provides invaluable diagnostic information, it is unusual for the contrast medium to permeate the very small terminal arteries (Fig. 20-7). Injection of the internal carotid artery usually permits visualization of the main branches of the anterior and middle cerebral arteries on the side of the injection. A radiographic technic for studying individual cerebral vessels and their branches in fresh cadaver brains has been developed by Kaplan ('56, '58, '61) and has been used extensively to study cerebral vessels (Salmon and Lazorthes, '71). The exquisite detail which can be brought out by this method is demonstrated in Figures 20-8 and 20-10.

The Central Branches

The Central or Ganglionic Arteries. These arteries which supply the diencephalon, corpus striatum and internal capsule, are arranged in four general groups: anteromedial, anterolateral, posteromedial and posterolateral (Fig. 20-9).

The *anteromedial arteries* arise from the domain of the anterior cerebral and anterior communicating arteries, but some twigs come directly from the terminal portion of the internal carotid (Fig. 20-9). They enter the most medial portion of the anterior perforated space and are distributed to the anterior hypothalamus, includ-

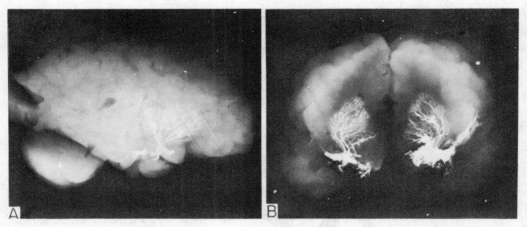

Fig. 20-10. Roentgenograms of fresh cadaver brains in which individual arteries have been injected with radiopaque material. A and B show lateral and frontal views, respectively, of the deep ganglionic branches of the middle cerebral artery that penetrate the brain in the anterior perforated substance. (Courtesy of Dr. Harry A. Kaplan.)

ing the preoptic and suprachiasmatic regions.

The *posteromedial arteries,* which enter the tuber cinereum, mammillary bodies and interpeduncular fossa, are derived from the most proximal portion of the posterior cerebral, and from the whole extent of the posterior communicating arteries. Some twigs come directly from the internal carotid artery just before its bifurcation. A rostral and caudal group may be distinguished. The rostral group supplies the hypophysis, infundibulum and tuberal regions of the hypothalamus. A number of vessels, the *thalamoperforating arteries,* penetrate more deeply and are distributed to the anterior and medial portions of the thalamus (Fig. 20-8*B*). The caudal group supplies the mammillary region of the hypothalamus, the subthalamic region, and sends small branches to the medial nuclei of the thalamus. Other vessels from the caudal group are distributed in the midbrain to the rapheal region of the tegmentum, the red nucleus and medial portions of the crus cerebri.

The *posterolateral (thalamogeniculate) arteries* arise more laterally from the posterior cerebral arteries (Figs. 20-9 and 20-11). They penetrate the lateral geniculate body and supply the larger caudal half of the thalamus, including the geniculate bodies, the pulvinar and most of the lateral nuclear mass.

The *anterolateral (striate) arteries,* which pierce the anterior perforated substance, arise mainly from the initial portion of the middle cerebral artery and, to a lesser extent, from the anterior cerebral (Figs. 20-4 and 20-9). As a rule, those from the anterior cerebral artery supply the rostroventral portion of the head of the caudate nucleus and adjacent portions of the putamen and internal capsule. The rest of the putamen, caudate nucleus and anterior limb of the internal capsule are supplied by branches from the middle cerebral artery, excepting only the most caudal tip of the putamen and the tail of the caudate nucleus (Figs. 20-10 and 20-11). These branches also nourish lateral parts of the globus pallidus and dorsal portions of the posterior limb of the internal capsule. In some instances all the striate arteries may be derived from the middle cerebral artery. One of the striate arteries, described as the cerebral vessel most prone to rupture, has been called the "artery of cerebral hemorrhage" (Charcot). Such an artery usually cannot be distinguished anatomically. While it appears doubtful that the striate arteries supply parts of the thalamus, vessels, referred to as lenticulo-optic arteries, have been described. The central perforating branches arising from the middle cerebral artery are shown radiographically in injected specimens in Figure 20-10.

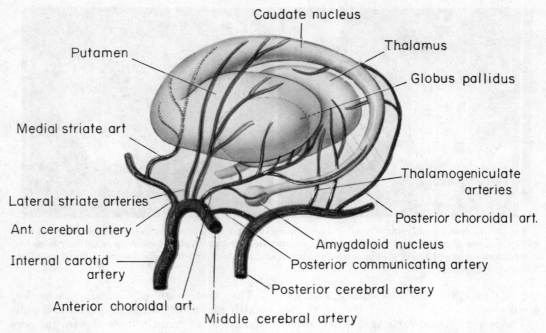

Caudate nucleus

Putamen

Thalamus

Globus pallidus

Medial striate art

Thalamogeniculate
arteries

Lateral striate arteries

Posterior choroidal art.

Ant. cerebral artery

Amygdaloid nucleus

Internal carotid
artery

Posterior communicating artery

Posterior cerebral artery

Anterior choroidal art.

Middle cerebral artery

FIG. 20-11. Diagrammatic representation of the arterial supply of the corpus striatum and thalamus (modified from Aitken, '09).

Choroidal Arteries. The anterior and posterior choroidal arteries may be regarded as distinctive central branches.

The *anterior choroidal artery* usually arises from the internal carotid artery distal to the origin of the posterior communicating artery, but it may arise from the middle cerebral artery (Carpenter et al., '54). This artery passes backward across the optic tract, to which it usually gives a few small branches, and then courses laterally toward the medial surface of the rostral part of the temporal lobe (Figs. 20-9 and 20-11). The vessel passes into the inferior horn of the lateral ventricle through the choroidal fissure where it supplies the choroid plexus. In addition the anterior choroidal artery supplies the hippocampal formation, portions of both segments of the globus pallidus (i.e., lateral parts of the medial pallidal segment and medial parts of the lateral pallidal segment), a large ventral part of the posterior limb of the internal capsule and the entire retrolenticular portion of the internal capsule (Fig. 20-12). Smaller branches of this vessel supply parts of the amygdaloid nuclear complex, ventral portions of the tail of the

caudate nucleus and extreme posterior parts of the putamen. A few branches of this artery enter lateral portions of the thalamus (Kaplan and Ford, '66). Alexander ('42) considered the anterior choroidal artery as a vessel highly susceptible to thrombosis because of its long subarachnoid course and its relatively small caliber. It appears significant that the globus pallidus and hippocampal formation, two of the most vulnerable structures of the brain, are both supplied by this artery.

The *posterior choroidal arteries* arising from the posterior cerebral artery (Fig. 20-11) consist of one medial posterior choroidal artery and at least two lateral posterior choroidal arteries (Galloway and Greitz, '60). The medial posterior choroidal artery arises from the proximal part of the posterior cerebral artery, curves around the midbrain and reaches the region lateral to the pineal body. This vessel gives off branches to the tectum, the choroid plexus of the third ventricle and the superior and medial surfaces of the thalamus (Fig. 20-8B). The lateral posterior choroidal arteries arise from the posterior cerebral artery as this vessel encircles the

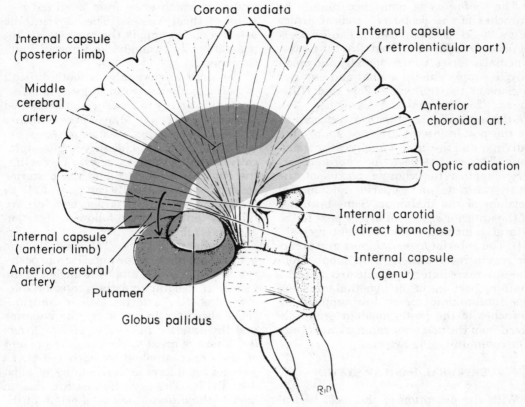

FIG. 20-12. Diagram of the blood supply of the internal capsule and corpus striatum. The putamen and globus pallidus are shown rotated ventrally away form their normal position adjacent to the internal capsule. Regions supplied by branches of the middle and anterior cerebral arteries are shown in *red;* portions of the internal capsule and corpus striatum supplied by the anterior choroidal artery are in *yellow*. Direct branches of the internal carotid artery supply the genu of the internal capsule (Alexander, '42).

brain stem. These vessels penetrate the choroidal fissure where they anastomose with branches of the anterior choroidal artery (Carpenter et al., '54).

BLOOD SUPPLY OF BASAL GANGLIA, INTERNAL CAPSULE AND DIENCEPHALON

The *striatum* is nourished mainly by the lateral striate arteries derived from the middle cerebral artery (Figs. 20-11 and 20-12). Rostromedial parts of the head of the caudate nucleus are supplied by the medial striate artery (Heubner), while the tail of the caudate nucleus and caudal parts of the putamen receive branches of the anterior choroidal artery. The lateral segment of the globus pallidus is supplied by branches of both the lateral striate and anterior choroidal arteries (Mettler et al.,

'56). The lateral part of the medial pallidal segment receives branches from the anterior choroidal artery, while branches of the posterior communicating artery nourish the most medial portions of this pallidal segment.

The *internal capsule,* both anterior and posterior limbs, is supplied primarily by the lateral striate branches of the middle cerebral artery (Fig. 20-12). The medial striate artery supplies a rostromedial part of the anterior limb of the internal capsule. As a rule, the genu of the internal capsule receives some direct branches from the internal carotid artery (Alexander, '42), while ventral parts of the posterior limb and its entire retrolenticular part are supplied by branches of the anterior choroidal artery (Salmon and Lazorthes, '71).

The *thalamus* is nourished mainly by branches of the posterior cerebral artery (Figs. 20-3*B*, 20-9 and 20-11). *Thalamoperforating branches,* referred to as the posteromedial arteries, course dorsally and medially to supply chiefly medial and anterior regions of the thalamus (Foix and Hillemand, '25; Salmon and Lazorthes, '71). *Thalamogeniculate branches,* referred to as the posterolateral arteries, supply the pulvinar and the lateral nuclei of the thalamus. The *medial posterior choroidal artery* supplies the choroid plexus of the third ventricle and superior and medial portions of the thalamus. Some branches of the anterior choroidal artery pass to the lateral geniculate body (Carpenter et al., '54). The anterior *hypothalamus* and preoptic region receive their blood supply from the anteromedian ganglionic arteries. Remaining portions of the hypothalamus and the subthalamic region are supplied by branches of the posteromedian group derived from the posterior cerebral and posterior communicating arteries.

VERTEBRAL BASILAR SYSTEM

With the exception of the most rostral portions of the crus cerebri, the entire blood supply of the medulla, pons, mesencephalon and cerebellum is derived from the vertebral basilar system.

Vertebral Artery. Each vertebral artery, as it passes over the anterior surface of the medulla, gives rise to: (1) a *posterior spinal artery,* (2) an *anterior spinal artery,* (3) a large *posterior inferior cerebellar artery,* and (4) a *posterior meningeal artery.* The two vertebral arteries unite to form the basilar artery at the lower border of the pons. This large vessel passes rostrally in the basilar sulcus and bifurcates at the upper border of the pons, forming the posterior cerebral arteries.

Basilar Artery. The basilar artery gives rise to: (1) the *anterior inferior cerebellar arteries,* (2) the *labyrinthine arteries,* (3) *numerous paramedian* and *circumferential pontine rami,* and (4) the *superior cerebellar arteries.* The *posterior cerebral arteries,* representing the terminal branches of the basilar artery, furnish the main blood supply to the midbrain via

branches which arise from proximal portions of these vessels. The labyrinthine arteries do not supply the brain stem, but pass laterally through the internal auditory meati.

Vertebral angiography is more difficult to perform than carotid angiography because this artery is smaller and contained within a bony canal. Many of the branches of the vertebral and basilar arteries are small and difficult to identify angiographically, but the anterior inferior cerebellar, the superior cerebellar and the posterior cerebral arteries usually can be seen. Both posterior cerebral arteries usually are filled by contrast media following injection of one vertebral artery.

Medulla and Pons. The medulla and pons are supplied by the anterior and posterior spinal arteries, and by branches of the vertebral, basilar and the posterior inferior cerebellar arteries. Minor contributions also may be made by the *superior* and the *anterior inferior cerebellar arteries.* There is great variation in the extent of the areas supplied by each vessel, as well as considerable overlapping of adjacent fields. These variations are due in part to the different levels of origin of the anterior spinal arteries, and to the varying level of fusion of the two vertebrals into the basilar artery. Not uncommonly one or another artery may be missing altogether and its place is taken by the vessel supplying the adjacent territory. Thus the area of the posterior spinal artery may be taken over by the posterior inferior cerebellar artery, or the latter may be replaced by branches from the vertebral artery. Since the vascular supply of this region has considerable clinical importance, the main structures normally supplied by the various arteries are summarized briefly (Figs. 20-13 and 20-14).

The *posterior spinal artery* supplies the gracile and cuneate fasciculi and their nuclei, and the caudal and dorsal portions of the inferior cerebellar peduncle (Figs. 20-1 and 20-13). When missing, its territory is taken over by the posterior inferior cerebellar artery.

The *anterior spinal artery* supplies the medial structures of the medulla, including the pyramids, pyramidal decussation, medial lemniscus, medial longitudinal fasciculus, predorsal bundle and hypoglossal nucleus, except its most cephalic portion. In addition, the artery supplies the medial accessory olive, the most caudal portions of the solitary nucleus and fasciculus and the dorsal motor nucleus of the vagus. In the upper medulla the distribution of the anterior spinal artery is reduced gradually, and it is replaced by branches of the vertebral and basilar arteries (Fig. 20-13).

The *bulbar branches of the vertebral artery* normally supply the pyramids at the lower border of the pons, the most cephalic part of the hypoglossal nucleus and large parts of the inferior olivary nucleus, including the dorsal accessory olive. The artery also supplies olivocerebellar fibers traversing the reticular formation, portions of the dorsal motor nucleus of the vagus and the solitary nucleus and fasciculus. At the level of the pyramidal decussation the most caudal branches are distributed to practically the whole lateral region of the medulla lying between the pyramids and the fasciculus cuneatus.

The *posterior inferior cerebellar artery* supplies the retro-olivary region, which contains the spinothalamic and rubrospinal tracts, the spinal trigeminal nucleus and tract, the nucleus ambiguus, the dorsal motor nucleus of the vagus and the emerging fibers of these nuclei. This artery also supplies ventral parts of the inferior cerebellar peduncle. Descending central autonomic tracts are found in this area of the medulla.

The ventral portion of the pons receives arterial blood from three series of branches, all derived from the *basilar artery* (Figs. 20-13, 20-14 and 20-15). These arterial branches are grouped into: (1) paramedian, (2) short circumferential, and (3) long circumferential.

Paramedian arteries leave the dorsal surface of the parent vessel to supply the most medial pontine area, including the pontine nuclei and the corticopontine, corticospinal and corticobulbar tracts. Smaller arterial twigs also penetrate dorsally to supply the most ventral part of the pontine tegmentum, including a portion of the medial lemniscus. Obstruction of the

paramedian arteries usually is followed by hemiplegia (at times a quadriplegia); pseudobulbar palsy, including dysarthria and dysphagia; transitory hemianesthesia; paresis of conjugate eye movements with deviation of the eyes to the side opposite the lesion (Frantzen and Olivarius, '57); or bilateral ophthalmoplegia (Masucci, '65).

Short circumferential arteries supply a wedge of tissue along the anterolateral pontine surface. Neural structures in this intermediate area of the pons include a variable number of fibers of the corticospinal tract and medial lemniscus, the pontine nuclei and pontocerebellar fibers and part of the nuclei and fibers of the trigeminal and facial nerves. Some of the circumferential branches may ascend to supply part of the superior cerebral peduncle. Obstruction of the short circumferential arteries on one side may result in ipsilateral cerebellar symptoms, contralateral hemianesthesia and disturbances of the sympathetic system, including an ipsilateral Horner's syndrome.

Long circumferential arteries pass laterally on the anterior surface of the pons to anastomose with smaller branches of the anterior inferior cerebellar and superior cerebellar arteries (Figs. 20-13 and 20-14). The long circumferential and *anterior inferior cerebellar arteries* supply most of the tegmentum in the caudal portion of the pons, whereas the long circumferential and *superior cerebellar arteries* supply a similar area in the more rostral levels of the pons. Important neural structures within this area of vascular distribution are the nuclei of cranial nerves III to VIII, the spinal trigeminal nucleus and tract, the medial longitudinal fasciculus, the medial lemniscus, the spinothalamic and spinocerebellar tracts, the superior cerebellar peduncle and the reticular formation. Obstruction of these vessels may produce injury to one or more of the cranial nerves mentioned, paresis of conjugate eye movements, contralateral hemianesthesia, ipsilateral cerebellar symptoms, nystagmus and sympathetic disturbances. Alterations in the individual's sensorium may increase until coma supervenes owing to anoxia or hemorrhage into the pontine tegmentum.

Complete or partial thrombosis of the

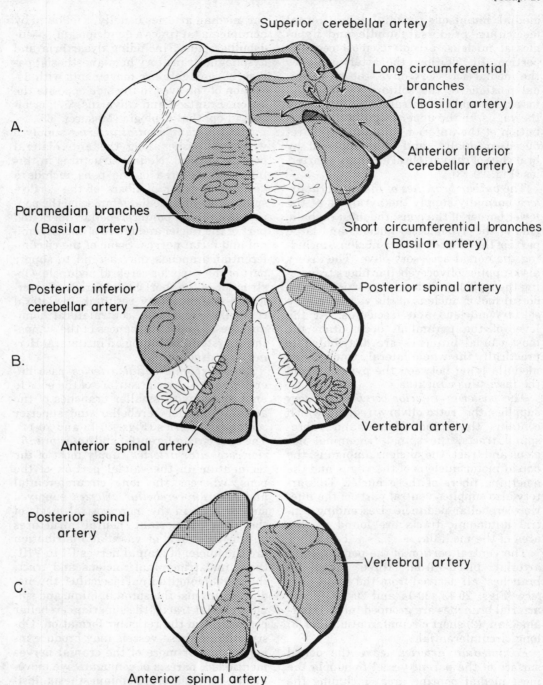

FIG. 20-13. Diagrams showing the arterial supply of the medulla and pons. Medullary levels shown are through the posterior column nuclei (C) and the inferior olivary nuclear complex (B) (based on Stopford, '15, '16). The pons (A) is supplied by paramedian and circumferential branches of the basilar artery (Frantzen and Olivarius, '57).

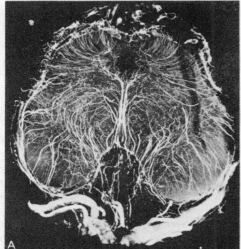

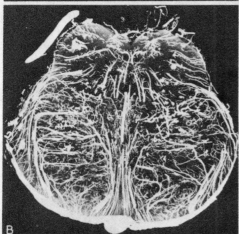

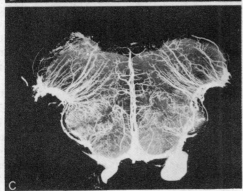

basilar artery may occur suddenly and is accompanied by severe headache, vomiting and a precipitous loss of consciousness. Complete thrombosis is generally fatal, although recoveries have been observed after partial occlusion (Haugsted, '56). Thrombosis of the basilar artery was once considered of purely academic interest. Today it is of great practical importance as well, for it can be recognized during life and this aids in the differential diagnosis and case prognosis. The symptoms of basilar artery occlusion (usually bilateral) are due to massive pontine damage and include a deep comatose state, generalized loss of muscular tone (flaccidity of limbs), dilated or pinpoint pupils that do not react to light and loss of superficial abdominal reflexes. Increased muscle tone and Babinski responses may be present within a variable period of time after such vascular accidents. There is often an intermingling of symptoms, depending upon the level, branches involved and degree of arterial occlusion. For example, thrombosis of the rostral part of the basilar artery, near its bifurcation into the two posterior cerebral arteries, may result only in visual defects (bilateral homonymous hemianopsia).

The venous drainage of the hindbrain has been demonstrated by stereomicroangiography (Hassler, '67). The paramedian veins which run near the midline to the ventral surface of the brain stem are inclined caudally in the upper pons, but are nearly perpendicular to the axis of the brain stem in more caudal regions. At the junction of pons and medulla a conspicuously large vein consistently drains the

Fig. 20-14. Microangiograms of the blood supply of the midbrain, pons and medulla made from 4 mm thick injected specimens. In the midbrain (A) the tegmentum is supplied mainly be branches of the posterior cerebral and superior cerebellar arteries, but it also receives contributions for the paramedian and both long and short circumferential arteries. The upper pons (B) receives paramedian and circumferential branches from the basilar artery, as well as branches of the superior cerebellar artery distributed to dorsal regions. The vascular pattern in the upper medulla (C) should be compared with the diagram (B) of Figure 20-13. (Courtesy of Dr. O. Hassler, '67.)

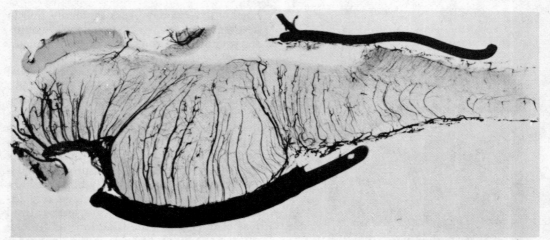

FIG. 20-15. Microangiogram of a 4 mm midsagittal section of the midbrain, pons and medulla made from an injected specimen. Paramedian arteries form different angles with the basilar artery at various levels. In the caudal midbrain and upper pons they are inclined caudally; in the upper medulla and caudal pons these vessels are inclined rostrally. (Courtesy of Dr. O. Hassler, '67.)

floor of the fourth ventricle. Veins draining ventral portions of the pons usually empty into paired longitudinal venous plexuses several millimeters lateral to the basilar artery. However, in some instances these veins enter a single unpaired vein situated between the basilar artery and the brain stem parenchyma. In the lower medulla posterior veins are larger than the anterior veins and penetrate deeper regions. Although the veins of the hindbrain seldom accompany the arterial branches in the same vascular sheath, the intraparenchymatous venous angioarchitecture resembles the arterial pattern. Anastomoses between intraparenchymatous veins occur mainly at the capillary level. Large veins draining the choroid plexus of the fourth ventricle, most of the pons, and the upper medulla, empty into the sigmoid sinus, or the superior or inferior petrosal sinuses. Veins draining caudal parts of the medulla empty into the anterior and posterior spinal veins (Hassler, '67).

Mesencephalon. The mesencephalon receives its blood supply principally from branches of the basilar artery, although branches of the internal carotid also contribute (Figs. 20-14 and 20-15). The main vessels supplying this portion of the brain stem include: (1) the *posterior cerebral artery,* (2) the *superior cerebellar artery,* (3)

branches of the *posterior communicating artery,* and (4) branches of the *anterior choroidal artery.* Branches from these arteries may be grouped, as in the case of the pons, into: (1) *paramedian arteries,* which nourish structures on both sides of the midline, and (2) *circumferential arteries,* both long and short, which wind laterally around the crus cerebri and supply lateral and dorsal regions of the midbrain (Fig. 20-14).

Paramedian branches are derived from the posterior communicating artery, from the basilar bifurcation and from proximal portions of the posterior cerebral arteries. These vessels form an extensive plexus in the interpeduncular fossa (Fig. 20-9) and enter the brain stem in the posterior perforated substance. They supply the rapheal region, the oculomotor complex, the medial longitudinal fasciculus, the red nucleus, medial parts of the substantia nigra and the crus cerebri. Branches of the anterior choroidal artery supply similar vessels which enter rostral portions of the interpeduncular fossa.

Short circumferential branches arise in part from both the interpeduncular plexus and from proximal portions of the posterior cerebral and superior cerebellar arteries. These arteries supply central and lateral parts of the crus cerebri, the substantia nigra and lateral portions of the midbrain tegmentum (Fig. 20-14). In the rostral mesencephalon some branches of the anterior choroidal artery are distributed to the interpeduncular fossa. Long circumferential arteries arise primarily from the posterior cerebral artery. The most important of these is the *quadrigeminal artery* which encircles the lateral surface of the midbrain and provides the main blood supply to the superior and inferior colliculi. Other vessels contributing to the blood supply of the tectum are branches of the medial posterior choroidal artery and the superior cerebellar artery.

Angiographic studies (Hassler, '67a) of the arterial pattern of the human brain stem clearly demonstrate the distribution of paramedian and circumferential arteries in the upper pons and midbrain (Figs. 20-14 and 20-15). Sagittal sections show that paramedian arteries entering the brain stem at various levels do so at different angles. At the junction of pons and medulla, these vessels are directed forward at an oblique angle, while at rostral pontine levels these vessels course obliquely in a caudal direction.

Numerous veins of the mesencephalon arise from capillaries and, in general, run near the arteries, but not directly with them. These veins form an extensive peripheral plexus in the pia and are collected by the basal veins which drain into either the great cerebral vein (Galen) or the internal cerebral veins.

Cerebellum. Each half of the cerebellum is supplied by one superior and two inferior cerebellar arteries passing, respectively, to the superior and inferior surfaces of the cerebellum (Figs. 20-5 and 20-6).

The *posterior inferior cerebellar artery* arises from the vertebral artery, courses rostrolaterally along the surface of the medulla and then curves upward onto the inferior surface of the cerebellum. This vessel supplies the inferior vermis, especially the uvula and nodulus, as well as the cerebellar tonsil and the inferolateral surface of the cerebellar hemisphere. Medial branches of this artery supply portions of the choroid plexus of the fourth ventricle.

The *anterior inferior cerebellar artery* is usually the most caudal large vessel arising from the basilar artery (Fig. 20-4), but it is highly variable both in its origin and area of distribution (Kaplan and Ford, '66). This vessel passed caudally and laterally to reach the inferior surface of the cerebellum where it supplies the pyramis, tuber, flocculus and portions of the inferior surface of the cerebellar hemisphere. It also sends branches to the deep portion of the corpus medullare and the dentate nucleus. In some cases, the flocculus and portions of the tonsil and biventer lobule may be supplied by an inconstant middle inferior cerebellar artery.

The *superior cerebellar artery* arises from the rostral part of the basilar artery (Fig. 20-9). On reaching the cerebellum, it divides into two main branches, a median one for the superior vermis and adjacent lateral portions, and a lateral one for the remaining hemispheral portions of the superior surface (Figs. 20-5 and 20-6). From these arteries numerous branches extend deeply into the cerebellum, supplying the superior medullary velum, middle and superior peduncles, deep portion of the corpus medullare and the intrinsic cerebellar nuclei, including parts of the dentate nucleus. Twigs also are given to the choroid plexus of the fourth ventricle.

The veins have a course generally similar to that of the arteries. A superior and an inferior median vein drain the respective portions of the vermis, adjacent paravermal regions and the deep cerebellar nuclei. The superior vein terminates in the *great cerebral vein (Galen)*, while the inferior vein drains into the straight and lateral sinuses (Fig. 20-20). Superior and inferior lateral veins drain blood from the hemispheres and flocculi to the lateral, and, in part, to the superior and petrosal sinuses.

ARTERIES OF THE DURA

The cranial dura mater is supplied by a number of meningeal arteries derived from several sources. The largest and most important is the *middle meningeal artery,* which supplies most of the dura and practically its entire calvarial portion. It is a branch of the maxillary artery which enters the cranial cavity through the foramen spinosum and then divides into an anterior and a posterior branch (Fig. 20-3). Each of the branches runs outward and upward and extends toward the superior sagittal sinus, giving off numerous branches which run forward and backward. A small *accessory meningeal artery* which may arise from the maxillary artery, or the middle meningeal artery, enters the middle fossa through the oval foramen. This vessel supplies the dura of the middle fossa and the trigeminal ganglion. Meningeal branches from the intracavernous portion of the internal carotid artery also supply the dura of the middle fossa.

In addition, the dura of the anterior and the posterior fossae receives a number of arteries, known respectively as the *anterior* and *posterior meningeal rami* or *arteries*. The anterior meningeal rami, usually two in number, are branches of the anterior and posterior ethmoidal arteries. The dura of the posterior fossa is supplied mainly by a variable number of posterior meningeal arteries. These include: (1) one or more meningeal branches from the occipital artery entering through the jugular and hypoglossal foramina, (2) meningeal branches of the vertebral artery reaching the posterior fossa through the foramen magnum, and (3) several branches of the ascending pharyngeal artery entering through the foramen lacerum and hypoglossal canal.

CEREBRAL VEINS AND VENOUS SINUSES

The cerebral veins of the brain do not run together with the arteries. Emerging as fine branches from the substance of the brain, they form a pial plexus from which arise the larger venous channels or cerebral veins. These veins run in the pia for a variable distance, pass through the subarachnoid space and empty into a system of intercommunicating endothelium-lined channels, the *sinuses of the dura mater,* located between the meningeal and periosteal layers of the dura (Figs. 1-1, 1-2, 1-3 and 20-3). The walls of these sinuses, unlike those of other veins, are composed of the tough fibrous tissue of the dura; hence, they exhibit a greater tautness and do not collapse when sectioned. The various venous sinuses converge at the internal occipital protuberance into two transversely running sinuses (Figs. 1-1 and 1-3), one for each side, which enter the juglar foramen to form the internal jugular vein. Besides draining the blood from the brain, the venous sinuses communicate with the superficial veins of the head by a number of small vessels which perforate the skull as *emissary veins* (Fig. 20-16).

The *superior sagittal sinus* extends from the foramen cecum to the internal occipital protuberance, lying along the attached border of the falx cerebri, and constantly increases in caliber as it proceeds caudally (Figs. 1-1 and 20-16). In its middle portion it gives off a number of lateral diverticula, the *venous lacunae,* into which the arachnoid villi protrude.

The *inferior sagittal sinus* extends caudally along the free border of the falx. On reaching the anterior border of the tentorium, it is joined by the *great cerebral vein (Galen),* which drains the deep structures of the brain, and the two veins form the *sinus rectus* (Figs. 1-3 and 20-16). The latter runs backward and downward along the line of attachment of the falx and tentorium and joins the superior sagittal sinus near the internal occipital protuberance (Fig. 20-3).

The two *transverse sinuses* arise from the confluens sinuum, and pass laterally and forward in a groove in the occipital bone (Figs. 1-3 and 20-3). At the occipitopetrosal junction each sinus curves downward and backward as the sigmoid sinus. The *sigmoid sinus* is drained by the internal jugular vein (Fig. 20-16).

The *confluens sinuum* is formed by the union of the superior, straight and transverse sinuses. A small unpaired *occipital sinus* from the region of the foramen magnum ascends in the falx cerebelli (Fig. 1-1) and joins the confluens. The confluens is asymmetrical and shows many individual variations (*arrow* in Fig. 20-3). In relatively few cases is there an actual union of the four sinuses. Most often the superior sagittal sinus turns to the right to become continuous with the right transverse sinus, while the straight sinus bends to the left as the left transverse sinus. In gen-

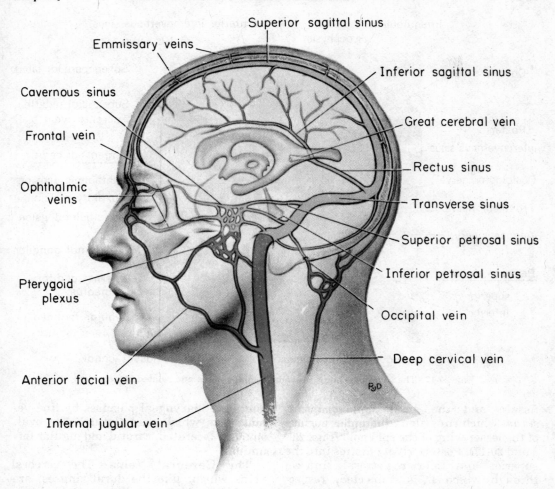

FIG. 20-16. The dural sinuses and their principal connections with extracranial veins.

eral, the venous blood of the superior cerebral veins and the superior sagittal, right transverse and right sigmoid sinuses is drained by the right internal jugular vein. Most of the venous blood of the Galenic vein, the straight sinus, left transverse and left sigmoid sinuses usually is drained by the left internal jugular vein.

The *cavernous sinus* is a large irregular space located on the side of the sphenoid bone, lateral to the sella turcica. It is a network of intercommunicating cavernous channels enclosing the internal carotid artery, the oculomotor, trochlear and abducens nerves, and the ophthalmic division of the trigeminal nerve (Fig. 20-17). The cavernous sinus of each side is connected with the other by venous channels which pass anterior and posterior to the hypophysis, and by the *basilar venous plexus*. The latter venous plexus extends along the basilar portion of the occipital bone as far caudally as the foramen magnum where it communicates with the venous plexuses of the vertebral canal (Fig. 20-17). The venous ring, surrounding the hypophysis and composed of the two cavernous sinuses and their connecting channels, often is designated as the *circular sinus*. Each cavernous sinus likewise may be regarded as a confluens sinuum. Rostrally it receives the two ophthalmic veins through the orbital

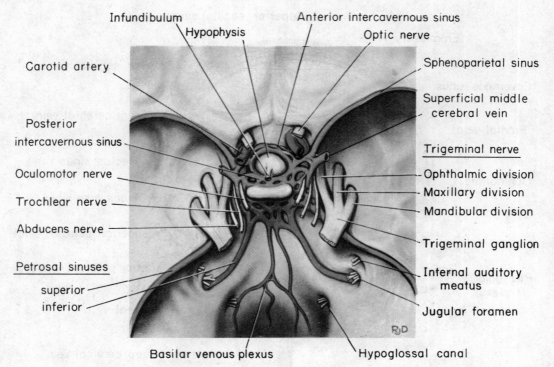

Infundibulum
Hypophysis
Anterior intercavernous sinus
Optic nerve
Carotid artery
Sphenoparietal sinus
Superficial middle cerebral vein
Posterior intercavernous sinus
Trigeminal nerve
Oculomotor nerve
Ophthalmic division
Maxillary division
Trochlear nerve
Mandibular division
Abducens nerve
Trigeminal ganglion
Petrosal sinuses
Internal auditory meatus
superior
inferior
Jugular foramen
Basilar venous plexus
Hypoglossal canal

FIG. 20-17. The cavernous sinus, its venous connections and related structures.

fissure and the small *sphenoparietal sinus,* which runs along the under surface of the lesser wing of the sphenoid (Figs. 20-3 and 20-17). Posteriorly it empties into the superior and inferior petrosal sinuses, through which it is connected, respectively, with the transverse sinus and the bulb of the internal jugular vein.

The dural sinuses communicate with the extracranial veins by a number of emissaries (Fig. 20-16). Thus the superior sagittal sinus is connected with the frontal and nasal veins and the emissaries of the foramen cecum (Fig. 20-3). It also sends a *parietal emissary* to the superficial temporal vein. The confluens sinuum usually gives off an *occipital emissary* to the occipital vein, which is connected also with the transverse sinus by the larger *mastoid emissary*. Smaller emissaries from the sigmoid sinus pass through the condyloid and hypoglossal foramina and communicate with vertebral and deep cervical veins. The cavernous sinus, besides receiving the ophthalmic veins, is connected with the internal jugular vein and with the ptery-

goid and pharyngeal plexuses by fine venous nets which pass through the oval, spinous, lacerated, carotid and jugular foramina.

The Cerebral Veins. The cerebral veins which, like the dural sinuses, are devoid of valves, usually are divided into superficial and deep groups. The superficial cerebral veins drain the blood from the cortex and subcortical medullary substance and empty into the superior sagittal sinus or into the several basal sinuses (Fig. 20-18). The deep veins, draining the deep medullary substance, the basal ganglia and dorsal portions of the diencephalon, ultimately terminate in the internal and great cerebral veins (Figs. 20-19 and 20-20). While the two groups of veins are anatomically distinct, they are interconnected by numerous anastomotic channels, both intracerebral and extracerebral. Thus large surface areas can be drained through the great cerebral vein (Galen). Conversely territories supplied by deep cerebral veins may be drained, when necessity arises, by surface vessels. This anasto-

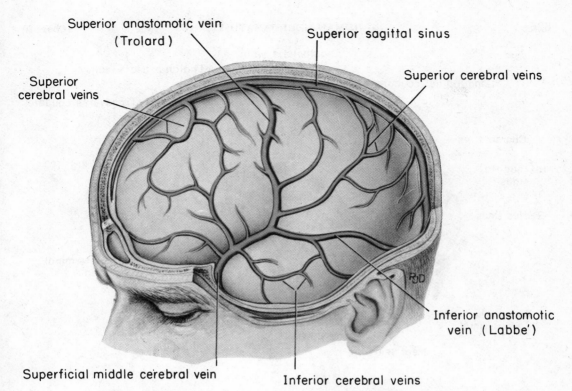

Superior anastomotic vein (Trolard)

Superior sagittal sinus

Superior cerebral veins

Superior cerebral veins

Inferior anastomotic vein (Labbe')

Superficial middle cerebral vein

Inferior cerebral veins

FIG. 20-18. The external cerebral veins on the convexity of the hemisphere.

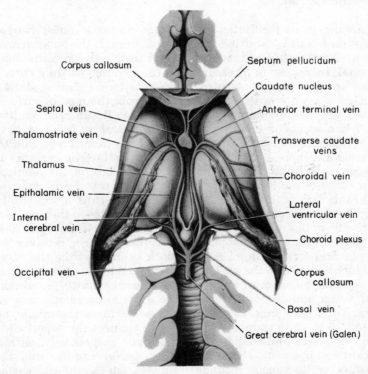

Corpus callosum

Septum pellucidum

Caudate nucleus

Septal vein

Anterior terminal vein

Thalamostriate vein

Transverse caudate veins

Thalamus

Choroidal vein

Epithalamic vein

Lateral ventricular vein

Internal cerebral vein

Choroid plexus

Occipital vein

Corpus callosum

Basal vein

Great cerebral vein (Galen)

FIG. 20-19. The internal cerebral veins and their tributaries (modified from Schwartz and Fink, '26).

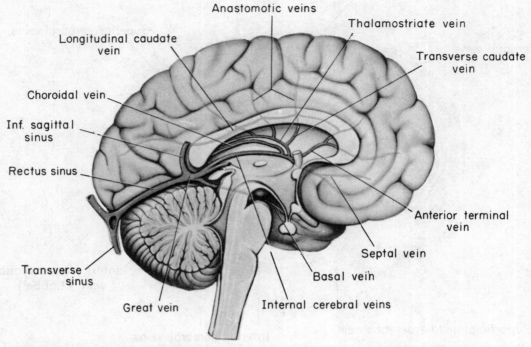

FIG. 20-20. Midsagittal view of the internal cerebral veins showing the relationship of the great vein to the rectus sinus (Schlesinger, '39).

motic venous arrangement facilitates the drainage of capillary beds by shifting the blood from one area to another and readily equalizes regional increases in pressure due to occlusion or other factors. As a result, the occlusion of even a large vein, if not too rapid, will produce slight and transitory effects. When occlusion or increase in pressure occurs suddenly, there will be marked hyperemia and more or less extensive hemorrhages, as in birth injuries and occasionally in cases of adult thrombosis (Schwartz and Fink, '26; Schlesinger, '39).

The Superficial Cerebral Veins. These veins arise from the cortex and subcortical medullary substance, anastomose freely in the pia and form a number of large vessels which empty into the various sinuses. They include the superior and inferior cerebral veins and the superficial middle cerebral vein. The *superior cerebral veins,* about 10 to 15 in number, collect blood from the convex and medial surfaces of the brain and open into the superior sagittal sinus, or its venous lacunae (Fig. 20-18). Many of them, especially the

larger posterior ones, run obliquely forward through the subarachnoid space and enter the sinus. The direction of blood flow in these veins, as they enter the sinus, is opposite to that in the sinus. Some of the veins from the medial surface of the brain drain into the inferior sagittal sinus. The *inferior cerebral veins* drain the basal surface of the hemisphere and the lower portion of its lateral surface. Those on the lateral surface of the hemisphere usually empty into the *superficial middle cerebral vein* which runs along the lateral sulcus and terminates in the cavernous or sphenoparietal sinus (Figs. 20-3, 20-17 and 20-18). The middle vein receives many anastomotic branches from the superior cerebral veins, and in many cases two of these channels become quite prominent. These are the *great anastomotic vein (Trolard)* and the *posterior anastomotic vein (Labbé),* which connect the superficial middle cerebral vein, respectively, with tributaries of the superior sagittal and the transverse sinuses. On the inferior surface, the small inferior cerebral veins arising from exten-

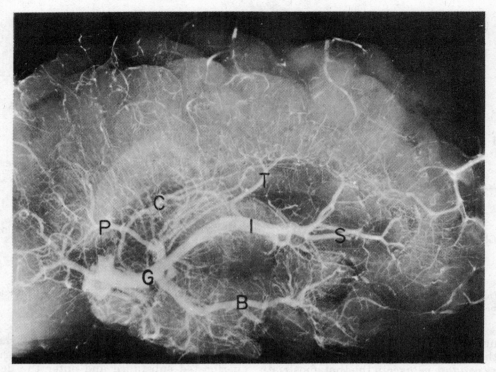

FIG. 20-21. Angiographic appearance of the deep venous system in one intact cerebral hemisphere. *Letters* indicate the following: *S*, septal vein; *T*, thalamostriate vein; *I*, internal cerebral vein; *B*, basal vein; *C*, choroidal vein; *G*, great cerebral vein (Galen); and *P*, occipital vein (vein of the posterior horn). (Courtesy of Dr. O. Hassler, '66.)

sive pial plexuses drain in part into the basal sinuses. Those from the tentorial surface of the brain empty into the transverse and superior petrosal sinuses (Figs. 20-3 and 20-17). Those from the anterior temporal lobe and from the interpeduncular regions drain partly into the cavernous and sphenoparietal sinuses, while some veins from the orbital region join the superior or the inferior sagittal sinus.

In addition, large cortical areas, especially on the inferior and medial surfaces, are drained by a number of vessels which empty into the great cerebral vein (Figs. 20-19 and 20-20). These are anastomotic veins which connect the superficial and deep venous systems. The more important ones include the occipital vein, the basal vein (Rosenthal) and the posterior callosal vein. Veins of this group are best considered in relation to the deep cerebral veins.

The Deep Cerebral Veins. The deep cerebral veins of major importance are: (1) the internal cerebral veins, (2) the basal vein (Rosenthal), and (3) the great cerebral vein (Galen).

The *internal cerebral veins* consist of two paired veins, situated just lateral to the midline in the tela choroidea of the roof of the third ventricle (velum interpositum; Figs. 20-19 and 20-20). The veins begin in the region of the interventricular foramina and extend caudally over the superior and medial surface of the thalamus. Caudally the veins enter the upper part of the quadrigeminal cistern where they join to form the great vein (Galen). Veins draining into the internal cerebral vein on each side include: (1) the thalamostriate vein (terminal vein), (2) the choroidal vein, (3) the septal vein, (4) the epithalamic vein, and (5) the lateral ventricular vein.

The *thalamostriate vein* runs forward in the terminal sulcus at the junction of the thalamus and caudate nucleus. This vein receives the *anterior terminal vein* which

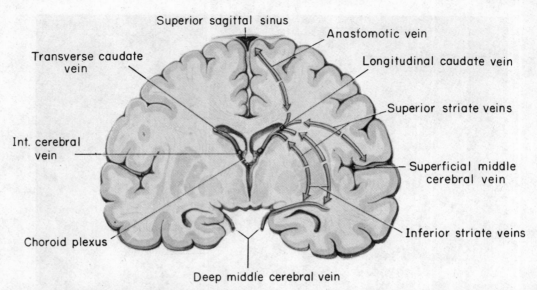

FIG. 20-22. Transverse section through the brain of the rhesus monkey showing diagrammatically the connections between deep and superficial veins (Schlesinger, '39).

drains the ventricular surface of the head of the caudate nucleus. Numerous *transverse caudate veins* join the thalamostriate throughout its course (Figs. 20-19 and 20-20). Distally the transverse caudate veins extend over the caudate nucleus to the lateral angle of the ventricle where they enter the adjacent white matter. In this area the smaller tributaries form the *longitudinal caudate veins* (Fig. 20-20). The latter veins divide at acute angles into a number of branches which fan out into the white matter, as a rule following the fibers of the corpus callosum (Figs. 20-20, 20-21 and 20-22). Some of the shorter branches drain the deep capillary plexuses of the white matter. Other longer branches, extending almost to the cortex, may be regarded as intracerebral anastomotic channels connecting ventricular and surface veins. In addition, the transverse and longitudinal caudate veins give rise to another group of branches known as the *superior striate veins* (Figs. 20-22 and 20-23). These veins pass ventrally through and around the caudate nucleus, perforate the internal capsule and break up into a number of smaller vessels which drain the dense capillary plexus of the lenticular nucleus (Fig. 20-22). This capillary plexus is

drained from below by the *inferior striate veins* which converge upon the anterior perforated substance and enter the deep middle vein.

The *choroidal vein* runs along the lateral border of the choroid plexus and distally extends into the inferior horn of the lateral ventricle (Fig. 20-19). This tortuous vessel drains portions of the choroid plexus and adjacent hippocampal regions. The choroid plexus also is drained by the choroidal branch of the basal vein and, to a lesser extent, through the lateral ventricular vein.

The *septal vein* drains the septum pellucidum and rostral portions of the corpus callosum. Distally branches of this vein extend beneath the head of the caudate nucleus into the medullary substance at the base of the frontal lobe (Figs. 20-19 and 20-20). The septal vein joins the internal cerebral vein in the region of the interventricular foramen.

The *epithalamic vein* is a small vessel which drains the dorsal part of the diencephalon. This vein enters the internal cerebral vein, or the great cerebral vein, near their junction. Blood from ventral portions of the thalamus and from the hypothalamus is drained by vessels which pass ventrally into the pial venous plexus of the interpeduncular fossa. From this plexus venous blood is conveyed into the cavernous or sphenoparietal sinuses or into tributaries of the basal vein.

The *lateral ventricular vein* courses over the superior caudal surface of the thalamus (Fig. 20-19) and enters the internal cerebral vein as this vessel joins the great cerebral vein. Occasionally this vein terminates directly in the great cerebral vein. Distally the lateral ventricular vein extends over the surface of the thalamus and the tail of the caudate nucleus and enters the medullary substance at the angle of the lateral ventricle. Small branches of this vein arise from the choroid plexus, and from the white matter of the parahippocampal gyrus.

The *great cerebral vein* (Galen) receives the two internal cerebral veins, the two basal veins, the two occipital veins and the posterior callosal vein (Figs. 20-19, 20-20 and 20-21). This very short vein extends posteriorly beneath the splenium of the corpus callosum and empties into the anterior part of the rectus sinus. The walls of this vein are delicate and easily torn, even in the adult.

The *basal vein* (Rosenthal) arises near the medial aspect of the anterior part of the temporal lobe where it receives tributaries from the medial surface and temporal horn (Figs. 20-20 and 20-21). This vein receives the anterior cerebral vein, the deep middle cerebral vein and the inferior striate veins. The *anterior cerebral vein* accompanies the anterior cerebral artery and drains the orbital surface of the frontal lobe, anterior portions of the corpus callosum and rostral parts of the cingulate gyrus. The *deep middle cerebral vein,* situated inferiorly in the depths of the lateral sulcus, drains insular and adjacent opercular cortex. The *inferior striate veins* drain ventral portions of the corpus striatum, emerge through the anterior perforated substance and empty into the deep middle cerebral vein (Figs. 20-21, 20-22 and 20-23). In the region of the anterior perforated substance these veins unite with the basal vein which courses caudally around the crus cerebri to join the great cerebral vein.

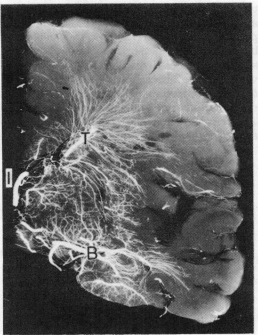

Fig. 20-23. Angioarchitecture of the deep cerebral venous system as shown in 1 cm thick coronal section. Anastomoses between deep and superficial veins are evident. *Letters* indicate the following: *T,* terminal vein; *B,* basal vein; *I,* internal cerebral vein. Compare with Figure 20-22. (Courtesy of Dr. O. Hassler, '66.)

The basal vein receives additional tributaries from the interpeduncular region, the midbrain and the inferior horn of the lateral ventricle. The hypothalamus, and ventral portions of the thalamus, are drained to a considerable extent by the basal veins.

The *occipital vein,* which drains the inferior and medial surface of the occipital lobe and adjacent parietal regions, empties directly into the great cerebral vein (Fig. 20-19). The posterior callosal vein, which extends around the splenium of the corpus callosum, enters the anterior part of the great cerebral vein. This vein drains the posterior part of the corpus callosum and adjacent medial surfaces of the brain.

Angiographic studies (Taveras and Wood, '64) of cerebral veins made by serial roentgenograms reveal that the superficial frontal veins fill slightly before the parietal veins. The deep veins usually are the last to fill and they retain sufficient concentrations of radiopaque material to be visualized for a longer time. From the standpoint of diagnostic radiology, the deep cerebral veins are more important than the superficial veins which exhibit extremely variable configurations. Visualization of the thalamostriate vein and some of its major tributaries can provide information concerning the position and size of the lateral ventricle.

It is evident from the above that the deep veins are concerned primarily with the drainage of the ventricular surface, the choroid plexuses, the deep medullary substance, the caudate nucleus and the dorsal portions of the lenticular nucleus and thalamus. All these structures also can be drained by surface vessels through numerous intracerebral and extracerebral anastomotic veins.

BIBLIOGRAPHY

ABELES, M., AND GOLDSTEIN, M. H., JR. 1970. Functional architecture in cat primary auditory cortex: Columnar organization and organization according to depth. J. Neurophysiol., 33: 172–187.

ABERCROMBIE, M., AND JOHNSON, M. L. 1947. The effect of reinnervation on collagen formation in degenerating sciatic nerves of rabbits. J. Neurol. Neurosurg. & Psychiat., 10: 89–92.

ADAL, M. N., AND BARKER, D. 1965. Intramuscular branching of fusimotor fibres. J. Physiol., 177: 288–299.

ADAMS, C. W. M. 1965. Disorders of neurons and neuroglia. In C. W. M. ADAMS (Editor), Neurohistochemistry. Elsevier Publishing Company, Amsterdam, Ch. 10, pp. 403–436. (See also, Ch. 1–8, pp. 1–332.)

ADAMS, C. W. M., IBRAHIM, M. Z. M., AND LEIBOWITZ, S. 1965. Demyelination. In C. W. M. ADAMS (Editor), Neurohistochemistry. Elsevier Publishing Company, Amsterdam, Ch. 11, pp. 437–487.

ADDISON, W. H. F. 1915. On the rhinencephalon of Delphinus delphis. J. Comp. Neurol., 25: 497–522.

ADES, H. W. 1941. Connections of the medial geniculate body in the cat. Arch. Neurol. & Psychiat., 45: 138–144.

ADES, H. W. 1943. A secondary acoustic area in the cerebral cortex of the cat. J. Neurophysiol., 6: 59–64.

ADES, H. W. 1959. Central auditory mechanisms. In J FIELD (Editor), Handbook of Physiology, Section I, Vol. I. American Physiological Society, Washington, D. C., Ch. 24, pp. 585–613.

ADES, H. W., AND BROOKHART, J. M. 1950. The central auditory pathway. J. Neurophysiol., 13: 189–205.

ADES, H. W., AND FELDER, R. 1942. The acoustic area of the monkey (Macaca mulatta). J. Neurophysiol., 5: 49–54.

ADEY, W. R. AND MEYER, M. 1952. Hippocampal and hypothalamic connexions of the temporal lobe in the monkey. Brain, 75: 358–384.

ADEY, W. R., SEGUNDO, J. P. AND LIVINGSTON, R. B. 1957. Corticofugal influences on intrinsic brain stem conduction in cat and monkey. J. Neurophysiol., 20: 1–16.

ADLER, A. 1933. Zur Topik des Verlaufes der Geschmackssinnsfasern und anderer afferenter Bahnen im Thalamus. Ztschr. ges. Neurol. u. Psychiat., 149: 208–220.

ADRIAN, E. D. 1940. Double representation of the feet in the sensory cortex of the cat. J. Physiol., 98: 16P–18P (abstract).

ADRIAN, E. D. 1941. Afferent discharges to the cerebral cortex from peripheral sense organs. J. Physiol., 100: 159–191.

ADRIAN, E. D. 1942. Olfactory reactions in the brain of the hedgehog. J. Physiol., 100: 459–473.

AFIFI, A., AND KAELBER, W. W. 1965. Efferent connections of the substantia nigra in the cat. Exper. Neurol., 11: 474–482.

AHLQUIST, R. P. 1948. A study of the adrenotropic receptors. Am. J. Physiol. 153: 586–600.

AITKEN, H. F. 1909. A report on the circulation of the lobar ganglia made to Dr. James B. Ayer (with a postscript by J. B. Ayer, M.D.). Boston Med. & Surg. J., 160: Suppl. 18.

AITKIN, L. M. AND WEBSTER, W. R. 1971. Tonotopic organization in the medial geniculate body of the cat. Brain Res., 26: 402–405.

AKELAITIS, A. J. 1943. Study of language function (tactile and visual lexia and graphia) unilaterally following section of the corpus callosum. J. Neuropath. & Exper. Neurol., 2: 226–262.

AKELAITIS, A. J., RISTEEN, W. A., HERREN, R. Y., AND VAN WAGENEN, W. P. 1942. Studies on corpus callosum; contribution to study of dyspraxia and apraxia following partial and complete section of corpus callosum. Arch. Neurol. & Psychiat., 47: 971–1008.

AKERT, K., POTTER, H. D., AND ANDERSON, J. W. 1961. The subfornical organ in mammals. I. Comparative and topographic anatomy. J. Comp. Neurol., 116: 1–14.

ALEXANDER, L. 1942. The vascular supply of the striopallidum. A. Res. Nerv. & Ment. Dis., Proc., 21: 77–132.

ALLEN, W. F. 1919. Application of the Marchi method to the study of the radix mesencephalica trigemini in the guinea pig. J. Comp. Neurol., 30: 169–216.

ALLEN, W. F. 1923. Origin and destination of the tractus solitarius in the guinea pig. J. Comp. Neurol., 35: 273–311.

ALLEN, W. F. 1925. Identification of the cells and fibers concerned in the innervation of the teeth. J. Comp. Neurol., 39: 325–343.

ALLEN, W. F. 1927. Experimental-anatomical studies on the visceral bulbospinal pathway in the cat and guinea pig. J. Comp. Neurol., 42: 393–456.

ALLEN, W. F. 1940. Effects of ablating the frontal lobes, hippocampi, and occipito-parieto-temporal (excepting pyriform areas) lobes on positive and negative olfactory conditioned reflexes. Am. J. Physiol., 128: 754–771.

ALLEN, W. F. 1941. Effect of ablating the pyriform-amygdaloid areas and hippocampi on positive and negative olfactory conditioned reflexes and on conditioned olfactory differentiation. Am. J. Physiol., 132: 81–92.

ALLISON, A. C. 1953. The morphology of the olfactory system in the vertebrates Biol. Rev. Cambridge Phil. Soc., 28: 195–244.

ALLISON, A. C. 1954. The secondary olfactory areas in the human brain. J. Anat., 88: 481–488.

ALLISON, A. C. AND WARWICK, R. 1949. Quantitative observations on the olfactory system of the rabbit. Brain, 72: 186–197.

ALPHEN, H. A. W. VAN. 1969. The anterior commissure of the rabbit. Acta anat., 74: Suppl. 57, 9–111.

ALTMAN, J. 1962. Some fiber projections to the superior colliculus in the cat. J. Comp. Neurol., 119: 77–95.

632 BIBLIOGRAPHY

ALTMAN, J. 1966. Proliferation and migration of undifferentiated precursor cells in the rat during postnatal gliogenesis. Exper. Neurol., 16: 263–278.

ALTMAN, J. AND CARPENTER, M. B. 1961. Fiber projections of the superior colliculus in the cat. J. Comp. Neurol., 116: 157–178.

AMBROGI, L. P. 1960. *Manual of Histologic and Special Staining Technics*, Ed. 2. McGraw-Hill Book Company, Inc., New York, pp. 157–174.

AMOORE, J. E., JOHNSTON, J. W., JR, AND RUBIN, M. 1964. The stereochemical theory of odor. Sc. Am., 210: 42–49.

AMOROSO, E. C., BELL, F. R. AND ROSENBERG, H. 1954. The relationship of the vasomotor and respiratory regions in the medulla oblongata of the sheep. J. Physiol., 126: 86–95.

ANAND, B. K., AND BROBECK, J. R. 1951. Hypothalamic control of food intake in rats and cats. Yale J. Biol. & Med., 24: 123–140.

ANAND, B. K., AND BROBECK, J. R. 1951a. Localization of a "feeding center" in the hypothalamus of the rat. Proc. Soc. Exper. Biol. & Med., 77: 323–324.

ANAND, B. K., AND BROBECK, J. R. 1952. Food intake and spontaneous activity of rats with lesions in the amygdaloid nuclei. J. Neurophysiol., 15: 421–430.

ANAND, B. K., AND DUA, S. 1956. Circulatory and respiratory changes induced by electrical stimulation of limbic system (visceral brain). J. Neurophysiol., 19: 393–400.

ANDÉN, N.-E., CARLSSON, A., DAHLSTRÖM, A., FUXE, K., HILLARP, N.-Å., AND LARSSON, K. 1964. Demonstration and mapping out of nigro-neostriatal dopamine neurons. Life Sc., 3: 523–530.

ANDERSSON, B. 1957. Polydipsia, antidiuresis and milk ejection caused by hypothalamic stimulation. In H. HELLER (Editor), *Neurohypophysis*. Butterworths Scientific Publications, London, pp. 131–140.

ANDERSSON, B., AND JEWELL, P. A. 1957. Studies on the thalamic relay for taste in the goat. J. Physiol., 139: 191–197.

ANDERSSON, S. 1962. Projection of different spinal pathways to the second somatic sensory area in cat. Acta physiol. scandinav., 56: Suppl. 194, 1–74.

ANDERSSON, S., AND GERNANDT, B. E. 1954. Cortical projection of vestibular nerve in cat. Acta oto-laryng., 116 (suppl.): 10–18.

ANDREW, J., AND NATHAN, P. W. 1964. Lesions of the anterior frontal lobes and disturbances of micturition and defecation. Brain, 87: 233–262.

ANDY, O. J., AND BROWN, J. S. 1960. Diencephalic coagulation in the treatment of hemiballismus. S. Forum, Proc. Clin. Cong. Am. Coll. Surgeons, 10: 795–799.

ANGAUT, P., AND BOWSHER, D. 1965. Cerebello-rubral connexions in the cat. Nature, 208: 1002–1003.

ANGAUT, P., AND BOWSHER, D. 1970. Ascending projections of the medial (fastigial) nucleus: An experimental study in the cat. Brain Res., 24: 49–68.

ANGAUT, P., AND BRODAL, A. 1967. The projection of the "vestibulocerebellum" onto the vestibular nuclei in the cat. Arch. ital. biol., 105: 441–479.

ANGEVINE, J. B. 1965. Time of neuron origin in the hippocampal region. An autoradiographic study in the mouse. Exper. Neurol., 2 (suppl): 1–70.

ANGEVINE, J. B., LOCKE, S., AND YAKOVLEV, P. I. 1962. Limbic nuclei of thalamus and connections of limbic cortex: IV. Thalamocortical projection of the ventral anterior nucleus in man. Arch. Neurol., 7: 518–528.

ANGEVINE, J. B., MANCALL, E. L., AND YAKOVLEV, P. I. 1961. *The Human Cerebellum. An Atlas of Gross Topography in Serial Sections*. Little, Brown & Company, Boston.

ANGEVINE, J. B., JR., AND SIDMAN, R. L. 1961. Auto-radiographic study of cell migration during histogenesis of the cerebral cortex in the mouse. Nature, 192: 766–768.

APPELBERG, B. 1960. Localization of focal potentials evoked in the red nucleus and ventrolateral nucleus of the thalamus by electrical stimulation of the cerebellar nuclei. Acta physiol. scandinav., 51: 356–370.

ARDUINI, A., AND ARDUINI, M. G. 1954. Effect of drugs and metabolic alterations on brain stem arousal mechanisms. J. Pharmacol. & Exper. Therap., 110: 76–85.

AREY, L. B. 1938. The history of the first somite in human embryos. Carnegie Inst. Washington, Contrib. Embryol., 27: 233–269.

ARONSON, L. R., AND PAPEZ, J. W. 1934. Thalamic nuclei of *Pithecus (Macacus) rhesus*. II. Dorsal thalamus. Arch. Neurol. & Psychiat., 32: 27–44.

ASHCROFT, D. W., AND HALLPIKE, C. S. 1934. On the function of the saccule. J. Laryng. & Otol., 49: 450–460.

ÅSTRÖM, K. E. 1967. On the early development of the cortex in fetal sheep. In C. G. BERNHARD AND J. P. SCHADÉ (Editors), *Developmental Neurology, Progress in Brain Research*, Vol. 26. Elsevier Publishing Company, New York, pp. 1–59.

AUER, J. 1956. Terminal degeneration in the diencephalon after ablation of frontal cortex in the cat. J. Anat., 90: 30–41.

BABKIN, B. P. 1950. Significance of the double innervation of the salivary glands. In B. P. BABKIN (Editor), *Secretory Mechanism of the Digestive Glands*, Ed. 2. P. B. Hoeber Company, New York, Ch. 27, pp. 733–766.

BAGSHAW, M. H., AND PRIBRAM, K. H. 1953. Cortical organization in gustation (*Macaca mulatta*). J. Neurophysiol., 16: 499–508.

BAILEY, P. 1948. *Intracranial Tumors*, Ed. 2. Charles C Thomas, Publisher, Springfield, Ill., p. 212.

BAILEY, P. AND VON BONIN, G. 1951. *The Isocortex of Man*. University of Illinois Press, Urbana.

BAILEY, P., VON BONIN, G., GAROL, H. W., AND McCULLOCH, W. S. 1943. Functional organization of temporal lobe of monkey (*Macaca mulatta*) and chimpanzee (*Pan satyrus*). J. Neurophysiol., 6: 121–128.

BAILEY, P., GAROL, H. W. AND McCULLOCH, W. S. 1941. Cortical origin and distribution of corpus callosum and anterior commissure in the chimpanzee (*Pan satyrus*). J. Neurophysiol., 4: 564–571.

BAKAY, L. 1952. Studies on blood-brain barrier with radioactive phosphorus. Arch. Neurol. & Psychiat., 68: 629–640.

BAKAY, L. 1956. *The Blood-Brain Barrier*. Charles C Thomas, Publisher, Springfield, Ill., pp. 1–30.

BAKAY, L. 1965. The movement of electrolytes and albumin in different types of cerebral edema. In E. D. P. DE ROBERTIS and R. CARREA (Editors), *Biology of Neuroglia, Progress in Brain Research*, Vol. 15. Elsevier Publishing Company, Amsterdam, pp. 155–183.

BAKER, A. B. 1961. Cerebrovascular disease. IX. The medullary blood supply and the lateral medullary syndrome. Neurology, 11: 852–861.

BAKER, J. R. 1960. *Cytological Technique. Methuen's Monographs on Biological Subjects*. John Wiley and Sons, New York.

BAPTISTA, A. P. 1963. Studies on the arteries of the brain. II. The anterior cerebral artery: Some anatomic features and their clinical implication. Neurology, 13: 825–835.

BARD, P. 1939. Central nervous mechanisms for emotional behavior patterns in animals. A. Res. Nerv. & Ment. Dis., Proc., 19: 190–218.

BARD, P. 1968. Regulation of the systemic circulation. In V. B. MOUNTCASTLE (Editor), *Medical Physiology*. Ed. 12. Vol. I. C. V. Mosby Company, St. Louis, Ch. 11, pp. 178–208.

BARD, P., AND MOUNTCASTLE, V. B. 1948. Some forebrain mechanisms involved in expression of rage with special reference to suppression of angry behavior. A. Res. Nerv. & Ment. Dis. Proc., 27: 362–404.

BARD, P., AND RIOCH, D. M. 1937. A study of 4 cats deprived of neocortex and additional portions of the forebrain. Bull. Johns Hopkins Hosp., 60: 73–147.

BARGMANN, W. 1966. Néurosecretion. Internat. Rev. Cytol., 19: 183–201.

BARGMANN, W., HILD, W., ORTHMANN, R. AND SCHIEBLER, T. H. 1950. Morphologische und experimentelle Untersuchungen über das hypothalamischhypophysäre System. Acta neuroveg., 1: 233–275.

BARKER, D. 1948. The innervation of the muscle-spindle. Quart. J. Microscop. Sci., 89: 143–186.

BARKER, D. 1967. The innervation of mammalian skeletal muscle. In A. V. S. DE REUCK AND J. KNIGHT (Editors), Myotatic, Kinesthetic and Vestibular Mechanisms. Little, Brown and Company, Boston, pp. 3–15.

BARKER, D., AND COPE, M. 1962. The innervation of individual intrafusal muscle fibres. In D. BARKER (Editor), Symposium on Muscle Receptors. Hong Kong University Press, Hong Kong, pp. 263–269.

BARKER, S. H., AND GELLHORN, E. 1947. Influence of suppressor areas on afferent impulses. J. Neurophysiol., 10: 133–138.

BARNES, S. 1901. Degenerations in hemiplegia: With special reference to a ventrolateral pyramidal tract, the accessory fillet and Pick's bundle. Brain, 24: 463–501.

BARNES, W. T., MAGOUN, H. W. AND RANSON, S. W. 1943. The ascending auditory pathway in the brain stem of the monkey. J. Comp. Neurol., 79: 129–152.

BARR, M. L. 1939. Some observations on the morphology of the synapse in the cat's spinal cord. J. Anat., 74: 1–11.

BARR, M. L., BERTRAM, L. F. AND LINDSAY, H. A. 1950. The morphology of the nerve cell nucleus according to sex. Anat. Rec., 107: 283–297.

BARRINGTON, F. J. F. 1921. The relation of the hind brain to micturition. Brain, 44: 23–53.

BARTON, A. A., AND CAUSEY, G. 1958. Electron microscopic study of the superior cervical ganglion. J. Anat., 92: 399–407.

BATES, J. A. V. 1953. Stimulation of the medial surface of the human cerebral hemisphere after hemispherectomy. Brain, 76: 405–447.

BAXTER, D. W., AND OLSZEWSKI, J. 1955. Respiratory responses evoked by electrical stimulation of pons and mesencephalon. J. Neurophysiol., 18: 276–287.

BEAMS, H. W. AND KING, R. L. 1935. The effect of ultracentrifuging the spinal ganglia cells of the rat, with special reference to Nissl bodies. J. Comp. Neurol., 61: 175–184.

VON BECHTEREW, W. V. 1900. Demonstration eines Gehirns mit Zerstörung der vorderen und inneren Theile der Hirnrinde beider Schläfenlappen. Neurol. Zentralbl., 19: 990–991.

BECK, E. 1929. Die myeloarchitektonische Felderung des in der Sylvischen Furche gelegenen Teiles des menschlichen Schläfenlappens. J. Psychol. u. Neurol., 36: 1–21.

BECK, E. 1950. The origin, course and termination of the prefronto-pontine tract in the human brain. Brain, 73: 368–391.

BÉDARD, P., LAROCHELLE, L., PARENT, A., AND POIRIER, L. J. 1969. The nigrostriatal pathway: A correlative study based on neuroanatomical and neurochemical criteria in the cat and the monkey. Exper. Neurol., 25: 365–377.

BÉKÉSY, G. VON. 1960. Experiments in Hearing. McGraw-Hill Book Company, New York.

BELL, C. C., AND DOW, R. S. 1967. Cerebellar circuitry.

Neurosc. Res. Progr. Bull., 5: (no. 2) 121–222.

BENDA, C. E., AND COBB, S. 1942. On the pathogenesis of paralysis agitans (Parkinson's disease). Medicine, 21: 95–142.

BENDER, M. B., AND WEINSTEIN, E. A. 1944. Effects of stimulation and lesion of the median longitudinal fasciculus in the monkey. Arch. Neurol. & Psychiat., 52: 106–113.

BENDER, M. B., AND WEINSTEIN, E. A. 1950. The syndrome of the median longitudinal fasciculus. A. Res. Nerv. & Ment. Dis., Proc. 28: 414–420.

BENJAMIN, R. M. 1963. Some thalamic and cortical mechanisms of taste. In Y. ZOTTERMAN (Editor), Olfaction and Taste. Macmillian Company, New York, pp. 309–329.

BENJAMIN, R. M., AND AKERT, K. 1959. Cortical and thalamic areas involved in taste discrimination in the albino rat. J. Comp. Neurol., 111: 231–260.

BENSLEY, R. R., AND GERSH, I. 1933. Studies on cell structure by the freezing-drying method. III. The distribution of cells of the basophil substances, in particular the Nissl substance of the nerve cell. Anat. Rec., 57: 369–385.

BERGER, H. 1929. Ueber das Elektrenkephalogramm des Menschen. Arch. Psychiat., 87: 527–570.

BERGER, H. 1930. Ueber das Elektrenkephalogramm des Menschen. J. Psychol. u. Neurol., 40: 160–179.

BERKE, J. J. 1960. The claustrum, the external capsule, and the extreme capsule of the Macaca mulatta. J. Comp. Neurol., 115: 297–331.

BERN, H. A., AND KNOWLES, F. G. W. 1966. Neurosecretion. In L. M. MARTINI AND W. F. GANONG (Editors), Neuroendocrinology. Academic Press, New York, Ch. 5, pp. 139–186.

BERN, H. A. AND YAGI, K. 1965. Electrophysiology of neurosecretory systems. In Proceedings of the Second International Congress of Endocrinology. Excerpta Medica, International Congress Section 83 (Part I), pp. 577–583.

BERNHARD, C. G. 1954. The corticospinal system. D. NACHMANSOHN AND H. H. MERRITT (Editors), Nerve Impulse, Transactions of the Fifth Conference, J. Macy, Jr. Foundation, New York, pp. 95–134.

BERNHARD, C. G., AND BOHM, E. 1954. Cortical representation and functional significance of the cortico-motoneuronal system. Arch. Neurol. & Psychiat., 72: 473–502.

BERNHARD, C. G., BOHM, E., AND PETERSEN, I. 1953. Investigations on the organization of the corticospinal system in monkeys. Acta physiol. scandinav., 29: 79–103.

BERNHARD, C. G., KOLMODIN, G. M., AND MEYERSON, B. A. 1967. On the prenatal development of function and structure in the somesthetic cortex of the sheep. In C. G. BERNHARD AND J. P. SCHADÉ (Editors), Developmental Neurology, Progress in Brain Research, Vol. 26. Elsevier Publishing Company, New York, pp. 78–91.

BERNHAUT, M., GELLHORN, E. AND RASMUSSEN, A. T. 1953. Experimental contributions to problems of consciousness J. Neurophysiol., 16: 21–35.

BERRY, C. M., ANDERSON, F. D. AND BROOKS, D. C. 1956. Ascending pathways of the trigeminal nerve in cat. J. Neurophysiol., 19: 144–153.

BERRY, C. M., HAGAMEN, W. D., AND HINSEY, J. C. 1952. Distribution of potentials following stimulation of olfactory bulb in cat. J. Neurophysiol., 15: 139–145.

BERRY, C. M., KARL, R. S., AND HINSEY, J. C. 1950. Course of spinothalamic and medial lemniscal pathways in the cat and rhesus monkey. J. Neurophysiol., 13: 149–156.

BERTRAND, G. 1956. Spinal efferent pathways from the supplementary motor area. Brain, 79: 461–473.

BESSOU, P., EMONET-DÉNAND, F., AND LAPORTE, Y. 1963. Occurrence of intrafusal muscle fibre innervation by branches of slow A motor fibres in the cat. Nature, 198: 594–595.

VAN BEUSEKOM, G. T. 1955. *Fibre Analysis of the Anterior and Lateral Funiculi of the Cord in the Cat.* Eduard Ijdo N.V., Leiden, pp. 1–136.

BIRD, E. D. AND IVERSEN, L. L. 1974. Huntington's chorea. Post-mortem measurements of glutamic acid decarboxylase, choline acetyltransferase and dopamine in the basal ganglia. Brain, 97: 457–472.

BISHOP, T. W., HEINBECKER, P., AND O'LEARY, J. L. 1933. The function of non-myelinated fibers of the dorsal roots. Am. J. Physiol., 106: 647–669.

BLACKSTAD, T. W. 1956. Commissural connections of the hippocampal region in the rat, with special reference to their mode of termination. J. Comp. Neurol., 105: 417–538.

BLAKEMORE, C. AND COOPER, G. F. 1970. Development of the brain depends on visual experience. Nature, 228: 477–478.

BLIX, M. 1884. Experimentelle Beiträge zur Lösung der Frage über die specifische Energie der Hautnerven. Ztschr. f. Biol. (München), 20: 141–156.

BLOMQUIST, A. J., BENJAMIN, R. M. AND EMMERS, R. 1962. Thalamic localization of afferents from the tongue in squirrel monkey (*Saimiri sciureus*). J. Comp. Neurol., 118: 77–87.

BLOOM, F. E., AND BARRNETT, R. J. 1966. Fine structural localization of noradrenaline in vesicles of autonomic nerve endings. Nature, 210: 599–601.

BLOOM, F. E., HOFFER, B. J. AND SIGGINS, G. R. 1971. Studies on norepinephrine containing afferent to Purkinje cells of rat cerebellum. I. Localization of the fibers and their synapses. Brain Res., 25: 501–521.

BLUM, M., WALKER, A. E., AND RUCH, T. C. 1943. Localization of taste in the thalamus of *Macaca mulatta*. Yale J. Biol. & Med., 16: 175–192.

BLUNT, J. J., WENDELL-SMITH, C. P., PAISLEY, P. B. AND BALDWIN, F. 1967. Oxidative enzyme activity in macroglia and axons of cat optic nerve. J. Anat., 101: 13–26.

BODIAN, D. 1936. A new method for staining nerve fibers and nerve endings in mounted paraffin sections. Anat. Rec., 65: 89–97.

BODIAN, D. 1937. The structure of the vertebrate synapse. A study of the axon endings on Mauthner's cell and neighboring centers in the goldfish. J. Comp. Neurology 68: 117–160.

BODIAN, D. 1940. Studies on the diencephalon of the Virginia opossum. II. The fiber connections in normal and experimental material. J. Comp. Neurol., 72: 207–297.

BODIAN, D. 1962. The generalized vertebrate neuron. Science, 137: 323–326.

BODIAN, D. 1963. Cytological aspects of neurosecretion in opossum neurohypophysis. Bull. Johns Hopkins Hosp., 113: 57–93.

BODIAN, D. 1966. Herring bodies and neuro-apocrine secretion in the monkey. An electron microscopic study of the fate of the neurosecretory product. Bull. Johns Hopkins Hosp., 118: 282–326.

BODIAN, D. 1967. Neurons, circuits and neuroglia. In G. C. QUARTON, T. MELNECHUK AND F. O. SCHMITT (Editors), *The Neurosciences. A Study Program.* Rockefeller University Press, New York, pp. 6–24.

BOK, S. T. 1928. Das Rückenmark. In W. VON MÖLLENDORFF (Editor), *Handbuch der mikroskopischen Anatomie des Menschen.* Julius Springer, Berlin, pp. 478–578.

BOLTON, B. 1939. The blood supply of the human spinal cord. J. Neurol. & Psychiat., 2: 137–148.

VON BONIN, G., AND SHARIFF, G. A. 1951. Extrapyramidal nuclei among mammals. J. Comp. Neurol., 94: 427–438.

BORG, E. 1973. On the neuronal organization of the acoustic middle ear reflex. A physiological and anatomical study. Brain Res., 49; 101–123.

BORISON, H. L., AND WANG, S. C. 1949. Functional localization of central coordinating mechanisms for emesis in cat. J. Neurophysiol., 12: 305–313.

BORISON, H. L., AND WANG, S. C. 1953. Physiology and pharmacology of vomiting. Pharmacol. Rev., 5: 193–230.

BÖRNSTEIN, W. S. 1940. Cortical representation of taste in man and monkey. I. Functional and anatomical relations of taste, olfaction and somatic sensibility. Yale J. Biol. & Med., 12: 719–736.

BÖRNSTEIN, W. S. 1940a. Cortical representation of taste in man and monkey. II. Localization of cortical taste area in man and method of measuring impairment of taste in man. Yale J. Biol. & Med., 13: 133–156.

BOVARD, E. W., AND GLOOR, P. 1961. Effect of amygdaloid lesions on plasma corticosterone response of the albino rat to emotional stress. Experientia, 17: 521.

BOWDEN, R. E. M., AND GUTMANN, E. 1944. Denervation and re-innervation of the human voluntary muscle. Brain, 67: 273–313.

BOWDEN, R. E. M., AND MAHRAN, Z. Y. 1956. The functional significance of the pattern of innervation of the muscle quadratus labii superioris of the rabbit, cat and rat. J. Anat., 90: 217–227.

BOWMAN, J. P., AND SLADEC, J. R. 1973. Morphology of the inferior olivary complex of the rhesus monkey (*Macaca mulatta*). J. Comp. Neurol:, 152: 299–316.

BOWSHER, D. 1957. Termination of the central pain pathway: the conscious appreciation of pain. Brain, 80: 606–622.

BOWSHER, D. 1958. Projections of the gracile and cuneate nuclei in *Macaca mulatta*: An experimental degeneration study. J. Comp. Neurol., 110: 135–155.

BOWSHER, D. 1961. The termination of secondary somatosensory neurons within the thalamus of Macaca mulatta: An experimental degeneration study. J. Comp. Neurol., 177: 213–227.

BOWSHER, D. 1966. Some afferent and efferent connections of the parafascicular-center median complex. In D. P. PURPURA AND M. D. YAHR (Editors), *The Thalamus.* Columbia University Press, New York, pp. 99–108.

BOYD, I. A. 1962. The nuclear-bag fibre and nuclear-chain fibre systems in the muscle spindles of the cat. In D. BARKER (Editor), *Symposium on Muscle Receptors.* Hong Kong University Press, Hong Kong, pp. 185–190.

BOYD, I. A. 1962a. The structure and innervation of the nuclear-bag fibre system and the nuclear-chain fibre system in mammalian muscle spindles. Phil. Tr. Roy. Soc. London ser. B, 245: 81–136.

BOYD, J. D. 1960. The embryology and comparative anatomy of the melanocyte. In A. ROOK (Editor), *Progress in the Biological Sciences in Relation to Dermatology.* Cambridge University Press, London, pp. 3–14.

BRADLEY, W. E., AND CONWAY, C. J. 1966. Bladder representation in the pontine-mesencephalic reticular formation. Exper. Neurol., 16: 237–249.

BRADY, J. V. 1960. Temporal and emotional effects related to intracranial electrical self-stimulation. In S. R. RAMEY AND D. S. O'DOHERTY (Editors), *Electrical Studies on the Unanesthetized Brain.* Paul B. Hoeber, Inc., New York, Ch. 3, pp. 52–77.

BRAIN, R. 1961. *Speech Disorders. Aphasia, Apraxia and Agnosia.* Butterworths, London, 184 pp.

BRAITENBERG, V., AND ATWOOD, R. P. 1958. Morphological observations on the cerebellar cortex. J. Comp. Neurol., 109: 1–27.

BRATTGÅRD, S. O., EDSTRÖM, J. E., AND HYDÉN, H. 1958. The productive capacity of the neuron in retrograde reaction. Exper. Cell Res., 5: (suppl.) 185–200.

BRAUS, H. 1932. In C. ELZE (Editor), *Anatomie des*

Menschen (Vol. 3). Verlag von J. Springer, Berlin.

BRAZIER, M. A. B. 1954. The action of anaesthetics on the nervous system, with special reference to the brain stem reticular system. In J. F. DELAFRESNAYE (Editor), *Brain Mechanisms and Consciousness* (Symposium). Blackwell Scientific Publications, Oxford, pp. 163–193.

BREMER, F. 1922. Contributions á l'étude de la physiologie de cervelet. La fonction inhibtrice du palaeocérébellum. Arch. internat. physiol., 19: 189–226.

BREMER, F. 1936. Nouvelles recherches sur le mécanisme dū sommeil. Comp. rend. Soc. biol., 122: 460–464.

BREMER, F. 1937. L'activité cérébrale au cours du sommeil et de la narcose. Contribution à l'étude du mecanisme du sommeil. Bull. Acad. Roy. Med., Belg., 2: 68–86.

BREMER, F., AND TERZUOLO, C. 1954. Contribution à l' étude des mécanismes physiologiques du maintien de l' activité vigile du cerveau. Interaction de la formation réticulée et de l'écorce cérébrale dans le processus du réveil. Arch. internat. physiol., 62: 157–178.

BRENDLER, S. J. 1968. The human cervical myotomes: Functional anatomy studied at operation. J. Neurosurg., 28: 105–111.

BRIGHTMAN, M. W., AND PALAY, S. L. 1963. The fine structure of ependyma in the brain of the rat. J. Cell Biol., 19: 415–439.

BRIZZEE, K. R., AND NEAL, L. M. 1954. A re-evaluation of the cellular morphology of the area postrema in view of recent evidence for a chemoreceptor function. J. Comp. Neurol., 100: 41–62.

BROCA, P. 1878. Anatomie comparée circonvolutions cérébrales. Le grand lobe limbique et la scissure limbique dans la série des mammifères. Rev. anthropol., ser. 2, 1: 384–498.

BRODAL, A. 1940. Experimentelle Untersuchungen über die olivocerebellare Lokalisation. Ztschr. ges. Neurol. u. Psychiat., 169: 1–153.

BRODAL, A. 1941. Die Verbindungen des Nucleus cuneatus externus mit dem Kleinhirn beim Kaninchen und bei der Katze. Experimentelle Untersuchungen. Ztschr. ges. Neurol. u. Psychiat., 171: 167–199.

BRODAL, A. 1947. The hippocampus and the sense of smell. Brain, 70: 179–222.

BRODAL, A. 1948. The origin of the fibers of the anterior commissure in the rat. Experimental studies. J. Comp. Neurol., 88: 157–205.

BRODAL, A. 1949. Spinal afferents to the lateral reticular nucleus of the medulla oblongata in the cat. An experimental study. J. Comp. Neurol., 91: 259–295.

BRODAL, A. 1953. Reticulo-cerebellar connections in the cat. An experimental study. J. Comp. Neurol., 98: 113–153.

BRODAL, A. 1954. Afferent cerebellar connections. In J. JANSEN AND A. BRODAL (Editors), *Aspects of Cerebellar Anatomy*. J. G. Tanum, Oslo, Ch. 2, pp. 82–188.

BRODAL, A. 1957. *The Reticular Formation of the Brain Stem. Anatomical Aspects and Functional Correlations.* Charles C Thomas, Publisher, Springfield, Ill., 87 pp.

BRODAL, A. 1963. General discussion of the terminology of the rhinencephalon. In W. BARGMANN AND J. P. SCHADÉ (Editors), *The Rhinencephalon and Related Structures*, (Editors), *Progress in Brain Research*, Vol. 3. Elsevier Publishing Company, Amsterdam, pp. 237–244.

BRODAL, A. 1969. *Neurological Anatomy in Relation to Clinical Medicine.* Oxford University Press, New York.

BRODAL, A., AND BRODAL, P. 1971. The organization of the nucleus reticularis tegmenti pontis in the cat in the light of experimental anatomical studies of its cerebral cortical afferents. Exper. Brain Res., 13: 90–110.

BRODAL, A., AND COURVILLE, J. 1973. Cerebellar corticonuclear projection in the cat. Crus II. An experimental

study with silver methods. Brain Řes., 50: 1–23.

BRODAL, A., AND GOGSTAD, A. C. 1954. Rubrocerebellar connections. An experimental study in the cat. Anat. Rec., 118: 455–486.

BRODAL, A., AND HØIVIK, B. 1964. Site and mode of termination of primary vestibulo-cerebellar fibres in the cat. Arch. ital. biol., 102: 1–21.

BRODAL, A., AND JANSEN, J. 1946. The ponto-cerebellar projection in the rabbit and cat. J. Comp. Neurol., 84: 31–118.

BRODAL, A., AND POMPEIANO, O. 1957. The vestibular nuclei in the cat. J. Anat., 91: 438–454.

BRODAL, A., AND POMPEIANO, O. 1957a. The origin of ascending fibers of the medial longitudinal fasciculus from the vestibular nuclei: An experimental study in the cat. Acta Morphol. Neerlando scandinav., 1: 306–328.

BRODAL, A., POMPEIANO O., AND WALBERG, F. 1962. *The Vestibular Nuclei and Their Connections, Anatomy and Functional Correlations.* Charles C Thomas, Publisher, Springfield, Ill.

BRODAL, A., AND ROSSI, G. F. 1955. Ascending fibers in brain stem reticular formation of cat. Arch. Neurol. & Psychiat., 74: 68–87.

BRODAL, A., SZABO, T., AND TORVIK, A. 1956. Corticofugal fibers to sensory trigeminal nuclei and nucleus of solitary tract. J. Comp. Neurol., 106: 527–555.

BRODAL, A., AND SZIKLA, G. 1972. The termination of the brachium conjunctivum descendens in the nucleus reticularis tegmenti pontis. An experimental study in the cat. Brain Res., 39: 337–351.

BRODAL, A., TABER, E., AND WALBERG, F. 1960. The raphe nuclei of the brain stem in the cat. II. Efferent connections. J. Comp. Neurol., 114: 239–259.

BRODAL, A., AND TORVIK, A. 1957. Über den Ursprung der sekundären vestibulo-cerebellaren Fasern bei der Katze. Eine experimentell-anatomische Studie. Arch. Psychiat., 195: 550–567.

BRODAL, A., AND WALBERG, F. 1952. Ascending fibers in the pyramidal tract of cat. Arch. Neurol. & Psychiat., 68: 755–775.

BRODAL, A., WALBERG, F., AND BLACKSTAD, T. 1950. Termination of spinal afferents to inferior olive in cat. J. Neurophysiol., 13: 431–454.

BRODAL, P. 1968. The corticopontine projection in the cat. I. Demonstration of a somatotopically organized projection from the primary sensorimotor cortex. Exper. Brain Res., 5: 212–237.

BRODAL, P. 1972. The corticopontine projection from the visual cortex in the cat. I. The total projection and the projection from area 17. Brain Res., 39: 297–317.

BRODAL, P. 1972a. The corticopontine projection from the visual cortex in the cat. II. The projection from areas 18 and 19. Brain Res., 39: 319–335.

BRODISH, A. 1964. Role of the hypothalamus in the regulation of ACTH release. In E. BAJUSZ AND G. JASMIN (Editors), *Major Problems in Endocrinology*. S. Karger, Basel.

BRODMANN, K. 1909. *Vergleichende Lokalisationlehre der Grosshirnrinde in ihren Prinzipien dargestellt auf Grund des Zellenbaues.* J. A. Barth, Leipzig, 324 pp.

BROUWER, B., AND ZEEMAN, W. P. C. 1926. The projection of the retina in the primary optic neuron in monkeys. Brain, 49: 1–35.

BROWN, J. O., AND MCCOUCH, G. P. 1947. Abortive regeneration of the transected spinal cord. J. Comp. Neurol., 87: 131–138.

BROWN-GRANT, K., AND RAISMAN, G. 1972. Reproductive function in the rat following selective destruction of afferent fibres to the hypothalamus from the limbic system. Brain Res., 46: 23–42.

BROWNSON, R. H. 1956. Perineuronal satellite cells in the motor cortex of aging brains. J. Neuropath. Exper.

Neurol., 15: 190–195.

BUCHER, V. M., AND BÜRGI, S. M. 1953. Some observations on the fiber connections of the di- and mesencephalon in the cat. III. The supraoptic decussations. J. Comp. Neurol., 98: 355–379.

BUCY, P. C. 1949. Effects of extirpation in man. In P. C. BUCY (Editor), *The Precentral Motor Cortex*, Ed. 2. University of Illinois Press, Urbana, Ch. 14, pp. 353–394.

BUCY, P. C. 1957. Principes physiologiques et résultats des interventions neurochirurgicales dans les affections dites extrapyramidales. I. Relationship of the "pyramidal tract" and abnormal involuntary movements. In *Premier Congrès International des Sciences Neurologiques. Première Journée Commune, Bruxelles, Juillet, 1957*. Pergamon Press, London, pp. 101–107.

BUCY, P. C. 1958. The cortico-spinal tract and tremor. In W. S. FIELDS (Editor), *Pathogenesis and Treatment of Parkinsonism*. Charles C Thomas, Publisher, Springfield, Ill., Ch. XI, pp. 271–293.

BUCY, P. C. 1959. The surgical treatment of abnormal involuntary movements. Neurologia, 1: 1–15.

BUCY, P. C. 1959a. The basal ganglia and skeletal muscular activity. In G. SCHALTENBRAND AND P. BAILEY (Editors), *Introduction to Stereotaxis, with an Atlas of the Human Brain*, Vol. I. Georg Thieme, Stuttgart, pp. 331–353.

BUEKER, E. D. 1948. Implantation of tumors in the hind limb field of the embryonic chick, and the developmental response of the lumbosacral nervous system. Anat. Rec., 102: 369–389.

BULL, J. W. D. 1961. Use and limitations of angiography in the diagnosis of vascular lesions of the brain. Neurology, 11: 80–85.

BULL, J. W. D., AND SUTTON, D. 1949. The diagnosis of paraphysial cysts. Brain, 72: 487–516.

BULLOCK, T. H., AND HORRIDGE, G. A. 1965. *Structure and Function in the Nervous Systems of Invertebrates*, Vols. 1 and 2. W. H. Freeman and Company, San Francisco.

BUNGE, M. B., BUNGE, R. P., AND PAPPAS, G. D. 1962. Electron microscopic demonstration of connections between glia and myelin sheaths in the developing mammalian central nervous system. J. Cell Biol., 12: 448–453.

BUNGE, M. B., BUNGE, R. P., PETERSON, E. R., AND MURRAY, M. R. 1967. A light and electron microscope study of long term organized cultures of rat dorsal root ganglia. J. Cell Biol., 32: 439–466.

BUNGE, M. B., BUNGE, R. P., AND RIS, H. 1961. Ultrastructural study of remyelination in an experimental lesion in adult cat spinal cord. J. Biophys. & Biochem. Cytol., 10: 67–94.

BUNGE, R. P. 1968. Glial cells and the central myelin sheath. Physiol. Rev., 48: 197–251.

BUNGE, R. P., AND GLASS, P. M. 1965. Some observations on myelin-glial relationships and on the etiology of the cerebrospinal fluid exchange lesion. Ann. New York Acad. Sci., 122: 15–28.

VAN BUREN, J. M., AND BORKE, R. C. 1972. *Variations and Connections of the Human Thalamus*. Springer-Verlag, New York, 2 vols.

BURGEN, A. S. V., AND EMMELIN, N. G. 1961. Innervation of the glandular elements. In A. S. V. BURGEN AND N. G. EMMELIN (Editors), *Physiology of the Salivary Glands*. Williams & Wilkins Company, Baltimore, Ch. III, pp. 38–71.

BÜRGI, S., AND BUCHER, V. M. 1960. *Markhaltige Faserverbindungen im Hirnstamm der Katze*. Julius Springer Verlag, Berlin.

BUSCH, H. F. M. 1961. *An Anatomical Analysis of the White Matter in the Brain Stem of the Cat*. Thesis, University of Leiden. Te Assen Bij Van Gorcum and Company, N.V., Leiden, 116 pp.

BUSER, P., AND BORENSTEIN, P. 1956. Donnés sur la répartition des réponses sensorielles corticales (somesthésiques, visuelles, auditives) chez le chat curarisé non anesthésie. J. physiol., Paris, 48: 419–421.

BUTLER, R. A., DIAMOND, I. T., AND NEFF, W. D. 1957. Role of auditory cortex in discrimination of changes in frequency. J. Neurophysiol., 20: 108–120.

CAIRNS, H. 1952. Disturbances of consciousness with lesions of the brain-stem and diencephalon. Brain, 75: 109–146.

CAJAL, S. RAMÓN Y 1909, 1911. *Histologie du système nerveux de l'homme et des vertébres*. Norbert Maloine, Paris. 2 vols.

CAJAL, S. RAMÓN Y 1913. Sobre un nuevo proceder de impregnación de la neuroglia y sus resultados in los centros nerviosos del hombre y animales. Trab. Lab. invest. biol., Univ. Madrid, 11: 219–237.

CAJAL, S. RAMÓN Y 1916. El proceder del oro-sublimado para la coloración de la neuroglia. Trab. Lab. invest. biol., Univ. Madrid, 14: 155–162.

CAJAL, S. RAMÓN Y 1928. *Degeneration and Regeneration of the Nervous System*, Vol. I. Translation by R. M. May. Oxford University, Press, London, pp. 27–40.

CALNE, D. B., AND PALLIS, C. A. 1966. Vibratory sense: A critical review. Brain, 89: 723–746.

CAMMERMEYER, J. 1947. Is the human area postrema a neuro-vegetative nucleus? Acta anat., 2: 294–320.

CAMMERMEYER, J. 1965. Histiocytes, juxtavascular mitotic cells and microglia cells during retrograde changes in the facial nucleus of rabbits of varying age. Ergebn. Anat. Entwickl.-Gesch., 38: 195–229.

CAMMERMEYER, J. 1966. Morphologic distinctions between oligodendrocytes and microglial cells in the rabbit cerebral cortex. Am. J. Anat., 118: 227–448.

CAMPBELL, A. W. 1905. *Histological Studies on the Localisation of Cerebral Function*. Cambridge University Press, New York, 360 pp.

CAMPBELL, J. B., BASSETT, C. A. L., HUSBY, J., AND NOBACK, C. R. 1957. Regeneration of adult mammalian spinal cord. Science, 126: 929.

CAMPBELL, J. B., BASSETT, C. A. L., HUSBY, J., AND NOBACK, C. R. 1958. Axonal regeneration in the transected adult feline spinal cord. S. Forum, Proc. Clin. Cong. Am. Coll. Surgeons, 8: 528–532.

CAMPBELL, M. F. 1957. Neuromuscular uropathy. In *Principles of Urology*. W. B. Saunders Company, Philadelphia, Ch. 9, pp. 337–378.

CAMPOS-ORTEGA, J. A., GLEES, P., AND NEUHOFF, V. 1968. Ultrastructural analysis of individual layers in the lateral geniculate body of the monkey. Ztschr. Zellforsch., 87: 82–100.

CANNON, W. B. 1929. *Bodily Changes in Pain, Hunger, Fear and Rage. An Account of Recent Researches into the Function of Emotional Excitement*. D. Appleton and Company, New York.

CANNON, W. B. 1939. A law of denervation. Am. J. M. Sc., 98: 737–750.

CANNON, W. B., AND ROSENBLUETH, A. 1933. Studies on activity in endocrine organs; sympathin E and sympathin I. Am. J. Physiol., 104: 557–574.

CANNON, W. B., AND ROSENBLUETH, A. 1937. *Autonomic Neuro-Effector Systems*. Macmillan Company, New York.

CANNON, W. B., AND ROSENBLUETH, A. 1949. *The Supersensitivity of Denervated Structures*. Macmillan Company, New York.

CARLSSON, A. 1965. Drugs which block the storage of 5-hydroxytryptamine and related amines. In O. EICHLER AND A. FARAH (Editors), *Handbuch der experimentellen Pharmakologie*, Vol. 19. Springer, Heidelberg, pp. 529–592.

CARLSSON, A., FALCK, B., AND HILLARP, N.-Å. 1962. Cellular localization of brain monoamines. Acta physiol. scandinav., 56: Suppl. 196, 1–28.

CARMAN, J. B., COWAN, W. M., AND POWELL, T. P. S. 1963. The organization of corticostriate connexions in the rabbit. Brain, 86: 525–562.

CARMAN, J. B., COWAN, W. M., AND POWELL, T. P. S. 1964. Cortical connexions of the thalamic reticular nucleus. J. Anat., 98: 587–598.

CARMAN, J. B., COWAN, W. M., POWELL, T. P. S., AND WEBSTER, K. E. 1965. A bilateral corticostriate projection. J. Neurol. Neurosurg. & Psychiat., 28: 71–77.

CARMEL, P. W. 1968. Sympathetic deficits following thalamotomy. Arch. Neurol., 18: 378–387.

CARMEL, P. W. 1970. Efferent projections of the ventral anterior nucleus of the thalamus in the monkey. Am. J. Anat., 128: 159–184.

CARMEL, P. W., AND STEIN, B. M. 1969. Cell changes in sensory ganglia following proximal and distal nerve section in the monkey. J. Comp. Neurol., 135: 145–166.

CARPENTER, F. W. 1918. Nerve endings of sensory type in the muscular coat of the stomach and small intestine. J. Comp. Neurol., 29: 553–560.

CARPENTER, M. B. 1950. Athetosis and the basal ganglia. Arch. Neurol. & Psychiat., 63: 875–901.

CARPENTER, M. B. 1956. A study of the red nucleus in the rhesus monkey. Anatomic degenerations and physiologic effects resulting from localized lesions of the red nucleus. J. Comp. Neurol., 105: 195–250.

CARPENTER, M. B. 1957. Functional relationships between the red nucleus and the brachium conjunctivum. Physiologic study of lesions of the red nucleus in monkeys with degenerated superior cerebellar brachia. Neurology, 7: 427–437.

CARPENTER, M. B. 1957a. The dorsal trigeminal tract in the rhesus monkey. J. Anat., 91: 82–90.

CARPENTER, M. B. 1958. The neuroanatomical basis of dyskinesia. In W. S. FIELDS (Editor), Pathogenesis and Treatment of Parkinsonism. Charles C Thomas, Publisher, Springfield, Ill., Ch. 2, pp. 50–85.

CARPENTER, M. B. 1959. Lesions of the fastigial nuclei in the rhesus monkey. Am. J. Anat., 104: 1–34.

CARPENTER, M. B. 1960. Fiber projections from the descending and lateral vestibular nuclei in the cat. Am. J. Anat., 107: 1–22.

CARPENTER, M. B. 1961. Brain stem and infratentorial neuraxis in experimental dyskinesia. Arch. Neurol., 5: 504–524.

CARPENTER, M. B. 1966. The ascending vestibular system and its relationship to conjugate horizontal eye movements. In R. J. WOLFSON (Editor), The Vestibular System and its Diseases. University of Pennsylvania Press, Philadelphia. pp. 68–98.

CARPENTER, M. B. 1967. Ventral tier thalamic nuclei. In D. WILLIAMS (Editor), Modern Trends in Neurology, Vol. 4. Butterworths, London. pp. 1–20.

CARPENTER, M. B. 1971. Upper and lower motor neurons. In J. A. DOWNEY and R. C. DARLING (Editors), Physiological Basis of Rehabilitation Medicine. W. B. Saunders Company, Philadelphia, Ch. 1, pp. 3–27.

CARPENTER, M. B. 1971a. Central oculomotor pathways. In P. BACH-Y-RITA et al. (Editors), The Control of Eye Movements. Academic Press, New York, Ch. 4, pp. 67–103.

CARPENTER, M. B. 1972. Core Text of Neuroanatomy. Williams & Wilkins Company, Baltimore, 269 pp.

CARPENTER, M. B., ALLING, F. A., AND BARD, D. S. 1960. Lesions of the descending vestibular nucleus in the cat. J. Comp. Neurol., 114: 39–50.

CARPENTER, M. B., BARD D. S., AND ALLING, F. A. 1959. Anatomical connections between the fastigial nuclei, the labyrinth and the vestibular nuclei in the cat. J. Comp. Neurol., 111: 1–26.

CARPENTER, M. B., AND BRITTIN, G. M. 1958. Subthalamic hyperkinesia in the rhesus monkey. Effects of secondary lesions in the red nucleus and brachium conjunctivum. J. Neurophysiol., 21: 400–413.

CARPENTER, M. B., BRITTIN, G. M., AND PINES, J. 1958. Isolated lesions of the fastigial nuclei in the cat. J. Comp. Neurol., 109: 65–90.

CARPENTER, M. B., AND CARPENTER, C. S. 1951. Analysis of somatotopic relations of the corpus Luysi in man and monkey. J. Comp. Neurol., 95: 349–370.

CARPENTER, M. B., AND CORRELL, J. W. 1961. Spinal pathways mediating cerebellar dyskinesia in the rhesus monkey. J. Neurophysiol., 24: 534–551.

CARPENTER, M. B., CORRELL, J. W., AND HINMAN, A. 1960. Spinal tracts mediating subthalamic hyperkinesia. Physiological effects of partial selective cordotomies upon dyskinesia in the rhesus monkey. J. Neurophysiol., 23: 288–304.

CARPENTER, M. B., FRASER, R. A. R., AND SHRIVER, J. E. 1968. The organization of pallidosubthalamic fibers in the monkey. Brain Res., 11: 522–559.

CARPENTER, M. B., AND HANNA, G. R. 1961. Fiber projections from the spinal trigeminal nucleus in the cat. J. Comp. Neurol., 117: 117–132.

CARPENTER, M. B., AND HANNA, G. R. 1962. Effects of thalamic lesions upon cerebellar dyskinesia in the rhesus monkey. J. Comp. Neurol., 119: 127–148.

CARPENTER, M. B., HARBISON, J. W., AND PETER, P. 1970. Accessory oculomotor nuclei in the monkey. Projections and effects of discrete lesions. J. Comp. Neurol., 140: 131–154.

CARPENTER, M. B., AND McMASTERS, R. E. 1963. Disturbances of conjugate horizontal eye movements in the monkey. II. Physiological effects and anatomical degeneration resulting from lesions in the medial longitudinal fasciculus. Arch. Neurol., 8: 347–368.

CARPENTER, M. B., AND McMASTERS, R. E. 1964. Lesions of the substantia nigra in the rhesus monkey. Efferent fiber degeneration and behavioral observations. Am. J. Anat., 114: 293–320.

CARPENTER, M. B., McMASTERS, R. E., AND HANNA, G. R. 1963. Disturbances of conjugate horizontal eye movements in the monkey. I. Physiological effects and anatomical degeneration resulting from lesions of the abducens nucleus and nerve. Arch. Neurol., 8: 231–247.

CARPENTER, M. B., AND METTLER, F. A. 1951. Analysis of subthalamic hyperkinesia in the monkey with special reference to ablations of agranular cortex. J. Comp. Neurol., 95: 125–158.

CARPENTER, M. B., NOBACK, C. R., AND MOSS, M. L. 1954. The anterior choroidal artery. Its origins, course, distribution and variations. A. M. A. Arch. Neurol. & Psychiat., 71: 714–722.

CARPENTER, M. B., AND NOVA, H. R. 1960. Descending division of the brachium conjunctivum in the cat: A cerebello-reticular system. J. Comp. Neurol., 114: 295–305.

CARPENTER, M. B., AND PETER, P. 1970/71. Accessory oculomotor nuclei in the monkey. J. Hirnforsch., 12: 405–418.

CARPENTER, M. B., AND PETER, P. 1972. Nigrostriatal and nigrothalamic fibers in the rhesus monkey. J. Comp. Neurol., 144: 93–116.

CARPENTER, M. B., AND PIERSON, R. J. 1973. Pretectal region and the pupillary light reflex. An anatomical analysis in the monkey. J. Comp. Neurol., 149: 271–300.

CARPENTER, M. B., STEIN, B. M., AND PETER, P. 1972. Primary vestibulocerebellar fibers in the monkey: Distribution of fibers arising from distinctive cell groups of the vestibular ganglia. Am. J. Anat., 135: 221–250.

CARPENTER, M. B., STEIN, B. M., AND SHRIVER, J.

E. 1968. Central projections of spinal dorsal roots in the monkey. II. Lower thoracic, lumbosacral and coccygeal dorsal roots. Am. J. Anat., 123: 75–118.

CARPENTER, M. B., AND STROMINGER, N. L. 1964. Cerebello-oculomotor fibers in the rhesus monkey. J. Comp. Neurol., 123: 211–230.

CARPENTER, M. B., AND STROMINGER, N. L. 1965. The medial longitudinal fasciculus and disturbances of conjugate horizontal eye movements in the monkey. J. Comp. Neurol., 125: 41–66.

CARPENTER, M. B., AND STROMINGER, N. L. 1967. Efferent fibers of the subthalamic nucleus in the monkey. A comparison of the efferent projections of the subthalamic nucleus, substantia nigra and globus pallidus. Am. J. Anat., 121: 41–72.

CARPENTER, M. B., STROMINGER, N. L., AND WEISS, A. H. 1965. Effects of lesions in the intralaminar thalamic nuclei upon subthalamic dyskinesia. A study in the rhesus monkey. Arch. Neurol., 13: 113–125.

CARPENTER, M. B., WHITTIER, J. R., AND METTLER, F. A. 1950. Analysis of choreoid hyperkinesia in the rhesus monkey. Surgical and pharmacological analysis of hyperkinesia resulting from lesions in the subthalamic nucleus of Luys. J. Comp. Neurol., 92: 293–332.

CARREA, R. M. E., AND GRUNDFEST, H. 1954. Electrophysiological studies of cerebellar inflow. I. Origin, conduction and termination of ventral spino-cerebellar tract in monkey and cat. J. Neurophysiol., 17: 208–238.

CARREA, R. M. E., AND METTLER, F. A. 1947. Physiologic consequences following extensive removals of the cerebellar cortex and deep cerebellar nuclei and effect of secondary cerebral ablations in the primate. J. Comp. Neurol., 87: 169–288.

CARREA, R. M. E., REISSIG, M., AND METTLER, F. A. 1947. The climbing fibers of the simian and feline cerebellum. J. Comp. Neurol., 87: 321–365.

CARREA, R., VOLKIND, R., FOLINS, J. C., COSARINSKY, D., SUAREZ, A. M., AND ALFONSO, J. 1970. Some physiological and statistical observations on single unit activity of the feline inferior olive. In W. S. FIELDS AND W. D. WILLIS (Editors), The Cerebellum in Health and Disease. Warren H. Green, Inc., St. Louis, Ch. 7, pp. 201–216.

CARRERAS, M., AND LEVITT, M. 1959. Microelectrode analysis of the second somatosensory cortical area in the cat. Fed. Proc., 18: 24.

CASAGRANDE, V. A., HARTING, J. K., HALL, W. C., AND DIAMOND, I. T. 1972. Superior colliculus of the tree shrew: A structural and functional subdivision into superficial and deep layers. Science, 177: 444–447.

CASPERSON, T. 1950. Cell Growth and Cell Function, a Cytological Study. W. W. Norton and Company, New York, 185 pp.

DE CASTRO, F. 1923. Contribution á la connaissance de l' innervation du pancréas. Y a-t-il des conducteurs specifigues pour les ilots de Langerhans, pour les acini glandulaires et pour les vaisseaux. Trab. Lab. rech. biol., Univ. Madrid, 21: 423–457.

CAUNA, N. 1965. The effects of aging on the receptor organs of the human dermis. In W. MONTAGNA (Editor), Advances in Biology of Skin, Vol. 6. Aging. Pergamon Press, New York, pp. 63–69.

CAUNA, N. 1966. Fine structure of the receptor organ and its probable functional significance. In A.V.S. DE REUCK AND J. KNIGHT (Editors), Touch, Heat and Pain. Ciba Foundation Symposium. Little, Brown and Company, Boston, pp. 117–127.

CAUNA, N., AND MANNAN, G. 1958. The structure of human digital pacinian corpuscles (Corpuscula lamellosa) and its functional significance. J. Anat., Part 1, 92: 1–20.

CAUNA, N., AND MANNAN, G. 1959. Development and postnatal changes of digital Pacinian corpuscles (Corpuscula lamellosa) in the human hand. J. Anat., 93: 271–286.

CAUNA, N., AND MANNAN, G. 1961. Organization and development of the preterminal nerve pattern in the palmar digital tissues of man. J. Comp. Neurol., 117: 309–328.

CAUSEY, G. 1960. The Cell of Schwann. E. and S. Livingston Ltd., Edinburgh.

CHAN-PALAY, V., AND PALAY, S. L. 1970. Interrelations of basket cell axons and climbing fibers in the cerebellar cortex of the rat. Ztschr. Anat. Entwickl.-Gesch., 132: 191–227.

CHAN-PALAY, V., AND PALAY, S. L. 1971. The synapse en marron between Golgi II neurons and mossy fibers in the rat's cerebellar cortex. Ztschr. Anat. Entwickl.-Gesch., 133: 274–287.

CHAN-PALAY, V., AND PALAY, S. L. 1971a. Tendril and glomerular collaterals of climbing fibers in the granular layer in the rat's cerebellar cortex. Ztschr. Anat. Entwickl.-Gesch., 133: 247–273.

CHARCOT, J. M. 1879. Lectures on the Diseases of the Nervous System. Translated by G. Sigerson. Henry C. Lea, Philadelphia, p. 390.

CHEATHAM, M. L., AND MATZKE, H. A. 1966. Descending hypothalamic medullary pathways in the cat. J. Comp. Neurol., 127: 369–380.

CHI, C. C., AND FLYNN, J. P. 1971. Neuroanatomical projections related to biting attack elicited from hypothalamus in cats. Brain Res., 35: 49–66.

CHRISTOFF, N., ANDERSON, P. J., NATHANSON, M., AND BENDER, M. B. 1960. Problems in anatomic analysis of lesions of the median longitudinal fasciculus. A. M. A. Arch. Neurol., 2: 293–304.

CHU, L. W. 1954. Cytological study of anterior horn cells isolated from human spinal cord. J. Comp. Neurol., 100: 381–413.

CHU, N.-S., AND BLOOM, F. E. 1973. Norepinephrine-containing neurons: Changes in spontaneous discharge patterns during sleeping and waking. Science, 179: 908–910.

CLARE, M. H. AND BISHOP, G. H. 1956. Potential wave mechanisms in the cat cortex. Electroencephalog. & Clin. Neurophysiol., 8: 583–602.

CLARK, W. E. L. 1926. The mammalian oculomotor nucleus. J. Anat., 60: 426–448.

CLARK, W. E. L. 1932. The structure and connections of the thalamus. Brain, 55: 406–470.

CLARK, W. E. L. 1936. The termination of ascending tracts in the thalamus of the macaque monkey. J. Anat., 71: 1–40.

CLARK, W. E. L. 1948. The connections of the frontal lobes of the brain. Lancet, 1: 353–356.

CLARK, W. E. L. 1951. The projection of the olfactory epithelium on the olfactory bulb in the rabbit. J. Neurol. Neurosurg. & Psychiat., 14: 1–10.

CLARK, W. E. L. 1956. Observations on the structure and organization of olfactory receptors in the rabbit. Yale J. Biol. Med., 29: 83–95.

CLARK, W. E. L. 1957. Inquiries into the anatomical basis of olfactory discrimination. Proc. Roy. Soc., London, ser. B, 146: 299–319.

CLARK, W. E. L., BEATTIE, J., RIDDOCH, G., AND DOTT, N. M. 1938. The Hypothalamus. Oliver and Boyd, Edinburgh.

CLARK, W. E. L., AND BOGGON, R. H. 1933. On the connections of the anterior nucleus of the thalamus. J. Anat., 67: 215–226.

CLARK, W. E. L., AND BOGGON, R. H. 1933a. On the connections of the medial cell group of the thalamus. Brain, 56: 83–98.

CLARK, W. E. L., AND BOGGON, R. H. 1935. The thalamic connections of the parietal and frontal lobes of the brain in the monkey. Phil. Tr. Roy. Soc., London, ser. B, 224: 313–359.

CLARK, W. E. L., AND MEYER, M. 1947. The terminal connexions of the olfactory tract in the rabbit's brain. Brain, 70: 304–328.

CLARK, W. E. L., AND MEYER, M. 1950. Anatomical relationships between the cerebral cortex and the hypothalamus. Brit. M. Bull., 6: 341–345.

CLARK, W. E. L., AND POWELL, T. P. S. 1953. On the thalamocortical connexions of the general sensory cortex of Macaca. Proc. Roy. Soc., London, ser. B, 141: 467–487.

CLARK, W. E. L., AND WARWICK, R. T. 1946. The pattern of olfactory innervation. J. Neurol. Neurosurg. & Psychiat., 9: 101–111.

CLARKE, R. H., AND HORSLEY, V. 1905. On the intrinsic fibers of the cerebellum, its nuclei and its efferent tracts. Brain, 28: 13–29.

COBB, S. 1948. Foundations of. Neuro-Psychiatry. Williams & Wilkins Company, Baltimore.

COERS, C. 1955. Les variations structurelles normales et pathologiques de la jonction neuromusculaire. Acta neurol. (belg.), 55: 741–866.

COERS, C., AND WOOLF, A. L. 1959. The Innervation of Muscle: A Biopsy Study. Blackwell Scientific Publications, Oxford.

COGAN, D. G. 1956. Neurology of the Ocular Muscles, (Ed. 2.) Charles C Thomas, Publisher, Springfield, Ill.

COGAN, D. G., KUBIK, C. S., AND SMITH, W. L. 1950. Unilateral internuclear ophthalmoplegia. Report of eight clinical cases with one postmortem study. Arch. Ophth., 44: 783–796.

COGGESHALL, R. E., AND FAWCETT, D. W. 1964. The fine structure of the central nervous system of the leech, Hirudo medicinalis. J. Neurophysiol., 27: 229–289.

COGHILL, G. E. 1929. Anatomy and the Problem of Behavior. Oxford University Press, London.

COHEN, B. 1971. Vestibulo-ocular relations. In P. BACH-Y-RITA et al. (Editors), The Control of Eye Movements. Academic Press, New York, pp. 105–135.

COHEN, B., HOUSEPIAN, E. M., AND PURPURA, D. P. 1962. Intrathalamic regulation of activity in a cerebellocortical projection pathway. Exper. Neurol., 6: 492–506.

COHEN, B., SUZUKI, J. I. AND BENDER, M. B. 1964. Eye movements from semicircular nerve stimulation in the cat. Ann. Otol. Rhin. & Laryng., 73: 153–169.

COHEN, D., CHAMBERS, W. W., AND SPRAGUE, J. M. 1958. Experimental study of the efferent projections from the cerebellar nuclei to the brain stem of the cat. J. Comp. Neurol., 109: 233–259.

COHEN, M. J., LANDGREN, S., STROM, L., AND ZOTTERMANN, Y. 1957. Cortical reception of touch and taste in the cat. Acta physiol. scandinav., 40: Suppl. 135, 50 pp.

COHEN, S. 1960. Purification of a nerve-growth factor promoting protein from the mouse salivary gland and its neuro-cytotoxic antiserum. Proc. Nat. Acad. Sc., 46: 302–311.

COLE, M., NAUTA, W. J. H. AND MEHLER, W. R. 1964. The ascending efferent projections of the substantia nigra. Tr. Am. Neurol. A. 89: 74–78.

COLONNIER, M. 1967. The fine structural arrangement of the cortex. Arch. Neurol., 16: 651–657.

COLONNIER, M. 1968. Synaptic patterns on different cell types in the different laminae of the cat visual cortex. An electron microscopic study. Brain Res., 9: 268–287.

COLONNIER, M. L., AND GUILLERY, R. W. 1964. Synaptic organization in the lateral geniculate nucleus of the monkey. Ztschr. Zellforsch., 62: 333–355.

COMBS, C. M. 1949. Fiber and cell degeneration in the albino rat brain after hemidecortication. J. Comp. Neurol., 90: 373–402.

COMBS, C. M. 1956. Bulbar regions related to localized cerebellar afferent impulses. J. Neurophysiol., 19: 285–300.

CONDE, H. 1966. Analyse électrophysiologique de la voie dentato-rubro-thalamique chez le chat. J. physiol., (Paris), 58: 218–219.

COOPER, E. R. A. 1946. The development of the substantia nigra. Brain, 69: 22–33.

COOPER, E. R. A. 1946a. The development of the human red nucleus and corpus striatum. Brain, 69: 34–43.

COOPER, I. S. 1956. Neurosurgical Alleviation of Parkinsonism. Charles C Thomas, Publisher, Springfield, Ill.

COOPER, I. S. 1957. Relief of juvenile involuntary movement disorders by chemopallidectomy. J. A. M. A., 164: 1297–1301.

COOPER, I. S. 1959. Dystonia musculorum deformans alleviated by chemopallidectomy and chemopallidothalamectomy. A. M. A. Arch. Neurol. & Psychiat., 81: 5–19.

COOPER, I. S. 1960. Neurosurgical relief of intention tremor due to cerebellar disease and multiple sclerosis. Arch. Phys. Med. & Rehab., 41: 1–4.

COOPER, I. S. 1960a. Neurosurgical alleviation of intention tremor of multiple sclerosis and cerebellar disease. New England J. Med., 263: 441–444.

COOPER, I. S. AND BRAVO, G. J. 1958. Anterior choroidal artery occlusion, chemopallidectomy and chemothalamectomy in parkinsonism: A consecutive series of 700 operations. In W. S. FIELDS (Editor), Pathogenesis and Treatment of Parkinsonism. Charles C Thomas, Publisher, Springfield, Ill., Ch. XV, pp. 325–352.

COOPER, I. S. AND POLOUKHINE, N. 1959. Neurosurgical relief of intention (cerebellar) tremor. J. Am. Geriatrics Soc., 7: 443–445.

COOPER, S., AND DANIEL, P. M. 1949. Muscle spindles in human extrinsic eye muscles. Brain, 72: 1–24.

COOPER, S., DANIEL, P. M., AND WHITTERIDGE, D. 1953. Nerve impulses in the brainstem of the goat. Short latency responses obtained by stretching the extrinsic eye muscles and the jaw muscles. J. Physiol., 120: 471–490.

COOPER, S., DANIEL, P. M., AND WHITTERIDGE, D. 1953a. Nerve impulses in the brainstem of the goat. Responses with long latencies obtained by stretching the extrinsic eye muscles. J. Physiol., 120: 491–513.

COOPER, S., DANIEL, P. M., AND WHITTERIDGE, D. 1955. Muscle spindles and other sensory endings in the extrinsic eye muscles; the physiology and anatomy of these receptors and their connections with the brain stem. Brain, 78: 564–583.

COOPER, S., AND SHERRINGTON, C. S. 1940. Gower's tract and spinal border cells. Brain, 63: 123–134.

COPENHAVER, W. M. 1964. Bailey's Textbook of Histology, Ed. 15. Williams & Wilkins Company, Baltimore, 633 pp.

COPENHAVER, W. M., BUNGE, R. P., AND BUNGE, M. B. 1971. Bailey's Textbook of Histology, Ed. 16. Williams & Wilkins Company, Baltimore.

CORBIN, K. B. 1940. Observations on the peripheral distribution of fibers arising in the mesencephalic nucleus of the fifth cranial nerve. J. Comp. Neurol., 73: 153–177.

CORBIN, K. B., AND HARRISON, F. 1940. Function of the mesencephalic root of the fifth cranial nerve. J. Neurophysiol., 3: 423–435.

CORNING, H. K. 1922. Lehrbuch der topographischen Anatomie für Studierende und Ärzte. J. F. Bergmann, Munich, pp. 609–614.

COURVILLE, J. 1966. Rubrobulbar fibres to the facial nucleus and the lateral reticular nucleus (nucleus of the lateral funiculus). An experimental study in the cat with silver impregnation methods. Brain Res., 1: 317–337.

COURVILLE, J. 1966a. Somatotopical organization of the projection from the nucleus interpositus anterior of the cerebellum to the red nucleus. An experimental study in the cat with silver impregnation methods. Exper. Brain Res., 2: 191–215.

COURVILLE, J. 1966b. The nucleus of the facial nerve; the relation between cellular groups and peripheral branches of the nerve. Brain Res. 1: 338-354.

COURVILLE, J., AND BRODAL, A. 1966. Rubrocerebellar connections in the cat: An experimental study with silver impregnation methods. J. Comp. Neurol., 126: 471-485.

COURVILLE, J., AND COOPER, C. W. 1970. The cerebellar nuclei of Macaca mulatta: A morphological study. J. Comp. Neurol., 140: 241-254.

COURVILLE, J., DIAKIW, N., AND BRODAL, A. 1973. Cerebellar corticonuclear projection in the cat. The paramedian lobule. An experimental study with silver methods. Brain Res., 50: 25-45.

COUTEAUX, R. 1958. Morphological and cytochemial observations on the postsynaptic membrane at motor end plates and ganglionic synapses. Exper. Cell Res., 5(suppl.): 294-322.

COWAN, W. M., GOTTLIEB, D. I., HENDRICKSON, A. E., PRICE, J. L., AND WOOLSEY, T. A. 1972. The autoradiographic demonstration of axonal connections in the central nervous system. Brain Res., 37: 21-51.

COWAN, W. M., AND POWELL, T. P. S. 1966. Strio-pallidal projection in the monkey. J. Neurol. Neurosurg. & Psychiat., 29: 426-439.

COWAN, W. M., RAISMAN, G., AND POWELL, T. P. S. 1965. The connexions of the amygdala. J. Neurol. Neurosurg. & Psychiat., 28: 137-151.

COXE, W. S., AND LANDAU, W. M. 1965. Observations upon the effect of supplementary motor cortex ablation in the monkey. Brain, 88: 763-772.

CRITCHLEY, M. 1953. The Parietal Lobes. Edward Arnold, London, 479 pp.

VAN CREVEL, H., AND VERHAART, W. J. C. 1963. The rate of secondary degeneration in the central nervous system. I. The pyramidal tract of the cat. J. Anat., 97: 429-449.

VAN CREVEL, H., AND VERHAART, W. J. C. 1963a. The rate of secondary degeneration in the central nervous system. II. The optic nerve of the cat. J. Anat., 97: 451-464.

CROSBY, E. C. 1950. The application of neuroanatomical data to the diagnosis of selected neurosurgical and neurological cases. J. Neurosurg., 7: 566-583.

CROSBY, E. C. 1953. Relations of brain centers to normal and abnormal eye movements in the horizontal plane. J. Comp. Neurol., 99: 437-480.

CROSBY, E. C., AND HUMPHREY, T. 1941. Studies of the vertebrate telencephalon. II. The nuclear pattern of the anterior olfactory nucleus, tuberculum olfactorum and the amygdaloid complex in adult man. J. Comp. Neurol., 74: 309-352.

CROSBY, E. C., HUMPHREY, T., AND LAUER, E. W. 1962. Correlative Anatomy of the Nervous System. Macmillan Company, New York, 731 pp.

CROUSE, G. S., AND CUCINOTTA, A. J. 1965. Progressive neuronal differentiation in the submandibular ganglia of a series of human fetuses. J. Comp. Neurol., 125: 259-272.

CROWE, S. J. 1935. Symposium on tone localization in the cochlea. Ann. Otol. Rhin. & Laryng., 44: 737-837.

CSERR, H. F. 1971. Physiology of the choroid plexus. Physiol. Rev., 51: 273-311.

CULLING, C. F. A. 1963. Handbook of Histopathological Techniques, Ed. 2 Butterworths, London, pp. 348-375.

CURRIER, R. D., GILES, C. L., AND DEJONG, R. N. 1961. Some comments on Wallenberg's lateral medullary syndrome. Neurology, 11: 778-791.

DAHLSTRÖM, A. 1965. Observation on the accumulation of noradrenaline in the proximal and distal parts of peripheral adrenergic nerves after compression. J.

Anat., 99: 677-689.

DAHLSTRÖM, A. 1971. Regional distribution of brain catecholamines and serotonin. In R. J. WURTMAN (Editor), Brain Monamines and Endocrine Function. Neurosc. Res. Bull., 9: 197-205.

DAHLSTRÖM, A., AND FUXE, K. 1964. Evidence for the existence of monoamine-containing neurons in the central nervous system. I. Demonstration of monoamines in the cell bodies of brain stem neurons. Acta physiol. scandinav., 62, Suppl. 232: 1-55.

DAITZ, H. M., AND POWELL, T. P. S. 1954. Studies of the connections of the fornix system. J. Neurol. Neurosurg. & Psychiat., 17: 75-82.

DALE, H. H. 1914. The action of certain esters and ethers of choline, and their relation to muscarine. J. Pharmacol. & Exper. Ther., 6: 147-190.

DANDY, W. E. 1933. Benign Tumors in the Third Ventricle of the Brain. Charles C Thomas, Publisher, Springfield, Ill.

DANDY, W. E. 1947. Intercranial Arterial Aneurysms. Comstock Publishing Company, Ithaca, N. Y., 147 pp.

DARIAN-SMITH, I., AND MAYDAY, G. 1960. Somatotopic organization within the brain stem trigeminal complex of the cat. Exper. Neurol., 2: 290-309.

DARIAN-SMITH, I., AND YOKOTA, T. 1966. Corticofugal effects on different neuron types within the cat's brain stem activated by tactile stimulation of the face. J. Neurophysiol., 29: 185-206.

DAVIDOFF, L. M., AND DYKE, C. G. 1951. The Normal Encephalogram, Ed. 3. Lea and Febiger, Philadelphia, pp. 167-170.

DAVIS, C. L. 1923. Description of a human embryo having 20 paired somites. Contrib. Embryol., 15: 1-51.

DAVIS, D. 1957. Radicular Syndromes With Emphasis on Chest Pain Simulating Coronary Disease. Year Book Publishers, Inc., Chicago, pp. 17-160.

DAVIS, H. 1961. Some principles of sensory receptor action. Physiol. Rev., 41: 391-416.

DAVSON, H. 1960. Intracranial and intraocular fluids. In J. FIELD (Editor), Handbook of Physiology, Section 1, Vol. III. Neurophysiology. American Physiological Society, Washington, D. C., Ch. 71, pp. 1761-1788.

DAVSON, H. 1967. Physiology of the Cerebrospinal Fluid. Little, Brown and Company, Boston.

DAVSON, H., AND BRADBURY, M. 1965. The extracellular space of the brain. In E. D. P. DE ROBERTIS AND R. CARREA (Editors), Biology of Neuroglia, Progress in Brain Research, Vol. 15. Elsevier Publishing Company, Amsterdam, pp. 124-134.

DEECKE, L., SCHWARZ, D. W. F., AND FREDRICKSON, J. M. 1973. The vestibular thalamus in the Rhesus monkey. Advances Oto-Rhino-Laryng., 19: 210-219.

DEECKE, L., SCHWARZ, D. W. F., AND FREDRICKSON, J. M. 1974. Nucleus ventroposterior inferior (VPI) as the vestibular thalamic relay in the Rhesus monkey. I. Field potential investigation. Exper. Brain Res., 20: 88-100.

DEITCH, A. D., AND MURRAY, M. R. 1956. Nissl substance of living and fixed spinal ganglion cells; phase contrast study. J. Biophys. & Biochem. Cytol., 2: 433-444.

DEJERINE, J. 1901. Anatomie des centres nerveux, Vol. 2. J. Rueff, Paris, 720 pp.

DEJONG, R. N. 1958. Neurologic Examination. Paul B. Hoeber, Inc., New York, pp. 664-683 and 834-867.

DELL, P. 1952. Corrélations entre le système vegetatif et le système de la vie de relation: mésencéphale, diencephale et cortex cerebral. J. Physiol., Paris, 44: 471-557.

DEKABAN, A. 1953. Human thalamus. An anatomical, developmental and pathological study. I. Division of the human adult thalamus into nuclei by use of the cyto-myelo-architectonic method. J. Comp. Neurol., 99: 639-683.

DEKABAN, A. 1954. Human thalamus. An anatomical developmental and pathological study. II. Development of the human thalamic nuclei. J. Comp. Neurol., 100: 63–97.

DE LONG, M. R. 1971. Activity of pallidal neurons during movement. J. Neurophysiol., 34: 414–427.

DEMPSEY, E. W. 1956. Variations in the structure of mitochondria. J. Biophys. & Biochem. Cytol., 2: Suppl. 4, 305–312.

DEMPSEY, E. W., AND LUSE, S. 1958. Fine structure of the neuropil in relation to neuroglia cells. In W. F. WINDLE (Editor), Biology of Neuroglia. Charles C Thomas, Publisher, Springfield, Ill., pp. 99–108.

DEMPSEY, E. W., AND MORISON, R. S. 1942. The production of rhythmically recurrent cortical potentials after localized thalamic stimulation. Am. J. Physiol., 135: 293–300.

DEMPSEY, E. W., AND MORISON, R. S. 1943. The electrical activity of a thalamocortical relay system. Am. J. Physiol., 138: 283–298.

DENNY-BROWN, D. 1946. Importance of neural fibroblasts in the regeneration of nerve. Arch. Neurol. & Psychiat., 55: 171–215.

DENNY-BROWN, D. 1951. The frontal lobes and their functions. In A. FEILING (Editor), Modern Trends in Neurology. Paul B. Hoeber, Inc., New York, pp. 13–89.

DENNY-BROWN, D. 1960. Motor mechanisms—Introduction: the general principles of motor integration. In J. FIELD (Editor), Handbook of Physiology, Section I, Vol. II. American Physiological Society, Washington, D. C. Ch. 32, pp. 781–796.

DENNY-BROWN, D. 1962. The Basal Ganglia and Their Relation to Disorders of Movement. Oxford University Press, London.

DENNY-BROWN, D., AND BOTTERELL, E. H. 1948. The motor functions of the agranular frontal cortex. A. Res. Nerv. & Ment. Dis., Proc., 27: 235–345.

DIAMOND, I. T., JONES, E. G., AND POWELL, T. P. S. 1969. The projection of the auditory cortex upon the diencephalon and brain stem in the cat. Brain Res., 15: 305–340.

DiBIAGIO, F., AND GRUNDFEST, H. 1955. Afferent relations of inferior olivary nucleus. II. Site of relay from hindlimb afferents into dorsal spino-olivary tract in cat. J. Neurophysiol., 18: 299–304.

DOGIEL, A. S. 1891. Die Nervenendkörperchen (Endkolben, W. Krause) in der Cornea und Conjuctiva Bulbi des Menschen. Arch. mikrosk. Anat., 37: 602–619.

DOGIEL, A. S. 1908. Der Bau der Spinalganglien des Menschen und der Säugetiere. Gustav Fischer, Jena.

DOHRMANN, G. J. 1970. The choroid plexus: A historical review. Brain Res., 18: 197–218.

DOTT, N. M. 1938. Surgical aspects of the hypothalamus. In W. E. L. CLARK et al. (Editors), The Hypothalamus. Oliver and Boyd, Edinburgh, pp. 131–185.

DOW, R. S. 1936. The fiber connections of the posterior parts of the cerebellum in the rat and cat. J. Comp. Neurol., 63: 527–548.

DOW, R. S. 1938. Efferent connections of the flocculonodular lobe in Macaca mulatta. J. Comp. Neurol., 68: 297–305.

DOW, R. S. 1942. Cerebellar action potentials in response to stimulation of the cerebral cortex in monkeys and cats. J. Neurophysiol., 5: 121–136.

DOW, R. S. AND MORUZZI, G. 1958. The Physiology and Pathology of the Cerebellum. University of Minnesota Press, Minneapolis.

DOWLING, J. E., AND BOYCOTT, B. B. 1966. Organization of the primate retina: Electron microscopy. Proc. Roy. Soc., London, ser. B., 166: 80–111.

DRACHMAN, D. A., AND ARBIT, J. 1966. Memory and the hippocampal complex. II. Is memory a multiple process? Arch. Neurol., 15: 52–61.

DREIFUSS, J. J., MURPHY, J. T., AND GLOOR, P. 1968. Contrasting effects of two identified amygdaloid efferent pathways on single hypothalamic neurons. J. Neurophysiol., 31: 237–248.

DRESEL, K., AND ROTHMAN, H. 1925. Völliger Ausfall der Substantia nigra nach Exstirpation von Grosshirn und Striatum. Ztschr. ges. Neurol. u. Psychiat., 94: 781–789.

DROOGLEEVER-FORTUYN, J., AND STEFENS, R. 1951. On the anatomical relations of the intralaminar and midline cells of the thalamus. Electroencephalog. & Clin. Neurophysiol., 3: 393–400.

DROZ, B., AND LEBLOND, C. P. 1962. Migration of protein along axons of the sciatic nerve. Science, 137: 1047–1048.

DRUCKMAN, R. 1952. A critique of "suppression" with additional observations in the cat. Brain, 75: 226–243.

DUSSER DE BARENNE, J. G. 1924. Experimental researches on sensory localization in the cerebral cortex of the monkey. Proc. Roy. Soc., London, ser. B, 96: 272–291.

DUSSER DE BARENNE, J. G., GAROL, H. W., AND MCCULLOCH, W. S. 1942. Physiological neuronography of the corticostriatal connections. A. Res. Nerv. & Ment. Dis., Proc., 21: 246–266.

DUSSER DE BARENNE, J. G., AND MCCULLOCH, W. S. 1939. Suppression of motor response upon stimulation of area 4S of the cerebral cortex. Am. J. Physiol., 126: 482.

EAGER, R. P. 1963. Efferent cortico-nuclear pathways in the cerebellum of the cat. J. Comp. Neurol., 120: 81–103.

EAGER, R. P. 1963a. Cortical association pathways in the cerebellum of the cat. J. Comp. Neurol., 121: 381–393.

EAGER, R. P. 1965. The mode of termination and temporal course of degeneration of cortical association pathways in the cerebellum of the cat. J. Comp. Neurol., 124: 243–257.

EAGER, R. P., AND BARRNETT, R. J. 1966. Morphological and chemical studies of Nauta-stained degenerating cerebellar and hypothalamic fibers. J. Comp. Neurol., 126: 487–510.

EARLE, K. M. 1952. The tract of Lissauer and its possible relation to the pain pathway. J. Comp. Neurol., 96: 93–111.

ECCLES, J. C. 1959. Neuron physiology—Introduction. In J. FIELD (Editor), Handbook of Physiology, Section I, Vol. I. American Physiological Society, Washington, D. C., Ch. 2, pp. 59–74.

ECCLES, J. C. 1966. Functional organization of the cerebellum in relation to its role in motor control. In R. GRANIT (Editor), Muscular Afferents and Motor Control. Almquist & Wiksell, Stockholm, pp. 19–36.

ECCLES, J. C., ITO, M., AND SZENTÁGOTHAI, J. 1967. The Cerebellum as a Neuronal Machine. Springer Verlag, New York.

ECCLES, J. C., LLINÁS, R., AND SASAKI, K. 1964. Excitation of cerebellar Purkinje cells by the climbing fibers. Nature, 203: 245–246.

ECCLES, J. C., LLINÁS, R., AND SASAKI, K. 1966. The excitatory synaptic action of climbing fibres on the Purkinje cells of the cerebellum. J. Physiol., 182: 268–296.

ECCLES, J. C., LLINÁS, R., AND SASAKI, K. 1966a. Parallel fibre stimulation and responses induced thereby in the Purkinje cells of the cerebellum. Exper. Brain Res., 1: 17–39.

ECCLES, J. C., LLINÁS, R., AND SASAKI, K. 1966b. The inhibitory interneurones within the cerebellar cortex. Exper. Brain Res., 1: 1–16.

ECCLES, J. C., LLINÁS, R., AND SASAKI, K. 1966c. The

mossy fibre-granule cell relay of the cerebellum and its inhibitory control by Golgi cells. Exper. Brain Res., 1: 82–101.

VON ECONOMO, C. F. 1911. Über dissoziierte Emphindungslähmung bei Ponstumoren und über die zentralen Bahnen des sensiblen Trigeminus. Jahrb. Psychiat. u. Neurol., 32: 107–138.

VON ECONOMO, C. F. 1929. *The Cytoarchitectonics of the Human Cerebral Cortex.* Oxford Medical Publications, London, 186 pp.

VON ECONOMO, C. F. AND KARPLUS, J. P. 1909. Zur Physiologie und Anatomie des Mittelhirns. Arch. Psychiat., 46: 275–356.

EDWARDS, S. B. 1972. The ascending and descending projections of the red nucleus in the cat: An experimental study using an autoradiographic tracing method. Brain Res., 48: 45–63.

ELDRED, E., AND FUJIMORI, B. 1958. Relations of the reticular formation to muscle spindle activation. In H. H. JASPERS et al. (Editors), *Reticular Formation of the Brain.* Little, Brown and Company, Boston, pp. 275–283.

ELDRED, E., GRANIT, R., AND MERTON, P. A. 1953. Supraspinal control of the muscle spindles and its significance. J. Physiol., 122: 498–523.

ELEFTHERIOU, B. E., ZOLOVICK, A. J., AND PEARSE, R. 1966. Effects of amygdaloid lesions on pituitary-adrenal axis in the deer-mouse. Proc. Soc. Exper. Biol. & Med., 122: 1259.

ELFVIN, L. G. 1958. The ultrastructure of unmyelinated fibers in the splenic nerve of the cat. J. Ultrastruct. Res., 1: 428–454.

ELLIOTT, K. A. C., AND JASPER, H. 1949. Measurement of experimentally induced brain swelling and shrinkage. Am. J. Physiol., 157: 122–129.

ELMAN, R. 1923. Spinal arachnoid granulations with especial reference to the cerebrospinal fluid. Bull. Johns Hopkins Hosp., 34: 99–104.

ELZE, C. 1932. Centrales Nervensystem. In H. BRAUS, *Anatomie des Menschen. Ein Lehrbuch für Studierende und Ärzte,* Vol. III. Julius Springer, Berlin.

EMMELIN, N. 1967. Nervous control of salivary glands. In C. F. CODE (Editor), *Handbook of Physiology,* Section 6, Vol. II, *Secretion.* American Physiological Society, Washington, D. C., Ch. 37, pp. 595–632.

EMMELIN, N., AND STROMBLAD, B. C. R. 1954. A method of stimulating and inhibiting salivary secretion in man. Acta physiol. scandinav., 31:Suppl. 114, 12–13.

EMMERS, R. 1964. Localization of thalamic projection of afferents from the tongue in the cat. Anat. Rec., 148: 67–74.

EMMERS, R. 1965. Organization of the first and second somesthetic regions (SI and SII) in the rat thalamus. J. Comp. Neurol., 124: 215–227.

EMMERS, R. 1966. Separate relays of tactile, thermal and gustatory modalities in the cat thalamus. Proc. Soc. Exper. Biol. & Med., 121: 527–531.

EMMERS, R. 1973. Interaction of neural systems which control body water. Brain Res., 49: 323–347.

EMMERS, R., BENJAMIN, R. M., AND BLOMQUIST, A. J. 1962. Thalamic localization of afferents from the tongue in albino rat. J. Comp. Neurol., 118: 43–48.

ERICKSON, T. C., AND WOOLSEY, C. N. 1951. Observations on the supplementary motor area of man. Tr. Am. Neurol. A., 76: 50–56.

ERLANGER, J., AND GASSER, H. S. 1937. *Electrical Signs of Nervous Activity.* University of Pennsylvania Press, Philadelphia, 221 pp.

ERULKAR, S. D., ROSE, J. C., AND DAVIES, P. W. 1956. Single unit activity in the auditory cortex of the cat. Bull. Johns Hopkins Hosp., 99: 55–86.

ESSNER, E., AND NOVIKOFF, A. B. 1960. Human hepatocellular pigments and lysosomes. J. Ultrastruct. Res., 3: 374–391.

VON EULER, U. S. 1956. *Noradrenaline.* Charles C Thomas, Publisher, Springfield, Ill.

VON EULER, U. S. 1961. Neurotransmission in the adrenergic nervous system. *The Harvey Lectures,* Ser. 55. Academic Press, New York, pp. 43–65.

VON EULER, U. S. 1966. Catecholamines in nerve and organ granules. In U. S. VON EULER et al. (Editors), *Mechanism of Release of Biogenic Amines,* Pergamon Press, New York, pp. 211–222.

EVANS, E. F., ROSS, H. F., AND WHITFIELD, I. C. 1965. The ειλ ial distribution of unit characteristic frequency in the primary auditory cortex of the cat. J. Physiol., 179: 238–247.

EVANS, E. F., AND WHITFIELD, I. C. 1964. Classification of unit responses in the auditory cortex of the unanesthetized. J. Physiol., 171: 476–493.

EVERETT, J. W. 1959. Neuroendocrine mechanisms in control of the mammalian ovary. In A. GORBMAN (Editor), *Comparative Endocrinology.* J. Wiley and Sons, New York, pp. 168–174.

EVERETT, J. W. 1964. Central neural control of reproductive functions of the adenohypophysis. Physiol. Rev., 44: 373–431.

FALCK, B. 1962. Observations on the possibilities of the cellular localization of monoamines by a fluorescence method. Acta physiol. scandinav., 56: Suppl. 197: 1–25.

FALCK, B., HILLARP, N.-Å., THIEME, G., AND TORP, A. 1962. Fluorescence of catecholamines and related compounds condensed with formaldehyde. J. Histochem. & Cytochem., 10: 348–354.

FALCK, B., AND TORP, A. 1962. A new evidence for localization of noradrenalin in adrenergic nerve terminals. Med. exp. (Basel) 6: 169–172.

FALCONER, M. A. 1948. Relief of intractable pain of organic origin by frontal lobotomy. A. Res. Nerv. & Ment. Dis., Proc., 27: 706–722.

FALCONER, M. A. 1949. Intramedullary trigeminal tractotomy and its place in treatment of facial pain. J. Neurol. Neurosurg. & Psychiat., 12: 297–311.

FARQUHAR, M. G., AND HARTMANN, J. F. 1957. Neuroglial structure and relationships as revealed by electron microscopy. J. Neuropath. & Exper. Neurol., 16: 18–39.

FAULL, R. L. M., AND CARMAN, J. B. 1968. Ascending projections of the substantia nigra in the rat. J. Comp. Neurol., 132: 73–92.

FEINDEL, W., AND GLOOR, P. 1954. Comparisons of electrographic effects of stimulation of the amygdala and brain stem reticular formation in cats. Electroencephalog. & Clin. Neurophysiol., 6: 389–402.

FEINDEL, W., AND PENFIELD, W. 1954. Localization of discharge in temporal lobe automatism. Arch. Neurol. & Psychiat., 72: 605–630.

FELTEN, D. L., LATIES, A. N., AND CARPENTER, M. B. 1974. Monamine-containing cell bodies in the squirrel monkey brain. Am. J. Anat., 139: 153–166.

FERNANDEZ, C., GOLDBERG, J. M., AND ABEND, W. K. 1972. Response to static tilts of peripheral neurons innervating otolith organs of the squirrel monkey. J. Neurophysiol., 35: 978–997.

FERRARO, A. 1925. Contributa sperimentale allo studio della substantia nigra normale e dei suoi rapporti con la corteccia cerebrale e con il corpo striato. Arch. Gen. Neurol. Psichiat., 6: 26–117.

FERRARO, A. 1928. The connections of the pars suboculomotoria of the substantia nigra. Arch. Neurol. & Psychiat., 19: 177–180.

FERRARO, A., AND BARRERA, S. E. 1935. Posterior column fibers and their terminations in the *Macacus rhesus.* J. Comp. Neurol., 62: 507–530.

FINK, R. P., AND HEIMER, L. 1967. Two methods for selective silver impregnation of degenerating axons and their synaptic endings in the central nervous system.

Brain Res., 4: 369–374.

FLECHSIG, P. 1905. Einige Bemerkungen über die Untersuchungsmethoden der Grosshirnrinde, insbesondere des Menschen. Arch. Anat. u. Entwicklungsgeschichte, 337–444.

FLOOD, S., AND JANSEN, J. 1961. On the cerebellar nuclei in the cat. Acta anat., 46: 52–72.

FLUUR, E. 1959. Influences of semicircular ducts on extraocular muscles. Acta Oto-laryng., 149(suppl.): 1–46.

FOERSTER, O. 1927. Die Leitungsbahnen des Schmerzgefühles und die chirurgische Behandlung der Schmerzzustände. Urban und Schwarzenberg, Berlin.

FOERSTER, O. 1929. Der Plexus lumbo-sacralis. In O. BUMKE AND O. FOERSTER (Editors), Handbuch der Neurologie, Suppl., Vol. 2. Julius Springer Verlag, Berlin, pp. 960–970.

FOERSTER, O. 1931. The cerebral cortex in man. Lancet, 2: 309–312.

FOERSTER, O. 1933. The dermatomes in man. Brain, 56: 1–39.

FOERSTER, O. 1936. Sensible cortical Felder. In O. BUMKE AND O. FOERSTER (Editors), Handbuch der Neurologie, Vol. 6. Julius Springer, Berlin, pp. 358–448.

FOERSTER, O. 1936a. Motor cortex in man in the light of Hughlings Jackson's doctrines. Brain, 59: 135–159.

FOERSTER, O. 1936b. Symptomatologie der Erkrankungen des Grosshirns. Motorische Felder und Bahnen. In O. BUMKE AND O. FOERSTER (Editors), Handbuch der Neurologie. Vol. 5. Julius Springer, Berlin, pp. 1–357.

FOERSTER, O. 1936c. Symptomatologie der Erkrankungen des Rückenmarks und seiner Wurzeln. In O. BUMKE AND O. FOERSTER (Editors), Handbuch der Neurologie, Vol. 5. Julius Springer, Berlin, pp. 1–400.

FOERSTER, O., AND GAGEL, O. 1932. Die Vorderseitenstrangdurchschneidung beim Menschen. Eine klinischpathophysiologisch-anatomische Studie. Ztschr. ges. Neurol. u. Psychiat., 138: 1–92.

FOERSTER, O., GAGEL, O., AND SHEEHAN, D. 1933. Veränderungen an den Endösen im Rückenmark des Affen nach Hinterwurzeldurchschneidung. Ztschr. Anat. Entwickl.-Gesch., 101: 553–565.

FOIX, C. 1921. Les lésions anatomiques de la maladie de Parkinson. Rev. neurol., 37: 593–600.

FOIX, C., AND HILLEMAND, J. 1925. Les artères de l'axe encéphalique jusqu'au diencéphale inclusivement. Rev. neurol., 44: 705–739.

FOIX, C. AND HILLEMAND, J. 1925a. Irrigation de la couche optique. Comp. rend. Soc. biol., 92: 52–54.

FOIX, C., AND NICOLESCO, J. 1925. Les Noyaux gris centraux et la région mesencephalo-sous-optique. Masson et Cie, Paris. pp. 581.

FOLEY, J. M., KINNEY, T. D., AND ALEXANDER, L. 1942. The vascular supply of the hypothalamus in man. J. Neuropath. & Exper. Neurol., 1: 265–296.

FOLEY, J. O., AND SCHNITZLEIN, H. N. 1957. The contributions of individual thoracic spinal nerves to the upper cervical sympathetic trunk. J. Comp. Neurol., 108: 109–120.

FONBERG, E. 1968. The role of the amygdaloid nucleus in animal behaviour. Prog. Brain Res., 22: 273–281.

FONBERG, E., AND DELGADO, J. M. R. 1961. Avoidance and alimentary reactions during amygdala stimulation. J. Neurophysiol., 24: 651–664.

FOX, C. A. 1940. Certain basal telencephalic centers in the cat. J. Comp. Neurol., 72: 1–62.

FOX, C. A. 1943. The stria terminalis, longitudinal association bundle and precommissural fornix fibres in the cat. J. Comp. Neurol., 79: 277–295.

FOX, C. A., ANDRADE, A. N., HILLMAN, D. E., AND SCHWYN, R. C. 1971. The spiny neurons in the primate striatum: A Golgi and electron microscopic study. J. Hirnforsch., 13: 181–201.

FOX, C. A., ANDRADE, A. N., LU QUI, I. J., AND RAFOLS, J. A. 1974. The primate globus pallidus: A Golgi and electron microscopic study. J. Hirnforsch., 15: 75–93.

FOX, C. A., ANDRADE, A. N., SCHWYN, R. C., AND RAFOLS, J. A. 1971/72. The aspiny neurons and the glia in the primate striatum: A Golgi and electron microscopic study. J Hirnforsch., 13: 341–362.

FOX, C. A., AND BARNARD, J. W. 1957. A quantitative study of the Purkinje cell, dendritic branchlets and their relationship to afferent fibres. J Anat., 91: 299–313.

FOX, C. A., FISHER, R. R., AND DeSALVA, S. J. 1948. The distribution of the anterior commissure in the monkey (Macaca mulatta). Experimental studies. J. Comp. Neurol., 89: 245–277.

FOX, C. A., HILLMAN, D. E., SIEGESMUND, K. A., AND DUTTA, C. R. 1967. The primate cerebellar cortex: A Golgi and electron microscope study. In C. A. FOX AND R. S. SNIDER (Editors), The Cerebellum, Progress in Brain Research, Vol. 25. Elsevier Publishing Company, Amsterdam.

FOX, C. A., HILLMAN, D. E., SIEGESMUND, K. A., AND SETHER, L. A. 1966. The primate globus pallidus and its feline and avian homologues: A Golgi and electron microscopic study. In R. HASSLER AND H. STEPHAN (Editors), Evolution of the Forebrain. Georg Thieme, Stuttgart, pp. 237–248.

FOX, C. A., McKINLEY, W. A., AND MAGOUN, H. W. 1944. An oscillographic study of olfactory system of cats. J. Neurophysiol., 7:1–16.

FOX, C. A., AND SCHMITZ, J. T. 1944. The substantia nigra and the entopeduncular nucleus in the cat. J. Comp. Neurol., 80: 323–334.

FOX, C. A., SIEGESMUND, K. A., AND DUTTA, C. R. 1964. The Purkinje cell dendritic branchlets and their relation with the parallel fibers: light and electron microscopic observations. In M. M. COHEN AND R. S. SNIDER, (Editors), Morphological and Biochemical Correlates of Neural Activity. Harper and Row, New York, Ch. 7, pp. 112–141.

FRANCOEUR, J., AND OLSZEWSKI, J. 1968. Axonal reaction and axoplasmic flow as studied by radioautography. Neurology, 18: 178–184.

FRANTZEN, E., AND OLIVARIUS, B. I. F. 1957. On thrombosis of the basilar artery. Acta psychiat. & neurol. scandinav., 32: 431–439.

FREDRICKSON, J. M., FIGGE, U., SCHEID, P., AND KORNHUBER, H. H. 1966. Vestibular nerve projection to the cerebral cortex of the rhesus monkey. Exper. Brain Res., 2: 318–327.

FREEMAN, L. W. 1952. Return of function after complete transection of the spinal cord of the rat, cat and dog. Am. Surgeon, 136: 193–205.

FREEMAN, W. AND WATTS, J. W. 1947. Retrograde degeneration of the thalamus following prefrontal lobotomy. J. Comp. Neurol., 86: 65–93.

FREEMAN, W., AND WATTS, J. W. 1948. The thalamic projection to the frontal lobe. A. Res. Nerv. & Ment. Dis., Proc., 27: 200–209.

FREEMAN, W., AND WATTS, J. W. 1949. Psychosurgery, Intelligence, Emotion and Social Behavior Following Prefrontal Lobotomy for Mental Disorders, Ed. 2. Charles C Thomas, Publisher, Springfield, Ill., 337 pp.

FRENCH, J. D., von AMERONGEN, F. K., AND MAGOUN, H. W. 1952. An activating system in the brain stem of monkey. A.M.A. Arch. Neurol. & Psychiat., 68: 577–590.

FRENCH, J. D., HERNANDEZ-PEON, R., AND LIVINGSTON, R. B. 1955. Projections from cortex to cephalic brain stem (reticular formation) in monkey. J. Neurophysiol., 18: 74–95.

FRENCH, J. D., AND MAGOUN, H. W. 1952. Effects of

chronic lesions in central cephalic brain stem of monkeys. A. M. A. Arch. Neurol. & Psychiat., 68: 591–604.

FRENCH, J. D., VERZEANO, M., AND MAGOUN, H. W. 1953. An extralemniscal sensory system in the brain. A. M. A. Arch. Neurol. & Psychiat., 69: 505–518.

FRIEDE, R. 1961. A histochemical study of DPN-diaphorase in human white matter; with some notes on myelination. J. Neurochem., 8: 17–30.

FRIEDE, R. L. 1962. The cytochemistry of normal and reactive astrocytes. J. Neuropath. & Exper. Neurol., 21: 471–478.

FRIEDMANN, U., AND ELKELES, A. 1932. Weitere Untersuchungen über die Permeabilität der Bluthirnschranke. Ztschr. ges. exper. Med., 80: 212–234.

FRIEND, D. S., AND FARQUHAR, M. G. 1967. Functions of coated vesicles during protein absorption in the rat vas deferens. J. Cell Biol., 35: 357–376.

FRIGYESI, T. L., AND PURPURA, D. P. 1964. Functional properties of synaptic pathways influencing transmission in the specific cerebello-thalamocortical projection system. Exper. Neurol., 10: 305–324.

FRY, W. J., KRUMINS, R., FRY, F. J., THOMAS, G., BORBELY, S., AND ADES, H. 1963. Origins and distribution of some efferent pathways from the mammillary nuclei of the cat. J. Comp. Neurol., 120: 195–258.

FUJITA, S. 1964. Analysis of neuron differentiation in the central nervous system by tritiated thymidine autoradiography. J. Comp. Neurol., 122: 311–327.

FULTON, J. F. 1949. Functional Localization in the Frontal Lobes and Cerebellum. Clarendon Press, Oxford.

FULTON, J. F., AND INGRAHAM, F. D. 1929. Emotional disturbances following experimental lesions of the base of the brain (pre-chiasmal). J. Physiol., 67: 27–28.

FULTON, J. F., AND KELLER, A. D. 1932. The Sign of Babinski. A Study of the Evolution of Cortical Dominance in Primates. Charles C Thomas, Springfield, Ill., 165 pp.

FULTON, J. F., AND KENNARD, M. A. 1934. A study of flaccid and spastic paralysis produced by lesions of the cerebral cortex in primates. A. Res. Nerv. & Ment. Dis. Proc., 13: 158–210.

FULTON, J. F., AND PI-SUÑER, J. 1927–28. A note concerning the probable function of various afferent end-organs in skeletal muscle. Am. J. Physiol., 83: 554–562.

FUXE, K., AND ANDÉN, N. E. 1966. Studies on the central monoamine neurons with special reference to the nigroneostriatal dopamine neuron system. In E. COSTA et al. (Editors), Biochemistry and Pharmacology of the Basal Ganglia. Raven Press, Hewlitt, N. Y., pp. 123–129.

FUXE, K., AND HÖKFELT, T. 1970. Central monaminergic systems and hypothalamic function. In L. MARTIN et al. (Editors), The Hypothalamus. Academic Press, New York, pp. 123–138.

FUXE, K., HÖKFELT, T., AND NILSSON, O. 1964. Observations on the cellular localization of dopamine in the caudate nucleus of the rat. Ztschr. Zellforsch. mikrosk. Anat., 63: 701–706.

GABE, M. 1966. Neurosecretion. Translated by R. Crawford. Pergamon Press, Ltd., Oxford, pp. 427–736.

GACEK, R. R. 1961. The efferent cochlear bundle in man. Arch. Otolaryng., 74: 690–694.

GALAMBOS, R. 1956. Suppression of auditory nerve activity by stimulation of efferent fibers to cochlea. J. Neurophysiol., 19: 424–437.

GALLOWAY, J. R., AND GREITZ, T. 1960. The medial and lateral choroid arteries: An anatomic and roentgenographic study. Acta radiol., 53: 353–356.

GAMBLE, H. J. 1964. Comparative electron-microscopic observations on the connective tissues of a peripheral nerve and a spinal nerve root in the rat. J. Anat., 98: 17–25.

GAMBLE, H. J., AND EAMES, R. A. 1964. An electron microscope study of the connective tissues of human peripheral nerve. J. Anat., 98: 655–663.

GARCIA-BENGOCHEA, F., CORRIGAN, R., MORGANE, P., RUSSELL, D., AND HEATH, R. 1951. Studies on the function of the temporal lobes: I. The section of the fornix. Tr. Am. Neurol. A., 76: 238–239.

GARDNER, E. 1944. The distribution and termination of nerve fibers in the knee joint of the cat. J. Comp. Neurol., 80: 11–32.

GAREY, L. J., JONES, E. G., AND POWELL, T. P. S. 1968. Interrelationships of striate and extrastriate cortex with the primary relay sites of the visual pathway. J. Neurol. Neurosurg. & Psychiat., 31: 135–157.

GARVEN, H. S. D. 1925. The nerve endings in the Panniculus carnosus of the hedgehog, with special reference to the sympathetic innervation of striated muscle. Brain, 48: 380–441.

GASKELL, W. H. 1916. The Involuntary Nervous System. Longmans, Green and Company, London.

GASSER, G. 1961. Basic Neuro-Pathological Technique. Blackwell Scientific Publications, Oxford pp. 39–74.

GASSER, H. A., AND GRUNDFEST, H. 1939. Axon diameters in relation to the spike dimensions and the conduction velocity in mammalian A fibers. Am. J. Physiol., 127: 393–414.

GASTAUT, H. 1954. The brain stem and cerebral electrogenesis in relation to consciousness. In J. F. DELAFRESNAYE (Editor), Brain Mechanisms and Consciousness. Blackwell Scientific Publications, Oxford, pp. 249–279.

GAZZANIGA, M. S. 1970. The Bisected Brain. Appleton-Century-Crofts, New York.

GAZZANIGA, M. S., BOGEN, J. E., AND SPERRY, R. W. 1965. Observations on visual perception after disconnexion of the cerebral hemispheres in man. Brain, 88: 221–236.

GAZZANIGA, M. S., AND SPERRY, R. W. 1967. Language after section of the cerebral commissures. Brain, 90: 131–148.

GEIGER, R. S. 1958. Subcultures of adult mammalian brain cortex in vitro. Exper. Cell Res., 14: 541–566.

GELFAN, S. 1964. Neuronal interdependence. In J. C. ECCLES AND J. P. SCHADÉ (Editors), Progress in Brain Research, Vol. 11. Elsevier Publishing Company, Amsterdam, pp. 238–260.

GENIEC, P., AND MOREST, D. K. 1971. The neuronal architecture of the human posterior colliculus. Acta otolaryng., 295(suppl.): 1–33.

GERARD, R. W., MARSHALL, W. H., AND SAUL, L. J. 1936. Electrical activity of the cat's brain. Arch. Neurol. Psychiat., 36: 675–738.

GEREBTZOFF, M. A. 1940. Recherches sur la projection corticale du labyrinth. I. Des effets de la stimulation labyrinthique sur l'activité électrique de l'écorce cérébrale. Arch. internat. physiol., 50: 365–378.

GEREN, B. B. 1954. The formation from the Schwann cell surface of the myelin in peripheral nerves of chick embryos. Exper. Cell Res., 7: 558–562.

GERSTMANN, J. 1940. Syndrome of finger agnosia; disorientation for right and left, agraphia and acalculia. Arch. Neurol. & Psychiat., 44: 398–408.

GESCHWIND, N. 1965. Disconnexion syndromes in animals and man. I. Brain, 88: 237–294.

GESCHWIND, N. 1965a. Disconnexion syndromes in animals and man. II. Brain, 88: 585–644.

GESCHWIND, N. 1970. The organization of language and the brain. Science, 170: 940–944.

GESCHWIND, N., AND KAPLAN, E. 1962. A human cerebral deconnection syndrome. Neurology, 12: 675–685.

GILBERT, G. J. 1960. The subcommissural organ. Neurology, 10: 138–142.

GILBERT, G. J., AND GLASER, G. H. 1961. On the nervous system integration of water and salt metabolism. Arch. Neurol., 5: 179–196.

GILLILAN, L. 1958. The arterial blood supply of the human spinal cord. J. Comp. Neurol., 110: 75–103.

GIOLLI, R. A., AND GUTHRIE, M. D. 1969. The primary optic projections in the rabbit. An experimental degeneration study. J. Comp. Neurol., 136: 99–126.

GIOLLI, R. A., AND GUTHRIE, M. D. 1971. Organization of subcortical projections of visual areas I and II in the rabbit. An experimental degeneration study. J. Comp. Neurol., 142: 351–376.

GIOLLI, R. A., AND TIGGES, J. 1970. The primary optic pathways and nuclei of primates. In C. R. NOBACK AND W. MONTAGNA (Editors), The Primate Brain, Advances in Primatology, Vol. 1. Appleton-Century-Crofts, New York, Ch. 2, pp. 29–54.

GLEES, P. 1945. The interrelation of the striopallidum and the thalamus in the macaque monkey. Brain, 68: 331–346.

GLEES, P. 1946. Terminal degeneration within the central nervous system as studied by a new silver method. J. Neuropath. & Exper. Neurol. 5: 54–59.

GLEES, P. 1955. Neuroglia. Morphology and Function. Charles C Thomas, Publisher, Springfield, Ill.

GLEES, P. 1961. Experimental Neurology. Oxford University, Press, London.

GLEES, P., AND GRIFFITH, H. B. 1952. Bilateral destruction of the hippocampus (cornu ammonis) in a case of dementia. Monatsschr. Psychiat. u. Neurol., 123: 193–204.

GLEES, P., AND NAUTA, W. J. H. 1955. A critical review of studies on axonal and terminal degeneration. Monatsschr. Psychiat. u. Neurol., 129: 74–91.

GLEES, P., AND WALL, P. D. 1946. Fibre connections of the subthalamic region and the centro-median nucleus of the thalamus. Brain, 69: 195–211.

GLOOR, P. 1955. Electrophysiological studies on the connections of the amygdaloid nucleus in the cat. Electroencephalog. & Clin. Neurophysiol., 7: 243–264.

GLOOR, P. 1960. Amygdala. In J. FIELD (Editor), Handbook of Physiology, Section 1, Vol. II. American Physiological Society, Washington, D. C., Ch. 57, pp. 1395–1420.

GLOOR, P. 1972. Temporal lobe epilepsy: Its possible contribution to the understanding of the functional significance of the amygdala and of its interaction with neocortical-temporal mechanisms. In B. E. ELEFTHERIOU (Editor), The Neurobiology of the Amygdala. Plenum Press, New York, pp. 423–457.

GLUSMAN, M. 1974. The hypothalamic "savage" syndrome. A. Res. Nerv. & Ment. Dis., Proc., 52: 52–92.

GOBEL, S., AND PURVIS, M. B. 1972. Anatomical studies of the organization of the spinal V nucleus: The deep bundles and the spinal V tract. Brain Res., 48: 27–44.

GOLDBERG, J. M., AND NEFF, W. D. 1961. Frequency discrimination after bilateral ablation of cortical auditory areas. J. Neurophysiol., 24: 119–128.

GOLDSTEIN, M. 1968. The auditory periphery. In V. B. MOUNTCASTLE (Editor), Medical Physiology, Ed. 12. C. V. Mosby Company, St. Louis, Ch. 64, pp. 1465–1498.

GOLGI, C. 1882–1885. Sulla fina anatomia degli organi centrali del sistema nervoso. Riv. sper. freniat. med. leg., 8: 165–195, 361–391; 9: 1–17, 161–192, 385–402; 11: 72–123, 193–220.

GOLGI, C. 1883. Recherches sur l'histologie des centres nerveux. Arch. ital. biol., 3: 285–317; 4: 92–123.

GOLGI, C. 1894. Untersuchungen über den feineren Bau des centralen und peripherischen Nervensystems. Gustav Fischer, Jena.

GOLGI, C. 1898. Sur la structure des cellules nerveuses. Arch. ital. biol., 30: 60–71.

GORDON, B. 1972. The superior colliculus of the brain. Sc. Am., 227: 72–82.

GORDON, G., AND JUKES, M. G. M. 1964. Dual organization of exteroceptive components of the cat's gracile nucleus. J. Physiol., 173: 263–290.

GORDON, G., AND JUKES, M. G. M. 1964a. Descending influences on the exteroceptive organization of the cat's gracile nucleus. J. Physiol., 173: 291–319.

GORDON, G., AND PAINE, P. H. 1960. Functional organization in nucleus gracilis of the cat. J. Physiol., 153: 331–349.

GRANIT, R. 1955. Receptors and Sensory Perception. Yale University Press, New Haven, Conn.

GRANIT, R., AND KAADA, B. R. 1952. Influence of stimulation of central nervous structures on muscle spindles in cat. Acta physiol. scandinav., 27: 130–160.

GRANT, G. 1962. Projection of the external cuneate nucleus onto the cerebellum in the cat: An experimental study using silver methods. Exper. Neurol., 5: 179–195.

GRANT, G. 1962a. Spinal course and somatotopically localized termination of the spinocerebellar tracts. An experimental study in the cat. Acta physiol. scandinav., 56: Suppl. 193: 1–45.

GRANT, G., AND OSCARSSON, O. 1966. Mass discharges evoked in the olivocerebellar tract on stimulation of muscle and skin nerves. Exper. Brain Res., 1: 329–337.

GRANT, G., AND REXED, B. 1958. Dorsal spinal root afferents to Clarke's column. Brain, 81: 567–576.

GRAY, E. G. 1961. The granule cells, mossy synapses and Purkinje spinal synapses of the cerebellum: Light and electron microscopic observations. J. Anat., 95: 345–356.

GRAY, E. G., AND GUILLERY, R. W. 1961. The basis for silver staining of synapses of the mammalian spinal cord: A light and electron microscope study. J. Physiol., 157: 581–588.

GRAY, E. G., AND GUILLERY, R. W. 1966. Synaptic morphology in the normal and degenerating nervous system. Internat. Rev. Cytol., 19: 111–182.

GRAY, J. A. B. 1959. Initiation of impulses at receptors. In J. FIELD (Editor), Handbook of Physiology, Section I, Vol. 1. American Physiological Society, Washington, D. C., Ch. 4, pp. 123–145.

GRAYBIEL, A. M. 1972. Some extrageniculate visual pathways in the cat. Invest. Ophth., 11: 322–332.

GRAZER, F. M., AND CLEMENTE, C. D. 1957. Developing blood-brain barrier to trypan blue. Proc. Soc. Exper. Biol. & Med., 94: 758–760.

GREEN, J. D. 1958. The rhinencephalon: Aspects of its relation to behavior and the reticular activating system. In H. H. JASPER et al. (Editors), Reticular Formation of the Brain. Henry Ford Hospital International Symposium. Little, Brown and Company, Boston, pp. 607–619.

GREEN, J. D. 1960. The hippocampus. In J. FIELD (Editor), Handbook of Physiology, Section I, Vol. II. American Physiological Society, Washington, D. C., Ch. 56, pp. 1373–1389.

GREEN, J. D. 1964. The hippocampus. Physiol. Rev., 44: 561–608.

GREEN, J. D., CLEMENTE, C. A., AND DE GROOT, J. 1957. Rhinencephalic lesions and behavior in cats. J. Comp. Neurol., 108: 505–545.

GREEN, J. D., AND HARRIS, G. W. 1949. Observation of the hypophysio-portal vessels of the living rat. J. Physiol., 108: 359–361.

GREEN, J. D., AND SHIMAMOTO, T. 1953. Hippocampal seizures and their propagation. Arch. Neurol. & Psychiat., 70: 687–702.

GREEN, J. R., DUISBERG, R. E. H., AND McGRATH, W. B. 1951. Focal epilepsy of psychomotor type. A preliminary report of observations on effects of surgical therapy. J. Neurosurg., 8: 157–172.

GREEN, J. R., DUISBERG, R. E. H., AND McGRATH, W. B. 1952. Orbitofrontal lobotomy with reference to effects on 55 psychotic patients. J. Neurosurg., 9: 579–587.

GREENE, J., AND JAMPEL, R.   1966.   Muscle spindles in the extraocular muscles of the Macaque. J. Comp. Neurol., 126: 547–550.

GREER, M. A., AND ERWIN, H. L.   1956.   Evidence of separate hypothalamic centers controlling corticotropin and thyrotropin secretion by the pituitary. Endocrinology, 58: 665–670.

GREVING, R.   1935.   Makroskopische Anatomie und Histologie des vegetativen Nervensystems. In O. BUMKE and O. FOERSTER (Editors), Handbuch der Neurologie, Vol. 1. Julius Springer, Berlin, pp. 811–886.

DE GROOT, J., AND HARRIS, G. W.   1950.   Hypothalamic control of the anterior pituitary gland and blood lymphocytes. J. Physiol., 111: 335–346.

GRUNDFEST, H.   1939.   The properties of mammalian B fibers. Am. J. Physiol. 127: 252–262.

GRUNDFEST, H.   1940.   Bioelectric potentials. Ann. Rev. Physiol., 2: 213–242.

GRUNSTEIN, A. M.   1911.   Zur Frage von den Leitungsbahnen des Corpus striatum. Neurol. Zentralbl., 30: 659–665.

GUILLERY, R. W.   1956.   Degeneration in the posterior commissural fornix and the mammillary peduncle of the rat. J. Anat., 90: 350–370.

GUILLERY, R. W.   1957.   Degeneration in the hypothalamic connexions of the albino rat. J. Anat., 91: 91–115.

GUILLERY, R. W.   1967.   A light and electron microscopic study of neurofibrils and neurofilaments at neuro-neuronal junctions in the lateral geniculate nucleus of the cat. Am. J. Anat., 120: 583–604.

GUTMANN, E., GUTTMANN, L., MEDAWAR, P. B., AND YOUNG, J. Z.   1942.   Rate of regeneration of nerve. J. Exper. Biol., 19: 14–44.

GUTMANN, E., AND YOUNG, J. Z.   1944.   The re-innervation of muscle after various periods of atrophy. J. Anat., 78: 15–43.

GUTTMANN, L.   1946.   Rehabilitation after injuries to spinal cord and cauda equina. Brit. J. Phys. Med., 9: 162–171.

GUTTMANN, L.   1952.   Studies on reflex activity of the isolated cord in the spinal man. J. Nerv. & Ment. Dis., 116: 957–972.

HA, H., AND LIU, C. N.   1968.   Cell origin of the ventral spinocerebellar tract. J. Comp. Neurol., 133:185–205.

HA, H., AND MORIN, F.   1964.   Comparative anatomical observations of the cervical nucleus, n. cervicalis lateralis, of some primates. Anat. Rec., 148: 374 (abstract).

HAGBARTH, K. E., AND KERR, D. I. B.   1954.   Central influences on spinal afferent conduction. J. Neurophysiol., 17: 295–307.

HÄGGQVIST, G.   1937.   Faseranalytische Studien über die Pyramidenbahn. Acta psychiat. et neurol., 12: 457–466.

HALL, E. A.   1963.   Efferent connections of the basal and lateral nuclei of the amygdala in the cat. Am. J. Anat., 113: 139–151.

HAMILTON, W. J., BOYD, J. D., AND MOSSMAN, H. W.   1962.   Human Embryology. Prenatal Development of Form and Function. Williams & Wilkins Company, Baltimore, Ch. XII, pp. 315–388.

HAMILTON, W. J., AND MOSSMAN, H. W.   1972.   Human Embryology. Williams & Wilkins Company, Baltimore.

HAMLYN, L. H.   1954.   The effect of preganglionic section on the neurons of the superior cervical ganglion in rabbits. J. Anat., 88: 184–191.

HAMMOND, W. A.   1871.   A Treatise on Diseases of the Nervous System. D. Appleton and Company, New York, pp. 655–662.

HÁMORI, J., AND SZENTÁGOTHAI, J.   1966.   Identification under the electron microscope of climbing fibers and their synaptic contacts. Exper. Brain Res., 1: 65–81.

HAMPEL, C. W.   1935.   The effect of denervation on the

sensitivity to adrenaline of the smooth muscle in the nictitating membrane of the cat. Am. J. Physiol., 61: 611–621.

HANAWAY, J.   1967.   Formation and differentiation of the external granular layer of the chick cerebellum. J. Comp. Neurol., 131: 1–14.

HANBERY, J., AJMONE-MARSAN, C., AND DILWORTH, M.   1954.   Pathways of non-specific thalamo-cortical projection system. Electroencephalog. & Clin. Neurophysiol., 6: 103–118.

HANBERY, J. AND JASPER, H.   1953.   Independence of diffuse thalamo-cortical projection system shown by specific nuclear destructions. J. Neurophysiol., 16: 252–271.

HAND, P. J.   1966.   Lumbosacral dorsal root terminations in the nucleus gracilis of the cat. Some observations on terminal degeneration in other medullary sensory nuclei. J. Comp. Neurol., 126: 137–156.

HARE, W. K., AND HINSEY, J. C.   1940.   Reaction of dorsal root ganglion cells to section of peripheral and central processes. J. Comp. Neurol., 73: 489–502.

HARRIS, G. W.   1948.   Electrical stimulation of the hypothalamus and the mechanism of neural control of the adenohypophysis. J. Physiol., 107: 418–429.

HARRIS, G. W.   1955.   Neural Control of the Pituitary Gland. Edward Arnold and Company, London.

HARRIS, G. W.   1956.   Hypothalamic control of the anterior lobe of the hypophysis. In W. S. FIELDS et al. (Editors), Hypothalamic-Hypophysial Interrelationships (Symposium). Charles C Thomas, Publisher, Springfield, Ill., pp. 31–42.

HARRIS, G. W., AND GEORGE, R.   1969.   Neurohumoral control of the adenohypophysis and regulation of the secretion of TSH, ACTH and growth hormone. In W. HAYMAKER et al. (Editors), The Hypothalamus. Charles C Thomas, Publisher, Springfield, Ill., Ch. 10, pp. 326–388.

HARRIS, G. W., AND WOODS, J. W.   1958.   The effect of electrical stimulation of the hypothalamus or pituitary gland on thyroid activity. J. Physiol., 143: 246–274.

HARTING, J. K., HALL, W. C., DIAMOND, I. T., AND MARTIN, G. F.   1973.   Anterograde degeneration study of the superior colliculus in Tupaia glis. Evidence for a subdivision between superficial and deep layers. J. Comp. Neurol., 148: 361–386.

HARTMANN, J. F.   1956.   Electron microscopy of mitochondria in the central nervous system. J. Biophys. & Biochem. Cytol., 2(suppl.): 373–378.

HASSLER, O.   1966.   Deep cerebral venous system in man. A microangiographic study on its areas of drainage and its anastomoses with the superficial cerebral veins. Neurology, 16: 505–511.

HASSLER, O.   1967.   Venous anatomy of human hindbrain. Arch. Neurol., 16: 404–409.

HASSLER, O.   1967a.   Arterial pattern of human brain stem. Normal appearance and deformation in expanding supratentorial conditions. Neurology, 17: 368–375.

HASSLER, R.   1939.   Zur pathologischen Anatomie des senilen und des parkinsonistischen Tremor. J. Psychol. u. Neurol., 49: 193–230.

HASSLER, R.   1950.   Über Kleinhirnprojektionen zum Mittelhirn und Thalamus beim Menschen. Deutsche Ztschr. Nervenh., 163: 629–671.

HATSCHEK, R.   1907.   Zur vergleichenden Anatomie des Nucleus ruber tegmenti. Arb. Neurol. Inst. Wiener Univ., 15: 89–135.

HAUGSTED, H.   1956.   Occlusion of the basilar artery. Diagnosis by vertebral angiography during life. Neurology, 6: 823–828.

HAY, E. D., AND REVEL, J. P.   1963.   The fine structure of the DNP component of the nucleus. An electron microscope study utilizing autoradiography to localize DNA synthesis. J. Cell Biol., 16: 29–51.

HAYMAKER, W. 1956. *Bing's Local Diagnosis in Neurological Diseases.* C. V. Mosby Company, St. Louis, pp. 57–62 and 105–112.

HAYMAKER, W. 1969. Hypothalamo-pituitary neural pathways and the circulatory system of the pituitary. In W. HAYMAKER et al. (Editors), *The Hypothalamus.* Charles C Thomas, Publisher, Springfield, Ill., Ch. 6, pp. 219–250.

HAYMAKER, W., AND WOODHALL, B. 1945. *Peripheral Nerve Injuries; Principles of Diagnosis.* W. B. Saunders Company, Philadelphia, 227 pp.

HEAD, H. 1905. The afferent nervous system from a new aspect. Brain, 28: 99–116.

HEAD, H. 1920. *Studies in Neurology.* Oxford University Press, London. 2 vols.

HEAD, H. AND HOLMES, G. 1911. Sensory disturbances from cerebral lesions. Brain, 34: 102–254.

HEATH, J. W. 1947. Clinicopathologic aspects of Parkinsonian states. A. M. A. Arch. Neurol. & Psychiat., 58: 484–497.

HEATH, R. G., MONROE, R. R., AND MICKEL, W. 1955. Stimulation of the amygdaloid nucleus in a schizophrenic patient. Am. J. Psychiat., 111: 862–863.

HEIMER, L. 1970. Selective silver-impregnation of degenerating axoplasm. In W. J. H. NAUTA and S. O. E. EBBESSON (Editors), *Contemporary Research Methods in Neuroanatomy.* Springer Verlag, New York, pp. 106–131.

HEIMER, L., AND NAUTA, W. J. H. 1967. The hypothalamic distribution of the stria terminalis in the rat. Anat. Rec., 157: 259.

HEIMER, L., AND NAUTA, W. J. H. 1969. The hypothalamic distribution of the stria terminalis in the rat. Brain Res., 13: 284–297.

HEINBECKER, P., BISHOP, G. H., AND O'LEARY, J. L. 1936. Functional and histologic studies of somatic and autonomic nerves of man. Arch. Neurol. & Psychiat., 35: 1233–1255.

HELLER, H. 1966. The hormone content of the vertebrate hypothalamo-neurohypophysial system. Brit. M. Bull., 22: 227–231.

HENDRICKSON, A. M., WILSON, M. E., AND TOYNE, M. J. 1970. The distribution of optic nerve fibers in *Macaca mulatta.* Brain Res., 23: 425–427.

HENNEMAN, E. 1968. Peripheral mechanisms involved in the control of muscle. In V. B. MOUNTCASTLE (Editor), *Medical Physiology.* C. V. Mosby Company, St. Louis, Ch. 73, pp. 1697–1716.

HENSCHEN, S. E. 1926. On the function of the right hemisphere of the brain in relation to the left in speech, music and calculation. Brain, 49: 110–123.

HERN, J. E. C., LANDGREN, S., AND PHILLIPS, C. G. 1960. Corticofugal discharges evoked by surface-anodal and surface-cathodal stimulation of the baboon's brain. J. Physiol., 154: 70P–71P.

HERN, J. E. C., AND PHILLIPS, C. G. 1959. Cortical thresholds for minimal synaptic action on cat motoneurons. J. Physiol., 149: 24P–25P.

HERNÁNDEZ-PEON, R., AND HAGBARTH, K. E. 1955. Interaction between afferent and cortically induced reticular responses. J. Neurophysiol., 18: 44–55.

HERNDON, R. M. 1964. The fine structure of the cerebellum. II. The stellate neurons, granule cells and glia. J. Cell Biol., 23: 277–293.

HERREN, R. Y., AND ALEXANDER, L. 1939. Sulcal and intrinsic blood vessels of human spinal cord. Arch. Neurol. & Psychiat., 41: 678–687.

HERRICK, C. J. 1948. *The Brain of the Tiger Salamander.* University of Chicago Press, Chicago, pp. 141–142 and 175.

HERRICK, C. J., AND COGHILL, G. E. 1915. The development of reflex mechanisms in Amblystoma. J. Comp. Neurol., 25: 65–85.

HERZ, E. 1931. Die amyostatischen Unruheerscheinun-

gen. J. Psychol. u. Neurol., 43: 3–182.

HESS, W. R. 1948. *Die Funktionelle Organisation des Vegetativen Nervensystems.* Benno Schwabe and Company, Basel.

HESS, W. R. 1954. *Diencephalon, Autonomic and Extrapyramidal Functions.* Grune & Stratton, Inc., New York, 79 pp.

HETHERINGTON, A. W., AND RANSON, S. W. 1940. Hypothalamic lesions and adiposity in the rat. Anat. Rec., 78: 149–172.

HEWITT, W. 1961. The development of the human internal capsule and lentiform nucleus. J. Anat., 95: 191–199.

HILD, W. 1956. Neurosecretion in the central nervous system. In W. S. FIELDS et al. (Editors), *Hypothalamic-Hypophysial Interrelationships.* Charles C Thomas, Publisher, Springfield, Ill., pp. 17–25.

HILLARP, N.-Å. 1959. The construction and functional organization of the autonomic innervation apparatus. Acta physiol. scandinav., 46: suppl. 157, 1–38.

HILLARP, N.-Å. 1960. Peripheral autonomic mechanisms. In J. FIELD et al. (Editors), *Handbook of Physiology,* Section I, Vol. II. American Physiological Society, Washington D. C., Ch. 38, pp. 979–1006.

HILTON, S. M., AND ZBROZYNA, A. 1963. Defence reaction from the amygdala and its afferent connections. J. Physiol., 165: 160–173.

HINES, M. 1936. The anterior border of the monkey's (*Macaca mulatta*) motor cortex and the production of spasticity. Am. J. Physiol., 116: 76.

HINES, M. 1937. The "motor" cortex. Bull. Johns Hopkins Hosp., 60: 313–336.

HINES, M. 1949. Significance of the precentral motor cortex. In P. C. BUCY (Editor), *The Precentral Motor Cortex.* University of Illinois Press, Urbana, Ch. 18, 461–494.

HINMAN, A., AND CARPENTER, M. B. 1959. Efferent fiber projections of the red nucleus in the cat. J. Comp. Neurol., 113: 61–82.

HIRSCH, H. V. B., AND SPINELLI, D. N. 1970. Visual experience modifies distribution of horizontally and vertically oriented receptive fields in cat. Science, 168: 869–871.

HOCHSTETTER, F. 1919. *Beiträge zur Entwicklungsgeschichte des menschlichen Gehirns,* Vol. I. F. Deuticke, Vienna and Leipzig.

HOFF, E. C. 1932. Central nerve terminals in the mammalian spinal cord and their examination by experimental degeneration. Proc. Roy. Soc., London, ser. B, 111: 175–188.

HOFF, E. C. 1932a. The distribution of the spinal terminals (boutons) of the pyramidal tract, determined by experimental degeneration. Proc. Roy. Soc. London, ser. B, 111: 226–237.

HOFF, E. C., AND HOFF, H. E. 1934. Spinal termination of the projection fibers from the motor cortex of primates. Brain, 57: 454–474.

HÖKFELT, T. 1967. The possible ultrastructural identification of tubero-infundibular dopamine-containing nerve endings in the median eminence of the rat. Brain Res., 5: 121–123.

HÖKFELT, T. 1967a. On the ultrastructural localization of noradrenaline in the central nervous system. Ztschr. Zellforsch. mikroskop. Anat., 79: 110–117.

HÖKFELT, T. 1967b. Ultrastructural studies on adrenergic nerve terminals in the albino rat iris after pharmacological and experimental treatment. Acta physiol. scandinav., 69: 125–126.

HÖKFELT, T., AND FUXE, K. 1969. Cerebellar monoamine nerve terminals: A new type of afferent fiber to the cerebellar cortex. Exper. Brain Res., 9: 63–72.

HÖKFELT, T., AND LJUNGDAHL, A. 1972. Application of cytochemical techniques to the study of suspected transmitter substances in the nervous system. In E. COSTA et *al.* (Editors), *Studies of Neurotransmitters at the Synaptic Level*. Raven Press, New York, pp. 1–36.

HÖKFELT, T., AND UNGERSTEDT, U. 1969. Electron and fluorescence microscopical studies on the nucleus caudatus putamen of the rat after unilateral lesions of ascending nigro-neostriatal dopamine neurons. Acta physiol. scandinav., **76**: : 415–426.

HÖKFELT, T., AND VAN ORDEN, L. S. 1972. Ultrastructure of amine-containing neurons In B. FALCK and R. Y. MOORE (Editors), *Fluorescence Histochemistry of Biogenic Amines*. Academic Press, New York.

HOLLÄNDER, H. 1972. Projection of the visual cortex to the lateral geniculate nucleus in the cat. In T. L. FRIGYESI *et al.* (Editors), *Corticothalamic Projections and Sensorimotor Activities*. Raven Press, New York, pp. 475–484.

HOLMES, G. 1901. The nervous system of the dog without a forebrain. J. Physiol., **27**: 1–25.

HOLMES, G. 1922. The Croonian Lectures on the clinical symptoms of cerebellar disease and their interpretation. Lancet, **1**: 1177–1182.

HOLMES, G. 1939. The cerebellum of man. Brain, **62**: 1–30.

HOLMES, G., AND MAY, W. P. 1909. On the exact origin of the pyramidal tract in man and other mammals. Brain, **32**: 1–43.

HOLMES, G., AND STEWART, T. G. 1908. On the connections of the inferior olive with the cerebellum in man. Brain, **31**: 125–137.

HOLMES, W. 1943. Silver staining of nerve axons in paraffin sections. Anat. Rec., **86**: 157–187.

HOLTZMAN, E., NOVIKOFF, A. B., AND VILLAVERDE, H. 1967. Lysosomes and GERL in normal and chromatolytic neurons of rat ganglion nodosum. J. Cell Biol., **33**: 419–435.

HONGO, T., JANKOWSKA, E., AND LUNDBERG, A. 1969. The rubrospinal tract. I. Effects on alpha-motoneurons innervating hindlimb muscles in cats. Exper. Brain Res., **7**: 344–364.

HONGO, T., JANKOWSKA, E., AND LUNDBERG, A. 1969a. The rubrospinal tract. II. Facilitation of interneuronal transmission in reflex paths to motor neurons. Exper. Brain Res., **7**: 365–391.

HOOKER, D. 1944. *The Origin of Overt Behavior*. University of Michigan, Ann Arbor.

HORNYKIEWICZ, O. 1966. Metabolism of brain dopamine in human parkinsonism: Neurochemical and clinical aspects. In E. COSTA *et al.* (Editors), *Biochemistry and Pharmacology of the Basal Ganglia*. Raven Press, Hewlett, N. Y., pp. 171–185.

HÖRSTADIUS, S. 1950. *The Neural Crest*. Oxford University Press, London.

HORSTMANN, E., AND MEVES, H. 1959. Die Feinstruktur des molekularen Rindengraues und ihre physiologische Bedeutung. Ztschr. Zellforsch., **49**: 569–604.

HOUK, J., AND HENNEMAN, E. 1967. Responses of tendon organs to active contractions of the soleus muscle of the cat. J. Neurophysiol., **30**: 466–481.

HOYT, W. F., AND LUIS, O. 1962. Visual fiber anatomy in the infrageniculate pathway of the primate. Arch. Ophth., **68**: 94–106.

HOYT, W. F., AND LUIS, O. 1963. The primate chiasm: Details of visual fiber organization studied by silver impregnation techniques. Arch. Ophth., **70**: 69–85.

HUBBARD, J. I., AND OSCARSSON, O. 1962. Localization of the cell bodies of the ventral spinocerebellar tract in lumbar segments of the cat. J. Comp. Neurol., **118**: 199–204.

HUBEL, D. H. 1963. The visual cortex of the brain. Sc. Am. **209**: (No. 5) 54–62.

HUBEL, D. H., AND WIESEL, T. N. 1959. Receptive fields of single neurons in the cat's striate cortex. J. Physiol., **148**: 574–591.

HUBEL, D. H., AND WIESEL, T. N. 1961. Integrative action in the cat's lateral geniculate body. J. Physiol., **155**: 385–398.

HUBEL, D. H., AND WIESEL, T. N. 1962. Receptive fields, binocular interaction and functional architecture in the cat's visual cortex. J. Physiol., **160**: 106–154.

HUBEL, D. H., AND WIESEL, T. N. 1963. Shape and arrangement of columns in cat's striate cortex. J. Physiol., **165**: 559–568.

HUBEL, D. H., AND WIESEL, T. N. 1963a. Receptive fields of cells in striate cortex of very young, visually inexperienced kittens. J. Neurophysiol., **26**: 994–1002.

HUBEL, D. H., AND WIESEL, T. N. 1965. Receptive fields and functional architecture in two non-striate visual areas (18 and 19) of the cat. J. Neurophysiol., **28**: 229–289.

HUBER, G. C., AND CROSBY, E. C. 1929. Somatic and visceral connections of the diencephalon. A. Res. Nerv. & Ment. Dis., Proc., **9**: 199–248.

HUMASON, G. L. 1961. *Animal Tissue Techniques*. W. H. Freeman and Company, San Francisco, pp. 189–217.

HUMPHREY, T. 1936. The telencephalon of the bat. The non-cortical nuclear masses and certain pertinent fiber connections. J. Comp. Neurol., **65**: 603–711.

HUMPHREY, T. 1966. Correlations between the development of the hippocampal formation and the differentiation of the olfactory bulbs. Alabama J. M. Sc., **3**: 235–269.

HUMPHREY, T. 1968. The development of the human amygdala during early embryonic life. J. Comp. Neurol., **132**: 135–166.

HUNSPERGER, R. W. 1956. Affektreaktionen auf elektrische Reizung im Hirnstamm der Katze. Helvet. physiol. et pharmacol. acta., **14**: 70–92.

HUNT, C. C., AND RIKER, W. K. 1966. Properties of frog sympathetic neurons in normal ganglia and after axon section. J. Neurophysiol., **29**: 1096–1114.

HUNT, J. R. 1915. The sensory field of the facial nerve: A further contribution to the symptomatology of the geniculate ganglion. Brain, **38**: 418–446.

HYDÉN, H. 1960. The neuron. In J. BRACHET AND A. E. MIRSKY (Editors), *The Cell: Biochemistry, Physiology, Morphology*, Vol. IV. Academic Press, New York, Ch. 5, pp. 215–323.

INGALLS, N. W. 1920. A human embryo at the beginning of segmentation with special reference to the vascular system. Contrib. Embryol., **11**: 61–90.

INGRAM, W. R. 1940. Nuclear organization and chief connections of the primate hypothalamus. A. Res. Nerv. & Ment. Dis., Proc., **20**: 195–244.

INGRAM, W. R. 1952. Brain stem mechanisms in behavior. Electroencephalog. & Clin. Neurophysiol., **4**: 397–406.

INGRAM, W. R., AND RANSON, S. W. 1932. Effects of lesions in the red nuclei in cats. Arch. Neurol. & Psychiat., **28**: 483–512.

ISHII, T., AND FRIEDE, R. L. 1968. Tissue binding of tritiated-norepinephrine in pigmented nuclei of human brain. Am. J. Anat., **122**: 139–144.

ITO, M., OBATA, K., AND OCHI, R. 1966. The origin of cerebellar-induced inhibition of Deiters' neurones. II. Temporal correlation between the trans-synaptic activation of Purkinje cells and the inhibition of Deiters' neurones. Exper. Brain Res., **2**: 350–364.

ITO, M., AND YOSHIDA, M. 1964. The cerebellar-evoked monosynaptic inhibition of Deiters' neurones. Experientia, **20**: 515.

ITO, M., AND YOSHIDA, M. 1966. The origin of cerebellar-induced inhibition of Deiters' neurones. I. Monosynaptic initiation of the inhibitory postsynaptic potentials. Exper. Brain Res., **2**: 330–349.

ITO, M., YOSHIDA, M., AND OBATA, K. 1964. Monosynaptic inhibition of the intracerebellar nuclei induced from the cerebellar cortex. Experientia, 20: 575–576.

IVERSEN, L. L. 1972. The uptake, storage, release and metabolism of GABA in inhibitory nerves. In S. H. SNYDER (Editor), Perspectives in Neuropharmacology. Oxford University Press, London, pp. 75–111.

JABBUR, S. J., AND TOWE, A. L. 1961. Cortical excitation of neurones in dorsal column nuclei of cat, including an analysis of pathways. J. Neurophysiol., 24: 499–509.

JACOBS, G. H. 1969. Receptive fields in visual systems. Brain Res., 14: 553–573.

JACOBSOHN, L. 1908. Über die Kerne des menschlichen Rückenmarks. Aus dem Anhang zu den Abhandlungen der königl. preuss. Akademie der Wissenschaften, p. 72.

JACOBSOHN, L. 1909. Über die kerne des menschlichen Hirnstamms. Aus dem Anhang zu den Abhandlungen der königl. preuss. Akademie der Wissenschaften, 1: 1–70.

JAKOB, A. 1923. Die Extrapyramidalen Erkrankungen. Julius Springer, Berlin.

JAKOB, A. 1925. The anatomy, clinical syndromes and physiology of the extrapyramidal system. Arch. Neurol. & Psychiat., 13: 596–620.

JAKOB, A. 1928. Das Kleinhirn. In W. VON MÖLLENDORFF (Editor), Handbuch der mikroskopischen Anatomie des Menschen, Vol. IV. Julius Springer, Berlin, pp. 674–916.

JANSEN, J. 1933. Experimental studies on the intrinsic fibers of the cerebellum. I. The arcuate fibers. J. Comp. Neurol., 57: 369–400.

JANSEN, J., AND BRODAL, A. 1940. Experimental studies on the intrinsic fibers of the cerebellum. II. The corticonuclear projection. J. Comp. Neurol., 73: 267–321.

JANSEN, J. AND BRODAL, A. 1942. Experimental studies on the intrinsic fibers of the cerebellum. The corticonuclear projection in the rabbit and in the monkey (Macacus rhesus). Norske Vid.-Akad. Avh. Mat.-Naturv., No. 3, 1–50.

JANSEN, J., AND BRODAL, A. 1958. Das Kleinhirn. In W. VON MÖLLENDORFF (Editor), Handbuch der mikroskopischen Anatomie des Mehschen, Vol. III. Julius Springer, Berlin, pp. 1–323.

JANSEN, J., AND JANSEN, J., JR. 1955. On the efferent fibers of the cerebellar nuclei in the cat. J. Comp. Neurol., 102: 607–632.

JASPER, H. H. 1949. Diffuse projection systems: The integrative action of the thalamic reticular system. Electroencephalog. & Clin. Neurophysiol., 1: 405–420.

JASPER, H. H. 1954. Functional properties of the thalamic reticular system. In J. F. DELAFRESNAYE (Editor), Brain Mechanisms and Consciousness (Symposium). Blackwell Scientific Publications, Oxford, pp. 374–395.

JASPER, H. H. 1958. Recent advances in our understanding of ascending activities of the reticular system. In H. H. JASPER et al. (Editors), Reticular Formation of the Brain. Henry Ford Hospital International Symposium. Little, Brown and Company, Boston, Ch. 15, pp. 319–331.

JASPER, H. H. 1960. Unspecific thalamocortical relations. In J. FIELD (Editor), Handbook of Physiology, Section I, Vol. II. American Physiological Society, Washington, D. C., Ch. 53, pp. 1307–1321.

JASPER, H. H., AJMONE-MARSAN, C., AND STOLL, J. 1952. Corticofugal projections to the brain stem. A. M. A. Arch. Neurol. & Psychiat., 67: 155–171.

JEFFERSON, G. 1950. Localization of function in the cerebral cortex. Brit. M. Bull., 6: 333–340.

JEFFERSON, G. 1958. Discussion: Ch. 2, SCHEIBEL, M. E., AND SCHEIBEL, A. B., Substrates for integrative patterns in the reticular core. In H. H. JASPER et al. (Editors), Reticular Formation of the Brain. Henry Ford Hospital International Symposium. Little, Brown and Company, Boston, pp. 65–68.

JENKINS, T. W., AND TRUEX, R. C. 1963. Dissection of the human brain as a method for its fractionation by weight. Anat. Rec., 147: 359–366.

JERGER, J. F. 1960. Observations on auditory behavior in lesions of the central auditory pathways. A. M. A. Arch. Otolaryng., 71: 797–806.

JOHNSON, F. H., AND RUSSELL, G. V. 1952. The locus caeruleus as a pneumotaxic center. Anat. Rec., 112: 348.

JOHNSON, T. N., AND CLEMENTE, C. D. 1959. An experimental study of the fiber connections between the putamen, globus pallidus, ventral thalamus and midbrain tegmentum in cat. J. Comp. Neurol., 113: 83–101.

JONES, E. G., AND LEAVITT, R. Y. 1974. Retrograde axonal transport and the demonstration of non-specific projections to the cerebral cortex and striatum from thalamic intralaminar nuclei in the cat, rat and monkey. J. Comp. Neurol., 154: 349–378.

JONES, E. G., AND POWELL, T. P. S. 1968. The ipsilateral cortical connexions of the somatic sensory areas in the cat. Brain Res., 9: 71–94.

JONES, E. G., AND POWELL, T. P. S. 1969. Connexions of the somatic sensory cortex of the rhesus monkey. I. Ipsilateral cortical connexions. Brain, 92: 477–502.

JONES, E. G., AND POWELL, T. P. S. 1969a. Connexions of the somatic sensory cortex of the rhesus monkey. II. Contralateral cortical connexions. Brain, 72: 717–730.

JONES, E. G., AND POWELL, T. P. S. 1970. Connexions of the somatic sensory cortex of the rhesus monkey. III. Thalamic connexions. Brain, 93: 37–56.

JONES, R. M. 1961. McClung's Handbook of Microscopical Technique, Ed. 3. Hafner Publishing Company, New York, pp. 346–431.

JOUVET, M. 1967. Neurophysiology of the states of sleep. Physiol. Rev., 47: 117–177.

JOUVET, M. 1968. Insomnia and decrease of cerebral 5-hydroxytryptamine after destruction of the raphe system in the cat. Advances Pharmacol., 6B: 265–279.

JOUVET, M. 1969. Biogenic amines and the states of sleep. Science, 163: 32–41.

KAADA, B. R. 1951. Somatomotor, autonomic and electrocorticographic responses to electrical stimulation of "rhinencephalic" and other structures in primates, cat and dog. Acta physiol. scandinav., 24: Suppl. 83, 285 pp.

KAADA, B. R. 1960. Cingulate, posterior orbital, anterior insular and temporal pole cortex. In J. FIELD (Editor), Handbook of Physiology, Section I, Vol. II. American Physiological Society, Washington, D. C., Ch. 55, pp. 1345–1372.

KAADA, B. R. 1972. Stimulation and regional ablation of the amygdaloid complex with reference to functional representations. In B. E. ELEFTHERIOU (Editor), The Neurobiology of the Amygdala. Plenum Press, New York, pp. 205–281.

KAADA, B. R., PRIBRAM, K. H., AND EPSTEIN, J. A. 1949. Respiratory and vascular responses in monkeys from temporal pole, insula, orbital surface and cingulate gyrus. J. Neurophysiol., 12: 347–356.

KAADA, B. R., RASMUSSEN, E. W., AND KVEINI, O. 1961. Effects of hippocampal lesions on maze learning and retention in rats. Exper. Neurol., 3: 333–355.

KAES, T. 1907. Die Grosshirnrinde des Menschen in ihren Massen und in ihrem Fasergehalt, Vol. I. Gustav Fischer, Jena, 64 pp., 92 plates.

KAPLAN, H. A. 1956. Arteries of the brain. Acta radiol., 46: 364–370.

KAPLAN, H. A. 1958. Vascular supply of the base of the brain. In W. S. FIELDS (Editor), *Pathogenesis and Treatment of Parkinsonism*. Charles C Thomas, Publisher, Springfield, Ill., Ch. 6, pp. 138–155.

KAPLAN, H. A. 1961. Collateral circulation of the brain. Neurology, 11: (No. 4, part 2) 9–15.

KAPLAN, H. A., AND FORD, D. H. 1966. *The Brain Vascular System*. Elsevier Publishing Company, Amsterdam, 230 pp.

KATZ, B. 1966. *Nerve, Muscle and Synapse*. McGraw-Hill Book Company, New York.

KEIBEL, F., AND MALL, F. P. 1912. *Manual of Human Embryology*, Vol. II. J. B. Lippincott Company, Philadelphia, Ch. XIV, pp. 1–144.

KELLER, A. D., AND HARE, W. K. 1934. The rubrospinal tracts in the monkey. Effects of experimental section. Arch. Neurol. & Psychiat., 32: 1253–1272.

KELLER, A. D., ROY, R. S., AND CHASE, W. P. 1937. Extirpation of the neocerebellar cortex without eliciting so-called cerebellar signs. Am. J. Physiol., 118: 720–733.

KELLER, J. H., AND MOFFETT, B. C., JR. 1968. Nerve endings in the temporomandibular joint of the Rhesus macaque. Anat. Rec., 160: 587–594.

KEMP, J. 1968. An electron microscopic study of the termination of afferent fibres in the caudate nucleus. Brain Res., 11: 464–467.

KEMP, J. 1968a. Observations on the caudate nucleus of the cat impregnated with the Golgi method. Brain Res., 11: 467–470.

KEMP, J. M., AND POWELL, T. P. S. 1970. The corticostriate projection in the monkey. Brain, 93: 525–546.

KEMPINSKY, W. H. 1951. Cortical projection of vestibular and facial nerves in cat. J. Neurophysiol., 14: 203–210.

KENNARD, M. A. 1949. Somatic functions. In P. C. BUCY (Editor), *The Precentral Motor Cortex*, Ed. 2. University of Illinois Press, Urbana, Ch. 9, pp. 243–276.

KENNARD, M. A., AND FULTON, J. F. 1933. The localizing significance of spasticity, reflex grasping and the signs of Babinski and Rossolimo. Brain, 56: 213–225.

KENNARD, M. A., VIETS, H. R., AND FULTON, J. F. 1934. The syndrome of the premotor cortex in man: Impairment of skilled movement, forced grasping, spasticity and vasomotor disturbances. Brain, 57: 69–84.

KERR, F. W. L. 1961. Structural relation of the trigeminal spinal tract to upper cervical roots and the solitary nucleus in the cat. Exper. Neurol., 4: 134–148.

KERR, F. W. L. 1962. Facial, vagal and glossopharyngeal nerves in the cat. Afferent connections. Arch. Neurol., 2: 264–281.

KERR, F. W. L. 1963. The divisional organization of afferent fibers of the trigeminal nerve. Brain, 86: 721–732.

KERR, F. W. L. 1969. Preserved vagal visceromotor function following destruction of the dorsal motor nucleus. J. Physiol., 202: 755–769.

KERR, F. W. L., AND O'LEARY, J. L. 1957. The thalamic source of cortical recruiting in the rodent. Electroencephalog. & Clin. Neurophysiol., 9: 461–476.

KERR, F. W. L., KRUGER, L. L., SCHWASSMANN, H. O., AND STERN, R. 1968. Somatotopic organization of mechanoreceptor units in the trigeminal nuclear complex of the monkey. J. Comp. Neurol., 134: 127–144.

KERR, F. W. L., AND PRESHAW, R. M. 1969. Secretomotor function of the dorsal motor nucleus of the vagus. J. Physiol., 205: 405–415.

KETY, S. S., AND SCHMIDT, C. F. 1948. The nitrous oxide method for the quantitative determination of cerebral blood flow in man: Theory, procedure and normal values. J. Clin. Invest., 27: 484–492.

KEY, A., AND RETZIUS, G. 1875. *Studien in der Anatomie des Nervensystems und des Bindegewebes*. Samson and Wallin, Stockholm.

KIEVIT, J., AND KUYPERS, H. G. J. M. 1972. Fastigial cerebellar projections to the ventrolateral nucleus of the thalamus and the organization of the descending pathways. In T. L. FRIGYESI *et al.* (Editors), *Corticothalamic Projections and the Sensorimotor Activities*. Raven Press, New York, pp. 91–111.

KILLAM, K. F., AND KILLAM, E. K. 1958. Drug action on pathways involving the reticular formation. In H. H. JASPER *et al.* (Editors), *Reticular Formation of the Brain*. Henry Ford Hospital International Symposium. Little, Brown and Company, Boston, Ch. 4, pp. 111–122.

KIMMEL, D. L. 1942. Nigro-striatal fibers in cat. Anat. Rec., 82: 425.

KIMMEL, D. L. 1959. The cervical sympathetic rami and the vertebral plexus in the human fetus. J. Comp. Neurol., 112: 141–162.

KIMMEL, D. L. 1961. Innervation of the spinal dura mater and dura mater of the posterior cranial fossa. Neurology, 9: 800–809.

KIMMEL, D. L., KIMMEL, C. B., AND ZARKIN, A. 1961. The central distribution of afferent nerve fibers of the facial and vagus nerves in the guinea pig. Anat. Rec., 139: 245.

KIMURA, R., AND WERSÄLL, J. 1962. Termination of the olivo-cochlear bundle in relation to the outer hair cells of the organ of Corti in guinea pig. Acta oto-laryng. 55: 11–32.

KING, J. S., SCHWYN, R. C., AND FOX, C. A. 1971. The red nucleus in the monkey (*Macaca mulatta*): A Golgi and an electron microscopic study. J. Comp. Neurol., 142: 75–108.

KIRKPATRICK, J. B. 1968. Chromatolysis in the hypoglossal nucleus of the rat: An electron microscopic analysis. J. Comp. Neurol., 132: 189–212.

KLATZO, I., MIGUEL, J., TOBIAS, C., AND HAYMAKER, W. 1961. Effects of alpha-particle irradiation on the rat brain, including vascular permeability and glycogen studies. J. Neuropath. & Exper. Neurol., 20: 459–483.

KLEITMAN, N. 1963. *Sleep and Wakefulness*. University of Chicago Press, Chicago.

KLING, A., AND SCHWARTZ, N. B. 1961. Effects of amygdalectomy on feeding in infant and adult animals. Fed. Proc., 20: 335.

KLÜVER, H. 1942. Functional significance of the geniculo-striate system. *Biological Symposia*, 7: 253–299.

KLÜVER, H. 1952. Brain mechanisms and behavior with special reference to the rhinencephalon. Lancet, 72: 567–574.

KLÜVER, H., AND BARRERA, E. 1953. A method for the combined staining of cells and fibers in the nervous system. J. Neuropath. & Exper. Neurol., 12: 400–403.

KLÜVER, H., AND BUCY, P. 1939. Preliminary analysis of functions of the temporal lobes in monkeys. Arch. Neurol. & Psychiat., 42: 979–1000.

KNIGHTON, R. S. 1950. Thalamic relay nucleus for the second somatic sensory receiving area in the cerebral cortex of the cat. J. Comp. Neurol., 92: 183–192.

KOELLA, W. P., AND GELLHORN, E. 1954. The influence of diencephalic lesions upon the action of nociceptive impulses and hypercapnia on the electrical activity of the cat's brain. J. Comp. Neurol., 100: 211–235.

KOELLE, G. B. 1970. Anticholinesterase agents. In L. S. GOODMAN AND A. GILMAN (Editors), *The Pharmacological Basis of Therapeutics*. Macmillan Company, New York, Ch. 22, pp. 442–465.

KOPELL, H. P., AND THOMPSON, W. A. L. 1963. *Peripheral Entrapment Neuropathies*. Williams & Wilkins Company, Baltimore.

KOSKOFF, Y. D., DENNIS, W., LAZOVIK, D., AND WHEELER, E. T. 1948. The psychological effects of frontal lobotomy performed for alleviation of pain. A. Res. Nerv. & Ment. Dis., Proc., 27: 723-753.

KREMER, W. F. 1947. Autonomic and somatic reactions induced by stimulation of the cingulate gyrus in dogs. J. Neurophysiol., 10: 371-379.

KRIEG, W. J. S. 1932. The hypothalamus of the albino rat. J. Comp. Neurol., 55: 19-89.

KRIEG, W. J. S. 1947. Connections of the cerebral cortex. I. The albino rat. C. Extrinsic connections. J. Comp. Neurol., 86: 267-394.

KRIEG, W. J. S. 1953. Functional Neuroanatomy. Blakiston Company, New York, 658 pp.

KRIEG, W. J. S. 1954. Connections of the cerebral cortex. II. The macaque. E. The postcentral gyrus. J. Comp. Neurol., 101: 101-165.

KRUGER, L., AND MAXWELL, D. S. 1966. Electron microscopy of oligodendrocytes in normal rat cerebrum. Am J. Anat., 118: 411-436.

KRUGER, L., AND MICHEL, F. 1962. A morphological and somatotopic analysis of single unit activity in the trigeminal sensory complex of the cat. Exper. Neurol., 5: 139-156.

KRUGER, L., AND MICHEL, F. 1962a. Reinterpretation of the representation of pain based on physiological excitation of single neurons in the trigeminal sensory complex. Exper. Neurol., 5: 157-178.

KRUGER, L., AND PORTER, P. 1958. A behavioral study of the functions of the Rolandic cortex in the monkey. J. Comp. Neurol., 109: 439-469.

KRUGER, L., SIMINOFF, R., AND WITKOVSKY, P. 1961. Single neuron analysis of dorsal column nuclei and spinal nucleus of trigeminal in cat. J. Neurophysiol., 24: 333-349.

KUFFLER, S. W. 1953. Discharge patterns and functional organization of mammalian retina. J. Neurophysiol., 16: 37-68.

KUFFLER, S. W., NICHOLLS, J. G., AND ORKAND, R. K. 1966. Physiological properties of glial cells in the central nervous system of amphibia. J. Neurophysiol., 29: 768-787.

KUFFLER, S. W., AND POTTER, D. D. 1964. Glia in the leech central nervous system: Physiological properties and neuron-glia relationships. J. Neurophysiol., 27: 290-320.

KUHLENBECK, H. 1948. The derivatives of the thalamus ventralis in the human brain and their relation to the so-called subthalamus. Mil. Surgeon, 102: 433-447.

KUHLENBECK, H. 1951. The derivatives of thalamus dorsalis and epithalamus in the human brain: Their relation to cortical and other centers. Mil. Surgeon, 108: 205-256.

KUHLENBECK, H. 1969. Derivation and boundaries of the hypothalamus, with atlas of hypothalamic grisea. In W. HAYMAKER et al. (Editors), The Hypothalamus. Charles C Thomas, Publisher, Springfield, Ill., Ch. 2, pp. 13-60.

KUHLENBECK, H., AND HAYMAKER, W. 1949. The derivatives of the hypothalamus in the human brain: Their relation to the extrapyramidal and autonomic systems. Mil. Surgeon, 105: 26-52.

KUHLENBECK, H., AND MILLER, R. N. 1949. The pretectal region of the human brain. J. Comp. Neurol., 91: 369-408.

KUHN, R. A. 1949. Topographical pattern of cutaneous sensibility in the dorsal column nuclei of the cat. Tr. Am. Neurol. A., 74: 227-230.

KUHN, R. A. 1950. Functional capacity of the isolated human spinal cord. Brain, 75: 1-51.

KUO, J.-S., AND CARPENTER, M. B. 1973. Organization of pallidothalamic projections in the rhesus monkey. J. Comp. Neurol., 151: 201-236.

KUYPERS, H. G. J. M. 1958. An anatomical analysis of cortico-bulbar connexions to the pons and lower brain-

stem in the cat. J. Anat., 92: 198-218.

KUYPERS, H. G. J. M. 1958a. Corticobulbar connexions to the pons and lower brain-stem in man. An anatomical study. Brain, 81: 364-388.

KUYPERS, H. G. J. M. 1958b. Some projections from the peri-central cortex to the pons and lower brain stem in monkey and chimpanzee. J. Comp. Neurol., 110: 221-256.

KUYPERS, H. G. J. M. 1958c. Pericentral cortical projections to motor and sensory nuclei. Science, 128: 662-663.

KUYPERS, H. G. J. M. 1960. Central cortical projections to motor and somato-sensory cell groups. Brain, 83: 161-184.

KUYPERS, H. G. J. M., HOFFMAN, A. L., AND BEASLEY, R. M. 1961. Distribution of cortical "feedback" fibers in the nuclei cuneatus and gracilis. Proc. Soc. Exper. Biol. & Med., 108: 634-637.

KUYPERS, H. G. J. M., AND LAWRENCE, D. G. 1967. Cortical projections to the red nucleus and the brain stem in the rhesus monkey. Brain Res., 4: 151-188.

KUYPERS, H. G. J. M., AND TUERK, J. D. 1964. The distribution of cortical fibres within the nuclei cuneatus and gracilis in the cat. J. Anat., 98: 143-162.

LAMMERS, H. J. 1972. The neural connections of the amygdaloid complex in mammals. In B. E. ELEFTHERIOU (Editor), The Neurobiology of the Amygdala. Plenum Press, New York, pp. 123-144.

LAMMERS, H. J., AND LOHMAN, A. H. 1957. Experimental anatomisch onderzoek naar de verbindingen van piriform cortex en amygdalakernen bij de kat. Nederld. tijdschr. geneesk., 101: 1-2.

LAND, L. J. 1973. Localized projection of olfactory nerves to rabbit olfactory bulb. Brain Res., 63: 153-166.

LANDGREN, S. 1957. Convergence of tactile, thermal and gustatory impulses on single cortical cells. Acta physiol. scandinav., 40: 210-221.

LANDGREN, S. 1961. The response of thalamic and cortical neurons to electrical and physiological stimulation of the cat's tongue. In W. A. ROSENBLITH (Editor), Sensory Communication. Massachusetts Institute of Technology Press, Cambridge, pp. 437-453.

LANDGREN, S., NORDWALL, A., AND WENGSTRÖM, C. 1965. The location of the thalamus relay in the spinocervico-lemniscal path. Acta physiol. scandinav., 65: 164-175.

LANDGREN, S., PHILLIPS, C. G., AND PORTER, R. 1962. Minimal synaptic actions of pyramidal impulses on some alpha motoneurones of the baboon's hand and forearm. J. Physiol., 161: 91-111.

LANDIS, C., ZUBIN, J., AND METTLER, F. A. 1950. The functions of the human frontal lobe. J. Psychol., 30: 123-138.

LANGLEY, J. N. 1921. The Autonomic Nervous System, Vol. 1. W. Heffer and Sons, Cambridge.

LANGMAN, J. 1963. Medical Embryology. Williams & Wilkins Company, Baltimore.

LANGMAN, J. 1968. Histogenesis of the central nervous system. In G. H. BOURNE (Editor), The Structure and Function of Nervous Tissue, Vol. 1. Academic Press, New York, pp. 33-65.

LANGMAN, J. 1969. Medical Embryology, Ed. 2. Williams & Wilkins Company, Baltimore.

LANGMAN, J., GUERRANT, R. L., AND FREEMAN, B. G. 1966. Behavior of neuroepithalial cells during closure of the neural tube. J. Comp. Neurol., 127: 399-411.

LANGMAN, J., AND HADEN, C. C. 1970. Formation and migration of neuroblasts in the spinal cord of the chick embryo. J. Comp. Neurol., 138: 419-432.

LARSELL, O. 1923. The cerebellum of the frog. J. Comp. Neurol., 36: 89-122.

LARSELL, O. 1947. The cerebellum of myxinoids and petromyzonts, including developmental stages in the lampreys. J. Comp. Neurol., 86: 395–446.

LARSELL, O. 1947a. The development of the cerebellum in man in relation to its comparative anatomy. J. Comp. Neurol., 87: 85–129.

LARSELL, O. 1951. Anatomy of the Nervous System, Ed. 2. Appleton-Century-Crofts, Inc., New York, 520 pp.

LARSELL, O., AND DOW, R. S. 1933. Innervation of the human lung. Am. J. Anat., 52: 414–438.

LARSELL, O., AND JANSEN, J. 1972. The Comparative Anatomy and Histology of the Cerebellum. The Human Cerebellum, Cerebellar Connections and Cerebellar Cortex. University of Minnesota Press, Minneapolis, 264 pp.

LASEK, R. 1970. Protein transport in neurons. Internat. Rev. Neurobiol., 13: 289–324.

LASSEK, A. M. 1940. The human pyramidal tract. II. A numerical investigation of the Betz cells of the motor area. Arch. Neurol. & Psychiat., 44: 718–724.

LASSEK, A. M. 1942. The human pyramidal tract. IV. A study of the mature, myelinated fibers of the pyramid. J. Comp. Neurol., 76: 217–225.

LASSEK, A. M. 1942a. The pyramidal tract. The effect of pre- and postcentral cortical lesions on the fiber components of the pyramids in monkey. J. Nerv. & Ment. Dis., 95: 721–729.

LASSEK, A. M. 1947. The pyramidal tract: Basic considerations of corticospinal neurons. A. Res. Nerv. & Ment. Dis., Proc., 27: 106–128.

LASSEK, A. M. 1953. Potency of isolated brachial dorsal roots in controlling muscular physiology. Neurology, 3: 53–57.

LASSEK, A. M. 1954. The Pyramidal Tract: Its Status in Medicine. Charles C Thomas, Publisher, Springfield, Ill., 166 pp.

LASSEK, A. M., AND EVANS, J. P. 1945. The human pyramidal tract. XII. The effect of hemispherectomies on the fiber components of the pyramids. J. Comp. Neurol., 83: 113–119.

LASSEK, A. M., AND RASMUSSEN, G. L. 1939. The human pyramidal tract. A fiber and numerical analysis. Arch. Neurol. & Psychiat., 42: 872–876.

LASSEK, A. M., AND RASMUSSEN, G. L. 1940. A comparative fiber and numerical analysis of the pyramidal tract. J. Comp. Neurol., 72: 417–428.

LAWRENCE, D. G., AND KUYPERS, H. G. J. M. 1968. The functional organization of the motor system in the monkey. I. The effects of bilateral pyramidal lesions. Brain, 91: 1–14.

LEÃAO, A. A. P. 1944. Spreading depression of activity in the cerebral cortex. J. Neurophysiol., 7: 359–390.

LEE, J. C. Y. 1963. Electron microscopy of Wallerian degeneration. J. Comp. Neurol., 120: 65–79.

LEMMEN, L. J., DAVIS, J. S., AND RADNOR, L. L. 1959. Observations on stimulation of the human frontal eye field. J. Comp. Neurol., 112: 163–168.

LEONARD, C. M., AND SCOTT, J. W. 1971. Origin and distribution of amygdalofugal pathways in the rat: An experimental neuroanatomical study. J. Comp. Neurol., 144: 313–330.

LEVI-MONTALCINI, R., AND ANGELETTI, P. V. 1961. Growth control of the sympathetic system by a specific protein factor. Quart. Rev. Biol., 36: 99–108.

LEVI-MONTALCINI, R., AND ANGELETTI, P. V. 1963. Essential role of the nerve growth factor in the survival and maintenance of dissociated sensory and sympathetic embryonic nerve cells in vitro. Develop. Biol., 7: 653–659.

LEVI-MONTALCINI, R., AND BOOKER, B. 1960. Excessive growth of the sympathetic ganglia evoked by a protein isolated from mouse. Proc. Nat. Acad. Sc., 46: 373–391.

LEVI-MONTALCINI, R., AND COHEN, S. 1960. Effects of the extract of the mouse submaxillary salivary glands on the sympathetic system of mammals. Ann. New York Acad. Sc., 85: 324–341.

LEVI-MONTALCINI, R., AND HAMBURGER, V. 1951. Selective growth stimulating effects of mouse sarcoma on the sensory and sympathetic nervous system of the chick embryo. J. Zool., 116: 321–362.

LEVI-MONTALCINI, R., MEYER, H., AND HAMBURGER, V. 1954. In vitro experiments on the effects of mouse sarcomas 180 and 37 on the spinal and sympathetic ganglia of the chick embryo. Cancer Res., 14: 49–57.

LEVIN, P. M. 1936. The efferent fibers of the frontal lobe of the monkey (Macaca mulatta). J. Comp. Neurol., 63: 369–419.

LEVIN, P. M. 1949. Efferent fibers. In P. C. BUCY (Editor). The Precentral Motor Cortex, Ed. 2. University of Illinois Press, Urbana, Ch. 5, pp. 133–148.

LEVIN, P. M., AND BRADFORD, F. K. 1938. The exact origin of the corticospinal tract in the monkey. J. Comp. Neurol., 68: 411–422.

LEVITT, M., CARRERAS, M., CHAMBERS, W. W., AND LIU, C. N. 1960. Pyramidal influence on unit activity in posterior column nuclei of cat. Physiologist, 3: 103.

LEWY, F. H., AND KOBRAK, H. 1936. Neural projection of cochlear spirals on primary acoustic centers. Arch. Neurol. & Psychiat., 35: 839–852.

LIDDELL, E. G. T., AND PHILLIPS, C. G. 1940. Experimental lesions in the basal ganglia of the cat. Brain, 63: 264–274.

LINDBLOM, U., AND LUND, L. 1966. The discharge from vibration-sensitive receptors in the monkey foot. Exper. Neurol., 15: 401–417.

LINDSLEY, D. B. 1960. Attention, consciousness, sleep and wakefulness. In J. FIELD (Editor), Handbook of Physiology, Section 1, Vol. III. American Physiological Society, Washington, D. C., pp. 1553–1593.

LIU, C. N. 1956. Afferent nerves to Clarke's and the lateral cuneate nuclei in the cat. Arch. Neurol. & Psychiat., 75: 67–77.

LIU, C. N., AND CHAMBERS, W. W. 1964. An experimental study of the corticospinal system in the monkey (Macaca mulatta). The spinal pathways and preterminal distribution of degenerating fibers following discrete lesions of the pre- and postcentral gyri and bulbar pyramid. J. Comp. Neurol., 123: 257–284.

LIVINGSTON, R. B. 1965. Mechanics of cerebrospinal fluid. In T. C. RUCH AND H. D. PATTON (Editors), Physiology and Biophysics. W. B. Saunders Company, Philadelphia, Ch. 47, pp. 935–940.

LLOYD, D. P. C. 1941. The spinal mechanisms of the pyramidal system in cats. J. Neurophysiol., 4: 525–546.

LLOYD, D. P. C. 1943. Conduction and synaptic transmission of reflex response to- stretch in spinal cats. J. Neurophysiol., 6: 317–326.

LLOYD, D. P. C., AND MCINTYRE, A. K. 1950. Dorsal column conduction of group I muscle afferent impulses and their relay through Clarke's column. J. Neurophysiol., 13: 39–54.

LOCKE, S., ANGEVINE, J. B., AND YAKOVLEV, P. I. 1961. Limbic nuclei of thalamus and connections of limbic cortex. II. Thalamo-cortical projections of the lateral dorsal nucleus in man. Arch. Neurol., 4: 355–364.

LOEWENSTEIN, W. R. 1959. The generation of electric activity in a nerve ending. Ann. New York Acad. Sc., 81: 367–387.

LOEWENSTEIN, W. R. 1960. Biological transducers. Sc. Am. 203: 99–108.

LOEWENSTEIN, W. R. 1971. Mechano-electric transduction in the Pacinian corpuscle. Initiation of sensory impulses in mechanoreceptors. In W. R. LOEWENSTEIN (Editor), Principles of Receptor Physiology. Springer Verlag, Berlin. Ch. 9, pp. 269–290.

LOEWENSTEIN, W. R., AND ALTAMIRANO-ORREGO, R. 1958. The refractory state of the generator and propagated potentials in a Pacinian corpuscle. J. Gen. Physiol., 41: 805–824.

LOEWENTHAL, M., AND HORSLEY, V. 1897. On the relations between the cerebellum and other centres (namely cerebral and spinal) with special reference to the action of antagonistic muscles. Proc. Roy. Soc., London, ser. B., 61: 20–25.

LOEWI, O. 1921. Über humorale Übertragbarkeit der Herznervenwirkung. Arch. ges. Physiol., 189: 239–242.

LOEWI, O. 1945. Chemical transmission of nerve impulses. Sc. Progr., 4: 98–119.

LOEWY, A. D., ARAUJO, J. C., AND KERR, F. W. L. 1973. Pupillodilator pathways in the brain stem of the cat: Anatomical and electrophysiological identification of a central autonomic pathway. Brain Res., 60: 65–91.

LOHMAN, A. H. M. 1963. The anterior olfactory lobe of the guinea pig. Acta anat. 53: Suppl. 49, 1–109.

LORENTE DE NÓ, R. 1924. Études sur le cerveau postérieur. Trav. Lab. rech. biol., Univ. Madrid, 22: 51–65.

LORENTE DE NÓ, R. 1928. Die Labyrinthreflexe auf die Augenmuskeln nach einseitiger Labyrinthexstirpation nebst einer kurzen Angabe über den Nervenmechanismus der vestibulären Augenbewegungen. Urban and Schwarzenberg, Vienna.

LORENTE DE NÓ, R. 1931. Ausgewählte Kapitel aus der vergleichenden Physiologie des Labyrinthes: Die Augenmuskelreflexe beim Kaninchen und ihre Grundlagen. Ergebn. Physiol., 32: 73–242.

LORENTE DE NÓ, R. 1933. Studies on the structure of the cerebral cortex. I. The area entorhinalis. J. Psychol. u. Neurol., 45: 381–438.

LORENTE DE NÓ, R. 1933a. Anatomy of the eighth nerve. The central projection of the nerve endings of the internal ear. Laryngoscope, 43: 1–38.

LORENTE DE NÓ, R. 1934. Studies on the structure of the cerebral cortex. II. Continuation of the study of the ammonic system. J. Psychol. u. Neurol., 46: 113–177.

LORENTE DE NÓ, R. 1949. The structure of the cerebral cortex. In J. F. FULTON (Editor), Physiology of the Nervous System, Ed. 3. Oxford University Press, New York, pp. 288–330.

LORENTE DE NÓ, R. 1953. Symposium discussion. In J. L. MALCOLM AND J. A. B. GRAY (Editors), The Spinal Cord. Ciba Foundation Symposium. Little, Brown and Company, Boston, pp. 40–41.

DE LORENZO, A. J. D. 1963. Studies on the ultrastructure and histophysiology of cell membranes, nerve fibers and synaptic junctions in chemoreceptors. In Y. ZOTTERMAN (Editor), Olfaction and Taste. Pergamon Press, Oxford, pp. 5–17.

LOWENSTEIN, O. 1954. Clinical pupillary symptoms in lesions of the optic nerve, optic chiasm and optic tract. Arch. Ophth., 52: 385–403.

LUK, G. D., MOREST, D. K., AND MCKENNA, N. M. 1974. Origins of the crossed olivocochlear bundle shown by an acid phosphatase method in the cat. Ann. Otol. Rhin. & Laryng. 83: 382–391.

LUNDBERG, A. 1958. Electrophysiology of the salivary glands. Physiol. Rev., 38: 21–40.

LUNDBERG, A. 1964. Ascending spinal hindlimb pathways in the cat. In J. C. ECCLES AND J. P. SCHADÉ (Editors), Physiology of Spinal Neurons, Progress in Brain Research, Vol. 12. Elsevier Publishing Company, Amsterdam, pp. 135–163.

LUNDBERG, A., AND OSCARSSON, O. 1962. Functional organization of the ventral spino-cerebellar tract in the cat. IV. Identification of units by antidromic activation from the cerebellar cortex. Acta physiol. scandinav., 54: 252–269.

LUSE, S. A. 1956. Electron microscopic observations of central nervous system. J. Biophys. & Biochem. Cytol., 2: 531–542.

LUSE, S. A. 1956a. Formation of myelin in the central nervous system of mice and rats, as studied with the electron microscope. J. Biophys. & Biochem. Cytol., 2: 777–783.

LUSE, S. A. 1958. Ultrastructure of reactive and neoplastic astrocytes. Lab. Invest., 7: 401–417.

LUSE, S. A. 1968. Microglia; neuroglia. In J. MINCKLER (Editor), Pathology of the Nervous System. McGraw-Hill Book Company, New York, pp. 531–553.

LYSER, K. M. 1964. Early differentiation of motor neuroblasts in the chick embryo as studied by electron microscopy. Develop. Biol., 10: 433–466.

LYSER, K. M. 1968. Early differentiation of motor neuroblasts in the chick embryo as studied by electron microscopy. II. Microtubules and neurofilaments. Develop. Biol., 17: 117–142.

MACLEAN, P. D. 1952. Some psychiatric implications of physiological studies on frontotemporal portions of limbic system (visceral brain). Electroencephalog. & Clin. Neurophysiol., 4: 407–418.

MACLEAN, P. D. 1954. The limbic system and its hippocampal formation: Studies in animals and their possible application to man. J. Neurosurg., 11: 29–44.

MACLEAN, P. D. 1957. Chemical and electrical stimulation of the hippocampus in unrestrained animals. I. Methods and electroencephalographic findings. A. M. A. Arch. Neurol. & Psychiat., 78: 113–127.

MACLEAN, P. D. 1957a. Chemical and electrical stimulation of the hippocampus in unrestrained animals. II. Behavioral findings. A. M. A. Arch. Neurol. & Psychiat., 78: 128–142.

MACLEAN, P. D. 1958. Contrasting functions of limbic and neocortical systems of the brain and their relevance to psycho-physiological aspects of medicine. Am. J. Med., 25: 611–626.

MACLEAN, P. D., AND DELGADO, J. M. R. 1953. Electrical and chemical stimulation of fronto-temporal portion of limbic system in the waking animal. Electroencephalog. & Clin. Neurophysiol., 5: 91–100.

McCOMAS, A. J. 1963. Responses of the rat dorsal column system to mechanical stimulation of the hind paw. J. Physiol., 166: 435–445.

McCULLOCH, W. S. 1949. Cortico-cortical connections. In P. C. BUCY (Editor), The Precentral Motor Cortex, Ed. 2. University of Illinois Press, Urbana, Ch. 8, pp. 214–242.

McCULLOCH, W. S., AND GAROL, H. W. 1941. Cortical origin and distribution of corpus callosum and anterior commissure in the monkey (Macaca mulatta). J. Neurophysiol., 4: 555–563.

McGEER, P. L., McGEER, E. G., WADA, J. A., AND JUNG, E. 1971. Effects of globus pallidus lesions and Parkinson's disease on brain glutamic acid decarboxylase. Brain Res., 32: 425–431.

McKINLEY, W. A., AND MAGOUN, H. W. 1942. The bulbar projection of the trigeminal nerve. Am. J. Physiol., 137: 217–224.

McLARDY, T. 1948. Projection of the centromedian nucleus of the human thalamus. Brain, 71: 290–303.

McLARDY, T. 1950. The thalamic projection to frontal cortex in man. J. Neurol. Neurosurg. & Psychiat., 13: 198–202.

McLENNAN, H. 1963. Synaptic Transmission. W. B. Saunders Company, Philadelphia, pp. 3–15.

McMANUS, J. F. A., AND MOWRY, R. W. 1960. Staining Methods. Histologic and Histochemical. Paul B. Hoeber Inc., New York, pp. 324–357.

McMASTERS, R. E., WEISS, A. H., AND CARPENTER, M. B. 1966. Vestibular projections to the nuclei of the extraocular muscles. Degeneration resulting from discrete partial lesions of the vestibular nuclei in the monkey. Am. J. Anat., 118: 163–194.

McMICHAEL, J. 1945. Spinal tracts subserving micturition in a case of Erb's spinal paralysis. Brain, 68: 162.

MACHNE, X., CALMA, I., AND MAGOUN, H. W. 1955. Unit activity of central cephalic brain stem in EEG arousal. J. Neurophysiol., 18: 547–558.

MACHNE, X., AND SEGUNDO, J. P. 1956. Unitary responses to afferent volleys in amygdaloid complex. J. Neuophysiol., 19: 232–240.

MADIGAN, J. C., JR., AND CARPENTER, M. B. 1971. Cerebellum of the Rhesus Monkey. Atlas of Lobules, Laminae, and Folia, in Sections. University Park Press, Baltimore, 137 pp.

MADONICK, M. J. 1957. Statistical control studies in neurology. 8. The cutaneous abdominal reflex. Neurology, 7: 459–465.

MAEDA, T., AND SHIMIZU, N. 1972. Projections ascendantes du locus coeruleus et d'antres neurones aminergiques pontiques au niveau du prosencéphale du rat. Brain Res., 36: 19–35.

MAFFEI, L., AND POMPEIANO, O. 1962. Cerebellar control of flexor motoneurons. Arch. ital. biol., 100: 476–509.

MAGOUN, H. W. 1952. An ascending reticular activating system in the brain stem. A. M. A. Arch. Neurol. & Psychiat., 67: 145–154.

MAGOUN, H. W. 1954. The ascending reticular system and wakefulness. In J. B. DELAFRESNAYE (Editor), Brain Mechanisms and Consciousness. Blackwell Scientific Publications, Oxford, pp. 1–20.

MAGOUN, H. W. 1963. The Waking Brain, Ed. 2. Charles C Thomas, Publisher, Springfield, Ill.

MAGOUN, H. W., ATLAS, D., INGERSOLL, E. H., AND RANSON, S. W. 1937. Associated facial, vocal and respiratory components of emotional expression. J. Neurol. & Psychopath., 17: 241–255.

MAGOUN, H. W., AND RANSON, S. W. 1935. The central path of the light reflex. A study of the effect of lesions. Arch. Ophth., 13: 791–811.

MAGOUN, H. W., AND RANSON, S. W. 1935a. The afferent path of the light reflex. A review of the literature. Arch. Ophth., 13: 862–874.

MAGOUN, H. W., RANSON, S. W., AND MAYER, L. L. 1935. The pupillary light reflex after lesions of the posterior commissure in the cat. Am. J. Ophth., 18: 624–630.

MAGOUN, H. W., AND RHINES, R. 1946. An inhibitory mechanism in the bulbar reticular formation. J. Neurophysiol., 9: 165–171.

MAGOUN, H. W., AND RHINES, R. 1947. Spasticity: The Stretch-reflex and Extrapyramidal Systems. Charles C Thomas, Publisher, Springfield, Ill.

MALMFÖRS, T. 1964. Release and depletion of the transmitter in adrenergic terminals produced by nerve impulses after the inhibition of noradrenalin synthesis or reabsorption. Life Sc., 3: 1397–1402.

MALONE, E. F. 1910. Über die Kerne des menschlichen Diencephalon. Aus dem Anhang zu den Abhandlungen der königl. preuss. Akademie der Wissenschaften, p. 92.

MANNI, E., BORTOLAMI, R., AND DESOLE, C. 1966. Eye muscle proprioception in the semilunar ganglion. Exper. Neurol., 16: 226–236.

MARBURG, O., AND WARNER, F. J. 1947. The pathways of the tectum (anterior colliculus) of the midbrain in cats. J. Nerv. & Ment. Dis., 106: 415–446.

MARCHI, V., AND ALGERI, G. 1885. Sulle degenerazioni discendenti consecutive a lesioni sperimentale in diverse zone della corteccia cerebrale. Riv. sper. freniat. meds leg., 11: 492–494.

MARIE, P. 1906. Revision de la question de l'aphasie: la troisième circonvolution frontale gauche ne joue aucun rôle special dans la fonction du langage. Semana méd., 26: 241–247.

MARK, V. H., ERVIN, F. R., AND SWEET, W. H. 1972. Deep temporal lobe stimulation in man. In B. E. ELEFTHERIOU (Editor), The Neurobiology of the Amygdala. Plenum Press, New York, pp. 485–507.

MARKEE, J. E., SAWYER, C. H., AND HOLLINSHEAD, W. H. 1946. Activation of the anterior hypophysis by electrical stimulation in the rabbit. Endocrinology, 38: 345–357.

MARKHAM, C. H., PRECHT, W., AND SHIMAZU, H. 1966. Effects of stimulation of interstitial nucleus of Cajal on vestibuular unit activity in the cat. J. Neurophysiol., 29: 493–507.

MARS, H. 1973. Modification of levodopa effect by systemic decarboxylase inhibition. Arch. Neurol., 28: 91–95.

MARSDEN, C. D. 1961. Pigmentation in the nucleus substantiae nigrae of mammals. J. Anat., 95: 256–261.

MARSHALL, W. H. 1950. The relation of dehydration of the brain to the spreading depression of Leão. Electroencephalog. & Clin. Neurophysiol., 2: 177–186.

MARSHALL, W. H. 1959. Spreading cortical depression of Leão. Physiol. Rev., 39: Suppl. 3, 239–279.

MARSHALL, W. H., AND ESSIG, C. F. 1951. Relation of air exposure of cortex to spreading depression of Leão. J. Neurophysiol., 14: 265–273.

MARSHALL, W. H., ESSIG, C. F., AND DUBROFF, S. J. 1951. Relation of temperature of cerebral cortex to spreading depression of Leão. J. Neurophysiol., 14: 153–166.

MARSHALL, W. R., WOOLSEY, C. N., AND BARD, P. 1941. Observations on cortical somatic sensory mechanisms of the cat and monkey. J. Neurophysiol., 4: 1–24.

MARTIN, J. P. 1927. Hemichorea resulting from a local lesion of the brain. (The syndrome of the body of Luys.) Brain, 50: 637–651.

MARTIN, J. P. 1959. Remarks on the functions of the basal ganglia. Lancet, 1: 999–1005.

MARTIN, J. P. 1960. Further remarks on the functions of the basal ganglia. Lancet, 1: 1362–1365.

MARTIN, J. P. 1967. The Basal Ganglia and Posture. Pitman Medical Publishing Company, Ltd., London, 152 pp.

MARTIN, J. P., AND ALCOCK, N. S. 1934. Hemichorea associated with lesions of the corpus Luysii. Brain, 57: 504–516.

MARTIN, J. P., AND HURWITZ, L. J. 1962. Locomotion and the basal ganglia. Brain, 85: 261–276.

MARTIN, J. P., HURWITZ, L. J., AND FINLAYSON, M. H. 1962. The negative symptoms of basal gangliar disease. A survey of 130 postencephalitic cases. Lancet, 2: 1–6 and 62–66.

MARTIN, J. P. AND McCAUL, I. R. 1959. Acute hemiballismus treated by ventrolateral thalamolysis. Brain, 82: 104–108.

MASSERMAN, J. H. 1943. Behavior and Neurosis. University of Chicago Press, Chicago.

MASSION, J. 1967. The mammalian red nucleus. Physiol. Rev., 47: 383–436.

MASUCCI, E. F. 1965. Bilateral ophthalmoplegia in basilar-vertebral artery disease. Brain, 88: 97–106.

MASUROVSKY, E. B., BUNGE, M. B., AND BUNGE, R. P. 1967. Cytological studies of organotypic cultures of rat dorsal root ganglia following X-irradiation in vitro. I. Changes in neurons and satellite cells. J. Cell Biol., 32: 467–496.

MATTHEWS, M. R., COWAN, W. M., AND POWELL, T. P. S. 1960. Transneuronal cell degeneration in the lateral geniculate nucleus of the macaque monkey. J. Anat., 94: 145–169.

MATTHEWS, P. B. C. 1964. Muscle spindles and their motor control. Physiol. Rev., 44: 219–288.

MATZKE, H. A. 1951. The course of fibers arising from

the nucleus gracilis and cuneatus of the cat. J. Comp. Neurol., 94: 439–452.

MAXWELL, D. S., AND KRUGER, L. 1965. The fine structure of astrocytes in the cerebral cortex and their response to focal injury produced by heavy ionizing particles. J. Cell Biol., 25: 141–157.

MAXWELL, D. S., AND KRUGER, L. 1965a. Small blood vessels and the origin of phagocytes in the rat cerebral cortex following heavy particle irradiation. Exper. Neurol., 12: 33–54.

MAXWELL, D. S., AND KRUGER, L. 1966. The reactive oligodendrocyte. An electron microscopic study of cerebral cortex following Alpha particle irradiation. Am. J. Anat., 118: 437–460.

MAYNARD, E. A., SCHULTZ, R. L., AND PEASE, D. C. 1957. Electron microscopy of the vascular bed of rat cerebral cortex. Am. J. Anat., 100: 409–434.

MEESEN, H., AND OLSZEWSKI, J. 1949. A Cytoarchitectonic Atlas of the Rhombencephalon of the Rabbit. S. Karger, Basel.

MEHLER, W. R. 1966. Further notes on the center median nucleus of Luys. In D. P. PURPURA AND M. D. YAHR (Editors), The Thalamus. Columbia University Press, New York, pp. 109–127.

MEHLER, W. R. 1966a. The posterior thalamic region. Confinia neurol., 27: 18–29.

MEHLER, W. R. 1966b. Some observations on secondary ascending afferent systems in the central nervous system. In R. S. KNIGHTON AND P. R. DUMKE (Editors), Pain. Little, Brown & Company, Boston, Ch. 2, pp. 11–32.

MEHLER, W. R., FEFERMAN, M. E., AND NAUTA, W. J. G. 1956. Ascending axon degeneration following anterolateral chordotomy in the monkey. Anat. Rec., 124: 332–333.

MEHLER, W. R., FEFERMAN, M. E., AND NAUTA, W. J. H. 1960. Ascending axon degeneration following anterolateral cordotomy. An experimental study in the monkey. Brain, 83: 718–750.

MEHLER, W. R., VERNIER, V. G., AND NAUTA, W. J. H. 1958. Efferent projections from the dentate and interpositus nuclei in primates. Anat. Rec., 130: 430–431.

MELTZER, S. J. 1906–07. The factors of safety in animal structure and animal economy. Harvey Lect., pp. 139–169.

MELZACK, R., AND WALL, P. D. 1965. Pain mechanisms: A new theory. Science, 150: 971–979.

MERKEL, F. 1875. Tastzellen und Tastkörperchen bei den Hausthieren und beim Menschen. Arch. mikrosk. Anat., 11: 636–652.

MERRILLEES, N. C. R. 1962. Some observations on the fine structure of a Golgi tendon organ of a rat. In D. BARKER (Editor), Symposium on Muscle Receptors. Hong Kong University Press, Hong Kong, pp. 199–206.

MERRILLEES, N., SUNDERLAND, S., AND HAYHOW, W. 1950. Neuromuscular spindles in the extraocular muscles in man. Anat. Rec., 108: 23–30.

MERTON, P. A. 1953. Speculations on the servo-control of movement. In G. E. W. WOLSTENHOLME (Editor), The Spinal Cord. Churchill, London, pp. 247–255.

MERZENICH, M. M. AND BRUGGE, J. F. 1973. Representation of the cochlear partition on the superior temporal plane of the Macaque monkey. Brain Res., 50: 275–296.

MERZENICH, M. M., KNIGHT, P. L., AND ROTH, G. L. 1973. Cochleotopic organization of primary auditory cortex in the cat. Brain Res., 63: 343–346.

METTLER, F. A. 1932. Connections of the auditory cortex of the cat. J. Comp. Neurol., 55: 139–183.

METTLER, F. A. 1942. Relation between pyramidal and extrapyramidal function. A. Res. Nerv. & Ment. Dis., Proc., 21: 150–227.

METTLER, F. A. 1943. Extensive unilateral cerebral removals in the primate. Physiologic effects and resultant degeneration. J. Comp. Neurol., 79: 185–243.

METTLER, F. A. 1944. The tegmento-olivary and central tegmental fasciculi. J. Comp. Neurol.; 80: 149–175.

METTLER, F. A. 1944a. On the origin of the fibers in the pyramid of the primate brain. Proc. Soc. Exper. Biol. & Med., 57: 111–113.

METTLER, F. A. 1947. The non-pyramidal motor projections from the frontal cerebral cortex. A. Res. Nerv. & Ment. Dis., Proc., 26: 162–199.

METTLER, F. A. 1947a. Extracortical connections of the primate frontal cerebral cortex. I. Thalamo-cortical connections. J. Comp. Neurol., 86: 95–117.

METTLER, F. A. 1947b. Extracortical connections of the primate frontal cerebral cortex. II. Corticofugal connections. J. Comp. Neurol., 86: 119–154.

METTLER, F. A. 1948. Neuroanatomy. C. V. Mosby Company, St. Louis, 536 pp.

METTLER, F. A. 1949. Selective Partial Ablation of the Frontal Cortex: A Correlative Study of the Effects on Human Psychotic Subjects. Paul B. Hoeber, Inc., New York, 527 pp.

METTLER, F. A. 1955. The experimental anatomophysiologic approach to the study of diseases of the basal ganglia. J. Neuropath. & Exper. Neurol., 14: 115–141.

METTLER, F. A. 1970. Nigrofugal connections in the primate brain. J. Comp. Neurol., 138: 291–319.

METTLER, F. A., COOPER, I. S., LISS, H., CARPENTER, M. B., AND NOBACK, C. R. 1954. Patterns of vascular failure in the central nervous system. J. Neuropath. & Exper. Neurol., 13: 528–539.

METTLER, F. A., LISS, H. R., AND STEVENS, G. H. 1956. Blood supply of the primate striopallidum. J. Neuropath., & Exper. Neurol., 15: 377–383.

METTLER, F. A., AND LUBIN, A. J. 1942. Termination of the brachium pontis. J. Comp. Neurol., 77: 391–397.

METUZALS, J. 1965. Ultrastructure of the nodes of Ranvier and their surrounding structures in the central nervous system. Ztschr. Zellforsch. mikrosk. Anat., 65: 719–759.

MEYER, A., BECK, E., AND McLARDY, T. 1947. Prefrontal leucotomy: A neuroanatomical report. Brain, 70: 18–49.

MEYER, D. R., AND WOOLSEY, C. N. 1952. Effects of localized cortical destruction upon auditory discriminative conditioning in the cat. J. Neurophysiol., 15: 149–162.

MEYER, M. 1949. Study of efferent connections of the frontal lobe in the human brain after leucotomy. Brain, 72: 265–296.

MEYERS, R. E. 1956. Function of corpus callosum in interocular transfer. Brain, 79: 358–363.

MIALE, I. L., AND SIDMAN, R. L. 1961. An autoradiographic analysis of histogenesis in the mouse cerebellum. Exper. Neurol., 4: 277–296.

MICKLE, W. A., AND ADES, H. W. 1952. A composite sensory projection area in the cerebral cortex of the cat. Am. J. Physiol., 170: 682–689.

MILLEN, J. W., AND WOOLLAM, D. H. M. 1961. Observations on the nature of the pia mater. Brain, 84: 514–520.

MILLEN, J. W., AND WOOLLAM, D. H. M. 1962. The Anatomy of the Cerebrospinal Fluid. Oxford University Press, New York, pp. 90–102.

MILLER, M. R., RALSTON, H. J., AND KASAHARA, M. 1958. The pattern of cutaneous innervation of the human hand. Am. J. Anat., 102: 183–218.

MILLER, M. R., RALSTON, H. J., AND KASAHARA, M. 1960. The pattern of cutaneous innervation of the human hand, foot, and breast. In W. MONTAGNA (Editor), Cutaneous Innervation. Advances in Biology of Skin, Vol. I. Pergamon Press, New York, pp. 1–47.

MILLER, S., AND OSCARSSON, O. 1970. Termination and functional organization of spino-olivocerebellar paths. In W. S. FIELDS AND W. D. WILLIS (Editors), The Cere-

bellum in Health and Disease. Warren H. Green, Inc., St. Louis, Ch. 6, pp. 172–200.

MINKOWSKI, M. 1913. Experimentelle Untersuchungen über die Beziehungen der Grosshirnrinde und der Netzhaut zu den primären optischen Zentren, besonders zum Corpus geniculatum externum. Arb. Hirnanat. Inst. Zürich, 7: 255–362.

MINKOWSKI, M. 1923–24. Etude sur les connections anatomiques des circonvolution rolandiques, parietales et frontales. Schweiz. Arch. Neurol. u. Psychiat., 12: 71–104 and 227–268; 14: 255–278; 15: 97–132.

MISCOLCZY, D. 1931. Über die Endigungsweise der spinocerebellaren Bahnen. Ztschr. Anat. Entwickl.-Gesch. 96: 537–542.

MISCOLCZY, D. 1934. Die Endigungsweise der olivocerebellaren Faserung. Arch. Psychiat., 102: 197–201.

MITCHELL, G. A. G. 1953. *Anatomy of the Autonomic Nervous System.* E. & S. Livingston, Ltd., Edinburgh.

VON MONAKOW, C. 1895. Experimentelle und pathologisch-anatomische Untersuchungen über die haubenregion, den Sehhügel und die Regio subthalamica. Arch. Psychiat., 27: 1–219.

VON MONAKOW, C. 1905. *Gehirnpathologie,* Ed. 2. Hölder, Wien, 1319 pp.

VON MONAKOW, C. 1909. Der rote Kern, die Haube und die regio subthalamica bei einigen Säaugetieren und beim Menschen. I. Anatomisches und Experimentelles. Arb. Hirnanat. Inst. Zurich, 4: 103–226.

MONIZ, E. 1931. *Diagnostic des tumeurs cérébrales et épreuve de l'encéphalographie artérielle.* Masson et Cie, Paris, 512 pp.

MONIZ, E. 1934. *L'Angiographie cérébrale, ses applications et resultats en anatomie, physiologie et clinique.* Masson et Cie, Paris, 327 pp.

MONIZ, E. 1936. *Tentatives opératoire dans le traitement de certaines psychoses.* Masson et Cie, Paris, 248 pp.

MONRAD-KROHN, G. H. 1924. On the dissociation of voluntary and emotional innervation in facial paresis of central origin. Brain, 47: 22–35.

MONRAD-KROHN, G. H. 1939. On facial dissociation. Acta psychiat. et neurol. scandinav., 14: 557–566.

MOORE, R. Y. 1973. Retinohypothalamic projection in mammals: A comparative study. Brain Res., 49: 403–409.

MOORE, R. Y., BHATNAGAR, R. K., AND HELLER, A. 1971. Anatomical and chemical studies of a nigro-neostriatal projection in the cat. Brain Res., 30: 119–135.

MOORE, R. Y., AND LENN, N. J. 1972. A retinohypothalamic projection in the rat. J. Comp. Neurol., 146: 1–14.

MOREL, F. 1947. La massa intermedia ou commissure grise. Acta anat., 4: 203–207.

MOREST, D. K. 1960. A study of the structure of the area postrema with Golgi methods. Am. J. Anat., 107: 291–303.

MOREST, D. K. 1964. The neuronal architecture of the medial geniculate body of the cat. J. Anat., 98: 611–638.

MOREST, D. K. 1965. The laminar structure of the medial geniculate body of the cat. J. Anat. 99: 143–159.

MOREST, D. K. 1967. Experimental study of the projections of the nucleus of the tractus solitarius and the area postrema in the cat. J. Comp. Neurol., 130: 277–299.

MORGAN, L. R. 1927. The corpus striatum. Arch. Neurol. & Psychiat., 18: 495–549.

MORIN, F. 1955. A new spinal pathway for cutaneous impulses. Am. J. Physiol., 183: 245–252.

MORIN, F., AND CATALANO, J. V. 1955. Central connections of a cervical nucleus (nucleus cervicalis lateralis of the cat). J. Comp. Neurol., 103: 17–32.

MORIN, F., AND GARDNER, E. D. 1953. Spinal pathways for cerebellar projections in the monkey (*Macaca mu-*

latta). Am. J. Physiol., 174: 155–161.

MORIN, F., SCHWARTZ, H. G., AND O'LEARY, J. L. 1951. Experimental study of the spinothalamic and related tract. Acta psychiat. et neurol. scandinav., 26: 371–396.

MORISON, R. S., AND DEMPSEY, E. W. 1942. A study of thalamocortical relations. Am. J. Physiol., 135: 281–292.

MORISON, R. S., AND DEMPSEY, E. W. 1942a. Mechanisms of thalamocortical augmentation and repetition. Am. J. Physiol., 138: 297–308.

MORRISON, L. R. 1929. *Anatomical Studies of the Central Nervous Systems of Dogs without Forebrain or Cerebellum.* De Erven F. Bohn, Haarlem. (Reviewed in Arch. Neurol. & Psychiat., 1930, 24: 218–220.)

MORUZZI, G. 1963. Active processes in the brain stem during sleep. Harvey Lec., ser. 58: 233–297.

MORUZZI, G., AND MAGOUN, H. W. 1949. Brain stem reticular formation and activation of the EEG. Electroencephalog. & Clin. Neurophysiol., 1: 455–473.

MORUZZI, G., AND POMPEIANO, O. 1956. Crossed fastigial influence on decerebrate rigidity. J. Comp. Neurol., 106: 371–392.

MOSKOWITZ, N., AND LIU, J.-C. 1972. Central projections of the spiral ganglion of the squirrel monkey. J. Comp. Neurol., 144: 335–344.

MOTT, F. W., AND SHERRINGTON, C. S. 1895. Experiments upon the influence of sensory nerves upon movement and nutrition of the limbs. Proc. Róy. Soc., London, 57: 481–488.

MOULTON, D. G., AND BEIDLER, L. M. 1967. Structure and function in the peripheral olfactory system. Physiol. Rev., 47: 1–52.

MOUNTCASTLE, V. B. 1957. Modality and topographic properties of single neurons of cat's somatic sensory cortex. J. Neurophysiol., 20: 408–434.

MOUNTCASTLE, V. B. 1962. Editor,*Interhemispheric Relations and Cerebral Dominance.* Johns Hopkins Press, Baltimore, 294 pp.

MOUNTCASTLE, V. B. 1974. Sensory receptors and neural encoding: Introduction to sensory processes. In V. B. MOUNTCASTLE (Editor), *Medical Physiology.* Vol. I. C. V. Mosby Company, St. Louis, pp. 285–306.

MOUNTCASTLE, V. B., AND HENNEMAN, E. 1949. Pattern of tactile representation in thalamus of cat. J. Neurophysiol., 12: 85–100.

MOUNTCASTLE, V. B., AND HENNEMAN, E. 1952. The representation of tactile sensibility in the thalamus of the monkey. J. Comp. Neurol., 97: 409–440.

MOUNTCASTLE, V. B., AND POWELL, T. P. S. 1959. Central nervous mechanisms subserving position sense and kinesthesis. Bull. Johns Hopkins Hosp., 105: 173–200.

MOUNTCASTLE, V. B., AND POWELL, T. P. S. 1959a. Neural mechanisms subserving cutaneous sensibility with special reference to the role of afferent inhibition in sensory perception and discrimination. Bull. Johns Hopkins Hosp., 105: 201–232.

MOUNTCASTLE, V. B., TALBOT, W. H., DARIAN-SMITH, I., AND KORNHUBER, H. H. 1967. The neural base for the sense of flutter vibration. Science, 155: 597–600.

MOZELL, M. M. 1964. Olfactory discrimination; electrophysiological spatio-temporal basis. Science, 143: 1336–1337.

MUGNAINI, E. 1972. The histology and cytology of the cerebellar cortex. In O. LARSELL AND J. JANSEN (Editors), *The Comparative Anatomy and Histology of the Cerebellum. The Human Cerebellum, Cerebellar Connections, and Cerebellar Cortex.* University of Minnesota Press, Minneapolis, pp. 201–262.

MUGNAINI, E., AND WALBERG, F. 1964. Ultrastructure of neuroglia. Ergebn. Anat. Entwickl.-Gesch., 37: 194–236.

MUGNAINI, E., AND WALBERG, F. 1967. An experimental electron microscopical study on the mode of termination of cerebellar corticovestibular fibres in the cat lateral vestibular nucleus (Deiters' nucleus). Exper. Brain Res., 4: 212–236.

MUGNAINI, E., WALBERG, F., AND BRODAL, A. 1967. Mode of termination of primary vestibular fibres in the lateral vestibular nucleus. An experimental electron microscopical study in the cat. Exper. Brain Res., 4: 187–211.

MULLAN, S., AND PENFIELD, W. 1959. Illusions of comparative interpretation and emotion. Arch. Neurol. & Psychiat., 81: 269–284.

MUNGER, B. L. 1965. The intraepidermal innervation of the snout skin of the opossum. A light and electron microscope study, with observations of the nature of Merkel's Tastzellen. J. Cell Biol., 26: 79–97.

MUNGER, B. L. 1966. In A. V. S. DE REUCK AND J. KNIGHT (Editors), Discussion of: Fine structure of the receptor organs and its possible significance (N. Cauna) Touch, Heat, and Pain. Ciba Foundation Symposium. Little, Brown and Company, Boston, pp. 129–130.

MURALT, A. V. 1946. Die Signalübermittlung im Nerven. Verlag Birkhäuser, Basel.

MURPHY, M. G., O'LEARY, J. L., AND CORNBLATH, D. 1973. Axoplasmic flow in cerebellar mossy and climbing fibers. Arch. Neurol., 28: 118–123.

MURRAY, M. R. 1957. Tissue culture studies of neural tissue. In W. F. WINDLE (Editor), New Research Techniques of Neuroanatomy. Charles C Thomas, Publisher, Springfield, Ill., Ch. 5, pp. 40–50.

MURRAY, M. R. 1958. Response of oligodendrocytes to serotonin. In W. F. WINDLE (Editor), Biology of Neuroglia. Charles C Thomas, Publisher, Springfield, Ill., pp. 176–180.

MURRAY, M. R. 1965. Nervous tissue in vitro. In E. N. WILMER (Editor), Cells and Tissues in Culture, Methods, Biology and Physiology, Vol. 2. Academic Press, New York, pp. 373–455.

MURRAY, M. R. 1966. Degeneration of some intralaminar thalamic nuclei after cortical removals in the cat. J. Comp. Neurol., 127: 344–368.

MURRAY, M. R., AND STOUT, A. P. 1947. Adult human sympathetic ganglion cells cultivated in vitro. Am. J. Anat., 80: 225–273.

MUSSEN, A. T. 1927. Experimental investigations on the cerebellum. Brain, 50: 313–349.

MYTILINEOU, C., ISSIDORIDES, M., AND SHANKLIN, W. M. 1963. Histochemical reactions of human autonomic ganglia. J. Anat., 97: 533–542.

NAGEOTTE, J. 1906. The pars intermedia or nervus intermedius of Wrisberg, and the bulbo-pontine gustatory nucleus in man. Rev. Neurol. Psychiat., 4: 473–488.

NAKAO, H. 1958. Emotional behavior produced by hypothalamic stimulation. Am. J. Physiol., 194: 411–418.

VON NAMBA, M. 1957. Cytoarchitektonische Untersuchungen am Striatum. J. Hirnforsch., 3: 24–48.

NAMBA, T., NAKAMURA, T., AND GROB, D. 1968. Motor nerve endings in human extraocular muscle. Neurology, 18: 403–407.

NANDY, K. 1968. Histochemical study of chromatolytic neurons. Arch. Neurol., 18: 425–434.

NARABAYASHI, H. 1972. Stereotaxic amygdalotomy. In B. E. ELEFTHERIOU (Editor), The Neurobiology of the Amygdala. Plenum Press, New York, pp. 459–483.

NARABAYASHI, H., NAGAO, T., SAITO, Y., YOSHIDA, M., AND NAGAHATA, M. 1963. Stereotaxic amygdalotomy for behavior disorders. Arch. Neurol., 9: 1–16.

NARABAYASHI, H., OKUMA, T., AND SHIKIBA, S. 1956. Procaine oil blocking of the globus pallidus. A. M. A. Arch. Neurol. & Psychiat., 75: 36–48.

NATHAN, P. W., AND SMITH, M. C. 1951. The centripetal pathway from the bladder and urethra within the spinal cord. J. Neurol. Neurosurg. & Psychiat., 14: 262–280.

NATHAN, P. W., AND SMITH, M. C. 1955. Spinocortical fibres in man. J. Neurol. Neurosurg. & Psychiat., 18: 181–190.

NATHAN, P. W., AND SMITH, M. C. 1955a. Long descending tracts in man. I. Review of present knowledge. Brain, 78: 248–303.

NATHANIEL, E. J. H., AND NATHANIEL, D. R. 1966. The ultrastructural features of the synapses in the posterior horn of the spinal cord in the rat. J. Ultrastruct. Res., 14: 540–555.

NATHANIEL, E. J. H., AND PEASE, D. C. 1963. Degenerative changes in rat dorsal roots during Wallerian degeneration. J. Ultrastruct. Res., 9: 511–532.

NATHANIEL, E. J. H., AND PEASE, D. C. 1963a. Regenerative changes in rat dorsal roots following Wallerian degeneration. J. Ultrastruct. Res., 9: 533–549.

NAUTA, W. J. H. 1956. An experimental study of the fornix in the rat. J. Comp. Neurol., 104: 247–272.

NAUTA, W. J. H. 1958. Hippocampal projections and related neural pathways to the midbrain in the cat. Brain, 81: 319–340.

NAUTA, W. J. H. 1961. Fibre degeneration following lesions of the amygdaloid complex in the monkey. J. Anat., 95: 515–531.

NAUTA, W. J. H. 1962. Neural associations of the amygdaloid complex in the monkey. Brain, 85: 505–520.

NAUTA, W. J. H. 1972. The central visceromotor system: A general survey. In C. H. HOCKMAN (Editor), Limbic System Mechanisms and Autonomic Function. Charles C Thomas, Springfield, Ill., Ch. 2, pp. 21–33.

NAUTA, W. J. H., AND BUCHER, V. M. 1954. Efferent connections of the striate cortex in the albino rat. J. Comp. Neurol., 100: 257–285.

NAUTA, W. J. H., AND GYGAX, P. A. 1951. Silver impregnation of degenerating axon terminals in the central nervous system: (1) technic; (2) chemical notes. Stain Technol., 26: 5–11.

NAUTA, W. J. H., AND GYGAX, P. A. 1954. Silver impregnation of degenerating axons in the central nervous system: A modified technic. Stain Technol., 29: 91–93.

NAUTA, W. J. H., AND HAYMAKER, W. 1969. Hypothalamic nuclei and fiber connections. In W. HAYMAKER et al. (Editors), The Hypothalamus. Charles C Thomas Publisher, Springfield, Ill., Ch. 4, pp. 136–209.

NAUTA, W. J. H., AND KUYPERS, H. G. J. M. 1958. Some ascending pathways in the brain stem reticular formation. In H. H. JASPER et al. (Editors), Reticular Formation of the Brain. Henry Ford Hospital International Symposium. Little, Brown and Company, Boston, Ch. 1, pp. 3–30.

NAUTA, W. J. H., AND MEHLER, W. R. 1966. Projections of the lentiform nucleus in the monkey. Brain Res., 1: 3–42.

NAUTA, W. J. H., AND WHITLOCK, D. G. 1954. An anatomical analysis of the non-specific thalamic projection system. In J. F. DELAFRESNAYE (Editor), Brain Mechanisms and Consciousness (Symposium), Blackwell Scientific Publications, Oxford, pp. 81–98.

NEFF, W. D. 1961. Neural mechanisms of auditory discrimination. In W. A. ROSENBLITH (Editor), Sensory Communications, Massachusetts Institute of Technology Press and John Wiley & Sons, New York.

NEFF, W. D., AND DIAMOND, I. T. 1958. The neural basis of auditory discrimination. In H. F. HARLOW AND C. N. WOOLSEY (Editors), Biological and Biochemical Bases of Behavior. University of Wisconsin Press, Madison, pp. 101–126.

NEFF, W. D., FISHER, J. F., DIAMOND, I. T., AND YELA,

M. 1956. Role of auditory cortex in discrimination requiring localization of sound in space. J. Neurophysiol., 19: 500–512.

NEUTRA, M., AND LEBLOND, C. P. 1969. The Golgi apparatus. Sc. Am., 220: 100–107.

NGAI, S. H., AND WANG, S. C. 1957. Organization of central respiratory mechanisms in the brain stem of the cat: Localization by stimulation and destruction. Am. J. Physiol., 190: 343–349.

NICKERSON, M. 1970. Drugs inhibiting adrenergic nerves and structures innervated by them. In L. S. GOODMAN AND A. GILMAN (Editors), The Pharmacological Basis of Therapeutics. The Macmillan Company, New York, Ch. 26, pp. 549–584.

NIEMER, W. T., AND MAGOUN, H. W. 1947. Reticulospinal tracts influencing motor activity. J. Comp. Neurol., 87: 367–379.

NIIMI, K., KATAYAMA, K., KANASEKI, T., AND MORIMOTO, K. 1960. Studies on the derivation of the centre median nucleus of Luys. Tokushima J. Exper. Med., 6: 261–268.

NOBACK, C. R., AND LAEMLE, L. K. 1970. Structural and functional aspects of the visual pathways of primates. In C. R. NOBACK AND W. MONTAGNA (Editors), The Primate Brain, Advances in Primatology, Vol. 1. Appleton-Century-Crofts, New York, Ch. 3, pp. 55–81.

NORBERG, K. A. 1967. Transmitter histochemistry of the sympathetic adrenergic nervous system. Brain Res., 5: 125–170.

NORRSELL, U., AND VOORHOEVE, P. 1962. Tactile pathways from the hindlimb to the cerebral cortex in cat. Acta physiol. scandinav., 54: 9–17.

NOVAK, J., AND SALAFSKY, B. 1967. Early electrophysiological changes after denervation of slow skeletal muscle. Exper. Neurol., 19: 388–400.

NYBERG-HANSEN, R. 1964. Origin and termination of fibers from the vestibular nuclei descending in the medial longitudinal fasciculus. An experimental study with silver impregnation methods in the cat. J. Comp. Neurol., 122: 355–368.

NYBERG-HANSEN, R. 1965. Sites and mode of termination of reticulospinal fibers in the cat. An experimental study with silver impregnation methods. J. Comp. Neurol., 124: 71–99.

NYBERG-HANSEN, R. 1966. Functional organization of descending supraspinal fibre systems to the spinal cord. Anatomical observations and physiological correlations. Ergebn. Anat. Entwicklungsgesch., 39: (no. 2) 1–48.

NYBERG-HANSEN, R., AND BRODAL, A. 1963. Sites of termination of corticospinal fibers in the cat. An experimental study with silver impregnation methods. J. Comp. Neurol., 120: 369–392.

NYBERG-HANSEN, R., AND BRODAL, A. 1964. Sites and mode of termination of rubrospinal fibres in the cat. An experimental study with silver impregnation methods. J. Anat., 98: 235–253.

NYBERG-HANSEN, R., AND MASCITTI, T. A. 1964. Sites and mode of termination of fibers of the vestibulospinal tract in the cat. An experimental study with silver impregnation methods. J. Comp. Neurol., 122: 369–387.

NYBY, O., AND JANSEN, J. 1951. An experimental investigation of the corticopontine projection in Macaca mulatta. Norske Vid.-Akad. Avh. Mat.-Naturv., 3: 1–47.

OLDS, J. 1960. Differentiation of reward systems in the brain by self-stimulation technics. In S. R. RAMEY AND D. S. O'DOHERTY (Editors), Electrical Studies on the Unanesthetized Brain. Paul B. Hoeber, Inc., New York, Ch. 2, pp. 17–51.

OLDS, J., AND MILNER, P. 1954. Positive reinforcement produced by electrical stimulation of septal area and other regions of the rat brain. J. Comp. & Physiol.

Psychol., 47: 419–427.

O'LEARY, J. L., DUNSKER, S. B., SMITH, J. M., INUKAI, J., AND O'LEARY, M. 1970. Termination of the olivocerebellar system in the cat. Arch. Neurol., 22: 193–206.

O'LEARY, J. L., KERR, F. W. L., AND GOLDRING, S. 1958. The relation between spinoreticular and ascending cephalic systems. In H. H. JASPERS et al. (Editors), Reticular Formation of the Brain. Henry Ford Hospital International Symposium. Little, Brown and Company Boston, Ch. 8, pp. 187–201.

OLIVECRONA, H. 1957. Paraventricular nucleus and the pituitary gland. Acta physiol. scandinav., 40: Suppl. 136, 1–178.

DE OLMOS, J. S. 1972. The amygdaloid projection field in the rat as studied with the cupric-silver method. In B. E. ELEFTHERIOU (Editor), The Neurobiology of the Amygdala. Plenum Press, New York, pp. 145–204.

OLSEN, L., AND FUXE, K. 1971. On the projections from the locus coeruleus noradrenalin neurons: The cerebellar innervation. Brain Res., 28: 165–171.

OLSZEWSKI, J. 1950. On the anatomical and functional organization of the spinal trigeminal nucleus. J. Comp. Neurol., 92: 401–413.

OLSZEWSKI, J. 1952. The Thalamus of the Macaca Mulatta. S. Karger, Basel, 93 pp.

OLSZEWSKI, J. 1954. Cytoarchitecture of the human reticular formation In J. F. DELAFRESNAYE (Editor), Brain Mechanisms and Consciousness (Symposium). Blackwell Scientific Publications, Oxford, pp. 54–80.

OLSZEWSKI, J., AND BAXTER, D. 1954. Cytoarchitecture of the Human Brain Stem. J. B. Lippincott Company, Philadelphia.

OOMURA, Y., ONO, T., AND OOYAMA, H. 1970. Inhibitory action of the amygdala on the lateral hypothalamic area in rats. Nature, 228: 1108–1110.

OPPENHEIMER, D. R., PALMER, E., AND WEDELL, G. 1958. Nerve endings in the conjunctiva. J. Anat., 92: 321–352.

ORBACH, J., AND CHOW, K. L. 1959. Differential effects of resection of somatic areas I and II in monkeys. J. Neurophysiol., 22: 195–203.

ORBACH, J., MILNER, B., AND RASMUSSEN, T. 1960. Learning and retention in monkeys after amygdala-hippocampus resection. Arch. Neurol., 3: 230–251.

ORIOLI, F. L., AND METTLER, F. A. 1956. The rubrospinal tract in Macaca mulatta. J. Comp. Neurol., 106: 299–318.

ORLOVSKY, G. N. 1972. Activity of vestibulospinal neurons during locomotion. Brain Res. 46: 85–98.

ORLOVSKY, G. N. 1972a. Activity of rubrospinal neurons during locomotion. Brain Res., 46: 99–112.

ORTMANN, R. 1960. Neurosecretion. In J. FIELD (Editor), Handbook of Physiology, Neurophysiology, Vol. II. American Physiological Society, Washington, D. C., Ch. 40, pp. 1039–1065.

OSCARSSON, O. 1964. Three ascending tracts activated from group I afferents in forelimb nerves of the cat. In J. C. ECCLES AND J. P. SCHADÉ (Editors), Physiology of Spinal Neurons, Progress in Brain Research, Vol. 12. Elsevier Publishing Company, Amsterdam, pp. 179–196.

OSCARSSON, O. 1964a. Integrative organization of the rostral spinocerebellar tract in the cat. Acta physiol. scandinav., 64: 154–166.

OSCARSSON, O. 1965. Functional organization of the spino- and cuneocerebellar tracts. Physiol. Rev., 45: 495–522.

OSCARSSON, O. 1967. Termination and functional organization of a dorsal spino-olivocerebellar path. Brain Res., 5: 531–534.

OSCARSSON, O. 1967a. Functional significance of information channels from the spinal cord to the cerebellum. In M. D. YAHR AND D. P. PURPURA (Editors), Neurophysiological Basis of Normal and Abnormal Motor Activities.

Raven Press, New York, pp. 93–113.

OSCARSSON, O., AND ROSÉN, I. 1966. Short-latency projections to the cat's cerebral cortex from skin and muscle afferents in the contralateral forelimb. J. Physiol., 182: 164–184.

OSCARSSON, O., AND UDDENBERG, N. 1964. Identification of a spinocerebellar tract activated from forelimb afferents in the cat. Acta physiol. scandinav, 62: 125–136.

OSEN, K. K. 1969. The intrinsic organization of the cochlear nuclei in the cat. Acta oto-laryng., 67: 352–359.

OZEKI, M., AND SATO, M. 1964. Initiation of impulses at the non-myelinated terminal in Pacinian corpuscles. J. Physiol., 170: 167–185.

OZEKI, M., AND SATO, M. 1965. Changes in the membrane potential and the membrane conductance associated with a sustained compression of the non-myelinated nerve terminal in Pacinian corpuscles, J. Physiol., 180: 186–208.

PALAY, S. L. 1945. Neurosecretion. VII. The preoptico-hypophysial pathway in fishes. J. Comp. Neurol., 82: 129–143.

PALAY, S. L. 1956. Synapses in the central nervous system. J. Biophys. Biochem. Cytol. 2 (suppl.): 193–201.

PALAY, S. L. 1957. The fine structure of the neurohypophysis. In H. WAELSCH (Editor), Ultrastructure and Cellular Chemistry of Neural Tissue. Paul B. Hoeber, Inc., New York, pp. 31–44.

PALAY, S. L. 1958. An electron microscopical study of neuroglia. In W. F. WINDLE (Editor), Biology of Neuroglia. Charles C Thomas, Publisher, Springfield, Ill., pp. 24–38.

PALAY, S. L. 1966. The role of neuroglia in the organization of the central nervous system. In K. RODAHL AND B. ISSEKUTZ, JR. (Editors), Nerve as A Tissue. Hoeber Med. Div. Harper and Row, New York, pp. 3–10.

PALAY, S. L., AND CHAN-PALAY, V. 1974. Cerebellar Cortex. Cytology and Organization. Springer Verlag, Berlin.

PALAY, S. L., AND PALADE, G. E. 1955. The fine structure of neurons. J. Biophys. Biochem. Cytol., 1: 69–88.

PAPEZ, J. W. 1927. Subdivisions of the facial nucleus. J. Comp. Neurol., 43: 159–191.

PAPEZ, J. W. 1936. Evolution of the medial geniculate body. J. Comp. Neurol., 64: 41–61.

PAPEZ, J. W. 1937. A proposed mechanism of emotion. Arch. Neurol. & Psychiat., 38: 725–743.

PAPEZ, J. W. 1938. Thalamic connections in a hemidecorticate dog. J. Comp. Neurol., 69: 103–119.

PAPEZ, J. W. 1942. A summary of fiber connections of the basal ganglia with each other and with other portions of the brain. A. Res. Nerv. & Ment. Dis., Proc., 21: 21–68.

PAPEZ, J. W. 1956. Central reticular path to intralaminar and reticular nuclei of thalamus for activating EEG related to consciousness. Electroencephalog. & Clin. Neurophysiol., 8: 117–128.

PAPEZ, J. W. 1956a. Path for projection of non-specific diffuse impulses to cortex for EEG, related to consciousness. Dis. Nerv. System, 17: 3–8.

PAPEZ, J. W., BENNETT, A. E., AND CASH, P. T. 1942. Hemichorea (Hemiballismus): Association with a pallidal lesion involving afferent and efferent connections of the subthalamic nucleus; curare therapy. Arch. Neurol. & Psychiat., 47: 667–676.

PAPEZ, J. W., AND FREEMAN, G. L. 1930. Superior colliculi and their fiber connections in the rat. J. Comp. Neurol., 51: 409–439.

PAPEZ, J. W., AND RUNDLES, W. 1937. The dorsal trigeminal tract and the centre median nucleus of Luys. J. Nerv. & Ment. Dis., 85: 509–519.

PAPPAS, G. D. 1966. Electron microscopy of neuronal junctions involved in transmission in the central nervous system. In K. RODAHL AND B. ISSEKUTZ, JR. (Editors), Nerve as a Tissue. Hoeber Med. Div., Harper and Row, New York, p. 49–87.

PARTRIDGE, M. 1950. Prefrontal Leucotomy: A Survey of 300 Cases Personally Followed over 1 1/2–3 Years. Blackwell Scientific Publications, Oxford, 496 pp.

PASS, I. J. 1933. Anatomic and functional relationship of nuc. dorsalis (Clarke's column). Arch. Neurol. & Psychiat., 30: 1025–1045.

PATTON, H. D. 1961. Reflex regulation of movement and posture. In T. C. RUCH et al. (Editors), Neurophysiology. W. B. Saunders Company, Philadelphia, Ch. 6, pp. 167–198.

PATTON, H. D. 1961a. Special properties of nerve trunks and tracts. In T. C. RUCH et al. (Editors), Neurophysiology. W. B. Saunders Company, Philadelphia, Ch. 3, pp. 66–95.

PATTON, H. D., AND RUCH, T. C. 1946. The relation of the foot of the pre- and postcentral gyrus to taste in the monkey and chimpanzee. Fed. Proc., 5: 79.

PATTON, H. D., RUCH, T. C., AND WALKER, A. E. 1944. Experimental hypogeusia from Horsley-Clarke lesions of the thalamus in Macaca mulatta. J. Neurophysiol., 7: 171–184.

PAYNE, F. 1924. General description of a 7-somite human embryo. Contrib. Embryol., 16: 115–124.

PEARSON, A. A. 1949. The development and connections of the mesencephalic root of the trigeminal nerve in man. J. Comp. Neurol., 90: 1–46.

PEARSON, A. A. 1949a. Further observations on the mesencephalic root of the trigeminal nerve. J. Comp. Neurol., 91: 147–194.

PEARSON, A. A. 1952. Role of gelatinous substance of spinal cord in conduction of pain. A. M. A. Arch. Neurol. & Psychiat., 68: 515–529.

PEARSON, A. A., SAUTER, R. W., AND BUCKLEY, T. E. 1966. Further observations on the cutaneous branches of the dorsal primary rami of the spinal nerves. Am. J. Anat., 118: 891–904.

PEELE, T. L. 1942. Cytoarchitecture of individual parietal areas in the monkey (Macaca mulatta) and distribution of the efferent fibers. J. Comp. Neurol., 77: 693–737.

PEELE, T. L. 1961. The Neuroanatomical Basis for Clinical Neurology. McGraw Hill Book Company, New York.

PENFIELD, W. 1920. Alterations of the Golgi apparatus in nerve cells. Brain, 43: 290–305.

PENFIELD, W. 1932. Neuroglia, normal and pathological. In W. G. PENFIELD (Editor), Cytology and Cellular Pathology of the Nervous System, Vol. II. Paul B. Hoeber, Inc., New York, pp. 423–479.

PENFIELD, W. 1957. Vestibular sensation and the cerebral cortex. Ann. Otol. Rhin. & Laryng., 66: 691–698.

PENFIELD, W., AND BOLDREY, E. 1937. Somatic motor and sensory representation in the cerebral cortex of man as studied by electrical stimulation. Brain, 60: 389–443.

PENFIELD, W., AND EVANS, J. 1934. Functional defects produced by cerebral lobectomies. A. Res. Nerv. & Ment. Dis., Proc., 13: 352–377.

PENFIELD, W., AND JASPER, H. H. 1954. Epilepsy and the Functional Anatomy of the Human Brain. Little, Brown and Company, Boston, 896 pp.

PENFIELD, W. G., AND McNAUGHTON, F. 1940. Dural headache and innervation of the dura mater. Arch. Neurol. & Psychiat., 44: 43–75.

PENFIELD, W., AND MILNER, B. 1958. Memory deficit produced by bilateral lesions in the hippocampal zone. Arch. Neurol. & Psychiat., 79: 475–497.

PENFIELD, W., AND RASMUSSEN, T. 1950. The Cerebral Cortex of Man. A Clinical Study of Localization of Function. Macmillan Company, New York, 248 pp.

PENFIELD, W. AND ROBERTS, L. 1959. Speech and Brain

Mechanisms. Princeton University Press, Princeton, N. J.

PENFIELD, W., AND WELCH, K. 1951. The supplementary motor area of the cerebral cortex. A clinical and experimental study. A. M. A. Arch. Neurol. & Psychiat., 66: 289–317.

PERL, E. R., AND WHITLOCK, D. G. 1961. Somatic stimuli exciting spinothalamic projections in thalamic neurons in the cat and monkey. Exper. Neurol., 3: 256–296.

PERL, E. R., WHITLOCK, D. G., AND GENTRY, J. R. 1962. Cutaneous projection to second-order neurons of the dorsal column system. J. Neurophysiol., 25: 337–353.

PETERS, A. 1960. The formation and structure of myelin sheaths in the central nervous system. J. Biophys. Biochem. Cytol., 8: 431–446.

PETERS, A. 1966. The node of Ranvier in the central nervous system. Quart. J. Exper. Physiol., 51: 229–236.

PETERS, A. 1968. An introduction to neuronal fine structure. M. & Biol. Illust., 18: 103–109.

PETERS, A., AND PALAY, S. L. 1965. An electron microscope study of the distribution and patterns of astroglial processes in the central nervous system. J. Anat., 99: 419.

PETERS, A., PALAY, S. L., AND WEBSTER, H. DeF. 1970. *The Fine Structure of the Nervous System*. Harper and Row, Publishers, New York.

PETERS, A., PROSKAUER, C. C., AND KAISERMAN-ABRAMOF, I. R. 1968. The small pyramidal neuron of the rat cerebral cortex: The axon hillock and initial segment. J. Cell Biol., 39: 604–619.

PETERS, A., AND VAUGHN, J. E. 1967. Microtubules and filaments in the axons and astrocytes of early postnatal rat optic nerve. J. Cell Biol., 32: 113–119.

PETERSON, E. R., AND MURRAY, M. R. 1955. Myelin sheath formation in cultures of avian spinal ganglia. Am. J. Anat., 96: 319–355.

PETRAS, J. M. 1964. Some fiber connections of the precentral cortex (areas 4 and 6) with the diencephalon in the monkey (*Macaca mulatta*). Anat. Rec., 148: 322.

PETRAS, J. M. 1965. Some fiber connections of the precentral and postcentral cortex with the basal ganglia, thalamus and subthalamus. Tr. Am. Neurol. A., 90: 274–275.

PETRAS, J. M. 1966. Fiber degeneration in the basal ganglia and diencephalon following lesions in the precentral and postcentral cortex of the monkey (*Macaca mulatta*); with additional observations in the chimpanzee. VII Internat. Congr. Anat. Wiesbaden.

PETRAS, J. M. 1967. Cortical, tectal and tegmental fiber connections in the spinal cord of the cat. Brain Res., 6: 275–324.

PETRAS, J. M. 1969. Some efferent connections of the motor and somatosensory cortex of simian primates and Felid, Canid and Procyonid carnivores. Ann. New York Acad. Sc., 167: 469–505.

PETRAS, J. M., AND CUMMINGS, J. F. 1972. Autonomic neurons in the spinal cord of the Rhesus monkey: A correlation of the findings of cytoarchitectonics and sympathectomy with fiber degeneration following dorsal rhizotomy. J. Comp. Neurol., 146: 189–218.

PETTIGREW, J. D., OLSON, C., AND HIRSCH, H. U. B. 1973. Cortical effects of selective visual experience: Degeneration or reorganization? Brain Res., 51: 345–351.

PFAFFMANN, C. 1939. Afferent impulses from the teeth resulting from a vibratory stimulus. J. Physiol., 97: 220–232.

PHALEN, G. S., AND DAVENPORT, H. A. 1937. Pericellular end-bulbs in the central nervous system of vertebrates. J. Comp. Neurol., 68: 67–81.

PICK, J. 1970. *The Autonomic Nervous System*. J. B. Lippincott Company, Philadelphia, 483 pp.

PICK, J., AND SHEEHAN, D. 1946. Sympathetic rami in man. J. Anat., 80: 12–20.

PICKFORD, M. 1969. Neurohypophysis-antidiuretic (vasopressor) and oxytocic hormones. In W. HAYMAKER *et al.* (Editors), *The Hypothalamus*. Charles C Thomas Publisher, Springfield, Ill., Ch. 13, pp. 463–505.

PIERSON, R. J., AND CARPENTER, M. B. 1974. Anatomical analysis of pupillary reflex pathways in the rhesus monkey. J. Comp. Neurol., 158: 121–143.

PIN, C., JONES, B., AND JOUVET, M. 1968. Topographie des neurones monoaminergiques du tronc cérébral du chat: étude par histofluorescence. Comp. rend. Soc. bic`., ¡62: 2137–2141.

PINDER, R. M. 1973. The pharmacology of Parkinsonism. In G. P. ELLIS AND G. B. WEST (Editors), *Progress in Medicinal Chemistry*, Vol. 9. Butterworths, London, pp. 191–274.

PINEDA, A., MAXWELL, D. S., AND KRUGER, L. 1967. The fine structure of neurons and satellite cells in the trigeminal ganglion of cat and monkey. Am. J. Anat., 121: 461–488.

PINES, I. L. 1925. Über die Innervation der Hypophysis cerebri. II. Mitteilung. Über die Innervation des Mittel- und Hinterlappens der Hypophyse. Ztschr. ges. Neurol. u. Psychiat., 100: 123–138.

PITTS, R. F. 1940. The respiratory center and its descending pathways. J. Comp. Neurol., 72: 605–625.

PITTS, R. F. 1946. Organization of the respiratory center. Physiol Rev., 26: 609–630.

PITTS, R. F., MAGOUN, H. W., AND RANSON, S. W. 1939. Localization of the medullary respiratory centers in the cat. Am. J. Physiol., 126: 673–688.

PLUM, F., AND POSNER, J. B. 1966. *The Diagnosis of Stupor and Coma*. F. A. Davis Company, Philadelphia.

POGGIO, G. F., AND MOUNTCASTLE, V. B. 1960. A study of the functional contributions of the lemniscal and spinothalamic systems to somatic sensibility. Bull. Johns Hopkins Hosp., 106: 266–316.

POIRIER, L. J. 1952. Anatomical and experimental studies on the temporal pole of the macaque. J. Comp. Neurol., 96: 209–248.

POIRIER, L. J., AND BERTRAND, C. 1955. Experimental and anatomical investigation of the lateral spinothalamic and spinotectal tracts. J. Comp. Neurol., 102: 745–757.

POIRIER, L. J., AND BOUVIER, G. 1966. The red nucleus and its efferent nervous pathways in the monkey. J. Comp. Neurol., 128: 223–244.

POIRIER, L. J., AND SOURKES, T. L. 1965. Influence of the substantia nigra on catecholamine content of the striatum. Brain, 88: 181–192.

POLAK, M. 1965. Morphological and functional characteristics of the central and peripheral neuroglia. (Light microscopic observations.) In E. D. P. DeROBERTIS AND R. CARREA (Editors), *Biology of Neurologia, Progress in Brain Research*, Vol. 15. Elsevier Publishing Company, Amsterdam, pp. 12–34.

POLIAK, S. 1924. Die Struktureigentümlichkeiten des Rückenmarkes bei den Chiropteren. Zugleich ein Beitrag zu der Frage über die spinalen Zentren des Sympatheticus. Ztschr. Anat. Entwickl-Gesch., 74: 509–576.

POLYAK, S. L. 1957. *The Vertebrate Visual System*. University of Chicago Press, Chicago, 1390 pp.

POMERAT, C. M. 1958. Functional concepts based on tissue culture studies of neuroglia cells. In W. F. WINDLE (Editor), *Biology of Neuroglia*. Charles C Thomas, Publisher, Springfield, Ill., pp. 162–175.

POMPEIANO, O. 1956. Sulle risposte posturali alla stimolazione elettrica del nucleo rosso nel gatto decerebrato. Boll. soc. ital. biol. sper., 32: 1450–1451.

POMPEIANO, O. 1957. Analisi degli effetti della stimolazione elettrica del nucleo rosso nel gatto decerebrato.

Rend. Accad. naz. Lincei, cl. sci. fis. mat. nat., 22: 100–103.

POMPEIANO, O. 1959. Organizzazione somatotopica delle risposte flessorie alla stimolazione elettrica del nucleo interposito nel gatto decerebrato. Arch. sc. biol., 43: 163–176.

POMPEIANO, O. 1960. Organizzazione somatotopica delle risposte posturali alla stimolazione elettrica del nucleo di Deiters nel Gatto cerebrato. Arch. sc. biol., 44: 497–511.

POMPEIANO, O. 1960a. Localizzazione delle risposte estensorie alla stimolazione elettrica del nucleo interposito nel gatto decerebrato. Arch. sc. biol., 44: 473–496.

POMPEIANO, O. 1967. The neurophysiological mechanisms of the postural and motor events during desynchronized sleep. A. Res. Publ. Nerv. Ment. Dis., Proc., 45: 351–423.

POMPEIANO, O., AND BRODAL, A. 1957. Experimental demonstration of a somatotopical origin of rubrospinal fibers in the cat. J. Comp. Neurol., 108: 225–251.

POMPEIANO, O., AND BRODAL, A. 1957a. Spinovestibular fibers in the cat. An experimental study. J. Comp. Neurol., 108: 353–382.

POMPEIANO, O., AND BRODAL, A. 1957b. The origin of the vestibulospinal fibres in the cat. An experimental-anatomical study, with comments on the descending medial longitudinal fasciculus. Arch. ital. biol., 95: 166–195.

POMPEIANO, O., AND MORRISON, A. R. 1965. Vestibular influences during sleep. I. Abolition of rapid eye movements of desynchronized sleep following vestibular lesions. Arch. ital. biol., 103: 569–595.

POMPEIANO, O., AND WALBERG, F. 1957. Descending connections to the vestibular nuclei. An experimental study in the cat. J. Comp. Neurol., 108: 465–502.

POOL, J. L. 1954. Neurophysiological symposium; visceral brain of man. J. Neurosurg., 11: 45–63.

POPA, G. T., AND FIELDING, U. 1930. A portal circulation from the pituitary to the hypothalamic region. J. Anat., 65: 88–91.

PORTER, J. C., AND JONES, J. C. 1956. Effect of plasma from hypophyseal-portal vessel blood on adrenal ascorbic acid. Endocrinology, 58: 62–67.

POTTS, T. K. 1924. The main peripheral connections of the human sympathetic nervous system. J. Anat., 59: 129–135.

POWELL, T. P. S. 1952. Residual neurons in the human thalamus following hemidecortication. Brain, 75: 571–584.

POWELL, T. P. S., AND COWAN, W. M. 1956. A study of thalamo-striate relations in the monkey. Brain, 79: 364–390.

POWELL, T. P. S., AND COWAN, W. M. 1962. An experimental study of the projection of the cochlea. J. Anat., 96: 269–284.

POWELL, T. P. S., AND COWAN, W. M. 1963. Centrifugal fibers in the lateral olfactory tract. Nature, 199: 1296–1297.

POWELL, T. P. S., AND COWAN, W. M. 1967. The interpretation of the degenerative changes in the intralaminar nuclei of the thalamus. J. Neurol. Neurosurg. & Psychiat., 30: 140–153.

POWELL, T. P. S., COWAN, W. M., AND RAISMAN, G. 1963. Olfactory relationship of the diencephalon. Nature, 199: 710–712.

POWELL, T. P. S., COWAN, W. M., AND RAISMAN, G. 1965. The central olfactory connexions. J. Anat., 99: 791–813.

POWELL, T. P. S., AND ERULKAR, S. D. 1962. Transneuronal cell degeneration in the auditory relay nuclei of the cat. J. Anat., 96: 249–268.

POWELL, T. P. S., GUILLERY, R. W., AND COWAN, W. M. 1957. A quantitative study of the fornix-mam-millo-thalamic system. J. Anat., 91: 419–432.

POWELL, T. P. S., AND MOUNTCASTLE, V. B. 1959. The cytoarchitecture of the postcentral gyrus of the monkey Macaca mulatta. Bull. Johns Hopkins Hosp., 105: 108–131.

POWELL, T. P. S., AND MOUNTCASTLE, V. B. 1959a. Some aspects of the functional organization of the cortex of the postcentral gyrus of the monkey: A correlation of findings obtained in a single unit analysis with cytoarchitecture. Bull. Johns Hopkins Hosp., 105: 133–162.

PREISIG, H. 1904. Le noyau rouge et le pédoncule cérébelleux superieur. J. Psychol. u. Neurol., 3: 215–230.

PRENTISS, C. W., AND AREY, L. B. 1920. A Laboratory Manual and Textbook of Embryology. W. B. Saunders Company, Philadelphia, Ch. XII, pp. 321–352.

PRESTON, J. B., AND WHITLOCK, D. G. 1960. Precentral facilitation and inhibition of spinal motoneurons. J. Neurophysiol., 23: 154–170.

PRESTON, J. B., AND WHITLOCK, D. G. 1961. Intracellular potentials recorded from motoneurons following precentral gyrus stimulation in primate. J. Neurophysiol., 24: 91–100.

PRIBRAM, K. H., AND BAGSHAW, M. 1953. Further analysis of the temporal lobe syndrome utilizing fronto-temporal ablations. J. Comp. Neurol., 99: 347–375.

PRIBRAM, K. H., AND FULTON, J. F. 1954. An experimental critique of the effects of anterior cingulate ablation in monkey. Brain, 77: 34–44.

PRIBRAM, K. H., ROSNER, B. S., AND ROSENBLITH, W. A. 1954. Electrical response to acoustic clicks in monkey: Extent of neocortex activated. J. Neurophysiol., 17: 336–344.

PURPURA, D. P. 1959. Nature of electrocortical potentials and synaptic organizations in cerebral and cerebellar cortex. In C. C. PFEIFFER AND J. R. SMYTHIES (Editors), International Review of Neurobiology, Vol. I. Academic Press, New York, pp. 47–163.

PURPURA, D. P. 1970. Operations and processes in thalamic and synaptically related neural subsystems. In F. O. SCHMITT (Editor), The Neurosciences. Second Study Program. Rockefeller University Press, New York, Ch. 42, pp. 458–470.

PURPURA, D. P., AND COHEN, B. 1962. Intracellular synaptic activities of thalamic neurons during evoked recruiting responses. In 22nd International Congress of Physiological Sciences, Excerpta Medica International Congress Series 48, Leiden.

PURPURA, D. P., FRIGYESI, T. L., McMURTRY, J. G., AND SCARFF, T. 1966. Synaptic mechanisms in thalamic regulation of cerebellocortical projection activity. In D. P. PURPURA AND M. D. YAHR (Editors), The Thalamus. Columbia University Press, New York, pp. 153–170.

PURPURA, D. P., AND GRUNDFEST, H. 1956. Nature of dendritic potentials and synaptic mechanisms in cerebral cortex of cat. J. Neurophysiol., 19: 573–595.

QUENSEL, F. 1910. Über den Stabkranz des menschlichen Stirnhirns. Folia neuro-biol. (Leipzig), 4: 319–334.

QUENSEL, W. 1944. Über die Faserspezifität in sensiblen Hautnerven. Arch. ges. Physiol., 248: 1–20.

QUILLIAM, T. A. 1966. Unit design and array patterns in receptor organs. In A. V. S. DeREUCK AND J. KNIGHT (Editors), Touch, Heat and Pain. Ciba Foundation Symposium. Little, Brown and Company, Boston, pp. 86–112.

RADEMAKER, G. G. T. 1926. Die Bedeutung der roten Kerne und des übrigen Mittelhirns für Muskeltonus, Körperstellung, und Labyrinthreflexe. Julius Springer, Berlin, pp. 64–222.

RAISMAN, G. 1966. Neural connexions of hypothalamus. Brit. M. Bull., 22: 197–201.

RAISMAN, G. 1966a. The connexions of the septum. Brain, 89: 317–348.

RAISMAN, G., COWAN, W. M., AND POWELL, T. P. S. 1965. The extrinsic afferent, commissural and association fibres of the hippocampus. Brain, 88: 963–996.

RAISMAN, G., COWAN, W. M., AND POWELL, T. P. S. 1966. An experimental analysis of the efferent projections of the hippocampus. Brain, 89: 83–108.

RAISMAN, G., AND FIELD, P. M. 1973. Sexual dimorphism in the neuropil of the preoptic area of the rat and its dependence on neonatal androgen. Brain Res., 54: 1–29.

RALSTON, H. J., III 1965. The organization of the substantia gelatinosa Rolandi in the cat lumbosacral spinal cord. Ztschr. Zellforschung, 67: 1–23.

RALSTON, H. J., III 1968. The fine structure of neurons in the dorsal horn of the cat spinal cord. J. Comp. Neurol., 132: 275–302.

ʼRALSTON, H. J., III 1968a. Dorsal root projections to the dorsal horn neurons in the cat spinal cord. J. Comp. Neurol., 132: 303–330.

RALSTON, H. R., III, MILLER, M. R., AND KASAHARA, M. 1960. Nerve endings in human fasciae, tendons, ligaments, periosteum, and joint synovial membrane. Anat. Rec., 136: 137–148.

RAMON-MOLINER, E. 1958. A tungstate modification of the Golgi-Cox method. Stain Technol., 33: 19–29.

RANSON, S. W. 1912. The structure of the spinal ganglia and of the spinal nerves. J. Comp. Neurol., 22: 159–175.

RANSON, S. W. 1913. The course within the spinal cord of the non-medullated fibers of the dorsal roots: A study of Lissauer's tract in the cat. J. Comp. Neurol., 23: 259–281.

RANSON, S. W. 1914. The tract of Lissauer and the substantia gelatinosa Rolandi. Am. J. Anat., 16: 97–126.

RANSON, S. W. 1939. Somnolence caused by hypothalamic lesions in the monkey. Arch. Neurol. & Psychiat., 41: 1–23.

RANSON, S. W., AND BILLINGSLEY, P. R. 1918. The superior cervical ganglion and the cervical portion of the sympathetic trunk. J. Comp. Neurol., 29: 313–358.

RANSON, S. W., AND INGRAM, W. R. 1932. The diencephalic course and termination of the medial lemniscus and brachium conjunctivum. J. Comp. Neurol., 56: 257–275.

RANSON, S. W., AND MAGOUN, H. W. 1933. The central path of the pupillo-constrictor reflex in response to light. Arch. Neurol. & Psychiat., 30: 1193–1204.

RANSON, S. W., AND RANSON, S. W., JR. 1942. Efferent fibers of the corpus striatum. A. Res. Nerv. & Ment. Dis. Proc., 21: 69–76.

RASMUSSEN, A. T. 1936. Tractus tecto-spinalis in the cat. J. Comp. Neurol., 63: 501–525.

RASMUSSEN, A. T., AND PEYTON, W. T. 1948. The course and termination of the medial lemniscus in man. J. Comp. Neurol., 88: 411–424.

RASMUSSEN, G. L. 1946. The olivary peduncle and other fiber projections of the superior olivary complex. J. Comp. Neurol., 84: 141–219.

RASMUSSEN, G. L. 1953. Further observations of the efferent cochlear bundle. J. Comp. Neurol., 99: 61–74.

RASMUSSEN, G. L. 1957. Selective silver impregnation of synaptic endings. In W. F. WINDLE (Editor), New Research Techniques in Neuroanatomy. Charles C Thomas, Publisher, Springfield, Ill., pp. 27–39.

RASMUSSEN, G. L. 1960. Efferent fibers of the cochlear nerve and cochlear nucleus. In G. L. RASMUSSEN AND W. F. WINDLE (Editors), Neural Mechanisms of the Auditory and Vestibular Systems. Charles C Thomas, Publisher, Springfield, Ill. Ch. 8, pp. 105–115.

RASMUSSEN, G. L. 1964. Anatomic relationships of the ascending and descending auditory systems. In W. S. FIELD AND B. R. ALFORD (Editors), Neurological Aspects of Auditory and Vestibular Disorders. Charles C Thomas, Publisher, Springfield, Ill., Ch. 1, pp. 1–14.

RAVIC, P., AND YAKOVLEV, P. I. 1968. Development of the corpus callosum and cavum septi in man. J. Comp. Neurol., 132: 45–72.

REGER, J. F. 1955. Electron microscopy of the motor end plate in rat intercostal muscle. Anat. Rec., 122: 1–10.

REGER, J. F. 1957. The ultrastructure of normal and denervated neuromuscular synapses in mouse gastrocnemius muscle. Exper. Cell Res., 12: 661–665.

REIS, D. J., AND OLIPHANT, M. C. 1964. Bradycardia and tachycardia following electrical stimulation of the amygdaloid region in monkey. J. Neurophysiol., 27: 893–912.

RENSHAW, B. 1940. Activity in the simplest spinal reflex pathways. J. Neurophysiol., 3: 370–387.

RENSHAW, B. 1941. Influence of discharge of motoneurons upon excitation of neighboring motoneurons. J. Neurophysiol., 4: 167–183.

RENSHAW, B. 1946. Central effects of centripetal impulses in axons of spinal ventral roots. J. Neurophysiol., 9: 191–204.

REXED, B. 1952. The cytoarchitectonic organization of the spinal cord in the cat. J. Comp. Neurol., 96: 415–495.

REXED, B. 1954. A cytoarchitectonic atlas of the spinal cord in the cat. J. Comp. Neurol., 100: 297–379.

REXED, B. 1964. Some aspects of the cytoarchitectonics and synaptology of the spinal cord. In J. C. ECCLES AND J. P. SCHADÉ (Editors), Organization of the Spinal Cord, Progress in Brain Research, Vol. II. Elsevier Publishing Company, Amsterdam, pp. 58–92.

REXED, B., AND BRODAL, A. 1951. The nucleus cervicalis lateralis: A spinocerebellar relay nucleus. J. Neurophysiol., 14: 399–407.

RHODIN, J. A. G. 1963. An Atlas of Ultrastructure. W. B. Saunders Company, Philadelphia, pp. 37–49.

RHOTON, A. L., O'LEARY, J. L., AND FERGUSON, J. P. 1966. The trigeminal, facial, vagal and glossopharyngeal nerves in the monkey. Arch. Neurol., 14: 530–540.

RICHTER, C. P., AND HINES, M. 1932. Experimental production of the grasp reflex in adult monkeys by lesions of the frontal lobe. Am. J. Physiol., 101: 87–88.

RICHTER, C. P., AND WOODRUFF, B. G. 1945. Lumbar sympathetic dermatomes in man determined by the electrical skin resistance method. J. Neurophysiol., 8: 323–338.

RICHTER, D. 1957. Editor, Metabolism of the Nervous System. Second International Neurochemical Symposium, Åarhus, Denmark, 1956. Pergamon Press, New York, 599 pp.

RICHTER, E. 1965. Die Entwicklung des Globus Pallidus und des Corpus Subthalamicum. Springer-Verlag, Berlin.

RIES, E. A., AND LANGWORTHY, O. R. 1937. A study of the surface structure of the brain of the whale (Balaenoptera physolus and Physeter catadon). J. Comp. Neurol., 68: 1–47.

RILEY, C. M. 1952. Familial autonomic dysfunction. J. A. M. A., 149: 1532–1535.

RILEY, C. M 1957. Familial dysautonomia. Advances Pediat., 9: 157–190.

RILEY, C. M., DAY, R. L., GREELEY, D. M., AND LANGFORD, W. S. 1949. Central autonomic dysfunction with defective lacrimation. Pediatrics, 3: 468–481.

RILEY, C. M., AND MOORE, R. H. 1966. Familial dysautonomia differentiated from related disorders. Pediatrics, 37: 435–446.

RILEY, H. A. 1943. An Atlas of the Basal Ganglia, Brain Stem and Spinal Cord. Williams & Wilkins Company, Baltimore, 708 pp.

RINVIK, E. 1966. The cortico-nigral projection in the cat. An experimental study with silver impregnation methods. J. Comp. Neurol., 126: 241–254.

RINVIK, E. 1968. The corticothalamic projection from the pericruciate and coronal gyri in the cat. An experimental study with silver-impregnation methods. Brain Res., 10: 79–119.

RINVIK, E., AND GROFOVÁ, I. 1970. Observations on the fine structure of the substantia nigra in the cat. Exper. Brain Res., 11: 229–248.

RINVIK, E., AND WALBERG, F. 1963. Demonstration of a somatotopically arranged cortico-rubral projection in the cat. An experimental study with silver methods. J. Comp. Neurol., 120: 393–407.

RINVIK, E., AND WALBERG, F. 1969. Is there a cortico-nigral tract? A comment based on experimental electron microscopic observations in the cat. Brain Res., 14: 742–744.

DEL RIO-HORTEGA, P. 1919. El "tercer elemento" de los centros nerviosus. Bol. Soc. espan. biol., 9: 69–120.

DEL RIO-HORTEGA, P. 1921. El Tercer elemento de los centros nerviosus. Histogenesis y evolucion normal; exoda y distribucion regional de microglia. Mem. Soc. espan. hist. nat., 11: 213–268.

DEL RIO-HORTEGA, P. 1921a. Estudios sobre la neuroglia. La glía de escasas radiaciones (oligodendroglia). Bol. R. Soc. espan. hist. nat., 21: 63–92.

DEL RIO-HORTEGA, P. 1932. Microglia. In W. G. PENFIELD (Editor), Cytology and Cellular Pathology of the Nervous System, Vol. II. Paul B. Hoeber, Inc., New York, pp. 483–534.

RISPAL-PADEL, L., MASSION, J., AND GRANGETTO, A. 1973. Relations between the ventrolateral thalamic nucleus and motor cortex and their possible role in the central organization of motor control. Brain Res., 60: 1–20.

RIVERA-DOMINGUEZ, M., AGATE, F. J., JR., AND NOBACK, C. R. 1973. Scanning electron microscopy of the spiral organ of Corti of the adult rhesus monkey. Brain Res., 65:159–164.

RIVERA-DOMINGUEZ, M., METTLER, F. A. AND NOBACK, C. R. 1974. Origins of cerebellar climbing fibers in the rhesus monkey. J. Comp. Neurol., 155: 331–342.

DE ROBERTIS, E. 1959. Submicroscopic morphology of the synapse. Internat. Rev. Cytol., 8: 61–96.

DE ROBERTIS, E. D. P. 1965. Some new electron microscopical contributions to the biology of neuroglia. In E. D. P. DE ROBERTIS AND R. CARREA (Editors), Biology of Neuroglia, Progress in Brain Research, Vol. 15. Elsevier Publishing Company, Amsterdam, pp. 1–11.

DE ROBERTIS, E. 1966. Synaptic complexes and synaptic vesicles as structural and biochemical units of the central nervous system. In K. RODAHL AND B. ISSEKUTZ, JR. (Editors), Nerve as a Tissue, Hoeber Med. Div. Harper and Row, New York, pp. 88–115.

DE ROBERTIS, E. 1967. Ultrastructure and cytochemistry of the synaptic region. Science, 156: 907–914.

DE ROBERTIS, E., AND BENNETT, H. S. 1954. Submicroscopic vesicular component in the synapse. Fed. Proc., 13: 35.

DE ROBERTIS, E., DE IRALDI, A. P., DE LORES, R., ARNAIZ, G., AND SALGANICOFF, L. 1962. Cholinergic and non-cholinergic nerve endings in rat brain. I. Isolation and subcellular distribution of acetylcholine and acetylcholinesterase. J. Neurochem., 9: 23–35.

DE ROBERTIS, E. D. P., NOWINSKI, W. W., AND SAEZ, F. A. 1965. The plasma membrane. In E. D. P. DE ROBERTIS et al. (Editors), Cell Biology. W. B. Saunders Company, Philadelphia, pp. 109–128.

ROBERTS, T. S. AND AKERT, K. 1963. Insular and opercular cortex and its thalamic projection in Macaca mulatta. Schweiz. Arch. Neurol. Neurochir. u. Psychiat., 92: 1–43.

ROBERTSON, D. M., AND VOGEL, F. S. 1962. Concentric lamination of glial processes in oligodendrogliomas. J. Cell Biol., 15: 313–334.

ROBERTSON, J. D. 1955. Ultrastructure of adult vertebrate peripheral myelinated nerve fibers in relation to myelinogenesis. J. Biophys. & Biochem. Cytol., 1: 271–278.

ROBERTSON, J. D. 1956. The ultrastructure of a reptilian myoneural junction. J. Biophys. & Biochem. Cytol., 2: 381–394.

ROBERTSON, J. D. 1958. The ultrastructure of Schmidt-Lantermann clefts and related shearing defects of the myelin sheath. J. Biophys. & Biochem. Cytol., 4: 39–46.

ROBERTSON, J. D. 1959. Preliminary observations on the ultrastructure of nodes of Ranvier. Ztschr. Zellforsch. u. mikroskop. Anat., 50: 553–560.

ROBERTSON, J. D. 1960. Electron microscopy of the motor end-plate and the neuromuscular spindle. Am. J. Phys. Med., 39: 1–43.

ROBERTSON, J. D. 1966. Current problems of unit membrane structure and contact relationships. In K. RODAHL AND B. ISSEKUTZ, JR. (Editors), Nerve as a Tissue. Hoeber Med. Div., Harper and Row, New York, pp. 11–48.

ROBINSON, B. W., AND MISHKIN, M 1962. Alimentary responses evoked from forebrain structures in Macaca mulatta. Science, 136: 260–261.

ROBINSON, B. W., AND MISHKIN, M. 1968. Alimentary responses to forebrain stimulation in monkeys. Exper. Brain Res., 4: 330–366.

RODRIGUEZ, L. A. 1955. Experiments on the histologic locus of the hemato-encephalic barrier. J. Comp. Neurol., 102: 27–46.

RODRIQUEZ, L. A. 1957. The role of the meningeal tissues in the hemato-encephalic barrier, J. Comp. Neurol., 107: 455–474.

RODRIGUEZ-ECHANDIA, E. L., PIEZZI, R. S., AND RODRIGUEZ, E. M. 1968. Dense-core microtubules in neurons and gliocytes of the toad Bufo arenarum Hensel. Am. J. Anat., 122: 157–168.

ROEDER, F., AND ORTHNER, H. 1956. Erfahrungen mit stereotaktischen Eingriffen. I. Mitteilung: Zur Pathogenese und Therapie extrapyramidal-motorischer Bewegungsstörungen. Erfolgreiche Behandlung eines Falles schwerem Hemiballismus mit gezielter Electrokoagulation des Globus pallidus. Deutsche Ztschr. Nervenh., 175: 419–434.

ROGER, A., ROSSI, G. F., AND ZIRONDOLI, A. 1956. Le rôle des nerfs craniens dans le maintien de l'état vigile de la preparation "encéphale isolé." Electroencephalog. & Clin. Neurophysiol., 8: 1–13.

ROGERS, D. C., AND BURNSTOCK, G. 1966. Multiaxonal autonomic junctions in smooth muscle of the toad (Bufo marinus). J. Comp. Neurol., 126: 625–652.

ROGERS, F. T. 1922. Studies of the brain stem. VI. An experimental study of the corpus striatum of the pigeon as related to various instinctive types of behavior. J. Comp. Neurol., 35: 21–59.

ROMANES, G. J. 1951. The motor cell columns of the lumbosacral spinal cord of the cat. J. Comp. Neurol., 94: 313–363.

ROOT, W. S. 1969. Physiology of micturition: A specific autonomic function. In V. B. MOUNTCASTLE (Editor), Medical Physiology, Ed. 12. C V. Mosby Company, St. Louis, Ch. 79, pp. 1831–1838.

ROSE, J. E. 1952. The cortical connections of the reticular complex of the thalamus. A. Res. Nerv. & Ment. Dis., Proc., 30; 454–479.

ROSE, J. E. 1960. Organization of frequency sensitive neurons in the cochlear complex of the cat. In G. L. RASMUSSEN AND W. F. WINDLE (Editors), Neural Mechanisms of the Auditory and Vestibular Systems. Charles C Thomas, Publisher, Springfield, Ill., Cht. 9, pp. 116–136.

ROSE, J. E., AND GALAMBOS, R. 1952. Microelectrode studies on the medial geniculate body of the cat. I. The thalamic region activated by click stimuli. J. Neurophysiol., 15: 343–357.

ROSE, J. E., GALAMBOS, R., AND HUGHES, J. R. 1959. Microelectrode studies of the cochlear nuclei of the cat. Bull. Johns Hopkins Hosp., 104: 211–251.

ROSE, J. E., GREENWOOD, D. B., GOLDBERG, J. M., AND HIND, J. E. 1963. Some discharge characteristics of single neurons in the inferior colliculus of the cat. I. Tonotopical organization, relation of spike-counts to tone intensity, and firing patterns of single elements. J. Neurophysiol., 26: 294–320.

ROSE, J. E., GROSS, N. B., GEISLER, C. D., AND HIND, J. E. 1966. Some neural mechanisms in the inferior colliculus of the cat which may be relevant to localization of a sound source. J. Neurophysiol., 29: 288–314.

ROSE, J. E., AND MOUNTCASTLE, V. B. 1952. The thalamic tactile region in rabbit and cat. J. Comp. Neurol., 97: 441–490.

ROSE, J. E., AND MOUNTCASTLE, V. B. 1959. Touch and kinesthesis. In J. FIELDS (Editor), Handbook of Physiology, Section I, Vol. I. American Physiological Society, Washington, D. C., Ch. 17, pp. 387–429.

ROSE, J. E., AND WOOLSEY, C. N. 1943. A study of thalamocortical relations in the rabbit. Bull. Johns Hopkins Hosp., 72: 65–128.

ROSE, J. E., AND WOOLSEY, C. N. 1943a. Potential changes in the olfactory brain produced by electrical stimulation of the olfactory bulb. Fed. Proc., 2: 42.

ROSE, J. E., AND WOOLSEY, C. N. 1949. The relation of thalamic connections, cellular structure and evocable electrical activity in the auditory region of the cat. J. Comp. Neurol., 91: 441–466.

ROSE, J. E., AND WOOLSEY, C. N. 1958. Cortical connections and functional organization of the thalamic auditory system of the cat. In H. F. HARLOW AND C. N. WOOLSEY (Editors), Biological and Biochemical Bases of Behavior. University of Wisconsin Press, Madison, pp. 127–150.

ROSE, M. 1935. Cytoarchitektonik und Myeloarchitektonik der Grosshirnrinde. In O. BUMKE AND O. FOERSTER, Handbuch der Neurologie, Vol. I. Springer, Berlin, pp. 588–778.

ROSEGAY, H. 1944. An experimental investigation of the connections between the corpus striatum and the substantia nigra in the cat. J. Comp. Neurol., 80: 293–310.

ROSENBLUTH, J. 1962. Subsurface cisterns and their relationships to the neuronal plasma membrane. J. Cell Biol., 13: 405–421.

ROSENBLUTH, J. 1968. Functions of glial cells. In O. T. BAILEY AND D. E. SMITH (Editors), The Central Nervous System. Williams & Wilkins Company, Baltimore, pp. 21–41.

ROSENZWEIG, M. R. 1954. Cortical correlates of auditory localization and of related perceptual phenomena. J. Comp. & Physiol. Psychol., 47: 269–276.

ROSS, L. L., BORNSTEIN, M. B., AND LEHRER, G. 1962. Electron microscope observations of rat and mouse cerebellum in tissue culture. J. Cell Biol., 14: 19–30.

ROSSI, G. F., AND BRODAL, A. 1956. Corticofugal fibers to the brain stem reticular formation. An experimental study in the cat. J. Anat., 90: 42–62.

ROSSI, G. F., AND BRODAL, A. 1956a. Spinal afferents to the trigeminal sensory nuclei and the nucleus of the solitary tract. Confinia neurol., 16: 321–332.

ROSSI, G. F. AND BRODAL, A. 1957. Terminal distribution of spinoreticular fibers in the cat. A. M. A. Arch. Neurol. & Psychiat., 78: 439–453.

ROSSI, G. F., AND ZIRONDOLI, A. 1955. On the mechanism of the cortical desynchronization elicited by volatile anesthetics. Electroencephalog. & Clin. Neurophysiol., 7: 383–390.

ROSSI, G. F., AND ZANCHETTI, A. 1957. The brain stem reticular formation. Anatomy and physiology. Arch. ital. biol., 95: 199–435.

RUBINSTEIN, L. J., KLATZO, I., AND MIQUEL, J. 1962. Histochemical observations on oxidative enzyme activity of glial cells in a local brain injury. J. Neuropath. & Exper. Neurol., 21: 116–136.

RUFFINI, A. 1894. Sur un nouvel Organe nerveux terminal et sur la présence des corpuscles Golgi-Mazzoni dans le conjunctif sous-cutane de la pulpe des doigts de l'homme. Arch. ital. biol., 21: 249–265.

RUNDLES, R. W., AND PAPEZ, J. W. 1937. Connections between the striatum and the substantia nigra in a human brain. Arch. Neurol. & Psychiat., 38: 550–563.

RUSSELL, G. V. 1954. The dorsal trigemino-thalamic tract in the cat. Reconsidered as a lateral reticulothalamic system of connections. J. Comp. Neurol., 101: 237–264.

RUSSELL, G. V. 1955. The nucleus locus coeruleus (dorsolateralis tegmenti). Texas Rep. Biol. & Med., 13: 939–988.

RUSSELL, G. V. 1955a. A schematic presentation of thalamic morphology and connections. Texas Rep. Biol. & Med., 13: 989–992.

RUSSELL, J. R., AND DEMYER, W. 1961. The quantitative cortical origin of pyramidal axons of Macaca rhesus. Neurology, 11: 96–108.

RUSSELL, W. R. 1948. Functions of the frontal lobes. Lancet, 254: 356–360.

RYLANDER, G. 1948. Personality analysis before and after frontal lobotomy. A. Res. Nerv. & Ment. Dis., Proc., 27: 691–705.

SACHS, E., JR., BRENDLER, S. J., AND FULTON, J. F. 1949. The orbital gyri. Brain, 72: 227–240.

SALAFSKY, B. AND JASINSKI, D. 1967. Early electrophysiological changes after denervation of fast skeletal muscle. Exper. Neurol., 19: 375–387.

SALMON, G., AND LAZORTHES, G. 1971. Atlas of the Arteries of the Human Brain. Sandoz, Paris.

VON SANTHA, K. 1928. Zur Klinik und Anatomie des Hemiballismus. Arch. Psychiat., 84: 664–678.

VON SANTHA, K. 1932. Hemiballismus und Corpus Luysi: (Anatomische und pathophysiologische Beiträge zur Frage des Hemiballismus nebst Versuch einer somatotopischen Lokalisation im Corpus Luysi.) Ztschr. ges. Neurol. u. Psychiat., 141: 321–342.

SASAKI, K., NAMIKAWA, A., AND HASHIRAMOTO, S. 1960. The effect of midbrain stimulation upon alpha motoneurones in lumbar spinal cord. Nippon Seirigaku Zassi, 3: 303–316.

SASAKI, K., TANAKA, T., AND MORI, K. 1962. Effects of stimulation of pontine and bulbar reticular formation upon spinal motoneurons of the cat. Jap. J. Physiol., 12: 45–62.

SAWYER, C. H. 1959. Nervous control of ovulation. In C. W. LLOYD (Editor), Endocrinology of Reproduction. Academic Press, New York, pp. 1–18.

SAWYER, C. H. 1969. Regulatory mechanisms of secretion of gonadotrophic hormones. In W. HAYMAKER et al. (Editors), The Hypothalamus. Charles C Thomas, Publisher, Springfield, Ill., Ch. 11, pp. 389–430.

SCALIA, F. 1972. The termination of retinal axons in the pretectal region of mammals. J. Comp. Neurol., 145: 223–257.

SCARFF, J. E. 1940. Primary cortical centers for movement of upper and lower limbs in man. Arch. Neurol. & Psychiat., 44: 243–299.

SCARFF, J. E. 1949. Unilateral prefrontal lobotomy for relief of intractable pain and termination of narcotic addiction. Surg. Gynec. & Obst., 89: 385–392.

SCHALTENBRAND, G. 1955. Plexus und Meningen. Saccus vasculosus. In W. VON MÖLLENDORFF (Editor), Hand-

buch der mikroskopisch. Anatomie des Menschen, Vol. IV, part 2. Springer, Berlin, pp. 94–98.

SCHARRER, B. 1965. Recent progress in the study of neuroendocrine mechanisms in insects. Arch. Anat. Microscop. Morph. Exper., 54: 331–342.

SCHARRER, E. 1944. The blood vessels of the nervous tissue. Quart. Rev. Biol., 19: 308–318.

SCHARRER, E. AND SCHARRER, B. 1940. Secretory cells within the hypothalamus. A. Res. Nerv. Ment. Dis., Proc., 20: 170–194.

SCHARRER, E., AND SCHARRER, B. 1945. Neurosecretion. Physiol. Rev., 25: 171–181.

SCHEIBEL, M. E.,, SCHEIBEL, A. B. 1954. Observations on the intracortical relations of the climbing fibers of the cerebellum. A Golgi study. J. Comp. Neurol., 101: 733–764.

SCHEIBEL, M. E., AND SCHEIBEL, A. B. 1958. Structural substrates for integrative patterns in the brain stem reticular core. In H. H. JASPER *et al.* (Editors), *Reticular Formation of the Brain*. Little, Brown & Company, Boston, Ch. 2, pp. 31–55.

SCHEIBEL, M. E., AND SCHEIBEL, A. B. 1958a. Neurons and neuroglial cells as seen with the light microscope. In W. F. WINDLE (Editor), *Biology of Neuroglia*. Charles C Thomas, Publisher, Springfield, Ill., pp. 5–23.

SCHEIBEL, M. E., AND SCHEIBEL, A. B. 1966. The organization of the nucleus reticularis thalami: A Golgi study. Brain Res., 1: 43–62.

SCHEIBEL, M. E., AND SCHEIBEL, A. B. 1966a. The organization of the ventral anterior nucleus of the thalamus. A Golgi study. Brain Res., 1: 250–268.

SCHEIBEL, M. E., AND SCHEIBEL, A. B. 1967. Structural organization of nonspecific thalamic nuclei and their projection toward cortex. Brain Res., 6: 60–94.

SCHLAG, J., AND FAIDLERBE, J. 1961. Recruiting responses in the brain stem reticular formation. Arch. ital. biol., 99: 135–162.

SCHLESINGER, B. 1939. Venous drainage of the brain, with special reference to Galenic system. Brain, 62: 274–291.

SCHMIDT, C. G. 1960. Central nervous system circulation, fluids and barriers—introduction. In J. FIELD (Editor), *Handbook of Physiology*, Section I, Vol. III. American Physiological Society, Washington, D. C., Ch. 70, 1745–1760.

SCHMITT, F. O., BEAR, R. S., AND PALMER, K. J. 1941. X-ray diffraction studies on the structure of the nerve myelin sheath. J. Cell. & Comp. Physiol., 18: 31–42.

SCHNEIDER, G. E. 1969. Two visual systems. Science, 163: 895–902.

SCHNITZLEIN, H. N., HOFFMAN, H. H., HAMLETT, D. M., AND HOWELL, E. M. 1963. A study of the sacral parasympathetic nucleus. J. Comp. Neurol., 120: 477–493.

SCHOULTZ, T. W., AND SWETT, J. E. 1972. The fine structure of the Golgi tendon organ. J. Neurocytol., 1: 1–26.

SCHREINER, L. H., AND KLING, A. 1954. Effects of castration on hypersexual behavior induced by rhinencephalic injury in cat. Arch. Neurol. & Psychiat., 72: 180–186.

SCHULTZ, R. L., MAYNARD, E. A., AND PEASE, D. C. 1957. Electron microscopy of neurons and neuroglia of cerebral cortex and corpus callosum. Am. J. Anat., 100: 369–407.

SCHULTZ, R. L., AND PEASE, D. C. 1959. Cicatrix formation in rat cerebral cortex as revealed by electron microscopy. Am. J. Path., 35: 1017–1041.

SCHÜTZ, H. 1891. Anatomische Untersuchungen über den Faserverlauf im zentralen Höhlengrau und den Nervenfaserschwund in demselben bei der progressiven Paralyse der Irren. Arch. Psychiat., 22: 527–587.

SCHWARTZ, P., AND FINK, L. 1926. Morphologie und Entstehung der geburtstraumatischen Blutungen im Gehirn und Schädel des Neugeborenen. Ztschr. Kinder., 40: 427–474.

SCHWYN, R. C. 1967. An autoradiographic study of satellite cells in autonomic ganglia. Am. J. Anat., 121: 727–740.

SCOTT, D., AND CLEMENTE, C. D. 1952. Mechanism of spinal cord regeneration in the cat. Fed. Proc., 11: 143–144.

SCOTT, D., JR. 1963. Influence of nerve growth factor on spinal regeneration in kittens. Anat. Rec., 145: 283.

SCOVILLE, W. B. 1954. Neurophysiological symposium; limbic lobe in man. J. Neurosurg., 11: 64–66.

SCOVILLE, W. B., AND MILNER, B. 1957. Loss of recent memory after bilateral hippocampal lesions. J. Neurol. Neurosurg. & Psychiat., 20: 11–21.

SEDDON, H. J. 1943. Three types of nerve injury. Brain, 66: 237–288.

SHANER, R. F. 1932. Development of nuclei and tracts of mid-brain. J. Comp. Neurol., 55: 493–512.

SHANER, R. F. 1936. Development of the finer structure and fiber connections of the globus pallidus, corpus of Luys and substantia nigra in the pig. J. Comp. Neurol., 64: 213–233.

SHANTHAVEERAPPA, T. R., AND BOURNE, G. H. 1962. The 'perineural epithelium', a metabolically active, continuous, protoplasmic cell barrier surrounding peripheral nerve fasciculi. J. Anat., 96: 527–537.

SHANTHAVEERAPPA, T. R., AND BOURNE, G. H. 1964. Arachnoid villi in the optic nerve of man and the monkey. Exper. Eye Res., 3: 31–35.

SHANTHAVEERAPPA, T. R., AND BOURNE, G. H. 1966. Perineural epithelium: A new concept of its role in the integrity of the peripheral nervous system. Science, 154: 1464–1467.

SHANZER, S., WAGMAN, I. H., AND BENDER, M. B. 1959. Further observations on the median longitudinal fasciculus. Tr. Am. Neurol. A., 14–17.

SHEALY, C. N., AND PEELE, T. L. 1957. Studies on amygdaloid nucleus of cat. J. Neurophysiol., 20: 125–139.

SHEEHAN, D. 1941. Spinal autonomic outflows in man and monkey. J. Comp. Neurol., 75: 341–370.

SHEEHAN, D. 1941a. The autonomic nervous system. Ann. Rev. Physiol., 3: 399–448.

SHENKIN, H. A., AND LEWEY, F. H. 1944. Taste aura preceding convulsions in a lesion of the parietal operculum. J. Nerv. & Ment. Dis., 100; 352–354.

SHEPS, J. G. 1945. The nuclear configuration and cortical connections of the human thalamus. J. Comp. Neurol., 83: 1–56.

SHERRINGTON, C. S. 1893. Experiments in examination of the peripheral distribution of the fibers of the posterior roots of some spinal nerves. Phil. Tr. Roy. Soc. London, ser. B, 184: 641–763.

SHERRINGTON, C. S. 1893a. Note on the spinal portion of some ascending degenerations. J. Physiol., 14: 255–302.

SHERRINGTON, C. S. 1898. Decerebrate rigidity, and reflex co-ordination of movements. J. Physiol., 22: 319–332.

SHERRINGTON, C. S. 1906. *The Integrative Action of the Nervous System*. Charles Scribner's Sons, New York. Reprinted, Yale University Press, New Haven, 1947.

SHOLL, D. A. 1956. *The Organization of the Cerebral Cortex*. John Wiley & Sons, Inc., New York.

SHOWERS, M. J. C. 1958. Correlation of medial thalamic nuclear activity with cortical and subcortical neuronal arc. J. Comp. Neurol., 109: 261–315.

SHOWERS, M. J. C. 1959. The cingulate gyrus: Additional motor area and cortical autonomic regulator. J. Comp. Neurol., 112: 231–301.

SHOWERS, M. J. C., AND CROSBY, E. C. 1958. Somatic and

visceral responses from cingulate gyrus. Neurology, 8: 561–565.

SHRIVER, J. E., STEIN, B. M., AND CARPENTER, M. B. 1968. Central projections of spinal dorsal roots in the monkey. I. Cervical and upper thoracic dorsal roots. Am. J. Anat., 123: 27–74.

SHUANGSHOTI, S., AND NETSKY, M. G. 1966. Histogenesis of choroid plexus in man. J. Comp. Neurol., 118: 283–316.

SHUANGSHOTI, S., AND NETSKY, M. G. 1970. Human choroid plexus: Morphologic and histochemical alterations with age. Am. J. Anat., 128: 73–96.

SIDMAN, R. L. 1970. Cell proliferation, migration and interaction in the developing mammalian central nervous system. In F. O. SCHMITT (Editor), *The Neurosciences.* Second Study Program. Rockefeller University Press, New York, pp. 100–116.

SIMPSON, D. A. 1952. The projection of the pulvinar to the temporal lobe. J. Anat., 86: 20–28.

SINCLAIR, D. C. 1967. *Cutaneous Sensation.* Oxford University Press, New York, pp. 35–80.

SINCLAIR, D. C., WEDDELL, G., AND FEINDEL, W. H. 1948. Referred pain and associated phenomena. Brain, 71: 184–211.

SJOQVIST, O. 1938. Studies on pain conduction in the trigeminal nerve. A contribution to surgical treatment of facial pain. Acta psychiat. neurol., Scandinav. 17 (suppl.): 1–139.

SJÖSTRAND, F. S. 1963. The structure and formation of the myelin sheath. In A. S. ROSE AND C. M. PEARSON (Editors), *Mechanisms of Demyelination.* McGraw-Hill Book Company, New York, pp. 1–43.

SKINNER, J. E., AND LINDSLEY, D. B. 1967. Electrophysiological and behavioral effects of blockage on the nonspecific thalamocortical system. Brain Res., 6: 95–117.

SLOAN, N., AND JASPER, H. 1950. The identity of spreading depression and "suppression." Electroencephalog. & Clin. Neurophysiol., 2: 59–78.

SLOPER, J. C. 1966. Hypothalmic neurosecretion. The validity of the concept of neurosecretion and its physiological and pathological implications. Brit. M. Bull., 22: 209–215.

SMIRNOW, A. 1895. Über die sensiblen Nervenendigungen im Herzen bei Amphibien und Säugetieren. Anat. Anz., 10: 737–749.

SMITH, C. A. 1967. Innervation of the organ of Corti. In S. IURATO (Editor) *Submicroscopic Structure of the Inner Ear,* Pergamon, Oxford, pp. 107–131.

SMITH, C. A., AND RASMUSSEN, G. L. 1963. Recent observations on the olivo-cochlear bundle. Ann. Otol., Rhin. & Laryng., 72: 489–507.

SMITH, C. A., AND RASMUSSEN, G. L. 1965. Degeneration in the efferent nerve endings in the cochlea after axonal section. J. Cell Biol., 26: 63–77.

SMITH, M. C. 1951. The use of Marchi staining in the later stages of human tract degeneration. J. Neurol. Neurosurg. & Psychiat., 14; 222–225.

SMITH, M. C. 1956. The recognition and prevention of artefacts of the Marchi method. J. Neurol. Neurosurg. & Psychiat., 19: 74–83.

SMITH, M. C. 1957. The anatomy of the spino-cerebellar fibers in man. I. The course of the fibers in the spinal cord and brain stem. J. Comp. Neurol., 108: 285–352.

SMITH, M. C. 1961. The anatomy of the spino-cerebellar fibers in man. II. The distribution of the fibers in the cerebellum. J. Comp. Neurol., 117: 329–354.

SMITH, O. A., JR., AND CLARKE, N. P. 1964. Central autonomic pathways. A study in functional neuroanatomy. J. Comp. Neurol., 122: 399–406.

SMITH, W. K. 1945. The functional significance of the rostral cingular cortex as revealed by its responses to electrical excitation. J. Neurophysiol., 8: 241–255.

SMYTH, G. E. 1939. The systemization and central connections of the spinal tract and nucleus of the trigeminal nerve. Brain, 62: 41–87.

SNIDER, R. S. 1936. Alterations which occur in mossy terminals of the cerebellum following transection of the brachium pontis. J. Comp. Neurol., 64: 417–435.

SNIDER, R. S. 1950. Recent contributions to the anatomy and physiology of the cerebellum. Arch. Neurol. & Psychiat., 64: 196–219

SNIDER, R. S., AND STOWELL, A. 1944. Receiving areas of the tactile, auditory, and visual systems in the cerebellum. J. Neurophysiol., 7: 331–357.

SNYDER, M., HALL, W. C., AND DIAMOND, I. T. 1966. Vision in tree shrews after removal of striate cortex. Psychoneurol. Sc., 6: 243–244.

SOKOLOFF, L. 1960. Metabolism in the central nervous system in vivo. In J. FIELD (Editor), *Handbook of Physiology,* Section I, Vol. III. American Physiological Society, Washington, D. C., Ch. 77, pp. 1845–1864.

SOSA, J. M., AND DEZORRILLA, N. B. 1966. Spinal ganglion cytological responses to axon and to dendrite sectioning. Acta anat., 65: 236–255.

SOTELO, C. 1967. Cerebellar neuroglia: Morphological and histochemical aspects. In C. A. FOX AND R. S. SNIDER (Editors), *The Cerebellum, Progress in Brain Research,* Vol. 25. Elsevier Publishing Company, Amsterdam, pp. 226–250.

SOTELO, C., AND PALAY, S. L. 1968. The fine structure of the lateral vestibular nucleus in the rat. I. Neurons and neurological cells. J. Cell Biol., 36: 151–179.

SPATZ, W. B., TIGGES, J., AND TIGGES, M. 1970. Subcortical projections, cortical associations and some intrinsic interlaminar connections of the striate cortex in the squirrel monkey (Saimiri). J. Comp. Neurol., 140: 155–174.

SPEIDEL, C. G. 1919. Gland cells of internal secretion in the spinal cord of the skates. Carnegie Inst. Wash. Publ., 13: 1–31.

SPERRY, R. W. 1961. Cerebral organization and behavior. Science, 133: 1749–1757.

SPERRY, R. W. 1962. Some general aspects of interhemispheric integration. In V. B. MOUNTCASTLE (Editor), *Interhemispheric Relations and Cerebral Dominance.* Johns Hopkins Press, Baltimore, Ch. 3, pp. 43–49.

SPIEGEL, E. A. 1929. Experimentalstudien am Nervensystem: XV. Der Mechanismus des labyrinthären Nystagmus. Ztschr. Hals-Nasen-u. Ohrenh., 25: 200–217.

SPIEGEL, E. A., KLETZKIN, M., AND SZEKELY, E. G. 1954. Pain reactions upon stimulation of the tectum mesencephali. J. Neuropath. & Exper. Neurol., 13: 212–220.

SPIEGEL, E. A., AND SOMMER, I. 1944. *Neurology of the Eye, Ear, Nose and Throat.* Grune & Stratton, Inc., New York, 667 pp.

SPIEGEL, E. A., AND WYCIS, H. T. 1950. Pallidothalamotomy in chorea. Arch. Neurol. & Psychiat., 64: 295–296.

SPIEGEL, E. A., AND WYCIS, H. T. 1954. Ansotomy in paralysis agitans. Arch. Neurol. & Psychiat., 71: 598–614.

SPIEGEL, E. A., AND WYCIS, H. T. 1958. Pallido-ansotomy: Anatomic-physiologic foundation and histopathologic control. In W. S. FIELDS (Editor), *Pathogenesis and Treatment of Parkinsonism.* Charles C Thomas, Publisher, Springfield, Ill., Ch. 3, pp. 86–105.

SPILLER, W. G. 1924. Ophthalmoplegia internuclearis anterior; a case with necropsy. Brain, 47: 345–357.

SPINELLI, D. N., HIRSCH, H. V. B., PHELPS, R. W., AND METZLER, J. 1972. Visual experience as a determinant of response characteristics of cortical receptive fields in cat. Exper. Brain Res., 15: 289–304.

SPOENDLIN, H. H. 1966. The organization of the cochlear receptor. Advances Oto-Rhino-Laryng., 13: 1–227.

SPOENDLIN, H. H., AND GACEK, R. R. 1963. Electronmicroscopic study of the efferent and afferent innervation of the organ of Corti in the cat. Ann. Otol. Rhin. & Laryn., 72: 660–686.

SPRAGUE, J. M. 1951. Motor and propriospinal cells in the thoracic and lumbar ventral horn of the Rhesus monkey. J. Comp. Neurol., 95: 103–124.

SPRAGUE, J. M. 1958. The distribution of dorsal root fibers on motor cells in the lumbosacral spinal cord of the cat, and the site of excitatory and inhibitory terminals in monosynaptic pathways. Proc. Roy. Soc., London, ser. B, 149: 534–556.

SPRAGUE, J. M. 1972. The superior colliculus and pretectum in visual behavior. Invest. Ophth., 11: 473–482.

SPRAGUE, J. M. AND CHAMBERS, W. W. 1953. Regulation of posture in intact and decerebrate cat. I. Cerebellum, reticular formation, vestibular nuclei. J. Neurophysiol., 16: 451–463.

SPRAGUE, J. M., AND CHAMBERS, W. W. 1954. Control of posture by reticular formation and cerebellum in the intact, anesthetized, unanesthetized and in the decerebrated cat. Am. J. Physiol., 176: 52–64.

SPRAGUE, J. M., AND HA, H. 1964. The terminal fields of dorsal root fibers in the lumbosacral spinal cord of the cat, and the dendritic organization of the motor nuclei. In J. C. ECCLES AND J. P. SCHADÉ (Editors), Organization of the Spinal Cord, Progress in Brain Research, Vol. 2. Elsevier Publishing Company, Amsterdam, pp. 120–152.

SPRAGUE, J. M., LEVITT, M., ROBSON, K., LIU, C. N., STELLER, E., AND CHAMBERS, W. W. 1963. A neuroanatomical and behavioral analysis of the syndromes resulting from midbrain lemniscal and reticular lesions in the cat. Arch. ital. biol., 101: 225–295.

SPRAGUE, J. M., AND MEIKLE, T. H., JR. 1965. The role of the superior colliculus in visually guided behavior. Exper. Neurol., 11: 115–146.

STAAL, A. 1961. Subcortical Projections on the Spinal Gray Matter of the Cat. Koninkl. Druk., Lankhout-Immig N.V., The Hague, 164 pp.

STARZL, T. E., AND MAGOUN, H. W. 1951. Organization of the diffuse thalamic projection system. J. Neurophysiol., 14: 133–146.

STARZL, T. E., TAYLOR, C. W., AND MAGOUN, H. W. 1951. Ascending conduction in reticular activating system, with special reference to the diencephalon. J. Neurophysiol., 14: 461–477.

STARZL, T. E., TAYLOR, C. W., AND MAGOUN, H. W. 1951a. Collateral afferent excitation of the reticular formation of the brain stem. J. Neurophysiol., 14: 479–496.

STARZL, T. E. AND WHITLOCK, D. G. 1952. Diffuse thalamic projection system in monkey. J. Neurophysiol., 15: 449–468.

STEIN, B. M., AND CARPENTER, M. B. 1965. Effects of dorsal rhizotomy upon subthalamic dyskinesia in the monkey. Arch. Neurol., 13: 567–583.

STEIN, M. B., AND CARPENTER, M. B. 1967. Central projections of portions of the vestibular ganglia innervating specific parts of the labyrinth in the rhesus monkey. Am. J. Anat., 120: 281–318.

STENGEL, E. 1926. Über den Ursprung der Nervenfasern der Neurohypophyse im Zwischenhirn. Arb. Neurol. Inst. Wiener Univ., 28: 25–37.

STENSAAS, L. J. 1968. The development of hippocampal and dorsolateral pallial regions of the cerebral hemisphere in fetal rabbits. J. Comp. Neurol., 132: 93–108.

STEPIEN, L. S., CORDEAU, J. P., AND RASMUSSEN, T. 1960. The effect of temporal lobe and hippocampal lesions on auditory and visual recent memory in monkeys. Brain, 83: 470–489.

STERLING, P., AND WICKELGREN, B. G. 1969. Visual receptive fields in the superior colliculus of the cat. J. Neurophysiol., 32: 1–15.

STERN K. 1938. Note on the nucleus ruber magnocellularis and its efferent pathway in man. Brain, 61: 284–289.

STEVENSON, J. A. F. 1949. Effects of hypothalamic lesions on water and energy metabolism in the rat. Recent Progr. Hormone Res., 4: 363–394.

STEVENSON, J. A. F. 1969. Neural control of food and water intake. In W. HAYMAKER et al. (Editors), The Hypothalamus. Charles C Thomas Publisher, Springfield, Ill., Ch. 15, pp. 524–621.

STOOKEY, B., AND SCARFF, J. 1943. Injuries of peripheral nerves. In Neurosurgery and Thoracic Surgery. National Research Council Committee on Surgery. W. B. Saunders Company, Philadelphia, pp. 81–184.

STOPFORD, J. S. B. 1915. The arteries of the pons and medulla oblongata. Part I. J. Anat. & Physiol., 50: 131–164.

STOPFORD, J. S. B. 1916. The arteries of the pons and medulla oblongata. Part II. J. Anat. & Physiol., 51: 255–280.

STOTLER, W. A. 1953. An experimental study of the cells and connections of the superior olivary complex of the cat. J. Comp. Neurol., 98: 401–423.

STROMINGER, N. L. 1969. Subdivisions of auditory cortex and their role in localization of sound in space. Exper. Neurol., 24: 348–362.

STROMINGER, N. L., AND STROMINGER, A. I. 1971. Ascending brain stem projections of the anteroventral cochlear nucleus in the rhesus monkey. J. Comp. Neurol., 143: 217–242.

STRONG, O. S. 1915. A case of unilateral cerebellar agenesia. J. Comp. Neurol., 25: 361–391.

SUGAR, O., AMADOR, L. V., AND GRIPONISSIOTES, B. 1950. Corticocortical connections of the walls of the superior temporal sulcus in the monkey (Macaca mulatta). J. Neuropath. & Exper. Neurol., 9: 179–185.

SUGAR, O., FRENCH, J. D., AND CHUSID, J. G. 1948. Corticocortical connections of the superior surface of the temporal operculum in the monkey (Macaca mulatta). J. Neurophysiol., 11: 175–184.

SUGAR, O., AND GERARD, R. W. 1940. Spinal cord regeneration in the rat. J. Neurophysiol., 3: 1–19.

SUH, T. H., AND ALEXANDER, L. 1939. Vascular system of the human spinal cord. Arch. Neurol. & Psychiat., 41: 659–677.

SULKIN, N. M. 1953. Histochemical studies of the pigments in the human autonomic ganglion cells. J. Gerontol., 8: 435–445.

SULKIN, N. M., AND SRIVANIJ, P. 1960. The experimental production of senile pigments in the nerve cells of young rats. J. Gerontol., 15: 2–9.

SUNDERLAND, S. 1950. Capacity of reinnervated muscles to function efficiently after prolonged denervation. Arch. Neurol. & Psychiat., 64: 755–771.

SUNDERLAND, S. 1952. Factors influencing the course of regeneration and the quality of the recovery after nerve suture. Brain, 75: 19–54.

SWANN, H. G. 1934. The function of the brain in olfaction. II. The results of destruction of olfactory and other nervous structures upon the discrimination of odors. J. Comp. Neurol., 59: 175–201.

SWANN, H. G. 1935. The function of the brain in olfaction. III. The effects of large cortical lesions on olfactory discrimination. Am. J. Physiol., 111: 257–262.

SWEET, W. H., TALLAND, G. A., AND ERVIN, F. R. 1959. Loss of recent memory following section of the fornix. Tr. Am. Neurol. A., 84: 76–82.

SYMONDS, C. 1966. Disorders of memory. Brain, 89: 625–644.

SZABO, J. 1962. Topical distribution of the striatal efferents in the monkey. Exper. Neurol., 5: 21–36.

SZABO, J. 1967. The efferent projections of the putamen

in the monkey. Exper. Neurol., 19: 463–476.

SZABO, J. 1970. Projections from the body of the caudate nucleus in the rhesus monkey. Exper. Neurol., 27: 1–15.

SZENTÁGOTHAI, J. 1950. The elementary vestibulo-ocular reflex arc. J. Neurophysiol., 13: 395–407.

SZENTÁGOTHAI, J. 1950a. Recherches experimentales sur les voies oculogyres. Semaine hôp. Paris, 26: 2989–2995.

SZENTÁGOTHAI, J. 1964. Neuronal and synaptic arrangement in the substantia gelatinosa Rolandi. J. Comp. Neurol., 122: 219–239.

SZENTÁGOTHAI, J. 1970. Glomerular synapses, complex synaptic arrangements, and their operational significance. In F. O. SCHMITT (Editor), The Neurosciences, Second Study Program. Rockefeller University Press, New York, Ch. 40, pp. 427–443.

SZENTÁGOTHAI, J., AND ALBERT, A. 1955. The synaptology of Clarke's column. Acta morphol. hungaricae, 5: 43–51.

SZENTÁGOTHAI, J., FLERKÓ, B., MESS, B., AND HALASZ, B. 1968. Hypothalamic Control of the Anterior Pituitary. An Experimental-Morphological Study. Akademiai Kiado, Budapest.

SZENTÁGOTHAI, J., AND RAJKOVITS, K. 1959. Über den Ursprung der Kletterfasern des Kleinhirn. Ztschr. Anat. Entwickl.-Gesch., 121: 130–141.

SZENTÁGOTHAI-SCHIMERT, J. 1941. Die Endigungsweise der absteigenden Rückenmarksbahnen. Ztschr. Anat. Entwickl.-Gesch., 111: 322–330.

TABER, E. 1961. The cytoarchitecture of the brain stem of the cat. I. Brain stem nuclei of cat. J. Comp. Neurol., 116: 27–70.

TABER, E., BRODAL, A., AND WALBERG, F. 1960. The raphe nuclei of the brain stem in the cat. I. Normal topography and cytoarchitecture and general discussion. J. Comp. Neurol., 114: 161–187.

TAIT, J., AND MCNALLY, W. J. 1925. Rotation and acceleration experiments, mainly on frogs. Am. J. Physiol., 75: 140–154.

TALAAT, M. 1937. Afferent impulses in the nerves supplying the urinary bladder. J. Physiol., 89: 1–13.

TALAIRACH, J., PAILLAS, J. E., AND DAVID, M. 1950. Dyskinésie de type hémiballique traitée par cortectomie frontale limitée, puis par coagulation de l'anse lenticulaire et de la portion interne du globus pallidus. Rev. neurol., 83: 440–451.

TALBOT, S. A., AND MARSHALL, W. H. 1941. Physiological studies on neuronal mechanisms of visual localization and discrimination. Am. J. Ophth., 24: 1255–1263.

TANG, P. C., AND RUCH, T. C. 1956. Localization of brain stem and diencephalic areas controlling the micturition reflex. J. Comp. Neurol., 106: 213–246.

TARKHAN, A. A., AND ABD-EL-MALEK, S. 1950. On the presence of sensory nerve cells on the hypoglossal nerve. J. Comp. Neurol., 93: 219–228.

TASAKI, I. 1954. Nerve impulses in individual auditory nerve fibers of guinea pig. J. Neurophysiol., 17: 97–122.

TAUB, A. 1964. Local, segmental and supraspinal interaction with a dorsolateral spinal cutaneous afferent system. Exper. Neurol., 10: 357–374.

TAUB, A., AND BISHOP, P. O. 1965. The spinocervical tract: Dorsal column linkage, conduction velocity, primary afferent spectrum. Exper. Neurol., 13: 1–21.

TAVERAS, J. 1961. Angiographic observation in occlusive cerebrovascular disease. Neurology, 11: 86–90.

TAVERAS, J. M., AND WOOD, E. H. 1964. Diagnostic Neuroradiology. Williams & Wilkins Company, Baltimore, 1960 pp.

TAYLOR, J., GREENFIELD, J. G., AND MARTIN, J.

P. 1922. Two cases of syringomyelia and syringobulbia, observed clinically over many years and examined pathologically. Brain, 45: 323–356.

TELLO, J. F. 1922. Die Entstehungen der motorischen und sensiblen Nervenendigungen. Ztschr. ges. Anat., 64: 348–440.

TENNYSON, V. M. 1962. Electron microscopic observations of the development of the neuroblast in the rabbit embryo. In S. S. BREESE (Editor), Fifth International Congress for Electron Microscopy (Philadelphia), Vol. 2. Academic Press, New York.

TENNYSON, V. M. 1965. Electron microscopic study of the developing neuroblast of the dorsal root ganglion of the rabbit embryo. J. Comp. Neurol., 124: 267–318.

TENNYSON, V. M. 1971. The differences in fine structure of the myelencephalic and telencephalic choroid plexuses in the fetuses of man and rabbit, and a comparison with the mature stage. In A. E. WALKER AND R. ARANA-IÑIGUEZ (Editors), Cerebrospinal Fluid in Health and Disease. Acta neurol. látinoam., 17: Suppl. 1, 11–52.

TENNYSON, V. M., BARRETT, R. E., COHEN, G., CÔTÉ, L., HEIKKILA, R., AND MYTILINEOU, C. 1973. Correlation of anatomical and biochemical development of the rabbit neostriatum. In D. FORD (Editor), Neurobiological Aspects of Maturation and Aging, Progress in Brain Research. Elsevier Publishing Company, Amsterdam, 40:203–217.

TENNYSON, V. M., AND PAPPAS, G. D. 1961. Electron microscope studies of the developing telencephalic choroid plexus in normal and hydrocephalic rabbits. In W. FIELDS AND M. DESMOND (Editors), Disorders of the Developing Nervous System. Charles C Thomas, Publisher, Springfield, Ill., Ch. 12, pp. 267–318.

TENNYSON, V. M., AND PAPPAS, G. D. 1964. Fine structure of the developing telencephalic and myelencephalic choroid plexus of the rabbit. J. Comp. Neurol., 123: 379–412.

TENNYSON, V. M., AND PAPPAS, G. B. 1965. Some aspects of the fine structure of the ependymal lining. In J. MINCKLER (Editor), Neuropathology. McGraw-Hill Book Company, New York.

TENNYSON, V. M., AND PAPPAS, G. D. 1968. The fine structure of the choroid plexus: Adult and developmental stages. In A. LAJTHA AND D. H. FORD (Editors), Brain Barrier Systems, Progress in Brain Research, Vol. 29. Elsevier Publishing Company, Amsterdam, pp. 63–86.

TERAYAMA, Y., AND YAMAMOTO, K. 1971. Olivo-cochlear bundle in the guinea pig cochlea after central transsection of the crossed bundle. Electron microscopic study on origin and distribution of unmyelinated efferent fibers by axonal degeneration. Acta oto-laryng. 72: 385–396.

TERRY, R. D. 1968. Electron microscopy of the central nervous system. In O. T. BAILEY AND D. E. SMITH (Editors). The Central Nervous System, Williams & Wilkins Company, Baltimore, pp. 335–347.

TERZIAN, H. 1958. Observations on the clinical symptomatology of bilateral partial or total removal of the temporal lobe in man. In M. BALDWIN AND P. BAILEY (Editors). Temporal Lobe Epilepsy. Charles C Thomas, Publisher, Springfield, Ill., pp. 510–529.

TERZIAN, H., AND ORE, G. D. 1955. Syndrome of Klüver and Bucy reproduced in man by bilateral removal of the temporal lobes. Neurology, 5: 373–380.

TERZUOLO, C., AND TERZIAN, H. 1953. Cerebellar increase of postural tonus after deafferentation and labyrinthectomy. J. Neurophysiol., 16: 551–561.

THACH, W. T. 1970. The behavior of Purkinje and cerebellar nuclear cells during two types of voluntary arm movement in the monkey. In W. S. FIELDS AND W. D. WILLIS (Editors), The Cerebellum in Health and Dis-

ease. Warren H. Green, Inc., St. Louis, Ch. 8, pp. 217–230.

THAEMERT, J. C. 1966. Ultrastructural interrelationships of nerve processes and smooth muscle cells in three dimensions. J. Cell Biol., 28: 37–49.

THAEMERT, J. C. 1966a. Ultrastructure of cardiac muscle and nerve contiguities. J. Cell Biol., 29: 156–162.

THIÉBLOT, L. 1965. Physiology of the pineal body. In J. ARIENS KAPPERS AND J. P. SCHADÉ (Editors), *Structure and Function of the Epiphysis Cerebri, Progress in Brain Research*, Vol. 10. Elsevier Publishing Company, Amsterdam, pp. 479–488.

THOMAS, D. M., KAUFMAN, R. P., SPRAGUE, J. M., AND CHAMBERS, W. W. 1956. Experimental studies of the vermal cerebellar projections in the brain stem of the cat (fastigiobulbar tract). J. Anat., 90: 371–385.

THOMAS, P. K. 1963. The connective tissue of peripheral nerve: An electron microscope study. J. Anat., 97: 35–44.

THOMPSON, J. M., WOOLSEY, C. N., AND TALBOT, S. A. 1950. Visual areas I and II of cerebral cortex of rabbit. J. Neurophysiol., 13: 277–288.

THOMPSON, R., AND HAWKINS, W. F. 1961. Memory unaffected by mammillary body lesions in the rat. Exper. Neurol., 3: 189–196.

THOMSON, A. F., AND WALKER, A. E. 1951. Behavioral alterations following lesions of the medial surface of the temporal lobe. A. M. A. Arch. Neurol. & Psychiat., 65: 251–252.

TONCRAY, J. E., AND KRIEG, W. J. S. 1946. The nuclei of the human thalamus. A comparative approach. J. Comp. Neurol., 85: 421–459.

TORVIK, A. 1956. Afferent connections to the sensory trigeminal nuclei, the nucleus of the solitary tract and adjacent structures. An experimental study in the rat. J. Comp. Neurol., 106: 51–142.

TORVIK, A. 1957. The ascending fibers from the main trigeminal sensory nucleus. An experimental study in the cat. Am. J. Anat., 100: 1–15.

TORVIK, A., AND BRODAL, A. 1957. The origin of reticulospinal fibers in the cat. An experimental study. Anat. Rec., 128: 113–137.

TOWER, D. B. 1960. Chemical architecture of the central nervous system. In J. FIELD (Editor), *Handbook of Physiology*, Section I, Vol. III. American Physiological Society, Washington, D. C., pp. 1793–1813.

TOWER, S. S. 1937. Function and structure in the chronically isolated lumbosacral spinal cord of the dog. J. Comp. Neurol., 67: 109–131.

TOWER, S. S. 1940. Pyramidal lesion in the monkey. Brain, 63: 36–90.

TOWER, S. S. 1949. The pyramidal tract. In P. C. BUCY (Editor), *The Precentral Motor Cortex*, Ed. 2. University of Illinois Press, Urbana, Ch. 6, pp. 149–172.

TRAVIS, A. M. 1955. Neurological deficiencies after ablation of the precentral motor area in *Macaca mulatta*. Brain, 78: 155–173.

TRAVIS, A. M. 1955a. Neurological deficiences following supplementary motor area lesions in *Macaca mulatta*. Brain, 78: 174–198.

TRETIAKOFF, C. 1919. Contribution à l'étude de l'anatomopathologie du locus niger de Sommering. Thèse, Université de Paris, Number 293. Jouve et Cie, Paris.

TRUEX, R. C. 1939. Observations on the chicken Gasserian ganglion with special reference to the bipolar neurons. J. Comp. Neurol., 71: 473–486.

TRUEX, R. C. 1940. Morphological alterations in the Gasserian ganglion cells and their association with senescence in man. Am. J. Path., 16: 255–268.

TRUEX, R. C. 1941. Degenerate versus multipolar neurons in sensory ganglia. Am. J. Path., 17: 211–218.

TRUEX, R. C. 1951. The sympathetic ganglions of hypertensive patients. Arch. Path., 51: 186–191.

TRUEX, R. C., AND KELLNER, C. E. 1948. *Detailed Atlas of the Head and Neck*. Oxford University Press, New York.

TRUEX, R. C., AND TAYLOR, M. 1968. Gray matter lamination of the human spinal cord. Anat. Rec., 160: 502.

TSCHIRGI, R. D. 1960. Chemical environment of the central nervous system. In J. FIELD (Editor), *Handbook of Physiology*, Section I, Vol. III. American Physiological Society, Washington, D. C., Ch. 78, pp. 1865–1890.

TSUKAHARA, N., TOYAMA, K., AND KOSAKA, K. 1964. Intracellular recorded responses of the red nucleus neurons during antidromic and orthodromic activation. Experientia, 20: 632–637.

TSUKAHARA, N., TOYAMA, K., AND KOSAKA, K. 1967. Electrical activity of red nucleus neurones investigated with microelectrodes. Exper. Brain Res., 4: 18–33.

TWITCHELL, T. E. 1954. Sensory factors in purposive movement. J. Neurophysiol., 17: 239–252.

TYLER, D. B., AND BARD, P. 1949. Motion sickness. Physiol. Rev., 29: 311–369.

UEMURA, T., AND COHEN, B. 1973. Effects of vestibular nuclei lesions on vestibulo-ocular reflexes and posture in monkeys. Acta oto-laryn. 315(suppl.): 1–71.

UNGERSTEDT, U. 1971. Stereotaxic mapping of the monoamine pathways in the rat brain. Acta physiol. scandinav., 367(suppl.): 1–48.

URSIN, H., AND KAADA, B. R. 1960. Functional localization within the amygdaloid complex in the cat. Electroencephalog. & Clin. Neurophysiol., 12: 1–20.

UZMAN, B. G., AND NOGUEIRA-GRAF, G. 1957. Electron microscope studies of the formation of nodes of Ranvier in mouse sciatic nerves. J. Biophys. & Biochem. Cytol., 3: 589–598.

UZMAN, L. L. 1960. The histogenesis of the mouse cerebellum as studied by its tritiated thymidine uptake. J. Comp. Neurol., 114: 137–159.

VALENSTEIN, E. S., AND NAUTA, W. J. H. 1959. A comparison of the distribution of the fornix system in the rat, guinea pig, cat and monkey. J. Comp. Neurol., 113: 337–363.

VALVERDE, F. 1965. *Studies on the Piriform Lobe*. Harvard University Press, Cambridge, 138 pp.

VELASCO, M., AND LINDSLEY, D. B. 1965. Role of orbital cortex in regulation of thalamo-cortical electrical activity. Science, 149: 1375–1377.

VELASCO, M. E., AND TALEISNIK, S. 1969. Release of gonadotropins induced by amygdaloid stimulation in the rat. Endocrinology, 84: 132–139.

VERHAART, W. J. C. 1935. Die aberrierenden Pyramidenfasern bei Menschen und Affen. Schweiz. Arch. Neurol. u. Psychiat. 36: 170–190.

VERHAART, W. J. C. 1950. Fiber analysis of the basal ganglia. J. Comp. Neurol., 93: 425–440.

VERHAART, W. J. C. 1954. The tractus trigeminalis of Wallenberg. Acta psychiat. et. neurol. scandinav., 29: 269–279.

VERHAART, W. J. C., AND KENNARD, M. A. 1940. Corticofugal degeneration following thermocoagulation of areas 4, 6, and 4S in *Macaca mulatta*. J. Anat., 74: 239–254.

VERHAART, W. J. C., AND KRAMER, W. 1952. The uncrossed pyramidal tract. Acta psychiat. et neurol. scandinav., 27: 181–200.

VERNEY, E. B. 1947. The antidiuretic hormone and factors which determine its release. Proc. Roy. Soc., London, ser. B, 135: 25–106.

VERSTEEGH, C. 1927. Ergebnisse partieller Labyrinthexstirpation bei Kaninchen. Acta oto-laryng., 11: 393–408.

VERZEANO, M., LINDSLEY, D. B., AND MAGOUN, H. W. 1953. Nature of recruiting response. J. Neurophysiol., 16: 183–195.

VICTOR, M. 1964. Functions of memory and learning in man and their relationship to lesions in the temporal lobe and diencephalon. In M. A. B. BRAZIER (Editor), Brain Function, RNA in Brain Function; Memory and Learning, Vol. III. American Institute of Biological Sciences, Washington, D. C.

VICTOR, M., ANGEVINE, J. B., MANCALL, E. L., AND FISHER, C. M. 1961. Memory loss with lesions of hippocampal formation. Arch. Neurol., 5: 244–263.

VIRCHOW, R. 1860. Cellular Pathology. Translated from the second German edition by F. Chance. Churchill, London.

VIZOSO, A. D. AND YOUNG, J. Z. 1948. Internode length and fibre diameter in developing and regenerating nerves. J. Anat., 82: 110–134.

VOGT, C., AND VOGT, O. 1919. Allgemeine Ergebnisse unserer Hirnforschung. Vierte Mitteilung: Die physiologische Bedeutung der architektonischen Rindenreizungen. J. Psychol. u. Neurol., 25: 279–462.

VONEIDA, T. J. 1960. An experimental study of the course and destination of fibers arising in the head of caudate nucleus in the cat and monkey. J. Comp. Neurol., 115: 75–87.

VOSS, H. 1956. Zahl und Anordnung der Muskelspindeln in den oberen Zungenbeinmuskeln, im M. trapezius und M. latissimus dorsi. Anat. Anz., 103: 443–446.

VRAA-JENSEN, G. F. 1942. The Motor Nucleus of the Facial Nerve, with a Survey of the Efferent Innervation of the Facial Muscles. Ejnar Munksgaard, Copenhagen. Thesis, 157 pp.

WAELSCH, H. 1957. Editor, Ultrastructure and Cellular Chemistry of Neural Tissue. Symposium, American Neurological Society and Medical School, Western Reserve University. Paul B. Hoeber, Inc., New York, 249 pp.

WAKSMAN, B. H. 1961. Experimental study of diphtheritic polyneuritis in the rabbit and guinea pig. III. The blood nerve barrier in the rabbit. J. Neuropath. & Exp. Neurol., 20: 35–77.

WALBERG, F. 1952. Lateral reticular nucleus in medulla oblongata in mammals; comparative-anatomical study. J. Comp. Neurol., 96: 283–343.

WALBERG, F. 1956. Descending connections to the inferior olive. An experimental study in the cat. J. Comp. Neurol., 104: 77–173.

WALBERG, F. 1957. Corticofugal fibres to the nuclei of the dorsal columns. An experimental study in the cat. Brain, 80: 273–287.

WALBERG, F. 1957a. Do the motor nuclei of the cranial nerves receive corticofugal fibres? An experimental study in the cat. Brain, 80: 597–605.

WALBERG, F. 1958. On the termination of rubrobulbar fibers. Experimental observations in the cat. J. Comp. Neurol., 110: 65–73.

WALBERG, F. 1958a. Descending connections to the lateral reticular nucleus. An experimental study in the cat. J. Comp. Neurol., 109: 363–389.

WALBERG, F. 1961. Fastigiofugal fibers to the perihypoglossal nuclei in the cat. Exper. Neurol., 3: 525–541.

WALBERG, F. 1972. Cerebellovestibular relations: Anatomy. Prog. Brain Res., 37: 361–376.

WALBERG, F. 1974. Descending connections from the mesencephalon to the inferior olive: An experimental study in the cat. Exper. Brain Res., 21: 145–156.

WALBERG, F., BOWSHER, D., AND BRODAL, A. 1958. The termination of primary vestibular fibers in the vestibular nuclei in the cat. An experimental study with silver methods. J. Comp. Neurol., 110: 391–419.

WALBERG, F., AND BRODAL, A. 1953. Spinopontine fibers

WALBERG, F., AND JANSEN, J. 1961. Cerebellar corticovestibular fibers in the cat. Exper. Neurol., 3: 32–52.

WALBERG, F., AND POMPEIANO, O. 1960. Fastigiofugal fibers to the lateral reticular nucleus. An experimental study in the cat. Exper. Neurol., 2: 40–53.

WALBERG, F., POMPEIANO, O., BRODAL, A., AND JANSEN, J. 1962. The fastigiovestibular projection in the cat. An experimental study with silver impregnation methods. J. Comp. Neurol., 118: 49–75.

WALD, G. 1968. Molecular basis of visual excitation. Science, 162: 230–239.

WALDEYER, W. 1891. Ueber einige neuere Forschungen im Gebiete der Anatomie des Centralnervensystems. Deutsche med. Wchnschr., 17: 1213–1218, 1244–1246, 1267–1269, 1287–1289, 1331–1332, 1352–1356.

WALKER, A. E. 1936. An experimental study of the thalamocortical projection of the macaque monkey. J. Comp. Neurol., 64: 1–39.

WALKER, A. E. 1938. The thalamus of the chimpanzee. IV. Thalamic projections to the cerebral cortex. J. Anat., 73: 37–93.

WALKER, A. E. 1938a. The Primate Thalamus. University of Chicago Press, Chicago.

WALKER, A. E. 1939. The origin, course and terminations of the secondary pathways of the trigeminal nerve in primates. J. Comp. Neurol., 71: 59–89.

WALKER, A. E. 1939a. Anatomy, physiology and surgical considerations of the spinal tract of the trigeminal nerve. J. Neurophysiol., 2: 234–248.

WALKER, A. E. 1942. Somatotopic localization of spinothalamic and secondary trigeminal tracts in mesencephalon. Arch. Neurol. & Psychiat., 48: 884–889.

WALKER, A. E. 1949. Afferent connections. In P. C. BUCY (Editor), The Precentral Motor Cortex, Ed. 2. University of Illinois, Urbana, Ch. 4, pp. 112–132.

WALKER, A. E. 1959. Normal and pathological physiology of the thalamus. In G. SCHALTENBRAND AND P. BAILEY (Editors), Introduction to Stereotaxis with an Atlas of the Human Brain, Vol. I. Georg Thieme, Stuttgart, pp. 291–330.

WALKER, A. E. 1966. Internal structure and afferent-efferent relations of the thalamus. In D. P. PURPURA AND M. D. YAHR (Editors), The Thalamus. Columbia University Press, New York, pp. 1–12.

WALKER, A. E., AND FULTON, J. F. 1938. Hemidecortication in chimpanzee, baboon, macaque, potto, cat and coati: A study in encephalization. J. Nerv. & Ment. Dis., 87: 677–700.

WALKER, A. E., AND WEAVER, T. A., JR. 1940. Ocular movements from the occipital lobe in the monkey. J. Neurophysiol., 3: 353–357.

WALKER, A. E., AND WEAVER, T. A., JR. 1942. The topical organization and termination of fibers of the posterior columns in Macaca mulatta. J. Comp. Neurol., 76: 145–158.

WALL, P. D. 1967. The laminar organization of dorsal horn and effects of descending impulses. J. Physiol., 188: 403–423.

WALL, P. D., AND TAUB, A. 1962. Four aspects of the trigeminal nucleus and a paradox. J. Neurophysiol., 25: 110–126.

WALLENBERG, A. 1905. Die secondären Bahnen aus dem frontalen sensiblen Trigeminus Kerne des Kaninchens. Anat. Anz., 26: 145–155.

WALLS, G. L. 1963. The Vertebrate Eye and Its Adaptive Radiation. Hafner Publishing Company, New York (reprinted from 1942).

WALSHE, F. M. R. 1942. The anatomy and physiology of cutaneous sensibility: A critical review. Brain, 65: 48–114.

WALTHER, J. B., AND RASMUSSEN, G. L. 1960. Descending connections of auditory cortex and thalamus of the cat. Fed. Proc., 19: 291.

WANG, S. C. 1955. Bulbar regulation of cardiovascular activity. In *Proceedings of the Annual Meeting of the Council for High Blood Pressure Research.* American Heart Association, pp. 145-158.

WARD, A. A., JR. 1948. The cingular gyrus: Area 24. J. Neurophysiol., 11: 13-24.

WARD, A. A., JR., AND McCULLOCH, W. S. 1947. The projection of the frontal lobe on the hypothalamus. J. Neurophysiol., 10: 309-314.

WARRINGTON, W. B., AND GRIFFITH, F. 1904. On the cells of the spinal ganglia and on the relationship of their histological structure to axonal distribution. Brain, 27: 297-326.

WARWICK, R. 1953. Representation of the extraocular muscles in the oculomotor nuclei of the monkey. J. Comp. Neurol., 98: 449-504.

WARWICK, R. 1953a. The identity of the posterocentral nucleus of Panegrossi. J. Comp. Neurol., 99: 599-612.

WARWICK, R. 1954. The ocular parasympathetic nerve supply and its mesencephalic sources. J. Anat., 88: 71-93.

WARWICK, R. 1955. The so-called nucleus of convergence. Brain, 78: 92-114.

WATERSTON, D. 1933. Observations on sensation. The sensory functions of the skin for touch and pain. J. Physiol., 77: 251-275.

WEBSTER, H. D. 1962. Transient, focal accumulation of axonal mitochondria during the early stages of Wallerian degeneration. J. Cell Biol., 12: 361-377.

WEBSTER, K. E. 1961. Cortico-striate interrelations in the albino rat. J. Anat., 95: 532-544.

WEBSTER, K. E. 1965. The cortico-striatal projection in the cat. J. Anat., 99: 329-337.

WEDDELL, G. 1941. The pattern of cutaneous innervation in relation to cutaneous sensibility. J. Anat., 75: 346-367.

WEDDELL, G., TAYLOR, D. A., AND WILLIAMS, C. M. 1955. Studies on the innervation of skin. III. The patterned arrangement of the spinal sensory nerves to the rabbit ear. J. Anat., 89: 317-342.

WEIL, A., AND LASSEK, A. 1929. A quantitative distribution of the pyramidal tract in man. Arch. Neurol. & Psychiat., 22: 495-510.

WEINBERGER, L. M., AND GRANT, F. C. 1941. Precocious puberty and tumors of the hypothalamus. Arch. Int. Med., 67: 762-792.

WEINBERGER, L. M., AND GRANT, F. C. 1942. Experiences with intramedullary tractotomy. III. Studies in sensation. Arch. Neurol. & Psychiat., 48: 355-381.

WEISS, P., AND HISCOE, H. B. 1948. Experiments on the mechanism of nerve growth. J. Exper. Zool., 107: 315-396.

WEISS, P., AND WANG, H. 1936. Neurofibrils in living ganglion cells of the chick, cultivated *in vitro*. Anat. Rec., 67: 105-117.

WELCH, W. K., AND KENNARD, M. A. 1944. Relation of cerebral cortex to spasticity and flaccidity. J. Neurophysiol., 7: 255-268.

WELKER, W. I., BENJAMIN, R. M., MILES, R. C., AND WOOLSEY, C. N. 1957. Motor effects of cortical stimulation in squirrel monkey (*Saimiri sciureus*). J. Neurophysiol., 20: 347-364.

WESTHEIMER, G., AND BLAIR, S. M. 1973. The parasympathetic pathways to the internal eye muscles. Invest. Ophth., 12: 193-197.

WHEATLEY, M. D. 1944. Hypothalamus and affective behavior in cats. Arch. Neurol. & Psychiat., 52: 296-316.

WHITE, J. C., OKELBERRY, A. M., AND WHITELAW, G. P. 1936. Vasomotor tonus of the denervated artery. Arch. Neurol. & Psychiat., 36: 1251-1276.

WHITE, L. E. 1965. Olfactory bulb projections of the rat.

Anat. Rec., 152: 465-480.

WHITFIELD, I. C. 1967. *The Auditory Pathway.* Williams & Wilkins Company, Baltimore.

WHITLOCK, D. G. 1952. A neurohistological and neurophysiological investigation of the afferent fiber tracts and the receptive areas of the avian cerebellum. J. Comp. Neurol., 97: 567-636.

WHITLOCK, D. G., AND NAUTA, W. J. H. 1956. Subcortical projections from the temporal neocortex in the Macaca mulatta. J. Comp. Neurol., 106: 183-212.

WHITLOCK, D. G., AND PERL, E. R. 1961. Thalamic projections of spinothalamic pathways in monkey. Exper. Neurol., 3: 240-255.

WHITTAKER, V. P. 1965. The application of subcellular fractionation techniques to the study of brain function. Progr. Biophys., 15: 39-96.

WHITTIER, J. R. 1947. Ballism and the subthalamic nucleus (nucleus hypothalamicus; Corpus Luysi). Arch. Neurol. & Psychiat., 58: 672-692.

WHITTIER, J. R., AND METTLER, F. A. 1949. Studies on the subthalamus of the rhesus monkey. I. Anatomy and fiber connections of the subthalamic nucleus of Luys. J. Comp. Neurol., 90: 281-317.

WHITTIER, J. R., AND METTLER, F. A. 1949a. Studies on the subthalamus of the rhesus monkey. II. Hyperkinesia and other physiologic effects of subthalamic lesions with special reference to the subthalamic nucleus of Luys. J. Comp. Neurol., 90: 319-372.

WICHMANN, R. 1900. *Die Rückenmarksnerven und ihre Segmentbezüge,* part 2. Viotto Salle, Berlin, pp. 151-279.

WICKELGREN, B. G., AND STERLING, P. 1969. Influence of visual cortex on receptive fields in the superior colliculus of the cat. J. Neurophysiol., 32: 16-32.

WIITANEN, J. T. 1969. Selective silver impregnation of degenerating axons and axon terminals in the central nervous system of the monkey (*Macaca mulatta*). Brain Res., 14: 546-548.

WILLIAMS, T. H. 1967. Electron microscopic evidence for an autonomic interneuron. Nature, 214: 309-310.

WILSON, M. E., AND TOYNE, M. J. 1970. Retino-tectal and cortico-tectal projections in Macaca mulatta. Brain Res., 24: 395-406.

WILSON, S. A. K. 1912. Progressive lenticular degeneration; a familial nervous disease associated with cirrhosis of the liver. Brain, 34: 295-509.

WILSON, S. A. K. 1914. An experimental research into the anatomy and physiology of the corpus striatum. Brain, 36: 427-492.

WILSON, S. A. K. 1925. Disorders of motility and muscle tone with special reference to the corpus striatum (Croonian Lectures). Lancet, 2: 215-291.

WILSON, S. A. K. 1928. *Modern Problems in Neurology.* Edward Arnold and Company, London.

WILSON, V. J., AND YOSHIDA, M. 1969. Monosynaptic inhibition of neck motoneurons by the medial vestibular nucleus. Exper. Brain Res., 9: 365-380.

WINDLE, W. F. 1926. Non-bifurcating nerve fibers of the trigeminal nerve. J. Comp. Neurol., 40: 229-240.

WINDLE, W. F. 1955. Editor, *Regeneration in the Central Nervous System.* Charles C Thomas, Publisher, Springfield, Ill., 311 pp.

WINDLE, W. F. 1957. Editor, *New Research Techniques of Neuroanatomy.* Charles C Thomas, Publisher, Springfield, Ill.

WINDLE, W. F. 1958. Editor, *Biology of Neuroglia.* Charles C Thomas, Publisher, Springfield, Ill., 340 pp.

WINDLE, W. F., AND CHAMBERS, W. W. 1950. Regeneration in the spinal cord of the cat and dog. J. Comp. Neurol., 93: 241-257.

WINKLER, C. 1918-1933. *Opera omnia,* Vols. 1 to 10. E. F. Bohn, Haarlem.

WINTER, D. L., 1965. N. gracilis of cat. Functional organization and corticofugal effects. J. Neurophysiol., 28: 48–70.

WISCHNITZER, S. 1960. The ultrastructure of the nucleus and nucleocytoplasmic relations. Internat. Rev. Cytol., 10: 137–162.

WISLOCKI, G. B., AND LEDUC, E. 1953. The cytology and histochemistry of the subcommissural organ and Reissner's fibers in rodents. J. Comp. Neurol., 97: 515–543.

WOLF, G., AND SUTIN, J. 1966. Fiber degeneration after lateral hypothalamic lesions in the rat. J. Comp. Neurol., 127: 137–156.

WOLF, G. A., JR. 1941. The ratio of preganglionic neurons to postganglionic neurons in the visceral nervous system. J. Comp. Neurol., 75: 235–243.

WOLFE, D. E., POTTER, L. T., RICHARDSON, K. C., AND AXELROD, J. 1962. Localizing tritiated norepinephrine in sympathetic axons by electron microscopic autoradiography. Science, 138: 440–442.

WOODBURNE, R. T. 1936. A phylogenetic consideration of the primary and secondary centers and connections of the trigeminal complex in a series of vertebrates. J. Comp. Neurol., 65: 403–501.

WOODBURNE, R. T., CROSBY, E. C., AND McCOTTER, R. E. 1946. The mammalian midbrain and isthmus regions. Part II. The fiber connections. A. The relations of the tegmentum of the midbrain with the basal ganglia in the Macaca mulatta. J. Comp. Neurol., 85: 67–92.

WOODBURY, D. M. 1958. Symposium discussion. In W. F. WINDLE, (Editor), Biology of Neuroglia. Charles C Thomas, Publisher, Springfield, Ill., pp. 120–127.

WOODBURY, D. M. 1965. Blood-cerebrospinal fluid-brain fluid relations. In T. C. RUCH AND H. D PATTON (Editors), Physiology and Biophysics. W. B. Saunders, Company, Philadelphia, pp. 942–950.

WOOLLARD, H. H. 1935. Observations on the terminations of cutaneous nerves. Brain, 58: 352–367.

WOOLLARD, H. H., AND HARPMAN, J. A. 1940. The connections of the inferior colliculus and dorsal nucleus of the lateral lemniscus. J. Anat., 74: 441–458.

WOOLSEY, C. N. 1947. Patterns of sensory representation in the cerebral cortex. Fed. Proc., 6: 437–441.

WOOLSEY, C. N. 1958. Organization of somatic sensory and motor areas of the cerebral cortex. In H. F. HARLOW AND C. N. WOOLSEY (Editors), Biological and Biochemical Bases of Behavior. University of Wisconsin, Madison, pp. 63–81.

WOOLSEY, C. N., AND FAIRMAN, D. 1946. Contralateral, ipsilateral, and bilateral representation of cutaneous receptors in somatic areas I and II of the cerebral cortex of pigs, sheep and other mammals. Surgery, 19: 684–

702.

WOOLSEY, C. N., SETTLAGE, P. H., MEYER, D. R., SENCER, W., HAMUY, T. P., AND TRAVIS, A. M. 1951. Patterns of localization in precentral and "supplementary" motor areas and their relation to the concept of a premotor area. A. Res. Nerv. & Ment. Dis., Proc., 30: 238–264.

WOOLSEY, C. N., AND WALZL, E. M. 1942. Topical projection of nerve fibers from local regions of the cochlea to the cerebral cortex of the cat. Bull. Johns Hopkins Hosp., 71: 315–344.

WOOLSEY, C. N., AND WANG, G. H. 1945. Somatic areas I and II of the cerebral cortex of the rabbit. Fed. Proc., 4: 79.

WYBURN, G. M. 1958. The capsule of spinal ganglion cells. J. Anat., 92: 528–533.

WYCIS, H. T., AND SPIEGEL, E. A. 1952. Ansotomy in paralysis agitans. Confinia neurol., 12: 245–246.

YAKOVLEV, P. I., LOCKE, S., AND ANGEVINE, J. B. 1966. The limbus of the cerebral hemisphere, limbic nuclei of the thalamus and the cingulum bundle. In D. P. PURPURA AND M. D. YAHR (Editors), The Thalamus. Columbia University Press, New York, pp. 77–97.

YOUNG, J. Z. 1942. The functional repair of nervous tissue. Physiol. Rev., 22: 318–374.

YOUNG, J. Z. 1949. Factors influencing the regeneration of nerves. Advances Surg., 1: 165–220.

ZACKS, S. I. 1964. The Motor Endplate. W. B. Saunders, Philadelphia, pp. 1–83.

ZANGWILL, O. L. 1960. Cerebral Dominance and Its Relation to Psychological Function. Charles C Thomas, Publisher, Springfield, Ill., 31 pp.

ZBROŻYNA, A. W. 1972. The organization of the defense reaction elicited from amygdala and its connections. In B. E. ELEFTHERIOU, The Neurobiology of the Amygdala, Plenum Press, New York, pp. 597–606.

ZIMMERMAN, E. A., CHAMBERS, W. W., AND LIU, C. N. 1964. An experimental study of the anatomical organization of the cortico-bulbar system in the albino rat. J. Comp. Neurol., 123: 301–324.

ZOLOVICK, A. J. 1972. Effects of lesions and electrical stimulation of the amygdala on hypothalamic-hypophyseal regulation. In B. E. ELEFTHERIOU (Editor), The Neurobiology of the Amygdala. Plenum Press, New York, pp. 643–683.

ZÜLCH, K. J. 1954. Mangeldurchblutung an der Grenzzone zweier Gefässgebiete als Ursache bisher ungeklärter Rückenmarksschädigungen. Deutsche Ztschr. Nervenh., 172: 81–101.

ATLAS OF BRAIN AND BRAIN STEM

SECTION I

Transverse sections of Brain Stem (A–1 to A–13).

SECTION II

Frontal sections cut transverse to the longitudinal axis of the Diencephalon (A–14 to A–18).

SECTION III

Frontal sections of Diencephalon and Basal Ganglia (A–19 to A–24).

SECTION IV

Parasagittal sections of Brain and Brain Stem (A–25 to A–32).

The following series of drawings of transverse sections of the brain stem taken at critical levels are reproduced in colors that faithfully reveal the definition of fiber tracts and cellular groupings characteristic of the original preparations. These sections, stained with Luxol Fast Blue and counterstained with cresyl violet (Klüver and Barrera, '53), appear particularly appropriate for laboratory instruction since the student is presented with a complete picture of cellular configurations in relationship with the myelinated fiber tracts in a single microscopic slide. The outline drawing of the brain stem indicates the levels and planes of section of the individual figures and should be used as a key. The magnification of the figures is noted in the legends.

Illustrations used in Sections I, II, and III were prepared by Miss Marjorie Stodgell, Medical Artist, of the Hahnemann Medical College and Hospital of Philadelphia. Photographs used in Section IV were made from original Weigert preparations of the late Professor Andrew T. Rasmussen of the University of Minnesota.

SECTION I

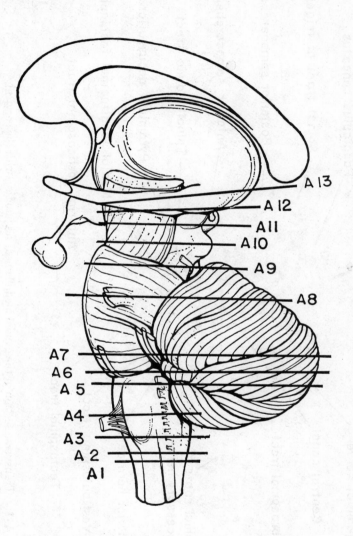

A 13
A 12
A11
A10
A9
A8
A7
A6
A 5
A4
A3
A 2
AI

Brain Stem Atlas

Drawing of the brain stem indicating the level and plane of sections A-1 through A-13.

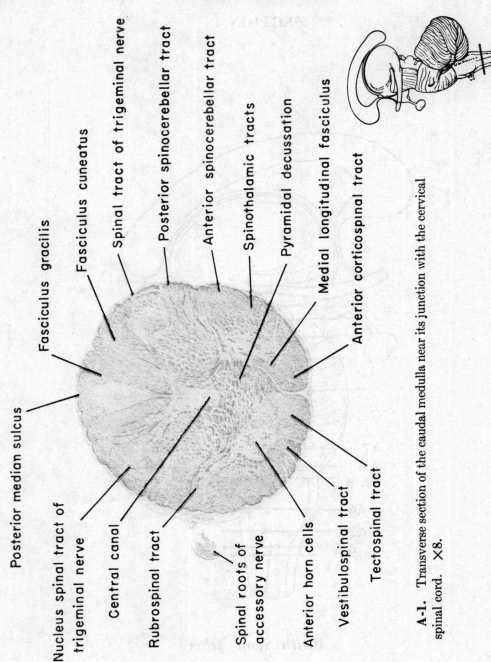

Posterior median sulcus

Fasciculus gracilis

Fasciculus cuneatus

Spinal tract of trigeminal nerve

Posterior spinocerebellar tract

Anterior spinocerebellar tract

Spinothalamic tracts

Pyramidal decussation

Medial longitudinal fasciculus

Anterior corticospinal tract

Nucleus spinal tract of trigeminal nerve

Central canal

Rubrospinal tract

Spinal roots of accessory nerve

Anterior horn cells

Vestibulospinal tract

Tectospinal tract

A-1. Transverse section of the caudal medulla near its junction with the cervical spinal cord. ×8.

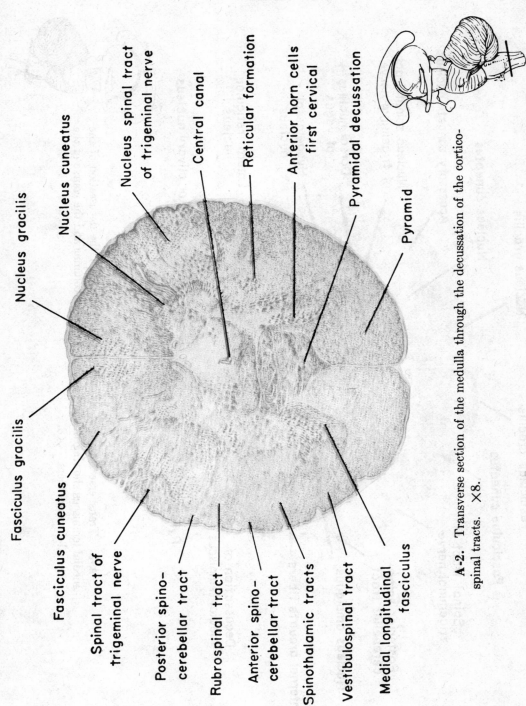

Nucleus gracilis

Nucleus cuneatus

Nucleus spinal tract
of trigeminal nerve

Central canal

Reticular formation

Anterior horn cells
first cervical

Pyramidal decussation

Pyramid

Fasciculus gracilis

Fasciculus cuneatus

Spinal tract of
trigeminal nerve

Posterior spino-
cerebellar tract

Rubrospinal tract

Anterior spino-
cerebellar tract

Spinothalamic tracts

Vestibulospinal tract

Medial longitudinal
fasciculus

A-2. Transverse section of the medulla through the decussation of the corticospinal tracts. ×8.

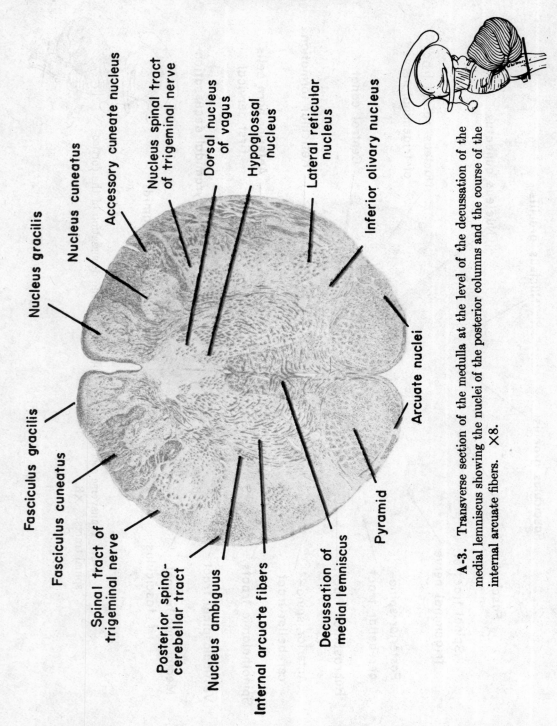

Nucleus gracilis

Nucleus cuneatus

Accessory cuneate nucleus

Nucleus spinal tract of trigeminal nerve

Dorsal nucleus of vagus

Hypoglossal nucleus

Lateral reticular nucleus

Inferior olivary nucleus

Fasciculus gracilis

Fasciculus cuneatus

Spinal tract of trigeminal nerve

Posterior spino-cerebellar tract

Nucleus ambiguus

Internal arcuate fibers

Decussation of medial lemniscus

Pyramid

Arcuate nuclei

A-3. Transverse section of the medulla at the level of the decussation of the medial lemniscus showing the nuclei of the posterior columns and the course of the internal arcuate fibers. ×8.

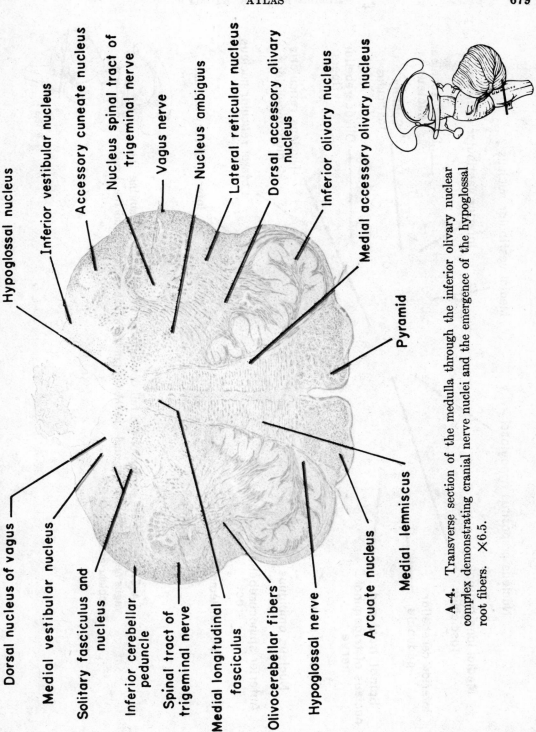

Hypoglossal nucleus

Inferior vestibular nucleus

Accessory cuneate nucleus

Nucleus spinal tract of trigeminal nerve

Vagus nerve

Nucleus ambiguus

Lateral reticular nucleus

Dorsal accessory olivary nucleus

Inferior olivary nucleus

Medial accessory olivary nucleus

Dorsal nucleus of vagus

Medial vestibular nucleus

Solitary fasciculus and nucleus

Inferior cerebellar peduncle

Spinal tract of trigeminal nerve

Medial longitudinal fasciculus

Olivocerebellar fibers

Hypoglossal nerve

Arcuate nucleus

Medial lemniscus

Pyramid

A-4. Transverse section of the medulla through the inferior olivary nuclear complex demonstrating cranial nerve nuclei and the emergence of the hypoglossal root fibers. ×6.5.

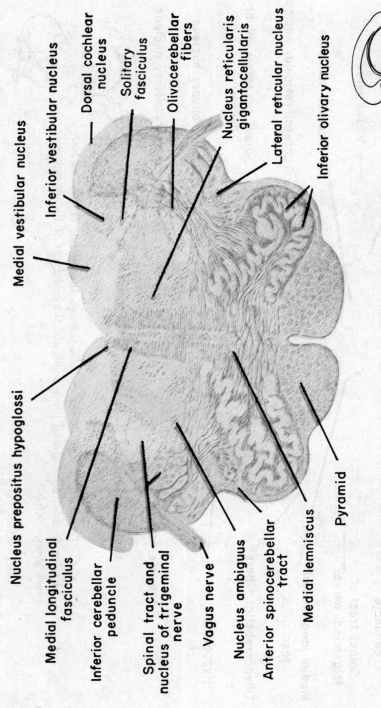

Medial vestibular nucleus

Inferior vestibular nucleus

Dorsal cochlear nucleus

Solitary fasciculus

Olivocerebellar fibers

Nucleus reticularis gigantocellularis

Lateral reticular nucleus

Inferior olivary nucleus

Nucleus prepositus hypoglossi

Medial longitudinal fasciculus

Inferior cerebellar peduncle

Spinal tract and nucleus of trigeminal nerve

Vagus nerve

Nucleus ambiguus

Anterior spinocerebellar tract

Medial lemniscus

Pyramid

A-5. Transverse section of the full development of the medulla showing the vagus nerve, the vestibular nuclei in the floor of the fourth ventricle, and the dorsal cochlear nuclei. ×6.5.

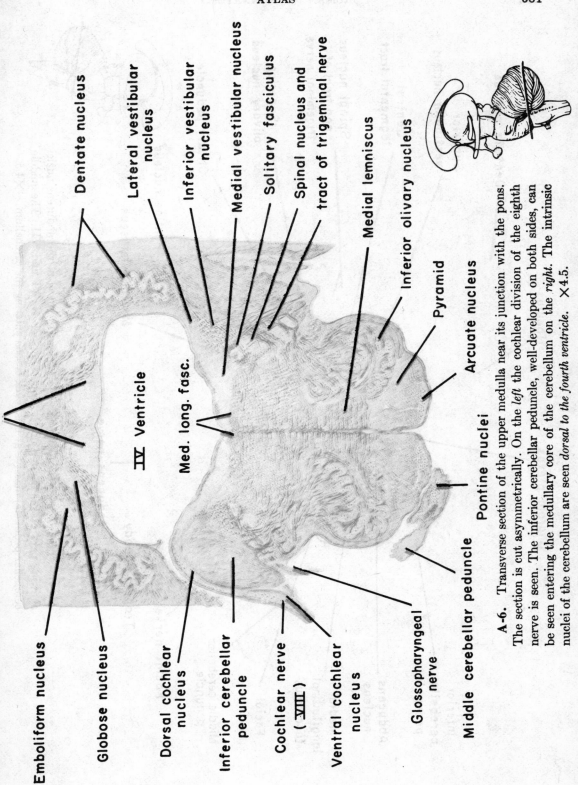

Fastigial nuclei

Emboliform nucleus

Globose nucleus

Dentate nucleus

Lateral vestibular nucleus

Inferior vestibular nucleus

Medial vestibular nucleus

Solitary fasciculus

Spinal nucleus and tract of trigeminal nerve

Medial lemniscus

Inferior olivary nucleus

Pyramid

Arcuate nucleus

IV Ventricle

Med. long. fasc.

Dorsal cochlear nucleus

Inferior cerebellar peduncle

Cochlear nerve (VIII)

Ventral cochlear nucleus

Glossopharyngeal nerve

Middle cerebellar peduncle

Pontine nuclei

A-6. Transverse section of the upper medulla near its junction with the pons. The section is cut asymmetrically. On the *left* the cochlear division of the eighth nerve is seen. The inferior cerebellar peduncle, well-developed on both sides, can be seen entering the medullary core of the cerebellum on the *right*. The intrinsic nuclei of the cerebellum are seen *dorsal to the fourth ventricle.* ×4.5.

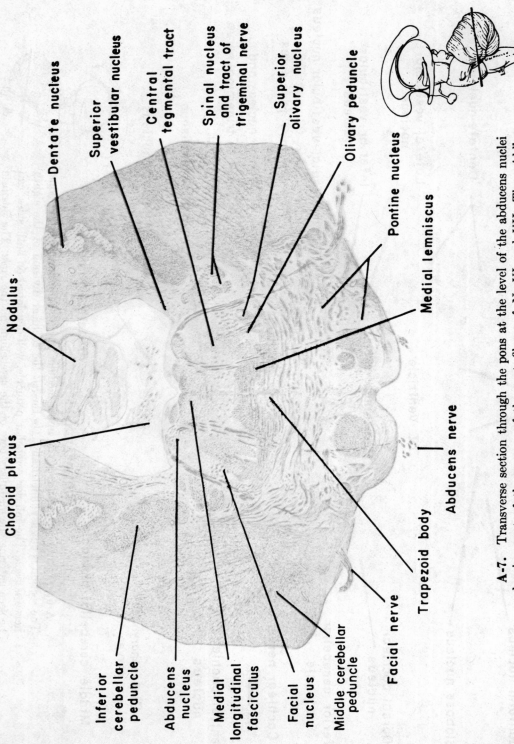

Dentate nucleus

Superior vestibular nucleus

Central tegmental tract

Spinal nucleus and tract of trigeminal nerve

Superior olivary nucleus

Olivary peduncle

Pontine nucleus

Medial lemniscus

Nodulus

Choroid plexus

Inferior cerebellar peduncle

Abducens nucleus

Medial longitudinal fasciculus

Facial nucleus

Middle cerebellar peduncle

Facial nerve

Trapezoid body

Abducens nerve

A-7. Transverse section through the pons at the level of the abducens nuclei showing part of the course of the root fibers of N. VI and VII. The middle cerebellar peduncle, massive at this level, is seen entering the cerebellum. ×4.5.

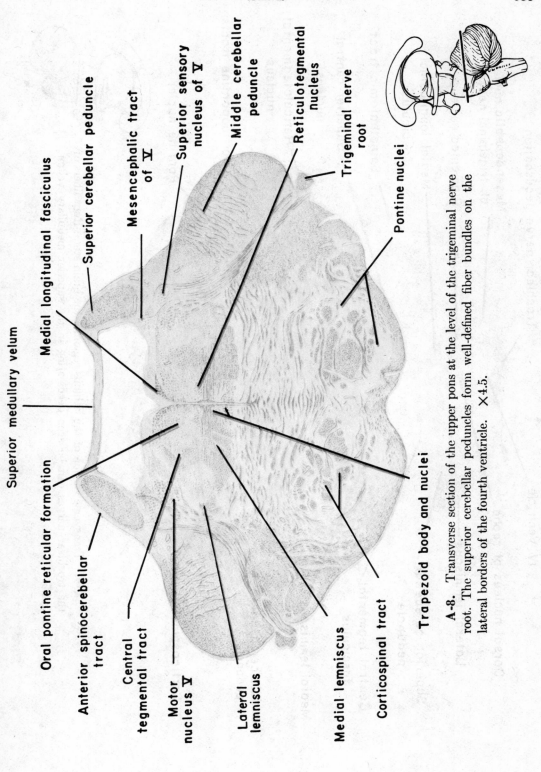

Superior medullary velum

Oral pontine reticular formation

Anterior spinocerebellar tract

Central tegmental tract

Motor nucleus V

Lateral lemniscus

Medial lemniscus

Corticospinal tract

Trapezoid body and nuclei

Medial longitudinal fasciculus

Superior cerebellar peduncle

Mesencephalic tract of V

Superior sensory nucleus of V

Middle cerebellar peduncle

Reticulotegmental nucleus

Trigeminal nerve root

Pontine nuclei

A-8. Transverse section of the upper pons at the level of the trigeminal nerve root. The superior cerebellar peduncles form well-defined fiber bundles on the lateral borders of the fourth ventricle. ×4.5.

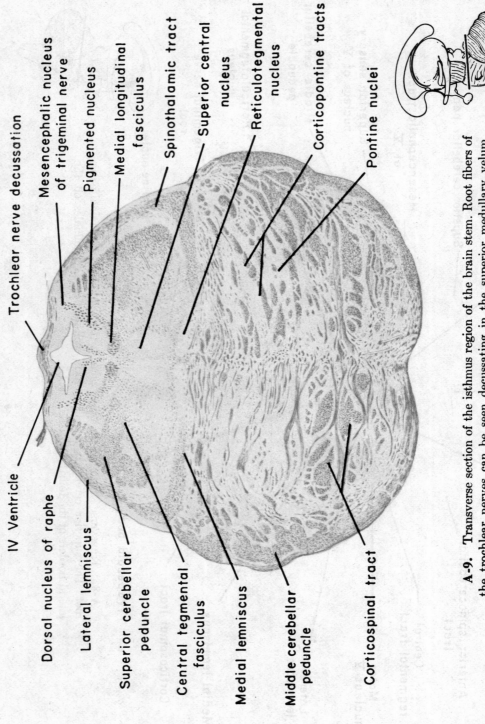

Trochlear nerve decussation

Mesencephalic nucleus of trigeminal nerve

Pigmented nucleus

Medial longitudinal fasciculus

Spinothalamic tract

Superior central nucleus

Reticulotegmental nucleus

Corticopontine tracts

Pontine nuclei

IV Ventricle

Dorsal nucleus of raphe

Lateral lemniscus

Superior cerebellar peduncle

Central tegmental fasciculus

Medial lemniscus

Middle cerebellar peduncle

Corticospinal tract

A-9. Transverse section of the isthmus region of the brain stem. Root fibers of the trochlear nerves can be seen decussating in the superior medullary velum. ×4.5.

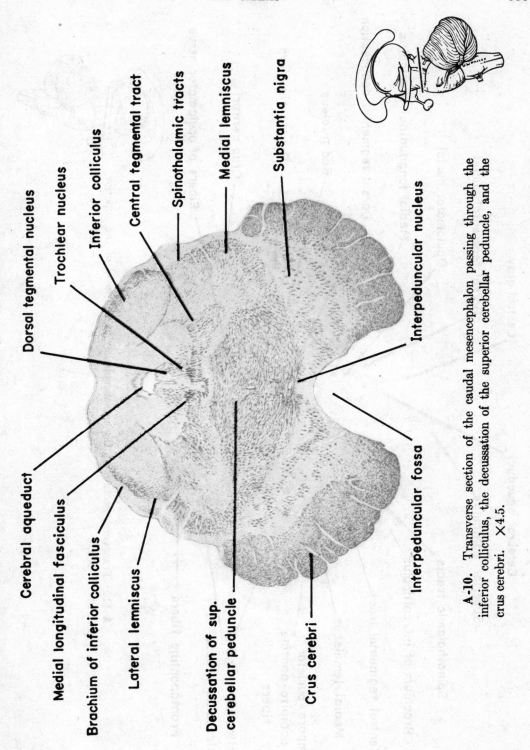

A-10. Transverse section of the caudal mesencephalon passing through the inferior colliculus, the decussation of the superior cerebellar peduncle, and the crus cerebri. ×4.5.

Cerebral aqueduct

Medial longitudinal fasciculus

Brachium of inferior colliculus

Lateral lemniscus

Decussation of sup. cerebellar peduncle

Crus cerebri

Interpeduncular fossa

Interpeduncular nucleus

Substantia nigra

Medial lemniscus

Spinothalamic tracts

Central tegmental tract

Inferior colliculus

Trochlear nucleus

Dorsal tegmental nucleus

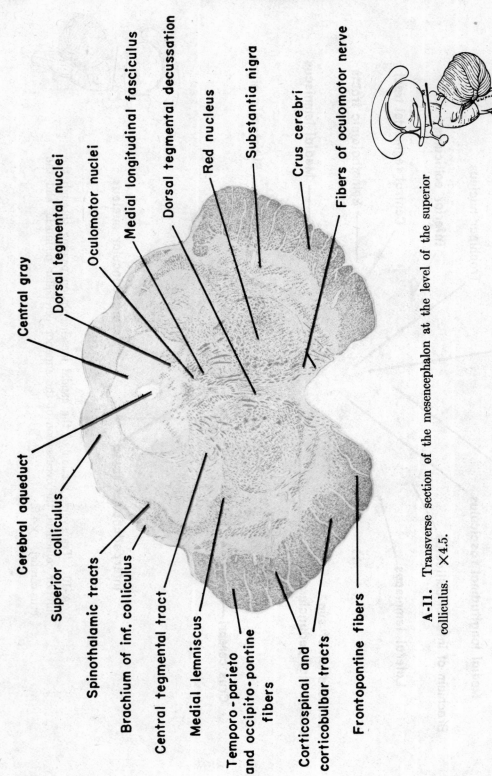

Cerebral aqueduct

Central gray

Dorsal tegmental nuclei

Oculomotor nuclei

Medial longitudinal fasciculus

Dorsal tegmental decussation

Red nucleus

Substantia nigra

Crus cerebri

Fibers of oculomotor nerve

Superior colliculus

Spinothalamic tracts

Brachium of inf. colliculus

Central tegmental tract

Medial lemniscus

Temporo-parieto and occipito-pontine fibers

Corticospinal and corticobulbar tracts

Frontopontine fibers

A-11. Transverse section of the mesencephalon at the level of the superior colliculus. ×4.5.

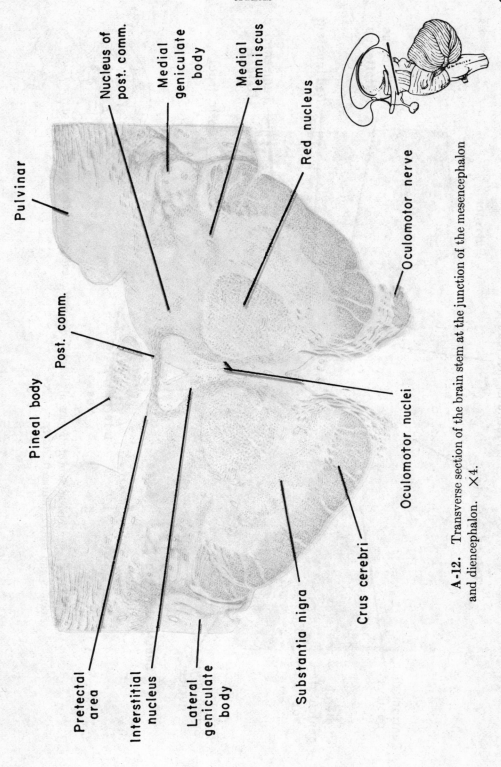

Pulvinar

Nucleus of post. comm.

Medial geniculate body

Medial lemniscus

Red nucleus

Oculomotor nerve

Post. comm.

Pineal body

Pretectal area

Interstitial nucleus

Lateral geniculate body

Substantia nigra

Crus cerebri

Oculomotor nuclei

A-12. Transverse section of the brain stem at the junction of the mesencephalon and diencephalon. ×4.

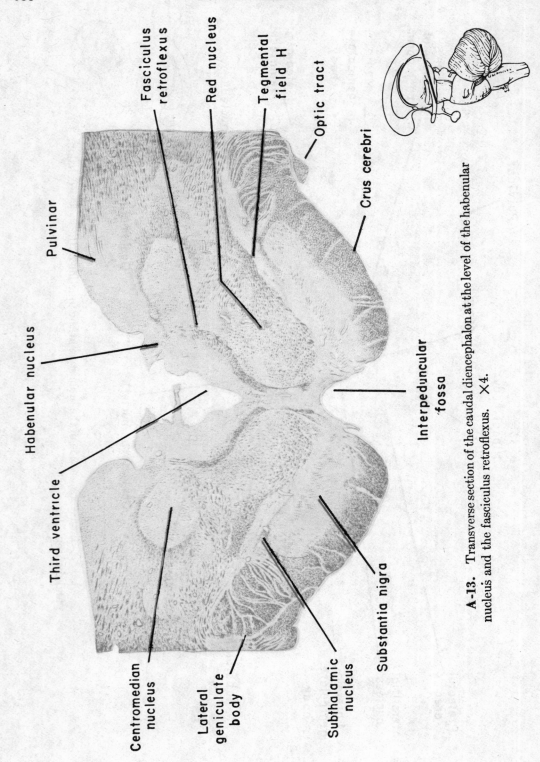

Pulvinar

Fasciculus retroflexus

Red nucleus

Tegmental field H

Optic tract

Crus cerebri

Habenular nucleus

Third ventricle

Interpeduncular fossa

Centromedian nucleus

Lateral geniculate body

Subthalamic nucleus

Substantia nigra

A-13. Transverse section of the caudal diencephalon at the level of the habenular nucleus and the fasciculus retroflexus. ×4.

SECTION II

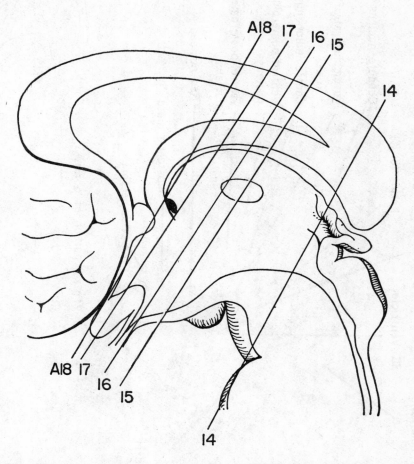

Outline of median sagittal surface of brain indicating level and plane of frontal sections A–14 to A–18.

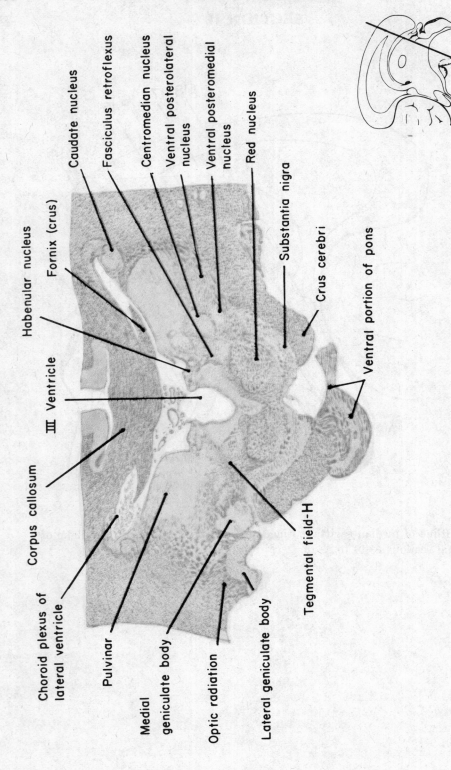

Choroid plexus of lateral ventricle

Corpus callosum

Habenular nucleus

Fornix (crus)

Caudate nucleus

Fasciculus retroflexus

Centromedian nucleus

Ventral posterolateral nucleus

Ventral posteromedial nucleus

Red nucleus

Substantia nigra

Crus cerebri

Ventral portion of pons

III Ventricle

Pulvinar

Medial geniculate body

Optic radiation

Lateral geniculate body

Tegmental field-H

A–14. Frontal section through the junction of the midbrain and the diencephalon at the level of the habenular nucleus. X2.5.

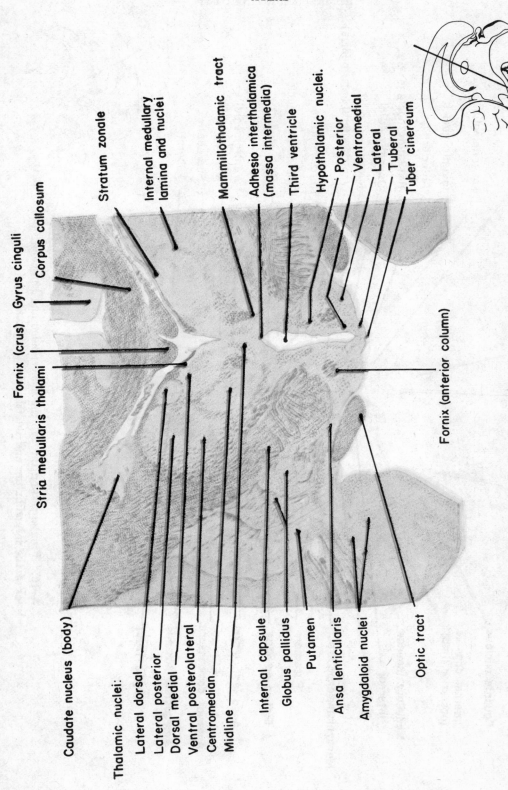

Caudate nucleus (body)

Thalamic nuclei:

Lateral dorsal
Lateral posterior
Dorsal medial
Ventral posterolateral
Centromedian
Midline
Internal capsule
Globus pallidus
Putamen
Ansa lenticularis
Amygdaloid nuclei
Optic tract

Stria medullaris thalami
Fornix (crus)
Gyrus cinguli
Corpus callosum

Stratum zonale
Internal medullary lamina and nuclei
Mammillothalamic tract
Adhesio interthalamica (massa intermedia)
Third ventricle
Hypothalamic nuclei.
Posterior
Ventromedial
Lateral
Tuberal
Tuber cinereum

Fornix (anterior column)

A–15. Frontal section through the diencephalon and lenticular nucleus at the level of the tuber cinereum and interthalamic adhesion. ×3.

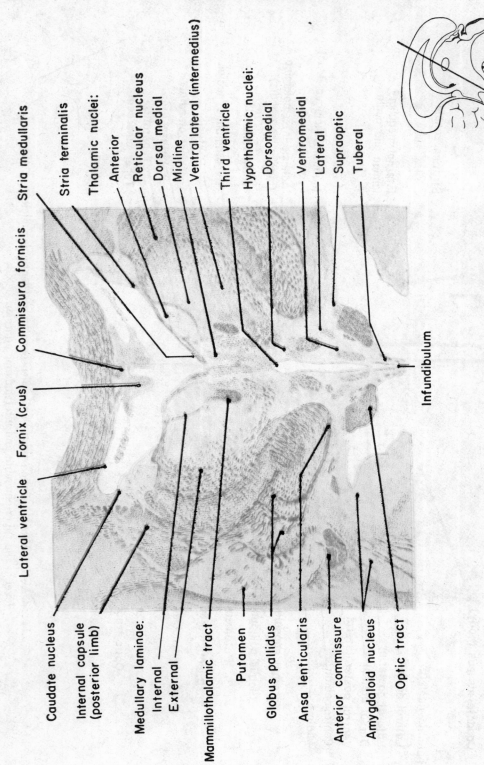

Stria medullaris

Stria terminalis

Thalamic nuclei:

Anterior

Reticular nucleus

Dorsal medial

Midline

Ventral lateral (intermedius)

Third ventricle

Hypothalamic nuclei:

Dorsomedial

Ventromedial

Lateral

Supraoptic

Tuberal

Commissura fornicis

Fornix (crus)

Lateral ventricle

Infundibulum

Caudate nucleus

Internal capsule (posterior limb)

Medullary laminae:

Internal

External

Mammillothalamic tract

Putamen

Globus pallidus

Ansa lenticularis

Anterior commissure

Amygdaloid nucleus

Optic tract

A–16. Frontal section through the diencephalon and lenticular nucleus at the level of the infundibulum and interthalamic adhesion. ×3.

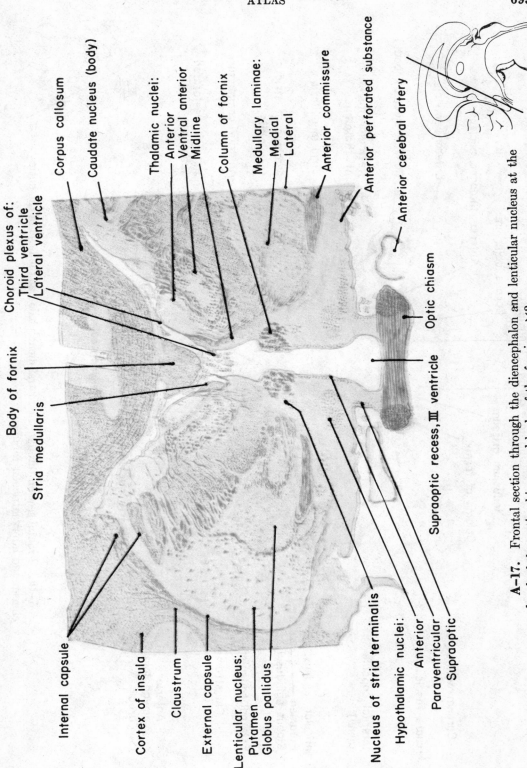

A–17. Frontal section through the diencephalon and lenticular nucleus at the level of the optic chiasm and body of the fornix. ×3.

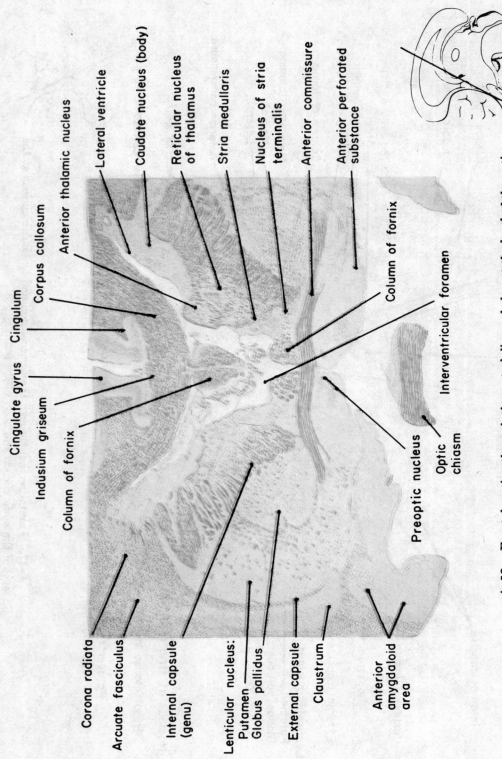

Cingulate gyrus   Cingulum

Corpus callosum

Indusium griseum

Column of fornix

Corona radiata

Arcuate fasciculus

Internal capsule (genu)

Lenticular nucleus:
Putamen
Globus pallidus

External capsule

Claustrum

Anterior amygdaloid area

Anterior thalamic nucleus

Lateral ventricle

Caudate nucleus (body)

Reticular nucleus of thalamus

Stria medullaris

Nucleus of stria terminalis

Anterior commissure

Anterior perforated substance

Column of fornix

Interventricular foramen

Optic chiasm

Preoptic nucleus

A–18. Frontal section through the rostral diencephalon at the level of the optic chiasm and interventricular foramen. ×3.

SECTION III

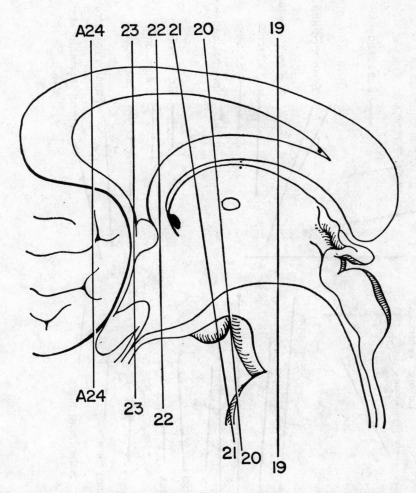

Outline of median sagittal surface of brain indicating level and plane of frontal sections A–19 to A–24.

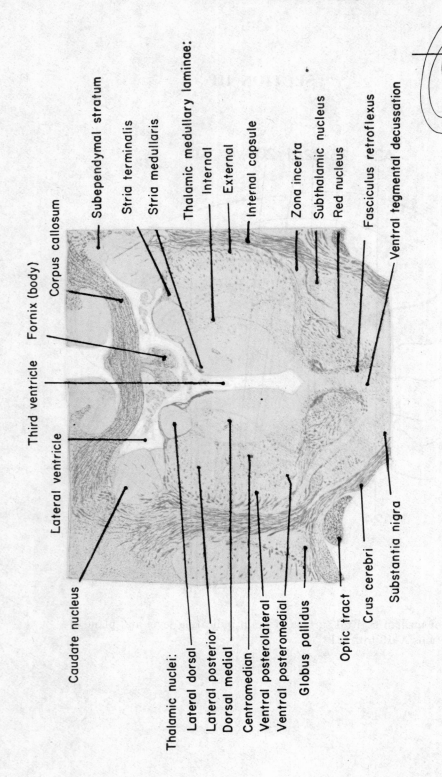

Caudate nucleus

Lateral ventricle

Third ventricle   Fornix (body)

Corpus callosum

Subependymal stratum

Stria terminalis

Stria medullaris

Thalamic medullary laminae:

Internal

External

Internal capsule

Zona incerta

Subthalamic nucleus

Red nucleus

Fasciculus retroflexus

Ventral tegmental decussation

Thalamic nuclei:

Lateral dorsal

Lateral posterior

Dorsal medial

Centromedian

Ventral posterolateral

Ventral posteromedial

Globus pallidus

Optic tract

Crus cerebri

Substantia nigra

A–19. Frontal section through midbrain and diencephalon at the level of red nucleus and posterior thalamic nuclei. ×2.5.

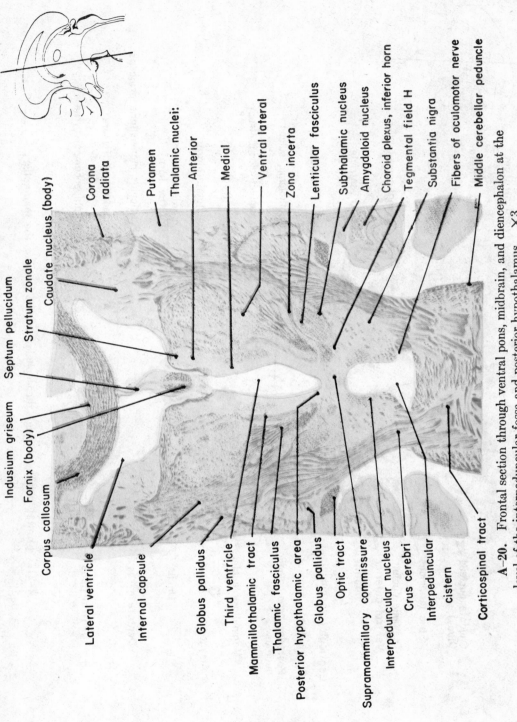

Indusium griseum
Septum pellucidum
Stratum zonale
Caudate nucleus (body)
Corona radiata
Putamen
Thalamic nuclei:
Anterior
Medial
Ventral lateral
Zona incerta
Lenticular fasciculus
Subthalamic nucleus
Amygdaloid nucleus
Choroid plexus, inferior horn
Tegmental field H
Substantia nigra
Fibers of oculomotor nerve
Middle cerebellar peduncle

Corpus callosum
Fornix (body)
Lateral ventricle
Internal capsule
Globus pallidus
Third ventricle
Mammillothalamic tract
Thalamic fasciculus
Posterior hypothalamic area
Globus pallidus
Optic tract
Supramammillary commissure
Interpeduncular nucleus
Crus cerebri
Interpeduncular cistern
Corticospinal tract

A–20. Frontal section through ventral pons, midbrain, and diencephalon at the level of the interpeduncular fossa and posterior hypothalamus. ×3.

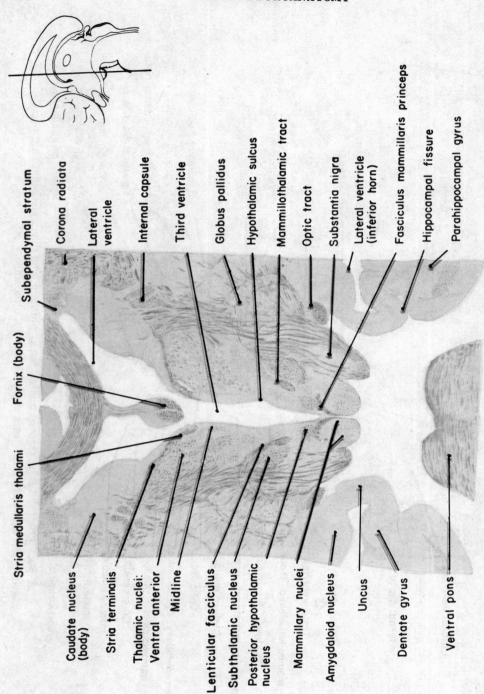

Subependymal stratum

Corona radiata

Lateral ventricle

Internal capsule

Third ventricle

Globus pallidus

Hypothalamic sulcus

Mammillothalamic tract

Optic tract

Substantia nigra

Lateral ventricle (inferior horn)

Fasciculus mammillaris princeps

Hippocampal fissure

Parahippocampal gyrus

Stria medullaris thalami

Fornix (body)

Caudate nucleus (body)

Stria terminalis

Thalamic nuclei: Ventral anterior

Midline

Lenticular fasciculus

Subthalamic nucleus

Posterior hypothalamic nucleus

Mammillary nuclei

Amygdaloid nucleus

Uncus

Dentate gyrus

Ventral pons

A–21. Frontal section through diencephalon at the level of the mammillary body. ×3.

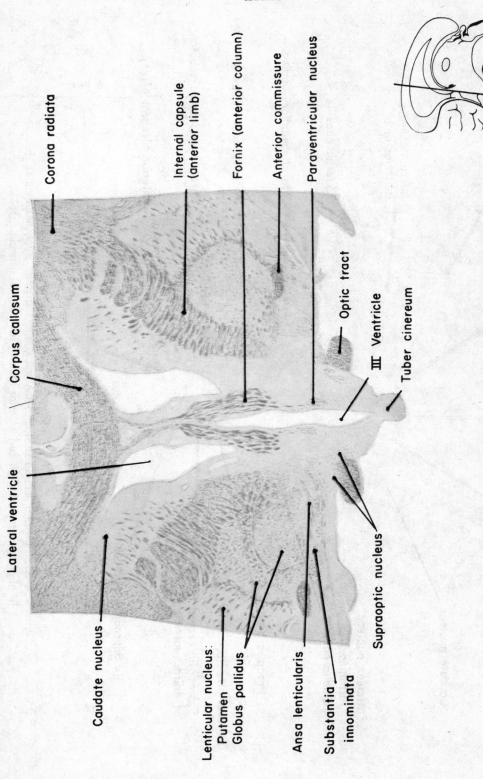

Corona radiata

Internal capsule (anterior limb)

Fornix (anterior column)

Anterior commissure

Paraventricular nucleus

Corpus callosum

Lateral ventricle

Optic tract

III Ventricle

Tuber cinereum

Caudate nucleus

Lenticular nucleus:
Putamen
Globus pallidus

Ansa lenticularis

Substantia innominata

Supraoptic nucleus

A–22. Frontal section through rostral hypothalamus and lenticular nucleus at the level of the tuber cinereum and column of the fornix. ×3.

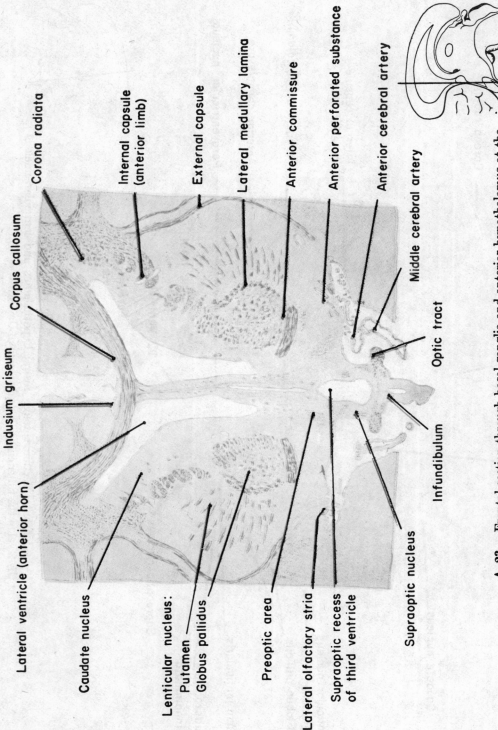

Corona radiata

Internal capsule (anterior limb)

External capsule

Lateral medullary lamina

Anterior commissure

Anterior perforated substance

Anterior cerebral artery

Corpus callosum

Indusium griseum

Middle cerebral artery

Optic tract

Lateral ventricle (anterior horn)

Infundibulum

Caudate nucleus

Lenticular nucleus:
Putamen
Globus pallidus

Preoptic area

Lateral olfactory stria

Supraoptic recess of third ventricle

Supraoptic nucleus

A–23. Frontal section through basal ganglia and anterior hypothalamus at the level of the infundibulum and anterior limb of the internal capsule. ×3.

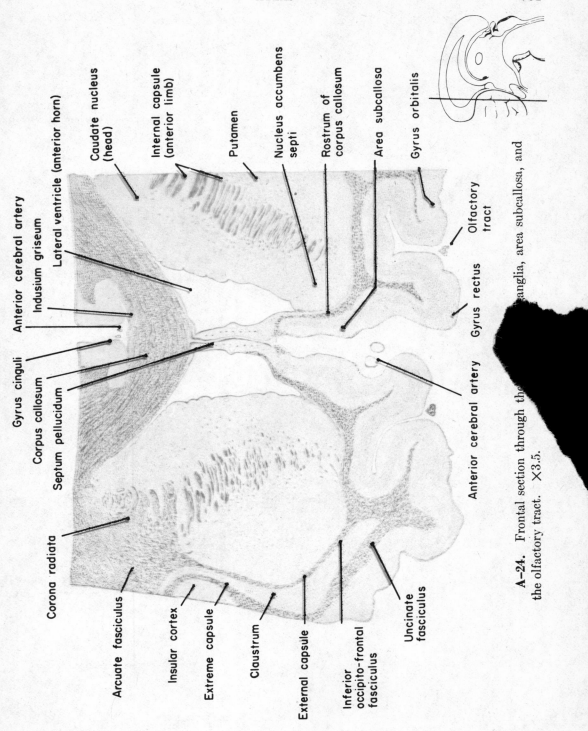

Caudate nucleus (head)

Internal capsule (anterior limb)

Putamen

Nucleus accumbens septi

Rostrum of corpus callosum

Area subcallosa

Gyrus orbitalis

Lateral ventricle (anterior horn)

Anterior cerebral artery

Indusium griseum

Olfactory tract

Gyrus rectus

Gyrus cinguli

Corpus callosum

Septum pellucidum

Anterior cerebral artery

Corona radiata

Arcuate fasciculus

Insular cortex

Extreme capsule

Claustrum

External capsule

Inferior occipito-frontal fasciculus

Uncinate fasciculus

A–24. Frontal section through the ...anglia, area subcallosa, and the olfactory tract. ×3.5.

SECTION IV

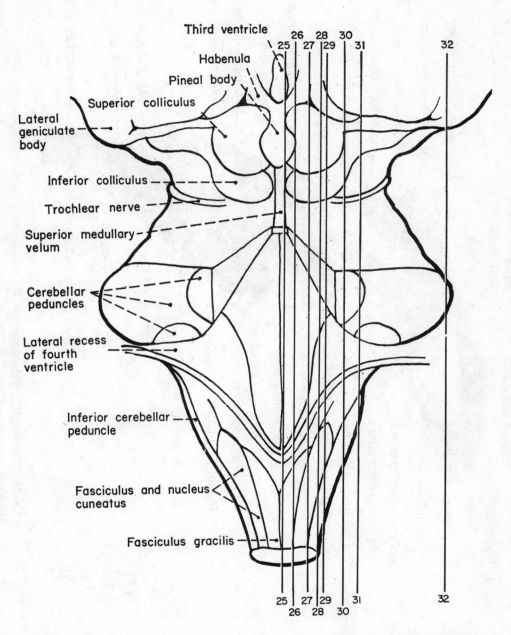

Outline of dorsal surface of brain indicating level and plane of parasagittal sections A–25 to A–32.

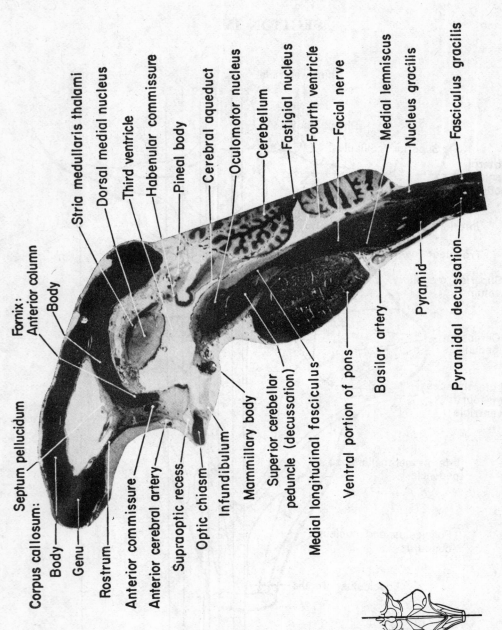

A–25. Parasagittal section through the ventricular system and brain stem at the level of the pineal body. × 1.5

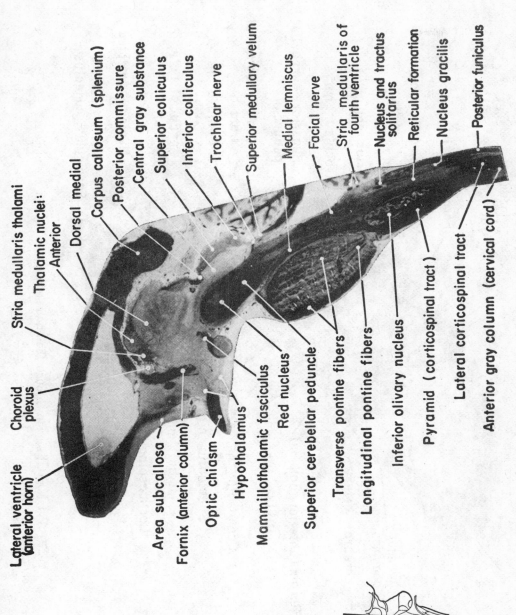

Lateral ventricle (anterior horn)
Choroid plexus
Stria medullaris thalami
Thalamic nuclei:
Anterior
Dorsal medial
Corpus callosum (splenium)
Posterior commissure
Central gray substance
Superior colliculus
Inferior colliculus
Trochlear nerve
Superior medullary velum
Medial lemniscus
Facial nerve
Stria medullaris of fourth ventricle
Nucleus and tractus solitarius
Reticular formation
Nucleus gracilis
Posterior funiculus

Area subcallosa
Fornix (anterior column)
Optic chiasm
Hypothalamus
Mammillothalamic fasciculus
Red nucleus
Superior cerebellar peduncle
Transverse pontine fibers
Longitudinal pontine fibers
Inferior olivary nucleus
Pyramid (corticospinal tract)
Lateral corticospinal tract
Anterior gray column (cervical cord)

A-26. Parasagittal section through brain stem at the level of the nucleus gracilis and emergence of the trochlear nerve. × 1.3

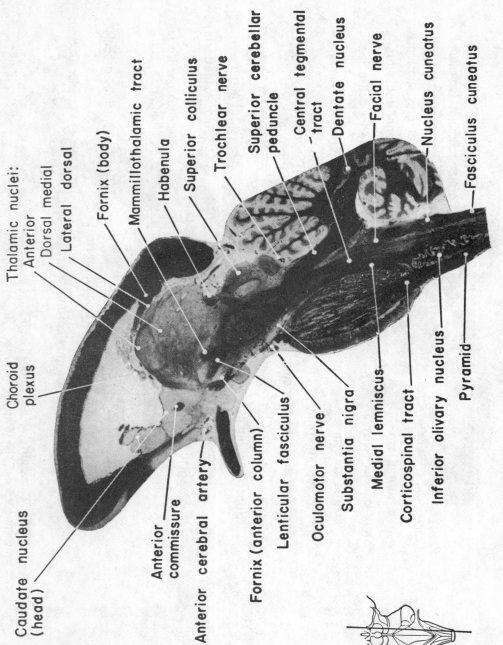

Caudate nucleus (head)

Choroid plexus

Thalamic nuclei:
Anterior
Dorsal medial
Lateral dorsal

Fornix (body)

Mammillothalamic tract

Habenula

Superior colliculus

Trochlear nerve

Superior cerebellar peduncle

Central tegmental tract

Dentate nucleus

Facial nerve

Nucleus cuneatus

Fasciculus cuneatus

Anterior commissure

Anterior cerebral artery

Fornix (anterior column)

Lenticular fasciculus

Oculomotor nerve

Substantia nigra

Medial lemniscus

Corticospinal tract

Inferior olivary nucleus

Pyramid

A-27.   Parasagittal section through the brain stem at the level of the nucleus cuneatus and habenula. × 1.3

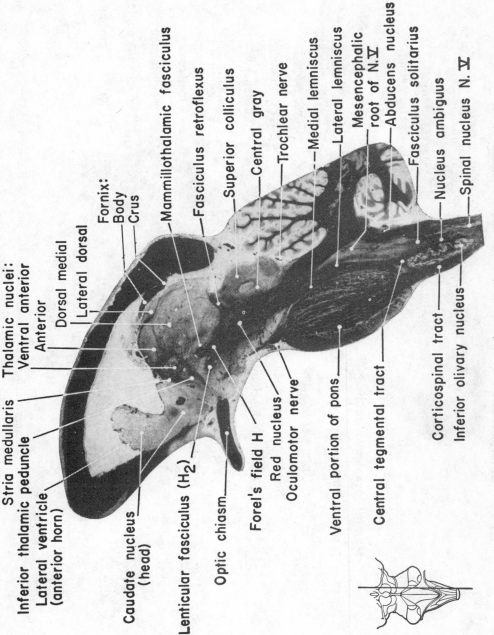

Stria medullaris

Inferior thalamic peduncle

Lateral ventricle
(anterior horn)

Thalamic nuclei:
Ventral anterior
Anterior
Dorsal medial
Lateral dorsal

Fornix:
Body
Crus

Mammillothalamic fasciculus

Fasciculus retroflexus

Superior colliculus

Central gray

Trochlear nerve

Medial lemniscus

Lateral lemniscus

Mesencephalic
root of N. V

Abducens nucleus

Fasciculus solitarius

Nucleus ambiguus

Spinal nucleus N. V

Caudate nucleus
(head)

Lenticular fasciculus (H₂)

Optic chiasm

Forel's field H

Red nucleus

Oculomotor nerve

Ventral portion of pons

Central tegmental tract

Corticospinal tract

Inferior olivary nucleus

A–28.   Parasagittal section through the brain stem at the level of the nucleus
ambiguus, lateral lemniscus, and fasciculus retroflexus. × 1.3

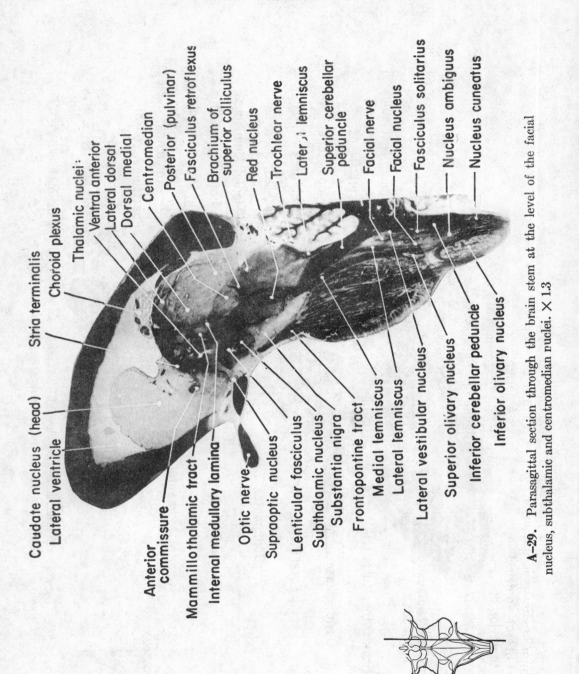

Caudate nucleus (head)
Lateral ventricle

Stria terminalis
Choroid plexus

Thalamic nuclei:
Ventral anterior
Lateral dorsal
Dorsal medial
Centromedian
Posterior (pulvinar)
Fasciculus retroflexus
Brachium of superior colliculus
Red nucleus
Trochlear nerve
Lateral lemniscus
Superior cerebellar peduncle
Facial nerve
Facial nucleus
Fasciculus solitarius
Nucleus ambiguus
Nucleus cuneatus

Anterior commissure
Mammillothalamic tract
Internal medullary lamina
Optic nerve
Supraoptic nucleus
Lenticular fasciculus
Subthalamic nucleus
Substantia nigra
Frontopontine tract
Medial lemniscus
Lateral lemniscus
Lateral vestibular nucleus
Superior olivary nucleus
Inferior cerebellar peduncle
Inferior olivary nucleus

A–29. Parasagittal section through the brain stem at the level of the facial nucleus, subthalamic and centromedian nuclei. × 1.3

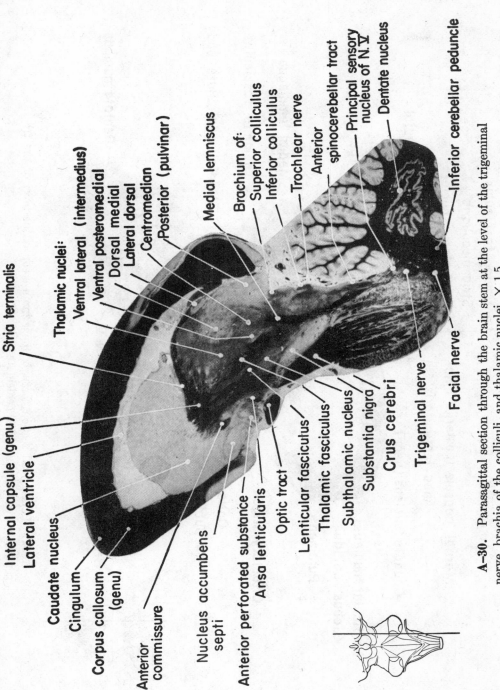

Internal capsule (genu)
Lateral ventricle

Stria terminalis

Caudate nucleus

Cingulum

Corpus callosum (genu)

Anterior commissure

Nucleus accumbens septi

Anterior perforated substance
Ansa lenticularis

Optic tract

Lenticular fasciculus

Thalamic fasciculus

Subthalamic nucleus

Substantia nigra

Crus cerebri

Trigeminal nerve

Facial nerve

Thalamic nuclei:
Ventral lateral (intermedius)
Ventral posteromedial
Dorsal medial
Lateral dorsal
Centromedian
Posterior (pulvinar)

Medial lemniscus

Brachium of:
Superior colliculus
Inferior colliculus

Trochlear nerve

Anterior spinocerebellar tract

Principal sensory nucleus of N. V

Dentate nucleus

Inferior cerebellar peduncle

A–30. Parasagittal section through the brain stem at the level of the trigeminal nerve, brachia of the colliculi, and thalamic nuclei. × 1.5

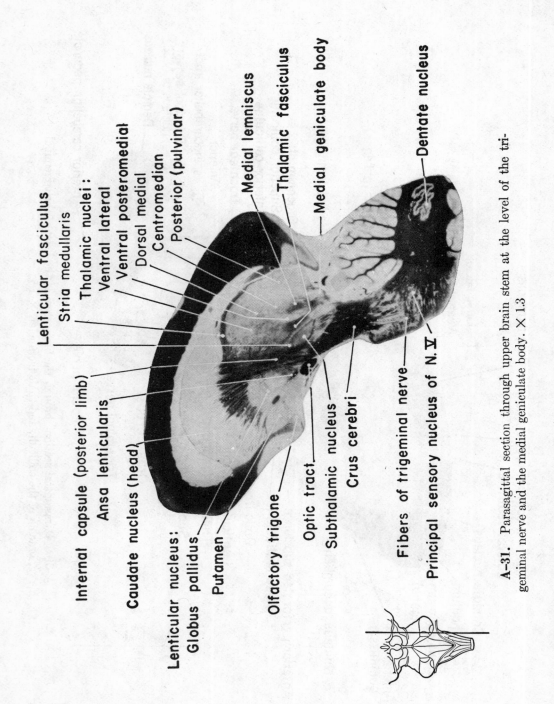

Lenticular fasciculus

Stria medullaris

Thalamic nuclei:
Ventral lateral
Ventral posteromedial
Dorsal medial
Centromedian
Posterior (pulvinar)

Medial lemniscus

Thalamic fasciculus

Medial geniculate body

Dentate nucleus

Internal capsule (posterior limb)
Ansa lenticularis

Caudate nucleus (head)

Lenticular nucleus:
Globus pallidus
Putamen

Olfactory trigone

Optic tract

Subthalamic nucleus

Crus cerebri

Fibers of trigeminal nerve

Principal sensory nucleus of N. V

A–31. Parasagittal section through upper brain stem at the level of the trigeminal nerve and the medial geniculate body. × 1.3

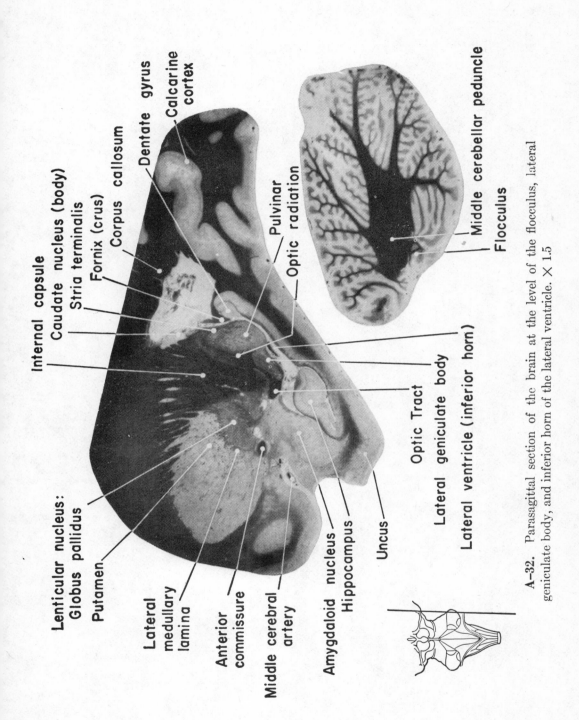

Internal capsule
Caudate nucleus (body)
Stria terminalis
Fornix (crus)
Corpus callosum
Dentate gyrus
Calcarine cortex

Pulvinar
Optic radiation

Middle cerebellar peduncle
Flocculus

Lenticular nucleus:
Globus pallidus
Putamen

Lateral medullary lamina

Anterior commissure

Middle cerebral artery

Amygdaloid nucleus
Hippocampus

Uncus

Optic Tract
Lateral geniculate body
Lateral ventricle (inferior horn)

A–32. Parasagittal section of the brain at the level of the flocculus, lateral geniculate body, and inferior horn of the lateral ventricle. × 1.5

Index

Abducens, *11-1*, *12-1*, *12-7*, 349–351,
  nerve, *12-7*, 349–351
    lesions, 349
  nucleus, *12-1*, *12-2*, *12-3*, 323, 349–351
    lesions, 349
  parabducens nucleus, 350–351
  paralysis of lateral gaze, 349, 350
  root fibers, 349
Aberrant pyramidal fibers, *12-17*, 398
Ablations, area 4, 260, 581–582
  area 6, 582–583
  cortex, 581, 585
  supplementary motor area, 584–585,
    19-21
Accessory nerve, *2-5*, *11-1*, *11-17*, *11-18*,
    11-19, 308–309
  nuclei, 308–309
Accessory oculomotor nuclei, *13-7*, *13-12*,
    13-13, *13-14*, 376, 379–380
Accommodation, 211, **383–384**
Acetylcholine, 91, 157, **200–202**, 595
Acetylcholine esterase, 201, 202
Acid, desoxyribonucleic (DNA), 84, 107,
    4-10
  gamma-aminobutyric (GABA), 91,
    205, 517
  ribonucleic (RNA), 82, 84–85
Acoustic nerve, *see* Cochlear nerve
Acoustic stria, *12-10*, **329–330**
  dorsal, 330
  intermediate, 330
  ventral, 329
Acoustic tubercle, 318, 327, *11-25*
Action potential, 101
Activity, pontogeniculate, 594
Adiadochokinesis, 430
Adipsia, 377, **493**
Adrenal medulla, 203
Adrenergic blocking agents, 204
Adrenergic nerves, **202–205**
Adrenergic transmitter, 203, 364, 366
Affective sensibility, 139, 155
  thalamic, 139, 472
  vital, 139
Afferent fibers, *9-22*, *9-23*, 159, 232–235,
    304–305, 325–329, 337, 347–
    348, 353–360, 465–470, 521–
    529
Afferents, flexor reflex, 251, 252, 419

  vesical, *8-11*, 211
Afterpotentials, negative and positive,
    101
Agenesia, cerebellum, *14-22*, **427–430**
Agnosia, 596
  auditory, 596
  tactile, 596
  visual, 596
Agranular cortex, *19-7*, *19-9*, 558, 578–
    583
Akenetic mutism, 393
Ala cinerea (trigonum vagi), *11-2*, 41,
    297
Alar plate, *3-10*, 53, 62, 64, 65, 66, *11-16*,
    304–305, 399
Alexia, 596
Allocortex, 547
Alveus, *18-8*, *18-9*, 531, 535
Amacrine cell, *15-19*, *15-20*, 465
Ambiguus nucleus, 11-9, *11-16*, *11-18*,
    297, 312
Amiculum, of dentate nucleus, *14-13*, 415
  of olive, *11-21*, 299
Amines, biogenic, 91, 104, 203–205,
    364–366, 397, 411, 489, 498,
    501, 517, 539, 593–595
Amphicyte (capsule cell), *4-1*, *7-3*, 55, 200
Ampullae, semicircular canals, *1-2*, *12-
    12*, 336
Amygdaloid nuclear complex, *2-6*, *2-14*,
    3-13, *17-4*, *18-4*, *18-6*, *18-12*, 32,
    33–34, 496, **539–543**
  connections, 539–541
  functional considerations, 541–543
  lesions, 542
  nuclear groups, 539
    basolateral, 539
    corticomedial, 539
Amyotrophic lateral sclerosis, *10-24*,
    280–281
Anesthesia, 277, 393, 566
Aneurysm, 600
Angiography, cerebral, *20-7*, 609
Angle, cerebellopontine, *11-19*, *12-2*, 41,
    326, 337, 347
Angular gyrus, *2-1*, *2-2*, *19-6*, 24, 598
Anisocoria, 383
Annulospiral endings, *6-11*, *6-12*, *6-13*,
    146–149, 235–237, 249–253

Anosmia, 521, 529
Ansa, cervicalis, 172
  lenticularis, *17-7*, *17-8*, *17-9*, 505–506
  peduncularis, *15-9*, 445
Ansiform lobule, 46, **400**, *14-1*
Anterior, cerebral artery, *20-4*, *20-5*, 605,
    606–607, **608–612**
  commissure, *see separate listing*
  communciating artery, *20-4*, 606, 608
  femoral cutaneous nerve, 182–183
  lobe of cerebellum, *14-1*, 46, **400**, 432–
    433
  median fissure, 55, 214, *9-2*, *9-6*
  meningeal arteries, *20-3*, 621–622
  olfactory nucleus, 522–523, *18-3*
  perforated substance, *2-6*, *18-2*, 29,
    524, 612, *20-3*, *20-9*
  rami of spinal cord, 168–169
  spinal artery, *20-1*, *20-2*, **600–602**,
    616–617
Anterior commissure, *2-10*, *2-13*, *18-7*, 32,
    69–70, **529–530**
  anatomy, 32, 529
    anterior part, 529
    posterior part, 32, 530
  origins of fibers, 32, 529
Anterior internuclear ophthalmoplegia,
    344, 512
Anticholinesterase drugs, 202
  "irreversible," 202
  "reversible," 202
Aphasia, 596
  defined, 596
  expressive, 596
  locations of lesions, 597
  receptive, 596
Apraxia, 597
  constructional, 597
  Gerstmann syndrome, 598
  ideational, 597
  ideomotor, 597
  kinetic, 597
  lesions, 597
Aqueduct, cerebral, *2-15*, *2-21*, *13-1*, 39,
    42, 60, 367
Arachnoid, *1-4*, *1-5*, *1-7*, *1-8*, *1-10*, 9–11
  granulations, *1-12*, *1-13*, 11
  villi, 11, 622
Arbor vitae, cerebellum, *2-26*, 48

Boldface numbers indicate principal references. *Italic* numbers refer to illustrations.

Archicerebellum, *14-1*, 63, 399, **431-432**
Archipallium, 65, 521, **530-535**,*18-6*, 547
Archistriatum, *see* Amygdaloid nuclear complex
Arcuate, fasciculus, *2-11*, **31**
  fibers, external, 296
    internal, *10-1, 11-8*, **240**, 291-293
  nucleus, *11-14, 11-21*, 296
  nucleus (hypothalomus), 92, 482, 489
Area(s), autonomic, **544-546**
  of Broca, 23, **590-592**, 596-597
  of Brodmann, *19-5*, **556-557**
  of cerebral cortex, **556-559**
  cutaneous, *7-11, 7-12, 7-13*, 165-166
  dentata, *18-10*, 531, 533
  of Economo, *19-7*, **558-559**
  entorhinal, *18-11, 19-5*, 525, 535
  exteroceptive, 138, *9-22*
  lateral hypothalamic, *16-2, 16-3*, **478-479**
  motor, nonpyramidal, *19-20*, **583-587**
    primary (area 4), *19-5, 19-19*, *23*, **578-582**
    supplementary, *19-21*, **583-585**
  olfactory, **525-526**
  parabigeminal, 369, *13-2*
  parastriate (area 18), *19-13*, **573-574**
  parolfactoria (subcallosal), 27, 525, *18-2*
  peristriate (area 19), *19-13*, 573
  postrema, *11-13*, 41, **296-297**
  precommissural (septal; paraterminal body), 525
  prefrontal, 23, **598-599**
  premotor, 23, *19-20*, **582-583**
  preoptic, *16-1*, **479**, 494, 541
  prepyriform, 525, *18-4*
  pretectal, *13-7*, **374-376**
  sensory, *19-11, 19-12*, **559-578**
    gustatory, 577
    primary, 559
      auditory, 24, **574-577**
      somesthetic, 24, **560-566**
      visual, *19-14*, 24, **566-574**
    secondary, 526, **559-560**
      auditory, *19-17, 19-18*, **574-577**
      somesthetic, 566
      visual, *19-13*, **573-574**
    somatic II, *19-13*, 566
    striate (area 17), *19-14, 19-15, 19-16*, 24, 470, 496, **566-574**
  subcallosal, 27, 525
  suppressor, 589
  ventral tegmental (Tsai), 396
  vestibularis, *11-12, 11-16*, 41, 297
Areflexia, 273, 277, 581
Argyll-Robertson pupil, 383
Arousal reaction, **390-393**, 476, **592-593**
Arterial, cerebral circle (of Willis), *20-3, 20-4*, **606-608**
  vasocorona, *20-2*, 601
Artery(ies)
  basilar, *20-1, 20-4, 20-5, 20-9*, 605, 609, **616-619**
  carotid, internal, *1-3, 1-10, 20-7*, **603-605**
  central (ganglionic), branches, 607, **612-615**
  cerebellar, anterior inferior, *10-5*, 605, **616**, 617, 621

  posterior inferior, *1-4*, 321, 617, 620, 621
    superior, **616**, 617, 620, 621
  cerebral, anterior, *20-4, 20-5*, 605, **606-607**, 608-609
    circle of Willis, *20-4*, **606-608**
    middle, *20-6*, 605, 607, **608**
    posterior, **609-612**
  choroidal, anterior, *20-9*, 604, **614**, 620
    posterior, *20-9*, **614-615**
  circumferential, **617-619**, *20-13*
    midbrain, *20-14*, **620-621**
    pons, short, *20-13*, 617
    long, **617-619**, *20-13*
  communicating, anterior, **605-607**, **608-612**, *20-4, 20-5*
    posterior, 604, 606, 620
  cortical branches, 607, **608-612**
  dural, *20-3*, **621-622**
  ganglionic (central), 607, **612-615**, *20-9, 20-10, 20-11, 20-12*
  labyrinthine, 616
  lenticulo-optic, 613
  lenticulostriate, *20-9*, 609, 613
  medial striate, *20-9*, **608**, 615
  meningeal, *20-3*, **621-622**
    accessory, 622
    anterior, 622
    middle, *20-3*, **621-622**
  ophthalmic, *20-4*, 604
  paramedian, *20-13*, **616-617**
  pontine, *20-13*, 617
  quadrigeminal, 621
  radicular, anterior, *20-2*, 601
    posterior, *20-2*, 601
  recurrent, of Heubner (*see* Anterior cerebral artery)
  spinal, anterior, *20-1, 20-2*, **600-602**, 616-617
    posterior, *1-4, 20-1*, **600-601**, 616
  striate, (anterolateral), 613
    medial (recurrent, of Heubner; anterior cerebral artery), *20-9*, 608, 615
  sulcal, 601
  thalamogeniculate (posterolateral), *20-11*, 613, 616
  thalamoperforating, *20-11*, 613, 616
  vertebral, *1-4, 1-10*, 600, **605-606**, 616
  vertebral basilar system, *20-9*, **616-621**
Ascending reticular activating system, **390-393**, 476-477, **592-593**
Ascending spinal pathways, *10-1, 10-7, 10-8, 10-10*, **238-255**
Association, areas (cortical)
  cells, *4-1C*, 53, **548-550**
  fibers, *2-11*, **31-32**, 549
    cingulum, *2-7, 2-12*, 31, 535, 537
    fasciculus, arcuate, *2-11*, 31
      inferior longitudinal (external sagittal stratum), 31, 467, 568
      inferior occipitofrontal, 31
      superior longitudinal, *2-11*, 31
      uncinate, *2-11*, 31
    intracortical, 31, **551-556**, *19-3*
    subcortical, 31
  nuclei, of thalamus, 45, *15-12*, 474
Associative memory, **595-596**, 597
Astereognosis, 240, 591
Astrocytes, *1-15, 5-1, 5-2, 5-3, 5-11*, **118-**

122
  fibrous, *3-5, 5-3, 5-4A, 5-12*, **119-120**
  protoplasmic (mossy), *3-5, 5-3, 5-4B, 5-12*, **120-122**
  reactive, 122, *5-6*
Asynergia, 430
Ataxia, cerebellar, **431**, 587
  posterior column, 241
Athetosis, 515
Atonia, 273, 277, **430**, 581
Auditory, cortex, *19-17, 19-18*, 24, 336, 457, **574-578**
  fibers, **327-329**, *15-18*, 436
    primary, 24, **327-329**, 574-578
    secondary, **329-332**, 574-576
  ganglion, *12-8*, **326-327**
  lesions, **335-336**, 576-577
  nuclei, accessory superior olive, 331
    dorsal cochlear, **326-327**, *11-25*
    inferior colliculus, *13-3*, 42, 64, 331, 367-369
    lateral lemniscus, *13-2*, 331, 368
    medial geniculate, *13-17*, 45, 331, **457-458**
    preolivary, 331
    superior olive, 331
    trapezoid, **330-331**, *12-3*
    ventral cochlear, *11-24*, 327
  pathways, *12-10*, **329-332**, **367-369**, **457-458**
    auditory radiations, *2-7, 15-18*, 331, 463, 574
    brachium of inferior colliculus, *2-19*, 331, *13-1*, 368
    descending, 333
    lateral lemniscus, 331, *12-23*, 368
    peduncle of superior olive (efferent cochlear bundle), *12-11*, **332-333**
    trapezoid body, 330, *12-7*
  receptors (hair cells of cochlea), *12-8, 12-9*, 329
  reflexes, **332-335**
    sharpening, 335
  system, **326-336**, 574-577
    transmission of impulses, 326
Autonomic, areas of cortex, *8-3, 18-13*, 544, 546
  ganglia, 55, **192-198**, *8-1, 8-3*, **199-200**, 313, 348, 379
    origin of, 50
    structure of, *8-1*, **199-200**
  nervous system, **191-212**, *8-1*
    afferent visceral fibers, 199
    descending pathways, 207, 271, 384, 487-488
    functional considerations, **208-212**, 364-366, 394-396, 491-495, 517, 544-546, 594-595
Autoradiography, 106, 533
  tracing technics, 106, 410, 482, 533
Axillary nerve, *7-17, 7-18*, 175
Axolemma, 94, *4-16*
Axon, *4-5, 4-14, 4-15, 4-18*, 77, 93-94, 108-113
  collaterals of, 97, 110
  hillock, 93
  myelinated, 93, **94-99**, 101-103
  primitive, 51
  remyelation of experimentally injured, 113, 188-190

Boldface numbers indicate principal references. *Italic* numbers refer to illustrations.

terminals, 103–105
  boutons terminaux (end feet), 93, 103
  neuropodia, 103
  unmyelinated, 93, 100–101
Axoplasmic flow, 88
  transport, *4-31*, 106, 111–112, 451, 592

Babinski's sign, 259, 275, 619
Baillarger, bands of, *19-1*, 550
Ballism, 515, 518
Band
  of Baillarger, *19-1*, 550
  diagonal, of Broca, *18-2*, *18-4*, 524
  of Gennari, *19-14*, 567
  of Giacomini, 532
  Kaes-Bechterew, 550
Barriers, 16–20, *1-16*
  blood-brain, *1-16*, 17–19, 116
  blood-cerebrospinal fluid, 19, 116
  brain-cerebrospinal fluid, 19–20
Bars, terminal, *3-4A*, 51
Basal, forebrain bundle, 513
  ganglia, *see separate listing*
  plate, 53, *3-3*, *3-10*
Basal ganglia, *2-14*, *17-1*, *17-2*, *17-4*, 32–
    34, 496–520
  amygdaloid nuclear complex, *2-6*, *2-14*,
    3-13, *17-4*, *18-4*, *18-6*, *18-12*,
    32, 33–34, 496, 539–543
  blood supply, 615–617
  caudate nucleus, *2-14*, *17-4*, 32, 33, 497
    connections, afferent, 499–504
    efferent, *17-6*, 504
    inhibitory responses, 517, 519
    lesions, 517, 518
  divisions, archistriatum (amygdaloid
      nuclear complex), *2-6*, *2-14*, *3-*
      13, *17-4*, *18-4*, *18-6*, *18-12*, 32,
      33–34, 496, 539–541
    neostriatum (striatum: caudate nu-
        cleus and putamen), *2-9*, *2-10*,
        2-13, *17-3*, *17-4*, *17-6*, 33, 66–
        67, 496–498, 499–504
    paleostriatum (pallidum), *17-3*, *17-*
        12, 33, 67, 496–499, 504–509
    corpus striatum (striatum and pal-
        - lidum), *17-3*, 66–67, 496–499
  dyskinesia, 514–520
    athetosis, 515
    ballism, 515, 517
    chorea, 515, 517
    experimental, 518–519
    pathology, 516–517
    torsion dystonia, 515
    treatment of, 517–519
    tremor, 514–515
  extrapyramidal system, 512–513
  syndromes, athetosis, 515
    ballism, 515
    chorea, 515
    paralysis agitans, 514–515
    pathological changes, 516–517
    phylogenetic development, 512–
      513
    surgical treatment, 518
    torsion dystonia, 515
  functional considerations, 512–520
  globus pallidus, *2-9*, *2-13*, *2-14*, *17-3*,

32, 33, 66–67, 498–499
  connections, 504–509
    striopallidal, 504
    subthalamopallidal, 504
    efferent, *17-7*, *17-8*, *17-15*, 505–509
      ansa lenticularis, 505
      descending, 507–508
      lenticular fasciculus, *17-10*, 505
  putamen, *2-14*, *17-6*, 33, 66, 497–498
    connections, afferent, 499–504
    strionigral, 504
    striopallidal, 504
  development, 66–67
    embryological, 66
    phylogenetic, 512–513
    inhibitory responses, 517, 519
    lesions, 518
    principal of physiological safety, 517
    release phenomena, 516
Basal nuclei of Meynert (*see* Substantia
    innominata)
Basal olfactory region, 382, 523
Basilar, artery, *20-1*, *20-4*, *20-5*, *20-9*,
    605, 609, 616–619
  membrane, 326
  sulcus, *2-17*, 41, 616
  venous plexus, *20-17*, 623
Basket cells, 401, *14-4*, 411–412, 533
  cerebellum, *14-4*, 401, 411–412
  hippocampus, 533
Basophilia, 84
Behavior, abnormal, 495, 541–543
  changes, 495
  emotional, 494–495
  goal directed, 495
Bell's palsy, 348
Betz cells, *19-9*, 255, 260, 548, 579
Biogenic monoamines, 91, 202, *8-6*, *8-7*,
    ·364–366, 593–595
  dopamine, *13-18*, 91, 204, 384, 394, 397,
    489, 498, 501, 517
  5-hydroxytryptamine, 91, 204, 366,
    593–595
  norepinephrine, *12-26*, 91, 202–203,
    364–365, 411, 593–595
Bipolar sensory nerve cells, 55, 77, *4-3*, *4-*
    6, 327, 337
Biventer lobule, *14-1*, 46, 400
Bladder, innervation, *8-11*, 211–212
  in nerve lesions, 279, 281
Blood-brain barrier, *1-16*, 17–19, 116
Blood supply, of brain, *20-4*, *20-5*, *20-6*,
    603–621
  cerebellum, 621
  cerebral cortex, 608–612
  corpus striatum, *20-10*, *20-11*, 613,
    615–616
  internal capsule, *20-12*, 615–616
  medulla and pons, *20-13*, 616–620
  mesencephalon, 620–621
  spinal cord, *20-1*, 600–603
  thalamus and hypothalamus, 612–615
  visual cortex, 568, 609, 611
Bodian method, 72
Body (*see also* Corpus)
  caudate nucleus, 497
  corpus callosum, *2-7*, 26, 591–592
  of fornix, 32, 535–537, *15-1*
  geniculate, lateral, 45, 64, 435, 458–
    461, 466–470, 569, *15-3*, *15-4*,

15-14, *15-18*, *15-21*, *19-15*
    medial, 45, 64, 457–458, *15-3*, *15-4*
  juxtarestiform, 342, 424, *12-6*
  mammillary, 37, 45, 64, 435, 478, 482–
    483, *2-14*, *2-17*, *2-19*, *15-1*, *15-*
    4, *16-1*
  paraterminal, 525, *18-2*, *18-4*
  pineal, 43, 438–440, *2-18*, *2-20*, *15-2*;
    15-7
  pituitary, 65, 478, 488–490, *1-11*, *16-1*,
    16-5, *16-7*, *16-9*
  psammomatous, 133
  restiform, *see* Inferior cerebellar
    peduncle,
  trapezoid, *12-1*, *12-4*, *12-10*, 330–331
  of ventricle, lateral, *2-15*, 34–35, 65
Boutons terminaux, 103, *4-25*
Brachial plexus, *7-14*, *7-15*, *7-17*, 173–
    175
  lesions of, 177–181
Brachium, conjunctivum, *see* Superior
    cerebellar peduncle
  pontis, *see* Middle cerebellar peduncle
  quadrigeminal, inferior, *see* Inferior
    collicular brachium
  superior, *see* Superior collicular brach-
    ium
Bradycardia, 209, *8-9*, 366
Brain barriers, *1-16*, 16–20
  blood-brain, *1-16*, 17–19, 116
  blood-CSF, 19, 116
  brain-CSF, 19–20
Brain cranial nerves, *1-4*, *11-1*, *11-16*, *11-*
    17, *11-18*, 39, 41, 42, 304–314,
    325–342, 346–351, 352–360,
    377–379, 469
  development, 57–71, *3-8*, *3-9*
  functional cell columns of brain stem,
    61, *11-17*, *11-18*, 304–305
  stem, *1-4*, *2-18*, *2-19*, *2-20*, *2-21*, *3-9*, *3-*
    14, 36–46, 385–398, 435–495
  suprasegmental structures, 21–36,
    314–318, 399
Brain metabolism, 600
  weight, 21
Branchial arches, 62, 305, 309–314,
    346–348, 352–362
Branchiomeric muscles, 62, 305, 309–
    314, 346–348, 352–362
Broca's, area, 23, 590–592, 596–597
  diagonal band of, *18-2*, 524
Brodmann's chart of cortical areas, *19-5*,
    556–557
Brown-Séquard syndrome, *10-23*, 279–
    280
Bulb, olfactory, *18-1*, *18-2*, 29, 522–523
Bulbar inhibitory center, 269, 388–389
Bundle, efferent cochlear, 332–333, *12-*
    11
  medial forebrain, *16-5*, 483, 487
  of Türck, 256
  of Vicq d'Azyr (mammillothalamic fas-
    ciculus), *16-6*, 444, 473, 488,
    16-8
  olivocochlear, *see* Efferent cochlear
    bundle
  Zuckerkandl's, 537
Bundles of dorsal root, *9-22*, 232–235
  lateral, 232
  medial, 232

Boldface numbers indicate principal references. *Italic* numbers refer to illustrations.

Cajal silver nitrate method, 72
Calamus scriptorius, 41
Calcar avis, *18-7*, 35
Calcarine sulcus, *2-4*, *15-21*, *19-14*, 24, **466–469**, **566–568**
Canals, semicircular, **336**, *1-2*, *12-12*
Capsule, of autonomic cells, 55, 200
  cells (amphicytes), *4-1*, *7-3*, 55, 200
  external, *2-9*, *2-13*, *2-14*, 32, 499
  extreme, 32, 499, 530, *2-9*, *2-13*, *2-14*
  internal, *2-8*, *15-17*, *15-18*, **462–465**
    anterior, limb, *2-9*, *15-17*, *15-18*, **29–30**, 464
    genu, *15-18*, 30, 464
    lesions of, **464–465**
    posterior limb, *2-9*, *15-17*, *15-18*, **30**, 464
      retrolenticular portion, *15-18*, **30**, 464
      sublenticular portion, 464
  of red nucleus, *13-4*, 384
  of spinal ganglion cells, *7-4*, **161–162**
Cardiac plexus, 196
Carotid, artery, **603–605**
  common, *20-7*, **603**
  internal, **603–605**, *20-7*
    branches, **604–605**
    segments, 603
  sinus nerve, 313
  siphon, 604
Catecholamines, *8-7*, 91, **202–205**, **364–366**, 411, 501, 517, **593–595**
Catechol-*o*-methyl transferase (COMT), 203
Cauda equina, *1-6*, 11, 55, 213, *9-1*
Caudate, nucleus, *2-9*, *2-10*, *2-13*, *17-4*, 33, 66, 496, 497, **499–504**
  veins, *20-19*, *20-20*, 628
Causalgia, 177, 184
Cavum, septum pellucidum, *2-13*, 525
Celiac, ganglion, *8-1*, 197
  plexus, *8-1*, 197
Cell, amacrine, *15-19*, *15-20*, 465
  amphicyte (capsule cell), *4-1*, *7-3*, 55, 200
  anterior horn, *3-6*, *4-1E*, *5-6*, *9-8*, *9-21*, 160, 215, **228–230**, **272–273**
  association, *4-1C*, 53, 221
  astroglia, **118–122**
  autonomic, **192–195**, **199–200**
  basket, 401, *14-4*, **411–412**, 533
  of Bergmann, *14-11*, **412–414**
  Betz, *19-9*, 255, 260, 548, 579
  of Cajal, 549, *19-3*
  capsule (amphicytes), *4-1*, *7-3*, 55, 200
  central, 53, 221
  chromaffin, 50
  chromatolysis, *7-5*, 107, 162
  chromophil, **84–85**
  column, *3-11*, **61–62**, 221
  commissural, 53, 221
  "complex" retina, **572–573**
  cone, of retina, *15-20*, 465
  ependymal, *3-5*, *3-6*, *5-13*, *5-14*, 15, **19–20**
  epiphysial, 349
  epithelial, *5-18*, 56
  of Fañanas, *14-11*, **412–414**
  fusiform, 549
  ganglion, *7-2*, *7-3*, *8-5*, **161–162**, 309, 313, 326, 337, 347

of dorsal root, *4-1A*, **161–162**
of retina, 465, *15-19*, *15-20*
of trigeminal, *7-4*, **353–354**
germinal, 50
giant pyramidal, of Betz, 80, 255, 260, *19-9*, 548, 579
giant stellate, of Meynert, 566
glia, 52, **115–128**, **412–414**, *5-1*, *5-3*
glioblast, *3-5*, 52
Golgi, of cerebellum, **403–404**, *14-5*
  of cortex, 548, *19-4*, 558
  type I, 80
  type II, 80, 401, **403–404**, 556
granule, of cerebellum, **402–403**, *14-2*, **406–407**
  of cortex, 548, *19-4* 558
  of olfactory bulb, *18-1*, *18-3*, **522–523**
horizontal, of Cajal, 549, *19-3*
"hypercomplex" retina, **572–573**
interfascicular, 125
intermediate (central), 53, 221
macroglia, 117, **118–125**
of Martinotti, 549, *19-3*
microglia, *3-5*, *5-3*, *5-10*, *5-11*, **125–128**
mitral, *18-1*, 522
neuroepithelial, *3-4A*, *3-4*, *3-5*, *6-5*, 51, 143
neuroglia, **115–125**, *5-1*, *5-3*
oligodendroglia, *5-7*, *5-8*, *5-9*, **122–125**
perivascular, 17, 19, 125
  mesenchymal, 117, **125–128**
pial, *3-4B*, 7
pineal, 439
posterior horn, 53, **231–232**
pseudounipolar, 55
Purkinje, *4-1D*, *4-5*, *4-9*, *14-7*, 63, **401–402**
pyramidal, of cortex, *4-5*, 255, 548, *19-1*, 550, **578–580**
Renshaw, *9-21*, 229
rod, of retina, 465, *15-19*, *15-20*
root, 221, **9–21**
satellite, 55
  perineuronal, 123
  Schwann sheath, **99–100**, *4-15*, 188
"simple (striate), *19-16*, **569–572**
spindle (cortex), **549–550**
star pyramid, 548
stellate, of cerebellum, 401, *14-4*
  of cerebral cortex, 548, *19-4*
  pyramidal, 548, *19-1*
  tufted, 522
  visual cortex, **572–574**, *19-15*, *19-16*
Cell groups of spinal cord, *9-18*, *9-21*, **221–229**
Center, facilitatory, reticular formation, 269, 389
  feeding, 494, 543
  genital, 167
    for ejaculation, 167
    for erection, 167
  inhibition, reticular formation, 269, 389
  lateral gaze, 350
  rectal, 168
  respiratory, 269
  satiety, 494, 543
  vesical, 167, 211
    micturition, 211
    retention of urine, 279
Central, autonomic pathways, **206–208**,

271, **487–488**
body of nerve cell (centrosome), 88
canal, 39, 215
  gray substance, 215, **217–218**
  sulcus, of Rolando, 23, **578–579**, *19-6*
  tegmental tract, *12-1*, *12-2*, 322, 351, 392, 450
  vision, *15-21*, *15-23*, 465, 469, 568
Central nervous system, 21
  blood supply, **600–630**, *20-1*, *20-4*
  metabolism, 600
Centromedian-parafascicular nuclear complex, *15-5*, *15-6*, *15-11*, *15-12*, **447–451**, **474–477**, **500–501**, *17-6*, **592–593**
Centrosome, 88
Centrum semiovale, *2-7*, 29
Cephalic flexure, *3-8*, 59
Cephalization, *3-14*, *3-15*, *3-16*, **67–69**, 300
Cerebellar, cortex, *14-2*, *14-3*, *14-4*, *14-5*, 63, **401–414**
  computer functions, 434
  disturbances, **430–433**
  nystagmus, 431
  peduncles, *2-19*, *2-25*, *10-10*, *11-2*, *11-22*, *11-24*, 39, 41, 42, 249, **303–304**, **324–325**, 363, **414–421**
  plate, 62
  stimulation, 432
  vermis, *2-26*, 46, 62, 399, 425, 431
Cerebello-oculomotor fibers, 421
Cerebelloreticular fibers, 363, 421, 425
Cerebellum, *2-1*, *2-2*, *2-23*, *2-24*, *2-25*, *2-26*, *3-14*, **46–48**, **399–434**
  anatomy, *2-23*, *2-24*, *2-25*, **46–49**, **62–63**, **399–401**
  arbor vitae, *2-26*, 48
  archicerebellum, 63, 399, **431–432**, *14-1*
  blood supply, 621
  corpus medullare, 414
  cortex, 46, 63, 399, **401–414**
    afferent fibers, **416–420**, *14-5*
    cells, **401–404**, *14-4*, *14-5*
    efferent fibers, **420–425**, *14-16*, *14-17*, *14-20*
    intracortical fibers, **404–412**
    layers, **401–404**, *14-2*
      external granular, *3-11*, 63
      granular, 63, **402–404**
      molecular, 401
      Purkinje, **401–402**
    nerve fibers, **404–412**
    structure, **401–404**, *14-4*, *14-5*
  cortical localization, 416, *14-14*, *14-15*, *14-20*
  crus I, *14-1*, 400
  crus II, *14-1*, 400
  development, *3-12A*, *3-12B*, **62–63**
  disturbances, **430–433**
  divisions, **399–401**
    archicerebellum, *14-1*, 399, **431–432**
    neocerebellum, *14-1*, 400, **430–431**
    paleocerebellum, *14-1*, 400, **432–433**
  exteroceptive areas, 416, *14-14*, *14-15*
  falx cerebelli, *1-2*, 1, 46
  fastigial efferent fibers, *14-19*, *14-20*, **421–425**
  feedback systems, 363, 418
  fibers, afferent, **416–420**

Boldface numbers indicate principal references. *Italic* numbers refer to illustrations.

climbing, 407–409, *14-5*
efferent, 420–425
intracortical, 414
mossy, 406–407, *14-7*, 409–411
fissures, *2-12, 2-24, 2-25, 2-26,* 46, *14-1,*
399–401
horizontal, 46, 399
posterior superior, 46, 399
prenodular, *14-1,* 46, 399
prepyramidal, 46, 399
primary, *14-1,* 46, 399–400
folia, 46, 399
functional considerations, 430–434
gemmules, *4-6,* 78, 402
glomeruli, 406–407, *14-9*
hemispheres, 46, 399
crus I, *14-1,* 46, 400
crus II, *14-1,* 46, 400
incisure, anterior, 46, *2-23*
posterior, 46, *2-23*
inner stellate cells, *see* Basket cells
lesions, 430–434
archicerebellar, 431–432
fastigial nucleus, 433
neocerebellar, 430–431
paleocerebellar, 433
lobes, anterior, *14-1,* 46, 400, 432–433
flocculonodular, 46, 399, 425
posterior, *14-1,* 46, 400
lobules, *2-26, 14-1,* 399–400
alar central, 46
anterior quadrangular, 46
ansiform, 46, 400
biventer, 46, 400
central, 46
flocculus, 46, 400, 425
gracile, 46, 400
inferior semilunar (crus II), 46, 400
posterior quadrangular, 46, 400
simple, 46, 400
superior semilunar (crus I), 46, 400
localization, 416
neocerebellum, *14-1,* 400, 430–431
neurolgia, 412–414, *14-11*
nuclei, *12-16, 14-13, 14-16,* 48, 414–
416, 420–425
deep, 414–416, *14-13*
dentate, 48, 414–415,
emboliform, 48, 415
fastigial, *14-19, 14-20,* 48, 415–416
globose, 48, 415
outer stellate cells, *14-4,* 401
paleocerebellum, 400, 432–433
parallel fibers, *14-4,* 403
peduncles, *2-26,* 46, 303–304, 324–325,
363, 414, 420–425
of flocculus, 318, *11-24*
inferior (restiform body), 39, 303–
304, 414, 416
middle (brachium pontis), 41, 324–
325, 414
superior (brachium conjunctivum),
42, 363, 414, 420–425
plate, 62
projection, corticonuclear, 425–430
structural mechanisms, 411–412
topographic representation, 416, *14-
14, 14-15*
uncinate fasciculus, 421–425
vallecula cerebelli, 46, *2-24*
vermis, *2-26, 14-1,* 46, 62, 399

central lobule, 46
culmen, 46
declive, 46
folium, 46
lingula, 46
nodulus, 46, 399
pyramis, 46, 399
tuber, 46
uvula, 46
zones, lateral, 425
paravermal, 425
vermal, 425
Cerebral, ambilaterality, 590
angiography, 611–612, *20-7*
aqueduct, 42, 367
arterial circle, *20-3, 20-4,* 606–608
blood flow, 600
blood supply, *20-4,* 606–616
cortex, *see separate listing*
decortication, 581
dominance, 23, 589–592
aphasia, 596–597
hemispheres, *see separate listing*
veins, 622–630
vesicles, *3-9, 3-14,* 57–60
Cerebral cortex, *19-1, 19-2, 19-3,* 67–69,
547–599
archipallium, 521, 530–535, *18-8*
areas, Brodmann, *19-5,* 556–557
Economo, *19-7,* 558–559
cell columns, 555–556, *19-11,* 564,
569–572, *19-15, 19-16,* 575
constituents,
cells, 548–550, *19-1*
fusiform (spindle), 549
giant pyramidal (Betz), 548, 579
Golgi type II, 556
granule (stellate), 548
star pyramids, 548
fibers, afferent, 462–464, 549–550
association areas, 559, 595–599
band of Kaes-Bechterew, 550
bands of Baillarger, *19-1,* 550
line of Gennari, *19-14,* 567
projection, 548
radial, *19-1,* 549
tangential, *19-1,* 549
efferent cortical areas, 578–589
nonpyramidal, 586–589
to basal ganglia, *17-6,* 451, 499–
500
corticobulbar, 314–318
corticofugal, 578–589
corticopontine, 324–325, 398,
419–420, 586–587
corticoreticular, 269, 302, 351,
391, 586
corticothalamic, 462–464, 587–
589
to secondary sensory relay nuclei,
315, 589
functional unit, 555–556
functioning of, 555, 559–586
histogenesis, 67–69, 547
homunculus, motor, *19-19,* 580–581
sensory, *19-12,* 563
interrelation of cortical neurons, *19-3,*
551–556
axodendritic terminations, 552
dendritic and axonal branchings,
552–555

elementary functional unit, 555–
556
Golgi type II cells, 63, 556
neuron chains, 556
nonspecific afferents, 551
specific afferents, *19-3,* 551
lamination, 547–551, *19-1, 19-2, 19-3,*
19-7, 19-9, 19-10
layers, 550–551
external granular, 550
infragranular, 551
internal granular, 550
molecular (plexiform), 550
multiform (fusiform), 550
pyramidal, 550
supragranular, 551
lesions, 565–566, 568, 576–577, 581–
585, 595–599
neopallium, 67–69, 521, 547–559
paleopallium, 521, 524–527
phenomenon of cortical suppression,
589
physical features, 547
area, 547
thickness, 547
variations, 547
physiology, premotor (area 6), *19-20,*
582–583
ablations, 583
efferent fibers, 582
histology, 582
stimulation of, 582
subdivisions of, 582
primary motor area (area 4), *19-19,*
23, 578–582
ablations, 581–582
comparisons of ablations and pyramidotomy, 581
histology, *19-9,* 578–579
lesions of, 581–582
origin of corticospinal tract, *10-12,*
10-13, 579–580
stimulation, 580–581
supplementary, motor area, *19-21,*
583–585
ablations, 584–585
location of, 583–584
neural pathways from, 585
somatic representation, 584
stimulation of, 584
sensory areas, 559–578
gustatory, 577
primary, 559
auditory, *19-17, 19-18,* 24, 574–
577
somesthetic, *19-11, 19-12,* 24,
560–566
visual, 24, 566–574, *19-14, 19-15,*
19-16
secondary, *19-13,* 559
auditory, 574–577
somesthetic, 566, *19-13*
visual, 573–574, *19-13*
vestibular, 578
types, allocortex (heterogenetic, heterotypical), 547
distribution, 556–559, *19-5, 19-8*
Economo, *19-7, 19-8,* 558–559
agranular, 558
frontal, 558
granulous (koniocortex), 558

Boldface numbers indicate principal references. *Italic* numbers refer to illustrations.

Cerebral—*Continued*
  parietal, 558
  polar, 558
  isocortex (neocortex, homogenetic, homotypical), **547**, **550–559**, *19-5*
Cerebral hemispheres, 21–32, 67, 547, *3-9, 3-14, 3-15, 3-16*
  association fibers, **31–32**, *2-11*, 547
  basal ganglia, *see separate listing*
  commissural fibers, *2-7*, 32, 69–70, 547
  convolutions, *2-1, 2-2, 2-4*, 22–29, 70
  development, 67
    formation of gyri, 70
  divisions, *2-1*, 21–29
  external features, *2-1*, 21–29
  fissures, *2-2, 2-4*, 21–29, 65–66, 70
  gyri, 22–29, 70
  inferior surface, 28–29, *2-6*
  lateral surface, *2-1, 2-2*, 22–26
  lateral ventricle, *2-15*, 34–36, 132
  lobes, 22–28
  medial surface, 26–28, *2-4*
  medullary substance, 29–32
  projection fibers, 29–31, 548
  rhinencephalon, 521
  sulci, *2-1, 2-2*, 22–29, 70
"Cerebral peduncular loop," 450, 454
Cerebral vesicles, 57–60, 65
Cerebrospinal fluid, *1-16*, 14–16, 19
  absorption, 15
  circulation, 15
  composition, **14–15**
  formation, **14–15**
  functions, 14
  overproduction, 15
  pressure, 14
  volume, 15
Cerveau isolé, 390
Cervical enlargement, *9-1*, 173, 216
  flexure, *3-8*, 59
  plexus, 169–173
  segments of spinal cord, *9-5*, 159, 213, 218–221
Chemoreceptors, emesis, *11-13*, 296–297
Chiasm, optic *1-3, 2-5, 2-6, 2-22, 15-16, 15-21*, 37, 64, 70, 461, 465–466
Cholinergic, nerve fibers, 157, **200–202**, 205
Chorda tympani, *12-15*, 348
Chorea, Huntington's, 517
Choreoathetoid movements, 515, 517
Choroid plexus, fourth ventricle, *1-11*, 9, 15, 41, *5-16*, 132, 297, 621
  lateral ventricle, *2-6, 2-15, 2-22, 15-16*, 34, 36, 132, 497, 530, 614
  third ventricle, 9, 37, 60, *1-11*, 132, *2-15*, 438, 616
Choroidal, arteries, *20-9*, 604, 614–615, 620
  anterior, *20-9, 20-11*, 604, 614, 620
  epithelial cells, *5-18*, 56, 132–136
  fissure, 65, *3-13, 19-8*, 530, 614
  posterior, 614–615, *20-9*
  vein, *20-19*, 628
Chromatolysis, *4-28*, 85, 107, 162
  central, *4-28*, 85, 107, 162
Chromophil substance, *4-1*, 84–85,
Ciliary ganglion, 197, *8-1*, 379, 382–384
Cingulate gyrus, *2-4*, 27–28, **544–546**, *18-13*

Cingulum, *2-7, 2-12*, 31, **537–538**
Circle of Willis (cerebral arterial) *20-3, 20-4*, **606–608**
Cisterna, ambiens, *1-11*, 11
  cerebellomedullaris, *1-10, 1-11*, 10, 41
  chiasmatica, 11
  interpeduncularis, 11
  lumbar, *1-6*, 11
  magna, *1-10*, 11, 41
  pontis, 11
  superior, 11
Cisterns, subsurface, 82,
Clarke's column, *9-7, 9-11, 9-24, 10-10*, 227, 231, 249, 252, 418
Claustrum, *2-9, 2-13, 2-14*, 32, 499
Clava, *see* Tubercle, gracilis
Climbing fibers, *14-4, 14-5*, **407–412**
Clunial nerves, inferior, 185
  medial, 169
  superior, 169
Coccygeal ligament, *1-6*, 7, 213
Cochlea, *12-8, 12-9*, 326
  tonotopic localization, 328–329
Cochlear, nerve, *11-24, 12-8, 12-10*, 318, **326–329**
  nuclei, 318, 326–327, *11-24, 11-25, 12-5, 12-10*, 330
  pathways, *12-10*, **329–332**
  primary fibers, 327–329
  secondary, 329–332
  reflex, connections, *12-11*, **332–335**
  lesions, **335–336**
Cochlear nucleus, dorsal, *11-12, 11-24, 11-25, 12-10*, 318, 327, 330
  ventral, *11-25, 12-5, 12-10*, 318, 327, 330
Collateral, sulcus, *2-4, 2-6*, 24, 28, *18-8*, 531, 625
  trigone, *2-15*, 35
Collaterals, distribution in spinal cord, *9-21, 9-23*, 232–235
  of nerve fibers, 77–78, 97, 234, 391
  of reflex, *9-23*, 234, 360
Colliculus, facial (abducens), *2-18, 11-2, 12-1, 12-7, 12-15*, 38, 41, 323, 347, 349, 350
  inferior, *13-2*, 37, 42, 64, 331, 332, **367–369**
  superior, *13-1, 13-5, 13-6*, 37, 63, 249, 261, **370–374**
Column, of anterior gray, 57, 228–230, *9-21*
  of Burdach (fasciculus cuneatus), *9-8*, 238–241, *10-1*
  of Clarke, *9-7, 9-11, 9-24, 10-10*, 227, 231, 249, 252, 418
  of fornix, *12-13*, 535–537, *18-6, 18-7*
  of Goll (fasciculus gracilis), *9-10, 10-1*, 218, 238–241, 289–291
  intermediolateral, *8-1, 9-10, 9-11, 9-12, 9-22*, 195, 227, 230–231
  posterior, gray, *1-8*, 231–232
    white, 218–221, *10-1*, 238–242
Coma, 393, 495
  vigil, 393
Combined system disease, *10-25*, 281–282
Comma tract of Schultze (fasciculus interfascicularis), *10-21*, 241
Commissural, fibers, 32, 69–70, 547, 591–592

plate, 69, *3-13*
Commissure, anterior (*see separate listing*), 2-10, 2-13, 18-7, 32, **69–70**, 529–530
  of cerebellum, 414
  corpus callosum, 32, 590–592
  of fornix, *2-13, 18-6, 32, 69*, 535
  of Ganser (anterior hypothalamic), *16-10*, 490–491, *17-9*
  gray, spinal, 215, *9-6*
  of Gudden (ventral supraoptic), *16-10*, 490–491
  habenular, 43, 64, 438, 439, *2-18, 2-22, 15-5*
  hippocampal, 32, 69, 535, *2-13, 18-6*
  hypothalamic, 490–491, *16-10*
  of Meynert (dorsal supraoptic), *16-10*, 490–491
  posterior, *13-7, 13-8, 13-13*, 64, **376–377**
  of spinal cord, anterior white, 215
    gray, anterior, 215
    posterior, 231
  of superior colliculi, *13–12*
Common nerve trunk, 159, 162
Common peroneal nerve, 185
Compartments, extracellular, 19, *1-16*, 115–116
  intracellular, 19, *1-16*
Complex, amygdaloid, *2-6, 2-14, 3-13, 17-4, 18-4, 18-6, 18-12*, 32, **33–34**, 496, 539–543
  centromedian-parafascicular, *15-5, 15-6, 15-11, 15-12*, **447–451**, 474–477, 500–501, 592–593, *17-6*
  inferior olivary, *2-19, 11-9, 11-13*, 11–14, *11-16, 11-21*, 37, 39, 61, 298–300, 418–419
  trigeminal, *see* Trigeminal nerve
  ventrobasal, 455
  vestibular, *12-13, 12-14*, 41, **337–339**
Computer functions, cerebellum, **434**
  cerebrum, 21, 599
Conduction deafness, **336**
Conduction of impulses, along nerve fiber, **101–103**
  across synapse, **103–105**
  velocity, 101–103
Cone cells, of retina, *15-19, 15-20*, 465
Confluens sinus, *1-1, 1-3*, **622–623**, *20-16*
Conjugate movements of eyes, 344, 350, 382
Connective tissue sheaths of nerves, *4-22*, 100, 164
  endoneurium (sheaths of Henle, of Key and Retzius), 100, 164
  epineurium, 100, 164, *1-7, 4-23*, 7-7
  perineurium, 100, 164, *4-22*, 7-7
Conscious proprioception, 240, 564
Consciousness, 393, 495
Contact receptors, *6-4*, 139
Controlled visual deprivation, 572–573
Conus medullaris, *1-6, 9-1*, 55, 213
  syndrome of, 279
Convergence, ocular, 383–384
Convolutions, *2-1, 2-2, 2-4*, 22–29, 70
Cordotomy, *10-22*, 245
Cords, brachial plexus, *7-14*, 173
  lateral, *7-14*, 173
  medial, *7-14*, 173
  posterior, *7-14*, 173
Corona radiata, *2-8*, 29, 464

Boldface numbers indicate principal references. *Italic* numbers refer to illustrations.

Corpus, callosum, *2-9*, *2-14*, 26, 32, 69, 591–592
   body, *2-7*, 26, 591–592
   forceps, anterior, *2-7*, *2-9*, 26
      posterior, 26, 592, *2-7*, *2-16*
   genu, *2-4*, *2-7*, *2-12*, 26, 30
   rostrum, 26
   splenium, *2-6*, *2-7*, *2-16*, 26, 592
cerebelli, 46, 63, 399–401
Luysi, *15-5*, *15-6*, *17-12*, *17-13*, 509–511
medullare, of cerebellum, 414
quadrigemia, *see* Colliculi
restiform, *see* Inferior cerebellar peduncle
striatum, 33, 66–67, 65, 496–499
   connections of, *17-6*, 499–504
   development, 66–67, *3-13*
subthalamicum, *see* Subthalamic nucleus
Corpuscles, genital, 144–146
   of Golgi-Mazzoni, *6-8*, 146
   of Meissner, *6-4*, *6-7*, 144–145
   of Pacini, *6-9*, *6-10*, 145–146
   of Ruffini, 143
Cortex, agranular, *19-7*, 558, *19-9*, 578–583
   association, 474, 595–599
   auditory, *19-17*, *19-18*, 24, 336, 457, 574–578
   classification, *19-7*, 556–559
   gustatory, 577
   lamination, *19-7*, *19-9*, *19-10*, 548–551
   motor, *19-19*, 23, 578–582
   prefrontal, 23, 598–599
   premotor, 23, 582–583, *19-20*
   primary olfactory, 24, 523
   secondary olfactory, 526
   sensory, *19-11*, *19-12*, 24, 470–473, 559–578
   somesthetic, *19-11*, *19-12*, 24, 456, 560–566
   vestibular, 456, 578
   visual, *19-13*, *19-14*, *19-15*, *19-16*, 24, 461, 466–470, 566–574
Corti, organ of, *12-8*, *12-9*, 326
Cortical eye fields, 585–586
Cortical, functioning, associative memory, 595–596, 597
   correlation, 595–596, 597
   discrimination, 559, 564
   mnemonic reactions, 595
   parasensory area, 595
   relay nuclei, 473
   symbolization, 596–597
Corticobulbar tracts, *11-23*, 314–318, 464, *15-18*, 580–582
   lesions of, 318
Corticofugal fibers, 462–464, 548, 578–589
   nonpyramidal, 464, 583–589
   pyramidal, 255–261, 462–464, 578–582
Corticopontine tracts, *13-1*, *14-21*, 324–325, 370, 419, 463–465, 586–587
Corticorubral tract, *15-18*, 263, 385, 464
Corticospinal tracts, *10-12*, *10-13*, *10-14*, *13-1*, *15-17*, *15-18*, 255–260, 275–276, 464–465, 578–582, *19-12*

Corticothalamic tracts, 462–464, *15-18*, 476, 587–589
Cranial nerve(s), *2-19*, *11-1*, *11-16*, *11-17*, *11-18*, 39, 41, 42, 60–61, 197–198, 304–314, 325–351, 352–362, 377–379
   abducens (VI), *12-1*, 349–351
   accessory (XI), *11-18*, 308–309
   branchiomeric, 304–305
   cochlear (VIII), *11-24*, 326–329
   facial (VII), *12-15*, 346–349
   functional components, 61, 304–305
   glossopharyngeal (IX), *11-19*, 312–314
   hypoglossal (XII), *11-14*, *11-16*, 305–308
   oculomotor (III), *13-1*, *13-4*, *13-11*, 377–379, 380–382
   olfactory (I), *18-1*, 521–527
   optic (II), *2-5*, *15-16*, *15-20*, *15-21*, 58, 465–466
   trigeminal (V), *12-19*, *12-20*, *12-21*, *12-22*, 352–362
   trochlear (IV), *12-23*, *13-11*, 369
   vagus (X), *11-15*, *11-16*, *11-17*, *11-18*, *11-19*, 309–312
   vestibular (VIII), *12-2*, *12-12*, *12-13*, *12-14*, 337–342
Cranial outflow, autonomic, *8-1*, 195, 197–198, 208, 311–312, 313–314, 348, 377–378, 382–384
Craniosacral outflow, *8-1*, *8-11*, 195, 197–198, 208–209, 311–312, 313–314, 348, 377–378, 382–384
Crista ampullaris, *12-12*, 336
"Crocodile tears," syndrome of, 348
Crura cerebri, *2-8*, *2-10*, *13-1*, 37, 42–43, 63, 367, 397–398
Crus of fornix, *18-6*, *18-7*, 535–537
Cuneate, fasciculus, *10-1*, *10-2*, 39, 218, 238–241, 288
   nucleus, *10-1*, *10-2*, *11-7*, 240, 288–293
   accessory, *11-8*, *11-10*, 252, 292, 418
   tubercle, 39, *2-18*, *11-2*, *11-3*, 288–289
Cuneus of hemisphere, *2-4*, *15-13*, *15-21*, 566
Cupula, 336
Cutaneous nerves, *7-11*, *7-12*, *7-13*, 137–146, 164–168
Cyanosis, 278
Cytoarchitectonic organization, cerebellar cortex, *14-2*, *14-4*, *14-5*, 401–404
   cerebral cortex, *19-7*, *19-8*, *19-9*, *19-10*, 549–559
   reticular formation, *10-20*, *11-9*, *12-1*, *12-3*, *13-10*, 296–297, 300–302, 351–352, 388–390
   spinal cord, *9-9*, *9-11*, *9-15*, *9-17*, *9-18*, 222–229
Cytoplasm, neuron, *4-7*, *4-8*, 82–84

Darkschewitsch, nucleus of, *13-7*, *13-12*, *13-14*, *13-15*, 376, 379–380, 388
Deafness, 355
   conduction, 336
   nerve, 335
   otosclerosis, 336
Decarboxylase, inhibitor (peripheral), 397, 517
Decerebrate rigidity, 345, 432–433

Decomposition of movement, 431
Decussation, corticospinal tract, *10-12*, *10-13*, *11-5*, *11-6*, 255, 287–288
   of Forel (ventral tegmental), *10-17*, *13-4*, 261, 386
   fountain, of Meynert (dorsal tegmental), *10-17*, 261, 374
   hypothalamic, anterior, *16-10*, 490–491
      dorsal, *16-10*, 490–491
   medial lemniscus, *10-1*, *11-8*, 240, 291–293
   optic nerve fibers, *15-16*, *15-21*, *15-23*, 465–466
   pyramidal, *10-12*, *10-13*, *11-5*, *11-6*, 255, 287–288
   superior cerebellar peduncle, *12-23*, *13-2*, *14-16*, *14-17*, 363, 367, 420–422
   supraoptic, *16-10*, 490–491
   tegmental, dorsal, *10-17*, 261, 374
      ventral, *10-17*, *13-4*, 261, 386
   of trochlear nerve, *2-18*, *11-18*, *12-23*, 42, 369
Degeneration, band fiber, *4-27*, 107
   cell body, *4-28*, 107, 162
   central fibers, 276
      ascending, *10-3*, *10-4*, *10-22*, 276, 279–280
      descending, *10-5*, *10-22*, 276, 279–280
   chromatolysis, *4-28*, 107, 162, 276
   nerve fibers, *4-27*, *4-30*, 105–107, 185–188, 277
   peripheral fibers, *4-27*, *4-29*, *4-31*, 105–107, 185–188, 277
   reaction of, 187
   retrograde, *4-28*, 107
   Schwann cells, *4-26*, 107, 189
   secondary (Wallerian), *4-27*, 88, 105–107, 276
Deiters' nucleus (lateral vestibular), *10-18*, *10-19*, *12-1*, *12-2*, *12-3*, *14-19*, *14-20*, 337–338, 421–425
Dendrites, *4-3*, *4-4*, *4-5*, *4-12*, *14-4*, *14-5*, *14-6*, *14-7*, *14-9*, 77–80, 88, 401–402, 500–501
   extracapsular, 200
   intracapsular, 200
   primitive, 51
Denervation sensitization, 205–206
Dentate nucleus, 48, *12-16*, *14-12*, *14-13*, *14-16*, *17-12*, 363, 414–415, 420–421, 454, 473
Dentatoreticular tract, *14-16*, 363, 421
Dentatorubral tract, *14-16*, 363, 385, 420
Dentatothalamic tract, *14-16*, 363, 421, 454
Denticulate ligament, *1-4*, *1-5*, *1-7*, 8, 308
Dermatome, *7-8*, *7-9*, *7-11*, *7-12*, 165–166, 277
   innervation of, *7-1*, *7-10*, *7-11*, *7-12*, 165–166, 277
Descending spinal pathways, *10-12*, *10-13*, *10-21*, 255–272
   long, *10-12*, *10-13*, *10-15*, *10-17*, *10-19*, *10-20*, *10-21*, 255–271
Desoxyribonucleic acid (DNA), 84, 107, *4-10*
Diabetes insipidus, 493

Boldface numbers indicate principal references. *Italic* numbers refer to illustrations.

Diagonal band, *18-2*, *18-4*, 524
Diaphragma sellae, 1, *1-3*, *20-3*, 529
Diencephalon, *2-22*, *3-8*, *3-9*, *15-1*, *15-7*, *15-12*, 21, 43–46, 64–65, 60, 435–477
  blood supply, *20-9*, *20-11*, 615–616
  caudal, *15-5*, 435–438
  development, *3-13B*, 64–65
  epithalamus, *15-4*, 43, 64, 438–440
  hypothalamus, *2-22B*, *15-10*, 45, 65, 478–495, *16-1*
  interthalamic adhesion, 45, *15-10*, 65, 446
  metathalamus, 45, 435
    geniculate body, lateral, *15-4*, *15-12*, *15-14*, 45, 435, 458–461, 466–470, 567–568
    medial, *15-4*, *15-12*, 45, 332, 368, 457–458, 574–575
  midbrain-diencephalic junction, *15-4*, *15-5*, 435–437
  subthalamus, *15-5*, *15-6*, 45, 509–512
  thalamus (*see also separate listing*), *2-22*, *15-6*, *15-12*, 440–462
  pulvinar, *15-3*, 440–462
  third ventricle, *2-15*, *2-18*, *2-22*, *15-6*, 15, 43, 45, 438
Dihydroxyphenylalanine (L-Dopa), 397, 517
Diplegia, 261, 608
Diplopia, 349, 369, 382
Discriminative sensibility, 139, 153–155, 240–242, 454–456, 472, 559, 564, 595
Disease, Reynaud's, 206
"Doctrine of specific energies," 137–138
Dominance, cerebral, 23, 589–592
Dopamine, *13-18*, *13-19*, *17-14*, 91, 204, 394, 397, 489, 498, 501, 517, 539
Dorsal, acoustic striae, 329–330, *12-10*
  cochlear nuclei, 318, 327, 330, *11-25*, *12-10*
  longitudinal fasciculus (Schütz), *11-14*, *16-7*, 308, 369–370, 488
  primary ramus, *7-1*, 162
  rami of spinal nerves, *7-1*, 162
  root of spinal nerve, *1-5*, *7-1*, 159–161
  scapular nerve, 173
  tegmental nucleus, *12-24*, 365, 369
  trigeminal tract, *11-13*, *11-16*, *12-20*, *12-21*, *12-22*, 361
Duchenne-Aran syndrome, 181
Duchenne-Erb syndrome, 181
Dura mater, *1-1*, *1-2*, *1-3*, *1-4*, *1-5*, *1-6*, *1-7*, *1-8*, *20-3*, 1–7, 621–624
  arteries of, *20-3*, 621–622
  innervation, 6, 353
  sinuses of, 1, *1-1*, *1-2*, *20-18*, 622–624
  spinal, *1-5*, *20-3*, 6–7, 213
Dynamic polarization, at synapse, 105
Dysarthria, 308
Dysautonomia, familial, 207
Dysesthesias, 282, 472, 565–566
Dyskinesia, 514–520
  experimental, 518–519
  pathology, 516–517
  release phenomenon, 516
  subthalamic, 518–519
  surgery of, 518–520
  types, athetosis, 515

ballism, 515, 517
  chorea, 515, 517
  torsion dystonia, 515
  tremor, 514, 518
Dysmetria, 430
Dysphagia, 312
Dysphonia, 312
Dyspnea, 312
Dystonia (torsion spasm), 515

Edinger-Westphal nucleus, 377, *13-11*, 382
Effectors somatic, *6-17*, 156–158, 229–230
  visceral, *6-18*, 158, 230–231
Effects, 201
  muscarinic, 201
  nicotinic, 201
Efferent, cochlear bundle, *12-11*, 332–333
  peripheral fibers, 156–158
Eighth cranial nerve, *1-4*, *2-5*, *2-17*, *2-18*, *11-24*, *12-2*, *12-10*, *12-11*, *12-12*, *12-13*, *12-14*, 39, 318, 319, 325–329, 336–342
Electron microscopy, 71, 85–90, 95–100, 103, 408, *14-9*, *14-10*
  axolemma, *4-16*, 94
  chromatolysis, *4-28*, 107, 162
  degeneration of nerve fibers, *4-27*, *10-22*, 105–107, 186–187
  myelin, *4-27*, *4-30*, *4-31*, 94–96
  Nissl bodies, *4-28*, 85
  node of Ranvier, *4-16*, 96–97
  perineural space, 19
  synapse, *4-12*, *4-23*, *4-24*, *4-25*, 103–105
Electronic brain, 21, 434, 599
Eleventh cranial nerve, *1-4*, *2-17*, *2-19*, *11-17*, *11-18*, *11-19*, 39, 308–309
Emboliform nucleus, *12-16*, *14-13*, *14-17*, 46, 63, 385, 415, 420, 425
Eminence, collateral, *2-16*, 35
  hypoglossal, *11-2*, 41, 297, 305
  medial, 482, 488
  olivary, 39, 298–300
Eminentia teres (medial eminence), 41, *11-2*, 297, 322
Emissary veins, *20-16*, 622, 624
  mastoid, 624
  occipital, 624
  parietal, 624
Encapsulated nerve endings, corpuscles of Golgi-Mazzoni, *6- 8*, 144
  of Ruffini, 143
  end bulbs, *6-8*, 145
  neuromuscular spindles, *6-11*, *6-12*, *6-13*, 146–149, 251, 252
  neurotendinous organ (Golgi), *6-15*, *6-16*, 149–153, 251, 252
  Pacinian corpuscles, *6-9*, *6-10*, 145–146, 155
  tactile corpuscles (Meissner), *6-4*, *6-7*, 144–145, 154
Encéphale isolé, 390
Endbrain, *see* Telencephalon
End bulbs, *6-8*, 145
End feet (boutons terminaux), *4-23*, 103–105
Endings, neuromuscular, *6-11*, 146–149, 156–158

en grappe, 157
en plaque, 157
Endocrine functions, 45, 91, 376, 478, 488–490, *16-9*, 493–494, 541–543
Endolymph, 336
Endoneurium, 100, *4-22*, *7-7*, 164
Endoplasmic reticulum, granular, 85, *4-10*, 107
Enophthalmos, 210, 384
Entorhinal area, *18-11*, *19-5*, 525–526, 535
Enzymes, 203
  catechol-o-methyl-transferase (COMT), 203
Ependyma, *5-12*, *5-13*, 19–20, 128–132
Ependymal layer, *3-3*, *3-6*, 19–20
Epineurium, *1-7*, *4-23*, *7-7*, 100, 164
Epiphysis (pineal body), *2-18*, *2-20*, *2-21*, *15-3*, *15-4*, *15-7*, 43, 439–440
Epithalamic vein, *20-17*, *20-19*, 628–629
Epithalamus, 37, 64, 438–440, *15-7*
Epithelial membrane, *5-16*, 132–136
Equilibrium, mechanism of, 336, 334–345
  disturbances, 345, 587
Experimental remyelination, 113–114, *4-30*, 189
External, capsule, *2-9*, *2-13*, *2-14*, 32, 499
  mesaxon, 96
  sagittal stratum (inferior longitudinal fasciculus), 31, *2-16*, 467, 568
External granular layer (cerebellum), *3-11*, 63
External preolivary nuclei, 331
Exteroceptors, 138, *9-22*
Extrafusal muscle fibers, 147, 160, *9-26*, *9-27*
Extraocular muscles, *13-11*, 343, 344, 350, 369, 377–379
  functional considerations, 344, 350, 369, 382
  nuclei of, *13-11*, 350, 369, 377–379
  stretch receptors, 360, 379
"Extrapyramidal," motor areas, *19-20*, 582–585
  system, 512–*513*, 520
Extreme capsule, *2-9*, *2-13*, *2-14*, 32, 499, 530
Eye fields, cortical, 585–586
  frontal, 585
  occipital, 585

Facial colliculus, *2-18*, *11-2*, *12-1*, *12-7*, *12-15*, 38, 41, 323, 347, 349, 350
Facial nerve, *2-5*, *12-15*, 346–349
  fibers, *11-17*, *11-18*, *12-1*, 347
    central course, *12-1*, 347
    motor, 347
    peripheral, *12-15*, 346
    root, *12-2*, 347
    sensory, *12-2*, 347
    visceral, 348, *12-15*
  ganglia, *12-15*, 347
    geniculate, 347
    genu, *11-17*, *11-18*, *12-1*, *12-7*, *12-15*, 323, 347, 350
    pterygopalatine, 348
    submandibular, 348
  hyperacusis, 348

Boldface numbers indicate principal references. *Italic* numbers refer to illustrations.

lesions, *12-15*, 348–349
  central, 349
  peripheral, 348
  nuclei, 346
    motor, 346
    superior salivatory, 348
  reflexes, corneal, 348, 361
Facilitation of neural activity, 264, 266, 389
Facilitatory center, 269, 389
Falx, cerebelli, *1-2*, 1, 46
  cerebri, *1-2*, *1-3*, *1-12*, 1, 622
Familial dysautonomia, 207
Fascia dentata (dentate gyrus), *18-6*, *18-8*, *18-9*, *18-10*, 28, 531–533
Fascicles, of dorsal root fibers, *1-8*, 232–235, *9-22*
Fasciculations, 188, 273
Fasciculus,
  arcuate, *2-11*, 31
  basal forebrain, 513
  central tegmental, *12-1*, *12-4*, 323, 351, 392, 450
  cuneatus, *10-1*, *10-2*, 39, 218, 238–241, 288
  dorsal longitudinal of Schütz, *11-4*, *16-7*, 308, 485, 488
  dorsolateral, *9-7*, *9-19*, 286
  gracilis, *9-10*, *10-1*, 218, 238–241, 289–291
  inferior longitudinal (external sagittal stratum), 31, 467, 568
  interfascicular, *10-21*, 241
  lenticular, *17-7*, *17-8*, *17-10*, *17-11*, 505
  mammillaris princeps, *16-5*, *16-6*, 488
  medial forebrain, *16-5*, 487, 541
  medial longitudinal, *10-18*, *10-19*, *12-14*, *13-2*, *13-4*, 269–270, 342–344
  occipitofrontal (inferior), 31
  pallidotegmental, *17-11*, 507–509
  predorsal (tectospinal), *10-17*, 261, 374
  proprii, *9-7*, *10-21*, 271–273
  retroflexus (habenulopeduncular tract), *15-5*, *16-5*, 64, 437, 438
  septomarginal, *10-21*, 241
  solitarius, *11-13*, *11-17*, *11-18*, 310, 347
  subcallosal, 500
  subthalamic, 508–509
  superior longitudinal, 31
  thalamic, *17-8*, *17-11*, *15-6*, 505–507
  uncinate, of hemisphere, *2-11*, 31
    of Russell, *14-18*, *14-19*, *14-20*, 422–425
    of Vicq d'Azyr (mammillothalamic tract), *15-1*, *15-6*, *16-5*, *16-7*, 444, 488
Fasciola cinerea, *see* Gyrus, fasciolar
Fastigial nucleus, *12-16*, *14-13*, *14-19*, *14-20*, 48, 63, 415–416, 422–425
  lesions of, 432–433
Fastigiobulbar tract, *see* Uncinate fasciculus of Russell
Fastigium, fourth ventricle, *2-26*, 41
Femoral nerve, *7-11*, 182–183
  lateral cutaneous, 183–184
Fibers, A, 101
  afferent, *9-22*, *9-23*, 159, 232–235, 304–305, 325–329, 337, 347–348, 353–360, 465–470, 521–529

brain stem reticular, 485
amygdalo-hypothalamic, *16-8*, 484, 540–541
B, 101, 193
C, *7-6*, 101, 193
cerebelloreticular, 363, 421, 425
cholinergic, 157, 200–202, 205
climbing, *14-4*, *14-5*, 407–412
collateral, 234, 302, 392
corticobulbar, *11-23*, 314–318, 464, 580, *15-18*
corticorubral, *15-18*, *263*, 385, 464
corticostriate, *17-6*, 499–500
corticotectal, 368, 373
corticothalamic, 462–464, 476, 587–589
cuneocerebellar, *10-10*, 293, 352–353, 417–418
external arcuate, *11-8*, 296
extrafusal, 147, 160, *9-26*, *9-27*
hippocampohypothalamic, 483
internal arcuate, *10-1*, *11-8*, 240, 292
intrafusal, *6-11*, 146–149
mossy, *14-4*, *14-5*, *14-8*, *14-9*, 406–412
nigrostriate, *13-19*, *17-6*, *17-14*, 396–397, 501–504
olivocerebellar, *11-14*, *11-21*, 298, 418, *14-22*
pallidosubthalamic, *17-8*, *17-11*, 504
pallidotegmental, *17-11*, 507–508
pallidothalamic, *17-8*, *17-11*, *17-15*, 454, 505–507
parallel of cerebellum, *14-4*, *14-5*, 403, 411
parasympathetic, 197–199, 211
physiological grouping, 101–103
pontocerebellar, *14-21*, 323–324, 419–420
postganglionic, *8-1*, *8-2*, 192–195
preganglionic, *8-1*, *8-2*, 192–195
  of Remak, 100–103
retinohypothalamic, 466, 486
rubrobulbar, 303, 386
rubrocerebellar, 386, 416
rubro-olivary, *14-21*, 386
secondary vestibular, 342
size, 101–102
strionigral, *17-4*, *17-6*, 396, 504
striopallidal, 504
subthalamopallidal, *17-8*, 504
tectocerebellar, *15-12*, *15-13*, 374
thalamocortical, *15-19*, 462–464, 466–476
thalamostriate, *17-6*, 500–501
trigeminocerebellar, 360, 420
ventral amygdalofugal, *16-8*, 484, 541
vestibulocerebellar, *12-14*, 341–342, 417
vestibulo-oculomotor, *12-14*, 342–344
visceral afferent, 80, 199, 309, 347
Fibrillations, 275
Field, H (*see also* Tegmental field of Forel), *15-5*, *15-6*, *15-10*, *17-8*, *17-11*, *17-14*, 437, 505
  H1 (*see also* Fasciculus, thalamic), *15-6*, *17-28*, *17-11*, 505–509
  H2 (*see also* Fasciculus, lenticular), *17-7*, *17-8*, *17-10*, *17-11*, 505
  visual, *15-21*, *15-23*, *19-15*, *19-16*, 466–470, 568
Fifth cranial nerve, *1-3*, *1-4*, *11-17*, *11-18*,

11-19, *12-17*, *12-20*, *12-21*, *12-22*, 41, 293–296, 352–362
Fila olfactoria, *18-1*, 521
Filum terminale, *1-6*, *9-1*, 7, 55
Fimbria, *18-6*, *18-7*, *18-8*, *18-9*, *18-10*, *18-11*, 35, 535–537
Final common pathway (*see also* Lower motor neuron), *9-21*, *9-22*, 156–158, 272
Fink and Helmer Method, 72, 277
First cranial nerve, *18-1*, *18-2*, 521
Fissure (*see also* Sulcus), anterior medial, *9-2*, *9-6*, 55, 214
  calcarine, *2-4*, *2-12*, *15-21*, *19-14*, 24, 466–469, 470, 568
  cerebellar, *2-12*, *2-24*, *2-25*, *2-26*, *14-1*, 46, 399–401
  choroidal, *3-13*, *18-8*, *18-11*, *19-8*, 65, 530
  collateral, *2-6*, 24, 28, 531
  development, 65–66, 70
  hippocampal, *18-8*, *18-11*, 28, 65–66, 530–532
  interhemispheric, 21–22
  lateral cerebral (Sylvian), *2-3*, *3-16*, 22, 566, 609, *20-7*
  longitudinal cerebral, 22
  posterolateral (prenodular), 63, 399
  primary, 46, 63, 399
  rhinal, *2-6*, 28, 524, 525
  transverse cerebral, *3-14*, 65
Fixation, nerve tissue, 71
Flaccidity, 273, 277, 581–582
Flexor reflex afferents, 251, 252, 419
Flexure, cephalic, *3-8*, 59
  cervical, *3-8*, 55, 59
  pontine, *3-8*, *3-9*, 59
Flocculonodular lobe, *2-24*, *2-26*, *14-1*, 46, 63, 399, 425, 431–432
Flocculus, *2-24*, *2-26*, *14-1*, 46, 63, 399, 425, 431–432
Floor plate, *3-3*, 53
Flower-spray endings (myotube), *6-11*, *6-12*, 148
Folia, cerebellar, *2-23*, *2-24*, *2-25*, *2-26*, *14-2*, 46, 399–401
Folium vermis, *2-26*, *14-1*, 46, 399, 425
Foot plates (perivascular feet), *5-2*, *5-3*, *5-4*, 118–119, 120
Foramen, cecum anterior, *13-3*
  cecum posterior, *11-25*, 320
  interventricular, *2-15*, 36, 60, 64
  of Luschka, *2-15*, *20-4*, 10, 41
  of Magendie, 10, 41
  magnum, *1-1*, *1-4*, *1-11*, 6, 308
  spinosum, *20-3*, 621–622
Forceps, corpus callosum, anterior, *2-7*, *2-9*, 26
  posterior, *2-7*, *2-16*, 26, 592
Forebrain (prosencephalon), *3-8*, 58, 547
Forel, tegmental field of, *15-5*, *15-6*, *15-10*, *17-8*, *17-9*, *17-10*, *17-11*, *17-14*, *17-15*, 437, 505
Fornix, *2-4*, *2-14*, *15-1*, *18-6*, *18-7*, 535–537
  body (cruca), *15-1*, 32, 535–537
  columns, *2-13*, *18-6*, *18-7*, 535–537
  commissure, *2-13*, *18-6*, 32, 69, 535
  fimbria, *18-6*, *18-7*, 535
  functions, 537–539
  postcommissural, 484, 536–537

Boldface numbers indicate principal references. *Italic* numbers refer to illustrations.

Fossa—*Continued*
  precommissural, **484**, **537**
Fossa, interpeduncular, *2-17*, *13-4*, *13-17*,
    42, 606
  lateral, *2-3*, *3-14*, *3-15*, *3-16*, **24–25**
  pituitary, *20-3*, 1, 529
  posterior, *1-2*, *1-3*, 1
  rhomboid, *1-4*, *2-18*, *11-18*, 41, 60, 297
Fourth cranial nerve, *1-3*, *1-4*, *2-18*, *2-19*,
    11-17, *11-18*, *12-23*, *13-11*, **369**
Fourth ventricle, *1-12*, *2-18*, *2-21*, *3-9*, *11-
    14*, *11-16*, *11-17*, **39–41**, 60,
    285, 297
  area, postrema, *12-13*, 296
    vestibularis, *11-2*, 41, 297
  calamus scriptorius, 41
  choroid plexus, *1-11*, 9, 15, 41, 132, 297,
    5-16
  facial colliculus, *2-18*, *11-18*, 41, 323,
    350
  fastigum, *2-26*, 41
  foramen, of Luschka, *2-15*, *20-3*, 41
    of Magendie, *2-15*, 41
  lateral recess, *11-24*, 41, **318**
  medial, eminence, *11-2*, 41, 297
  median sulcus, *2-18*, 41, 297
  rhomboid fossa, *2-18*, *11-18*, 41, 297
  striae medullares, *2-18*, 41
  sulcus limitans, *11-16*, 41, 305
  superior cerebellar peduncles, *2-19*, *11-
    2*, **363**, 385, 420
  tela choroidea, *1-11*, 41, 297,
  trigonum, hypoglossi, *11-2*, 41, 297
    vagi, *11-2*, 41, 297
  velum, inferior medullary, *2-26*, 41
    superior medullary, *2-25*, 41, 362,
    369
Fovea centralis, 465
Free nerve endings, *6-1*, *6-3*, *6-6*, 142–144
Frontal eye fields (area 8), *19-20*, 585
Frontal lobe, *2-6*, *19-5*, *19-6*, *19-20*, 23,
    67, **444–446**, 598–599
Frontopontine tract, *13-1*, *15-18*, 324,
    398, 419, 464, **586–587**
Functional components of nerves, 9-22,
    11-16, *11-18*, 56–57, **304–305**
Funiculus, anterior, *9-6*, *10-21*, 216
  anterolateral, *9-16*, *10-21*, 216
  lateral, *1-8*, *9-6*, *10-21*, 216
  posterior, *9-6*, *10-21*, 216

Gamma-aminobutyric acid (GABA), 91,
    205, 517
Ganglion (ganglia), aorticorenal, 197
  autonomic, *8-1*, *8-3*, 55, 192–198, 199–
    200, 313, 348, 379
    origin of, 50
  basal, of hemisphere, *see* Basal gan-
    glia
  celiac, *8-1*, 197
Ganglion cells of retina, *15-19*, *15-20*,
    465, **568–569**, *19-15*
  cervical, inferior, *8-1*, *8-10*, 195, 196
    middle, *8-1*, 195, 196
    superior, *8-1*, *8-10*, 195, 196
  ciliary, 197, 379, *8-1*, **382–384**
  coccygeal, 195
  colateral, 193
  dorsal root, *1-4*, *3-6*, 56, 161–162, 232
  Gasserian, *see* trigeminal
  geniculate, 347

glossopharyngeal, inferior (petrosal),
    11-19, 313
  superior, *11-19*, 313
habenular, *15-1*, *15-5*, 43, **437–438**
inferior mesenteric, *8-3*, 197
inferior ganglion (Nodose), 199
otic, 198, 314
parasympathetic, *8-3*, **197–198**
paravertebral, *8-2*, 193
phrenic, 196
prevertebral, *8-2*, 193, 195
pterygopalatine, *12-15*, 198, 348,
  of Scarpa (vestibular), *12-13*, **337**
semilunar, *see* trigeminal
sphenopalatine (pterygopalatine), *12-
    15*, 198, 348
spinal, *1-5*, *1-7*, *3-6*, *3-7*, *7-1*, *7-3*, *7-10*,
    161–162, 232
spiral, *12-8*, **326–327**
stellate, *8-1*, *8-10*, 195
submandibular, 198, 348
superior mesenteric, *18-3*, 197
terminal, 193
thoracic (stellate), *8-1*, 195
trigeminal, *1-3*, *2-19*, *11-19*, **353–354**
vagus, inferior (nodosal), *11-19*, 199,
    309
  superior (jugular), *11-19*, 199, 309
vestibular (Scarpa), *12-13*, **337**
Ganglionated, cords, *8-1*, **195–196**
  plexuses, 198,
  of Auerbach, 198
  of Meissner, 198
Ganglionic arteries (central), *20-9*, *20-10*,
    20-11, *20-12*, 607, **612–615**
Ganglionic crest, *see* Neural crest
Ganser's commissure (anterior hypotha-
    lamic), *16-10*, **490**, *17-9*
Gasserian ganglion, *see* Ganglion, tri-
    geminal
Gelatinous substance of Rolando, *9-7*, *9-
    8*, *9-14*, *9-17*, *9-19*, 78, **223–
    224**, 231
Gemmules, *4-5*, 78, 103, **402**
Geniculate, body, lateral, *15-3*, *15-4*, *15-
    14*, *15-18*, *15-21*, 45, 64, 435,
    458–461, 466–470, **569**, *19-15*
  functional properties, cells, 469–
    470, 568–569
  glomeruli, *15-15*, **458–461**
  lamination, *15-14*, 458
  medial, *13-17*, *15-3*, *15-4*, 45, 64, 435,
    457–458
  organization, 457
  projection, *15-18*, 457, 472, **574–575**
Geniculocalcarine tract (optic radiation),
    15-21, *15-23*, 30, **466–470**,
    566–568
Geniculotemporal tract (auditory radia-
    tions), *12-10*, *15-18*, **457–458**,
    463–465, **574–576**
Genitofemoral nerve, *7-19*, 181, 183
Gennari, band of, *19-14*, 567
Genu, corpus callosum, *2-4*, *2-7*, *2-12*, 26,
    30
  facial nerve, *11-17*, *11-18*, *12-1*, *12-15*,
    323, 347, 350
  internal capsule, *2-9*, *15-17*, *15-18*, 30,
    464–465
Germ layers, 3–2, 50
  ectoderm, *3-2*, 49–50, 165
  entoderm, *3-2*

mesoderm, *3-2*, 49, 164
Germinal cells, *3-4*, *3-5*, 50–52, 533, 547
  layer, 50
  zone, 67
Giacomini, band of, 532
Glees method, 72, 277
Glia, *5-2*, *5-3*, *5-4*, *5-5*, *5-8*, *5-9*, 52, 115–
    128, **412–414**
Glial membrane, *1-9*, 8, 129
  scars, *5-6*, 116
  staining technics, *4-1*, 115
Glioblasts, *3-5*, 52
Gliofibrils, *5-6*, 119
Gliosomes, *5-4*, 120
Globose nucleus, *12-16*, *14-13*, 48, 63, 415
Globus pallidus, *2-9*, *2-13*, *2-14*, *17-3*, 33,
    66–67, 496, 498, **504–509**
  blood supply, *20-11*, **614–615**, *20-12*
  connections, afferent, 504
    efferent, *17-7*, *17-8*, *17-9*, *17-10*, *17-
    11*, **505–509**
  medullary lamina lateral, *17-7*, 498
    medial, *17-7*, 498, 505
  segments, lateral, *17-3*, *17-7*, *17-8*,
    498, 508
    medial, *17-7*, *17-8*, *17-11*, 498, **505–
    508**
Glomeruli, of autonomic ganglia, *8-5*,
    200
  cerebellar, *14-4*, *14-5*, *14-9*, *14-10*, **406–
    407**
  lateral geniculate body, *15-15*, **458–
    461**
  olfactory, *18-1*, **522**
Glossopharyngeal nerve, *11-1*, *11-17*, *11-
    18*, *11-19*, *11-21*, **312–314**
  ganglion, inferior (petrosal), *11-19*, 313
    superior, *11-19*, 313
  lesions, 314
  nuclei, 314
Glutamic acid decarboxylase (GAD),
    504, 517
Gluteal nerve, inferior, 185
  superior, 185
Gnosis, 139, **595–596**
Gnostic disturbances, 596
Golgi, apparatus, *4-8*, *5-14*, **88–91**
  classification of nerve cells, *4-3*, 80
  studies, climbing fibers, cerebellum,
    407–408, *14-4*
    inferior colliculus, 368
    medial geniculate, 457
    pallidum, 498
    reticular formation, 301
    striatum, *17-6*, **497–498**
  technic, 72, *4-5*, 368, 408, 457, 462, 497,
    17-5, 551
  tendon organs, *6-15*, *6-16*, **149–153**
Gracile nucleus, *10-1*, *11-6*, *11-7*, *11-8*, *11-
    12*, 240, **289–290**
Granulous cortex, *19-7*, *19-8*, 558
Gray, commissure, *9-6*, 215
  substance, *9-6*, **217–218**
Great, auricular nerve, *7-13*, 169
  cerebral vein, *20-19*, *20-20*, 629
Greater occipital nerve, *7-13*, 169
Gudden's commissure (ventral supra-
    optic), *16-10*, **490–491**
Gustatory,
  cortical area, **577–578**
  fibers, 310
  nucleus, 310, 313

receptive area, 577
thalamic representation, 456
Gyrus (gyri), 22
angular, *2-1, 2-2, 19-6*, 24, 598
breves, *2-3*, 26
cingulate, *2-4*, 27–28, 544–546, *18-13*
isthmus of, *2-4*, 28, 544, *18-13*
cuneus, *2-4*, 566
dentate, *18-6*, *18-8*, *18-9*, *18-10*, 28, 531–533
development, 70
diagonal, 524, *18-2*
fasciolar, 532
frontal, inferior, *2-1, 2-2*, 23, 596–597
middle, *2-1, 2-2*, 23, 585
superior, *2-1, 2-2, 2-4*, 23, 583
fusiform (see occipitotemporal)
of Heschl (see temporal, transverse) *2-7, 12-10*, 24, 331, 457, 574–576
intralimbic, 532
lingual, *2-6*, 24
longus, 26
marginal (see frontal, superior), *2-4*, 23
occipital, lateral, *2-2*, 24
occipitotemporal, *2-6*, 28, 18-8, 525
orbital, *2-2, 2-5, 2-6*, 28, 453, 475
parahippocampal, *2-6*, *18-8*, *18-9*, *18-13*, 24, 27, 525
paraterminal, *18-2*, *18-4*, 525
postcentral, *2-1, 2-2*, 23, 24, 560–566
precentral, *2-1, 2-2*, 23, 578–582
rectus, *2-6*, 29, *18-2*
subcallosal, *18-2*, 27, 525
supracallosal, *2-7*, 532, *18-6*
supramarginal, *2-1, 2-2*, 24, 595–597
temporal, inferior, *2-1*, *2-2*, *2-6*, 24, 530
middle, *2-1*, *2-2*, 24, 530
superior, *2-1, 2-2, 2-3*, 24, 575
transverse, *2-3*, 24, 331, *12-10*, 457, 574–576
uncus, *2-5, 2-6, 2-12, 18-6*, 24, 539

Habenular, commissure, *2-18, 2-22, 15-5*, 43, 64, 438–439
ganglion, *15-1, 15-5*, 43, 438
nuclei, *15-5*, 43, 438
Habenulopeduncular tract (fasciculus retroflexus), *15-5, 16-5*, 438
Hair cells, of cochlea, *12-8, 12-9*, 326
crista, ampullaris, 336
macula saccule, 336
macula utricle, 336
Hallucinations, olfactory, 529
Hemianalgesia, 296, 464
Hemianesthesia, 296, 464
Hemianopsia, *15-23*, 470, 568
binasal, *15-23*, 470
bitemporal, *15-23*, 470
heteronymous, 470
homonymous, 470, 568
quadrantic, 470, 568
Hemiathetosis, 517
Hemiballism, 517
Hemihypacusis, 465
Hemihypesthesia, 464
Hemiparesis, *10-22, 10-23*, 261, 275–276, 279–280, 308, 351, 382, 464–465, 581–582
Hemiplegia, 261, 275–276, 464–465, 581–582

inferior alternating, *10-13, 20-13*, 308, 351
middle alternating, *10-13, 20-13*, 351
superior alternating (Weber), *10-13, 20-14*, 382
Hemisection of spinal cord, *10-23*, 279–280
Hemisphere, cerebellar, *2-23, 2-24, 2-25, 14-1*, 46–48, 63, 399–401
cerebral, *3-9, 3-14, 3-15, 3-16*, 21–32, 547
dominant, 23, 589–592, 598
nondominant, 24, 589–592
Hemispherectomy, 585
Hemispheric, independence, 591–592
sulcus, *3-9*, 60
vesicles, 58
Hemithermo-anesthesia, 296
Henle, sheath of, 100, 164
endoneurium, 100, 164, *4-22, 7-7*
Herpes zoster, 166
Herring bodies, 92
Heschl, gyri of (see Gyri, temporal, transverse), *2-7*, *12-10*, *19-5*, 24, 331, 457, 464, 574–576
Heterogenetic cortex, 524, 530–535, 547, 551, *18-9*
Heteronymous defects, visual, *5-23*, 470
Heterotypical cortex, 524, 530–535, 547, 551, *18-9*
Hexamethonium, 201
Hindbrain (rhombencephalon; see also Medulla oblongata, Pons, and Cerebellum),
development, *3-8, 3-9, 3-10, 3-11, 3-12*, 59–63
venous drainage, 619–620
Hippocampal formation, *2-6, 18-6, 18-7, 18-8, 18-9*, 28, 35, 65, 530–539
alveus, *18-8, 18-9*, 531, 535
anatomy, 530–533
anosmatic cetaceans, 521
connections, afferent, *16-8, 18-11*, 535
efferent, *18-11*, 535–537
fornix, *18-1, 18-6, 18-7*, 535–537
commissure, see Commissure of fornix
development, *3-15*, 66, 69, 530–532
fissure, *18-8, 18-11*, 28, 65–66, 530–532
functional considerations, 537–539
behavior, 537–538
emotion, 537–538
experimental studies, 537
lesions, 537
memory, 538
seizure discharge, 537
histology, *18-10, 18-11*, 530–535
layers, cells, *18-20*, 532–533
ridge, *3-15*, 65, 530
sectors, *18-20*, 533–535
Histofluorescence technics, *8-6, 8-7*, 202, 364, 366, 394–395, 501, 594–595, *13-18*
Histogenesis, autonomic ganglia, *3-7*, 50, 55
cerebral cortex, 67–69, 70, 547
neural tube, *3-1, 3-2, 3-3, 3-4*, 50–51
neuroglia, *3-5*, 53
neurons, *3-5*, 51–52
olfactory bulb, 522
spinal ganglia, *3-6, 3-7*, 55
Holmes silver technic, 72
Homogenetic cortex (isocortex), *19-9, 19-*

10, 547
Homonymous visual defects, *15-23*, 470, 568
Homotypical cortex, 547, *19-1*
Hormone, ACTH, 489, 490, 493–494, 542
antidiuretic, 488, *16-9*, 492–493
FSH, 490
gonadotropic, 490, 493–494, 542
neurosecretory, 91–93, 488–490, 493–494
oxytocin, 488, 493
releasing factors, 92, 489, 490, 493–494
TSH, 490, 493–494
Horn, of lateral ventricle, *2-15*, 34–36, 497
anterior, *2-15, 17-1*, **34**, 497
inferior, *2-15, 18-6, 18-9*, 35, 467, 497, 530
posterior, *2-15, 2-16, 18-7*, 35, 568
of spinal cord, anterior gray, *9-6, 9-7, 9-21*, 215, 229–230
lateral gray, *9-6, 9-7*, 215, 230–231
posterior gray, *9-6, 9-7, 9-18*, 215, 231–232
Horner's syndrome, 210–211, 283, *10-26*, 384
Horseradish peroxidase (HRP), 451, 501, 592
retrograde transport, 451, 501, 592
Hydroxytryptamine (5-) (5-HT, serotonin), 204, 366, 594–596
Hyperacusis, 348
Hyperesthesia, 166, 472
Hyperkinetic state, 518
Hyperphagia, 494, 543
Hyperpyrexia, 492
Hyperreflexia, 276, 581–582
Hypertonus, 275, 516, 583–584
Hypesthesia, 166, 277, 472
Hypogastric plexus, *8-11*, 197, 211
Hypoglossal nerve (XII), *2-5, 2-17, 2-19, 11-14, 11-17, 11-18, 11-19*, 305–308
lesions, 308
nucleus of, *11-15, 11-16*, 305
Hypokinetic state, 387, 518
Hypophysial portal system, *16-9*, 490, 493–494
Hypophysis, *2-5, 2-19, 2-21, 16-1, 16-5, 16-7, 16-9*, 64, 92, 490, 493–494, 613
Hypothalamus, *16-1, 16-2, 16-3, 16-4*, 37, 45, 64, 206–207, 478–495
anatomy, 37, 45, 478–491
blood supply, *20-9*, 490, 612–615
connections, *16-5*, *16-6*, *16-7*, *16-8*, 483–490
afferent, 483–487
cortex, 483, 486–487, 535–537
descending, *16-7*, 485
efferent, 487–490
hypophysis, *16-9*, 490, 493–494
olfactory, *16-8*, 482, 541
decussations, 490–491
anterior (Ganser), 16–10, 490–491
dorsal supraoptic (Meynert), 16–10, 490–491
ventral supraoptic (Gudden), 16–10, 490–491
divisions, lateral, 478–479

Boldface numbers indicate principal references. *Italic* numbers refer to illustrations.

Hypothalamus—*Continued*
  medial, 478–479
  functional considerations, 491–495
    anterior pituitary, 493–494
    autonomic regulation, 492
    diabetes insipidus, 493
    emotion, 493–495
    endocrine, 493–494
    feeding, 494
    homeostatic, 492
    metabolic, 492–493, 543
    "pseudoaffective" reactions, 495
    rage, 492, 495
    regulation, temperature, 492
    satiety, 494, 543
    sleep, 491, 492, 495
    stimulation, 491–493
    water balance, 491, 493
  hormones, 488–490, 493–494
  lesions, 492–495
  nuclei, *16-1, 16-2, 16-3, 16-4, 16-8,*
      478–483
    lateral group, 478–483
    medial group, 479–482
      arcuate, 482, *16-1*
      mammillary bodies, 482–483
      posterior area, 482, 492
      suprachiasmatic, 482
      supraoptic region, 479–482
      tuberal region, 482
  preoptic, *16-1,* 479
  portal system, *16-9,* 490
  sulcus, *2-23, 15-6,* 45, 478
  tracts, corticomammillary, *16-6,* 383–
      385
    mammillary peduncle, *16-5,* 485
    mammillotegmental, *16-5,* 488
    mammillothalamic, *16-5, 16-6,* 488
    supraopticohypophysial, *16-7, 16-9,*
      488
    tuberohypophysial, *16-9,* 488–490
Hypotonia, 273, 515, 581

Iliohypogastric nerve, *7-19,* 181
Ilioinguinal nerve, *7-19,* 181
Iliopsoas nerve *7-19,* 181
Implantation cone, 93,
Incisures, of Schmidt-Lantermann, *4-15,*
    4-20, 97–99
Inclusion, bodies, 90–91, 482
Indusium griseum (supracallosal gyrus),
    2-7, 18-6, 532
Inferior, cerebellar peduncle (restiform
    body), *2-19, 10-10, 11-2, 11-22,*
    11-24, 39, 249, 303–304, 319,
    324–325, 363, 414–421
  collicular brachium, *2-19, 12-10, 13-17,*
    37, 331, 368
  colliculus, *2-18, 2-19, 12-10, 13-2,* 42,
    64, 331, 367–369
  frontal gyrus, parts, *2-1, 2-2,* 23
  gluteal nerve, 185
mesenteric, ganglion, *8-3,* 197
  plexus, *8-11,* 197
olive *see* Inferior olivary complex
Inferior olivary complex, *2-19, 11-9, 11-*
    13, 11-14, 11-15, 37, 61, 298–
    300, 319, 418–419
  afferent fibers, 299, 386
    central tegmental tract, 299, 322,
      392, 450
    cortex, 299

spinal cord, 299, 419
  amiculum, *11-21,* 299
  efferent fibers, *11-21,* 299, 303, 418
    olivocerebellar, 298, 303, 418
  nuclei, dorsal accessory, *11-15,* 298
    medial accessory, 298
    principal, 298
Inferior surface of hemisphere, 28–29
Inferior vestibular nucleus, 337, 417 *11-*
    21, 12-13, 12-14
Infragranular layers, cortex, 551
Infundibulum, *2-6, 15-5, 16-1, 16-5, 16-7,*
    16-9, 45, 64, 438, 478, 482,
    488–490, 493–494, 613
Inhibition, of neural activity, 269
  cochlea, *12-11,* 332–333
  reticular formation, 269, 388–389
Innervation, autonomic, *8-1, 8-3,* 192–
    212
  arrector pili muscles, *6-2,* 196
  bladder, 8–11, 211–212
  cutaneous blood vessels, *8-2,* 196
  dura, 6, 353
  eye, 210–211, 382 384
  gastrointestinal tract, 196–199, 8-1
  heart, 196, 198, 312
  lungs and bronchi, 196, 198
  rectum, 197–198
  submandibular and lacrimal glands,
    198, 348
  sweat glands, 205
motor, anal sphincter, 168
  diaphragm, 167
  facial muscles, *12-15,* 348–349
    pyramidal (corticobulbar), 316,
      348
    nonpyramidal, 349, 586–587
  larynx and pharynx, 312
  lower extremity, *7-16,* 180–181
  masticatory muscles, *12-17,* 360
  neck, 167, 308–309
  peripheral, *7-15, 7-19, 7-20,* 168–185,
    segmental, *7-16, 7-17, 7-18,* 164–168
  shoulder, 167, 175, 309
  tongue, 305–308
  upper extremity, *7-14, 7-15,* 167
peripheral of, plexus, brachial, *7-14, 7-*
    15, 173–177
  cervical, 169–173
  lumbar, *7-19,* 181
  lumbosacral, *7-20,* 181–185
  sacral, 181
rami, dorsal, 162
  ventral, 162
Insula (island of Reil), *2-11, 3-16,* 24–26,
    577, 609
Interbrain, *see* Diencephalon
Interhemispheric, commissure, *2-4, 2-7,*
    2-12, 32, 591–592
  fissure, *21-22*
  transfer, 591–592
  gnostic activity, 591
    interocular transfer, 591
  learning, 591–592
    memory, 591–592
    motor, 591
    somesthetic, 591
    visual, 591–592
  visual discrimination, 591–592
Intermediate, acoustic stria, 330
  gray (substance), *9-7,* 226–227, 231
  nerve (Wrisberg), *2-5, 12-2, 12-15,* 347

Intermediolateral cell column, *8-1, 9-10,*
    9-11, 9-12, 9-22, 195, 227,
    230–231
Internal, arcuate fibers, *10-1, 11-8,* 240,
    292
  cerebral veins, *20-19, 20-20,* 627–630
  facial genu, *12-1, 12-7, 12-15,* 323, 347,
    350
Internal capsule, *2-8, 2-9, 2-13, 2-14, 15-*
    17, 15-18, 29–31, 66–67, 462–
    465, 615–616
  blood supply, 615–616, *20-12*
  genu, *2-9,* 30, 464, *15-17, 15-18*
  lesions, 463–465
  limb anterior, *2-9, 15-17, 15-18,* 29, 30,
    67, 464
    posterior, *2-9, 15-17, 15-18,* 29, 30, 67,
      464–465
  optic radiation, *15-18, 15-21, 15-22,* 30,
    463, 466–469, 566–568
  retrolenticular portion, *15-18,* 464
  sublenticular portion, *15-18,* 464
  tapetum, *2-7, 2-16,* 32, 568
Internode, nerve fibers, 97
Interoceptors, 138
Interpeduncular, fossa, *2-17, 13-4, 13-17,*
    42, 379, 620
  nucleus, *13-3, 13-4, 13-10, 13-17,* 369,
    438
Intersegmental reflexes, *9-23,* 272
Interstitial nucleus, Cajal, 264, 270,
    379–380, *13-12, 13-13, 13-14,*
    13-15
  of vestibular nerve, 339, *12-14*
Interthalamic adhesion, *15-10,* 45, 64, 446
Interventricular foramen, *2-15,* 43
Intralaminar nuclei, thalamus, *15-5, 15-*
    6, 15-11, 15-12, 17-6, 17-8, 45,
    446–451, 474–477, 592–593
Intraparietal sulcus, *2-2,* 24
Intraperiod line, 96
Intrinsic, eye muscles, 209–210, 382–
    384
  nuclei of cerebellum, *12-16, 14-13,* 399,
    414–416
Island of Reil, *see* Insula
Isocortex (homogenetic cortex), *19-9, 19-*
    10, 547, 550–559
Isthmus, of gyri cinguli, *2-4,* 28, 544, *18-*
    13
  rhombencephali, *3-8, 3-9,* 362

Junction, medullary pontine, *11-24, 11-*
    25, 41, 318–321
  midbrain-diencephalon, *15-3, 15-4, 15-*
    5, 435–437
  spinomedullary, *11-4, 11-5, 11-6,* 286–
    297
Juxtallocortex, *18-13,* 544
Juxtarestiform body, *12-6,* 342, 424

Kaes-Bechterew, band of, 550
Kinesthetic sense (kinesthesis), 138,
    155, 240–241, 455, 472, 564
Klumpke's syndrome, 181
Klüver-Bucy syndrome, 543–545
Koniocortex, *19-7, 19-10B, 19-11,* 558
Korsakoff's psychosis, 538
  syndrome, 538

Labyrinth, *see* Vestibular end organ
Lamina, affixa, *15-6,* 45

Boldface numbers indicate principal references. *Italic* numbers refer to illustrations.

accessory medullary of pallidum, *17-7*, 498
choroidea epithelialis, 132–136
medullary of pallidum, lateral, 33, 498
medial, *17-7*, 33, 498
of thalamus, external, *15-6*, *15-12*, 442, 461
internal, *15-12*, 45, 441
of Rexed, *9-9*, *9-11*, *9-15*, *9-17*, *9-18*, 222–229
of septum pellucidum, *2-4*, *2-20*, *2-21*, 34, 525
terminalis, *2-20*, *2-21*, 49, 64, 69
Laminae of Rexed (*see also* Spinal cord cytoarchitecture), *9-9*, *9-11*, *9-15*, *9-17*, *9-18*, *9-19*, 222–229
Lamination of cerebral cortex, *19-1*, *19-2*, *19-3*, *19-7*, *19-9*, *19-10*, 547–551
Lateral, antebrachial cutaneous nerve, 176
brachial cutaneous nerve, 175
cerebral sulcus, *2-3*, *3-16*, 22, 566
femoral cutaneous nerve, 183–184
gaze, mechanism of, 350
gaze paralysis, 349, 350
geniculate body, *15-3*, *15-4*, *15-14*, *15-18*, *15-21*, 45, 435, 458–461, 466–470, 566–568
lemniscus, *12-10*, *12-23*, *13-2*, 329, 331, 368
recess of fourth ventricle, 10, 39–41
sural cutaneous nerve, 184
tracts, corticospinal, *10-13*, 255–261
spinothalamic, *10-7*, *10-8*, 245–249
ventricle, *2-6*, *2-15*, *2-22*, 34, 36, 132, 497, 530, *15-16*
Lateral surface of hemisphere, 22–26, *2-1*, *2-2*
Lateral vestibular nucleus, 264–266, *10-19*, 337, 424–425, *12-14*
Layer(s) of cerebellar cortex, *14-2*, *14-3*, *14-4*, *14-5*, 401–404
granular, *3-11*, *14-3*, 402–404
molecular, *14-4*, 401
Purkinje, *14-6*, 401–402
of cerebral cortex, *19-1*, *19-2*, *19-3*, *19-7*, *19-9*, *19-10*, 550–551
fusiform, 550
ganglionic, 550
granular, external, 550
internal, 550
infragranular, 551
molecular, 550
multiform, 550
plexiform, 550
pyramidal, 550
supragranular, 551
neural tube, 50–51
ependymal (nuclear), *3-3A*, *3-3B*, 50
mantle, *3-3A*, *3-3B*, 50, 51
marginal, *3-3A*, *3-3B*, 50, 51
retina, *15-19*, *15-20*, 465
superior colliculus, *13-5*, *13-6*, 370–372
Lemniscal system(s), 391
Lemniscus, lateral, *12-10*, *12-23*, *13-2*, 329–331, 368, 398
nucleus of, *13-2*, 331, 362
medial, *10-1*, *11-8*, *11-13*, *12-1*, *12-4*, *13-1*, 240, 291–293, 360, 398, 455
lesions of, 292

Lemnocytes, *see* Neurolemma
Lenticular, fasciculus, *17-7*, *17-8*, *17-10*, *17-11*, 505
nucleus, *2-9*, *2-14*, 33, 66, 497–499, *17-4*
Leptomeninges (leptomenix), *1-5*, *1-8*, *1-9*, *1-10*, *1-12*, *9-2*, 1, 7–11, 115, 465
Lesions, abducens nerve, 349,
abducens nucleus, 349–350
axillary nerve, 175
brachial plexus, 177–181
cerebellum, 430–433
cerebral cortex, 559, 565, 568, 576–577, 581–585
cervical sympathetic trunk, 205–206, 209–210, *8-10*
cochlear, nerve, 335
pathway, 336
common peroneal nerve, 185
corpus striatum, 517–518
corticobulbar tract, *11-23*, 318, 348–349
corticospinal tract, *10-22*, 259–261, 275–276, 581–582
cutaneous nerves, lower extremity, 183–184, 185
upper extremity, 175–177
dorsal roots, *10-22*, 186, 277
facial nerve, 12–15, 348–349
fastigial nucleus, 433
femoral nerve, 183
glossopharyngeal nerve, 314
hypoglossal nerve, 308
inferior gluteal nerve, 185
internal capsule, 464–465
lemniscal systems, 392
medial lemniscus, 292
median nerve, 176
medulla, 308, 321
medullary pyramids, 308
mesencephalon, 369, 374, 382, 387, 392, 397
motor area of cortex, 581–582
musculocutaneous nerve, 176
neocerebellum, 430–431
obturator nerve, 182
oculomotor nerve, 382
optic pathway, 470, *15-23*
pons, 335, 344–345, 348–350, 357, 366
posterior white column, 241
prefrontal lobe, 598–599
premotor cortex, 583
radial nerve, 175–176
red nucleus, 387–388
reticular formation, 392–393
sciatic nerve, 184
sensory areas of cortex, 559, 565, 568, 576
spinal cord, *10-22*, *10-23*, *10-24*, *10-25*, *10-26*, 276–284
spinal nerve, 185–188
spinal trigeminal tract, 296, 357
spinothalamic tract, 245–248
substantia nigra, 397
superior gluteal nerve, 185
supplementary motor area, 584–585
thalamus, 445, 456, 470, 472
tibial nerve, 184
trigeminal nerve, 166, 356–357
ulnar nerve, 177
vagus nerve, 312
ventral roots, *10-22*, 167, 186–187,

277–278
vestibular mechanism, 344–345
visual pathways, *15-23*, 470, 568
Lesser occipital nerve, 169, *7-13*
Leucotomy, 598–599
Ligament, coccygeal, *1-6*, 7, 213
denticulate, *1-4*, *1-5*, *1-7*, 8, 308
Light reflex, pupillary, 382–384
Limbic, lobe, *18-13*, 27–28, 544
structures, 544
amygdaloid nuclear complex, *2-6*, *2-14*, *18-6*, *18-9*, *18-12*, 539–543
orbital-insular-temporal cortex, 33–34, 545–546
system, 543–546
concept, 28, 543
functions, autonomic, 545
behavioral, 545
emotion, 545
endocrine, 542
hypersexuality, 543
Klüver-Bucy syndrome, 543, 545
self-stimulation, 545
somatic, 545
lesions, 545
phylogeny, 544
Limen of insula, 26
Lingual gyrus, *2-6*, 24
Lingula, cerebellum, *14-1*, 46
Lipochrome pigment, *4-1B*, 90
Lipofuscin, *4-1B*, *8-4*, 90
Lissauer, zone of, *see* Fasciculus, dorso-lateral
Lobe(s), cerebellar, *2-23*, *2-24*, *2-25*, *2-26*, *14-1*, 46–48
flocculonodular, *2-24*, *2-26*, *14-1*, 46, 63, 399, 425, 431–432
frontal, *2-1*, *2-2*, 23, 324, 444–446, 598–599
insular, *2-3*, 24–26
limbic, *18-13*, 27, 544
occipital, *2-4*, 24, 324, 452, 566–574
olfactory, 524–527
parietal, *2-2*, 23–24, 324, 451, 454–456, 560–566
pyriform, *18-3*, 24, 524–525
temporal, *2-2*, *2-4*, *18-6*, *18-11*, 24, 28, 324, 445, 574–577
Lobotomy, 445, 598–599
Lobule (lobulus), ansiform *14-1*, 46, 400
biventer, 46
centralis, 46
insula (island of Reil), *2-3*, 24–26
paracentral, 27, 560, 578
parietal, inferior, *2-2*, 24, 595
superior, *2-2*, 24
precuneus (quadrate), *2-4*, 27
quadrangular, *14-1*, 46
semilunar, *14-1*, 46, 400
simple, *14-1*, 46, 400
Localization, somatotopic, 263, 264, 455, 563, 580
tonotopic, 328, 368, 574
topographic, 295, 298, 451, 454, 568
Locus ceruleus (nucleus pigmentosus pontis), *2-24*, *2-25*, *2-26*, 364–365, 594
Long thoracic nerve, *7-18*, 173
Longitudinal cerebral fissure, 23
Lower motor neuron, 156–158, 186, 228–230, 260, 272
lesions of, 186–188, 272–275

Boldface numbers indicate principal references. *Italic* numbers refer to illustrations.

Lumbar, cistern, *1-6*, 11
  enlargement, *9-1*, 213, 216
  plexus, *7-19*, 181–185
  puncture, 11
  segments of spinal cord, *9-1*, *9-3*, *9-5*, 220–221
Lumbosacral, plexus, *7-20*, 181–185
Luschka, foramen of, *2-15*, *20-3*, 10, 41
Luxol fast blue, 72
Lysosome, 90

Macroglia, *5-1*, *5-2*, *5-3*, *5-4*, *5-5*, 52, 117–125, 412–414
Macula, lutea, 373, 465
  sacculi, *12-12*, 336, 337
  utriculi, *12-12*, 336, 337
Magendie, foramen of, 10, 41
Major dense lines, 96, *4-19*
Mammillary, body, *2-14*, *2-17*, *2-19*, *15-1*, *15-4*, *16-1*, 37, 45, 64, 435, 478, 482–483
  connections of, *16-5*, 444, 488
  nuclei, 482–483
  peduncle, *16-5*, 485
  princeps, 488, *16-5*
Mammillotegmental tract, *16-5*, 488
Mammillothalamic tract (fasciculus of Vicq d'Azyr), *15-1*, *16-5*, *16-7*, 444, 488
Mandibular nerve, *1-10*, *2-19*, *7-13*, *12-21*, 355
Mantle layer, *3-3*, *3-6*, 50, 52, 54, 68–69, 547
Marchi, method, 71, *10-5*, 277, *14-18*
Marginal, glia, 8, 218
  layer, *3-3*, 51, 68, 547
Massa intermedia, *see* Interthalamic adhesion,
Maxillary nerve, *1-10*, *2-19*, *7-13*, *12-21*, 353
Medial, antebrachial cutaneous nerve, 173, 179, *7-18*
  brachial cutaneous nerve, 179–180, 173
  eminence, hypothalamus, 482, *16-1*, 488
  forebrain bundle, *16-5* 487–488, 541
  geniculate body, 45, 368, 457–458, *15-4*, *15-12*, 574–575
  lemniscus, *10-1*, *11-8*, *11-13*, *12-1*, *12-4*, *13-1*, 240, 291–293, 360, 367, 391, 399, 454–455, 564
    lesions of, 292
  longitudinal fasciculus, *10-21*, *11-6*, *11-14*, *12-14*, 269–270, 288, 342–344
    lesions of, 344
Medial surface of hemisphere, 26–28, *2-4*, *2-12*, *2-20*
Medial vestibular nucleus, 319, 338, *12-4*, 417
Median nerve, *7-17*, *7-18*, 176–177
Medulla oblongata (myelencephalon), *2-2*, *2-17*, *3-9*, *11-1*, *11-2*, *11-18*, 21, 60–61, 285–321
  amiculum of inferior olive, *11-21*, 299
  anatomy, 38–39, 59, 60, 285–304
  area, postrema, *11-13*, 296–297
    vestibularis, *11-2*, 297
  blood supply, *20-13*, *20-14*, 616–620
  corticospinal decussation, *11-5*, 287–

288
cranial nerves, *11-17*, *11-18*, 285, 304–314
  cochlear, *11-24*, 318, 326–329
development, *3-8*, *3-9*, 60–61, 304
functional components, *11-16*, 304–305
  glossopharyngeal, 312–314, *11-19*, *11-22*
  hypoglossal, 305–308, *11-1*, *11-14*
  spinal accessory, 308–309
  vagus, 309–312, *11-13*, *11-19*
fibers, arcuate, external, *11-8*, 253, 293
  internal, *10-1*, *11-8*, 240, 291–293
  internal, *10-1*, *11-8*, 240, 291–293
form and length, *11-1*, *11-2*, 285
fourth ventricle (see Fourth ventricle), *2-15*, *2-26*, 39–41, 60, 297
  choroid plexus, *1-11*, 132, 297
  foramen, cecum posterior, 320, *11-25*
    Luschka, *2-15*, *20-3*, 10, 41
    Magendie, 10, 41
  inferior, cerebellar peduncle, *2-19*, *10-10*, *11-13*, *11-22*, *11-24*, 41, 303–304, 414
    olivary complex, *2-19*, *11-9*, *11-13*, *11-14*, *11-15*, 297, 298–300, 418–419
  lesions, 296, 308, 318, 321
    lateral medullary syndrome, 296, 321, 617, *20-13*
    vascular, 296, 308
  levels, junction of spinal cord and medulla, *11-4*, *11-5*, *11-6*, 286–297
    midolivary, *11-22*, 297–303
    pons-medulla, *11-24*, *11-25*, 318–321
    transition from spinal cord, *11-4*, *11-5*, *11-6*, 38–39, 286–297
    upper medulla, *11-24*, 318–321
  medial lemniscus, descussation, *11-8*, 291–293
    formation, *10-1*, 240, 292
  nuclei, accessory, cuneate, *11-9*, *11-10*, *11-12*, 252, 292–293
    ambiguus, *11-9*, *11-15*, 312
    arcuate, *11-13*, *11-15*, 296
    cochlear, *11-24*, *11-25*, 318, 326–327
    cuneatus, *11-8*, *11-9*, 240, 289–291
    dorsal motor vagus, *11-9*, *11-17*, *11-18*, 311–312
    dorsal sensory vagus, *11-8*, 310
    gracilis, *11-8*, *11-9*, 240, 289–291
    intercalatus, *11-15*, 308
    lateral reticular, *11-15*, 296, 301, 418
    olivary, *see* Inferior olivary complex
    pontobulbar, *11-15*, 304
    prepositus, *11-21*, 308
    reticular formation, *11-9*, *11-15*, 296–297, 300–303
    solitarius (ventral sensory), 310, *11-20*
    vestibular, inferior, *11-21*, 297, 319, 337
      medial, *11-21*, 297, 319, 338
  obex, *11-2*, 41, 296
  perihypoglossal nuclei, 308
  pseudobulbar palsy, 318
  rhomboid fossa, *11-2*, 41, 297
  striae medullares, *11-2*, 41
  sulci, anterior median, 285
    anterolateral, 305

postolivary, 296
tract, dorsal longitudinal, *11-14*, 308
  solitarius, *11-14*, *11-16*, 310
  spinal trigeminal, 293–296, 354–357, *12-21*
trigonum, hypoglossi, *11-2*, 41, 297
  vagi, *11-2*, 41, 297
  tuberculum, cinereum, *11-2*, 289
  cuneatum, *11-2*, *11-8*, 39, 289
Medulloblastoma, 431
Meissner's corpuscle (tactile corpuscles), *6-4*, *6-7*, 144–145
  plexus (submucosal), 198
Melanin granules, 90, 364–365, 393
  pigment, *13-10*, 90, 311, 364–365, 393
Meltzer's principle, 517
Membrane, basilar, 326,
  external glial limiting, *1-9*, *3-4A*, *3-4B*, 51, 218
  internal limiting, 51, 129
  of nerve cell, *4-8*, 82–84
  perivascular limiting, 119
  plasma, 82–84
  pump, 203
  subsynaptic, 103
  superficial glial limiting, 8, 119, 218
  vestibular (Reissner's), *12-8*, 326,
Memory, 538
  associative, 595
Meningeal arteries, *20-3*, 621–622
Meninges, *1-1*, *1-2*, *1-3*, *1-4*, *1-5*, 1–14
  arachnoid, *1-5*, 9–11
  blood supply, *20-3*, 621–622
  dura mater, *1-2*, *1-3*, *1-4*, *1-5*, *1-7*, 353, 622–624, *20-16*
  innervation, 6, 353
  pia mater, *1-5*, 7–9
Mesencephalic, nucleus of N.V., *12-17*, *12-19*, *12-20*, *12-21*, *12-22*, 359–360
  tract of N.V., *12-20*, *12-21*, *12-22*, 359–360
  tract of trigeminal nerve, 352, 359
Mesencephalon (midbrain), *2-17*, *3-8*, *3-9*, *13-1*, 21, 42–43, 63–64, 367–398
  anatomy, *13-1*, 42–43, 58, 60
  blood supply, *20-14*, 620–621
  colliculi inferior, *13-2*, 42, 367–369
    superior, *13-1*, *13-5*, *13-6*, 42, 370–374
  crura cerebri, *13-1*, 42–43, 397–398
  development, 63–64
  lesions, 369, 374, 382, 384, 387, 390, 393, 396
  nerves, *13-1*, *13-11*, 42, 367, 369, 377–379
    oculomotor, *13-11*, 377–379
    trochlear, *13-3*, 369
  nuclei, cuneiformis, 388
    Darkschewitsch, *13-7*, *13-12*, *13-14*, *13-15*, 380
    dorsal tegmental, *16-5*, 369, 485
    interpeduncular, *13-3*, *13-4*, *13-10*, *13-17*, 369, 438
    interstitial (Cajal), *13-12*, *13-13*, *13-14*, *13-15*, 379–380
    oculomotor, *13-1*, *13-4*, *13-10*, *13-11*, *13-12*, *13-13*, 377–379
    anterior median, *13-11*, *13-12*, *13-13*, 378

Boldface numbers indicate principal references. *Italic* numbers refer to illustrations.

caudal central, *13-10*, **377**
Edinger-Westphal, 377
extraocular muscles, representation, *13-11*, 377
Perlia, *13-11*, 379
visceral, 377–378, *13-11*, 382–383
posterior commissure, *13-7*, *13-8*, *13-9*, *13-13*, 376–377, 437
red, *13-1*, *13-4*, *13-10*, 261–264, 384–388, 420–421
subcommissural organ, *13-9*, 129, 376
subcuneiformis, *13-9*, 388
substantia nigra, *13-18*, *13-19*, 43, 63, 393–397, 501–504, 517
pedunculopontine, *12-24*, *13-2*, 363, 389, 507–508, *17-11*
trochlear, *13-2*, *13-11*, 42, 369
ventral tegmental, *16-5*, 369, 485
posterior perforated substance, *2-17*, *20-9*, 620
pretectum, *13-7*, 374–376
reflexes, 382–384
accommodation, 383
pupillary, 382
reticular formation, 389
functional considerations, 390–395
nuclei, 389–390
superior, cerebellar peduncle, 367, 385, 420–421, *14-16*
colliculus, 370–374
syndrome, Benedikt, 387
Weber, 382
tectum, 42, 63, 367–369, 370–374
tegmentum, 42, 63, 367, 369–370, *13-1*
Mesenchyme, *see* Mesoderm
Mesocortex, 544
Mesoderm, 49, *3-2*, 164
Metameres, 164
Metathalamus, geniculate bodies, 435
lateral, *15-3*, *15-4*, *15-14*, *15-18*, *15-21*, 45, 458–461, 466–470, 567, 569, *19-15*
medial, *13-7*, *15-3*, *15-4*, 45, 457–458, 574–575
Metencephalon, *see* Pons
Method, Bodian, 72
Cajal silver, 72
Golgi, 72, *4-5*, 368, 408, 457, 462, 497, *17-5*, 551
Marchi, 71, 276, *10-5*, 14-18
Ranvier's gold chloride, 72
Weigert, 71, 276, *9-10*, *10-13*, *11-4*
Meynert's commissure (dorsal supraoptic), *16-10*, 490–491
Microcentrum, *see* Central body
Microglia, *5-3*, *5-10*, *5-11*, 117, 125–128, 412–414
Microsmatic mammals, 521, 537
Microvilli, *5-14*, *5-18*, 134
Micturition, *8-11*, 211–212
automatic, 279
overflow, 279
paralytic incontinence, 279
Midbrain, *see* Mesencephalon
Middle, cerebellar peduncle, *2-5*, *2-17*, *2-19*, *12-1*, *12-2*, *12-4*, *14-21*, 41, 324–325, 419–420
cerebral artery, *20-4*, *20-5*, *20-6*, 609, *20-7*
meningeal artery, *20-3*, 621–622
superficial cerebral *20-18*, 626

Midline nuclei of thalamus, *15-10*, *15-11*, 446–447
Mimetic facial paralysis, 349
Miosis, 210, 383
Mitochondria, *4-10*, *4-12*, *5-18*, *6-17*, 88
Mitral cells, *18-1*, *18-3*, 522–523
Mixed spinal nerve, *7-1*, 162–164
Mnemonic reactions, 595
Monoamine(s), 202
oxidase (MAO), 203
pathways, 204, 364–366, 394–396, 411, 489, 498, 501, 517, 594–595
Monoplegia, 261, 582
Mossy fibers, *14-4*, *14-5*, 406–407
rosettes, *14-5*, *14-8*, 406
Motion sickness, 345, 431
Motor, area, cortex, *19-9*, *19-12*, *19-19*, *19-20*, *19-21*, *19-23*, 578–583
end plate, *6-17*, 156–158
neuron lesions, lower (anterior horn cell), 186–188, 272–275
upper (corticospinal tract), 259–261, 275–276, *10-22*, 578–583
nuclei of anterior horn, *9-9*, *9-15*, *9-21*, 156–158, 186, 228–230, 260, 272
pathway, 255–261, *10-13*, 287–288, 397, 398, 578–583
unit, 157–158
Movement, involuntary, 514–516
voluntary, 255–261, 430–431, 578–586
Multiple sclerosis, 284, 344
Muscle(s), special visceral (*see also* Branchiomeric muscles), fibers, extrafusal 147, 160
intrafusal, *see* Muscle spindle
spindle, *6-11*, *6-12*, *6-13*, *6-14*, *9-26*, 146–149, 160, 228, 235–237, 251, 344
tone, *9-26*, *9-27*, 149, 271–272, 277, 345, 389–390, 430, 514, 516, 581–585
Musculocutaneous nerve, 176, *7-18*
Mydriasis, *8-9*, 382–384
Myelencephalon, *see* Medulla oblongata
Myelin, chemical structure, 94–96
electron microscopy, *4-17*, *4-18*, *4-20*, *4-21*, 94–96
formation, *4-19*, 96
intraperiod lined, 96, *4-19*
major dense lines, *4-19*, 96
mesaxon, external, *4-18*, 96
internal, *4-18*, 96
nodes of Ranvier, *4-15*, *4-16*, *4-17*, 96–97
remyelination, *4-30*, *4-31*, 107–114
Schmidt-Lantermann incisures, *4-15*, *4-20*, 97–99
sheath, *4-15*, 94–96
stains, *4-2*, 71–72, *9-8*, *10-4*, 276–277
Myelinated axons, 93–96, *4-18*
Myelinated nerve fibers, *4-15*, *4-16*, *4-18*, *4-19*, *4-21*, *5-5*, 93–100, 105–107, 110–114
Myenteric plexus (of Auerbach), 198
Myotatic reflex, *9-27*, 235–237, 276, 277, 281, 362, 389, 430, 581–585
Myotomes, *3-2*, 164, 166–168

Nauta-Gygax technic, 72, 277, *9-24*, *9-25*, *13-15*

Necrosis, 600, 601
Neocerebellum, 63, 400–401
lesions of, 430–431
Neopallium, 67–69, 521, 547–599, *19-1*, *19-6*
Neostriatum, *17-3*, *17-4*, *17-6*, 33, 66–67, 396, 451, 496–504, 589
Nerve, abducens (VI), *12-1*, *12-7*, 349–351
accessory (XI), *2-5*, *11-1*, *11-17*, *11-18*, *11-19*, 308–309
acoustic (VIII), *12-8*, *12-10*, *11-24*, 318, 326–329
ansa cervicalis, 172
axillary, *7-17*, *7-18*, 175
calcaneal, lateral, 184
medial, 184
cardiac, inferior cervical, 196
middle cervical, 196
superior cervical, 196
carotid sinus, 313
cell, *see separate listing*
chorda tympani, *12-15*, 347
clunial, inferior, 185
medial, 169
superior, 169
cochlear (VIII), *11-24*, *12-10*, 318, 326–329
common peroneal, 185
conduction, 101–103
cutaneous, anterior femoral, 182, *7-11*, *7-12*, *7-13*
lateral antebrachial, 176
lateral brachial, 175
lateral femoral, 183–184
lateral sural, 184
dorsal, scapular, 173
eighth, *see* cochlear
eleventh, *see* accessory
endings, *see separate listing*
facial (VII), *2-5*, *12-15*, 346–349
fascicles, 162–164
femoral, 182–183, *7-11*
fibers, *see separate listing*
fifth, *see* trigeminal
first, *see* olfactory
fourth, *see* trochlear
genitofemoral, 181, 183, *7-19*
glossopharyngeal (IX), *2-5*, *11-1*, 11–17, 11–18, 11–19, *11-21*, 312–314
great auricular, 169, *7-13*
greater occipital, 169, *7-13*
greater splanchnic, 197
growth factor, 113
to hamstrings, 184
hypoglossal (XII), *2-5*, *2-17*, *2-19*, *11-1*, *11-14*, *11-17*, *11-18*, *11-19*, 305–308
iliohypogastric, 181, *7-19*
ilioinguinal, 181, *7-19*
iliopsoas, 181, *7-19*
inferior, gluteal, 185
laryngeal, 308
intercostobrachial, 177
intermediate (of Wrisberg), *2-5*, *12-2*, *12-15*, 347
lateral femoral cutaneous, 183–184
lesser occipital, 169, *7-13*
lesser splanchnic, 197
long thoracic, 173
mandibular, 353, **360**

Boldface numbers indicate principal references. *Italic* numbers refer to illustrations.

Nerve—*Continued*
maxillary, 353, *7-13*
medial, antebrachial cutaneous, 173
  brachial cutaneous, 173
median, 176–177, *7-15*
mixed, 162–164, *7-1*
musculocutaneous, 176
ninth, *see* glossopharyngeal
obturator, 182
oculomotor (III), 2–5, *13-11*, 377–379
olfactory, (I), *2-5, 18-1*, 521–522
ophthalmic, 353, 360
optic (II), *2-5, 2-6, 15-21*, 465–466
pectoral, lateral, 173
  medial, 173
pelvic, *8-11*, 198, 211
peroneal, common, 185
  superficial, 185
phrenic, 169
plantar, lateral, 184
  medial, 184
posterior, antebrachial cutaneous, 175
  brachial cutaneous, 175
  femoral cutaneous, 185
pudendal (pudic), 211
radial, *7-17, 7-18*, 175–176
  superficial, 176
recurrent laryngeal, 312
saphenous, 182
sciatic, *7-7, 7-20*, 184
second, *see* optic
seventh, *see* facial
sinus, 313
sixth, *see* abducens
splanchnic, 197,
  smallest, 197
spinal, *7-1*, 159–164
subclavius, 173
suboccipital, 169
subscapular, 173
superficial ramus, of radial, 175
  of ulnar, 177
superior gluteal, 185
supraclavicular, *7-13*, 169
suprascapular, 173
sural, 184
tenth, *see* vagus
third, *see* oculomotor
thoracodorsal, 173
tibial, 184–185, *7-20*
transverse colli, 169
trigeminal (V), *2-5, 12-17, 12-19, 12-20, 12-21*, 352–360
trochlear (IV), *2-5, 11-18*, 42, 369
twelfth, *see* hypoglossal
ulnar, 177, *7-15*
vagus (X), *2-5, 11-16, 11-17, 11-18*, 198, 309–312
vestibular (VIII), *12-12, 12-13, 12-14*, 336–342
vestibulocochlear, *2-5, 11-18, 12-12*, 325–345
of Wrisberg (intermediate), *12-2, 12-15*, 347–348
Nerve cell (*see also* Neuron), *4-1, 4-3, 4-4, 4-5*, 71–93
  body, 82–91, *4-4, 4-5*
  nucleus, *4-9*, 84
  plasma membrane, *4-8*, 82–84
  reaction of degeneration, 187
  structure, *4-8*, 71–93
Nerve endings (*see also* Receptor and Ef-

fector), afferent fibers, *6-2, 6-3*, 137–155
corpuscles, of Golgi-Mazzoni, 144–146
  of Meissner, 144–145
  of Ruffini, 143
efferent fibers, 156–158
  motor end plates, *6-17, 6-18*, 156
  somatic efferent, *6-17, 6-18*, 156–158
  visceral efferent, *6-18*, 158
encapsulated, 144–146
end bulbs, *6-8*, 143, 145
free, 142–143
genital corpuscles, 145
intraepithelial, *6-5*, 142
Meissner's corpuscles, *6-4, 6-7*, 144–145
neuromuscular spindles, *6-12, 6-13, 6-14, 9-26, 9-17*, 146–149, 235–237
neurotendinous organs (Golgi), 149–153, *6-15, 6-16*
Pacinian corpuscles, *6-9, 6-10*, 145–146

peritrichial, 6–2, 142
tactile discs, *6-4*, 143
Nerve fibers, adrenergic, *8-7*, 202–204
arcuate, of cerebral cortex, *2-11*, 31
dorsal, external, 253
  internal, *10-1*, 240, 291–293
association, *2-11*, 29, 31–32, 547
autonomic, *10-21, 10-26*, 192–200
  descending, *10-26*, 207, 271, 488
branchiomeric, 60–61, 304–305
climbing, *14-4, 14-5*, 407–411
collaterals of, 110, 232–235, 301
commissural, of hemisphere, *2-7, 2-16*, 29, 32, 69–70, 590–592
conduction of impulses by, 97, 101
  action potential, 101
  afterpotential, negative, 101
    positive, 101
  saltatory transmission, 97
  spike potential, 101
degeneration of, *4-26, 4-27*, 105–107
  chromatolysis, *4-28*, 107
  Schwann cells, *4-21*, 107, 188
  secondary (Wallerian), 105–107, *4-26*, 276–277, *10-22*
efferent, peripheral, 159–161
  somatic, *3-7, 9-21*, 57, 229–230
  visceral, *3-7*, 57, 230–231
    postganglionic, *3-7, 8-1*, 57, 192–195
    preganglionic, *3-7, 8-1*, 57, 192–195
functional types of, *9-22*, 57, 229–231, 304–305, *11-16, 11-17, 11-18*
internuclear, 350
intrafusal, 146–149, *6-11*
length of, 241
mossy, 406–407, *14-8*
myelinated, *4-16, 4-20, 4-21*, 93–100, 105–107, 110–114
noradrenergic, *4-13, 8-6, 8-7*, 202–203, 205, 209, 364–365, 411, 594–595
peripheral, 168–185
physiological grouping, 101–103
postganglionic, *8-1, 8-2*, 193–195
preganglionic, *8-1, 8-5*, 193–195
projection, 29, 548,
radial, of cerebral cortex, *19-1*, 549,

555, 578–585
regeneration of, *4-31*, 107–114, 188–190
nervous system, central, 112
  peripheral, 107–114, 188–190
of Remak, 100–103
root, dorsal, *7-6*, 159–162
  ventral, *7-6*, 160, 162–164
sheath of, 99–100, 164
size of, 101
somatic, *3-7*, 57, 159–164, 229–235
spinal, *7-1*, 56, 159–164
tangential, of cerebral cortex, *19-1*, 549
types of, 100–103
unmyelinated, *7-6*, 100–101, 193
of vagus, *11-16*, 309–312
visceral, *3-7*, 57, 192–206, *8-1*
Nervous system, autonomic, *8-1*, 191–212
afferent fibers, 199
central nuclei, 206–207
  brain stem, 207, 487–488
  hypothalamus, *16-1*, 207, 478–495
  innervation of urinary bladder, *8-11*, 211–212
  spinal cord, *9-2, 9-5, 9-6*, 230–231
central pathways, *10-1, 10-7, 10-8, 10-10, 10-13*, 206–207
chemical transmitters, 200–205, *8-6*, 364–366, 394–396, 411, 489, 517, 594–595
functional considerations, 208–212, 364–366, 394–396, 517, 544–546, 594–595
ganglia, structure of, 199–200
nerve fibers, adrenergic, 202–204
  cholinergic, *8-7*, 201–202
  postganglionic, 192–195
  preganglionic, 192–195
  rami communicantes, *8-1*, 195–196
    gray, *8-2*, 196
    white, *8-2*, 195
outflow, cranial, *8-1, 11-17, 11-18*, 197–198
  facial nerve, *12-1, 12-15*, 348
  glossopharyngeal nerve, *11-17, 11-18*, 313–314
  oculomotor, *13-11*, 377–379, 382–384
  vagus, *11-17, 11-18*, 311–312
  sacral, *8-1*, 198
  thoracolumbar (sympathetic), *8-1*, 195–197
  parasympathetic (craniosacral), *8-1*, 197–198
  peripheral ganglia and nerve fibers, 192–199
  sympathetic, *8-1*, 195–197
central, 21,
ganglia, autonomic, *8-1, 8-3*, 192–199
  parasympathetic (craniosacral), *8-1*, 197–198
  ciliary, 197, 379
  otic, 197, 314
  pterygopalatine, *12-15*, 197, 348
  sacral, 198
  submandibular, *12-15*, 348
  terminal, 193
  sympathetic, 195–197
  celiac, 197

Boldface numbers indicate principal references. *Italic* numbers refer to illustrations.

cervical, 196
  inferior, 196
  middle, 196
  superior, 196
inferior mesenteric, 197
  paravertebral, 193, 196, 8-2
  prevertebral, 193, 195, 8-2
  stellate, 8-1, 195
nerves, inferior mesenteric, 197
  pelvic, 8-11, 211
  splanchnic, 197
    greater, 197
    lesser, 197
neurons, postganglionic, 192–197
  preganglionic, 192–195, 230–231,
    311–312, 314, 348, 377–378
peripheral, 21, 137, 161–190
plexus, celiac, 197
  enteric, 198
  hypogastric, 197
  myenteric (Auerbach) 198
  pelvic, 198
  submucosal (Meissner), 198
regeneration (central), 112–114
synapses, 103–105, 4-25
  adrenergic fibers, 202–204
  chemical mediation 200–205
  cholinergic, 200–202
syndrome, Horner's, 10-26, 210–283,
    384
vegetative, 191–212, 8-1
visceral, 191–212, 8-1, 230–231
Networks, 204, 8-7
  neurokeratin, 99
  terminals, 204
Neural, crest, 3-2, 49–50
  folds, 3-1C, 49
  groove, 3-1B, 3-2B, 3-2C, 49,
  plate, 3-1A, 3-2A, 49
  tube, 3-1C, 3-2D, 3-2E, 49–51
Neuroanatomical methods, 4-1, 4-2, 71–
    77
Neuroblast, 3-4B, 3-5, 51
  apolar, 51
  bipolar, 51
  multipolar, 51
Neuroepithelial cell, 3-4A, 3-4B, 51, 143
Neurofibrils, 4-11, 85–88
Neurofilaments, 86
Neuroglia, 115–128, 412–414
  astrocyte, 1-15, 5-1, 5-2, 5-3, 5-11, 118–
    122
    fibrous, 119–120, 3-5, 5-3, 5-4A, 5-12
    protoplasmic, 120–122, 3-5, 5-3, 5-
      4B, 5-12
    velate, 412
  of cerebellum, 14-11, 412–414
  ependyma, 5-12, 5-13, 5-14, 128–132
  fibers, 119
  functions, 116, 121
  gliosomes, 120, 5-4
  Golgi epithelial cell, 5-18, 56, 412
  histogenesis, 3-5, 52
  macroglia
    astrocytes, 5-1, 5-2, 118–122
    oligodendrocytes, 5-7, 5-8, 5-9, 122–
      125
  microglia, 5-10, 125–128
Neurohypophysis, 16-1, 16-9, 64, 488, 493
Neurokeratin, network, 99, 4-15
Neurolemma, see Schwann sheath
Neuroma, traumatic, 4-29, 188

Neuromuscular, junction, 103, 156–158
  spindles, 6-11, 146–149, 9-26, 9-27
Neuron(s), 4-1, 4-3, 4-4, 4-5, 8-6, 51–52,
    77–100
  afferent peripheral, 161
  anterior horn, 57, 228–230, 9-21
  association, 55, 221
  autonomic, 8-3, 50, 55, 192–198, 230–
    231
  axon, 4-5, 4-11, 4-15, 4-18, 77, 80, 84,
    93–94
    hillock, 93
  binucleated, 199
  bipolar, 55, 77, 199, 4-3, 4-6, 327, 337
  bi- and trinucleated, 84
  body, (perikaryon), 4-1, 4-4, 4-5, 4-6, 4-
    7, 82–84
  central (intermediate), 55, 221
  collaterals, 9-23, 229, 301–302
  commissural, 55, 69–70, 221, 547
  dendrite, 4-4, 4-5, 77, 103–105
  differentiation, 55–56, 3-5
  doctrine, 71,
  efferent peripheral, 53, 160, 229–231
  form of, 77–82
  functional concept, 77
  functional types, 9-23, 11-16, 11-18, 56–
    57, 304–305
  gamma motor, 9-21, 147–148, 229, 9-
    22, 235, 9-27
  gemmules of, 78, 402
  histogenesis, 3-5, 51–52, 55–57
  internuncial, 221
  lower motor, 156–158, 186, 228–230,
    260, 272–275
  multipolar, 4-1B, 4-1C, 51, 77
  neurofibrils, 4-11, 85–88
  neurosecretory, 91, 482, 488, 493
  Nissl bodies, 4-10, 82–84, 85
  nucleus, 4-9, 84
  plasma membrane of, 4-18, 82
  posterior horn, 9-6, 9-7, 223–226, 231
  postganglionic, 192–195, 8-1, 195–199
  preganglionic, 192–195, 8-1, 198, 230–
    231
  relationship, 71, 77, 103–105
  sensory, 7-4, 55, 161–162, 223–226,
    231
  shape and size of, 4-4, 77–82
  somatic efferent, 80, 228–230
  structure, 4-6, 4-7, 4-8, 71–105
  trinucleated, 84,
  unipolar, 4-1A, 77, 161
  upper motor, 260, 275–276, 314–318,
    11-23
  varieties, 4-3, 77–82
  visceral, 80, 199–200, 230–231
Neuronophagia, 126–128, 5-11
Neuropil, 5-1, 115–125
Neuroplasm (axoplasm), 4-26, 4-31, 82,
    86–88, 93–94, 111–114
Neuropodia (end feet) (boutons termi-
    naux), 4-23, 103–105
Neuropore, anterior, 3-1C, 49
  posterior, 3-1, 49
Neurosecretion, 91, 200–205, 482, 488–
    490, 493–494
Neurotendinous organs (Golgi), 6-15, 6-
    16, 9-26, 9-27, 149–153, 251–
    252
Neurotransmitter, 91, 200–205, 364–
    366, 394–396, 411, 489, 517,

593–595
Neurotubules, 4-17, 86–87, 111
Nigral efferent fibers, 396–397, 501–
    504
  nigrostriatal, 13-19, 17-6, 17-14, 396–
    397, 501–504
  nigrothalamic, 13-19, 397
Ninth cranial nerve, 1-4, 11-1, 11-16, 11-
    17, 11-18, 11-21, 312–314
Nissl bodies, 4-1, 4-9, 4-10, 84–86, 90
  chromatolysis, 107
  electron microscopic study, 85
  granules, 4-10, 85–86
  material, 84–86
Node of Hensen, 3-1, 49
Node of Ranvier, 4-15, 93, 96–97
  electronmicroscopy of, 4-16, 96–97
  internodal length, 97, 110
Nodosal ganglion (see Ganglion, vagus,
    inferior), 11-19, 199, 309
Nodulus, 4-26, 14-1, 46, 63, 399, 431
Nonspecific thalamocortical relation-
    ships, 451, 474–477, 592–593
  association cortex, 474, 595–599
  cortical electrical activity, 451, 453,
    473
    local, 593, 595
    microelectrical analysis, 593
    recruiting response, 453, 474–477,
      592–593
    dendritic activity, 592–593
    sleep, 593–595
Noradrenalin, 91, 202–204, 364–366,
    411, 594–595
Norepinephrine, 91, 202–204, 364–366,
    411, 594–595
  containing neurons, 366, 411, 594–595
Notch, preoccipital, 2-2, 24
  tentorial, 1-2, 1
Nuclear complex, amygdaloid, 18-12, 33–
    34, 539–543
  oculomotor, 13-11, 42, 377–379
  trigeminal, 12-20, 12-21, 12-22, 354–
    360
  vestibular, 12-13, 12-14, 337–339
Nuclear pores, 84
Nuclei reticularis pontis, pars caudalis,
    267, 322, 351, 389, 12-1
  pars oralis, 267, 322, 351, 389, 12-19
Nucleolar satellite, 4-7, 84
Nucleolus, 4-7, 84
Nucleus (nuclei), 84
  abducens nerve, 12-1, 12-2, 12-3, 323,
    349–351
  accessory cuneate, 11-8, 11-10, 292,
    417–418
  accessory nerve, 11-17, 11-18, 308–309
  accessory oculomotor, 13-7, 13-12, 13-
    13, 13-14, 376, 379–380
  accumbens septi, A-24, 394, 483
  ambiguus, 11-9, 11-16, 11-18, 297, 312
  amygdaloid (nuclear complex), 2-6, 2-
    14, 18-6, 18-12, 33–34, 539–
    543
  ansa lenticularis, 17-10, 511
  anterior horn, 3-6, 4-1E, 5-6, 9-8, 9-21,
    228–230
  anterior median, 13-11, 13-12, 378
  anterior, of thalamus, 15-1, 15-8, 15-12,
    443–444, 473
  anterior olfactory, 18-3, 523
  arcuate, 11-14, 11-21, 92, 296, 482, 489

Nucleus—*Continued*
hypothalamus, 92, 482, *16-1*, 488–490
association, of thalamus, 45, 474, *15-12*
basal magnocellular, *9-12*, 231
Bechterew (superior vestibular nucleus) *12-7*, 338–339
branchiomotor, of facial nerve, *11-17, 11-18, 12-15*, 347
caudal, central, *13-10*, 377
caudate, *2-9, 2-10, 2-13, 17-4*, 33, 66, 496–497, 499–504
central, magnocellular, of thalamus, *see* centromedian
centrodorsal, 231
centromedian-parafascicular nuclear complex, *15-5, 15-6, 15-11, 15-12*, 447–451, 474–477, 592–593
cochlear, dorsal, *11-12, 11-24, 11-25, 12-10*, 318, 327, 330
ventral, *11-25, 12-5, 12-10*, 327, 330
commissural, of vagus nerve, *11-9*, 310
cornucommissural, 231
cuneate, *10-1, 10-2, 11-7*, 240, 289–293
accessory, *11-8, 11-10*, 241, 292–293
Darkschewitsch, *13-7, 13-12, 13-14, 13-15*, 379–380, 388
Deiters' (lateral vestibular), *10-18, 10-19, 12-1, 12-2, 12-3, 14-19, 14-20*, 264–267, 337–338, 421–425
dentate, *12-16, 14-12, 14-13, 14-16, 17-2*, 48, 63, 363, 414–415, 420–421, 454, 473
dorsal cochlear, 318, 327, 330
dorsal, of Clarke, *9-7, 9-11, 9-24, 10-10*, 227, 231, 249, 252
motor, of vagus nerve, *11-9, 11-14, 11-15, 11-17, 11-18*, 198, 311–312
paramedian reticular, *11-15*, 301, 418
raphe, *12-4*, 365–366
sensory, or vagus nerve, *11-14*, 310
tegmental, *12-24*, 365, 369–370
dorsomedial, of thalamus, *15-6, 15-9, 15-10, 15-12*, 444–446, 474, 598
Edinger-Westphal, *13-11*, 377–378, 382
emboliform, *12-16, 14-13, 14-17*, 46, 63, 385, 415, 420, 425
eminentiae teretis, 297, 322, *11-2*
external preolivary, 331
facial nerve, *12-1, 12-15*, 346–347
fasciculus solitarius, *11-13, 11-17, 11-18, 11-20*, 310, 347
fastigial, *12-16, 14-13, 14-19, 14-20*, 48, 63, 415–416, 422–425, 433
Forel's field (prerubral), *17-8, 17-9, 17-10, 17-11*, 437, 508, 511–512
gelatinous substance, *9-7, 9-8, 9-14, 9-17, 9-19*, 223–224, 231
geniculate, lateral, *15-3, 15-4, 15-14, 15-18, 15-21*, 45, 435, 458–461, 466–470, 569
medial, *13-7, 15-3, 15-4*, 45, 435, 457–458, 574
globose, *12-16, 14-13*, 48, 63, 415
gracilis, *10-1, 11-6, 11-7, 11-8, 11-12*, 240, 289–290

gustatory, 310, 313, 347
habenular, *2-18, 2-22, 15-5, 16-5*, 43, 64, 437, 438, 439
hypoglossal nerve, *11-1, 11-14, 11-17, 11-18*, 305–308
hypothalamic, anterior, *16-1*, 482
arcuate, 92, 482, *16-1*, 488–490
dorsomedial, *16-1, 16-2*, 482
lateral, *16-1, 16-2*, 478–479, 488
paraventricular, 482, 493
posterior, 482, *16-1, 16-2, 16-3*, 492
suprachiasmatic, *16-1*, 482
supraoptic, *16-1, 16-2, 16-3*, 479–482, 488, 493
ventromedial, *16-3*, 482, 494
inferior central (of raphe), *11-24*, 365,
inferior colliculus, *2-18, 2-19, 12-10, 13-2*, 42, 332, 367–369
inferior vestibular, 337, *11-22*
intercalatus, *11-15*, 308
intermediolateral, *8-1, 9-10, 9-11, 9-12, 9-22*, 227, 230–231
intermediomedial, 227
interpeduncular, *13-3, 13-4*, 369–370
interposed, 63, 415
interstitial (of Cajal), *13-12, 13-13, 13-14, 13-15*, 270, 379–380
intralaminar, *15-5, 15-6, 15-11, 15-12, 17-6, 17-8*, 447–451, 474–477, 592–593
lateral cervical, *10-9*, 248
lateral lemniscus, *12-10, 12-23, 13-2*, 362–363
lateral reticular medulla, *11-8, 11-9, 11-13*, 296, 301
lateral, of thalamus, *15-12*, 451–452
dorsal, 451
posterior, 452
lateral vestibular, 264–267, 337
lenticular, *2-9, 2-14, 17-3, 17-4*, 33, 66, 497–499
magnocellularis, 231
basalis, 231
centralis, 231
pericornualis, 251
mammillary, *2-5, 2-6, 2-17, 15-1, 15-5, 16-1, 16-5*, 45, 444, 478, 482
intercalatus, *16-2*, 482
lateral, *16-2*, 482
medial, *16-2*, 482
medial eminence, *2-5*, 92, 482, 488
medial vestibular, 269–270, 338
median central, 447
mesencephalic, of V, *12-17, 12-19, 12-20, 12-21, 12-22*, 359–360
midline, of thalamus, 446
motor, of facial nerve, *12-1, 12-3, 12-4*, 347
of N.VII, 323, 347
of spinal cord, *9-9, 9-11, 9-15, 9-22*, 228–230
of trigeminal nerve, *12-17, 12-19, 12-20, 12-21, 12-22*, 41, 352–360
oculomotor complex, *13-11*, 377–379
olfactory, anterior, *18-3*, 522–523
olivary, inferior, *2-19, 11-9, 11-13, 11-14, 11-15*, 298–300
accessory, dorsal, *11-14*, 298
medial, *11-14*, 298
superior, *12-3, 12-4, 12-10*, 330–331
parabducens, 350–351

parabigeminal, *13-1*, 369
paracentralis, *15-10*, 447, 451, 500,
parafascicularis, *15-11*, 447–448, 500–501
paratenial, 446
paraventricular of thalamus, *15-11*, 446, 482
pedunculopontine, *12-24, 13-3, 363*, 507
pericornualis anterior, 251
perihypoglossal, *11-15*, 308
periolivary, lateral, 333
medial, 333
peripeduncular, *13-10*, 394
Perlia, 379
pigmentosus pontis (locus ceruleus) *12-24, 12-25, 12-26*, 364–365, 411, 594
pontine, *12-1, 12-2, 12-3, 12-4*, 62, 324–325, 419–420, 586–587
pontobulbar, *11-15*, 304
posterior commissure, *13-7, 13-13*, 375–376
posteromarginal, *9-8, 9-9, 9-14*, 223, 231
pregeniculate, 458
preolivary, 331
preoptic periventricular, 479, *16-1*, 541
lateral, 479
medial, 479
prepositus, *11-12*, 308
prerubral field (tegmental) *17-8, 17-10, 17-11*, 437
principal sensory N.V. *12-17, 12-19, 12-20, 12-21*, 357–359
proper sensory, *9-8, 9-10, 9-12*, 224, 231
proprius, of anterior horn, 228–230
of posterior horn, *9-8, 9-10, 9-12*, 231–232
pulvinar, *15-4, 15-5, 15-12*, 451–452, 474
raphe, *11-24*, 365–366, 594
dorsal, 365,
pontis, 365,
red, *see separate listing*
relay, of thalamus, *15-12, 15-13*, 470–474
reticular, see Reticular formation
reticular of thalamus, *15-6, 15-10, 15-11*, 461–462
reticularis pontis oralis, 267, 351, *12-19*
reticularis tegmenti pontis, 267, 351
reticulotegmental, *12-24*, 363, 419
reuniens, *15-10*, 446
rhomboidal, 446
Roller, *11-15*, 308
ruber, *see* Red nucleus
sacral autonomic, 198, 211–212, 230–231
salivatory, inferior, *11-17, 11-18*, 314
superior, *11-17, 11-18*, 348
sensorius principalis, 357–359, *12-19*
septal, *16-5, 16-8, 18-4*, 483, 525
spinal trigeminal, *12-20, 12-21*, 288, 294–296, 354–357
spinal vestibular, *11-21, 12-13, 12-14*, 337
subceruleus, 364
subthalamic, *15-5, 15-6, 17-8, 17-12, 17-13*, 67, 509–511
superior, central, *12-24*, 352, 365,

Boldface numbers indicate principal references. *Italic* numbers refer to illustrations.

salivatory, **348**
sensory (principal N.V.), *12-19, 12-20, 12-21*, **357-359**
vestibular, **337-339**, *12-13*
suprachiasmatic, *16-1*, **466**, 482
supraoptic, of hypothalamus, *16-1, 16-3*, **482**, 493
supraspinal, *11-5*, 287
tegmental, dorsal, *16-5*, **365**, 369
peduncolopontine, *12-24, 13-3*, **363**, **507-508**
ventral, *16-5*, **369**
tegmental field (subthalamic reticular), 512
thalamic, *15-10, 15-11, 15-12*, 45, **440-462**, 470-477
thoracicus, *9-7, 9-11, 9-24, 10-10*, **227**, **231**
trapezoid, *12-3*, 331
triangular, *see* vestibular, medial
trigeminal, mesencephalic, *12-17, 12-19, 12-20, 12-21, 12-22*, **359-360**
motor, *12-17*, **360**
spinal, *12-20, 12-21, 12-22*, **294-296**, **354-357**
superior sensory (principal N.V.), *12-17, 12-19, 12-20*, **357-359**
trochlear nerve, *13-3*, 369
tuberal, *16-7*, 478
tuberomammillary, *16-7*, 478
ventral cochlear, 318, 327
ventral, of thalamus, *15-12*, **452-456**
anterior, *15-8*, **452-454**
lateral, *15-9*, 454
posterior, *15-6*, **454-456**
posterior inferior, 456
posterolateral, **454-455**, 561
posteromedial, **455-456**, 561
Nucleus, red (ruber), *10-17, 13-1, 13-4, 13-10*, **261-264**, **384-388**
cytology, 261, **384-385**
fibers, afferent, *14-17*, 263, 385
efferent, *10-17, 14-17*, **261-264**, **385-387**
lesions, experimental, 387
syndrome of Benedikt, 387
somatotopic features, 263, **385-386**
vagus nerve, *11-17, 11-18*, **309-312**
ventral tegmental decussation, *10-17*, 261, 386
vestibular, inferior, *11-21, 12-13, 12-14*, **337**, 417
lateral, *10-18, 10-19, 12-6, 12-13, 12-14*, **264-267**, **337-338**, **423-424**
cell group *f*, 337
medial, *12-4, 12-13, 12-14*, **269-270**, 338
superior, *12-13, 12-14, 12-16*, **338-339**
Nystagmus, 344, 345
monocular, 344

Obturator nerve, *7-19*, **181-182**
Occipital, lobe, *2-2, 2-4, 2-6, 2-10, 2-12*, 24, *15-21*, 463, **466-470**, **566-574**
vein, *20-19*, 629
Occipitopontine tract, *13-1*, 324, **586-587**
Ocular movements, 344, **349-350**, 368, **377-379**

Oculomotor nerve, *1-10, 13-1, 13-4, 13-11, 13-12, 13-13*, 42, **377-379**
lesions of, 382
nuclei, anterior median, *13-12, 13-13*, 378
caudal central, *13-4*, 377
Edinger-Westphal, *13-11*, 377
extraocular muscles, representation, *13-11*, 377
lateral cell columns, 377, *13-11*
Perlia, 379
reflexes, **382-384**
root, *13-4*, 379
Oculomotor nuclear complex, *13-1, 13-4, 13-11, 13-12, 13-13*, **377-379**
extraocular muscles, *13-11*, 305, 316, **377-379**
intrinsic eye muscles, **382-384**
Olfactory, bulb, histology, *18-1, 18-2*, 29, **522-523**
glomeruli, *18-1*, 522
mitral cells, *18-1*, 522
tufted cells, 522
cortex, primary, 523
secondary, 526
pathways, *18-1, 18-2, 18-3, 18-4, 18-5, 18-11*, **521-529**
receptors, *18-1*, **521-522**
reflex connections, *18-4, 18-5*, **525-526**
tract, *18-2*, 29, 523
structures, basal, *see separate listing*
system, clinical considerations, **527-529**
hallucinations, 529
hallucinate fits, 529
lesions, 529
pathways, **523-527**, *18-4*
Olfactory structures, basal, *18-2*
amygdaloid nuclear complex, *2-6, 2-14, 18-6, 18-12*, 33-34, 496, **539-543**
anterior olfactory nucleus, *18-1, 18-3*, 523
anterior perforated substance, *18-2, 20-9*, 29, 483, 524, 612
archipallium, *18-6*, **521**, **530-539**
diagonal band of Broca, *18-2, 18-4*, 524
entorhinal area, *18-11*, **525-526**
fila olfactoria, *18-1*, 521
hippocampal formation, *18-6, 18-7, 18-8, 18-9, 18-10, 18-11*, 66, **530-539**
mammillary peduncle, *18-5*, 485
medial forebrain bundle, *18-5*, 29, **487-488**, 541
olfactory, bulb, *18-1*, **522-523**
gyri, lateral, 523
medial, 523
lobe, 24, **524-527**
nerve, **521-522**, *18-1*
stria, lateral, *18-2*, 29, 523
medial, *18-2*, 29, 523
tract, 29, **523-524**
trigone, *18-2*, 29, 524
tubercle, 525
paraterminal tyrus (subcallosal gyrus), *18-2, 18-4*, 525
pryiform lobe, 24, **524-525**
entorhinal area, *18-11, 19-5*, **525-526**
periamygdaloid region, *18-4*, 525

prepyriform area, *18-4*, 525
septal, area (paraterminal body), *18-4*, **482-483**, 525
nuclei, lateral, 483, 525
medial, 483, 525
subcallosal area (parolfactory area), *18-4*, 27, 525
uncus, *2-6, 2-12, 18-6*, 24, 28, 525
Oligodendroglia, *5-7, 5-8, 5-9*, **122-125**
interfascicular cells, 125 *5-3*
juxtavascular cells, 125
perineuronal satellite cells, *5-3 5-7*, 123
Olivary nucleus, inferior, *2-19, 11-9, 11-13, 11-14, 11-15*, 39, **298-300**, **418-419**
accessory, *11-14*, 298, 419
superior, *12-7, 12-10, 12-11*, **329-331**
peduncle of, *12-11*, **332-333**
Olive, superior, **329-331**, *12-16*
Olivocerebellar tract, *11-21*, 298, **418-419**, *14-22*
Olivocochlear bundle, **332-333**, *12-11*
Olivospinal tract (of Helweg), 271
Operculum, frontal, *2-3*, 23
parietal, *2-3*, 23, 577
temporal, *2-3*, 23
Ophthalmic nerve, *1-10, 7-13*, 353
Ophthalmoplegia, anterior internuclear, 344, 382
Optic, chiasm, *1-3, 2-5, 2-6, 2-22, 15-16, 15-21*, 37, 64, 70, 461, **465-466**
cup, 58
lobe, **566-567**, *19-13, 19-14*
nerve, 59, 461, **465-466**
pathways, *15-16, 15-21, 15-23*, **465-470**, **566-568**
clinical considerations, *15-23*, 470, 568
radiations, *2-7, 2-16, 15-21, 15-22*, 30, **466-470**, **567-568**
reflexes, **370-376**, **382-384**
tract, *2-6, 15-16, 15-21*, 466
vesicles, *3-8D*, 58
Orbital muscle of Müller, 210
Organ, of Corti, *12-8*, 326
subcommissural, *13-9*, 129
subfornical, 129
Osmoreceptors, 493
Otic ganglion, *8-1*, 198, 314
Otoliths, *12-12*, 336
organ, 336
Otosclerosis, 336
Ovulation, 494, 542

Pacchionian bodies, *see* Arachnoid villi
Pachymeninx, *1-1, 1-2, 1-3*, **1-7**
Pain, *10-8*, 140, **245-249**, **456-457**, **564-566**
loss of, **245-248**, 249, **356-357**
phantom, 188
referred, **155-156**
relief of, 199, 245
visceral, 191, 199
Paleocerebellum, *14-1*, 46, 63, 400, **432-433**
Paleocortex, *2-6*, 24, 521, **524-527**
Paleopallium, *2-6*, 24, 521, **524-527**
Paleostriatum, *17-3*, 17-12, 33, 67, 496, 498, 499, **504-508**
Paleothalamus, 446
Pallidosubthalamic fibers, *17-8, 17-11*, **508-509**

Boldface numbers indicate principal references. *Italic* numbers refer to illustrations.

Pallidotegmental fibers, *17-11*, **507–508**
Pallidothalamic fibers, *17-8*, *17-11*, *17-15*, 454, **505–507**
Pallidum, 33, 67–69, 496, 498–499
  blood supply, *20-4*, *20-5*, *20-6*, **608–612**
Pallium, **21–27**, **547–559**
  development, *3-9*, *3-13*, *3-14*, 67–69
Palsy, bulbar, 308, 312
  facial, **348–349**
  pseudobulbar, 318
Papez, theory of emotion, **538–539**
Parabducens nucleus, **350–351**
Parabigeminal, area, *13-2*, 369
  nucleus, 369, *13-1*
Paracentral lobule, *2-4*, *2-12*, 27, 560, 563, 578, 581
Parahippocampal gyrus, *2-4*, *2-6*, *18-8*, *18-11*, 27, **525–527**, 531, 544
  presubiculum, *18-8*, 532
  prosubiculum, *18-8*, 532
  subiculum, *18-8*, 532
Paralysis, agitans, 64, 397, 514, **516–517**
  facial, central, 349,
    mimetic, 349,
    peripheral, 348,
  flaccid, 273,
  inferior alternating, 308, 351
  of lateral gaze, 349,
  lower motor neuron, 260, **272–275**
  middle alternating, 324, 351
  spastic, **275–276**
  superior alternating (Weber), 382
  supranuclear, 316
  upper motor neuron, 260, **275–276**, **314–318**
Paraplegia, 261, **278–279**
Parasensory areas, **595–598**
Parasympathetic, ganglia, *8-1*, *8-11*, *11-17*, *11-18*, *12-15*, 197–198, **377–379**, **382–384**
  fibers to the eye, 197, 211, **377–379**, **382–384**
  neurons, 208, 211
  pathways, **197–198**, 211, **382–384**
  responses, regulation of, 208–209, **211–212**
Paraterminal body, *18-2*, *18-4*, 525
Paraventricular nucleus, 482, 488, 493
  of thalamus, *15-10*, 446
Paresthesia, 282, 472, 565
Parietal, lobe, **23–24**, **451–452**, 471, **559–566**, 577–578, **595–598** *19-6*
  lobules, *2-2*, 24, *19-6*, **596–597**
Parieto-occipital sulcus, *2-4*, *2-12*, 24, *19-6*
Parkinson's disease, 397, 514, 517
Parolfactory area (subcallosal), *18-2*, 27, 525
Past-pointing, 345, 430
Pathway(s) auditory, *12-10*, **329–332**, 367–369, 457–458, **574–577**
  autonomic, *8-6* **191–212**
    central, **206–208**, **487–488**
    descending, *10–12* *10-13*, 271
  cochlear, secondary, *12-10*, **329–332**
  corticobulbar, *11–23*, **314–318**
  corticopontocerebellar, *14–21*, 323–325 **419–420**, 586–587
  corticospinal, *10-12*, *10-13*, **255–261**, 578–582
  anterior, 258
  lateral, **255–258**
  discriminative sensibility, *10-1*, **238–242**, 454–456, **560–566**
  fasciculus proprius, **271–272**, *10-21*
  gustatory, 310, 313, 347, 455–456
  lemniscal, *10-1*, *12-10*, **238–242**, 391, 470–473
  lemniscus, lateral *12-10*, 329, 331, 362, 368
    medial, *10-1*, 240, **289–293**, 391, 454–455, **560–566**
  medial longitudinal fasciculus, *12–14*, **269–270**, 286, **342–344**
  monoamine, 91, 204–205, **264–266**, 394–396, 411, 489, 501, 516–517, **594–595**
  olfactory, *18-1*, **521–529**
  olivocerebellar, 299, 418
  olivospinal, 271
  optic, *15-16*, *15-21*, *15-22*, *15-23*, **465–470**, **566–568**
  pain and temperature (lateral spinothalamic), *10-8*, **245–249**, 454–455, 456–457, 564
  pallidal (efferent), *17-7*, *17-8*, *17-11*, **505–509**
  posterior white column, *10-1*, **238–242**, 289–291, 454
  reticular, **267–271**, **301–303**, 388–393, **474–477**
  reticulospinal, *10-11*, *10-20*, **267–271**
  rubroreticular, 386
  rubrospinal, *10-17*, **261–264**, 385–386
  spinocerebellar, anterior, *10-10*, 251–252, 363, 417
    posterior, *10-10*, **249–251**, 303–304, 417
    rostral, 253, 418
  spinocortical, 253,
  spino-olivary, 255, 299
  spinoreticular, 253, **301–302**, 391
  spinothalamic, anterior, *10-7*, **242–244**, 302, *13-4*, 454–455, *14-18*
    lateral, *10-8*, **245–249**, 302, *13-4*, 454–455
  tectobulbar, 374
  tectospinal, 261, 374
  trigeminal, secondary, *12-22*, **360–361**
  vagal, **310–312**
  vestibular, *12-14*, 242
  vestibulospinal, *10-18*, *10-19*, **264–267**, 442–443
  visual, *15-16*, *15-21*, *15-22*, *15-23*, **465–470**
Peduncle(s), cerebellar, inferior (restiform body), *2-19*, *2-25*, *10-10*, *11-2*, *11-22*, *11-24*, 39, 41, 249, 303–304, 414, 416
  middle (brachium pontis) *2-5*, *2-17*, *2-19*, *2-25*, *12-1*, *12-2*, *12-4*, *14-21*, 41, 62, **324–325**, 419–420, 586–587
  superior (brachium conjunctivum), *see separate listing*
  cerebral, *2-8*, *13-1*, 367, **397–398**
  of flocculus, 318 399 *11-24*
  inferior thalamic, *15-9*, 445, 463–464
  of mammillary body, *16-5*, 485
  of superior olive (efferent cochlear bundle), *12-11*, **332–333**
  thalamic, *15–17*, *15–18*, **463–465**
Peduncle, superior cerebellar, *2-25*, *12-23*, *13-2*, *14-16*, *14-17*, 42, 252, 253, 363, **420–422**
  course, 252, 253, 363, 367, **420–422**
  divisions, *14–16*
    ascending, **420–421**
    descending, 421
  functional considerations, 430
  lesions, 430
  origin, 420
  projections, *14-16*, 421
    red nucleus, 385, 421, *14–17*
    reticular formation, 363, 418, 421
    thalamus, 421, 450, 454
Pelvic nerve, *8-11*, 198, 211
Periamygdaloid area, *18-4*, 483, 525
Periaqueductal gray, *13-1*, *13-2*, *13-4*, 207, 367
Perikaryon, *4-1*, *4-3*, *4-4*, *4-5*, *4-6*, *4-7*, **82–93**
  shape, 82,
  size, 82,
Perineurium, *4-22*, *7-7*, 100, 164
Perineuronal, satellite cells, 123
  space, 19, 115
Periosteum, 1, 167, 622
Peripheral nerves *7-11*, *7-12*, *7-13*, *7-18*, *7-19*, *7-20*, **159–190**
  connective tissue sheaths, *4-22*, **100**, **159**, 164
  degeneration, *4-26*, **105–107**
  functional components, *9-27*, *11-16*, 57, **304–305**
  functional considerations, **186–188**
  injuries, 172–173, 175–181
  regeneration of *4-31*, **107–114**, 188–190
  segmental arrangement of, *7-14*, *7-15*, *7-16*, **159–190**
  system, **159–190**
Peripheral, nervous system, *7-1*, *7-11*, *7-12*, 21, **159–190**
  receptive field, *7-10*, 137
Peritrichial endings, *6-2*, 142
Perivascular, feet (foot plates), *5-2*, *5-3*, *5-4*, **118–119**, 120
  limiting membrane, 129
  satellites, 125
  spaces, *1-14*, 115
Periventricular, fibers, 308, 446
  tracts, *16-7*, 308, 488
Perlia, central nucleus of, 379
Peroneal nerve, common, *7-20*, **185–186**
  superficial, 185
Pes, cavus, 185
  lemniscus, *12-10*, *12-23*, *13-2*, **329–331**, 398
    lateral, 398
    medial, *13-1*, 398
Petrosal ganglion, *see* Ganglion, inferior glossopharyngeal
Phagocytosis, **127–128**, 136
Phrenic, ganglion, 196
  nerve, **169–172**
Pia-glia membrane, *1-9*, *1-16*, **11–14**, 116
Pia mater, *1-7*, *1-8*, *1-9*, *1-12* **7–9**, 115, 213
  epipial layer, *7-8*, 7

Boldface numbers indicate principal references. *Italic* numbers refer to illustrations.

intima pia, 7–8, 7
Pigment, lipochrome (lipofuscin), *4-1B*, 90
  melanin, *12-26*, *13-18*, 90, 311, 364–365, 393–394
Pineal, body (epiphysis), *2-18*, *2-20*, *2-21*, *15-2*, *15-3*, *15-7*, 43, **438–440**
  gland, 64, **439–440**
  recess, *15–4*, 43
Pinocytosis, 134
Pituitary, body, *1-11*, *16-1*, *16-5*, *16-7*, *16-9*, 65, 478, **488–490**, 493–494
  fossa (sella turcica), *1-3*, *20-3*, 1
Plasma membrane, 82–84, *4-8*
Plate, alar, *3-10*, 53, 62, 64, 65, 66, *11-16*, 304–305, 399
  basal, *3-3*, *3-10*, 53
  cerebellar, *3-10*, *3-11*, *3-12* 62
  commissural, *3-13*, 69
  cribriform, 521, *18-1*
  floor, *3-3*, 53
  neural, *3-2*, 49
  quadrigeminal, *3-9*, 63, 367
  roof, *3-10*, *3-11*, 53
Plexus, abdominal aortic, 197
  basilar venous, *20-17*, 623
  brachial, *7-14*, *7-17*, *7-18*, **173–175**
  cardiac, 196
  carotid, external, 196
    internal, 196
  celiac, *8-1*, 197
  cervical, 196
  choroid, of fourth ventricle, *1-11*, *5-16*, *5-18*, 41, 132, 621
    of lateral ventricles, *3-13B*, 36, 132, **614–615**
    of third ventricle, *1-11*, *3-13A*, *3-13B*, 64, 132, 614
  enteric, 198
  formation of spinal nerves, *3-6*, *3-7*, **159–161**
  ganglionated, 198
  gastric, 198
  hepatic, 197
  hypogastric, *8-11*, 197, 211
  inferior mesenteric, 197
  internal vertebral venous, **602–603**
  lumbar, *7-19*, **181–185**
  lumbosacral, *7-20*, **181–185**
  myenteric, of Auerbach, 198
  pelvic, 197
  phrenic, **169–172**, 197
  postfixed, 173
  prefixed, 173
  sacral, 198
  spermatic, 197
  splenic, 197
  submucous, of Meissner, 198
  superior mesenteric, 197
  suprarenal, 197
Polarized light technic, 97
Pole, frontal *2-2*, *2-4*, 23, 558
  occipital, *2-2*, *2-4*, 24, 558
  temporal, *2-2*, *2-4*, 24, 525
Pons, *2-17*, *3-9*, *3-11*, *12-1*, *12-4*, 21, 41, 61–63, **322–366**
  anatomy, 21, 59, 60, 61, **322–366**,
  basilar portion (ventral), *12-1*, **323–325**
  fibers, afferent, 324–325
    corticopontine, *13-1*, 324, 419,

586–587
  spinopontine, 255
  tectopontine, 325
  efferent, brachium pontis (Middle cerebellar peduncle), *12-1*, *12-4*, *12-7*, *14-21*, 41, 324, **419–420**
    longitudinal, 323
    transverse, 323, 419
  nuclei, *3-11*, *12-3*, 325, 419
  blood supply, *20-13*, *20-14*, **616–620**
  brachium pontis, *12-1*, *12-4*, *12-7*, *14-21*, 41, 62, **323–325**, **419–420**
  development, *3-11*, 62,
  dorsal portion, 41, 62, 322–324
  internal structure, *12-1*, **322–366**
  lesions of, 335, 344, 348, 349, 357
  tegmentum, *12-1*, 41, **322–323**
  nuclei, 362–366, 369–370
  upper, 12–23, 362–365
    cranial nerves, abducens, *12-3*, 349–351
    cochlear, *12-10*, **326–329**
    facial, *12-15*, **346–349**
    trigeminal, *12-20*, *12-21*, *12-22*, **352–360**
    vestibular, *12-14*, **336–342**
  dorsal, paramedian, 62
  of raphe, 365,
  medial eminence, 41, 322,
  reticularis pontis caudalis, *12-3*, 302, 322
  reticularis pontis oralis, *2-19*, 303, 322, 351, 389, 391
  reticulotegmental, *12-19*, 363, 421
  pedunculopontine tegmental, *12-24*, 363, 388, *13-3*, **507–508**, *17-11*
  superior central, *12-24*, 365, *16-5*
  ventral portion, *12-1*, *12-3*, 41, 62, **323–325**
Pontine, branches of basilar artery, *20-1*, *20-4*, *20-9*, **617–619**, *20-13*, *20-14*
  flexure, *3-8*, *3-9*, 59
  nuclei, *12-3*, **324–325**
Pontobulbar nucleus, *11-15*, 304
Pontocerebellar tract, *14-21*, **419–420**
Pontogeniculo-occipital (PGO) activity, 594
Postcentral gyrus, *2-1*, *2-2*, *19-11*, 24, 456, **560–566**
  sulcus, *2-2*, 24, *19-11*
Posterior, antebrachial cutaneous nerve, 175
  brachial cutaneous nerve, 175
  cerebral artery(ies), *20-4*, *20-9*, **609–612**
  commissure, 43, **376–377**, 437
  femoral cutaneous nerve, **183–184**
  inferior cerebellar artery, *20-1*, 321, **616–617**
  lobe of cerebellum, *14-1*, 46, 400
  medium septum, 55, *9-2*, *9-6*, 214
  meningeal artery, *20-3*, 622
  rami of spinal nerve, **162–163**
  spinal artery, *20-1*, *20-2*, 601
Postganglionic visceral efferent fibers, *8-1*, *8-2*, *8-3*, **193–198**
Posture and movement regulation, **146–153**, 336, 344–345, 399, 425,

518
Potential, action, 101
  spike, 101
Precentral, gyrus, *2-1*, *2-2*, 23, 255, 260–261, **314–318**, *11-23*, 454, **578–583**
  sulcus, *2-2*, 23, 579, *19-6*, *19-9*
Precuneus (quadrate lobule), *2-4*, *2-12*, 27, 451
Prefrontal area, 23, **598–599**
  cortex, **598–599**
    functions, 445, 599
    pain, 445, 598
    relationships to thalamus, *15-13*, **444–446**, 474
  surgery of, 445, **598–599**
    emotional changes, 445, 599
    evaluation, 445, 599
    intellectual changes, 599
    leucotomy, 598
    lobotomy, 445, 598
    topectomy, 599
Preganglionic visceral efferent fibers, *8-1*, *8-2*, *8-11*, **192–195**
Premotor area, *19-20*, 23, **582–583**
Preoccipital notch, *2-2*, 24
Preoptic area, *16-1*, 479, 494, 541
Preoptic nuclei, 479, *16-1*, 541
Prepyriform area, *18-4*, 525
Prerubral field, *17-8*, *17-11*, 437, **511–512**
Presubiculum, *18-8*, 532
Pretectal area, *13-7*, **374–376**
  nuclei, *13-7*, *13-8*, 374–376
  pupillary light reflex, *13-13*, **382–384**
Prevertebral ganglia, *8-1*, *8-2*, 193, **195–196**
Priapism, 279
Primary, auditory area, *19-5*, *19-7*, *19-18*, 24, 331, **574–577**
  auditory fibers, 327–329
  motor area, *19-5*, *19-19*, *19-20*, 23, **578–582**
  olfactory area, *19-5*, 24, 525–526, 547
  sensory area, *19-5*, *19-11*, *19-12*, 24, **560–566**
  vestibular fibers, 337, 339–342
  vestibulocerebellar fibers, **341–342**
  visual area, *19-5*, *19-10C*, *19-14*, 24, **566–574**
Primitive streak, *3-1*, 49
Projection fibers, cortex, **29–31**, 464–465, **578–589**
Projections, ventral, amygdalofugal, *16-8*, 541
Proprioceptive, **138–139**, **336–337**
  pathways, *10-1*, **238–242**, 339–344
  receptors, *6-7*, *6-9*, *6-10*, **138–139**, 336
  sense, 138
Prosencephalon (forebrain), *3-8*, 58
Prosubiculum, *18-8*, 532
Proteinaceous neurosecretory material (NSM), 92
Protopathic sensibility, 139
  system, 139
Psalterium (*see* Commissure of fornix), *18-6*, 69, 535
Psammoma bodies, 133
Pseudobulbar palsy, 318, 349
Pseudopregnancy, 489
Pterygopalatine ganglion, 198, 348, *12-15*

Boldface numbers indicate principal references. *Italic* numbers refer to illustrations.

Ptosis, eyelid, 209–210, 382
Pulvinar, *15-3, 15-4, 15-5, 15-12*, 45, 435, 451–452, 474, 595
Pupil, Argyll-Robertson, 383
    constriction (miosis), 210, 383
    dilatation (mydriasis), 382
    reflexes, 382–384
Pupillography, infrared, 376
Purkinje cells, *4-5, 4-9, 14-4, 14-5, 14-6, 14-7*, 63, 78, 401–402, 425, 434
Putamen, *2-11, 17-4, 17-6*, 33, 66, 451, 497–498, 499–504
Pyramid of medulla, *2-8, 2-17, 10-12, 10-13, 11-1, 11-5, 11-6, 11-13*, 37, 255–256, 287–288, 581
Pyramidal, decussation, *10-13, 11-1, 11-5, 11-6*, 287–288
Pyramidotomy, 581
Pyramis of cerebellum, *2-26, 14-1, 14-6*, 46
Pyriform lobe, *18-4*, 24, 525–527

Quadrangular lobule, anterior, *14-1*, 46
    posterior, *14-1*, 46, 400
Quadrigeminal brachium, inferior, *see* Inferior collicular brachium
    superior, *see* Superior collicular brachium
    plate, *3-9*, 64
Quadriplegia, 261
"Quermembran," 97

Radial nerve, *7-17, 7-18*, 175–176
Radiations, auditory, *12-10, 15-18*, 457, 463–464, 574
    internal capsule, *2-8, 2-9, 2-13, 2-14, 10-12, 15-8, 15-9, 15-17, 15-18*, 29–31, 462–465
    optic, *15-21, 15-22*, 30, 461, 463, 466–469, 470, 566–568
    thalamic, *15-18*, 462–465
Radicular, arteries, *20-1, 20-2*, 600–601
    veins, *20-2*, 602
Rage, reactions, 494–495, 541–542
    triggering mechanisms, 495
Ramus, communicans, *1-7, 8-2*, 56, 195
    gray, *1-7, 8-2*, 196
    white, *1-7, 8-2*, 195
    dorsal (posterior), *1-7, 3-7*, 56, 162
    meningeal, 162
    ventral (anterior), *1-7, 3-7*, 56, 162
Ranvier's gold chloride method, 72
    nodes of, 93, 96–97
Raphe nuclei, 365–366, 594–595
    dorsal nucleus, *13-3*, 365
    inferior central, *11-24*, 365
    pontine, *12-24*, 365
    superior central, *12-24*, 365
    transmitter substance, 366, 594
Rapid eye movements (REM) 366, 594
Rasmussen technic, 72
Rathke's pouch, 64
Reaction(s), arousal, 390–393, 476, 592–593
    arrest, 541
    of degeneration, 187
    mnemonic, 595
    past-pointing, 430
    pseudoaffective, 495
    recruiting, 453, 475, 592–593
    righting, 444

Rebound phenomenon, 431
Receptive fields, 355, 568
    axis of orientation, *19-15, 19-16*, 470
    cutaneous, 137
    lateral geniculate, *19-15*, 469, 569
    retina, *19-15*, 469, 568–569
    striate cortex, *19-15, 19-16*, 469–470, 569–574
Receptors, alpha (α), 203
    auditory, *12-8, 12-9*, 329
    beta (β), 203
    chemoreceptors, *11-13*, 296–297
    classification, 138–142
    contact, *6-4*, 139
    diffuse endings, *6-3*, 143–144
    encapsulated endings, *6-4*, 144–146
    exteroceptors, 138, *9-22*
    free endings, *6-3*, 142–143
    gustatory, *6-5*, 143
    hair cells of cochlea, *12-8, 12-9*, 326
    interoceptors, 138
    mechanoreceptors, *6-9, 6-10*, 140
    nicotinic, 201
    nociceptors, 139–140
    olfactory, *18-1*, 521–522
    pain, 139–140
    photoreceptors, 465, *15-19, 15-20*
    of position and movement, 138, *6-9, 6-10*, 143–144, 146
    pressure, 139, 146
    proprioceptors, 138, *6-9, 6-10, 6-11, 6-13*
    quick adapting, 138
    slow adapting, 138
    structure of, 142–146
    teloreceptors, 138
    temperature, 140, *6-8, 10-8*
    thermoreceptors, 140
    touch, 139, 143, *6-9, 6-10, 10-7*
    vestibular, *12-12*, 336–337
    visceroceptors, 139
    visual, *15-19, 15-20*, 465
Recess, infundibular, *2-15*, 438, *15-5*
    lateral, of fourth ventricle, *2-15*, 41, 318, *11-2*
    optic, *15-6*, 479, *16-1*
    pineal, *2-15, 15-4*, 439
Rectum, innervation, *8-3*, 198
Red nucleus, *see also* Nucleus, red, 42, 64, 261–263, 384–388, *13-17*, 420–421, *14-16, 14-17*
Referred pain, 199
Reflex(es), abdominal, 259
    accommodation, 211, 383
    Achilles (ankle jerk), 167
    anal, 168
    arc, 235–237
    auditory, 332–335
    Babinski, 259, 275, 582
    biceps, 167
    bulbocavernosus, 168
    carotid sinus, 313
    cochlear, *12-11*, 335
    consensual, 361, 382
    corneal, 361
    cough, 212
    cremasteric, 167
    cutaneous, *9-23*, 237, 275
    deep tendon, *see* myototic
    disynaptic, *9-23*, 237
    facial, 347
    flexor afferent 251, 252, 419

    gluteal, 167
    grasp, 585
    intersegmental, 271–272, *9-23*
    intrasegmental, *9-23*, 235–237
    jaw jerk, 362
    kinetostatic, 345
    lacrimal, *12-15*, 361
    laryngeal, 312
    light, 382–383
    mass, 278,
    monosynaptic, *9-23*, 235–237
    multisynaptic, *9-23*, 237
    myotatic (stretch), *9-27*, 235–237, 279, 282
    optic, 382–384
    patellar (knee jerk), *9-27*, 167, 235–237
    periosteal, 167
    pharyngeal, 312
    plantar, 167, 259, 275
    postural, 241, 344–345
    proprioceptive, 271–272, 344
    pupillary 382–384
    radial, 167
    righting, 344–345
    salivary, 212, 348
    segmental, *9-23*, 103, 167–168
    sneezing 212, 361
    spinal, 235–237, *9-27*, 273–276
    static, 344
    stretch, *see* myotatic
    superficial, 259, 275
    tendon, *see* myotatic
    triceps, 167
    trigeminal, 361–362
    vagal, 212, 312
    vestibular, 344–345
    visceral, 191, 199
        somatic, 199
    visual, 374, 382–383
    vomiting, 361,
    wrist, 167
Regeneration of nerve fibers, 107–114, 188–190
    nervous system, central, 3, 112
    of peripheral nerves, *4-20, 4-31*, 107–114, 188–190
Region, basal olfactory, *18-2*, 482, 523
    mammillary, 482–483
    preoptic, *16-1*, 479, 494, 540–541
    pretectal, *13-7*, 374–376
    septal, *18-4*, 482, 525
    supraoptic, 479–482, *16-4*
    tuberal, 478, 482, *16-3*
Reil, island of (*see* Insula), *2-11, 3-16*, 24–26, 499, 577, 609
Relationship of neurons, 103–105, *4-3*
Relay nuclei of thalamus, *15-12*, 470–473, 559
    cortical, 473, 559
    specific sensory, 470–473, 559
Release phenomena, 516
Releasing factors, *16-9*, 92, 489–490, 493–494
Remak, fibers of (unmyelinated peripheral nerve fibers), 100–103
Remyelination of experimentally injured axons, 113–114, 189–190
Respiratory center, 269, 311, 321
Response, arousal, 390–393, 476
    augmenting, 473
    cholinomimetic, 201

Boldface numbers indicate principal references. *Italic* numbers refer to illustrations.

EEG arousal, 390–393, 476
muscarinic, 201,
recruiting, 453, 475–476, 592–593
Restiform body, see Inferior cerebellar
    peduncle
Reticular formation, 267–269, 296, 300–
    303, 315–316, 322, 351–352,
    388–393
  areas, 269, 301, 351,
    "effector," 302–303, 388
    "sensory," 302, 388
  ascending activating system, 390–393,
    476–477, 592–593
  cell types, 301
  cortical activity, 390–393, 476, 592–
    593
  cytoarchitecture, 300–301, 351–352,
    388
  descending projections, 267–269
  electrophysiological studies, 388–393
  facilitation, 269, 389
  fibers, afferent, 269, 296, 301–302,
    351–352, 390–392
    collaterals, 302, 388–391
      cranial nerves, 302, 390
      secondary sensory, 302, 390–391
    corticoreticular, 302, 391
    fastigioreticular, 14–19, 422, 424
    spinoreticular, 253, 391
  efferent, 267–269, 302–303, 322,
    351, 392
    ascending, 303, 323, 351, 390–393,
      449–450
      central tegmental tract, 12-1,
        12-4, 322, 386, 393, 450
    cerebellopedal, 302, 363, 418
    descending, 267–269, 303, 351,
      389
      medulla, 267–269, 302
      pons, 267–269, 322–323, 351–
        352
    reticulospinal, 267–269
  functional considerations, 269, 388–
    393
    ascending influences, 390–393
    anesthetic states, 394
    arousal response, 390–393
    ascending reticular activating sys-
      tem, 390–393
    coma, 393
    consciousness, 393
    electroencephalogram, 390–393,
      476
    intralaminar thalamic nuclei,
      392, 448–450
    relation to lemniscal systems,
      391, 474
    sleep, 366, 393, 593–595
    synaptic transmission, 392
  descending influences, 10-11, 10-20,
    267–269, 389–390
    autonomic effects, 206–207, 269,
      389, 488
    decerebrate animal, 345
    facilitation, 269, 389
    gamma motor neuron, 269, 390
    inhibition, 267, 389
    muscle spindle, 269, 390
    reflex, activity, 267, 389
    sensory impulses, 390
  inhibition, 267, 388–389

lesions, 391, 393
medulla, 300–304
midbrain, 64, 388
nuclei, cuneiformis, 388
  Darkschewitsch, 13-16, 380
  dorsal nucleus raphe, 322–323, 365
  dorsal tegmental, 12-24, 365, 369,
    485
  interstitial (Cajal), 13-16, 379
  lateral reticular medulla, 11-15, 296,
    301, 418
  paramedian reticular, 11-15, 12-3,
    301, 418
  pedunculopontine tegmental, 12-14,
    363, 388, 507–508, 17-11
  posterior commissure, 376–377
  reticularis, gigantocellularis, 11-5,
    267, 301
    parvicellularis, 301
    pontis caudalis, 12-3, 267, 322
    pontis oralis, 12-19, 267, 322, 351
    tegmenti pontis (reticulotegmen-
      tal), 12-24, 363, 419
    ventralis, 301
  subcuneiformis, 388
  superior central, 12-24, 365, 18-5,
    488
  ventral tegmental, 18-5, 388, 488
phylogeny, 300
pons, 322, 351–352, 389
process (spinal cord), 9-7, 225
relation to intralaminar thalamic
    nuclei, 392–392, 476
relation to lemniscal systems, 391
synaptic transmission, 301, 392, 393
Reticulocerebellar tracts, 14-16, 363, 418
Reticulospinal tracts, 10-11, 10-20, 267–
    269
Retina, cell organization, 15-19, 15-20,
    465, 568–569
  cells, 15-19, 465, 568–569
  fovea centralis, 465
  layers, 15-19, 15-20, 465
Retinohypothalamic fibers, 466
Retisolution, 88
Retispersion, 88
Reverberating circuits, 434
Rhinal sulcus, 2-6, 28, 524
Rhinencephalon, 521
  components of, 521
Rhizotomy, dorsal, 9-24, 9-25, 10-2, 10-6,
    10-22, 166, 186, 277
Rhombencephalon (hindbrain), 3-8, 3-9,
    11-1, 11-2, 21, 38–42, 58, 285–
    366
  blood supply, 20-14, 616–619
  isthmus, 12-23, 12-24, 362–363
Rhombic lip, 3-11, 3-12, 3-14, 21, 62, 399
Rhomboid fossa, 2-18, 3-14, 11-2, 41, 285,
    297
Ribonucleic acid (RNA) 82, 84–85
Righting reactions, 344–345, 387
Rigidity, decerebrate, 345
  of extrapyramidal disease, 516
Rod cells, retina, 15-19, 15-20, 465
Rolando, gelatinous substance of, 9-7, 9-
    8, 9-14, 9-17, 223–224, 231,
    242, 245
  sulcus of, see Central sulcus
Roots, of spinal nerve, 7-1, 8-1, 8-2, 9-1, 9-
    2, 9-3, 9-6, 159–161, 165–166,

213
  dorsal, 1-5, 1-7, 3-6, 9-6, 159, 165,
    232–235
  ventral, 1-5, 1-7, 3-6, 9-6, 160, 166,
    229–231
  of trigeminal nerve, 12-20, 12-21, 354,
    357, 359–360
    motor, 360
    sensory, 354, 357, 359
Rostrum of corpus callosum, 2-7, 2-12, 26,
    32
Rubroreticular tract, 263, 386
Rubrospinal tract, 10-17, 261–264, 384–
    386, 421, 14-17

Saccule (sacculae), 12-12, 336
Sacral, outflow, 195, 8-1
  plexus, 7-20, 181
  preganglionic fibers, 198
  segments of spinal cord, 9-1, 9-2, 9-3, 9-
    5, 9-6, 218–221
Salivatory nucleus, inferior, 11-17, 11-18,
    314
  superior, 11-17, 11-18, 348
Saltatory transmission, 97
Saphenous nerve, 183
Satellite cells, nucleolar, 4-7, 84
  perineuronal, 123
  perivascular, 125
Scala media, 326, 12-8
Scala tympani, 326, 12-8
Scala vestibuli, 326, 12-8
Schmidt-Lantermann clefts, 97–99, 4-15
    4-20
Schütz, bundle of (dorsal longitudinal fas-
    ciculus), 11-4, 16-7, 308, 488
Schwann cell, membrane, 4-18, 4-19,
    4-21, 99–100
  mesaxon, external, 4-18, 96
    internal, 4-18, 96
  sheaths of (neurolemma), 4-15, 93, 99–
    100
Sciatic nerve, 7-20, 184–185
Sclerotome, 164
Secondary, auditory area, 19-17, 574–
    576
  degeneration (Wallerian), 4-27, 106,
    276
  olfactory area, 18-11, 526
  sensory area, 19-13, 471, 559–560, 566
  vestibular fibers, 342
  visual area, 19-13, 573–574
Segmental, innervation, 7-10, 7-14, 7-15,
    7-16, 164–168
  reflexes, 9-23, 9-27, 103, 167–168,
    235–237
Segmentation, 3-1, 3-7, 9-1, 9-2, 9-3, 9-5,
    9-6, 159
Self-stimulation brain, 545–546
Sella turcica, 1-3, 203, 529
Semicircular canals, 1-2, 12-12, 336
Semilunar, ganglion, see Trigeminal gan-
    glion
  lobules, 14-1, 400
Sensations, cortical, 139, 559–578
  gnostic, 139, 596
Sensibility, 137–138
  affective, 139, 155, 472
  deep, 139, 472
  discriminative, 139, 153–155, 240–
    242, 454–456, 472, 559, 564,

Boldface numbers indicate principal references. *Italic* numbers refer to illustrations.

Sensibility—*Continued*
   595
   epicritic, 139
   kinesthetic, 138, 240–242, 564
   protopathic, 139
   superficial, 139, 244
   vibratory, 139, 241
Sensory, endings, *6-1, 6-2, 6-3, 6-4,* 138–146
   innervation, 137–138
   modalities, relation to receptors, *6-2, 6-3, 6-4,* 137, 153–155
   nerve fibers, 162–164
   neurons, 161–162, 231–232
Septal, nuclei, *16-8, 18-4,* 483, 525
   region, *18-4,* 482, 525
   vein, *20-19, 20-20,* 628
Septo-hypothalamo-mesencephalic continuum, 207, 544
Septomarginal fasciculus, *10-21,* 241
Septum, pellucidum, *2-4, 2-20, 2-21,* 34, 525
   posterior intermediate, *9-6,* 214
   posterior median, *9-6, 9-7, 9-12,* 55, 214
Serotonin (5-hydroxytryptamine), 204, 366, 594–595
Seventh cranial nerve, *1-4, 2-5, 2-17, 2-19, 12-1, 12-15,* 346–349
Sham rage, 494–495, 541–542
Sheath, cell, *4-15, 4-16, 4-18, 4-19, 4-21,* 99–100
   of Henle; of Key and Retzius, 100, 164
   of Schwann, *4-15, 4-16, 4-18, 4-19, 4-21,* 99–100
   neurolemma, 99–100
Sign of Babinski, 259, 275, 582
Sinus(es), cavernous, *20-16, 20-17,* 623
   circular, *20-17,* 623
   confluens, *1-1, 1-3,* 622, *20-16*
   of dura mater, *1-1, 1-2, 1-12, 20-16,* 1, 622–624
   nerve, 313
   occipital *1-1, 20-19,* 622
   petrosal, *1-10, 20-16,* 624
   rectus, *1-3, 20-16, 20-20,* 622
   sagittal, inferior, *20-16,* 622
      superior, *1-1, 1-12, 20-16,* 622
   sigmoid, *1-2, 1-3, 1-4,* 622
   sphenoparietal, *20-17,* 624
   transverse, *1-1, 1-2, 1-3, 1-10, 20-16, 20-20,* 622
Sixth cranial nerve, *1-3, 11-17, 11-18, 12-1, 12-7,* 349–351
Sleep, 365–366, 495, 593–595
   biogenic amines, 366, 489, 593–595
   deep, 366, 593
   locus ceruleus, 364–365, 594–595
   norepinephrine, 364–366, 594–595
   paradoxical, 366, 594
   rapid eye movements in, 366, 594
   REM, 366, 594
   slow, 366, 593
   slow wave, 366, 593
   triggering mechanisms, 366, 594
Solitarius, fasciculus, *11-13, 11-14, 11-17, 11-18,* 310, 313, 347
   nucleus, *11-20,* 310, 313, 347
Somatic, afferent fibers, *6-6, 9-22,* 80, 161–163, 232–235
   efferent fibers, *9-21, 9-22,* 160, 228–230

Somatoceptors, 137–146
Somatotopic organization, anterior horn, *9-21,* 230
   cerebellum, *14-14, 14-15,* 416
   nuclei, accessory cuneate, *11-12,* 292
      cuneate, *11-11,* 291
      facial, 346–347
      lateral vestibular, *10-18,* 264, 342
      red, *10-17,* 263, 384–386
Somesthetic cortex, reciprocal connections, 564–565
Somesthetic sensory areas, *19-11, 19-12, 19-13,* 471, 560–566
   primary, *19-12,* 471, 560–566
   secondary, *19-13,* 472, 566
Somite formation, *3-1A, 3-1B, 3-1C,* 49
Somnolence, 393
Space, epidural, 1, 6, 622
   extracellular, 14, *1-16,* 19, 115–116
   perivascular, *1-14,* 11, 125
   subarachnoid, *1-6, 1-7, 1-10, 1-11, 1-12, 1-14,* 10–11
   subdural, *1-7,* 6
   Virchow-Robins, 11
Spasticity, 260, 276, 579, 583, 584–585
Special types of nerve fibers, 57, *9-22, 11-16,* 304–305
   somatic afferent, 57, 304–305
   visceral afferent, 57, 304–305, 347
   visceral efferent, 57, 304–305, 346
Speech centers, 23, 596–597
Sphenopalatine ganglion, *see* Pterygopalatine ganglion
Spike potential, 101
Spinal arteries, *20-1, 20-2,* 600–603
Spinal cord, *3-6, 3-8, 9-1, 9-2, 9-5, 9-6,* 53–57, 213–284
   anatomy, 213–221
   anterior white commissure, 215
   arrangement of fibers, *9-19, 9-21, 9-22,* 232–235
   blood supply, *20-1, 20-2,* 600–603
   cauda equina, *1-6, 9-1,* 213
   corticospinal tract, *10-13,* 255–261
   cytoarchitectural lamination (Rexed) *9-9, 9-11, 9-15, 9-17, 9-18, 9-19,* 222–229
   degeneration, *10-22, 10-23, 10-24, 10-25, 10-26,* 276–284
      method of study, 276–278
   disturbances, 272–284
      anesthesia, 278–280
      autonomic, 279, 282–283
      bladder, *8-11,* 211, 279
      muscle tone, 272–279
      paresis, 272–276
      reflexes, 272–276
      spasms, 278
      vasomotor, 279
   enlargements, *9-1, 9-3,* 213
      cervical, 213
      lumbosacral, 213
   fibers, afferent, *9-22,* 232–235
      collaterals, 232–234
      medial bundle, 232
      lateral bundle, 232
      efferent, somatic, *9-21,* 228–230
      visceral, *9-22,* 230–231
   fissure, anterior median, *9-6,* 214
   form and size, *9-1, 9-5,* 213–221
   funiculi, *9-6,* 215–216

   anterior, 215
   lateral, 215
   posterior, 216
   general topography, *9-6, 9-7,* 216–221
   gray and white substance, *9-6,* 217–218, 219–221
   lesions, *10-22, 10-23, 10-24, 10-25, 10-26,* 272–284
      hemisection (Brown-Séquard), *10-23,* 279–280
      lower motor neuron, 272–275
      transection, 278–279
   neuroglia, 217
   neuropil, 217
   nuclear, groups, 9-18, 9-21, 221–232
      associational, 221
      central, 221
      commissural, 221
      internuncial, 221
      lamination, *9-18,* 221–229
      pericornualis, anterior 251
   anterior, horn, *9-21,* 228–230
      cornucommissuralis, 231
   lateral horn, 230–231
   posterior horn, *9-6, 9-7, 9-8,* 223–226, 231–232
      dorsal nucleus (Clarke), *9-7, 9-11, 9-24, 10-10,* 227, 231, 249
      intermediomedialis, 227
      posterior cornucommissuralis, 231
      posteromarginalis, *9-8,* 223, 231
      proprius cornu dorsalis, 231
      substantia gelatinosa, *9-7, 9-8, 9-14, 9-17, 9-19,* 223–224, 230
   somatic efferent, *9-22,* 228–230
      gamma, 228
   visceral efferent, *9-22,* 230–231
      intermediolateral, 231
      sacral autonomic, *8-11,* 231–232
   reflex centers, 167–168
   Renshaw cells, *9-21,* 229
   reticular process, 220, 225
   roots, dorsal, 159, 213, 232–235
      ventral, 159, 213, 229–231
   segments, cervical, *9-1, 9-3, 9-5,* 159, 213, 218
      lumbar, 159, 220
      sacral, 159, 221
      thoracic, *9-7,* 159, 220
   septum, posterior median, *9-6,* 214
   superficial glial limiting membrane, 8, 218
   tracts, ascending, 238–255
      anterior spinocerebellar, *10-10,* 251–252
      anterior spinothalamic, *10-7,* 242–244
      cuneocerebellar, *10-10,* 252–253
      fasciculus cuneatus, *10-1,* 238–242
      fasciculus gracilis, *10-1,* 238–242
      lateral spinothalamic, *10-8,* 245–249
      posterior spinocerebellar, *10-10,* 249–251
      rostral spinocerebellar, 253
      spinocortical, 253–255
      spino-olivary, 255, 299
      spinopontine, 255
      spinoreticular, 253, *10-11*
      spinotectal, 249
      spinovestibular, 255

Boldface numbers indicate principal references. *Italic* numbers refer to illustrations.

descending, arms of dorsal roots, *9-23*, 241
  autonomic, 271
  corticospinal, *10-13*, **255–261**
    anterior (uncrossed), 256
    lateral (crossed), 256–260
  medial longitudinal fasciculus, *10-18, 10-19*, 269–270
  olivospinal (of Helweg), 271
  reticulospinal, *10-11, 10-20*, **267–269**, 388–390
    medullary, 267–269
    pontine, 267
  rubrospinal, *10-17*, **261–264**
  tectospinal, 261
  vestibulospinal, *10-18, 10-19*, **264–267**
  upper motor neuron, 260, 275
    fasciculi proprii, *10-21*, 271–272
  variations at different levels, *9-5*, **218–221**
  zone of Lissauer (dorsolateral fasciculus), *9-7, 9-14*, 233
Spinal, ganglia, *7-1, 7-2, 7-3, 7-10*, **161–162**
  cells, clear, 161
    obscure, 161
    satellite, 161
  nerve, *see separate listing*
  shock, 278
  veins, 601–603
Spinal nerve, *7-1*, **159–161**
  components, 159–161
  dermatome, *7-11, 7-12*, 165–166
  distribution, *7-10*, 165
  functional considerations, *7-10*, 166, 185–188, 276–278
  plexus formation, *7-17, 7-18*, **163–165**
  primary ramus, 162
    communicantes, *8-2*, 196
    dorsal, 162
    meningeal, 162
    ventral, 160–161
  roots, 162–164, 277–278
  structure, 159–161
Spinocerebellar tract, anterior, *10-10*, **251–252**, 417
  posterior, *10-10*, **249–251**, 417
  rostral, 253, 418
Spino-olivary tract, 255, 419
Spinoreticular tract, *10-11*, 253, 391–392
Spinotectal tract, 249, 373
Spinothalamic tract, anterior, *10-7*, **242–244**, 455–456
  lateral, *10-8*, **245–249**, 455–456, 566
Spiral ganglion, *12-8*, 326
Spireme, 84
Splanchnic nerves, *8-1*, 197
Splenium of corpus callosum, *2-16*, 26, 32, 592
Split-brain preparation, 589–591
Spread depression, 589
Stain technic, **71-77**
  Bodian, 72
  Fink-Heimer, 72
  Glees, 72
  Golgi, *4-1D, 4-4, 4-5*, 72
  Luxol fast blue (Klüver-Barrera), 72, *see Atlas*
  Marchi, *10-5*, 71
  Nauta-Gygax, *9-24*, 72

Nissl, *4-1E, 10-6*, 71
  Rasmussen, 72
  Weigert, *10-3*, 71
  Wiitanen, *4-1F*, 72
Stellate cells of cerebellum, *14-4*, 401
Stereognosis, 566, 591
Stimulation of labyrinth, 345
Strabismus, external, 382
  internal, 349
Stratum cinereum, *13-5*, 372
  external sagittal (inferior longitudinal fasciculus), 30, *2-16*, 467, 568
  intermedium, 394
  internal sagittal, 568
  lemnisci, 372
  opticum, 372
  zonale, of midbrain, *13-5*, 372
    of thalamus, *15-6*, 45, 435
Stria, dorsal acoustic, 330, *12-10*
  intermediate acoustic, 330
  Lancissi, *2-7, 1-6*, 532
  longitudinal, *2-7, 18-6*, 532
  medullaris, *2-18, 11-2*, 37
    of thalamus, *16-5*, 45, 439
  olfactory, *18-2*, 29, 523
  terminalis (semicircularis), *2-18, 15-6, 15-7*, 34, 45, 69, 436, 484, 540–541
  ventral acoustic, 329
Striate, arteries, *20-9*, 608, 613, 615
  cortex, *19-14*, 467–470, 566–574
  veins, *20-21, 20-22*, 627–628
Striatum (caudate nucleus and putamen), 33, 67, **497–504**, *3-13, 17-4, 17-6*, 517–518
  blood supply, *20-11*, 615–616
  neurons, *17-5*, 497–498
  projections, 504
Strionigral fibers, *17-6, 17-14*, 396, 504
Subacute combined degeneration, *10-25*, 281–282
Subarachnoid, cisterns, *1-10, 1-11*, **10-11**
  space, *1-7, 1-8, 1-9, 1-14*, 10
Subdural space, *1-7, 1-14*, 6
Subependymal astrocytes, *5-13*, 128
Subiculum, *18-8*, 532
Submandibular ganglion, *12-15*, 198, 348
Suboccipital nerve, 169, *7-13*
Subscapular nerve, 173
Substance (substantia), gelatinosa, of Rolando, *9-7, 9-8, 9-14, 9-17, 9-19*, 78, 223–224, 231
  innominata, *17-11, 17-14, 18-12, A-22*, 483
  nigra, *see* separate listing
  perforated, anterior, *2-6, 20-3, 20-9*, 29, 524, 612
    posterior, *2-17*, 620
Substantia nigra, *13-1, 13-4, 13-10, 13-18, 13-19*, 43, 63, 64, 367, **393–397**, 501–504
  fibers
    afferent, *17-14*, 396, 504
    efferent, *13-19, 17-14*, 396–397, 501–504
  lesions, 397, 516–517
  melanin, astrocytes, 394
  paralysis agitans, 397, 517
  pars compacta, 393–395
  pars reticulata, 393–395
Subsurface cisterns, 82

Subsynaptic membranes, 103
Subthalamic nucleus, *15-5, 15-6, 15-10, 17-8, 17-11, 17-12*, 45, **508–511**, 515, 517
  comparative features, 509
  connections, 510–511
  experimental studies, 518–519
  hemiballism, 515, 517
  reticular nucleus, 512
Subthalamus, *17-8, 17-9, 17-10, 17-11*, 45, **508–511**
  connections, 509–512
  functional considerations, 511, 515, 517, 518–519
  nuclei, corpus Luysii, 510–511
    zona incerta, 511
  syndromes of, 511, 515, 517, 518–519
Sudomotor, innervation, 205, 279
Sulcal artery, *20-2*, 601
Sulcus, anterolateral, of medulla, *11-13*, 312
  of spinal cord, *9-6*, 214
  basilar, *217*, 41, 616
  calcarine, *2-4, 2-12*, 24, **466–469**, 566–568, *19-14*
  callosomarginal, *2-4*, 27, 608
  central, *2-1, 2-2, 2-3*, 23, *19-6*, 578
  cinguli, *2-4, 2-12*, 27, 543, *18-13*
  collateral, *2-4, 2-6*, 24, 28, *18-8*, 531
  development, *3-16*, 70
  frontal, inferior, *2-2*, 23, 597
    middle, *2-2*, 23
    superior, *2-2*, 23, 585
  hemispheric, *3-9*, 60
  hippocampal, *2-4*, 27, 28, 66, 530, *18-8*
  hypothalamic, *15-6*, 45, 64, 478
  intraparietal, *2-2*, 24
  lateral, *2-1, 2-2*, 22, 70, 566
  limitans, *3-10, 3-11, 11-16*, 53, 305
  longitudinal, 22
  marginal, 27
  median, of rhomboid fossa, *3-10*, 41, 297
  occipital, lateral, *2-2*, 24
  olfactory, *2-5*, 29
  paracentral, *2-4*, 27, 578
  parieto-occipital, *2-2*, 24
  parolfactory, anterior, 525
    posterior, 525
  postcentral, *2-2, 2-4, 2-12*, 24, 563
  posterior, intermediate, *9-6*, 214
    median, of spinal cord, *9-6*, 214
  posterolateral, of spinal cord, *9-6*, 214, 232–233
  precentral, *2-1, 2-2*, 23, 582
  prenodular, *14-1*, 46, 399
  prepyramidal, of cerebellum, *2-26, 14-1*, 46, 399
  primary, *2-26, 14-1*, 46, 399
  rhinal, *2-6*, 28, 524
  of Rolando, *see* central sulcus
  temporal, inferior, 24
    middle, 24,
    superior, 24, 575
  terminal, 45,
  transverse rhombencephalic, *3-9*, 60
Superficial glial limiting membrane, 8, *1-9*, 218
Superficial middle cerebral veins, *20-18*, 626
Superior, cerebellar peduncle, *2-18, 2-19*,

Boldface numbers indicate principal references. *Italic* numbers refer to illustrations.

Superior, cerebellar peduncle—*Continued*
    12-23, *13-2*, *14-12*, *14-16*, 42,
    252, 318, **363**, 367, **420–421**,
    454
  cervical ganglion, *8-1*, 195, 196
  collicular brachium, *2-19*, *13-17*, 37,
    372, 466
  colliculus, *see* separate listing
  ganglion, of glossopharyngeal nerve,
    11-19, 313
  gluteal nerve, 186
  longitudinal fasciculus, *2-11*, 31
  mesenteric ganglion, 197
    plexus, 197
  olive, *12-10*, **329–331**,
  quadrigeminal brachium, *2-19*, *13-17*,
    37, 372, 466
  salivatory nucleus, 348
Superior colliculus, *2-18*, *2-19*, *13-1*, *13-5*,
    13-6, *13-7*, 37, 42, **307–374**
  afferent fibers, 370–374
  EEG arousal, 374
  efferent fibers, 373–374
  functional considerations, 374
  macular representation, 372–373
  movement detection, 374
  stratum, cinereum, *13-5*, *13-6*, 372
    lemnisci, *13-5*, *13-6*, 372
    opticum, *13-5*, *13-6*, 372
    zonale, *13-5*, *13-6*, 372
  stimulation of, 374
  visual fields, 374
  visual pathways, *15-21*, 373
Supplementary, motor area, *19-21*, **583–585**
  connections, 585
Suppression, cortical, 589
  centers of brain stem, 332–335, 388–389
Supraclavicular nerve, 169
Supragranular layers, 551
Supramarginal gyrus, *2-1*, *2-2*, 24, **595–596**
Supraoptic, decussations, *16-10*, 490–491
  nucleus, *16-1*, *16-4*, **479–482**, 488
  region, *16-1*, 479–482
Supraopticohypophysial tract, *16-9*, 92,
    488, 493
Suprascapular nerve, *7-15*, 173
Suprasegmental levels of nervous sys-
    tem, 159, **164–168**, 213–232,
    9-1, 399
Sural nerve, 185
Surgery, stereotaxic, 518, 543
Sylvian, aqueduct, *2-15*, *13-1*, *13-4*, 42,
    367
  sulcus (lateral), *2-1*, *2-2*, 22, *3-16*, 566
  triangle, *3-16*, *20-7*, 609
Sympathectomy, 206
Sympathetic, ganglia, *8-1*, *8-3*, **192–198**
  nervous system, 191–212
  nuclei, *8-3*, 195–197, 230
  pathways, 192–198
  plexuses, 195–198
  responses, regulation of, **209–212**
  trunks, 193
Synapse, **103–105**, 200–205
  axoaxonic, 103, 461, *15-15*
  axodendritic, 103, 461, 501, 523
  axosomatic, 103, 523
  chemical, 91–92, 104, 200–205

cleft, 103, 201
dynamic polarization, 105
electrical, 104
electron microscopic study of, *4-24*, *4-25*, 103
membranes, 103
physiological peculiarities of, 104
synaptic vesicles, *4-24*, *4-25*, *8-8*, 82,
    104
Syndrome, archicerebellar, **431–432**
  basilar artery, 616–621, *20-15*
  Benedikt, 387
  Brown-Séquard, *10-23*, **279–280**
  carotid sinus, 313
  conus medullaris, 279
  cord transection, 278–279
  "crocodile tears," 348
  disconnection, 592
  dorsal root, *10-22*, 277
  Duchenne-Aran, 181
  Duchenne-Erb, 181
  Gerstmann, 598
  Horner's, 210, 283, *10-26*, 384
  inferior alternating hemiplegia, 308
  Klüver-Bucy, 542
  Klumpke, 181
  Korsakoff's, 538
  lateral medullary, 321
  lower motor neuron, *10-22*, **272–275**
  middle alternating hemiplegia, 351
  posterior white column, 241
  pseudobulbar palsy, 318
  Riley-Day, 207
  superior alternating hemiplegia (We-
    ber), 382
  upper motor neuron, pyramidal, **275–276**, 578–582
Synergic action of muscle groups, 430,
    580–581
Synergy, 430
Syringobulbia, 282, 366
Syringomyelia, *10-26*, **282–283**
System, auditory, **326–336**, 574–577
  corticospinal, *10-12*, *10-13*, **255–261**,
    287–288, 578–582
  epicritic, 139
  hypophysial portal, *16-9*, 490, **493–494**
  limbic, *18-13*, **543–546**
  parasympathetic (or craniosacral), *8-3*,
    8-11, 197–198
  protopathic, 139
  sympathetic (or thoracolumbar), *8-2*, *8-11*, **195–197**

Tactile discs, 143
Tapetum, *2-7*, *2-16*, 32, 568
Taste, receptors, *6-5*, 143
  secondary pathways, 310, 313, 347,
    455–456
Technic, autoradiographic tracing, 106,
    410, 482, 533
  axonal transport, 333, 451, 501
  evoked potential, 276
  Fink and Heimer, 72, 277
  fluorescent, *4-13*, *8-6*, *8-7*, *13-18*, 91,
    202, 364, 366, 394
  Glees, 72, 277
  Golgi silver, 72, *4-5*, 368, 408, 457, 462,
    497, *17-5*, 551
  histochemical, 202
  histofluorescence, *8-6*, *8-7*, 302, 364,

    366, 394, *13-18*, 501, 594–595
  histological, 71–77
  Holmes silver, 72
  Nauta and Gygax, 72, 277, *9-24*, *9-25*,
    13-15
  polarized light, 97
  Rasmussen, 72,
  silver impregnation, *4-1F*, *13-15*, 276
  Wiitanen, 72, 277, *4-1F*
Tectal tracts, tectobulbar, 374
  tectopontine, 374
  tectoreticular, 374
  tectospinal, *10-17*, 261, 374
  tectothalamic, 373
Tectum, *3-9*, *3-12*, 42, 64, **367–374**
Tegmental, decussations, of Forel, *10-17*,
    261, 386, *15-5*, *15-6*, *15-10*, *17-8*, *17-11*, *17-14*, 437
  nucleus, dorsal, *10-17*, 261, 374
    ventral, 261, 386
  tract, central, *12-1*, *12-2*, 322, 351, 392,
    450
Tegmentum, of midbrain, *13-1*, 42, 63,
    367, 369
  of pons, *12-1*, 41, **322–323**
Tela choroidea, development, *3-9*, 132
  fourth ventricle, 9, 41, 132
  lateral ventricle, *3-13*, 9, 36, 132
  third ventricle, *3-13*, 9, 132
Telencephalon, *3-8*, *3-9*, *3-13B*, **21–36**, 60,
    65–70
  subcortical derivatives, *see* Basal gan-
    glia
Telodendria, 77
Teloreceptors, 138
Temperature, pathways, *10-8*, **245–249**,
    566
  receptors, 140
  regulation, 492
Temporal lobe, *2-1*, *2-2*, *2-4*, *2-5*, *2-6*, *18-8*,
    18-11, 24, 28, **524–529**, 574
Temporopontine tract, *13-1*, 324, 586
Tenia of thalami, 438
Tenth cranial nerve, *1-4*, *11-1*, *11-15*, *11-16*, *11-17*, *11-18*, 309–312
Tentorium, cerebelli, *1-2*, *1-3*, *2-1*, 1, 24
  incisure, 1, *1-3*
Terminal, ganglia, 193
  networks, 204
  sulcus, 34
  veins, 34, 627–628
Tests for vestibular function, 345
Tetraethylammonium, 201
Tetraplegia, 261
Thalamic, fasciculus, *17-8*, *17-11*, 454,
    505–507
  nuclei, *2-22B*, *15-12*, **440–461**
  peduncles, *15-19*, 462–464
  radiations, *15-19*, 462–465
  reticular nucleus, 461–462, *15-6*
Thalamocortical radiations, *15-19*, 30,
    462–465
Thalamus, *2-14*, *15-5*, *15-6*, *15-7*, *15-12*,
    37, 64, 440–462, 470–477
  adhesion (massa intermedia), *15-10*,
    45, 446
  anatomy, 43–45, *2-22*, **440–443**
  association nuclei, 474
  blood supply, *20-11*, 612–615
  connections, *15-12*, *15-13*, 443–462
    afferent, *15-12*, 242–249, 331, 343,

Boldface numbers indicate principal references. *Italic* numbers refer to illustrations.

360–361, 363
basal ganglia, *17-6*, **446–451**, 505–507, *17-8*
cerebellar, *14-6*, 363, **420–425**
cortical, *15-13*, **470–477**, 587–589, 592–593
corticothalamic fibers, 587–589, 592–593
striatal, 446–451, *17-6*, **500–501**
subcortical, 451, **452–453**, 461–462
development, 64
divisions, **442–443**
functional considerations, **470–477**
affective sensation, 472
association nuclei, 474
consciousness, 470
cortical activity, 473, 474–476, 592–593
dysesthesia, 472
electroencephalogram, 470, 474–475
emotion, 472
nonspecific nuclei, 475–477, 592–593
sensation, **470–473**
specific relay nuclei, 473–474
cortical, 473–474
sensory, 470–473
systems, auditory, 45, 457–458, 574–577
somesthetic, 454–457, 560–566
visual, *15-14*, 45, 458–461, 566–574
lamina, external medullary, *15-12*, 441
internal medullary, 45, 442, 446–450
lesions, 445, 458, 470
metathalamus, 45, 435
geniculate body, lateral, *15-14*, *15-15*, 45, 458–461, 568
medial, *13-17*, *15-4*, 45, 457–458, 574–575
nonspecific system, **447–451**, 474–477, 592–593
nuclear groups, **443–462**, *15-12*
anterior, *2-14*, **443–444**
intralaminar, 45, 446–451
centromedian, 447, 450, 500–501
parafascicular, 447, 500–501
lateral, **451–452**
lateral dorsal, 451
lateral posterior, 451
pulvinar, *15-5*, 451–452
midline, 446
dorsomedial, *15-6*, **444–446**
ventral, **452–456**
anterior, *15-8*, 452–454
lateral, 454, 473, 505–507
posterior inferior, 456
posterolateral, 454–455
posteriomedial (arcuate; semilunar) 15-11, 455–456
reticular, *15-11*, 461–462
peduncles, **462–465**
anterior, 463
inferior, 463
posterior, 463
superior, 463
radiations, 464–465
relationships, ascending reticular system, 475–476

consciousness, 470
response, augmenting, 473
EEG arousal, 476
recruiting, 453, 475–476, 592–593
reticular nucleus, 461–462
specific thalamic nuclei, 470–473
Thermoanesthesia, 245, 282
Third, cranial nerve, *1-3*, *2-5*, *2-17*, *2-19*, *13-1*, **377–382**
ventricle, 9, *1-11*, *2-15*, 37, 60, 432, 438
recesses, *2-15*, *15-5*, 438
Thirst, 139, 493
Thoracic segments of spinal cord, *7-1*, *9-5*, *9-7*, *9-10*, *9-11*, *9-12*, 195, 220
Thoracordorsal nerve, *7-15*, *7-17*, 173
Thoracolumbar outflow, *8-1*, *8-3*, 195–197
Thrombosis, 600, 619
Tibial nerve, 185
Tigroid bodies, *see* Nissl bodies
Tonotopic localization, 328
cerebral cortex, *19-17*, *19-18*, 574–576
cochlea, 328–329
cochlear nuclei, 328
inferior colliculus, 368
medial geniculate body, 457
Tonsil, cerebellar, *2-24*, 46, 400
Tonus, *see* Muscle tone
Torsion spasm, 515
Torticollis, 172
Tracers, horseradish peroxidase, 451, 592
radioactive, 19, 410
Tract(s), autonomic, descending, 207, 271, 488
of Burdach (fasciculus cuneatus), *10-1*, 238–242
central tegmental, 322, 392, 450
comma, of Schultze, 241
corticobulbar, *11-23*, **314–318**, 464, *15-18*, 580–582
corticomammillary, *15-1*, *18-7*, **483–484**
corticopontine, *13-1*, *14-21*, 324–325, 370, **419–420**, 463–465, 586–587
frontal, 325, 419
temporoparietal, 325, 419
corticorubral, *15-18*, 263, 385, 464
corticospinal, *10-13*, **255–261**, 578–582
anterior, 256
anterolateral, 256
lateral, 256–259, 286–287, 578–582
corticostriate, *17-6*, 499–500
corticotectal, 373
corticothalamic, **462–465**, 476, 587–589, *15-18*
cuneocerebellar, *10-10*, 418
dentatoreticular, 363, 421, *14-16*
dentatorubral, *14-16*, 363, 385, 420
dentatothalamic, *14-16*, 363, 421, 454
descending vestibular, *10-18*, *10-19*, 264–267, 269–270, 342–343
dorsal trigeminal, *12-22*, 361
fastiglobular, (*see* Uncinate fasciculus of Russell), *14-19*, *14-20*, 422–425
frontopontine, *13-1*, *15-18*, 324–325, 398, 419, 464, 586–587
of Gall (fasciculus gracilis), *10-1*, 238–242

geniculocalcarine, *15-21*, *15-22*, 30, 466–470, 566–568
geniculotemporal, *12-10*, *15-18*, *15-19*, 457, 463–465, 574–576
habenulopeduncular (retroflexus), *15-5*, 437
of Helweg (olivospinal), 271
interstitiospinal, *10-21*, 270, 380
lateral lemniscus, *12-10*, *12-23*, 329, 331, 368
of Lissauer, *9-7*, 233
mammillotegmental, *16-5*, 488
mammillothalamic, *16-5*, 444, 488
medial lemniscus, *10-1*, 359–360, 454–455
mesencephalic of N.V., *12-21*, 359
nigrostriatal, *17-6*, 396–397, 501–504
olfactory, *18-1*, *18-2*, 29, 523–524
olivocerebellar, *14-21*, 303, 418
optic, *15-21*, *15-22*, 466
pallidosubthalamic, *17-8*, 508
pallidotegmental, *17-11*, 507–508
pallidothalamic, *17-8*, *17-11*, 454, 505–507
periependymal, *16-7*, 488
pontocerebellar, *14-21*, 324–325, 419–420
pyramidal, *see* Corticospinal
reticulocerebellar, *14-16*, 418
reticulospinal, *10-11*, *10-20*, 267–269
rostral spinocerebellar, 253, 418
rubrobulbar, 386
rubro-olivary, 299, 386
rubroreticular, *10-17*, 386
rubrospinal, *10-17*, **261–264**, 385–386
Schütz, *11-14*, 308, 488
spinal trigeminal (spinal V), *12-21*, 288, 293–294, 354–357
spinocerebellar, anterior, *10-10*, 251–252, 417
posterior, *10-10*, 249–251, 417
spinocervical, 248, *10-9*
spinocortical, 253
spino-olivary, 255
spinopontine, 255
spinoreticular, 253, 391
spinospinal, *10-21*, 271–272
spinotectal, 249, 373
spinothalamic, anterior, *10-7*, 242–245
lateral, *10-8*, 245–249, 454–455, 456, 566
spinovestibular, 255
strionigral, *17-14*, 396, 504
striopallidal, 504
supraopticohypophysial, *16-9*, 488
tectobulbar, 374
tectopontine, 374
tectoreticular, 374
tectospinal, *10-17*, 261, 374
tegmentocerebellar, 420
temporopontine, *13-1*, 324–325, 419, 586–587
thalamocortical, *15-13*, *15-17*, *15-18*, 470–477
thalamostriate, *17-6*, 450–451, 500–501
trigeminocerebellar, 420
trigeminothalamic, *12-22*, 360–361, 455–456
dorsal, 360

Boldface numbers indicate principal references. *Italic* numbers refer to illustrations.

Tract(s)—*Continued*
  ventral, 360
  tuberohypophysial, 488–490
  tuberoinfundibular, *16-9*, 488–490
  ventral trigeminal, *12-22*, 360
  vestibulocerebellar, 341, 342
  vestibulospinal, *10-18, 10-19*, 264–267, 342
Tractotomy, trigeminal, 357
Transection of spinal cord, 278–279
Transfer, interhemispheric, 591–592
Transmitters, acetylcholine, 200–202, 517
  dopamine, 204, 394, 397, 489, 498, 501, 517
  gamma-aminobutyric acid (GABA), 91, 205, 517
  glutamic acid decarboxylase (GAD), 517
  norepinephrine, 104, 202–203, 364–365, 411, 594–595
  neurohumoral, 200
  serotonin, 204, 366, 594
Transverse, cerebral fissure, *3-13*, 65
  colli, 169
  rhombencephalic sulcus, *3-9*, 60
  temporal gyri, *2-1, 2-2, 2-5, 2-6, 18-9, 18-11*, 24, 28, 331, 457, 574–575
Trapezoid, body, *12-1, 12-4, 12-10*, 330–331
  nucleus, *12-3*, 330–331
Tremor, cerebellar, 431
  parkinsonism, 514–515
Triangle of Phillippe-Gombault, *10-21*, 241
Trigeminal nerve, *2-5, 2-19, 11-17, 11-18, 12-17, 12-20, 12-21, 12-22*, 352–362
  divisions,
    mandibular, *7-13, 12-20*, 353
    maxillary, *7-13, 12-20*, 353
    ophthalmic, *7-13, 12-20*, 353
  ganglion, *1-10*, 353–354
  lesions, 356–357
  mesencephalic tract of, *12-20*, 352
  motor nucleus, 360
  nuclei, mesencephalic, *12-20*, 359–360
    principal sensory, *12-19*, 357–359
    spinal, *11-14*, 354–357
  peripheral distribution, *7-13*, 165, 352–353
  reflexes, 361–362
  roots of, *11-17, 11-18*, 352, 359
  secondary pathways, *12-22*, 360–361
    dorsal trigeminal, 361, 555–556
    ventral trigeminal, 360, 555–556
  sensory functions, 352–353, 359
  spinal nucleus, 294–296, *11-19, 11-15*, 354–357
  spinal tract, *12-20*, 293–294, 354–357
  tractotomy, 357
Trigeminocerebellar tract, 360, 420
Trigeminothalamic tracts, *12-22*, 360–361, 455–456
Trigone (trigonum), collateral, *2-15*, 35
  habenular, *2-18, 15-7*, 43, 438
  hypoglossal, *11-2*, 41, 297
  lemnisci, 362
  olfactory, *18-2*, 29, 524
  vagi, *11-2*, 41, 297

Trochlear nerve, *2-5, 2-18, 2-19, 13-3*, 42, 369
  nucleus, *13-3*, 369
  lesions, 369
Tuber, of vermis, *2-26, 14-1*, 46
Tuberal nuclei, *16-2, 16-3, 16-7*, 478–479
Tubercle, acoustic, 318, 327, *11-25*
  acusticum, *12-24, 12-25*, 318, 327
  anterior (thalamus), *15-8*, 444
  cuneate, *2-18, 11-2, 11-3*, 39, 288–289
  gracilis, *2-18, 11-2*, 39, 288–289
  olfactory, *18-4*, 525
Tuberohypophysial tract, *16-9*, 488–490
Tubocurarine-*d*, 201
Twelfth cranial nerve, *11-1, 11-13, 11-16, 11-17, 11-18*, 39, 305–308
Tyrosine hydroxylase (T-OH), 517

Ulnar nerve, 177
Ultrastructural studies, 71, 82–91, 94–99, *4-8, 4-9, 4-10, 4-12, 4-17, 4-18, 14-10*, 458–461, 497–498
Uncinate bundle of Russell, *14-18, 14-19, 14-20*, 422–425
  fasciculus, of cerebral hemisphere, 31
Unconsciousness, 393, 495
Uncus, *2-4*, 24, 28, 525
Unipolar neuron, *4-3*, 55, 161–162
Unit, motor, *4-3*, 156, 160, 229–230
  sensory, 137
Unmyelinated axons, 93
Unmyelinated nerve fibers (fibers of Remark), 100–103
  C fibers, 103
Upper motor neuron, 360, 375, 578–582
  lesion, 359, 375–376
Utricle, 336
Uvula, cerebellum, *2-26, 14-1, 14-20*, 46, 417

Vagus nerve, *2-5, 2-17, 2-19, 11-9, 11-13, 11-15, 11-16, 11-17, 11-18*, 309–312
  ganglion, inferior, *11-19*, 309
    superior, *11-19*, 309
  lesions, 312
  nuclei, *11-17, 11-18*, 198, 310–312
  reflexes, 312
  secondary fibers, 310
Vallecula cerebelli, *2-24*, 46
Vascular, lesions, 321, 350, 600, 608, 611–612
  malformations, 600
    aneurysms, 600
    arteriovenous, 600
Vein(s), anastomotic, great (of Trolard), *20-18*, 626
  posterior (of Labbé), *20-18*, 626
  basal (of Rosenthal), *20-19, 20-20*, 629
  caudate, *20-19, 20-20*, 628
  cerebral, 622–630
    great (of Galen), *20-19, 20-20*, 621–622, 624, 627, 629
    inferior, 626
    internal, 626–627, *20-19, 20-20*
    middle, deep, *20-22*, 627–630,
      superficial, *20-18*, 626–627,
    superior, 627
  choroidal, *20-19*, 628
  emissary, *20-16*, 622, 624
  epithalamic, *20-17, 20-19*, 628–629

  lateral ventricular, 629
  occipital, *20-19*, 629
  posterior callosal, 629
  radicular, anterior, *20-2*, 601
    posterior, *20-2*, 601
  septal, *20-19, 20-20*, 628
  striate, inferior, *20-22*, 628, 629
    superior, *20-22*, 628
  terminal, anterior, *20-19*, 627–628
  thalamostriate, *20-19, 20-20*, 627
Velum, inferior medullary, *2-21*, 41, 431
  interpositum, *2-22*, 9, 43, 65, 627
  superior medullary, *2-25, 12-23*, 41, 362, 369
Vena radicularis magna, 602
Venous, drainage, *1-1*, 601–603, 619–620, 621, 622–630
  lacunae, *1-12*, 622
  sinuses, *1-1, 1-2, 1-3, 20-16, 20-17*, 622–630
  vasocorona, *20-2*, 602
Ventral acoustic stria, 329
  cochlear nuclei, 318, 327
  nuclei of thalamus, *15-12*, 452–456
  portion pons 322, 324–325
  primary ramus, *7-1*, 162
  rami of spinal nerves, *7-1*, 162
  tegmental decussation, *10-17, 13-4*, 261, 386
  tier thalamic nuclei, 452–456
Ventral tegmental area (Tsai), 396
Ventricles of brain, fourth, *2-15, 2-18, 2-21*, 39–41, 60, 132, 297–298
  lateral, *2-15*, 34–36, 60, 132
    body of, *2-15*, 34–35, 65
    calcar avis, *18-7*, 35
    collateral eminence, *2-16*, 35
    collateral trigone, *2-15*, 35
    horns, *2-15*, 34–36, 530
  third, *2-15, 15-6, 16-2, 16-4*, 37, 132, 438
    recesses, *2-15*, 438
Ventricular system, *2-15, 3-13A, 3-13B*, 34–36, 39–41, 132
Vermis, of cerebellum, *2-26, 14-1*, 46, 62, 399
Vertebral artery, *1-7, 20-1, 20-4, 20-5, 20-6, 20-9, 20-15*, 600, 605–606
Vertigo, 345, 578
Vesical afferents, *8-11*, 211
Vesicles, 203
  "dense-cored," 203
  synaptic, 82, 103–104
Vestibular, end organ (*see also* Receptors), *12-12*, 336
  fibers, primary (root), *12-13*, 339–342
    secondary, *12-14*, 342–344
    vestibulocochlear anastomosis, *12-11*, 333
  functional considerations, 344–345
    decerebrate rigidity, 345
    equilibrium, 344
    eye movements, 344
    gravity, 336, 345
    motion sickness, 431–432
    muscle tone, 345
    nystagmus, 345
    orientation in space, 336
    posture, 344–345
    rotation, 345
    stimulation (of semicircular canals),

Boldface numbers indicate principal references. *Italic* numbers refer to illustrations.

345
  tests for, 345,
  vertigo, 345
ganglion (Scarpa), *12-13*, **341**
lesions, 341
membrane, 326
nerve, **337-342**
  central distribution of fibers, *12-13*, **339-342**
    cerebellum, *12-14*, 341-342, 416-417
    vestibular nuclei, *11-12*, *12-1*, *12-3*, *12-4*, 339-341
  divisions, 341
  peripheral branches, *12-13*, 341
nuclei, *14-20*, **337-339**
  cell group *f*, 337
  inferior, *11-12*, 337
  interstitial of vestibular nerve, *12-14*, 339
  lateral (Deiters'), *12-3*, 337-338
  medial, *11-12*, 338
  superior, 12-16, **338-339**
receptors, labyrinth, *1-2*, *12-12*, 336
  saccule, *12-12*, 336
  semicircular canals, 336
  utricle, *12-12*, 336
representation cortex, 456, 578
secondary fibers, 342
system, **336-345**
tracts, *10-18*, *10-19*, 264-267, 269-270
  medial longitudinal fasciculus, *12-14*, 269-270, 342-344
  vestibulocerebellar, *12-14*, 341-342, 417
  secondary, 342

vestibulospinal, *10-18*, *10-19*, 264-267, 342
Vestibulocerebellar fibers, *12-14*, 341-342, 417
  primary, 341-342
Vestibulocochlear anastomosis, *12-11*, 333
Vestibulocochlear nerve, *11-17*, *11-18*, **325-345**
  pars cochlearis, *11-25*, 326-336
  pars vestibularis, *12-2*, 336-345
Vestibulo-oculomotor fibers, *12-14*, 342-344
Vestibulospinal tracts, *10-18*, *10-19*, 264-267, 345
Vibratory sense, 139, 241, 337
Vicq d'Azyr, bundle of, *see* Mammillothalamic tract
Virchow-Robins spaces, 11
Visceral, afferent fibers, 80, **199**, 309, 347
  brain, 545
  efferent fibers, 192-198
  reflex, 208-211
Visceroceptor, **139**
Vision, binocular, 572-573
  monocular, 572
Visual, agnosia, **596**
  areas of cortex, *19-13*, *19-14*, 24, 566-574
    complex cells, 572-573
    hypercomplex cells, 573
    simple cells, *19-15*, *19-16*, 569
  deprivation, 572-573
  experience, 572-573
  fields, *15-21*, *15-23*, 470, 568

receptive-field orientation, *19-15*, *19-16*, 569-574
  orientation, *19-15*, *19-16*, 344-345
  pathways, 15-16, *15-21*, *15-22*, 465-470
  lesions, *15-23*, 470
  receptors, *15-19*, *15-20*, 465
  reflexes, 374, 382-384

Wallerian degeneration (secondary degeneration), *4-26*, *4-31*, 88, 105-107, 276
Weber's syndrome (superior alternating hemiplegia), 382
Weigert, method, 71, 276, *9-10*, *10-13*, *11-4*
Wernicke's zone, *15-3*, 436
White matter, 29-32, 462-465
  semioval center, 29
Wiitanen method, 72, 277, *4-1F*
Word, blindness, 596
  deafness, 596

X-ray diffraction, 94

Zona incerta, *15-6*, *17-8*, *17-11*, 505, 511
  intermedia (spinal cord), *9-7*, 226-228
Zone, cortical, 67, 547
  dendritic, 77
  germinal (matrix), 67, 547
  intermediate, 67, 547
  of Lissauer, (fasciculus dorsolateralis), 233
  of Wernicke, *15-3*, 436
Zonula adhaerens, *5-15*, 132
Zonulae occludens, *5-15*, 132

Boldface numbers indicate principal references. *Italic* numbers refer to illustrations.

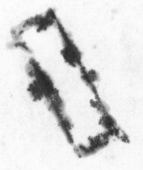